PASS
CEN®!

PASS
CEN®!

Robin Donohoe Dennison, DNP, RN, CCNS, CEN, CNE
Associate Professor of Clinical Nursing
College of Nursing, University of Cincinnati
Cincinnati, Ohio

Jill Johnson, DNP, APRN, FNP-BC, CCRN, CEN, CFRN
Market Manager
Clinic Operations for Take Care Health
Louisville, Kentucky
Emergency Department Staff Nurse
Saint Joseph Hospital
Lexington, Kentucky

Meg Blair, PhD, MSN, RN, CEN
Associate Professor of Nursing
Nebraska Methodist College
Omaha, Nebraska

ELSEVIER
MOSBY

3251 Riverport Lane
St. Louis, Missouri 63043

PASS CEN©!

ISBN: 978-0-323-04879-8

ISBN: 978-0-323-04879-8

Acquisitions Editor: Maureen Iannuzzi
Developmental Editor: Robin Richman
Publishing Services Manager: Deborah Vogel
Project Manager: Pat Costigan
Design Direction: Maggie Reid

Printed in the United States of America

Last digit is the print number: 9 8 7 6 5 4 3 2

To Russell, my husband of 31 years. Not only is he a wonderful husband but, as an emergency medicine physician, he has served as an always-willing-to-answer-questions consultant to me during the writing and editing of this book.

Robin Donohoe Dennison

To all of my friends and colleagues in the emergency department and critical care transport who have dedicated their life to caring for others. Your compassion, expertise, and commitment to nursing are an inspiration. I hope this book will provide emergency and transport nurses with the tools to prepare for certification success. A special thanks to my Mom and Dad for always being there and believing in me.

Jill Johnson

This book is dedicated to all nurses everywhere who wish to improve their practice through the certification process. Patients and colleagues everywhere will benefit from your knowledge and expertise. I also dedicate this to my family for being so supportive and to my coauthors Robin Dennison and Jill Johnson for working so hard to ensure the success of this book.

Meg Blair

Contributor

Cornelia Wilson, EdD, RN, FAAN
Professor
College of Nursing
University of Cincinnati
Cincinnati, Ohio

Reviewers

Patricia Ann Bemis, RN, CEN
National Nurses in Business Association, Inc.
Rockledge, Florida

Sherri Denise Caldwell, RN, BSN, CEN
Chesapeake Regional Medical Center
Chesapeake, Virginia

Patricia L. Clutter, RN, MEd, CEN, FAEN
St. John's Hospital — Lebanon and Springfield
Lebanon, Missouri
Springfield, Missouri

Sara Duvall, MSN, RN, FNP-BC, ENP, CEN
Baylor University Medical Center
Dallas, Texas

Joyce Foresman-Capuzzi, BSN, RN, CEN, CPN, CCRN, CTRN, CPEN, SANE-A, EMT-P
Lankenau Hospital
Wynnewood, Pennsylvania

Lisa Hollett, RN, BSN, MA, MICN
Division of Trauma, Acute Care and Critical Care Surgery
Penn State Milton S. Hershey Medical Center
Hershey, Pennsylvania

Cathy McJannet, RN, MN, CEN, HTCP/I
Director of Nursing and Health Occupations Programs
Southwestern College
San Diego, California

Jeff Solheim, RN, CEN, CFRN, FAEN
President
Solheim Enterprises
President
Project Helping Hands
Keizer, Oregon

Preface

Welcome to *Pass CEN®!* And congratulations—you have chosen the most up-to-date, comprehensive review of emergency nursing available on the market today. If you are a registered nurse planning to take the CEN® examination for certified emergency nursing practice offered by the Board of Certification for Emergency Nursing (BCEN®), this book is the tool that you need to prepare for the examination with confidence.

Who will Benefit from this Book?

This book is written for nurses who are preparing to take the CEN® examination. The goal is to provide a pertinent content review, fun but challenging learning activities, realistic practice questions, and comprehensive mock examinations that reflect the content and complexity of the CEN® examination.

Although this book is written based on the CEN® examination, a majority of the content is also found on the blueprints for the CFRN®, CTRN®, and FP-C® examinations. Recognizing that transport nurses and paramedics would benefit from *Pass CEN®!*, we incorporated some additional information specific to transport nurses and paramedics preparing for their transport certification examination. This bonus content can be found on the Evolve Exam Review website at http://evolve.elsevier.com/Dennison/passCEN/.

Organization and Unique Features

Pass CEN®! is unlike other review books. At any time in the emergency department (ED), a patient can present with minor to life-threatening emergencies, requiring the emergency nurse to be knowledgeable and prepared for the unexpected. A collaborative team approach, essential to providing appropriate patient care, provides the basis for the format and organization of *Pass CEN®!* The succinct and easy-to-read outline format fosters comprehension and retention of information. Figures and tables further clarify content, highlight key concepts, and enhance written explanations.

Information is organized according to the blueprint for the latest CEN® examination, the summary of which is located on the inside back cover for quick reference. This test plan, issued by the BCEN®, identifies the content areas tested and the percentage of the examination devoted to each. Content included in the CEN® test blueprint is the primary focus of this book, eliminating extraneous, distracting information. The latest blueprint for the CFRN® and CTRN® examinations along with additional transport information specific to the transport certification examinations and a detailed blueprint of the FP-C® examination (Appendix F) appear on the Evolve Exam Review website at http://evolve.elsevier.com/Dennison/passCEN/.

Chapter 1: Preparing for the CEN® Exam

Chapter 1 focuses on how to prepare for and perform on the CEN® exam. A comprehensive discussion of test-taking strategies is included, along with test-taking strategies for all of the practice questions located in the Exam Review Course on the EVOLVE website for the book.

Chapters 2-14: CEN® Exam Test Plan

Components of each chapter are:
- Introduction to chapter content and number of items on the CEN® exam
- Age-related considerations across the life span
- Selected concepts in anatomy and physiology
- Physical assessment
- System-specific tasks, including laboratory studies and radiographics
- Selected references and bibliography for each chapter
- Specific examples of emergencies in detailed Learning Activities at the end of each chapter, followed by Answers to the Learning Activities

Examples of Specific Emergencies

Each emergency starts with a **definition** and brief description followed by **predisposing factors**. **Pathophysiology** provides a better understanding a of the disease process. The **clinical presentation** includes specific **subjective** and **objective assessment** findings and indicated **diagnostic studies**, which provide the building blocks to critically think through examination questions and understand the processes. The **collaborative management** section for each emergency begins with continued assessment items that should be monitored throughout the patient's stay in the ED. Then management priorities, including **medical and nursing interventions**, are provided. **Major complications** are listed, some of which may not be evident in the ED when caring for the patient, but which are still an important part of understanding the specific emergency and treatment. **Evaluation outcomes** are stated in measurable terms and typical **patient disposition** upon discharge or admission is explained.

Unique Appendixes in *Pass CEN®!*

The following appendixes are unique to *Pass CEN®!* and provide a wealth of pertinent information for nurses taking the CEN® Exam.
- Appendix A is a list of common abbreviations and acronyms used in this book and common to emergency care.

Available on the Evolve Exam Review website:
- Appendix B lists signs, syndromes, and triads used in *Pass CEN®!* along with a brief description of each.
- Appendix C is a table of mnemonics/memory aids to help you remember processes such as ABCD for

Primary Survey (Airway, Breathing, Circulation, Disability).

- In Appendix D, you will find normal laboratory values used in emergency care.
- Appendix E includes selected medications used in the ED.
- Appendix F includes a detailed outline of the flight paramedic certification exam blueprint with complete information on resources within *Pass CEN®!* and other options for preparing for each item on the FP-C®.

Learning Aids

Sometimes we learn best when information is organized and accessed in unfamiliar ways—that's the principle at work behind the diverse **Learning Activities** in this book. Every chapter features a range of activity styles, including matching, fill-in-the-blank, comparison, and crossword puzzles, to test comprehension and improve recall for readers with a variety of learning styles.

You won't be asked to complete a crossword puzzle or a matching exercise when you take the CEN® examination, but doing so when practicing for it helps you learn and retain an astonishing amount of information. It also makes your study sessions more enjoyable, encouraging you to stick to the timetable that you have set for yourself. We hope that working through these activities will be a pleasurable way to review terminology, anatomy and physiology, and pharmacology as well as link concepts.

Evolve Exam Review Course

The Evolve Exam Review Course on the accompanying website contains more than 700 review questions written in a format that represents the actual CEN® examination. The practice exam reflects the percentages set forth for each content area on the most recent test blueprint. The Exam Review Course offers two modes: (1) a quiz mode in which practice questions are arranged by body system and (2) a test mode that offers realistic practice CEN® examinations.

The quiz mode allows you to select topic areas in which you need additional review and creates quizzes that target those areas. The practice test mode, on the other hand, replicates the actual CEN® exam as closely as

possible. It draws questions from all content areas in the number and proportion called for in the latest CEN® exam blueprint. The program will reshuffle the questions randomly (but retaining the correct percentages in each content area) to create as many practice tests as you like. Both modes are self-scoring. **Instant rationales** are given to explain which answer is correct and why it is the best answer among the possible choices. **Test-taking strategies** are provided as appropriate to show you how to think through the questions if you are not sure of the content. Both of these features will boost your confidence and make you a better test taker on the important day of the CEN® examination. Analyzing your performance on several practice exams will help you focus your final preparation on your weakest areas.

Emergency nursing has never been more exciting. For those of us who thrive on this challenge, keeping up with new research and clinical developments is a continual test of our professionalism. CEN® certification is a prestigious credential for those of us who specialize in emergency nursing. We are confident that you will pass the examination if you study this book and use the Evolve Exam Review Course to practice your test-taking skills.

We would love to hear from you about your success with the examination, how this book helped you, and how you feel it could be even more useful. E-mail us at rddennison@aol.com or write to:

Robin Donohoe Dennison, DNP, RN, CCNS
c/o Nursing Editorial
Elsevier, Inc.
1600 JFK Boulevard
Suite 1800
Philadelphia, PA 19103

We believe that this book will be your most valuable resource in preparing for the CEN® examination. Good luck!

Robin Donohoe Dennison
Jill Johnson
Meg Blair

Contents

CHAPTER 1

Preparing and Performing on the CEN Examination

Certification

Definition: A "voluntary credentialing process that [is] designed to elevate professional standards and enhance individual performance" (BCEN, 2010)

Purpose: Certification has been advocated as one method of assurance of competence

1. Competence is the "the application of knowledge and the interpersonal, decision-making, and psychomotor skills expected for the nurse's practice role, within the context of public health, welfare, and safety" (National Council of State Boards of Nursing, 1996, p. 5)
2. Continued competence refers to the maintenance of adequate knowledge and skills for safe ongoing practice that occurs after the initial demonstration of competence at the time of licensure (National Council of State Boards of Nursing, 1996)

Benefits of achieving professional certification

1. For the nurse
   a. Self-satisfaction and validation of your knowledge and clinical judgment in your chosen nursing specialty
   b. Motivation to update and maintain your knowledge base
   c. Career mobility: National certification is as prestigious in one state as another
   d. Clinical advancement and promotion
      1) Most unit nurse managers encourage their nursing staff to become certified
      2) Certification is often recommended or required for promotion up a clinical career ladder
   e. Financial remuneration
      1) Some hospitals offer a bonus for professional certification
      2) Some hospitals offer an hourly differential for professional certification
      3) Some hospitals prefer certified nurses for clinical or administrative promotion
      4) Many hospitals reimburse the nurse for the expense of taking the test if a passing score is attained
2. For the institution
   a. Assurance to the general public that the nurse is competent (ENA, 2008)
   b. Evidence of excellence for marketing and awards such as American Nurses Credentialing Center (ANCC) Magnet Recognition Program (ANCC, 2010)
   c. Financial incentives by insurance carriers

3. For patients and their families
   a. Assurance that the nurse is currently competent and knowledgeable regarding emergency nursing

The CEN Examination (ENA, 2008)

The Board of Certification for Emergency Nursing (BCEN), a nonprofit organization, administers the certification for emergency nurses (CEN) as well as the certification for flight registered nurses (CFRN), and the certification for transport registered nurses (CTRN), which is specific to critical care ground transport

The examination is based on a role delineation study so that the examination reflects the current national practice of emergency nursing; the test is usually revised approximately every 4 years

Eligibility and testing process

1. Current unrestricted RN license in the United States or in any of its territories that use the NCLEX for RN licensure is required; a nursing certificate that is equivalent to a registered nurse in the United States is also acceptable (ENA, 2008)
2. Clinical practice in emergency nursing for 2 years is recommended but not required
3. Application for eligibility to take the examination
   a. To obtain an application
      1) Telephone: 800-900-9659, ext. 2630
      2) Web: www.ena.org/bcen/application
4. The computerized form of the test is administered by Applied Measurement Professionals (AMP) at their testing centers nationwide; note that paper-and-pencil examinations can be administered at a local site if minimum attendance requirement is met
5. Schedule the examination
   a. Complete the application and send it to BCEN
   b. BCEN will send you an authorization letter indicating that you meet the requirements to take the examination, along with instructions on how to schedule the examination
   c. Call the testing service to schedule your examination date and time; you must schedule the examination within 90 days of the date printed on your authorization letter
      1) Computer-based testing is available most weekdays year-round with two testing times daily

2) Schedule the time of the examination according to when you do your best thinking or are most productive: Schedule for the morning if you are a lark or the afternoon if you are an owl

3) This flexibility in scheduling allows you to avoid scheduling conflicts between the examination and major life events such as a family wedding, graduation, or birth

   d. DO SCHEDULE THE EXAM so that you have a target date; you can reschedule up to 1 business day prior to the scheduled test day if something comes up that interferes with your ability to complete the examination on the scheduled day

6. Requirements on the day of the examination
   a. Testing authorization letter with your authorization number
   b. Two pieces of identification, one of which must have a current photograph
7. A score report will be given to you before you leave the testing center

The CEN examination

1. Basic information about the CEN examination
   a. The test is designed to evaluate your understanding of the common body of knowledge needed to function effectively in an emergency setting
      1) The test consists of 175 multiple-choice questions to be completed within 3 hours; 25 of these items are not scored but are test items for the development of future examinations
   b. Blueprint for the CEN examination (Table 1-1)
      1) The blueprint identifies the categories tested and the percentage of questions in each category
      2) The blueprint identifies what percentage of questions is in each task area
2. Cognitive levels of questions
   a. Knowledge questions require you to remember previously learned information
   b. Comprehension questions require you to understand the information
   c. Application questions require you to use information
   d. Analysis questions require you to break down information into its component parts and recognize commonalities, differences, and interrelationships
   e. Synthesis questions require you to put parts of information together to form a new conclusion
   f. Evaluation questions require you to judge the value of information
   g. Questions on the examination are distributed across these cognitive levels
3. Distribution of questions related to the nursing process: All phases of nursing process are included on the examination
4. Passing score
   a. The passing score for the examination is approximately 75% (ENA, 2010)
   b. About 70% of nurses taking the CEN examination pass (ENA, 2010)
5. For more specific information about these examinations, the application and application process, and the testing process, visit www.ena.org or call ENA at 800-900-9659, ext. 2630

Preparation to Improve Performance on the these Examination

1. Be positive!
2. Avoid negative self-talk; "I'll never pass this examination" can be a self-fulfilling prophecy because you begin to believe it
3. Practice positive self-talk
   a. Write down some affirmations (positive statements) related to your preparation and performance on this examination; suggested affirmations are listed in Box 1-1
   b. Say these and other affirmations that you have written over and over again throughout your preparation time; say them like you believe them and you will!
   c. Record your affirmations on audiotape and play them often; play them in the car, while you walk or do dishes, or any other time when you can listen and repeat them

TABLE 1-1 Blueprint for the CEN Examination Indicating Distribution of Questions on Each Section		
Content	**No. of Items**	**Percentage**
Cardiovascular	21	14
Respiratory	18	12
Neurological	15	10
Medical emergency	15	10
Orthopedic/wound	13	9
Shock/multisystem	11	7
Genitourinary, gynecology, obstetric	10	6.5
Substance abuse/toxicological/ environmental	10	6.5
Gastrointestinal	9	6
Patient care management	9	6
Professional issues	7	5
Maxillofacial/ocular	6	4
Psychological/social	6	4
Total	150	100

BOX 1-1 Affirmations
■ I am a knowledgeable emergency nurse.
■ I understand the information important for this examination.
■ I am an excellent test-taker.
■ I feel prepared for this examination.
■ I will pass this examination.

Prepare for the test

1. Establish a realistic schedule for your preparation; 1- to 2-hour time slots are probably the most helpful
   a. Study examination content: Plan to review a system per evening, day, or weekend, depending on how much time you have left before the examination
      1) Set priorities
         a) Study your weak areas first
         b) Study the large percentage content areas even if you feel confident about them
      2) Review content using this review book
         a) Highlight areas that you do not feel confident about; you may need to refer to more comprehensive texts or articles when you need additional clarification
         b) Complete the learning activities at the end of each chapter to consolidate your knowledge by looking at the information in another way
      3) Practice using your test-taking skills by doing practice questions
         a) In addition to looking at the answer, read the rationale; remember that the question may not be written exactly the same as the practice question, but the concept may be on the examination
         b) If you still do not understand why you missed the question, refer back to the section in this book or an emergency nursing text to understand why the correct answer is better than your answer
         c) In addition to looking at the answer and the rationale, read the test-taking strategy included with questions on the Review Course for the CEN Examination on the Evolve website; this information will help you identify how to approach a similar question to which you do not know the answer
         d) Analyze why you missed a question. Consider:
            i) Did you not know the content? Study this content again
            ii) Did you misread the question? Slow down and read the question more thoroughly
            iii) Did you misread the options? Slow down and read all of the options and select the best one
            iv) Did you miss an important element such as age, diagnosis, or parameter? Again, slow down and read the question carefully; mentally highlight the critical points in the case study that you feel are important
            v) Did you read into the question?
               (a) Do not assume information that is not given; take the question at face value
               (b) Do not assume that the question is intended to "trick" you; there are no "trick" questions on the practice examination questions on the Evolve site Review Course or on professional certification examinations

4) Study in a quiet place with minimal distractions
   a) Turn off the television, radio, and stereo; let the answering machine and voice mail pick up telephone calls
   b) Avoid getting too comfortable; sit upright at a desk or table so that you can spread out your study materials; avoid trying to study while in bed or a recliner
   c) Ensure adequate lighting
   d) Reading, repeating, and writing are methods that improve remembering
   e) Use margins to write down memory joggers or additional thoughts

2. If you like study groups, organize a study group of nurses who are also preparing for the CEN examination
   a. Include only members who will fulfill their obligation to participate
   b. Establish guidelines for the group
      1) When will you meet?
      2) What will you do at the meetings?
         a) A selected member may present essential content related to their specific area of interest
         b) Members may collect resource materials related to the specified content area and distribute them to fellow members
         c) Members may discuss review questions related to the specified content area
      3) What are the group members' expectations?

3. Create memory joggers
   a. Almost everyone knows "On Old Olympus' Towering Tops A Fin and German Viewed Some Hops" to remember the 12 cranial nerves; establish others that help you identify things that you have trouble remembering

4. Remember case study links. For example, you remember a patient with a triglyceride level over 2000 mg/dl who presented with boring epigastric pain helps you remember that a major risk factor for acute pancreatitis is hypertriglyceridemia and that a common symptom of acute pancreatitis is boring epigastric pain

Take a practice test 1 week before the examination; use this test to identify weak areas for final study time

1. Analyze which categories (systems) are your weakest and which are your strongest
2. Analyze which cognitive level question is the most difficult for you
3. Analyze which component of the nursing process is most difficult for you

Final preparations

1. Do not cram the night before the examination; cramming usually just decreases your self-confidence and increases your anxiety
2. Go to bed at your usual time; if you go to bed early, you probably will not go to sleep anyway and will just worry about the test

3. Do not consume alcohol or other sedating drugs the night before or the day of the examination
4. Choose comfortable clothes that allow layering so you can remove or add clothing in response to the room temperature; wear bright colors (e.g., yellow red, hot pink, orange) to project a more optimistic image
5. Take a watch, a sweater, tissue, and hard candy; do not forget your glasses if you wear them
6. Eat a healthy but light meal before the examination; avoid simple carbohydrates such as a doughnut or Danish; instead, eat peanut butter on whole wheat toast or an egg sandwich to sustain you through the examination
7. Be sure to take two forms of identification with one of them being a government-issued photograph identification that contains a signature
8. Make sure that you know where the testing site is located and how long it will take you to get there considering traffic at the time your test is scheduled; getting lost or just having to rush to arrive on time causes anxiety and may affect your performance
9. Plan to arrive 15 minutes before your scheduled appointment; if you arrive later than 15 minutes after the scheduled testing time, you may not be admitted
10. Take the time to visit the restroom before you check in

Performance During the Examination

Control of anxiety

1. Remember that some anxiety improves your performance; panic does not
2. Feeling adequately prepared decreases anxiety; take the time to prepare for this examination, including practicing your test-taking strategies
3. Use visualization: See yourself receiving your passing score
4. Use deep breathing and/or progressive muscle relaxation
   a. Deep breathing is performed by putting your hand below your costal margin and breathing deeply enough to raise your hand; focus on your breathing instead of anything else
      1) Use this method at anytime during the examination when you feel frustrated or stressed
   b. Progressive muscle relaxation is performed by contracting a group of muscles and then relaxing it: leg, leg, arm, arm, back, face
      1) Use this techniques in the car before you go in to take the examination and at anytime during the examination that you feel tense
5. Use meditation or prayer depending on your religious beliefs: These techniques are also helpful in verbalizing your goals and desires
6. Do not allow a memory lapse or a difficult question to affect your attitude or throw you into panic mode; move on to the next question, for which you are likely to know the answer, rather than letting it affect your performance on the entire examination

Take the time to read the directions at the beginning of the examination

Test-taking skills

1. Reading questions thoroughly
   a. Mentally highlight key points as you read the question
      1) Age and gender of the patient
      2) Setting: prehospital, emergency, critical care, progressive care, home care
      3) Medical diagnosis and other coexisting diagnoses
      4) Timeframe in relation to admission, trauma, surgery, pain, visitation
   b. Look for qualifying word
      1) Such as:
         a) *All, most, some, few, none*
         b) *Always, usually, frequently, seldom, never*
         c) *First, last*
         d) *Best, worst*
         e) *Most, least*
         f) *Smallest, largest*
         g) *Acute, chronic*
         h) *Partial, total*
         i) *Early, late*
      2) Answers that include global answers such as *all, always, never,* or *none* are seldom the correct answer
   c. Look for negative words such as *not, except, contraindicated,* or *inappropriate*
   d. Read all the options as well as the stem
   e. After you read the stem, answer the question without looking at the options; if your answer is there, it is probably right; however, go ahead and read all options—there may be one better than your answer
2. Choosing the correct answer
   a. Make sure that you understand what the question really is; answer *the* question, not just *a* question
   b. Always choose the best answer; even if there are two answers that you consider correct, choose the one that best answers the question being asked
      1) If more than one option appears correct, look for the most comprehensive option
   c. Assumptions
      1) Do not assume information that is not given; the only assumption is an ideal situation unless the question indicates otherwise
      2) All important information is included
         a) Do not read into the question additional information such as "maybe she's a diabetic" or "maybe he has COPD"; if information is important to the question, it will be included
      3) Included information is probably important
         a) Extraneous information is not usually included, so if the case study or question gives you information that you feel is extraneous or superfluous, ask yourself why this information was given and how it is important to this situation

d. Answer questions according to national standards of care and national guidelines rather than regional, local, or specific physician's practices

e. Select options that are therapeutic based on evidence and show respect and acceptance for the patient and the family; eliminate options that are based on tradition rather than science and options that are inappropriate, disrespectful, or punitive

f. Repetition of a word or a synonym of the word in the stem and an option may help you to identify the correct answer

g. If the answers are numbers or number ranges, the extremes are less likely to be the correct option than the middle number or number range

h. This examination is computerized and answers are random; therefore, C is no more likely to be the correct answer than A, B, or D; also, there are no patterns to the answers so do not look for one

3. Answering priority questions
   a. Priority one is always whatever must be done to prevent death; always follow the ABC order: airway, then breathing, and finally circulation
   b. Priority two is whatever must be done to prevent disability or serious complication; consider this D for disability
   c. Priority three is pain or discomfort; if nothing in the case study or question could cause death or disability, pain should be considered the priority
   d. Actual problems always take precedence over potential problems; for example, actual hypoxemia takes precedence over potential oxygen toxicity
   e. If there are two potential problems, the priority is the one that is more likely to cause death or disability

4. Answering questions where the answers have multiple answers (also referred to as multiple/multiples)
   a. If the option has more than one answer (such as x and y or even w, x, y, and z), both or all of the answers must be correct for the option to be correct
   b. Elimination works well with this type of question; if there is one answer in the option that is incorrect, that option is eliminated

5. Guessing
   a. Do not leave any question blank; unanswered questions are counted as incorrect, so you should never not answer a question even if you must guess
   b. You are not penalized for guessing but it should be used only as a last resort
   c. First eliminate any choices that you can; it is better to guess between two choices than to guess between four
      1) Eliminate clearly wrong answers
      2) Eliminate any response that has no relationship to the question
      3) Eliminate similar options that say essentially the same thing because they cannot both be correct
      4) *All, always, never, none,* or *only* options are *usually* incorrect

d. If you cannot even eliminate answers down to two, then look for the option that is different from the others; for example:
   1) Three antibiotics and an antifungal—choose the antifungal option
   2) Three beta-blockers and a calcium channel blocker—choose the calcium channel blocker
   3) Three very specific and one very comprehensive option—choose the comprehensive option

e. Bookmark questions of which you are unsure and want to return to; at the end of the test, the computer allows you to go back to these marked items and review them before unmarking them and continuing to the end of the examination

6. Changing answers
   a. You may have been told to never change answers and you should not change an answer unless you have a good reason for changing it; one good reason is that you missed a negative qualifier, such as *not, except,* or *contraindicated,* when you read it the first time
   b. It may be helpful to change answers in a different color when doing a practice test; then evaluate how many you changed from wrong to right and how many you changed from right to wrong
      1) If you change more from wrong to right, you most likely miss questions because you do not read them thoroughly, so when realize that you misread a question, then by all means change your answer
      2) If you change more from right to wrong, do not change your initial answer (unless you realize in this case that you had misread the question) because first impressions tend to be correct more often than not

7. Answering math questions
   a. Math questions are usually drug calculations, such as dopamine in micrograms per kilogram per minute, but could be other emergency calculations
   b. You are provided with scratch paper and pencil
   c. Recheck your math if you have time

8. Maintaining concentration
   a. Write down formulas, normal values, toxic levels, etc. that you think you might forget on your scratch paper before you do the first question
   b. Change your process of reading the case study, the question, and the options
      1) Read the options in reverse order from option *d* to option *a*. Use this action especially when you suspect that option *a* or *b* is the correct option
      2) Make this change every 25 to 50 questions OR
         a) When you are physically tired, mentally anxious, or lose your concentration abilities
         b) When you come to the easier or the more difficult questions
   c. Rephrase the question rather than rereading the question over and over

  d. Use three slow deep breaths to regroup and get refocused at any time

  e. Sign out and go to the restroom and splash water on your face if you are losing your ability to concentrate, but remember that the clock does not stop during this time—so consider this if you are a slow test-taker

9. Budgeting your time

  a. If you are a slow test-taker, you may run short on time but more likely you will run out of mental energy because maintaining concentration for a 2- to 3-hour period is very difficult

  b. You should try to be at least halfway through the examination in 75 minutes; this halfway point will leave you some time to recheck your math and go back to items where you used a bookmark

  c. One helpful technique to save time is to read the question (at the end of the case study) and then go back and read the case study; because we frequently read the case study, then the question at the end of the case study, and then reread the case study, this technique saves you time by knowing what you are looking for in the case study

  d. Do not be distressed by people finishing before you; we all take examinations at different speeds, and the others may not even be taking the CEN examination because several examinations are given at the same place and same time

Reasons for Failing the Examination

Knowledge deficit

1. Prepare to take the examination even if you feel that you are an experienced emergency nurse because we all have our chosen areas of interest and our weak areas

2. Use this book to review the content for the examination and complete the learning activities at the end of each chapter

3. Take a practice examination 1 week before the examination to identify your weak areas; use your final study time focusing on those weak areas

Testing errors

1. Practice using your test-taking skills with the questions on the Evolve site and pay close attention to both the rationale and the test-taking strategy included with each question

2. Use the learned test-taking strategies during the CEN examination

Test anxiety and negative thinking: Believe in your ability to pass the examination and control your anxiety with prayer, meditation, deep breathing, and/or progressive relaxation

Test Results

You will be given your test results at the completion of computerized testing and within 6 to 8 weeks by mail for pencil and paper testing
Congratulate yourself on having the initiative to take the examination
If you pass, flaunt it!

1. You should display your credential on your hospital name badge

2. You should proudly write it after RN when you sign your name; Your Name, RN, CEN

3. Encourage others to become certified; offer to tutor, mentor, share study materials to assist your colleagues to become certified, too

If you fail, try again!

1. The fear of the unknown is now gone

2. You know clearly what your weak areas are from the score breakdown that was given to you as you left the testing site

3. You can now prepare by focusing on your weak areas and then reapply to take the test again; there is a 90-day waiting period before retesting

4. You can do it!

Maintaining Your CEN Certification

Certification is for a 4-year period
Recertification is achieved by retaking the examination, or by providing evidence of continuing education (i.e., 100 contact hours over the 4-year period), or by successfully completing the Internet-based test

References and Selected Readings

American Nurses Credentialing Center. (March 26, 2010). *Magnet Recognition Program Overview*. Retrieved from http://www.nursecredentialing.org/Magnet/ProgramOverview.aspx

Board of Certification for Emergency Nursing. (March 20, 2010). *Purpose of certification*. Retrieved from http://www.ena.org/bcen/exams/Purpose/Pages/default.aspx

National Council of State Boards of Nursing. (1996). *Assuring competence: A regulatory responsibility*. Chicago: Author.

LEARNING ACTIVITIES

1. What are your personal reasons for taking the CEN examination?

_____
_____
_____
_____

2. List your top five life priorities for the next year. Is CEN certification on this list? What is the ranking for CEN certification?

1st _____
2nd _____
3rd _____
4th _____
5th _____

3. Prioritize this list from 1 (least comfortable) to 13 (most comfortable). Use this list to schedule your preparation with 1 being first and 13 being last.

Content	Comfort Level
Cardiovascular	
Respiratory	
Neurological	
Medical emergency	
Orthopedic/wound	
Shock/multisystem	
Genitourinary, gynecology, obstetric	
Substance abuse/toxicological/ environmental	
Gastrointestinal	
Patient care management	
Professional issues	
Maxillofacial/ocular	
Psychological/social	

4. Describe your plan to prepare for the CEN examination.

_____
_____
_____
_____

5. List three new test-taking strategies that you have learned from this chapter and will use while taking the CEN examination.

A. _____
B. _____
C. _____

CHAPTER 2

Patient Care Management

Introduction

Patient care management constitutes 6% (9 items) of the CEN examination

It is comprised of a wide variety of content

Much of the content of this section overlaps with other content areas of the CEN examination

1. General pharmacology and the administration of fluids and medications are considered part of patient care management, but, in each chapter, you will find medications that pertain to the relevant content; in addition, Appendix D describes medications that are frequently used in an emergency setting
2. Patient safety is listed in patient care management, but patient safety is covered in each chapter as it pertains to each specific content area
3. Primary and secondary assessment are covered in this chapter, but you will find more specific information in other chapters

Triage and Priority Setting

An essential component of emergency care

A framework in which patients are sorted with the use of an acuity system to determine their priority for treatment

1. Triage systems typically classify patients into one of three or five categories on the basis of the severity of their complaints
2. Triage should be completed before financial information is obtained

Roles of the triage nurse

1. Assess, prioritize, categorize, and monitor patients who present to the emergency department (ED) for treatment
2. Ensure that all patients receive an initial triage assessment within 5 minutes of arrival
3. Initiate appropriate interventions and transfer patients to the appropriate care areas if, at any time during the triage process, a life-threatening problem is identified
4. Maintain confidentiality with all patients
5. Maintain focus and objectivity when making triage decisions and acuity assignments
   a. Avoid being distracted by noise and the number of patients waiting
   b. Avoid making judgments on the basis of a patient's appearance and the frequency of his or her prior ED visits

Components of triage

1. Across-the-room look
   a. Visually assess to determine the stability of ABCD: *A*irway, *B*reathing, *C*irculation, and *D*isability; this begins as soon as the triage nurse first sees the patient walk through the door
   b. Observe for the following:
      1) Airway patency
      2) Respiratory distress
      3) Use of oxygen
      4) Obvious bleeding, wounds, or deformities
      5) Level of consciousness
      6) Signs of pain
      7) Skin color
      8) General appearance
      9) General behavior
      10) Posture and gait
      11) Weight
   c. Listen for the following:
      1) Any abnormal airway sounds
      2) Breathing
      3) Speech pattern, tone, and language
      4) Interaction with others
   d. Smell for the following:
      1) Alcohol
      2) Body odor, secretions: stool, urine, and vomit
      3) Cigarettes or smoke
      4) Chemicals
      5) Infection
   e. Note anything that would indicate that immediate care is required (e.g., lethargic pediatric patient)
2. Chief complaint
   a. Record why the patient has come to the ED in the patient's own words; do not convert to a medical diagnosis
   b. If the complaint or condition is not new, then ask what made the patient come to the ED today for treatment of the complaint
   c. The across-the-room look and the rapid assessment of the chief complaint should take <60 seconds
3. Focused assessment
   a. Symptoms: what are the symptoms that the patient is experiencing?
   b. Onset of symptoms: when did the symptoms first start?
   c. Precipitating events: what events, if any, led up to the symptoms or injury?

d. Mechanism of injury (if applicable)
  1) MIVT (Emergency Nurses Association [ENA], 2004)
    a) M: mechanism of injury
    b) I: injuries sustained
    c) V: vital signs
    d) T: treatment before arrival; did this treatment help or make the situation worse?
e. Pain assessment: PQRST format for describing complaint (Sullivan, 1989)
  1) P
    a) Provocation: what provokes or worsens the pain?
    b) Palliation: what relieves the pain? (also include what treatments were used that did not relieve the pain)
  2) Q
    a) Quality: what does the pain feel like?
  3) R
    a) Region: where is the pain?
    b) Radiation: if the pain radiates, to what area?
  4) S
    a) Severity: how severe is the pain?
      i) 0 to 10 scale with 0 being no pain and 10 being the most severe pain
      ii) Faces scale, especially for children
  5) T
    a) Timing: is the pain intermittent or continuous, and what is the relationship of the pain to other events or activities?
f. AMPLE history (American College of Surgeons, 2004)
  1) A: allergies
    a) Medications
    b) Environmental exposures
  2) M: medications
    a) Prescription
    b) Over the counter
    c) Vitamins and herbal remedies
  3) P: past or pertinent medical history
  4) L: last oral intake
  5) E: events or environment surrounding the patient's current situation
g. The Pediatric Assessment Triangle (ENA, 2007) (Figure 2-1)
  1) Appearance
    a) Muscle tone
    b) Intractability/consolability
    c) Look or gaze
  2) Work of breathing
    a) Nasal flaring
    b) Retractions
    c) Abnormal airway sounds
    d) Position of comfort
    e) Altered respiratory rate
  3) Circulation or skin
    a) Pallor
    b) Mottling
    c) Cyanosis
h. Pediatric focused assessment (Table 2-1)

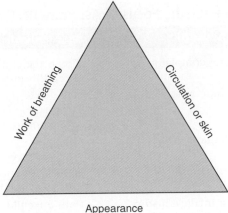

Work of breathing

Circulation or skin

Appearance

Figure 2-1 Pediatric assessment triangle.

4. Assigning acuity level
  a. Three-level acuity (ENA, 2005)
    1) Emergent
      a) Go directly back into the treatment area; triage is finished in that area
      b) Examples: cardiac arrest; myocardial infarction; respiratory failure; major trauma; and threat to life, limb, or organ
    2) Urgent
      a) Requires prompt care, but patient may wait safely in the waiting room, if necessary
      b) Needs to be reassessed every 30 minutes to be sure acuity has not changed
      c) Examples: abdominal pain, kidney stone, and fracture
    3) Nonurgent
      a) Requires care, but patient can wait safely, if needed
      b) Needs to be reassessed every 1 hour to check for acuity changes
      c) Examples: sore throat, toothache, sexually transmitted infection, and suture removal
  b. Five-level acuity (ENA, 2005)
    1) Critical
      a) Requires immediate treatment and constant monitoring
      b) Examples: cardiac arrest, respiratory failure, airway compromise, multiple trauma, myocardial infarction, and suicidal thoughts with a plan
    2) Unstable or emergent
      a) Requires treatment and reassessment every 15 mintues
      b) Examples: angina, open fracture, neurovascular compromise, acute asthma attack, severe pain, suspected cerebrovascular accident, and pregnancy with active bleeding
    3) Urgent or potentially unstable
      a) Requires treatment and reassessment every 30 to 60 minutes
      b) Examples: noncardiac or minor chest pain, kidney stone, and closed fracture

TABLE 2-1 Pediatric Focused Assessment: CIAMPEDS

	Mnemonic	Assessment
C	Chief complaint	Why is the child here today? (Keep this information in the child's or parent's own words.)
I	Immunizations, isolation	Is the child up to date on all immunizations for his or her age? If not, why? Any possible communicable diseases (e.g., measles, mumps, chicken pox)? Any exposure that may require isolation (e.g., meningitis)?
A	Allergies	Any hypersensitivities or allergies to medications? Any food or environmental allergies?
M	Medications	Is the child currently taking any medications, either prescription or over the counter? (If yes, record the dosage, frequency, last dose, and duration of use.)
P	Past medical history	Does the child have a history of surgeries, illnesses, hospitalizations, injuries, chronic or physical illnesses, substance abuse, sexually activity, or sexually transmitted infection? If the patient is an infant, were there any maternal complications? Was the child born prematurely? Were there any congenital abnormalities?
E	Events leading to injury or illness	When was the onset of the child's illness or injury? Has any treatment been initiated before arrival at the emergency department? What were the results? If the child was injured, what were the date, time, and mechanism of the injury? Was any treatment initiated before arrival at the emergency department?.
D	Diet, diapers	What are the child's diet and eating patterns? When was his or her last meal? Does the child have any food restrictions? When did the child last void or have his or her diaper changed? What has been the frequency of urination during the last 24 hours? When was the last bowel movement? What was the color and consistency?
S	Symptoms associated with illness or injury	What are the child's symptoms? How have they progressed since the time of onset of the illness or injury?

Adapted from Emergency Nurses Association (2010). *Sheehy's emergency nursing: principles and practice* (6th ed.). St. Louis: Mosby, pp. 66-67.

4) Stable or nonurgent
   a) Requires treatment and reassessment every 1 to 2 hours.
   b) Examples: sore throat, minor burn, strain, sprain, constipation, and urinary tract infection without fever
5) Minor
   a) Stable and requires reassessment every 4 hours
   b) Examples: wound check, staple or suture removal, and viral illness without fever

Telephone triage (ENA, 2001)

1. Telephone triage involves assessment of a patient's health through a telephone interview with a triage nurse; the assessment is done by a phone interview and then provides recommendations for treatment or referral
2. It is a way to assess patients and direct them to appropriate care without causing overcrowding or unneeded emergency department visits
3. Registered nurses must have competency assessment training and continuing education to demonstrate proficiency and competency in telephone triage
4. "Telephone triage should only be done by registered nurses who have had specialized training in telephone triage, assessment, communication, and documentation skills." (ENA, 2010)

5. Emergency departments utilizing telephone triage should have policies and procedures that clearly define the triage protocols and decision making
6. Advice should not be given by phone when there are no established telephone triage protocols and guidelines
7. In situations where there are no established protocols or guidelines, the nurse answering the phone should inform the patient that an appropriate assessment cannot be made over the phone and the person needs to call their primary care provider or come into the emergency department for further evaluation
8. In any situation that may be life threatening, the nurse should instruct the caller to call 911
9. Careful documentation should be maintained of any conversation involving patient recommendations

Triage documentation

1. The triage nurse must document a brief subjective and objective assessment on the basis of the patient's chief complaint and physical status
   a. Subjective assessment: what the patient describes or tells the triage nurse; includes the chief complaint
   b. Objective assessment: what the triage nurse sees, hears, and feels during the triage assessment that is relevant to the patient's complaint
   c. Reportable occurances: mandated by law to be reported to the health department, social services,

or law enforcement; examples include but are not limited to the following:

1) Abuse or neglect (child or elder)
2) Animal bites
3) Assualt
4) Communicable diseases
5) Domestic violence
6) Gun or knife wounds
7) Sexual assualt
8) Suicide attempt

d. Triage red flags (Table 2-2)

Primary Assessment

Introduction

1. Rapid and organized systematic assessment to detect and manage life-threatening conditions

TABLE 2-2	Triage Red Flags
Airway	• Apnea • Choking • Drooling • Audible airway sounds • Positioning
Breathing	• Grunting • Sternal retractions, increased work of breathing • Irregular respiratory patterns • Respiratory rate >60 breaths/min • Respiratory rate <20 breaths/min for children <6 years old • Respiratory rate <15 breaths/min for children <15 years old • Absence of breath sounds • Cyanosis
Circulation	• Cool or clammy skin • Tachycardia, bradycardia • Heart rate >200 beats/min • Heart rate <60 beats/min • Hypotension • Diminished or absent peripheral pulses • Decreased tearing, sunken eyes
Disability	• Altered level of consciousness • Inconsolability • Sunken or bulging fontanel
Exposure	• Petechiae • Purpura • Signs and symptoms of maltreatment or abuse
Vital signs	• Hypothermia • Temperature >100.4° F (38° C) in infant <3 months old • Temperature >104° F (40° C) at any age
Pain	• Severe pain
History	• History of a chronic illness • History of a family crisis • Return visit to emergency department within 24 hours

Adapted from Emergency Nurses Association. (2005). *Sheehy's manual of emergency care* (6th ed.). St Louis: Mosby.

2. Initial assessment that should be performed on all patients who present to the ED
3. Mnemonic for the primary assessment: ABCD
   a. A: airway
   b. B: breathing
   c. C: circulation
   d. D: disability

Airway

1. Open and clear
   a. Good air exchange is noted; the patient is able to speak clearly
   b. Intervention
      1) Supplemental oxygen as appropriate
      2) Stabilization of cervical spine (if there is an indication of possible cervical injury)
2. Obstructed
   a. Assessment for cause
      1) Tongue (most common cause)
      2) Blood
      3) Loose tooth or foreign body
      4) Vomitus or secretions
      5) Edema
   b. Intervention
      1) Supine position
      2) Stabilization and immobilization of cervical spine in trauma patients
      3) Establishment of open and clear airway
         a) Jaw thrust for trauma patients
         b) Chin lift
         c) Head tilt/chin lift for nontrauma patients
         d) Removal of loose objects or debris
         e) Suctioning of airway as required
         f) Insertion of an airway adjunct as required
            i) Oropharyngeal airway if gag reflex absent
            ii) Nasopharyngeal airway if gag reflex present
            iii) Consideration of endotracheal intubation

Breathing

1. Rise and fall of chest: symmetry, depth, and use of accessory muscles
2. Rate and pattern of respirations
   a. Regular
   b. Irregular
   c. Kussmaul: regular, rapid, deep, and labored
   d. Cheyne-Stokes: alternating periods of hyperventilation and apnea (injury to the cerebrum)
   e. Biot: three to four breaths of identical rate and depth followed by apnea (injury of lower pons or upper medulla)
   f. Ataxic: no respiratory pattern, mostly apneic (injury of medulla)
3. Presence of bilateral breath sounds
4. SpO_2 via pulse oximetry
5. Any chest injury
6. Skin color and mucosa: pink, dusky, pale, or cyanotic
7. Indications of ineffective ventilation
   a. Chest excursion: shallow, asymmetric, or paradoxic
   b. Skin color: pale, ashen, or cyanotic

c. Increased work of breathing: labored, nasal flaring, or accessory muscle use

d. Abnormal breath sounds: stridor, wheezing, crackles, rhonchi, or absent

e. Presence of injury
   1) Sucking chest wound (i.e., obvious wound, sucking noise)
   2) Flail chest (i.e., paradoxic chest movement, chest wall tenderness)
   3) Pneumothorax and tension pneumothorax (i.e., jugular venous distention, absent or diminished breath sounds, hyperresonance to percussion, tracheal deviation [late sign])
   4) Hemothorax (i.e., flat neck veins, absent or diminished breath sounds, dullness to percussion)
   5) Pulmonary contusion (i.e., ecchymoses on chest wall)
   6) Impaled object

8. Interventions for ineffective ventilation
   a. Supplemental oxygen to maintain SpO_2 >90%
      1) Nonrebreather (NRB) mask at 12 to 15 L per minute (L/min) if patient has spontaneous respirations
      2) Positive-pressure ventilation with a bag-valve-mask (BVM) device with 100% oxygen or a liter flow of at least 15 L/min if no spontaneous respirations
   b. Airway adjuncts as indicated (oropharyngeal or nasopharyngeal airway; progress to endotracheal intubation as indicated)
   c. Management of injuries
      1) Open pneumothorax (i.e., sucking chest wound)
         a) Petroleum gauze dressing secured on three sides; removal and reapplication if tension pneumothorax develops
         b) Chest tube
      2) Flail chest
         a) Stabilization of the flail portion with a bulky dressing
         b) Mechanical ventilation may be required for internal stabilization
      3) Tension pneumothorax: needle decompression followed by chest tube
      4) Hemothorax
         a) Chest tube
         b) Surgical exploration and repair may be required
      5) Impaled object
         a) Stabilization of object
         b) Removal by surgeon

Circulation

1. Assessment of circulation
   a. Central pulses versus peripheral pulses
      1) Peripheral pulses present or absent bilaterally
      2) Quality of pulse: normal, weak, strong, thready, or absent
   b. Heart rate: normal, bradycardia, or tachycardia
      1) 60 to 100 beats per minute in uncompromised adults (Seidel, Ball, Dains, & Benedict, 2007)
      2) 90 to 170 beats per minute in uncompromised infants (ENA, 2007)
      3) 80 to 160 beats per minute in uncompromised 1-year-old children (ENA, 2007)
      4) 70 to 110 beats per minute in uncompromised children between the ages of 8 and 12 years (ENA, 2007)
   c. Systolic blood pressure of >90 mm Hg in adults or within normal limits for age and weight
      1) Brachial or radial: systolic blood pressure is at least 80 mm Hg if palpable (ACS, 2004)
      2) Femoral: systolic blood pressure is at least 70 mm Hg if palpable (ACS, 2004)
      3) Carotid: systolic blood pressure is at least 60 mm Hg if palpable (ACS, 2004)

2. Bleeding
   a. Assessment
      1) No visible active bleeding
      2) Visible bleeding is minimal: oozing or low in volume, and dark red in color
      3) Bleeding that requires immediate intervention
         a) Uncontrolled, pulsating bleeding
         b) Pallor of lips, skin, or nail beds
         c) Large amounts of blood or clots in emesis, urine, or stool or from any orifice
         d) Distended, rigid abdomen
         e) Gross swelling of an injured extremity
   b. Interventions for bleeding
      1) Control of bleeding with direct pressure to site or over arterial pressure points
      2) Monitoring of hemodynamics and vital signs
      3) Other interventions depend on cause and location of bleeding but could include transfusion, chest tubes, and so on; specific interventions will be discussed in later chapters

3. Perfusion
   a. Assessment
      1) Level of consciousness and orientation to person, place, time, and event
      2) Skin color: pink, pale, ashen, mottled, cyanotic, or flushed
      3) Skin temperature: warm, cool, cold, or diaphoretic
      4) Capillary refill
         a) Normal: <1 to 2 seconds in a warm environment (Jarvis, 2008)
         b) Delayed: >2 seconds in a warm environment
      5) Peripheral pulses in all extremities
      6) Urine output: at least 1 ml/kg/hour
   b. Interventions for hypoperfusion
      1) Supplemental oxygen
      2) Vascular access with two large-bore intravenous catheters
      3) Fluids as indicated (i.e., normal saline (NS) or lactated Ringer (LR) solution for boluses)
      4) Pharmacologic agents as prescribed
      5) Flat positioning

a) Do not use Trendelenburg or modified Trendelenburg
   i) Not effective
   ii) May cause respiratory distress
   iii) May cause increased intracranial pressure
b) Although modified Trendelenburg has been used in the emergency setting, current research shows that it is not beneficial (Bridges and Jarquin-Valdivia, 2005.)

Disability: brief neurologic assessment

1. Level of consciousness
   a. AVPU format (ENA, 2007)
      1) A: alert; patient is alert and responsive
      2) V: verbal; patient responds to verbal stimulus
      3) P: pain; patient responds to painful stimulus
      4) U: unresponsive; patient does not respond to painful stimulus
   b. Glasgow Coma Scale score (GCS) (Table 2-3)
   c. Pupil assessment
      1) Size in millimeters
      2) Reaction to light
      3) Shape
      4) Gaze: conjugate (i.e., normal movement of both eyes together in the same direction) or disconjugate

Exposure or environment

1. Removal of clothing to prepare for the secondary assessment
2. Adequate coverage for privacy and prevention of heat loss

Secondary Assessment

Introduction

1. Begins after primary assessment and any lifesaving interventions
2. Systematic process to assess the patient from head to toe to discover abnormalities or injuries that are not life threatening
   a. Techniques include inspection, auscultation, percussion, and palpation
3. Mnemonic for the secondary assessment: FGHI
   a. F: full set of vitals, focused adjuncts, and family presence
   b. G: give comfort measures

c. H: history not obtained during primary assessment; then head-to-toe assessment
d. I: inspect posterior surfaces

Full set of vital signs

1. Pulse: rate, quality, and rhythm
2. Respirations: rate, depth, and quality
3. Blood pressure
4. Temperature

Focused adjuncts

1. Cardiac monitoring if indicated
2. End-tidal carbon dioxide ($ETCO_2$) monitoring for intubated patients
3. Gastric tube if endotracheally intubated and as indicated
4. Foley catheter as indicated to monitor urine output and to decompress bladder
   a. Do not insert if there is blood at meatus, scrotal hematoma, or perineal ecchymosis
   b. Male trauma patients should have a rectal examination before the insertion of a Foley catheter to rule out urethral injury or trauma
5. Diagnostic evaluations pertinent to illness and injury
   a. Electrocardiogram (ECG)
   b. Radiographic studies
   c. Computerized tomography studies
   d. Magnetic resonance imaging (MRI) studies
   e. Laboratory blood work
   f. Arterial blood gases (ABG)
   g. Focused assessment sonogram for trauma (FAST)

Facilitate family presence

1. Determination of family's desire to be present with the patient
2. Family support and comfort
3. Explanation of all procedures and events to the family in terms that they can understand
4. Honesty and openness with family

Give comfort measures

1. Assessment of pain
   a. Use mnemonic PQRST
   b. Use pain scale
      1) 1 to 10 scale for adults
      2) Faces scale for children and nonverbal adults

TABLE 2-3 Glasgow Coma Scale Score

Eye-Opening Response	Verbal Response	Motor Response
4 = Opens eyes spontaneously 3 = Opens eyes to voice 2 = Opens eyes to pain 1 = Does not open eyes	5 = Oriented 4 = Confused 3 = Uses inappropriate words 2 = Makes incomprehensible sounds 1 = No vocalization	6 = Obeys commands 5 = Localizes pain 4 = Withdraws from pain 3 = Abnormal flexion to pain 2 = Abnormal extension to pain 1 = No movement

Note: The lowest possible score on this scale is 3, and the best possible score is 15.

2. Positioning for comfort if not contraindicated
3. Rest, ice, splint or compression, and elevation of extremity injury as indicated
4. Pharmacologic agents as prescribed
5. Evaluation of effectiveness of intervention and documentation

History

1. Review of triage note before obtaining more detailed history
2. Review of patient's current health status, risk factors for illness, behavior, occupation, hobbies, support system, access to care, living accommodations, and implications of present illness
3. Developmental age assessment for pediatric patients (Jarvis, 2008)
   a. Infants
      1) Task: develop trust
      2) Fears: separation and strangers
   b. Toddlers
      1) Task: autonomy and self-control
      2) Fears: separation and loss of control
   c. Preschool-aged children
      1) Task: creating a sense of initiative
      2) Fears: bodily injury and mutilation, loss of control, the unknown, the dark, and being left alone
   d. School-aged children
      1) Task: developing a sense of industry
      2) Fears: loss of control, bodily injury and mutilation, failure to live up to expectations of important others, and death
   e. Adolescents
      1) Task: separation from parents, adaptation to a rapidly changing body, development of a sexual identity and a sense of who they are, and autonomous function; privacy is extremely important
      2) Fears: loss of control, altered body image, and separation from peer group

Head-to-toe assessment: performed on most injured or ill patients unless the problem is very isolated

1. General appearance
   a. Note the following:
      1) Behavior and affect
      2) Odors
      3) Gait
      4) Hygiene
      5) Level of distress
2. Head and face
   a. Inspect head and face, and note the following:
      1) Deformities
      2) Contusions
      3) Abrasions or avulsions
      4) Lacerations
      5) Penetrating injuries
      6) Burns
      7) Swelling or edema
      8) Ecchymoses or hematomas
   b. Palpate the head, scalp, and face, and note the following:
      1) Crepitus
      2) Symmetry
      3) Instability
      4) Step offs
3. Eyes: assess for the following
   a. Abrasions, avulsions, or lacerations around the eyes
   b. Penetrating injuries or impaled objects
   c. Burns
   d. Lid edema or lesions
   e. Ptosis (i.e., drooping of eyelids)
   f. Blepharospasm (i.e., inability to open eyes)
   g. Impairment in visual acuity (i.e., injury to cranial nerve II)
   h. Pupil changes, such as inequality and absence of reaction to light (i.e., injury to cranial nerve III)
   i. Impairment of extraocular movement (i.e., injury to cranial nerves III, IV, or VI)
   j. Absence of corneal reflexes (i.e., injury to cranial nerves V [sensation] or VII [motor])
   k. Bruising around the eyes (e.g., raccoon sign, which is indicative of a basal skull fracture)
   l. Presence of contact lenses (remove if present)
4. Ears, nose, and mouth
   a. Inspect for the following:
      1) Drainage from the nose, ears, and mouth
         a) Clear fluid may be a cerebrospinal fluid (CSF) leak (i.e., rhinorrhea or otorrhea) associated with basal skull fracture; do not pack or insert anything into the nose
         b) Bloody drainage indicates possible maxillofacial fracture
      2) Loose teeth or debris that could compromise airway
      3) A change in the color or moisture of the mucous membrane
      4) Bruising behind the ear (i.e., Battle sign): indicates possible basal skull fracture but may not be evident immediately after injury
   b. Palpate for the following:
      1) Crepitus
      2) Deformities
      3) Symmetry
      4) Instability of midface
      5) Malocclusion of teeth and trismus (i.e., inability to open mouth completely)
5. Neck
   a. Inspect for the following:
      1) Obvious wounds or penetrating trauma
      2) Abrasion, avulsions, or lacerations
      3) Ecchymoses or hematomas
      4) Edema or swelling
      5) Tracheal deviation from midline
      6) Jugular neck veins
         a) Flat veins when the patient's position is flat indicate hypovolemia
         b) Distended veins when the patient's position is elevated may indicate hypervolemia, right

ventricular failure, cardiac tamponade, or tension pneumonia

b. Palpate for the following:
1) Instability of the cervical spine and step offs
2) Subcutaneous emphysema
3) Tenderness or pain
4) Presence of carotid pulses
5) Nuchal rigidity (i.e., neck stiffness)

c. Auscultate carotid arteries for bruits

d. Assist with diagnostic studies as indicated
1) Cervical spine radiographs: cross-table lateral, anterior, posterior, and open mouth odontoids
2) Spinal column radiographs

6. Chest
a. Inspect for the following:
1) Obvious wounds or penetrating trauma
2) Abrasion, avulsions, or lacerations
3) Ecchymosis or hematomas
4) Edema or swelling
5) Puncture wounds or impaled objects
6) Scars

b. Palpate for the following:
1) Expansion and stability
2) Subcutaneous emphysema
3) Crepitus of the clavicles, sternum, or ribs
4) Tenderness or pain

c. Percuss the chest to determine if there are changes from normal resonance
1) Hyperresonance: hyperinflated lung or air-filled thoracic cavity
2) Dullness: fluid-filled or consolidated lung tissue

d. Auscultate the following:
1) Breath sounds: presence or absence and any abnormal sounds
2) Heart sounds: note any extra sounds (e.g., S_3, S_4, friction rub) or murmurs

e. Assist with diagnostic studies as indicated
1) Chest radiograph
2) Computed tomography (CT) scan of chest
3) Focused assessment sonogram for trauma (FAST)

7. Abdomen and flanks
a. Inspect for the following:
1) Obvious wounds or penetrating trauma
2) Abrasion, avulsions, or lacerations
3) Ecchymoses or hematomas
4) Edema or swelling
5) Puncture wounds or impaled objects
6) Evisceration
7) Contour of abdomen: flat, distended, or pregnant
8) Scars
9) Bruising in flank area (i.e., Grey-Turner sign): suggestive of retroperitoneal bleeding
10) Bruising of periumbilical area (i.e., Cullen sign): suggestive of intraperitoneal bleeding

b. Auscultate for the following:
1) Presence or absence of bowel sounds; listen in all four quadrants
2) Presence or absence of bruits, which indicate turbulent flow

c. Percuss the abdomen for the following:
1) Deviation from normal tympany over abdomen
a) Dullness
i) Normal over solid organs (e.g., liver)
ii) Fluid
iii) Mass
2) Fluid wave (i.e, ascites)

d. Palpate for guarding, masses, rigidity, tenderness, and pain

e. Assist with diagnostic studies as indicated:
1) Peritoneal lavage
2) Ultrasound (US)
3) Computed tomography (CT) scans
4) Gastric occult blood testing
5) Intravenous pyelography (IVP)

8. Pelvis/perineum
a. Inspect for the following:
1) Obvious wounds or penetrating trauma
2) Abrasion, avulsions, or lacerations
3) Ecchymoses or hematomas
4) Edema or swelling
5) Puncture wounds or foreign bodies
6) Bleeding
7) Priapism
8) Genital lesions or discharge

b. Palpate for the following:
1) Instability or tenderness over the iliac crests and the symphysis pubis
2) Pelvic instability: push the pelvis in and press down but do not rock it

c. Assist with diagnostic studies as indicated
1) Radiography
2) Urine dipstick or urinalysis
3) Fecal occult blood testing
4) Retrograde urethrography

9. Extremities
a. Inspect the extremities for the following:
1) Skin color and bilateral symmetry
2) Abrasion, avulsions, or lacerations
3) Bleeding
4) Ecchymoses or hematomas
5) Edema or swelling
6) Puncture wounds or impaled objects
7) Angulations and deformity
8) Impaired movement, muscle strength, or symmetry of strength
a) Spontaneous movement of extremities
b) Range of motion
c) Grip and pedal-push strength and symmetry
9) Clubbing of fingertips

b. Palpate for the following:
1) Abnormal skin temperature
2) Impaired capillary refill (i.e., >2 seconds)
3) Diminished pulse amplitude, especially distal to injury
4) Diminished sensation (i.e., paresthesia), especially distal and proximal to any injury
5) Deformities, step offs, and crepitus
6) Tenderness or pain

c. Assist with diagnostic studies as indicated
  1) Radiographic studies
  2) Angiography

Inspection of posterior surfaces

1. Logroll the patient while maintaining cervical spine stabilization as indicated; splint injured extremities and do not roll the patient onto any injuries
2. Inspect the posterior side for the following:
   a. Exit or entrance wounds
   b. Abrasion, avulsions, or lacerations
   c. Bleeding
   d. Ecchymoses or hematomas
   e. Edema or swelling
   f. Puncture wounds or impaled objects
   g. Scars
3. Palpate for deformities, crepitus, step offs, muscle spasms, or tenderness along the entire spinal column
4. Auscultate posterior lung sounds
5. Assist with or conduct a rectal examination

Documentation

1. Assessment findings from the primary and secondary assessments
2. All interventions and patient responses
3. Reassessments
4. Vital signs and neurologic assessments
5. Fluids and medications administered, including dosage, route, and patient's response

Age-specific assessment considerations for pediatric and geriatric patients (Table 2-4)

Pain Management

Introduction

1. Pain is subjective; objectivity and a nonjudgmental attitude are crucial for the effective management of pain
2. The role of the emergency nurse is to provide comfort and to assist with managing the patient's pain through pharmacologic and nonpharmacologic methods

Pain theories (Jarvis, 2008)

1. Specific theory: specific sensation independent of other sensations
2. Gate theory: inputs in the spinal dorsal horns and brain act as a gate mechanism
3. Neuromatrix theory: there is a network of neurons between the thalamus and the cortex and the cortex and the limbic system; neural processes can trigger this network with or without stimuli from the body

Types of pain (Table 2-5)

1. Acute: caused by injury to body tissue
2. Chronic: caused by body tissue
3. Nociceptive: caused by a noxious stimulus that is damaging or that can damage tissue if it is not removed
4. Neuropathic: caused by damage to peripheral or central nerve cells

Management

1. Assessment of pain as previously described
2. Differentiation between chronic and acute pain
   a. If the patient has chronic pain, it needs to be determined whether the current pain is different from the pain that is usually felt with the condition
3. Nonpharmacologic interventions as appropriate
   a. Positioning
   b. Ice or heat
   c. Massage
   d. Relaxation or distraction
   e. Music
   f. Aromatherapy
4. Pharmacologic interventions as prescribed
   a. Agents
      1) Nonopioids (e.g., acetaminophen [Tylenol], aspirin, ibuprofen [Motrin], naproxen [Naprosyn], ketorolac [Toradol], indomethacin [Indocin])
      2) Opioids
         a) Agonists (e.g., codeine, hydrocodone, morphine, propoxyphene [Darvon], oxycodone)
         b) Partial agonists (e.g., butorphanol [Stadol], nalbuphine [Nubain])
         c) Agonist-antagonists (e.g., buprenorphine [Buprenex], pentazocine hydrochloride [Talwin])
      3) Adjuvants
         a) Antidepressants
         b) Antiemetics
         c) Sedatives
         d) Corticosteroids
         e) Local anesthetics
   b. Routes (note that not all agents may be given via all routes)
      1) Oral
      2) Intravenous
         a) Infusion
         b) Injection
         c) Patient-controlled analgesia
      3) Intramuscular
      4) Topical
      5) Rectal

Transfer and Stabilization

Patients in the ED may be transferred within the hospital or to another medical facility if their conditions warrant transfer
1. Applicable policy and procedures for boarding, admitting, or transferring patients to other facilities must be followed

Interfacility stabilization and transport: the transport of a patient to another medical facility must follow Emergency Medical Treatment and Active Labor Act (EMTALA) and Consolidated Omnibus Budget Reconciliation Act (COBRA) laws (National Highway Traffic Safety Administration, 2006)
1. Responsibility for interfacility transport is shared by both the transferring and receiving personnel and the transport program

TABLE 2-4   **Age-Specific Assessment Considerations**

Assessment Parameter	Pediatric	Geriatric
History	Consider mother's health during pregnancy; parent-child interactions; developmental level; childhood diseases; and child's ability to give pertinent data.	History may be influenced by patient's attitudes about aging; patient may respond slowly to questions; history may be influenced by deterioration of the senses.
Vital signs	Child may have faster heart and respiratory rates; blood pressure about [70 + (2 × age in years)] mm Hg; and be prone to hypothermia.	Cardiac irregularities may be a normal variable; vital signs are influenced by many medications; seniors are prone to hypothermia.
Cardiovascular	Consider potential congenital heart problems; murmur and third heart sound may be normal variants.	Cardiac output at rest decreases; development of coronary artery disease may occur; heart is less able to adapt to stress.
Respiratory	Infants are obligate nose breathers; abdominal breathing occurs until age 6 or 7; infants more susceptible to respiratory infections; airway is smaller and more easily occluded.	Elderly adults experience increased anteroposterior chest diameter, decreased pulmonary function, and decreased surface area for gas exchange.
Neurologic	Must consider developmental stage; use pediatric coma scale.	Degenerative changes occur; nerve transmission slows and may be affected by changes in other systems.
Head, ears, eyes, nose, and throat	Visual acuity of 20/20 not obtained until age 7; anatomic differences in eustachian tube predispose to ear infection; hearing develops fully at age 5 years.	Conjunctiva is thinner and yellow; arcus senilis may appear; pupil is smaller; lens loses transparency; seniors are prone to hearing loss.
Gastrointestinal	Abdominal guarding is more common in child with pain; air swallowed with crying causes abdominal distention.	Digestion, gastrointestinal tract motility, and anal sphincter tone decrease with age; seniors are prone to loss of appetite and constipation.
Genitourinary	Ability to control urination is gained between 2 and 3 years old; consider age of puberty.	Renal function decreases after age 40; incomplete bladder emptying occurs.
Musculoskeletal	Bones are flexible, increasing risk of greenstick fractures; subluxation is common.	Elderly adults have decreased muscle mass and are prone to fractures; degenerative joint disease may occur.
Integumentary	Consider diaper rash, susceptibility to contact dermatitis.	Decreased mobility leads to stasis dermatitis and ulcers.
Endocrine	Growth hormone abnormalities may occur.	Thyroid disorders may occur.
Hematopoietic	Anemias, leukemias, clotting disorders may occur during childhood.	Vitamin B_{12} absorption decreases; levels of hemoglobin and hematocrit decrease.
Immune	Child has passive immunity at birth.	Decreased antibody response occurs with age.

From Emergency Nurses Association (2010). *Sheehy's emergency nursing: principles and practice* (6th ed.). St. Louis: Mosby, p. 85.

2. Referring physician must give a report to the receiving physician who has agreed to accept the patient

3. Emergency nurse from the referring facility must call and give a report to the nurse who is receiving the patient

4. Patient must be stabilized before transport (i.e., the patient cannot be deteriorating when leaving the referring institution)

5. Correct patient materials, documents, charts, radiographs, images, angiograms, and films should be sent with the patient or transmitted to the receiving facility

6. Transfer forms must be completed with appropriate signatures and must include information regarding the certification and justification of the transfer

7. Reports and copies of the patient's chart are to be provided to the transporting agency

8. It is the responsibility of the referring hospital to make sure that the transport mode that is used is appropriate and that the agency called is qualified to assume the care of the patient and to continue the care established and given in the ED; it is an EMTALA violation to turn patient care over to a

TABLE 2-5 Physiologic Sources of Pain

Type of Pain	Physiologic Structures	Mechanism of Pain	Characteristics of Pain	Sources of Acute Pain	Sources of Chronic Pain Syndromes
Somatic pain	Cutaneous: skin and subcutaneous tissues Deep somatic: bone, muscle, blood vessels, connective tissues	Activation of nociceptors	Well localized Constant and achy	Incisional pain, pain at insertion sites of tubes and drains, wound complications, orthopedic procedures, skeletal muscle spasms	Bony metastases, osteoarthritis and rheumatoid arthritis, low back pain, peripheral vascular disease
Visceral pain	Organs and the linings of the body cavities	Activation of nociceptors	Poorly localized Diffuse, deep, cramping, or splitting	Chest tubes, abdominal tubes and drains, bladder distention or spasms, intestinal distention	Pancreatitis, liver metastasis, colitis
Neuropathic pain	Nerve fibers, spinal cord, and central nervous system	Nonnociceptive Injury to the nervous system structures	Poorly localized Shooting, burning, fiery, shocklike, sharp, and painful numbness	Phantom limb pain, postmastectomy pain, and pain from nerve compression	Diabetes, human immunodeficiency virus, chemotherapy-induced neuropathies, postherpetic neuralgia, cancer-related nerve injury

From Ignatavicius, D. & Workman, M. L. (2010). *Medical-surgical nursing: patient-centered collaborative care* (6th ed.). St. Louis, W.B. Saunders, p.

provider who cannot provide the appropriate level of skill and care

Intrafacility (ENA, 2005)

1. Admissions
   a. When a patient is admitted to the hospital, a report should be given to the receiving nurse
   b. A copy of the patient's chart should be sent with the patient
   c. Patients are to be stabilized before they leave the ED; any immediate orders should be completed before transfer
2. Patients who are boarding in the ED
   a. It is the responsibility of the emergency nurse to ensure that the same level of care is provided to patients who have been boarding in the ED as they would receive if a bed was available (e.g., a patient who would be sent to the critical care unit receives the same level of care that they would receive in the critical care unit if boarding in the ED)

Cultural Diversity

Introduction

1. The ENA has a position statement regarding diversity in emergency care (ENA, 2003)
2. The ENA believes that it is a basic human right for every patient to access culturally congruent and culturally competent care in the ED setting (ENA, 2003)

3. Emergency nurses are encouraged to support cultural awareness and competence in the ED
4. Emergency nurses should have the sensitivity to recognize, appreciate, and incorporate differences during the provision of care

Definitions

1. Diversity: those differences that make each person unique, including (but not limited to) national origin, religion, age, gender, sexual orientation, race, ethnicity, education, socioeconomic status, abilities, and disabilities
2. Culture: the learned, shared, and transmitted values, beliefs, and practices of a particular group that guide thinking, actions, behaviors, interactions with others, emotional reactions to daily living, and one's world view; subculture: a recognizable segment of a larger cultural group that shares some characteristics of the larger group but that has unique features of its own
3. Cultural sensitivity: a learned skill that involves a person having an awareness of and appreciation for another's cultural uniqueness; also referred to as *ethnosensitivity*
4. Cultural competence: "a set of congruent behaviors, attitudes, and policies that come together in a system, agency, or among professionals that enables effective work in cross-cultural situations" (U.S. Department of Health and Human Services, 2001)

5. Culturally congruent nursing care: the use of cognitively based nursing techniques that incorporate an individual's cultural values, beliefs, and lifestyles; these techniques facilitate, assist, support, or enable an individual to develop health and well-being or to face illness and death in culturally meaningful ways
6. Race: a group of people related by common descent or heredity who have similar physical characteristics, such as skin color, facial form, and eye shape
7. Ethnic group: a subset of a culture; a smaller group that identifies itself as distinct because of shared characteristics, such as culture, language, traditions, appearance, or social heritage
8. Nationality: an identifying factor of people from a place with specified political and geographic boundaries
9. Customs: patterns and practices within a cultural group that encompass collective learned behaviors, including diet and health behaviors
10. Rituals: culturally prescribed codes of behavior that may guide practices and decisions, including those that involve health and wellness
11. Values: personal standards of what is good or useful in relationship to oneself and to others
12. Norms: commonly shared customs and standards of behavior that are acceptable within a given group of people
13. Cultural paradigms: abstract explanations used by a cultural group to account for major life events
14. Enculturation: the process by which culture is transmitted from one generation to the next by means of social learning
15. Acculturation: the process by which an individual or a group takes on the behaviors and practices of the dominant culture; factors that influence the degree and pace of an individual's acculturation include the length of time in the new culture, the individual's age and economic or educational status, and the discriminatory practices of the dominant culture
16. Ethnocentrism: the belief that one's own ethnic group, way of life, beliefs, values, and so on are superior to those of others
17. Cultural imposition: the practice of imposing one's cultural beliefs on others with the belief that yours are best or superior
18. Cultural relativism: the attitude that different ways of doing things have equal validity
19. Cultural pain: the discomfort or suffering experienced by an individual or group as a result of the insensitivity of others who have different beliefs or cultural norms

Significance

1. Of the developed countries of the world, the United States experiences the greatest increase in population and diversity of inhabitants; immigration accounts for at least one third of the increase
   a. The percentage of whites of European origin (i.e., the dominant culture in the United States) will continue to decline, thereby creating a more multicultural power base
2. Nurses must be aware that issues of culture, race, gender, and socioeconomics strongly influence health status and the use of the health care system
   a. Culturally inappropriate care and inattention to cultural differences in care may negatively affect health outcomes
   b. Individuals from different cultures and illegal immigrants often delay seeking medical attention because of language, cost, and cultural barriers; these delays often result in more serious conditions
3. Health care reform is resulting in cultural competence guidelines and enforcement by state agencies

Aspects of cultural sensitivity

1. Acknowledgment that cultural diversity exists
2. Avoidance of stereotypes; appreciation of the uniqueness of each patient, with culture as one aspect that enhances his or her uniqueness
3. Respect for the unfamiliar
4. Appreciation that cultural values are ingrained and difficult to change
5. Modification of care to include consistency with the patient's culture
6. Examination of personal cultural beliefs and values
7. Realization that the patient's health practices may be very different from one's own but that each cultural group has health practices that attempt to improve health and temper illness
8. Recognition that all people within a cultural group do not respond to illness in the same way; there is diversity within cultures

Cultural assessment

1. Assess the patient's degree of acculturation (e.g., how well the language of the dominant culture is spoken, the language spoken in the home, the length of time in the country, food preferences)
2. Encourage the patient to discuss cultural beliefs and practices; definitions of health and illness, ideas about the origin of illnesses, and so on may differ within cultures
3. Make an effort to respect and understand different communication styles
4. Honor time and value orientation
5. Provide privacy according to each individual's needs; be aware that, in many cultures, it is extremely important for family members to be present during assessments
6. Identify the decision maker within the patient's family; it may be someone other than the patient
7. Recognize that a patient's reactions to pain are culturally driven
8. Be aware of biologic variations among cultures, such as body structure, skin and hair color, population-specific diseases, and psychologic coping characteristics
9. Recognize that dietary practices, religious practices, and cultural taboos have important implications that relate to nursing care

10. Identify the patient's hobbies
11. Note the patient's cultural practices and modify care as necessary

Cultural phenomena that affect nursing care (Table 2-6)
Cultural aspects of pain
1. Pain is not purely a neurophysiologic response; cultural, social, and psychologic factor influence a patient's perception of pain
2. Pain intensity, expression, tolerance, and expected responses from caretakers are influenced by culture
3. A patient's attitude and beliefs about pain are determined by culture
4. Each culture has its own language of distress:
   a. Facial expressions
   b. Sounds
   c. Changes in activity
   d. Words to describe feelings
5. Nurses must always remember that, regardless of the patient's cultural background, pain is what the patient says it is, and it occurs when the patient says that it does
   a. All pain should be considered to be real and treated compassionately
   b. Be aware that patients who do not verbally express the presence of pain may not be pain free

Drug polymorphism
1. Age, drug, gender, body size, and body composition affect an individual's response to drugs
2. Factors that influence drug polymorphism vary among ethnic groups and can be categorized as environmental, genetic, and cultural; these do not include all of the aspects that affect a patient's response to drugs, but they raise awareness of possible differences in responses
3. Drug metabolism is genetically determined
4. Race may affect a patient's response; this is also called *genetic polymorphism*
5. Environmental factors include diet, alcohol, smoking, malnutrition, vitamin deficiencies, stress, fever, and physiologic rhythms; each of these can affect drug absorption
6. Cultural factors include values, beliefs, compliance, family influence, and prior drug experience; patients may be taking herbal or homeopathic remedies that can alter the response to drug absorption
7. Nurses must become familiar with drugs that affect patients of different ethnicities; one example of this is that angiotensin-converting enzyme inhibitors (e.g., captopril) are ineffective or minimally effective in African Americans (the new angiotensin II blocker valsartan [Diovan], a calcium-channel blocker, or a β-blocker is more likely to be used for hypertension in these patients)

Cultural behaviors relevant to nursing care (Table 2-7)
1. Respect and embrace diversity among patients and health care team members

2. Have a cultural reference available on your unit
3. Have a list of contact information for employees who speak other languages and who are willing to assist with translation

Problems with providing culturally congruent health care; all of the following issues can lead to poor health outcomes
1. Stereotyping, prejudice, ignoring blind spots, and labeling
2. Personal biases and bigotry
3. Cultural differences
4. Patients being labeled by nurses as being difficult or as having a difficult family
5. Lack of interpreters and educational materials in the patient's native language
6. Lack of diversity among nursing staff
7. Lack of time (when providing culturally congruent care, listening to patients' stories is important)
8. Lack of flexibility of teaching methods

Religious diversity
1. Definitions
   a. Spirituality: a basic human phenomenon that helps create meaning in the world
      1) It encompasses a person's ideology, view of the world, and meaning of life
      2) It gives an individual a sense of inner peace and harmony
   b. Spiritual distress: a disruption in the life principle that pervades a person's entire being and that integrates and transcends one's biologic and psychosocial nature
   c. Religion: a specific unified system of an expression of the belief in and the reverence for a supernatural power accepted as the creator and governor of the universe
   d. Religious symbols: symbols used in the expression of faith (e.g., rosary, prayer cloth, prayer rug, medicine bundles, red ribbon, charms, "the garment")
   e. Meditation: a devotional exercise of contemplation
   f. Prayer: an intimate conversation between an individual and God or another higher being
   g. Hope: a wish for something that includes expectation of the wish's fulfillment
   h. Faith: a confident belief in the truth of a person, idea, or thing (e.g., God); a belief that is not based on logical proof or material evidence
2. Significance
   a. The exclusion of the important role of spirituality for patients and families can affect recovery and health
   b. The care of the whole person enhances healing and health
   c. The spiritual beliefs of the providers may be an important consideration for many patients when selecting a health care provider
3. Causes of spiritual distress
   a. Separation from religious and cultural ties
   b. Challenged belief and value systems

TABLE 2-6   Phenomena That Affect Nursing Care

Communication	Space	Time Orientation	Social Organization	Environmental Control	Biological Variation
• National language preference • Dialects, written characters • Use of silence • Nonverbal and contextual cuing	• Noncontact people	• Present	• Family; hierarchical structure, loyalty • Devotion to tradition • Many religions, including Taoism, Buddhism, Islam, and Christianity • Community social organizations	• Traditional health and illness beliefs • Use of traditional medicines • Traditional practitioners: Chinese doctors and herbalists	• Liver cancer • Stomach cancer • Coccidioidomycosis • Hypertension • Lactose intolerance
• National languages • Dialect: pidgin, Creole, Spanish, and French	• Close personal space	• Present over future	• Family: many female, single parent • Large, extended family networks • Strong church affiliation within community • Community social organizations	• Traditional health and illness beliefs • Folk medicine tradition • Traditional healer: root-worker	• Sickle cell anemia • Hypertension • Cancer of the esophagus • Stomach cancer • Coccidioidomycosis • Lactose intolerance
• National languages • Many learn English immediately	• Noncontact people • Aloof • Distant • Southern countries: closer contact and touch	• Future over present	• Nuclear families • Extended families • Judeo-Christian religions • Community social organizations	• Primary reliance on modern health care system • Traditional health and illness beliefs • Some remaining folk medicine traditions	• Breast cancer • Heart disease • Diabetes mellitus • Thalassemia
• Tribal languages • Use of silence and body language	• Space very important and has no boundaries	• Present	• Extremely family oriented • Biological and extended families • Children taught to respect traditions • Community social organizations	• Traditional health and illness beliefs • Folk medicine tradition • Traditional healer: medicine man	• Accidents • Heart disease • Cirrhosis of the liver • Diabetes mellitus
• Spanish or Portuguese primary language	• Tactile relationships • Touch • Handshakes • Embracing • Value physical presence	• Present	• Nuclear family • Extended families • Compadrazza: godparents • Community social organizations	• Traditional health and illness beliefs • Folk medicine tradition • Traditional healers: curandero, espiritisco, portera, señoro	• Diabetes mellitus • Parasites • Coccidioidomycosis • Lactose intolerance

Compiled by Rachel Spector, in Potter, P. A. & Perry, A. G. (1997). *Fundamentals of nursing: concepts, process, and practice* (4th ed.). St. Louis: Mosby.

TABLE 2-7 Cultural Behaviors That Are Relevant to Nursing Care

Cultural Group	Cultural Variations (Common Belief/Practice)	Nursing Implications
African Americans	• Dialect and slang terms require careful communication to prevent error (e.g., "bad" may mean "good").	• Question the client's meaning or intent.
Mexican Americans	• Eye behavior is important. An individual who looks at and admires a child without touching the child has given the child the "evil eye"	• Always touch the child you are examining or admiring.
Native Americans	• Eye contact is considered a sign of disrespect and is thus avoided.	• Recognize that the client may be attentive and interested even though eye contact is avoided.
Appalachians	• Eye contact is considered impolite or a sign of hostility. Verbal patter may be confusing.	• Avoid excessive eye contact. • Clarify statements.
American Eskimos	• Body language is important. The individual seldom disagrees publicly with others. Client may nod yes to be polite, even if not in agreement.	• Monitor own body language closely, as well as client's to detect meaning.
Jewish Americans	• Orthodox Jews consider excess touching, particularly from members of the opposite sex, offensive.	• Establish whether client is an Orthodox Jew and avoid excessive touch.
Chinese Americans	• Individual may nod head to indicate yes or shake head to indicate no. • Excessive eye contact indicates rudeness. • Excessive touch is offensive.	• Ask questions carefully and clarify responses. • Avoid excessive eye contact and touch.
Filipino Americans	• Offending people is to be avoided at all cost. • Nonverbal behavior is important.	• Monitor nonverbal behaviors of self and client, being sensitive to physical and emotional discomfort or concerns of the client.
Haitian Americans	• Touch is used in conversation. • Direct eye contact is used to gain attention and respect during communication.	• Use direct eye contact when communicating.
East Indian Hindu Americans	• Women avoid eye contact as a sign of respect.	• Be aware that men may view eye contact by women as offensive. Avoid eye contact.
Vietnamese Americans	• Avoidance of eye contact is a sign of respect. • The head is considered sacred; it is not polite to pat the head. • An upturned palm is offensive in communication.	• Limit eye contact. • Touch the head only when mandated and explain clearly before proceeding to do so. • Avoid hand gesturing.

From Giger, J. & Davidhizer, R. (1995). *Transcultural nursing* (2nd ed.). St. Louis: Mosby. (Originally from Kozier, B., et al. [1993]. *Techniques in clinical nursing* [2nd ed.]. Reading, MA: Addison-Wesley.

c. Sense of meaninglessness or purposelessness
d. Remoteness from God
e. Disrupted spiritual trust
f. Moral or ethical nature of therapy
g. Sense of guilt and shame
h. Intense suffering
i. Unresolved feelings about death
j. Anger toward God
4. Aspects of spiritual sensitivity include the following:
   a. Performing self-exploration of your own values and beliefs
   b. Acknowledging that you may not agree with every aspect of the patient's spiritual beliefs and practices; being nonjudgmental and respecting the patient's right to worship the supreme being of his or her choice
   c. Developing good listening skills and encouraging patients to discuss their spiritual concerns

d. Knowing your limits; if you are uncomfortable discussing spiritual needs or praying with the patient, contact the patient's personal spiritual advisor or consult the hospital chaplain service as requested by the patient or the patient's family
   e. Scheduling physical care to allow time for religious rituals and practices
   f. Respecting the patient's rights and privacy
   g. Increase your knowledge of different faiths (Table 2-8 identifies selected faiths and their nursing implications)
5. Performance of a spiritual needs assessment
   a. Assess the patient's spiritual or religious beliefs, values, and practices
   b. Listen for verbal cues regarding spirituality (e.g., referring to God, talking about religious services)
   c. Note the presence of religious symbols (e.g., crucifix, Star of David, Bible, Torah, Quran, other spiritual

TABLE 2-8   Religious Beliefs of Selected Religions and Appropriate Nursing Interventions

Religion	Belief	Interventions
Catholicism	• God does not cause suffering but allows it to further human growth • Baptism is necessary for salvation	• Inform the patient that Holy Communion is available • Have a Catholic priest or deacon available to perform the Anointing of the Sick • If the patient is close to death and a Catholic religious representative is not available, any Christian may perform a baptism; the priest should then be notified immediately • Make all efforts to leave religious symbols (e.g., a rosary) in place
Christian Scientist	• Sin, sickness, and death can be overcome by a full understanding of the divine principle of Jesus' teachings and healing • Disease and illness are delusions of the nonspiritual mind and can be overcome by prayer	• Be aware that medical care may be refused • These patients may use the services of physicians for the purposes of setting bones, treating malignancies, and delivering babies • Pain medications may be accepted for severe pain only • There is no clergy or priesthood in this religion
Hinduism	• Illness may result from the misuse of the body or from the sins of a previous lifetime • Meditation and prayer must be performed at specific times throughout the day • Females cannot be left in the presence of unfamiliar males	• Plan care around the timing of religious practices • Provide same-sex caregivers • Provide vegetarian meals as requested • These patients may refuse medications that are in capsule form because many capsules are made from beef • Allow the family to wash the family member's body after death if desired; do not remove any sacred threads that are placed on the body
Islam (Muslim)	• Followers of this religion submit to Allah's will in matters of health • Prayer and washing are required five times a day • The left hand is considered unclean; food will not be handled with the left hand	• Provide privacy and plan care to accommodate prayer times • Educate the patient about pain-reducing techniques • Provide a diet that reflects any requested dietary restrictions • Pork and some other foods are prohibited • These patients may refuse medications that are in capsule form because many capsules are made from pork • Follow patient and family wishes regarding therapies; prolonging life by life support machinery is often considered unacceptable to these patients • Allow the family to stay with the patient during the process of dying • Allow the family to wash the body after death • Turn deceased person's face toward the right
Jehovah's Witnesses	• These individuals are opposed to transfusions of blood obtained from a blood bank and to some blood products because the source of the soul is believed to be in the blood • They are opposed to eating foods to which blood has been added • They do not celebrate national holidays (including Christmas) or birthdays, and they do not salute flags; it is believed that those who violate these restrictions will spend an eternity in nothingness	• Assess the patient's religious beliefs and practices before administering blood or blood products • Most Jehovah's Witnesses carry cards that indicate the acceptable types of transfusions • According to Jehovah's Witness standards, "mature minors" may refuse blood transfusions • Be aware that the patient may refuse surgical or medical interventions that will require the transfusion of blood • Consider the use of volume expanders such as saline, lactated Ringer solution, and hetastarch (Hespan) • Implement blood-conservation strategies, especially for children • Consult hematologists and medical centers that are familiar with bloodless medicine and surgery management if needed • Respect patient and family decisions to refuse blood products • Avoid giving these patients foods to which blood has been added to (e.g., certain sausages, lunch meats) • Avoid attempts to involve these patients in preparations for the celebration of national holidays

continued

TABLE **2-8** Religious Beliefs of Selected Religions and Appropriate Nursing Interventions—cont'd

Religion	Belief	Interventions
Judaism	• Sabbath begins at sundown on Friday and ends at sundown on Saturday • There is hope for recovery until death is imminent • Orthodox Jews: may not eat non-Kosher foods • Orthodox Jews: work of any kind is prohibited on the Sabbath, including driving or using the telephone • Orthodox Jews: prayer required three times a day • A person must stay with a critically ill or dying family member until death so that the soul will not feel alone.	• Provide a kosher diet if requested • Provide privacy and plan care to accommodate prayer times • Allow a relative to stay with the dying patient • Notify a rabbi/rebbe according to the family's wishes • Caregivers should leave the body untouched for approximately 30 minutes after death to allow the soul to depart • After death, according to Judaic law, the body cannot be left alone • Autopsies are generally not allowed unless required by law • Assist and respect the practices of the Sabbath • Do not shave the body hair of Hasidic Jews • Provide same-sex caregivers for Hasidic/orthodox Jews
Seventh-Day Adventist	• Sabbath begins at dusk on Friday and continues until dusk on Saturday • The body is a temple of God and should be kept healthy	• Provide a diet that reflects requested dietary restrictions • This faith encourages a vegetarian diet • Be aware that the patient may avoid seafood, meat, caffeine, alcohol, drugs, and tobacco • Protein and iodine deficiency may occur in these patients • Be aware that the patient may refuse procedures (medical or surgical) that occur on the Sabbath

From Dennison, R. D. (2007). *Pass CCRN!* (3rd ed.). St. Louis: Mosby.

books, prayer cloth) in the room during the interview
   d. Listen for expressions of spiritual distress (e.g., expressed hopelessness or guilt, crying, sleep disturbances, disrupted spiritual trust, loss of meaning and purpose in life)
   e. Be alert to comments related to spiritual concerns or conflicts (e.g., "Why me, God?"; "I'm being punished for my sins")
   f. Determine if there are religious or spiritual practices (e.g., communion) that the patient wishes to participate in during his or her hospitalization
   g. Identify specific religious concerns (e.g., dietary needs, refusal of blood transfusions)
6. Provision of care that is sensitive to the patient's spiritual and religious needs
   a. Convey a caring, nonjudgmental attitude
   b. Inform the patient and the patient's family about the availability of spiritual and religious services (e.g., pastoral care, chapel, religious services, religious books, communion, baptism, last rites)
   c. Inform the patient and the patient's family about policies related to clergy visitation
   d. Provide privacy and opportunities for religious practices (e.g., prayer, meditation)
   e. Prepare the patient for desired religious rituals
   f. Join the patient in prayer or the reading of scripture if comfortable doing so
      1) If you are comfortable praying with the patient and the patient's family, the following suggestions may be helpful:

      a) Trust God or another higher power to enable you to know what to do and what to say
      b) Really listen to the patient so that you know what the patient's and the family's greatest concerns are
      c) Explore the spiritual needs of the patient; ask the patient what he or she would like for God or another higher power to do
      d) Keep prayers realistic (e.g., comfort versus miraculous healing)
      e) Be sensitive and respectful
      f) Hold the patient's hand or stroke his or her arm if culturally appropriate
      2) If you are not comfortable praying with or providing other spiritual support for the patient and the patient's family, call the patient's own spiritual advisor or a representative of pastoral care to pray with or comfort the patient and the patient's family
   g. With the patient's permission, notify the hospital chaplain or the patient's own spiritual advisor of the patient's spiritual distress
   h. Provide honest information to help with informed decision making when spiritual beliefs and therapeutic regimens are in conflict
7. Problems with providing spirituality sensitive health care
   a. Avoiding or minimizing the role of spirituality in patient healing
   b. Treating religious beliefs as mental illness
   c. Failing to involve the patient and the patient's family in decision making

d. Providing information that can lead to false hope
e. Not allowing the patient to have an opportunity to work through grief

Organ and Tissue Donation

Introduction

1. Emergency nurses can play a vital role in helping support families through the organ donation decision-making process
2. "The Uniform Anatomical Gift Act of 1968 allows individuals 18 years and older to give consent for removal of organs or tissue after their death by signing a donor card" (ENA, 2006, p. 129)
3. The Omnibus Reconciliation Act of 1986 requires hospitals that receive Medicare and Medicaid reimbursement to make patients and families aware of organ and tissue donation options

Sources of transplantable organs (Table 2-9)
Organ and tissue candidate criteria (Table 2-10)
Classification and characteristics of rejection response (Table 2-11)

TABLE 2-9 Sources of Transplantable Organs

Donor Source	Description	Organ Types
Deceased: donation occurs after brain death but while the heart is still beating	The patient is declared brain dead; cardiovascular circulation is maintained until the organs are removed	Kidney Pancreas Liver Intestines Heart Lung
Deceased: donation occurs after cardiac death	Nonrecoverable injury without brain death has occurred, and the removal of life support is being considered; the organs are removed immediately after the cessation of cardiopulmonary function	Kidney Pancreas Liver Lung
Living	These donations come from related family members or nonrelated donors with compatible organs; donors are living volunteers who have consented to donation	Kidney Pancreas portion Liver segment Lung lobe Intestine portion Heart*

*A patient who needs a lung transplant has a better prognosis if he or she also receives a new heart. The living heart and lung recipient can donate his or her original healthy heart at the time of surgery to a recipient who needs a heart transplant. This procedure is known as a *domino transplant*, and it is rarely performed.
Adapted from Emergency Nurses Association. (2007). *Emergency nursing core curriculum* (6th ed.). Philadelphia: Saunders.

TABLE 2-10 Organ and Tissue Donor Criteria

	Age	Qualifications	Exclusions
Deceased: brain dead	Newborn to 70 years	Brain dead and on ventilator; no prolonged cold ischemia	Suspected or history of intravenous drug use during the past year; sepsis; transmissible disease; metastatic cancer (except for primary brain tumor)
Deceased: donation immediately after cardiac death	Age varies depending on organ, up to 60 years	Nonrecoverable injury; no organ trauma or dysfunction; no prolonged warm ischemia	Cardiac death more than 1 hour after the removal of life support; other exclusions; same exclusion criteria as for "Deceased: brain death" above
Expanded or marginal	>60 years	Variable	None; weigh the risks of dying while on the transplant waiting list against those of living with a less-than-ideal organ
Eyes	Any	Acceptable condition; no malignancy or transmissible disease	Viral meningitis; systemic infection; intravenous drug use
Heart valves	38 weeks' gestation (1800 g) to 55 years	No malignancy or transmissible disease	Systemic infection; intravenous drug use
Skin and bone	16 to 75 years	No malignancy or transmissible disease	Systemic infection; intravenous drug use

Adapted from Emergency Nurses Association. (2007). *Emergency nursing core curriculum* (6th ed.). Philadelphia: Saunders.

TABLE 2-11   Classification and Characteristics of Rejection Responses

	Hyperacute	Acute	Chronic
Occurrence time frame	Within minutes to hours after transplant	1 week to 1 year after transplant	Months to years after transplant
Outcome	Organ function deteriorates rapidly	Acceleration in organ function deterioration	Organ function deteriorates gradually as a result of progressive fibrotic changes in the vascular supply to the organ
Immune response	Antibodies react quickly to class I human leukocyte antigen (HLA) donor tissue	T-cell response and antibody activation produce inflammatory and immune response	Actual cause unknown; thought to be T-cell action and immune mediators (i.e., interleukins and lymphocytes)
Confirm rejection	Tissue necrosis confirmed by laboratory studies	Loss of organ function confirmed by laboratory studies and organ biopsy but may not appear until the process has advanced	Presence of infiltrates of inflammatory cells and vascular and tissue damage that lead to organ failure; specific changes related to graft type
Treatment	None; can be prevented with improved cross matching and screening	Immunosuppressive therapy	Retransplantation

Adapted from Emergency Nurses Association. (2007). *Emergency nursing core curriculum* (6th ed.). Philadelphia: Saunders.

Clinical indications of brain death

1. Criteria: irreversible cessation of all functions of the entire brain, including the brainstem; note that specific requirements for the declaration of brain death may be affected by state laws and hospital policies
   a. Recognizable cause of coma (e.g., severe traumatic brain injury, intracranial hemorrhage or infarction, anoxic encephalopathy after cardiac arrest, drowning, asphyxiation)
   b. Exclusion of potentially reversible causes of coma (e.g., sedative drugs [including alcohol], neuromuscular blocking agents, hypothermia, metabolic or endocrine disturbances)
      1) Blood pressure >90 mm Hg
      2) Temperature >32° C (90° F)
   c. Clinical examination
      1) Absence of responsiveness to noxious stimuli
      2) Absence of movement, including posturing, shivering, and seizures, either spontaneously or to control pain stimulation in the absence of sedation and neuromuscular blockade; spinal reflexes and Babinski reflex may be present even in the presence of brain death
      3) Absence of brainstem function
         a) No pupillary light reflex
         b) No corneal reflex
         c) No oculocephalic reflex (i.e., doll's eyes)
         d) No oculovestibular reflex (caloric)
         e) No gag or cough reflexes
      4) Absence of spontaneous ventilation when tested for a sufficient time (usually 3 to 5 minutes of $PaCO_2$ of >60 mm Hg); apnea testing is performed by doing the following:
         a) Disconnecting the mechanical ventilator
         b) Delivering 100% oxygen

c) Monitoring for ventilatory effort
d) Measuring arterial blood gases to confirm $PaCO_2$ of >60 mm Hg
e) Reconnecting the ventilator
   d. Diagnostic and laboratory studies
      1) Electroencephalography: no electrical activity during a period of at least 30 minutes
      2) Cerebral angiography: no intracerebral filling in circle of Willis or at carotid bifurcation
      3) Cerebral blood flow scan: no uptake of radionuclide in brain parenchyma (this indicates that there is no cerebral blood flow)
      4) Transcranial Doppler: reverberating flow signals
2. A repeat evaluation 6 hours later is recommended
3. The signature of two physicians required for the determination of brain death, with one of the physicians not being involved in the care of the patient; note that neither of the two physicians should be involved in organ transplantation

Discharge Planning

Introduction

1. Discharge planning involves education; it provides a critical link between the treatment received and the care provided to the patient after discharge
2. Discharge planning includes an assessment of the patient's physiologic, psychologic, and social and cultural needs
3. Nurses are responsible for patient education and for making sure that the patient understands the information
   a. Teaching is an ongoing process that begins at triage
   b. Written and verbal instructions should be provided to the patient
   c. Family and friends should be involved in the process

4. Communication is a key factor; instructions should have the following characteristics:
   a. Clear and specific
   b. Age appropriate
   c. Adapted to the patient's culture and ethnicity
   d. Read through with the patient
   e. Followed by an opportunity for the patient to ask questions
5. Referrals are provided as needed, and arrangements are made for follow up

Emergency Preparedness

Introduction
1. Disaster
   a. A disaster is a catastrophic event that overwhelms local resources
   b. It may be a result of natural hazards, environmental hazards, industrial hazards, or acts of terrorism
2. Disaster preparedness (Goolsby and Kulkarni, 2006)
   a. Disaster preparedness involves the readiness of individual staff, the department, and the institution to constructively react to disaster events while reducing the negative effects on the health and safety of the staff, the patients, and the community as well as on the integrity and functioning of physical structures and systems
   b. The achievement of preparedness occurs through the process of planning, training staff, and implementing a disaster plan
   c. The goals of preparedness are to be able to respond, to mitigate damage, and to recover from a disaster if and when one occurs
3. Disaster planning: a cyclic process that is ongoing

Disaster phases (ENA, 2007)
1. Warning: the probability that a disaster is going to occur or is approaching
2. Impact: damage that occurs during the actual disaster
3. Isolation: time from when impact and damage occurs until outside help arrives

4. Rescue: assistance from outside sources becomes available
5. Restoration: emergency operations will begin to diminish as normal function returns to the community

Preplanning
1. Disaster response involves extensive preplanning of the event and the role of each specialty in the disaster response
2. ED staff participates in drills on the local and regional levels to prepare for possible disasters

Disaster management stages (ENA, 2007)
1. Preparedness
   a. Having a plan before a disaster occurs
   b. Informing the community
   c. Training for disasters
   d. Performing and evaluating disaster exercises
2. Mitigation
   a. Minimizing the effects of the disaster (e.g., moving people out of the way of a hurricane before it hits)
3. Response
   a. Activating and implementing of plan
4. Recovery
   a. Returning to predisaster functioning
   b. Debriefing after a critical incident

Multiple-casualty incident
1. Makes use of various systems to rapidly triage and sort patients into categories
   a. START (simple triage and rapid transport) (Figure 2-2)
   b. Patient priority established on the basis of respiratory, hemodynamic, and mental statuses
   c. METTAG system (medical emergency triage tag) (ENA, 2007)
      1) Red: critical injuries: rapid transport
      2) Yellow: less serious injuries: delayed transport
      3) Green: no or mild injuries: transport not needed
      4) Black: dead or not salvageable

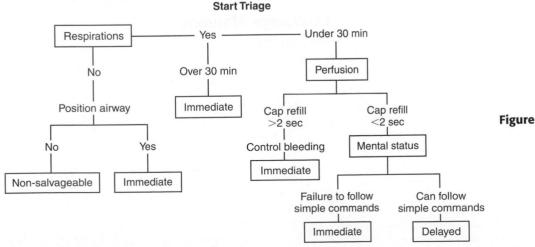

Figure 2-2 START triage.

Weapons of mass destruction include the following:

1. Explosives
2. Chemical weapons
3. Biologic weapons
4. Radiation or nuclear weapons

Bioterrorism

1. The deliberate use of a microorganism to cause disease for a purpose
2. ED procedures during chemical hazard emergencies follow the recommendations of the Centers for Disease Control and Prevention (2005):
   a. When the patient presents, try to determine the identity of the agent
   b. Use personal protection equipment; decontaminate supplies, and obtain antidotes
   c. If a chemical hazard certain or very likely, ED personnel should put on their personal protective equipment, and the ED should set up a hotline
   d. Clear and secure all areas that could become contaminated
   e. Secure the hospital entrances and grounds
   f. Notify local emergency management authorities if required
   g. If the chemical is a military agent and the army has not been informed, call them (www.cdc.gov/nceh/demil/articles/initialtreat.htm)
   h. If an organophosphate is involved, notify the hospital pharmacy that large amounts of atropine and pralidoxime (2-PAM) chloride may be needed.
   i. Keep in mind that a contaminated patient may present at an ED without warning
   j. Determine whether a chemical hazard exists
   k. If the patient is grossly contaminated or if there is any suspicion of contamination, decontaminate the patient before he or she enters the building
3. More specific information about certain agents, patient assessments, and treatments is discussed in Chapter 12

LEARNING ACTIVITIES

1. DIRECTIONS: Complete the following crossword puzzle related to patient care management.

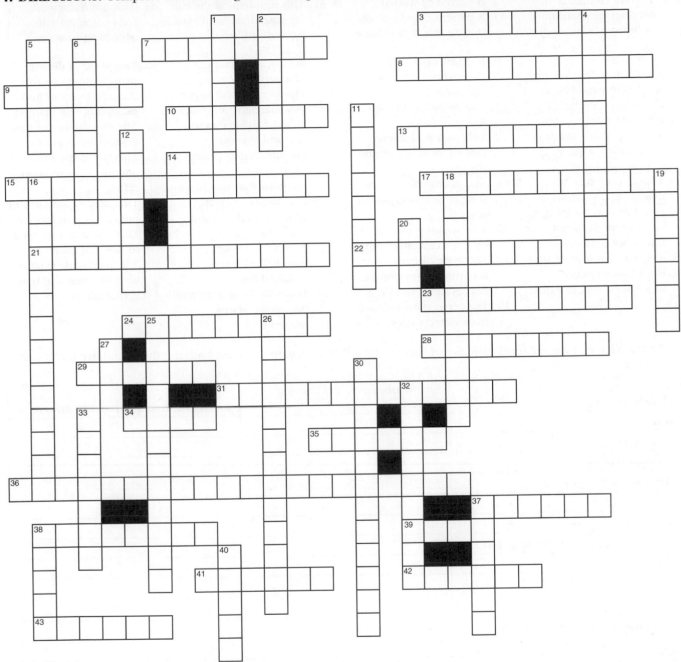

ACROSS

3. Suture removal would be at this level in the three-level acuity system
7. A patient with a myocardial infarction would be at this level in the three-level acuity system
8. This type of chest movement is characteristic of flail chest

9. A drooping eyelid
10. An initial assessment that consists of ABCD
13. This type of planning includes an assessment of the patient's physiologic, psychologic, social, and cultural needs
15. This is why the patient is seeking help in his or her own words (2 words)

17. This type of pain is caused by damage to nerve cells
21. The belief that one's own ethnic group, way of life, beliefs, and values are superior to those of others
22. The differences that make each person unique

23. This is indicative of an intact oculocephalic reflex (2 words)
24. The phase during a disaster from when impact and damage occur until outside help arrives
28. This respiratory pattern is regular, rapid, deep, and labored

29. Triage rating systems are based on this
31. The inability to open the eyes
34. This mnemonic is used for mechanism of injury

DOWN

1. A patient with myocardial infarction would be rated at this level in the five-level acuity system
2. This system for triage is used during a mass-casualty incident
4. This type of pain is caused by a noxious stimulus that is damaging or that can damage tissue if it is not removed
5. The law that forbids turning a patient over to a lower level of care

35. This is the damage phase of a disaster
36. These are situations that are mandated to be reported (2 words)
37. A patient of any age can donate this organ/tissue

6. A catastrophic event that overwhelms local resources
11. The pediatric focused assessment
12. This sign is characterized by bruising around the eyes
14. The mnemonic that is used to describe patient history
16. This sound is produced by a hyperinflated lung
18. This type of movement is controlled by cranial nerves III, IV, and VI
19. The learned, shared, and transmitted values,

38. A persistent penile erection
39. A mnemonic for a brief neurologic assessment
41. This sign behind the ear indicates that basal skull fracture is likely

beliefs, and practices of a particular group
20. This occurs with hypervolemia, right ventricular failure, cardiac tamponade, and tension pneumothorax (abbrev)
25. This is a basic human phenomenon that helps individuals to create meaning in the world
26. This type of transfer must be consistent with EMTALA and COBRA laws
27. This scale is used to rate neurologic status (abbrev)

42. This color tag would be given to patients in a disaster whose transportation can be delayed
43. This is a framework for sorting patients according to acuity
30. This stage of disaster management involves the development and practicing of a plan
32. The mnemonic for this assessment is *FGHI*
33. This test is used to evaluate the oculovestibular reflex
37. This sign is indicative of intraperitoneal bleeding
38. This mnemonic is used to describe pain
40. This pain scale is used with children and nonverbal adults

2. DIRECTIONS: Rate the level of acuity of each of the following situations using both the three- and five-level acuity systems.

Situation	Rating on three-level acuity system	Rating on five-level acuity system
Sore throat		
Cardiac arrest		
Multiple trauma		
Need for staple removal		
Anaphylaxis		
Abruptio placentae		
Urinary tract infection without fever		
Traumatic amputation		
Kidney stone		
Need for wound check		
Open fracture with good pulses		
Acute arterial occlusion		
Closed fracture		
Sexually transmitted disease exposure		
Toothache with abscess		
Possible pregnancy		
Dehydration with mild tachycardia		
Acute asthma attack		
Sprained ankle		

3. DIRECTIONS: List the functions of the triage nurse.

1	
2	
3	
4	
5	
6	

4. DIRECTIONS: Describe the components of the MITV assessment.

M	
I	
V	
T	

5. DIRECTIONS: List the "triage red flags."

Airway	• • • • •
Breathing	• • • • • • • •
Circulation	• • • • • • •
Disability	• • •
Exposure	• • •
Vital signs	• • •
Pain	•
History	• • •

6. DIRECTIONS: Briefly describe the treatment for each of the following problems that affect breathing during the primary survey.

Open pneumothorax	
Flail chest	

Tension pneumothorax	
Hemothorax	
Impaled objects	

7. DIRECTIONS: List the five focused adjuncts.

8. DIRECTIONS: Describe the AVPU mnemonic that is used to assess neurologic status

A	
V	
P	
U	

9. DIRECTIONS: A trauma patient is being assessed in the ED. Place each of the patient's assessments into either the primary assessment column or the secondary assessment column in the table. The patient arrives in the ED screaming in pain: "It hurts! It hurts where I fell from the car." The patient is alert but combative, and the abdomen is rigid. There is obvious deformity of the right lower extremity without bleeding. The right lower extremity is elevated, and ice is applied. There are no bleeding, loose teeth, or vomitus in the oral cavity. There are multiple scrapes to all four extremities. The neurovascular status in the right lower limb is as follows: pulses, 2; capillary refill, 2 seconds; patient can move toes. The respiratory rate is 28 breaths per minute.

Primary Survey	Secondary Survey

10. DIRECTIONS: List nonpharmacologic interventions for pain.

11. DIRECTIONS: Identify the following as true or false.

a. The nurse's own values and beliefs will not affect his or her sensitivities toward his or her patients.	True	False
b. Pain is influenced by culture.	True	False
c. Race is not a factor in drug absorption and action.	True	False

d. It is never appropriate for a nurse to pray with a patient; he or she should call the chaplain.	True	False
e. Decisions regarding medical care should be made by the physician alone.	True	False
f. Physical care should always take precedence over psychosocial and spiritual care.	True	False
g. The inability to speak English is an indication of ignorance.	True	False

12. DIRECTIONS: Match the religion with the implication.

___Islam (Muslim)	a. Provide a kosher diet as requested
___Catholicism	b. Opposed to blood transfusions
___Judaism	c. Provide same-sex caregivers
___Hinduism	d. Medical care may be refused; prayer is used as the primary treatment of illness
___Christian Scientist	e. The patient must be baptized before death
___Seventh-Day Adventist	f. Procedures may be refused between dusk on Friday and dusk on Saturday
___Jehovah's Witnesses	g. The patient's head is turned to the right after death

13. DIRECTIONS: Describe the sources of a disaster.

14. DIRECTIONS: Describe the color coding of the METTAG system.

LEARNING ACTIVITIES ANSWERS

1.

Crossword puzzle answers:

3 Across: NONURGENT
7 Across: EMERGENT
8 Across: PARADOXICAL
9 Across: PTOSIS
10 Across: PRIMARY
13 Across: DISCHARGE
15 Across: CHIEF COMPLAINT
17 Across: NEUROPATHIC
21 Across: ETHNOCENTRISM
22 Across: DIVERSITY
23 Across: DOLLS EYES
24 Across: ISOLATION
28 Across: KUSSMAUL
29 Across: ACUITY
31 Across: BLEPHAROSPASM
35 Across: IMPACT
36 Across: REPORTABLE OCCURRENCE
37 Across: CORNEA
38 Across: PRIAPISM
39 Across: AVPU
41 Across: BATTLE
42 Across: YELLOW
43 Across: TRIAGE

2.

Situation	Rating on three-level acuity system	Rating on five-level acuity system
Sore throat	3	4
Cardiac arrest	1	1
Multiple trauma	1	1
Need for staple removal	3	5
Anaphylaxis	1	1

Abruptio placentae	2	2
Urinary tract infection without fever	3	4
Traumatic amputation	1	1
Kidney stone	2	3
Need for wound check	3	5
Compound fracture with good pulses	2	3
Acute arterial occlusion	1	1
Closed fracture	2	3
Sexually transmitted disease exposure	3	5
Toothache with abscess	2	3
Possible pregnancy	3	5
Dehydration with mild tachycardia	2	3
Acute asthma attack	1	2
Sprained ankle	3	4

3.

1. Assess, prioritize, categorize, and monitor patients who present to the Ed for treatment
2. Ensure that all patients receive an initial triage assessment within 5 minutes of arrival
3. Initiate appropriate interventions and transfer the patient to the care area if at any time during the triage process a life-threatening problem is identified
4. Maintain confidentiality with all patients
5. Maintain focus and objectivity when making triage decisions and acuity assignments

4.

M	Mechanism of injury
I	Suspected injuries
V	Vital signs
T	Treatment on scene and patient response

5.

Airway	• Apnea • Choking • Drooling • Audible airway sounds • Positioning
Breathing	• Grunting • Sternal retractions, increased work of breathing • Irregular respiratory patterns • Respiratory rate >60 breaths/min • Respiratory rate <20 breaths/min for children <6 years old • Respiratory rate <15 breaths/min for children <15 years old • Absence of breath sounds • Cyanosis
Circulation	• Cool or clammy skin • Tachycardia, bradycardia • Heart rate >200 beats/min • Heart rate <60 beats/min • Hypotension • Diminished or absent peripheral pulses • Decreased tearing, sunken eyes

Disability	• Altered level of consciousness • Inconsolability • Sunken or bulging fontanel
Exposure	• Petechiae • Purpura • Signs and symptoms of maltreatment or abuse
Vital signs	• Hypothermia • Temperature >100.4° F (38° C) in an infant <3 months old • Temperature >104° F to 105° F (40° C to 40.6° C) at any age
Pain	• Severe pain
History	• History of chronic illness • History of family crisis • Return visit to ED within 24 hours

6.

Open pneumothorax	• Petroleum gauze dressing secured on three sides; removal and reapplication if tension pneumothorax develops • Chest tube
Flail chest	• Stabilization of the flail portion with a bulky dressing • Mechanical ventilation frequently required for internal stabilization
Tension pneumothorax	• Needle decompression followed by chest tube
Hemothorax	• Chest tube • Surgical exploration and repair
Impaled objects	• Stabilization of object • Removal by surgeon

7.

Attach cardiac monitor
Obtain pulse oximeter
Consider inserting urinary catheter if no contraindications
Insert gastric tube if patient intubated or if condition warrants
Facilitate laboratory studies if not already performed

8.

A	Alert
V	Responds to verbal stimulation
P	Responds only to painful stimulation
U	Unresponsive

9.

Primary Survey	Secondary Survey
Vocalizing Alert Combative No uncontrolled bleeding Oral cavity: no bleeding, loose teeth, or vomitus Respiratory rate of 28 breaths/minute	Rigid abdomen Obvious deformity of right lower extremity Multiple scrapes on all four extremities Neurovascular status of right lower limb

10.

Positioning
Ice or heat
Massage
Relaxation or distraction
Music
Aromatherapy

11.

a. False
b. True
c. False
d. False
e. False
f. False
g. False

12.

g. Islam (Muslim)
e. Catholicism
a. Judaism
c. Hinduism
d. Christian Scientist
f. Seventh-Day Adventist
b. Jehovah's Witnesses

13.

Natural hazards
Environmental hazards
Industrial hazards
Acts of terrorism

14.

Red: critical injuries: rapid transport
Yellow: less serious injuries: delayed transport
Green: no or mild injuries: transport not needed
Black: dead or not salvageable

References and Selected Readings

American College of Surgeons. (2004). *Advance trauma life support manual.* (7th ed.). Chicago: Author.

Bridges, N., & Jarquin-Valdivia, A.A. (2005). Use of the Trendelenburg Position as the Resuscitation Position: To T or Not to T? *Am J Crit Care, 14(5),* 364–368.

Centers for Disease Control and Prevention. (2005). *Emergency room procedures in chemical hazard emergencies.* Retrieved August 9, 2008, from www.cdc.gov/nceh/demil/articles/initialtreat.htm.

Dennison, R.D. (2007). *Pass CCRN!* (3rd ed.). St. Louis: Mosby.

Emergency Nurses Association. (2007). *Emergency nursing core curriculum* (6th ed.). Philadelphia: Saunders.

Emergency Nurses Association. (2003). *Emergency nursing pediatric course provider manual* (3rd ed.). Park Ridge, IL: Author.

Emergency Nurses Association. (2003). *Position statement: Diversity in emergency care.* Retrieved August 14, 2008, from http://www.ena.org/about/position/PDFs/Diversity-in-Emergency-Care.pdf.

Emergency Nurses Association. (2005). *Sheehy's manual of emergency care* (6th ed.). St. Louis: Mosby.

Fultz, J., & Sturt, P.A. (2005). *Mosby's emergency nursing reference* (3rd ed.). St. Louis: Mosby.

Giger, J. & Davidhizer, R. (1995). *Transcultural nursing* (2nd ed.). St. Louis: Mosby.

Goolsby, C.A., & Kulkarni, R. (2006). *Disaster planning. Emedicine.* Retrieved August 14, 2008, from www.emedicine.com/emerg/topic718.htm.

Ignatavicius, D. & Workman M.L. (2010). *Medical-surgical nursing: patient-centered collaborative care* (6th ed.). St. Louis: W.B. Saunders.

Jarvis, C. (2008). *Physical examination and health assessment* (5th ed.). St. Louis: Saunders.

National Highway and Transportation Safety Administration. (2006). *Guidelines for interfacility patient transfer.* Retrieved August 10, 2008. from http://www.nhtsa.dot.gov/people/injury/ems/Interfacility/images/Interfacility.pdf.

Ostrow, L., Hupp, E., & Topjian, D. (1994). The effect of Trendelenburg and modified Trendelenburg positions on cardiac output, blood pressure, and oxygenation: A preliminary study. *American Journal of Critical Care, 3,* 382.

Price, S.A., & Wilson, L.M. (2003). *Pathophysiology: Clinical concepts of disease process* (6th ed.). St. Louis: Mosby.

Seidel, H.M., Ball, J.W., Dains, J.E., & Benedict, G.W. (2007). *Mosby's guide to physical examination* (6th ed.). Philadelphia: Mosby

Sullivan, R. (1989). Triage: A subspecialty of emergency nursing. *Emphasis: Nursing, 3,* 26–33.

National Conference Of Commissioners On Uniform State Laws. (2008). *The Uniform Anatomical Gift Act of 1968, amended 1987.* Retrieved August 14, 2008, from www.law.upenn.edu/bll/archives/ulc/fnact99/uaga87.htm.

U.S. Department of Health and Human Services, Health Resources and Services Administration. (2001). *Cultural competence works.* Retrieved August 15, 2008, from ftp://ftp.hrsa.gov/financeMC/cultural-competence.pdf.

Zimmerman, P.G., & Herr, R. (2006). *Triage nursing secrets.* St. Louis: Mosby.

Professional Issues in Emergency Nursing

Introduction to the Professional Issues in Emergency Nursing Chapter

Constitutes 5% (seven items) of the CEN examination

Comprised of a wide variety of content

Delegation

Delegation involves "the transfer of responsibility for the performance of a task from one individual to another while remaining accountable for the outcome" (Bonalumi and King, 2007, p. 1047)

1. Communication must be clear
2. Ongoing assessment of the delegated task is necessary

Delegation of specific elements of care using the "Five Rights of Delegation" (American Nurses Association [ANA], 2005)

1. Right task
2. Right circumstances
3. Right person
4. Right direction and communication
5. Right supervision and evaluation

Process of delegation (ANA, 2005)

1. Identify desired outcome
2. Identify necessary skills and competencies
3. Select the individual or team most capable to accomplish the desired outcome
4. Communicate clearly the desired outcome but do not dictate how to get there
5. Empower the delegate to complete the task
6. Set deadlines and monitor progress along the way
7. Provide guidance through the process
8. Evaluate performance and reward accomplishment

Guidelines for delegation

1. Recognize what may not be delegated (ANA, 2005)
   a. Initial and subsequent nursing assessments requiring the professional judgment of a registered nurse
   b. Determination of nursing diagnoses, care goals, care plans, and progress
   c. Interventions that require the knowledge and skill of a registered nurse
2. Be aware of the job description, skills, and knowledge of the individual to whom you have delegated a task

Critical Incident Stress Management

Critical incident
Definition

1. Any event that causes a team member to experience overwhelming emotions and may interfere with personal or professional functioning
2. Examples (Mitchell and Bray, 1990)
   a. Death of a coworker
   b. Death of a child
   c. Event that led to excessive media coverage
   d. When team members know their patients
   e. Mass casualty disasters
   f. Incidents that threaten the safety of the team
   g. Any incident that has unusual circumstances

Critical incident stress management
Definition

1. Set of interventions designed to assist emergency medical services personnel with dealing with the stress from critical incidents
   a. Specific signs and symptoms can occur as a reaction to a critical incident and are a normal reaction to an abnormal event (Emergency Nurses Association [ENA], 2007)
   b. Interventions include the following:
      1) Ongoing education on stress management
      2) Specific services, such as debriefing, to assist personnel in dealing with a specific critical incident
2. Debriefing (Mitchell and Bray, 1990)
   a. Purpose: allows emergency personnel to discuss their perceptions of the incident and their feelings and emotions in a supportive environment
   b. Timing: done soon after an event (hopefully within 72 hours) and conducted by a mental health provider and one or two peers who have received special training in the process
   c. Goal: personnel to return to their previous level of functioning and not suffer the effects of cumulative stress
   d. Phases in the debriefing process
      1) Initial phase: introductions and ground rules
      2) Fact phase: individuals discuss their role in the incident and what they experienced through their five senses
         a) Note: this is the only mandatory part of the debriefing; after this, individuals do not have to speak

3) Thought phase: individuals who are willing to share at this point explain their thoughts and feelings during the incident

4) Reaction phase: a typical question asks what the worst part of the incident was for each participant

5) Symptom phase: individuals discuss physical, cognitive, emotional, and behavioral symptoms they may be experiencing

6) Teaching phase: Critical Incident Stress Management (CISM) members teach participants about stress management techniques and ways of supporting one another

7) Reentry phase: opportunity to ask questions is followed by a summary of the event and debriefing
    a) The mental health provider can make referrals if needed
    b) Debriefing process is often followed by food, the universal symbol of caring

Preservation of Evidence for Legal/Forensic Situations

Preservation of evidence is an important aspect of forensics; medical forensics is the "collection, analysis, and interpretation of medical evidence in legal cases" (Johnson, 2005, p. 28)

Nurses need to understand how to collect and preserve evidence and the chain of custody of the evidence

1. Most crime laboratories follow Federal Bureau of Investigation (FBI) laboratory standards for collecting evidence

2. Locard's principle is that: "when a person or object comes in contact with another person or object, there exists a possibility that an exchange of material will take place" (Saferstein, 2006, p. 101)
   a. This is an important principle to remember as evidence that comes into contact with other evidence or other items can become "contaminated" and the evidence can be called into question

3. Commercial evidence kits and preprinted forms should be used whenever possible for consistency

There are many situations in which the nurse should collect evidence, including cases that involve the following:

1. Child/disabled adult/elder abuse or neglect
2. Sexual assault
3. Crimes (e.g., homicide)
4. Trauma or other unexpected deaths

Guidelines for preserving evidence collected in the emergency department include the following (Saferstein, 2006):

1. Do not delay lifesaving measures in an attempt to collect evidence; the priority is patient care and lifesaving interventions
2. Do not throw away clothing; place wet or bloody clothes in a paper bag after they have air-dried

   a. Do not give personal items to family members without checking with local authorities first
   b. Never use plastic bags or airtight containers
   c. Place each piece of clothing in a separate bag
   d. Do not fold items if possible; if items must be folded, place paper between the folds
   e. If clothing must be cut, carefully cut around gunshot holes or knife wounds; try to cut along seams

3. Place the hands of a person involved in a shooting incident in paper bags without washing them to preserve gunpowder evidence if present; it does not matter if the person is a victim or the alleged shooter

4. Document what the patient says about the incident exactly; also document behavior carefully and objectively

5. Carefully and objectively document wound assessments; if allowed, take photographs of wounds
   a. Use a body diagram or commercial drawings to identify location of wounds
   b. Use photographs to supplement the documentation
      1) Attempt to get patient or family permission before taking photographs
      2) Obtain three views (ENA, 2007)
         a) Show orientation of injury
         b) Show location
         c) Show size; include ruler or coin in photograph
      3) Label appropriately (ENA, 2007)
         a) Do not write directly on photograph
         b) Identify patient's name and photographer's name
         c) Identify date and time the photograph was taken
      4) Place photograph in envelope, seal envelope, and keep with medical record
   c. Accurately measure wounds
   d. Use correct terminology
   e. Do not make judgments about wounds (i.e., do not classify bullet wounds as "entrance" or "exit")

6. Avoid cleaning wounds until after the police investigation if possible

7. Do not handle evidence removed from the patient (i.e., a bullet); place the object in a sealed container and label with location found, date and time, and the initials of the person who found the item

8. Be aware of state and local laws and facility policies pertaining to consent for specimen collection (e.g., blood, urine, etc.)

9. Follow institutional procedure, procedures developed by local law enforcement, or other guidelines

Chain of custody

1. Refers to ensuring that evidence has not been tampered with and will be considered valid in a court of law
2. Consists of documentation of how the evidence was collected and labeled, by whom, and how that evidence was transferred to law enforcement officials
   a. Documentation includes the name of the person who obtained the evidence with date and time and the person who took the evidence with affiliation, date, and time

b. Best to use preprinted chain of custody forms
c. The fewer people who handle evidence, the better

Ethical Decision Making

Definitions and concepts related to ethical decision making

1. Altruism: acting in a way that benefits others
2. Values: "ideals, beliefs, and patterns of behaviors that are prized and chosen by a person, group, or society" (Harkreader, Hogan, and Thobaben, 2007, p. 17)
3. Morals: "standards of conduct that represent the ideal in human behavior" (Harkreader et al., 2007, p. 17)
4. Bioethics: considers ethics in light of new discoveries and advances in science

Nurses, guided by ethics, must consciously act in a way that considers the consequences of their action on others
Decision making in nursing combines knowledge of legal standards plus altruism, values, morals, and ethical standards
The ANA has delineated a Code of Ethics for Nurses (Box 3-1)

Ethical Principles

1. Autonomy: an individual's obligation to respect a person's the right of self-determination, independence, and freedom
   a. The nurse must be willing to respect the patient's right to make decisions about his or her own care, even if the nurse does not agree with those decisions
   b. Limitations to autonomy include the following:
      1) When the rights of one person interfere with another individual's rights, health, or well-being
      2) When there is a high probability that a person may injure himself or others
2. Beneficence: an individual's obligation to do good and not harm
   a. Conflicts that may occur include the following decisions:
      1) What is best for another person
      2) Who should make the decision
      3) Long-term or short-term benefit (a temporary harm may eventually produce a greater good)
3. Nonmaleficence: an individual's obligation to do no harm, intentionally or nonintentionally
   a. It includes protecting mentally incompetent persons, nonresponsive persons, children, and any other person who cannot protect himself
   b. This principle is not absolute; an example of a conflict related to nonmaleficence is when surgical trauma causes an ultimate cure or improvement in the patient's condition
4. Veracity: an individual's obligation to tell the truth and to not intentionally deceive or mislead the patient
   a. This principle is not absolute; an example of a conflict related to veracity is when telling the patient the truth may cause harm

---

BOX 3-1   American Nurses Association (ANA) Code of Ethics for Nurses

1. The nurse, in all professional relationships, practices with compassion and respect for the inherent dignity, worth, and uniqueness of every individual, unrestricted by considerations of social or economic status, personal attributes, or the nature of health problems.
2. The nurse's primary commitment is to the patient, whether an individual, family, group, or community.
3. The nurse promotes, advocates for, and strives to protect the health, safety, and rights of the patient.
4. The nurse is responsible and accountable for individual nursing practice and determines the appropriate delegation of tasks consistent with the nurse's obligation to provide optimum patient care.
5. The nurse owes the same duties to self as to others, including the responsibility to preserve integrity and safety, to maintain competence, and to continue personal and professional growth.
6. The nurse participates in establishing, maintaining, and improving health care environments and conditions of employment conducive to the provision of quality health care and consistent with the values of the profession through individual and collective action.
7. The nurse participates in the advancement of the profession through contributions to practice, education, administration, and knowledge development.
8. The nurse collaborates with other health professionals and the public in promoting community, national, and international efforts to meet health needs.
9. The profession of nursing as represented by associations and their members, is responsible for articulating nursing values, for maintaining the integrity of the profession and. its practice, and for shaping social policy.

From the American Nurses Association. (2001). *Code of ethics for nurses with interpretive statements.* Washington, D.C.: Author.

---

5. Justice: an individual's obligation to be fair to all people
   a. Individuals have the right to be treated fairly and equally regardless of race, sex, marital status, medical diagnosis, social standing, economic level, or religious belief; also includes equal access to health care for all
6. Paternalism: an individual's obligation to assist an individual to make a decision when they do not have sufficient data or expertise
   a. Undesirable when the entire decision if taken away from the patient
7. Fidelity: an individual's obligation to be faithful or loyalty to agreements and responsibilities that the individual has accepted
   a. It is one of the key elements of accountability
   b. A conflict may occur between fidelity to patients and fidelity to employer, government, and society

Ethical approaches: vary in the basis for ethical decisions

1. Deontology: actions are right or wrong based on a set of morals or rules
   a. Emphasizes duty or obligation to another person
   b. Only acceptable ethical theory for decision making in health care
2. Teleology: actions are right or wrong based on the action's consequences and usefulness; looks at outcome; the end justifies the means
3. Utilitarianism: the morally right thing to do is whatever produces the greatest good for the greatest number; it is derived from teleology
4. Egoism: actions are right or wrong based on self-interest and self-preservation
5. Paternalism: beneficence should take precedence over autonomy
6. Social contract theory: actions are considered with distributive justice with each person having equal right to the greatest degree of liberty possible
7. Natural law: actions are morally or ethically right when they are in accord with human nature

Moral distress: when one knows the right thing to do but cannot pursue the right action; obstacles may be internal or external

1. Four As model to rise above moral distress (American Association of Critical-Care Nurses [AACN], 2004)
   a. Ask: determine whether the nurse is experiencing moral distress
      1) Expressions of anger, resentment, frustration
      2) Statements such as "why are we doing this?"
      3) Physical symptoms such as change in weight, sleep patterns, depression
   b. Affirm
      1) Affirm the distress
      2) Affirm professional obligations as described in the ANA Code of Ethics for Nurses
   c. Assess
      1) Identify sources and severity of moral distress
      2) Identify barriers, risks, strengths
   d. Act: based on self-exploration regarding obligations, responsibilities, risks

Ethical dilemma: situation that requires a choice between two or more equally undesirable alternatives

1. Characteristics of an ethical dilemma (Curtin, 1982)
   a. The problem cannot be solved using only empirical data
   b. The problem is so perplexing that it is difficult to decide what facts and data should be used to make the decision
   c. There are far-reaching effects to the decision
2. Conflicts related to rights of the individual: autonomy versus paternalism
   a. Informed consent
   b. Technology versus quality of life
   c. Resuscitate versus do-not-resuscitate (DNR)

   d. Behavior control
      1) Behavior control may be misused to suppress personal freedom (e.g., use of restraints or sedating drugs)
      2) Individual's right to freedom may conflict with society's obligation to maintain social order
3. Conflicts related to resource allocations: justice versus utilitarianism
   a. Triage decisions
   b. Quality-of-life decisions
   c. Inability to pay and/or lack of health insurance
   d. Organ transplantation decisions
      1) Living donors: rights of donor, recipient, families, society
      2) Choice of one recipient over another: potential for elitism
      3) Utilization of health care resources: tremendous cost of organ transplantation
      4) Designation of death: when can an organ or organs be removed
4. Conflicts related to the role of the nurse: veracity versus fidelity
   a. Withholding therapy
   b. Right to die
      1) Positive euthanasia (also referred to as active euthanasia or mercy killing): life support systems are withdrawn or a medication, treatment, or procedure is used to cause death (e.g., assisted suicide)
      2) Negative euthanasia (also referred to as passive euthanasia): no extraordinary or heroic life-support measures are used to save a person's life (e.g., DNR orders)
5. Conflicts related to personal values: professional integrity versus personal ethical and moral beliefs
   a. Nurse participation in treatments or therapies against his or her ethical or moral beliefs (e.g., abortion)
   b. Nurse providing care for patients whose practices are against his or her ethical or moral beliefs (e.g., domestic violence)

Factors affecting ethical issues and ethical decision making (Figure 3-1)
Steps in the ethical decision making process (Harkreader et al., 2007, p. 23)
1. Identify the ethical dilemma [situation]
2. Gather pertinent data
3. Examine the dilemma for ethical principles
4. Examine all solutions
5. Choose solution
6. Evaluate solutions chosen

Patient Confidentiality
Confidentiality is both a legal and an ethical issue
1. Health Insurance Portability and Accountability Act of 1996 (HIPAA) ensures confidentiality by outlining how a patient's medical information can be used
   a. Personally identifiable information is protected
      1) Access is limited to those with a "need to know"

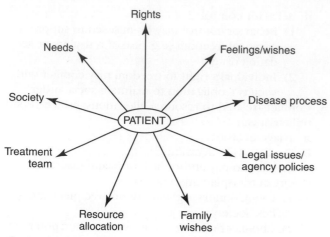

Figure 3-1 Factors affecting ethical issues and ethical decision making in nursing. (From Kinney, M., et al. [1998]. *AACN clinical reference for critical care nursing* (4th ed.). St. Louis: Mosby.)

     2) Anyone else wishing to view a patient's record must obtain the patient's permission

  b. Specific constraints mandated on electronic records

  c. Violations can incur both civil and criminal penalties

2. Common ways in which confidentiality is breached in emergency departments (EDs)

  a. Status board listing patient's names and/or initials and complaints

  b. Staff conversations in crowded ED spaces or in open bays

  c. Conversations by non-ED personnel, such as police or emergency medical technicians

3. Nurses must be extremely vigilant to not breach the confidentiality of their patients

  a. Never share passwords

  b. Never leave computer terminals unattended

  c. Do not allow anyone else to view patient information on the computer screen

  d. Do not view things you do not have a need to know

Notification of authorities of reportable situations

1. Certain conditions require breaching patient confidentiality and reporting to local or state authorities; state law determines what conditions are reportable

  a. Situations that require reporting in most states (ENA, 2005)

    1) Any death in the ED and deaths within 28 hours of hospital admission

    2) Child abuse

    3) Disabled adult abuse

    4) Elder abuse

    5) Elopement of psychiatric patients

    6) Extensive burns

    7) Gunshot and stab wounds

    8) Homicide

    9) Infectious outbreaks

    10) Internal disasters

    11) Rape/sexual assault

    12) Serious injury, illness, or death reasonably suggested to be related to the use of a medical device

    13) Sexually transmitted infections

    14) Suicide (including attempted suicides)

2. Nurses should understand who, in their department, has the duty to report these situations

  a. Ultimate responsibility lies with the nurse

3. All 50 states have child abuse/neglect reporting laws

4. Other general situations that may require reporting include violence/crime, vulnerable person abuse/neglect, and communicable diseases

5. In some states, psychiatric issues are also reportable

Legal Concepts Important to Emergency Nursing

Legal issues

1. Sources of law

  a. A *constitution* establishes the basis of a governing system

  b. *Statutes* are laws that govern

    1) Made, voted on, and passed by legislative bodies

    2) Nurse practice acts are statutes

      a) Define and limit the practice of nursing

      b) May vary state to state but all must be consistent with federal provisions and statutes

  c. Administrative agencies (e.g., state boards of nursing) create rules and regulations that enforce statutory laws

    1) Each state has a Nurse Practice Act, which is the legal document spelling out nursing responsibilities and scope of practice

  d. Court decisions are made when the courts interpret legal issues that are in dispute

  e. Common law consists of broad and comprehensive principles based on justice, reason, and common sense rather than rules and regulations

2. Types of court cases

  a. Criminal: charges filed by the state or federal attorney general for crimes committed against an individual or society

    1) Burden of proof is on the filing agency; the defendant is presumed innocent and must be proven guilty beyond reasonable guilt

    2) Consequences if found guilty are imprisonment or even death

    3) An example would be a nurse who intentionally administered drugs that causes a patient's death

  b. Civil: one individual sues another

    1) Burden of proof to be found guilty is a preponderance of the evidence

    2) Consequences are monetary

    3) An example would be a nurse sued for wrongful death because she or he failed to do something that would have prevented the death

    4) Intentional torts

      a) Definition: a tort is a legal wrong committed against a person or property, independent of a contract, which renders the person who commits it liable for damages in a civil action; an intentional tort is a direct invasion of someone's legal rights

  b) Examples include assault, battery, false imprisonment, invasion of privacy, defamation, slander

c. Administrative: charges filed by a state or federal government agency (e.g., state board of nursing)
  1) Burden of proof to be found guilty if a preponderance of the evidence
  2) Consequences may be monetary, disciplinary, or loss of privileges (e.g., professional license)
  3) An example would be failure to obtain a new license at the predetermined time

3. Malpractice (i.e., professional negligence)
  a. Definition: the omission to do something that a reasonable and prudent professional would do or as doing something that a reasonable and prudent professional would not do; an unintentional tort
    1) Reasonable and prudent: average judgment, foresight, intelligence, and skill that would be expected of a person with similar training and experience
  b. Elements that must be present for a professional to be held liable for malpractice
    1) Duty: the nurse had a duty to provide care and follow an acceptable standard of care
    2) Breach: there was be a breach of duty (i.e., the nurse failed to adhere to the standard of care)
    3) Causation: the failure to meet the standard of care must have caused injury to the patient
    4) Damages: the patient must have suffered injuries as a result of the nurse's breach of duty
  c. Avoidance of malpractice claims (Marquis and Huston, 2006)
    1) Practice within the scope of your state's Nurse Practice Act
    2) Follow your institution's policies and procedures
    3) Model your practice after established practice standards
    4) Make patients' rights and welfare the priority
    5) Make rational decisions based on the biological, psychological, and social sciences and be aware of laws and legal doctrines
    6) Practice within your area of competence
    7) Continue to update and upgrade your technical skills and seek specialty certification
    8) Purchase professional liability insurance and know the limits of your policy
    9) Document thoroughly in the patient's record and incident reports
      a) Document
        i) Patient status with factual observations along with time, date, and signature (may be electronic signature)
        ii) Any deviations from standard practice and reasons for such deviations
        iii) Notification of physician for changes in status and the physician's response
      b) Common problems made in documentation
        i) Omissions without explanation
        ii) Vague and ambiguous language
        iii) Unapproved abbreviations
        iv) Error correction
        v) Spelling and grammar errors
        vi) Illegibility
  d. Remember that patients are health care consumers and they want good service; try to exceed your patients' expectations

Consent
1. General concepts
  a. Supported by the 1975 Patient Bill of Rights and 2003 Patient Care Partnership documents
  b. Driven by self-determination and autonomy
2. Informed consent (Harkreader et al., 2007)
  a. Elements of informed consent
    1) The client has received the following information:
      a) Diagnosis
      b) Name of procedure, test, or medication
      c) Explanation of procedure, test, or medication
      d) Reasons for recommending the procedure, test, or medication
      e) Anticipated benefits
      f) Major risks of the procedure, test, or medication
      g) Alternative treatments
      h) Prognosis if treatment is refused
    2) The nurse has performed the following duties:
      a) Assessed barriers that could influence the client's understanding of the information
      b) Assessed the influence of education, age, developmental level, and emotional status on the client's ability to understand the information
      c) Ensured that information was provided in a manner that facilitated understanding
      d) Determined that the client is voluntarily giving informed consent
    3) Informed consent is generally required for invasive procedures, surgery, blood transfusions, and participation in research projects
      a) The physician who is performing the procedure is generally expected to obtain consent
3. Other consent issues
  1) Minors
    a) Age at which person can give informed consent varies by state
    b) Exceptions are made for certain conditions: pregnancy, treatment of sexually transmitted diseases, drug/alcohol abuse treatment, birth control

2) Persons in custody of law enforcement
  a) Patient generally still has the right to consent or refuse
    i) Including cases where patient has ingested or inserted drugs; if physician believes patient is in danger, may obtain court order
  b) Complications occur when consent is regarding collection of forensic evidence; court order may be obtained
    i) For example, blood alcohol from patient who caused a motor vehicle collision
3) Implied consent
  a) Consent is assumed
    i) Life- or limb-threatening condition
    ii) Patient is unable to expressly consent for treatment
    iii) ED staff should make all possible attempts to obtain consent from either patient or family
4) Life support issues
  a) Patient Self-Determination Act of 1991
    i) Federal law
    ii) Patients must be given information regarding advance directives if they do not already have one
    iii) Copies of existing advanced directives must be placed in chart
  b) Living wills
    i) Describe care measures patients want or expressly do not want
    ii) Check with state law as to legal status; may need to provide power of attorney
  c) Power of attorney for health care matters
    i) Legal document giving a named person the right to make care decisions for the patient who is not competent or no longer able to make decisions

Refusal of treatment/leaving against medical advice (AMA)

1. The patient can refuse treatment even if it will lead to that person's death if the patient:
  a. Has received all information necessary to make an informed decision
  b. Is of legal age to consent
  c. Is mentally competent to understand the information
2. Facilities should have clear policies regarding patients who refuse treatment or leave AMA
  a. Failure to follow policies and holding a patient against his will could result in legal claims such as false imprisonment or even assault and battery
3. Recommended action to follow if a patient wants to leave AMA (Austin, 2006)
  a. Try to find out why the patient wishes to leave
  b. Attempt to remedy the patient's concerns, using hospital resources as appropriate, such as a social worker
  c. Tell the physician the patient wants to leave AMA

  d. Inform the patient of the risks he is incurring by leaving
  e. Document the situation carefully, including what the patient was told and how the patient responded

Evidence-Based Practice, Research, and Quality Improvement

Three interrelated processes crucial to quality care (Figure 3-2)
Evidence-based practice
Definition
1. The integration of the following (Straus, Richardson, Glasziou, and Haynes, 2005):
  a. Best evidence
  b. Clinician expertise
  c. Patient values
  d. Circumstances
2. The deliberate use of identified best practices when making decisions about patient care; shift away from basing interventions on tradition
3. Five-step process for ensuring that clinical decisions are based on best evidence (Straus et al., 2005)
  a. Converting information into clear questions
    1) PICO format frequently used (Melnyk and Fineout-Overholt, 2005)
      a) P: problem or population
      b) I: intervention
      c) C: comparison intervention
      d) O: outcome
  b. Seeking evidence to answer those questions
    1) Systematic reviews of research reports
    2) Published research reports
      a) Use search engines such as CINAHL, PubMed/MEDLINE, Google Scholar
      b) Scour the bibliographies of the articles that you found helpful
    3) Unpublished research reports
      a) Consult known researchers regarding the issue
      b) Important because research studies with statistically nonsignificant results are frequently not published; either the researcher chooses not to publish or the report is rejected for publication (i.e., publication bias)
  c. Evaluating (critically appraising) the evidence for its validity (truthfulness) and usefulness
    1) Grading the evidence
      a) Quality: the aggregate of quality ratings for individual studies, predicated on the extent to which bias was minimized (i.e., level of evidence)
        i) Study designs
          (a) Traditional hierarchy of evidence based on study designs; note that all grading systems include all of these as valid evidence especially manufacturer's recommendations and expert

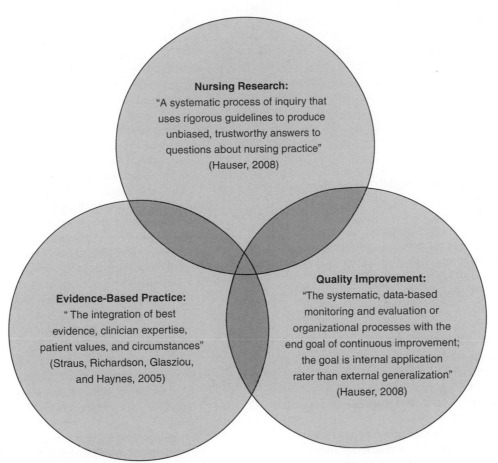

Nursing Research:
"A systematic process of inquiry that uses rigorous guidelines to produce unbiased, trustworthy answers to questions about nursing practice" (Hauser, 2008)

Evidence-Based Practice:
" The integration of best evidence, clinician expertise, patient values, and circumstances" (Straus, Richardson, Glasziou, and Haynes, 2005)

Quality Improvement:
"The systematic, data-based monitoring and evaluation or organizational processes with the end goal of continuous improvement; the goal is internal application rater than external generalization" (Hauser, 2008)

Figure 3–2 Nursing research, evidence-based practice, and quality improvement.

opinion since they are more likely to be biased
  (i) Randomized controlled trials (double-blinded)
  (ii) Nonblinded randomized clinical trials
  (iii) Nonrandomized clinical trials
  (iv) Prospective cohort studies
  (v) Case-control studies
  (vi) Case reports
  (vii) Expert opinion (including consensus groups)
  (viii) Manufacturer's recommendations
  (b) Randomized controlled trials are considered the "gold standard" but many nursing questions are not answered using quantitative techniques
  ii) Sample size
  iii) Control of extraneous variables
  b) Quantity: the magnitude of effect, numbers of studies, and sample size or power (i.e., strength of evidence)
  c) Consistency: the extent to which similar findings are reported using similar and different study designs

  d) Relevance: the study question's similarity to the clinical question and the extent to which the findings from the study can be applied in other clinical settings to different patients
  d. Integrating findings with clinical expertise, patient values, and circumstances and, if appropriate, applying these findings
  e. Evaluating performance and the outcomes of the clinical practice

The cycle of knowledge transformation using the ACE Star Model of Knowledge Transformation (Stevens, 2005) (Figure 3-3)

1. Knowledge discovery: research
  a. Primary goal of nursing research: develop a specialized, scientifically based body of nursing knowledge to facilitate improvement in patient care
  b. Definitions
    1) Nursing research: "a systematic process of inquiry that uses rigorous guidelines to produce unbiased, trustworthy answers to questions about nursing practice" (Hauser, 2008, p. 5)
    2) Scientific method: systematic approach to solving problems which controls variables and biases

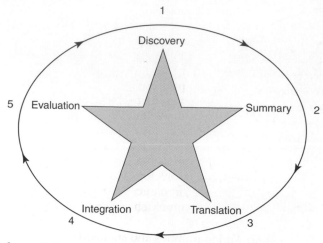

Figure 3–3 ACE Star Model of Knowledge Transformation. (From Stevens, K. R. [2005]. ACE Star Model of Knowledge Transformation. Retrieved Aug. 6, 2006, from http://www. acestar.uthscwsa.edu/Learn_model.htm.)

3) Basic research: research to advance knowledge; helps in understanding relationships among phenomena
4) Applied research: research to solve a particular problem; helps in making decisions or evaluating techniques
5) Variable: a measurable concept that varies among the subjects in a research study
   a) Independent variable: the variable that is being observed, introduced or manipulated in a research study; may be referred to as the treatment variable
   b) Dependent variable: the variable that is being observed for a change after the intervention
   c) Extraneous variables: variables that are not being studied but may or may not be relevant to the results of the study; these variables can affect the dependent variable and interfere with research results
6) Hypothesis: statement that predicts a relationship among two or more variables; may be simple, complex, directional, nondirectional, or null
c. Research types
   1) Quantitative research: deductive process that tests hypotheses and examines cause and effect relationships to examine specific phenomena; emphasizes facts and data to validate or extend existing knowledge
      a) Experimental: uses randomization and a control group to test the effects of an intervention
      b) Quasi-experimental: involves manipulation of variables but lacks a comparison group or randomization
      c) Nonexperimental
         i) Descriptive: describes situations, experiences, and phenomena as they exist
         ii) Ex post facto (correlational): describes relationships between variables

2) Qualitative: inductive process used to understand phenomena in a define contest; emphasizes development of new insights, theory, and knowledge
   a) Relies less on numbers and measurements and more on nursing strategies, interpersonal communication techniques, intuition, and collaboration between nurse and patient to discover underlying relationships
   b) Includes case studies, open-ended questions, field studies, and participant observation
d. Steps in the research process
   1) Formulate the research problem
   2) Review related literature
   3) Formulate the hypothesis
   4) Select the research design
   5) Identify the population to be studied
   6) Specify methods of data collection
   7) Design the study
   8) Conduct the study
   9) Analyze the data
   10) Interpret the results
   11) Communicate the findings
   12) Use the findings to improve patient care
e. Ethical responsibilities related to nursing research studies
   1) Protect the rights of research subjects
   2) Ensure that the potential benefits of the study outweigh any potential risk to the subjects
   3) Submit the proposed study for review by the investigational review committee
   4) Obtain informed consent from each subject
f. Nursing responsibilities related to research
   1) Identify problem areas and research questions for investigation
   2) Find existing evidence and read and interpret reports of nursing research
   3) Assess the body of evidence and applicability to practice
   4) Apply findings to change clinical practice and improve patient care
   5) Design and conduct nursing research
   6) Assist in collection of data as requested
   7) Share research findings with peers
g. While nurses with a doctorate are expected to be active researchers, some responsibility exists at each level of educational preparation for using research or participating in research projects; all levels of nurses are responsible for the ethical conduct of research (ANA, 1994)
   1) Nurses with an associate degree can help identify problems that may benefit from research, assist in data collection, and use research findings in practice
   2) Nurses with a baccalaureate degree can independently identify clinical issues that would benefit from research, assist the investigators in gaining access to clinical sites,

assist in data collection, and use research findings in practice

   3) Nurses with a master's degree are often active members of research teams and collaborate throughout the research process, assess the relevance of the findings for their clinical area, and take a leadership role in incorporating the findings into practice

2. Evidence synthesis: systematic reviews
   a. Definition: a summary of all evidence related to a specific research question using a rigorous method
      1) Quantitative systematic reviews are conducted using meta-analysis statistical techniques
      2) Qualitative systematic reviews are a descriptive summary of the review of existing studies
   b. Advantage to using systematic reviews (Stevens, 2005)
      1) Preappraised so in more usable form
         a) For clinicians making clinical decisions
         b) For policy makers making policy decisions
         c) For administrators making economic decisions
         d) For researchers making decisions about future research designs
      2) Shortens time between research and clinical implementation
      3) Provides a distillation of large quantities of information into a manageable form with an answer
   c. Finding systematic reviews
      1) Agency for Healthcare Research and Quality (www.ahrq.gov)
      2) The Cochrane Collaborative (www.cochrane.org)
      3) The Campbell Collaborative (www.campbellcollaborative.org)
      4) The Joanna Briggs Institute (www.joannabriggs.edu/au)
3. Translation into practice recommendations: clinical practice guidelines (CPGs)
   a. Definition: a "systemically developed statement designed to assist clinician and patient decisions about appropriate health care for specific clinical circumstances" (Straus et al., 2005)
      1) Evidence-based CPGs: explicitly articulate the link between the clinical recommendation and the strength of supporting evidence (Stevens, 2005)
   b. Advantage of CPG: "can help to overcome the barriers to research use because they eliminate the need to search for journal and articles, overcome nurses' limited skills in critical analysis, and minimize the impact of research jargon and unfamiliar terminology because most guidelines are published as clinical application documents" (Ciliska, Pinelli, DiCenso, and Cullum, 2001, p. 524)
      1) CPGs may be incorporated into standards of care, care MAPS, policies and procedures, and protocols

   c. Topic of a clinical guideline
      1) A condition (e.g., myocardial infarction)
      2) A symptom (e.g., chest pain)
      3) A clinical procedure (e.g., percutaneous coronary intervention)
   d. Clinical guidelines: purpose
      1) Encourage treatment that offers individual patients maximum likelihood of benefit and minimum harm and is acceptable in terms of cost
      2) Reduce inappropriate variations in practice
         a) Common reasons for variations
            i) Variations in clinical decision making
            ii) Differing approaches to problem solving
            iii) Varied routines and standards
            iv) Availability of resources
            v) Lack of consensus related to appropriate treatment for given conditions
      3) Promote the delivery of evidence-based health care
      4) Provide ready evaluation criteria by which health care professionals can be made accountable for clinical performance
      5) May reduce the cost of health care
   e. Finding clinical practice guidelines
      1) Government agencies
         a) National Guidelines Clearing House (www.guidelines.gov)
         b) Scottish Intercollegiate Guideline Network (SIGN) (www.sign.ac.uk/guidelines/index.html)
      2) Professional associations
         a) Sigma theta tau (www.stti.org)
         b) American Association of Critical-Care Nurses (www.aacn.org)
         c) Registered Nurses Association of Ontario (www.rnao.org/bestpractices/index.asp)
      3) Evidence-based practice (EBP) centers
         a) Joanna Briggs Institute (www.joannabriggs.edu.au)
   f. Tool for evaluation of guidelines: Appraisal of Guidelines for Research and Evaluation (AGREE) Instrument (www.agreecollaboration.org)
   g. Toolkit for implementation of a guideline: Registered Nurses Association of Ontario Toolkit for Implementation of CPG Registered Nurses Association of Ontario Toolkit for Implementation of CPG (www.rnao.org/bestpractices/completed_guidelines/BPG_Guide_C1_Toolkit.asp)
4. Implementation into practice
   a. Select an EBP change model (e.g., Iowa model, Stetler model, Rosswurm-Larrabee model)
   b. Consider organizational barriers to EBP
   c. Use organizational strategies to facilitate EBP
      1) Foster an environment that values inquiry and critical thinking
         a) Encouragement of formal education
         b) Provision of time to read research and evaluate applicability to setting

    c) Provision of access to Internet, e-journals, library, and photocopying

    d) Provision of opportunities to attend conferences, continuing education, and inservice education including education regarding critical appraisal of research

    e) Addition of scholarship to the nurse's role so that dissemination through local, regional, and national presentations and publication is encouraged and expected

    f) Establishment of nursing leadership to spearhead EBP activities, such as a nurse researcher, clinical nurse specialist, or nurse practitioner

    g) Encouragement of the questioning of the "status quo" and nursing rituals

    h) Development of collaborative teams across disciplines: "EBP is a multi-disciplinary practice" (Gray, 1997)

2) Communicate the expectation of EBP

    a) Incorporation of EBP activities in job descriptions, performance appraisals, merit raises, and career ladder promotions

    b) Leaders ask, "Why are you doing that?" "Why are you doing that in that way?" "What is the evidence?"

3) Increase nurse autonomy over practice

    a) Decentralization of administration

    b) Establishment of shared governance with appropriate nursing department council and committee structures

    c) Establishment of unit-level EBP committees

4) Eliminate the gap between theory and practice

    a) Establishment of more joint appointments between academic and practice settings

    b) Appointment of a nurse researcher on staff

    c) Utilization of expert consultants as necessary

    d) Provision of support for EBP committees and research activities

    e) Development of research presentations (e.g., Nursing Research Grand Rounds)

    f) Establishment of journal clubs

    g) Publication of a monthly research newsletter

5) Use resources appropriately

    a) Commitment of expertise, money, and time to EBP activities including have adequate staffing

    b) Use of systematic reviews and implementation of clinical practice guidelines

5. Evaluation of the impact of EBP

  a. Patient health outcomes

  b. Patient satisfaction

  c. Staff satisfaction

  d. Cost-benefit analysis

Quality improvement

1. Definition: "the systematic, data-based monitoring and evaluation or organizational processes with the end goal of continuous improvement; the goal is internal application rather than external generalization" (Hauser, 2008, p. 11)

2. Quality improvement (QI) is a local process in which people work together to improve systems and processes within an organization

  a. Important in improving patient outcomes; may also be used to reduce the costs of delivering health care and improve competitiveness; may also reduce liability and the costs of legal action

  b. Used in conjunction with EBP to improve practice

  c. Includes incident reporting and risk management programs

3. Incident or adverse occurrence reports

  a. An incident or adverse event is "any untoward incident, therapeutic mishap, iatrogenic injury, or other undesirable occurrence arising out of medical care and treatment" (Department of Veterans Affairs, 2005, as cited in Monson, 2006)

  b. An incident report is "a tool used by health care facilities to document situations that have caused harm or have the potential to cause harm to clients, employees, or visitors" (Harkreader et al., 2007, p. 39)

    1) Common examples of situations that generate incident reports are patient falls and medication errors

  c. An incident report is filled out by the person discovering the situation and is not part of a patient's chart

    1) A physician might complete the report if called to examine a person if there was an actual injury or potential for injury

    2) Incident report forms might also have a section for the person filling it out to try to identify causative factors

  d. The incident report is reviewed to determine if there are system problems that lead to the incident and to determine if there is a pattern of such incidents that needs to be addressed to prevent further incidents in the future

  e. The objective nature of the report makes it a valuable record if the incident leads to a court case

  f. Since 2001, disclosing adverse events to patients has been mandated by The Joint Commission (TJC; formerly Joint Commission on Accreditation of Healthcare Organizations [JCAHO])

4. Risk management programs

  a. Attempts to reduce liability by designing programs to address known risks and problems

  b. Includes a comprehensive assessment of "all matters and issues that might impact on an area of clinical practice" and is considered "part of the methodology whereby nurses . . . ensure that their practice is clear, rationale, and evidence-based . . . " (Fulbrook, 2007, pp. 112-113)

  c. Frequently includes designated risk managers

  d. Tools for risk management include the following:

    1) Failure mode effects analysis (Day, Dalto, Fox, and Turpin, 2006)

a) Used to anticipate what could happen when a change is implemented; use of the concept of Murphy's Law (whatever can happen, will happen) to resolve issues before the change to prevent an incident with a true adverse outcome

b) Often used after a "near miss" situation

c) Helps meet new TJC regulations that hospitals perform risk assessments for at least one high-risk process each year

2) Crew resource management: modeled on changes in the air transportation industry

3) Tools for communication

a) SBAR: tool adapted from military use, to standardize communication between professionals and units

i) S: situation: describe the current situation

ii) B: background: provide pertinent background information about the patient

iii) A: assessment: current clinical condition

iv) R: recommendations: recommendations, or requests for further action

b) Research shows using a standardized tool promotes better and more timely communication (American Association of Critical-Care Nurses, 2007, September; Woodhall, Vertacnik, and McLaughlin, 2008)

Documentation of Assessment, Intervention, and Evaluation of Patient Care

Documentation expectations related to TJC core processes (ENA, 2005)

1. General activities related to core elements
   a. Providing access to appropriate levels of care and disciplines for patients
   b. Providing interventions based on the plan for care, treatment, and services
   c. Teaching patients what they need to know about their care, treatment, and services
   d. Coordinating care, treatments, and services, if needed, when the patient is referred, transferred, or discharged
2. Documentation components related to core elements (Harkreader et al., 2007)
   a. Initial assessments as defined by the organization; reassessment as needed; physical assessment as appropriate; psychological and social assessment as appropriate
   b. Symptoms associated with a disease, condition, and treatment
   c. Nutritional status, when warranted by patient condition
   d. Functional assessment, when warranted by patient condition
   e. Pain assessment and treatment provided
   f. Diagnostic testing, including laboratory and radiologic studies

g. Physical, developmental, visual, communication, behavioral, and emotional disorders

h. Alcohol and substance abuse assessments, as needed

i. Medication administration

j. Education and training specific to patient needs

k. Screening for victims of abuse; focuses screening of those identified as potential victims

l. Conscious sedation: preassessment and monitoring during the procedure to include heart rate, respiratory status, and oxygen saturation

m. Interdisciplinary and collaborative care rendered

n. The patient's position should be documented

o. Restraint/seclusion; TJC requirements for documentation of restraint and/or seclusion (ENA, 2005)

1) Decision to restrain/seclude patients must be based on the patient's condition at the time

2) Alternative therapies attempted before restraint must be documented

3) Explanations to patient and family must be documented

4) Less restrictive approaches must be attempted first

5) The least restrictive device should be used first

6) A physician's order must have the date and time and must indicate the type of restraint and purpose for the restraint and must specify a time limit within established guidelines. As-needed orders or restraint/seclusion for the duration of the ED visit are not acceptable

7) The first hour of restraint requires continuous face-to-face observation

8) Assessment of the patient must occur at specified intervals; for example, every 15 minutes while in seclusion or nondisposable restraints

9) The patient must be offered food, toileting, and hydration every 3 hours while awake

10) The patient's condition and response to treatment must be documented

11) Condition of the patient's limb before restraint must be documented

12) Condition of the patient's skin in the area of the restraints must be documented

13) Restraint must be loosened at regular intervals

Purposes of documentation

1. Communication
2. Quality assurance
3. Legal accountability
4. Reimbursement
5. Research

Good documentation (Harkreader et al., 2007)

1. Is brief but contains enough detail to be complete
2. Uses proper terminology and acceptable abbreviations
3. If handwritten, is legible
4. Be done in a sequential order
5. Show all elements of the nursing process: assessment, diagnosis, planning, intervention, goals/outcomes, and evaluation

6. Has corrections that are done properly
7. If written, cross out error with a single line, write "edit" and initial, write the correct information, add the date and time, and sign [do not ever write "error"]
8. Computer charting systems have specific directions for the correction of errors
9. Is signed correctly: first initial, last name, credentials
10. Is factual and clear without opinions or judgments
11. Must include an admission note, ongoing assessments, teaching, and transfer notes; any unusual incidents should be documented on an incident report form
   a. Documentation must reflect compliance with state law (e.g., evidence of request for organ donation upon death)
   b. If the patient is critically ill, charting must show evidence that the standard of care for a critically ill patient was provided

Documentation via an electronic record

1. Must be done carefully without the following:
   a. Simply saving the previous nurse's charting
   b. Simply checking the "normal" or "within normal limits" box

Documentation should be thorough enough so that if the patient's case goes to court, the record can paint a clear picture of what happened even several years later

Orientation/Continuing Education/Inservice Programs

Orientation to nursing in the ED differs from institution to institution but is likely to include the following:

1. Critical care and/or emergency nursing course
2. Advanced cardiac life support (ACLS)
3. Pediatric advanced life support (PALS)
4. Trauma nursing core course (TNCC)
5. Preceptorship with an experienced emergency nurse

Two types of ongoing education for nurses: continuing education and inservice education

1. Continuing education (CE) is vital to practicing nurses and to the public they serve
   a. Purposes include the following:
      1) "Enhance knowledge and skills in practice, administration, research, and education" (Harkreader et al., 2007, p. 11)
      2) Improve quality and safety for patients and the public
      3) Meet requirements for licensure renewal in many states
      4) Fulfills a professional obligation whether or not it is mandated in a specific area
         a) Staying competent in nursing requires lifelong learning
         b) Staying up-to-date also reduces legal liability
   b. CE is offered by professional organizations, health care organizations, institutions of higher learning

such as colleges and universities, or commercial companies
      1) Live continuing education programs or conferences
      2) Distance learning programs offered through reading or web-based programs
      3) College courses
2. Inservices are generally offered by specific institutions in order to provide care for their specific patient population in their setting
   a. An example might be inservice training on the new computer system or a new piece of equipment in the hospital where you work
Lifelong learning is required of all nurses

Patient Education
Definitions

1. Teaching: the process of facilitating learning; an interaction designed to help a person learn to do something that he is currently unable to do; two-way interaction
2. Learning: the process by which a person becomes capable of doing something he could not do before including a wide range of behavior, from motor skills to intellectual skills; an emotional experience which can be negative or positive, traumatic, or pleasant
3. Patient education: the process of teaching patients and their families about the illness, treatment, and other health-related matters, including how to adhere to the regimen and helping them change their behavior.

Reasons for patient education

1. Because the patient has a need and a right to know those things that are relevant to his condition, disease, or situation
2. To produce changes in knowledge, skills, attitudes, appreciation, and understanding
3. To promote and improve health
4. To encourage the patient to assume responsibility for disease management
5. To prevent illness and complications
6. To aid in coping with illness and adaptation to change
7. To promote compliance with the therapeutic regimen
8. To reduce anxiety (including family stress and anxiety)
9. To reduce number of physician's office and/or ED visits and number and length of hospitalizations

Principles of adult education

1. Qualities of the adult learner: a self-directed independent person who becomes ready to learn when the need to know or to perform is experienced; characteristics of the adult learner include the following:
   a. Goal oriented
   b. Less flexible
   c. Requires longer to perform learning tasks
   d. Impatient in the pursuit of objectives

e. Finds little use for isolated facts

f. Strives for recognition and success

g. Has multiple responsibilities, all of which draw upon his time

h. Experienced in the "school of life"

i. Requires a more constant and ideal learning environment

j. Usually comes to the teaching program on a voluntary basis

k. Wishes to be involved in mutual planning of learning experiences

l. Likes to participate in diagnosing needs for learning, formulating learning objectives, and evaluating learning

m. Expects a climate of mutual respect, trust, and collaboration that supports learning

2. Educational concepts useful with adults

a. Pacing

1) Allow adults to set their own pace, if possible

2) Tasks or methods involving significant time pressure are likely to be difficult for adults

b. Arousal anxiety

1) Some degree of arousal is necessary for learning; however, older adults may become anxious in a learning situation

2) Allow individuals an opportunity to become familiar with the situation

3) Minimize the role of competition and evaluation

c. Dealing with fatigue

1) Some tasks may produce considerable mental or physical fatigue, a problem that is likely to particularly affect older adults

2) Shorten the instruction sessions or provide frequent rest breaks

d. Difficulty: arrange materials from the simple to the complex to build individual's confidence and skills

e. Errors: structure the tasks so errors are avoided and do not have to be unlearned

f. Practice: provide an opportunity for practice on similar but different tasks; such practice helps to develop generalizable skills

g. Feedback: provide information on the adequacy of previous responses

h. Cues

1) Materials should be presented to compensate for the potential sensory problems of older adults

2) Direct attention toward the relevant aspects of the task

3) Reduce the level of irrelevant information to a minimum

i. Organization

1) Learning and remembering often require that information be grouped or related in some way

2) Instruct individuals in the use of various mnemonic techniques (mental images, verbal associations, etc.) which may be used to elaborate or organize the material

j. Relevance/experience

1) People learn and remember what is important to them

2) Attempt to make the task relevant to individual's concerns

3) Performance is likely to be facilitated to the extent that the individuals are able to integrate the new information with known information

Barriers to teaching/learning

1. Nurse factors: lack of time; lack of knowledge; consideration of teaching as a lower priority than physical care

2. Physician interference

a. Some physicians do not want their patients educated because they may then question the authority of the physician

b. Lack of communication regarding the physician's plan for the patient may impair educational process because time may not be available for adequate teaching

3. Patient factors

a. Physiologic instability

b. Psychological factors (e.g., anxiety, pain)

c. Poor language or reading skills

d. Sensory deficits: vision, hearing

e. Poor manual dexterity for psychomotor skills

4. Environmental factors

a. Noise

b. Lack of privacy

c. Need to move patient out of ED to make room for more seriously ill patients

Teaching/learning process

1. Assessment

a. Readiness to learn

1) Desire to know (e.g., asking questions)

2) Absence of acute distress (e.g., pain, dyspnea)

3) Adequate energy

b. Sensory deficits (e.g., use of eyeglasses, hearing aid)

c. Educational level and reading ability

d. Learning style

e. Attitudes and beliefs that conflict with teaching

f. Age and developmental level; cultural considerations

g. Priority teaching-learning need: teaching in the ED will be a one-time activity

2. Plan

a. Identify objectives; parts of the objective should include the following:

1) What should be learner be able to do? (behavior)

a) Cognitive: being able to learn material intellectually, factual knowledge

b) Affective: related to attitude and motivation to learn

c) Psychomotor: being able to do the skills required

2) How well should he be able to do it? (the criteria)

3) Under what conditions should he be able to do it? (the condition)

b. Identify content to teach, examples include:
   1) Language and terminology
   2) Health care system: personnel; organization and structure; routines and procedures; norms and expectations; immediate environment
   3) Basic anatomy and physiology of affected body system
   4) Diagnosis, disease process
   5) Therapy: treatments, medications, diet, activity, personal health habits
   6) Prevention of complications
   7) Skills (e.g., insulin administration, pulse taking)
   8) Community resources
3. Implement
   a. Keep teaching short and to the point
      1) Time constraints and rapid turnover in the ED will necessitate quick teaching
      2) Patients in the ED will rapidly develop information overload
   b. Always use written material to supplement what you are teaching
      1) May use commercially available preprinted teaching guidelines
      2) May need age-appropriate material (i.e., coloring books for children)
   c. Learner must be able to understand material with little effort
      1) Be specific: instead of "Practice safe sex," state "Use a condom each time you have sex"
   d. Must include information that will keep patient safe and provide information on follow up appointments needed
      1) Examples of safety-related information are crutch-walking, safety with an eye patch, driving restrictions for a patient on narcotic analgesics
      2) Tell patient if he or she needs to make a follow-up appointment or if one was made for the patient
      3) Provide telephone numbers for follow-up appointments
      4) Always provide telephone number for ED with instructions to call at any time if there are questions
   e. May need to consult with a specialty educator (i.e., diabetic educator)
   f. Use a professional interpreter if needed; avoid using children for teaching if at all possible
4. Evaluation
   a. Ask patient questions to determine understanding
   b. Have patient do return demonstration for psychomotor skills
   c. Ask patient/family if there are any questions
5. Documentation should include:
   1) Objectives
   2) Content outline
   3) Method used
   4) Evaluation of learning
   5) Comments
   6) Signature of patient and nurse who provided the teaching

Education for low-literacy individuals

1. Significance: While one of five American adults reads at the fifth-grade level or below and the average American reads at the eighth- to ninth-grade level, most health care materials are written above the 10th-grade level (National Patient Safety Foundation, 2008)
2. Definitions
   a. Low-literacy individuals: adults with poorly developed skills in reading, writing, listening, and/or speaking
   b. Health literary: ability to read, understand, and act on health information
   c. Low or limited health literary: inability to adequately understand and act on basic health information
3. Assessing literacy level
   a. Individuals reading at a fifth-grade or higher level are considered literate; hand-printed instructions and asking the patient to read them back to you is a nonthreatening way to assess reading ability
   b. Incongruent behavior may signal a literacy problem; be alert for behavior that does not match the reported level of understanding
   c. Low-literacy materials are preferred for the low-literacy individuals
4. Teaching strategies for low-literacy patients
   a. Identify and eliminate or minimize stress, anxiety, or other distractions before teaching
   b. Correct misconceptions that affect learning
   c. Personalize the health message and explain the need for the information
   d. Relate information to patient's past experiences and actively involve the patient and family in discussions
   e. Consider qualities of poor readers and use teaching strategies that are helpful (Table 3-1)

Stress Management

Stress

1. Originally referred to as general adaptation syndrome by Selye
2. Two types include the following:
   a. Distress (to noxious stimuli) such as physical or emotional strain
   b. Eustress (to nonthreatening stimuli)
3. Physiologic response to stress; frequently referred to as "flight or fight"
   a. Increase in heart rate, cardiac contractility, blood pressure
   b. Dilation of pupils
   c. Bronchodilation
   d. Perspiration
   e. Dry mouth
   f. Frequent urination

Common causes of stress pertinent to emergency setting

1. Sudden change in personal health or health of a loved one

TABLE

3-1 Qualities of Poor Readers and Appropriate Teaching Strategies

Qualities of Poor Readers	Teaching Strategies
Takes words literally	Explain the meaning of all words
Reads slowly; miss meaning	Use common words and examples
Skips over uncommon words	Use examples, review content frequently
Misses content	Describe content first, use verbal heading and visuals
Tires quickly	Use short segments

From Dennison, R. D. (2007): *Pass CCRN!* 3rd ed. St, Louis, Mosby.

2. Terminal phase of a chronic illness with the need to make end-of-life decisions
3. Sensory deprivation and sensory overload; note that these can coexist
4. Feelings of powerlessness
5. Guilt related to personal contribution to injury or illness

Interventions to decrease or eliminate stress

1. Maintain a calm, restful environment
2. Provide for as much independence of the patient as possible
3. Provide contact with reality and outside world
4. Encourage use of coping mechanisms (Table 3-2) while assessing for defense mechanisms (Table 3-3)

Crisis

1. Definition: an acute state of stress in which the person feels overwhelmed by stressors
   a. Involves an attempt to regain equilibrium
   b. Self-limited and allows for growth
2. May be maturational, adventitious, or situational in focus; admission to an ED is often unexpected and without warning

3-2 Coping Mechanisms to Stress

Type of Mechanism	Example
Action	Taking walks, cleaning house, gardening, singing
Cognitive	Problem solving, reading about issue
Spiritual	Prayer
Interpersonal	Talking with support person
Emotional	Use of psychological defense mechanisms

From Dennison, R. D. (2007): *Pass CCRN!* 3rd ed. St, Louis, Mosby.

   a. Maturational: arises as a result of growth and development and involve changes in self-concept and roles
   b. Adventitious: follows accidental and uncommon events leading to major environmental changes (e.g., natural disasters)
   c. Situational: follows an external event or experience and its associated losses and changes
3. Stages
   a. Shock and disbelief
   b. Disorganization: may be demanding, irrational, angry
   c. Reorganization: difficulty making decisions, forced to confront critical questions
   d. Resolution
4. Interventions to assist the patient in crisis
   a. Listen to the patient's perception of the situation
   b. Encourage the patient to express his feelings about the situation
   c. Assist the patient to gain an understanding of the situation by discussing losses and positive outcomes
   d. Assist the patient in developing a viable solution
5. Fear/anxiety
   a. Definition: fear is an unpleasant feeling specific to a known threat; anxiety is an unpleasant feeling to an unknown threat
   b. Anxiety can produce both psychological and physiologic symptoms; manifestations may include

3-3 Psychological Defense Mechanisms

Defense Mechanism	Description
Suppression	Conscious, deliberate forgetting of unacceptable or painful thoughts, impulses, feelings, or acts
Repression	Unconscious, involuntary forgetting of unacceptable or painful thoughts, impulses, feelings, or acts
Denial	Treating obvious reality factors as though they do not exist because they are consciously intolerable
Rationalization	Attempting to justify feelings, behavior, & motives that would otherwise be intolerable, by offering a socially acceptable, intellectual, & apparently logical explanation for an act or a decision
Compensation	Making extra effort to achieve in one area to offset real or imagined deficiencies in another area
Sublimation	Directing energy from unacceptable drives into socially acceptable behavior
Projection	Unconsciously attributing one's unacceptable qualities and emotions to others
Regression	Going back to an earlier level of emotional development and organization
Withdrawal	Separating oneself from interpersonal relationships to avoid emotional expression or responsiveness

From Dennison, R. D. (2007): *Pass CCRN!* 3rd ed. St, Louis, Mosby.

restlessness, irritability, increase in questions, insomnia, tachycardia, tremors

  c. Interventions to decrease feelings of fear and anxiety

    1) Communicate honestly and empathetically

    2) Refer to psychologist, psychiatric liaison nurse, chaplain if appropriate

    3) Identify adaptive and maladaptive coping mechanisms being used

    4) Encourage expression of fears and concerns

    5) Reduce sensory overload

    6) Teach relaxation and imagery techniques

    7) Encourage the patient to ask questions

    8) Encourage the patient to participate in his care

    9) Explore the patient's desire for spiritual or psychological counseling

6. Loneliness

  a. Definition: discomfort caused by separation from significant relationships, places, events, and objects

  b. Manifestations may include crying, withdrawal

  c. Interventions to decrease loneliness

    1) Encourage participation in decision making and self-care

    2) Encourage discussion of fears and to ask questions

    3) Encourage the patient to talk about his life, his family, his work, his pet, etc.

7. Powerlessness

  a. Definition: a perceived lack of control over the outcome of a specific situation or problem and the patient's perception that any action he takes will not affect the outcome

  b. May be manifested by apathy, withdrawal, resignation, fatalism, lack of decision making, aggression, anger

  c. Interventions to decrease feelings of powerlessness

    1) Recognize of the potential for feelings of powerlessness; particularly at risk are individuals who are usually in a position of power or control in their daily life or those who are suffering from an unanticipated medical condition. Also at risk are the families of those with sudden health crises

    2) Support the patient's sense of control by offering alternatives for care as much as possible

    3) Keep the patient informed about his treatment

    4) Encourage the patient's involvement in decision making related to his or her treatment

    5) Increase the patient's control as warranted; often teaching about self-care measures will give patients some sense of control

8. Anger

  a. Definition: feeling of great displeasure, hostility, exasperation

  b. May be manifested by clenching of teeth or muscles, avoidance of eye contact, sarcasm, insulting comments, screaming, argumentativeness, demanding behavior

  c. Interventions to decrease feelings of anger

    1) Assist in identifying the cause of anger

    2) Give the patient permission to be angry

    3) Assist the patient in identifying appropriate ways to express the anger

    4) Violence in the ED is a real issue requiring vigilance

9. Depression

  a. Definition: feeling of sadness, hopelessness

  b. May be manifested by loss of interest in people, dissatisfaction, difficulty making decisions, crying; patient may say that he is a failure, that he is being punished, or that he is considering hurting himself

  c. Interventions to decrease feelings of depression

    1) Provide information necessary to identify his needs and to realistically visualize the future

    2) Inspire hope and facilitate coping

10. Denial

  a. Definition: refusal to acknowledge the truth; allows the patient to come to grips with reality a little at a time

  b. Denial may be manifested by shrugging off symptoms; refusing to discuss the illness; appearing cheerful; and verbalizing the illness while ignoring restrictions

  c. Interventions

    1) Allow the patient to express his or her feelings

    2) Do not confront the patient with the truth

11. Interventions to assist the family

  a. Allow the family to be with the patient

    1) The ENA supports family presence during resuscitation

    2) EDs wishing to allow family presence during resuscitation should have written policies and a designated staff person to be the facilitator for the family

    3) Research shows that families appreciate the opportunity to be with their loved ones during this time.

  b. Encourage the family to participate in the care of the patient as appropriate

  c. Reassure the family of the patient's analgesia and comfort

  d. Provide information about the patient's status frequently, especially the patient's imminent death

  e. Encourage ventilation of anxiety, fears, concerns

  f. Ensure a private, comfortable area for the family

  g. Refer the family to other sources of support, such as the chaplain, social worker, support group

LEARNING ACTIVITIES

1. DIRECTIONS: Complete the following crossword puzzle related to professional issues in emergency nursing.

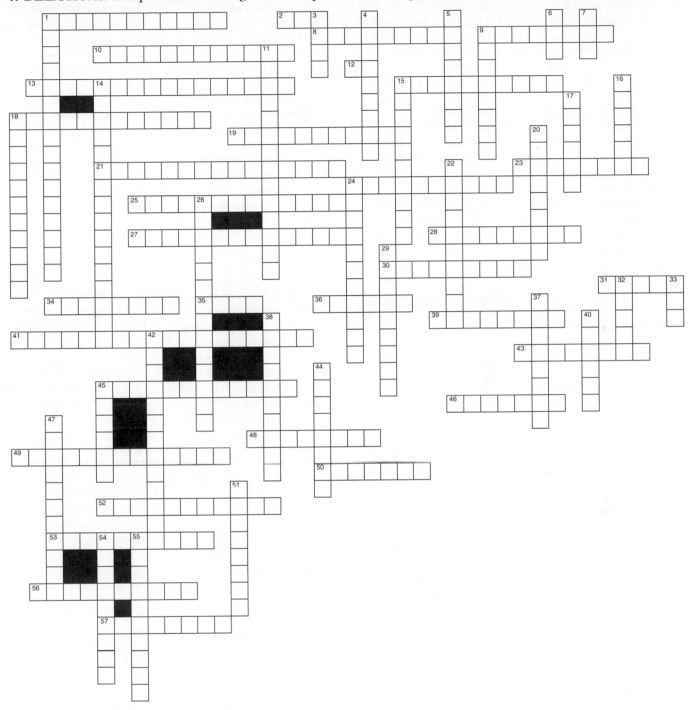

ACROSS

1. Directing energy from unacceptable drives into socially acceptable behavior

2. Integration of best evidence, clinician expertise, patient values, and circumstances (abbrev)

8. Hour-long program regarding a new infusion pump illustrates this type of education

9. Self-determination

10. Type of research that used randomization and a control group to test the effects of an intervention

12. Day-long program regarding care of a patient on therapeutic hypothermia illustrates this type of education (abbrev)

13. Collection, analysis, and interpretation of medical evidence in legal cases (2 words)
15. Approach to ethical decision making based on moral rules and unchanging principles
18. This type of research is a deductive process
19. Doing good
21. Respecting privileged information
23. Concept examined in a research study
24. This aids in documentation of wounds
25. Situation that requires a choice between two or more equally undesirable alternatives (two words)

DOWN
1. Summary of all evidence related to a specific research question using a rigorous method (two words)
3. Commonly used format to frame clinical questions for searching for evidence in ebp (abbrev)
4. Type of variable which is the response or outcome the research would like to explain or predict
5. Process by which a person becomes capable of doing something he could not previously do
6. This professional association developed the code of ethics for nurses (abbrev)
7. When a patient leaves without being discharged (abbrev)
9. Respecting and supporting the basic values, rights, and beliefs of the patient
11. Answerability or responsibility

27. Doing no harm
28. Approach to ethical decision-making based on "the end justifies the means"
30. This discipline considers ethics in light of new discoveries and advances in science
31. This type of research is intended to advance knowledge
34. Keeping promises
35. This phase of debriefing would allow participants to discuss their role in the incident
36. Ideals, beliefs, and patterns of behaviors that are prized and chosen by a person, group, or society

14. Any event that causes a team member to experience overwhelming emotions and may interfere with personal or professional functioning (two words)
15. Transfer of responsibility for the performance of a task from one individual to another while remaining accountable for the outcome
16. Treating obvious reality factors as though they do not exist because they are consciously intolerable
17. Acute state of stress in which the person feels overwhelmed by stressors
18. This type of research is an inductive process
20. This phase of debriefing might include questioning each participant to identify the worst part of the incident
22. Unconsciously attributing one's own unacceptable qualities and emotions to others

39. This type of consent must be obtained prior to procedures and inclusion in study groups
41. Systematic, data-based monitoring and evaluation of organizational processes with the goal of continuous improvement
43. Truth telling
45. Quantitative systematic review using statistical methods
46. Treating people fairly
48. Stress response to noxious stimuli
49. Perceived lack of control over the outcome of a specific situation or problem

24. Approach to ethical decision-making when beneficence takes precedence over autonomy
26. Process used to ensure that evidence has not been tampered with and that the evidence will be considered valid in a court of law (three words)
29. Includes the desired behavior, criteria, and conditions
32. This type of learner is motivated by the need for application
33. These are developed and used during the translation phase of the cycle of knowledge translation (abbrev)
37. Knowledge discovery phase of the cycle of knowledge transformation
38. This process allows emergency personnel to discuss their perceptions of the incident and their feelings and emotions in a supportive environment

50. This phase of debriefing would allow participants to discuss their reaction to the incident
52. Type of variable that is the presumed cause manipulated by the researcher to observe the effect in a cause-and-effect relationship
53. Going back to an earlier level of emotional development
56. Statement that predicts a relationship among two or more variables
57. Acting in a way that benefits others

40. ____'s principle states that when a person or object comes in contact with another person or object
42. When one knows the right thing to do but cannot pursue the right action; obstacles may be internal or external (two words)
44. Stress response to non-threatening stimuli
45. Standards of conduct that represent the ideal in human behavior
47. Adults with poorly developed skills in reading, writing, listening, and speaking (2 words)
51. Process of facilitating learning
54. This intervention mandates special documentation requirements
55. This method is a systematic approach to solving problems that controls variables and biases

2. DIRECTIONS: Describe the process of and considerations in delegation.

a.

b.

c.

d.

e.

f.

3. DIRECTIONS: Describe the phases in a debriefing.

a.

b.

c.

d.

e.

f.

g.

4. DIRECTIONS: A patient has been brought to the ED by squad after a shooting. List four things you should do to preserve evidence in this case.

a.

b.

c.

d.

5. DIRECTIONS: Match the ethical standard with its description or definition

Descriptions		Terms	
a.	To do good	_____ 1.	Autonomy
b.	To do no harm	_____ 2.	Fidelity
c.	Telling the truth	_____ 3.	Beneficence
d.	Self-determination	_____ 4.	Nonmaleficence
e.	Right to privacy	_____ 5.	Veracity
f.	Honoring promises	6.	Confidentiality

6. DIRECTIONS: List the six steps in the ethical decision-making process.

a.

b.

c.

d.

e.

f.

7. DIRECTIONS: Answer each of the following True or False.

True	False	A minor can generally consent to treatment for a sexually transmitted infection
True	False	Implied consent means that the person has consented to this type of procedure or treatment before
True	False	When obtaining consent for a radiograph, a simple verbal agreement is sufficient to proceed
True	False	If a suicidal person refuses treatment, there is no recourse to force it upon that person
True	False	Alternatives to the proposed treatment should be explained as part of the informed consent process
True	False	The nurse should assess for barriers to understanding the material presented when obtaining a signature for informed consent
True	False	If a patient refuses treatment and the physician thinks that refusing will harm the patient, that patient can be forced to undergo the treatment
True	False	Institutions should avoid policies on patients leaving AMA because it will encourage them to do so

8. DIRECTIONS: Correct the following chart entries with proper documentation.

a. Patient arrives by squad. Belligerent and obviously drunk. Removed dirty clothes and a large diamond ring. MBlair

b. Child brought in by hysterical mother who reports child was mauled by dog. Large wound to thigh covered with bloody gauze.

c. Patient complains of stomach pain for a long time. Given IV morphine and sent to x-ray. On return, patient says pain is better.

9. DIRECTIONS: List at least five things the nurse must do for a patient who is in restraints.

a.

b.

c.

d.

e.

10. DIRECTIONS: List five strategies for teaching a person who has a low literacy level.

a.

b.

c.

d.

e.

11. DIRECTIONS: List five barriers to teaching-learning and ways to overcome them.

a.

b.

c.

d.

e.

12. DIRECTIONS: A patient is near death in the emergency department. List interventions you can do to provide caring and comfort for the family.

a.

b.

c.

d.

e.

13. DIRECTIONS: Match the following signs and symptoms of stress to their category. Categories may be used more than once.

Category		Symptom of stress	
a.	Physical	_____ 1.	Fatigue
b.	Cognitive	_____ 2.	Nightmares
c.	Emotional	_____ 3.	Uncertainty
d.	Behavioral	_____ 4.	Withdrawal from relationships
		_____ 5.	Change in sexual functioning
		_____ 6.	Intense anger
		_____ 7.	Memory problems
		_____ 8.	Headaches
		_____ 9.	Elevated blood pressure
		_____ 10.	Difficulty making decisions
		_____ 11.	Apprehension
		_____ 12.	Alcohol consumption

LEARNING ACTIVITIES ANSWERS

1.

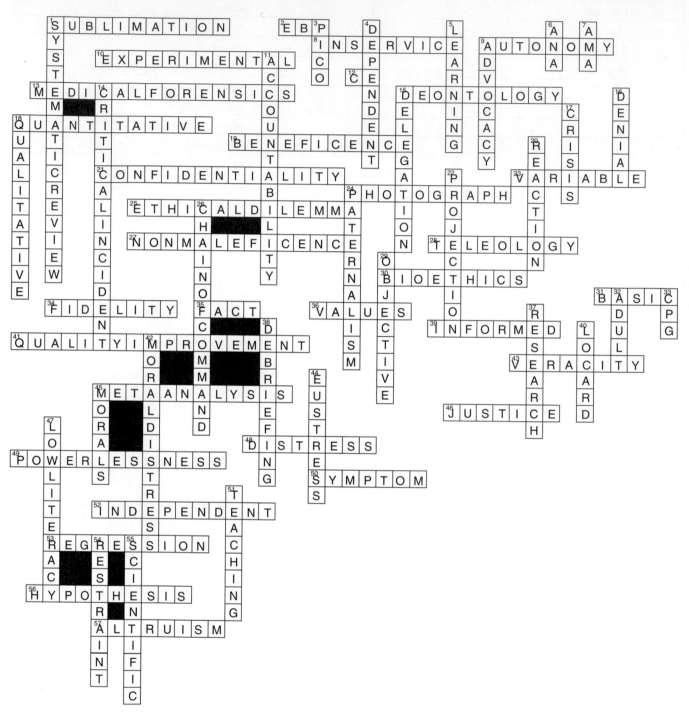

2.

a. Use the five rights of delegation
b. Identify desired outcomes and the skills/competencies needed to achieve them
c. Communicate clearly
d. Empower the person so she or he can accomplish the job
e. Supply deadlines, monitor progress, give rewards
f. Evaluate the process and outcomes

3.
a. Initial
b. Fact
c. Thought
d. Reaction
e. Symptom
f. Teaching
g. Reentry

4.
a. Cut clothing off carefully, avoiding bullet holes
b. Wrap patient's hands in paper bags
c. Put clothing in paper bags
d. Use official chain of custody forms to document

5.

Descriptions	Terms
a. To do good	_d_ 1. Autonomy
b. To do no harm	_f_ 2. Fidelity
c. Telling the truth	_a_ 3. Beneficence
d. Self-determination	_b_ 4. Nonmaleficence
e. Right to privacy	_c_ 5. Veracity
f. Honoring promises	_e_ 6. Confidentiality

6.
a. Identify the ethical dilemma [situation]
b. Gather pertinent data
c. Examine the dilemma for ethical principles
d. Examine all solutions
e. Choose solution
f. Evaluate solutions chosen

7.

True	False	A minor can generally consent to treatment for a sexually transmitted infection
True	**False**	Implied consent means that the person has consented to this type of procedure or treatment before
True	False	When obtaining consent for a radiograph, a simple verbal agreement is sufficient to proceed
True	**False**	If a suicidal person refuses treatment, there is no recourse to force it upon that person
True	False	Alternatives to the proposed treatment should be explained as part of the informed consent process
True	False	The nurse should assess for barriers to understanding the material presented when obtaining a signature for informed consent
True	**False**	If a patient refuses treatment and the physician thinks that refusing will harm the patient, that patient can be forced to undergo the treatment
True	**False**	Institutions should avoid policies on patients leaving AMA because it will encourage them to do so

8.

a. Patient arrives by squad. Belligerent and obviously drunk. Removed dirty clothes and a large diamond ring. MBlair

> Suggested answer: (Date and Time): Patient arrived per (city) Squad 21. Sitting upright on gurney. Yelling and trying to hit EMS personnel. Smells of alcohol. States "I have been drinking all night!" Clothes removed and placed in bag; see patient belonging list. One ring with large clear stone removed and given to security. M. Blair, RN

b. Child brought in by hysterical mother who reports child was mauled by dog. Large wound to thigh covered with bloody gauze.

> Suggested answer: (Date and time): 8-year-old child carried into ED by mother. Mother screaming, "She was bit by a big dog! Help her! Help her!" 8X10 cm ragged laceration to upper left thigh covered with blood-soaked 4X4 gauze. M. Blair, RN

c. Patient complains of stomach pain for a long time. Given IV morphine and sent to x-ray. On return, patient says pain is better.

> Suggested answer: (Date and time): Patient complains of right upper quadrant pain, 8 on a scale of 10, X3 days. Made worse by eating, no relieving factors. Abdomen normal on inspection. Bowel sounds present, pain to right upper quad on palpation, percussion not done because patient refused. No rebound tenderness. M. Blair, RN
> (Time) Dr. Smith aware, examined patient, orders received. M. Blair, RN (Time) Patient given 10 mg morphine IV push. M. Blair, RN
> (Time) Vital signs _____, patient now reports pain 2/10. Sent to x-ray by cart. M. Blair, RN

9.

a. Offer food/fluids at specified regular intervals
b. Offer toileting at specified regular intervals
c. Assess limb distal to restraint at specified regular intervals
d. Try alternatives to restraints before applying them
e. Clearly document behavior requiring restraints

10.

a. Identify/eliminate stress, anxiety, or other distractions before teaching
b. Correct misconceptions that affect learning
c. Personalize the health message and explain the need for the information
d. Relate information to patient's past experiences and actively involve the patient and family in discussions
e. Consider qualities of poor readers and use teaching strategies that are helpful

11.

a. Physician interference: involve physician in planning and delivering teaching
b. Lack of time on nurse's part: delegate other patient care duties for a specified amount of time to work with patient
c. Psychological factors, i.e., pain or fear: address and control issues, give pain meds, discuss reason for anxiety with patient
d. Sensory deficits: adapt teaching materials to sensory limitation
e. Attitudes and beliefs that conflict with teaching (patient): discuss patient's beliefs regarding role in health care, amount of power he/she has over problem, specific tasks patient is willing to do; identify reasons why it would be important for patient to learn

12.

a. Allow family presence
b. Encourage family to express concerns and ask questions
c. Encourage family to participate in patient's care as they are able
d. Consult with social worker, chaplain, to provide support for family
e. Keep family informed as to patient's condition

13.

Category		Symptom of stress
a. Physical	a	1. Fatigue
b. Cognitive	b	2. Nightmares
c. Emotional	c	3. Uncertainty
d. Behavioral	d	4. Withdrawal from relationships
	d	5. Change in sexual functioning
	c	6. Intense anger
	b	7. Memory problems
	a	8. Headaches
	a	9. Elevated blood pressure
	b	10. Difficulty making decisions
	c	11. Apprehension
	d	12. Alcohol consumption

References and Suggested Readings

American Association of Critical-Care Nurses. (2007). SBAR techniques help EDs comply with handoff regs. *ED Management (Supplement)*, 3–4.

American Association of Critical-Care Nurses. (2004). *The four As to rise above moral distress.* Aliso Viejo, CA: Author.

American Nurses Association. (1994). *Education for participation in nursing research.* Retrieved February 22, 2008, from http://www.nursingworld.org/readroom/position/research/rseducat.htm

American Nurses Association. (2001). *Code of ethics for nurses with interpretive statements.* Washington, D.C.: Author.

American Nurses Association. (2005). *Principles for delegation.* Silver Spring, MD: Author.

Austen, S. (2006). Walk a fine line if your patient wants to leave AMA. *Nursing 2006, 36(12)*, 48–49.

Bonalumi, N. M., & King, D. (2007). Professionalism and leadership. In K. S. Hoyt & J. Selfridge-Thomas (Eds.), *Emergency nursing core curriculum* (6th ed.). St. Louis: Elsevier-Saunders.

Ciliska, D. K., Pinelli, J., DiCenso, A., & Cullum, N. (2001). Resources to enhance evidence-based nursing practice. *AACN Clinical Issues, 12(4)*, 520–528.

Curtin, L. (1982). Ethics in nursing administration. In A. Marriner (Ed.). *Contemporary nursing management.* St. Louis: CV Mosby.

Day, S., Dalto, J., Fox, J., & Turpin, M. (2006). Failure mode and effects analysis as a performance improvement tool in trauma. *Journal of Trauma Nursing, 13(3)*, 111–117.

Dennison, R. D. (2007). *Pass CCRN!* (3rd ed.). St. Louis: Mosby.

Donaldson, N. E., Rutledge, D. N., & Pravikoff, D. S. (1999). Principles of effective adult-focused patient education in nursing. *The Online Journal of Clinical Innovations, 2(2)*, 1–22.

Doucette, J. N. (2006). View from the cockpit: What the airline industry can teach us about patient safety. *Nursing 2006, 36(1)*, 50–53.

Emergency Nurses Association. (2006). *Position statement: Violence in the emergency care setting.* Des Plaines, IL: Author.

Emergency Nurses Association. (2007). *Trauma nursing core course provider manual* (6th ed.). Des Plaines, IL: Author.

Emergency Nurses Association. (2005). *Sheehy's manual of emergency care.* St. Louis: Elsevier Mosby.

Fulbrook, S. (2007). The duty to care 2: Risk assessment and risk management. *British Journal of Nursing, 16(2)*, 112–113.

Gray, J. A. M. (1997). *Evidence based health care: How to make health policy and management decisions.* London: Churchill Livingstone.

Harkreader, H., Hogan, M. A., & Thobaben, M. (2007). *Fundamentals of nursing: Caring and clinical judgment* (3rd ed.). St. Louis: Elsevier-Saunders.

Hauser, J. (2008). *Nursing research: Reading, using, & creating evidence.* Sudbury, MA: Jones & Bartlett.

Johnson, K. P. (2005). Basic legal issues for emergency nurses. In L. Newberry & L. M. Criddle (Eds.), *Sheehy's manual of emergency care* (6th ed.). St. Louis: Elsevier Mosby.

Lynch, A., & Cole, E. (2006). Human factors in emergency care: The need for team resource management. *Emergency Nurse, 14(2)*, 32–35.

Melnyk, B. M., & Fineout-Overholt, E. (2002). Putting research into practice. *Reflections on Nursing Leadership, 28(2)*, 22–25.

Mitchell, J. T., & Bray, G. P. (1990). *Emergency services stress.* Englewood Cliffs, NJ: R. J. Brady/Prentice Hall.

Monson, M. S. (2006). Disclosing adverse events: You said it, now write it. *Nursing Management, 37(8)*, 16–17, 55.

National Patient Safety Foundation. (2008). *Health literary: Statistics at-a-glance.* Retrieved October 11, 2008, from http://www.npsf.org/askme3/pdfs/STATS_GLANCE_EN.pdf

Newhouse, R. P. (2007). Diffusing confusion among evidence-based practice, quality improvement, & research. *Journal of Nursing Administration, 37(10)*, 432–435.

Saferstein, R. (2006). Evidence collection and preservation. In V. A. Lynch (Ed.), *Forensic nursing.* St. Louis: Elsevier-Mosby.

Stevens, K. R. (2005). *ACE Star Model of Knowledge Transformation.* Available at http://www.acestar.uthscsa.edu/Learn_model.htm. Last retrieved March 30, 2010.

Straus, S. E., Richardson, W. S., Glasziou, P., & Haynes, R. B. (2005). *Evidence based medicine* (3rd ed.). London: Churchill Livingstone.

Woodhall, L. J., Vertacnik, L., & McLaughlin, M. (2008). Implementation of the SBAR communication technique in a tertiary center. *Journal of Emergency Nursing, 34(4)*, 314–317.

CHAPTER 4

Cardiovascular Emergencies

Introduction

This content constitutes 14% (21 items) of the CEN examination

The focus is on cardiovascular conditions that are commonly encountered in an emergency department setting

The continuum of age needs to be considered from infancy to old age

Age-Related Considerations

Neonates, infants, and children

1. Cardiovascular deterioration in neonates and infants may be caused by congenital heart defects
2. Dysrhythmias, heart failure (HF), and cardiogenic shock in a neonate, an infant, or a child is usually related to a congenital cardiac problem (Emergency Nurses Association [ENA], 2007)
3. Pediatric patients have a decreased vascular tone that causes decreased venous return and that limits their ability to increase stroke volume to raise cardiac output; if cardiac output is decreased, these patients compensate with tachycardia
4. Bradycardia or cardiac arrest is more frequently caused by respiratory problems rather than cardiac causes
5. A new murmur with a fever in a child is likely to be rheumatic fever, which may be the cause of significant valvular disease, especially later in life
6. Tachycardia in the pediatric patient may be related to underlying conduction system anomalies, such as accessory pathways (e.g., Wolff-Parkinson-White syndrome [WPW], Lown-Ganong-Levine [LGL] syndrome) (ENA, 2007)
7. Cardiac signs and symptoms may be caused by accidental drug ingestion

Older adults

1. Cardiac output at rest decreases and cardiac reserve is limited, so older adults are less able to adapt to cardiac stressors
2. Vascular changes with aging cause an increase in diastolic blood pressure (BP) and may make it difficult to feel peripheral pulses
3. Geriatric patients may have multiple underlying medical problems (i.e., comorbidities) that can confound cardiac symptoms (ENA, 2007)

4. Symptoms of myocardial ischemia in the older adult may include weakness, shortness of breath, syncope, confusion, dysrhythmias, and stroke (ENA, 2007)
5. Older adults are more likely to have silent myocardial infarction (MI) than younger patients
6. The effects of aging on the liver and kidneys alter drug metabolism; this may cause cumulative effects if one dose has not been metabolized and eliminated when the next dose is administered
7. Extra caution is warranted with the administration of cardiac drugs in older adults; lower doses and longer intervals between doses are frequently needed
8. Polypharmacy in older adults predisposes these patients to adverse effects caused by drug interactions
9. Older adults' desires after they are given information about their treatment and consequences of the treatment must be considered as part of resuscitation efforts and end-of-life care

Selected Concepts in Anatomy and Physiology

General information about the cardiovascular system

1. The cardiovascular system is a continuous, fluid-filled elastic circuit with a pump
2. The cardiovascular system provides communication among all body parts via the transportation of oxygen, nutrients, hormones, water, enzymes, vitamins, minerals, buffers, leukocytes, antibodies, and wastes; these functions maintain dynamic equilibrium to provide homeostasis
3. The cardiovascular system consists of the heart and the vascular system

The heart

1. Four-chambered muscular organ that provides the forward propulsion of blood into the vascular system
2. Size of a closed fist: usually approximately 9 cm wide and 12 cm long; weighs approximately 4 g/kg of ideal body weight
3. Lies in the mediastinum between the sternum (anterior) and the spine (posterior), with two thirds to the left of the body's midline and one third to the right of the midline (Figure 4-1)
4. Shaped like a blunt cone
   a. Apex
      1) Inferior, anterior, and to the left

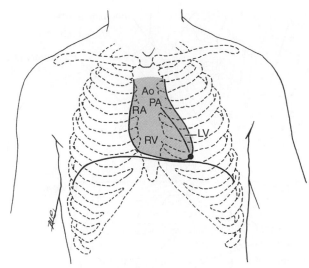

Figure 4-1 Location and orientation of the heart within the thorax. *Ao,* Aorta; *LV,* left ventricle; *PA,* pulmonary artery; *RA,* right atrium; *RV,* right ventricle. (From Price, S., & Wilson, I. [1996]. *Pathophysiology: Clinical concepts of disease processes* [5th ed.] St. Louis: Mosby.)

2) Normally at the fifth left intercostal space at the midclavicular line (MCL)
3) On the upper surface of the diaphragm
   b. Base
      1) Superior, posterior, and to the right
      2) Normally at level of the second intercostal space
5. Layers of the cardiac wall (Figure 4-2)
   a. Pericardium: maintains the heart in a stationary position
      1) Fibrous: loose-fitting, white, fibrous layer that acts as a barrier against infection and neoplastic invasion

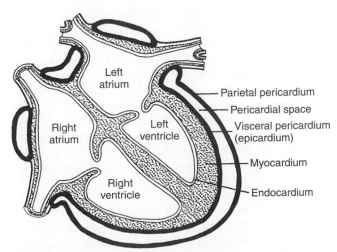

Figure 4-2 Layers of the cardiac wall. (From Copstead, I. [1995]. *Perspectives on pathophysiology.* Philadelphia: W. B. Saunders.)

2) Serous
   a) Parietal layer: lines the inner surface of the fibrous pericardium
   b) Visceral layer: lines the surface of the heart; synonymous with *epicardium*
3) Pericardial space: located between the parietal and visceral layers of the serous pericardium and contains 10 to 30 ml of lubricating fluid
   a) Protects the heart against friction and erosion
   b) Provides a well-lubricated sac in which the heart moves during contraction
   b. Epicardium: visceral layer of serous pericardium
   c. Myocardium: largest portion of the cardiac wall, which consists of specialized conduction fibers and interlacing cardiac muscle fibers
   d. Endocardium: consists of connective tissue, elastic fibers, and endothelial cells, which form a smooth surface for blood contact and the deterrence of clot formation
      1) Contiguous with the lining of the great vessels
      2) Lines the heart chambers and valves
6. Cardiac chambers
   a. Atria
      1) Act as reservoirs and booster pumps for the ventricles
         a) Passive ventricular filling: 70% to 75% of ventricular filling is passive as blood falls through the atrium into the ventricle
         b) Active ventricular filling: 25% to 30% of ventricular filling is active as the atrium contracts at the end of ventricular diastole
      2) Right atria
         a) Inflow tracts: superior vena cava, inferior vena cava, coronary sinus, and Thebesian veins
         b) Outflow tract: through the tricuspid valve to the right ventricle
      3) Left atria
         a) Inflow tracts: four pulmonary veins (this is the only case of veins carrying oxygenated blood)
         b) Outflow tract: through the mitral valve to the left ventricle
   b. Ventricles
      1) Act as pumps that receive blood from the atria and that pump blood into the great vessels
      2) Right ventricle: thin walled and low pressure
         a) Inflow tract: from the right atria via the tricuspid valve and the Thebesian veins
         b) Outflow tract: pulmonary artery (PA) (this is the only case of an artery carrying deoxygenated blood)
      3) Left ventricle: thick-walled and high-pressure
         a) Inflow tract: left atria via the mitral valve and the Thebesian veins
         b) Outflow tract: aorta
7. Cardiac valves (Figure 4-3)
   a. Purpose: to maintain unidirectional flow

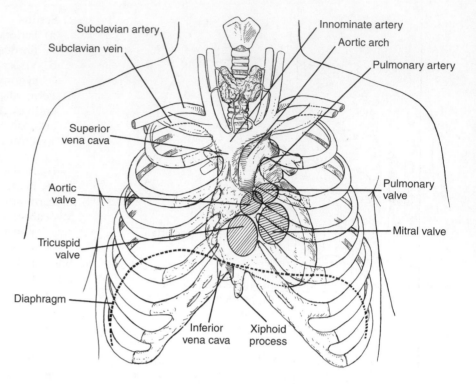

Figure 4-3 Position of the cardiac valves. (From Seifert, P. C. [1994]. *Mosby's perioperative nursing series. Cardiac surgery.* St. Louis: Mosby.)

1) To permit antegrade flow; the narrowing of the valvular orifice to prevent normal antegrade flow is referred to as *stenosis*
2) To prevent retrograde flow: the inadequate closure of the valvular orifice, which allows for retrograde flow, is referred to as *regurgitant, incompetent,* or *insufficient*

b. Atrioventricular (AV) valves: the tricuspid and mitral valves
1) Located between the atria and the ventricles
a) The tricuspid valve is between the right atria and the right ventricle
b) The mitral valve is between the left atria and the left ventricle
2) These valves cause the first heart sound, S_1, when they close

c. Semilunar valves: the aortic and pulmonic valves
1) Located between the ventricles and the great vessels
a) The pulmonic valve is located between the right ventricle and the PA
b) The aortic valve is located between the left ventricle and the aorta
2) These valves cause the second heart sound, S_2, when they close

8. The pathway of blood through the heart and the vascular system is as follows: vena cavae (superior and inferior) → right atrium → tricuspid valve → right ventricle → pulmonic valve → PA → pulmonary capillary bed → pulmonary veins → left atrium → mitral valve → left ventricle → aortic valve → aorta → arteries → arterioles → capillaries → venules → veins → vena cavae (Figure 4-4)

9. Coronary vasculature
a. The coronary arteries are the first branch off of the aorta, immediately outside of the aortic valve
b. Coronary artery perfusion
1) The left ventricle is perfused primarily during diastole
2) The right ventricle is perfused throughout the cardiac cycle, but perfusion is greater during diastole
3) Myocardial oxygen consumption (Figure 4-5)
a) Determinants of myocardial oxygen demand include the following:
i) Heart rate: the number of times per minute that the ventricles contract
ii) Preload: the stretch on the myofibrils at the end of diastole; the degree of myofibril stretch is affected by the ventricular volume
iii) Afterload: the pressure against which the ventricle must pump to open the semilunar valve; this is affected by vascular resistance, ventricular diameter, and the mass and viscosity of the blood
iv) Contractility: the contractile force of the heart independent of preload and afterload
b) Determinants of myocardial oxygen supply include the following:
i) Patent arteries
ii) Diastolic pressure
iii) Diastolic time
iv) Oxygen extraction
(a) Hemoglobin
(b) Oxygen saturation in arterial blood (SaO_2)

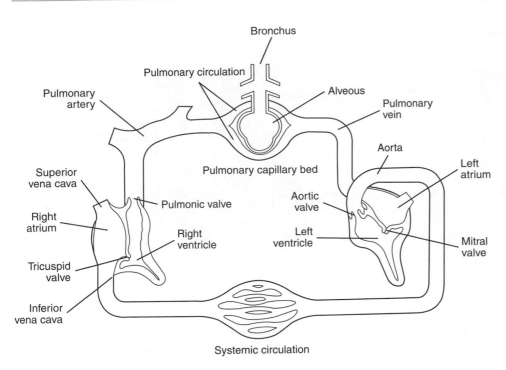

Figure 4-4 Pathway of blood through the heart and the vascular system. (Reproduced with permission of Edwards Lifesciences, Irvine, CA.)

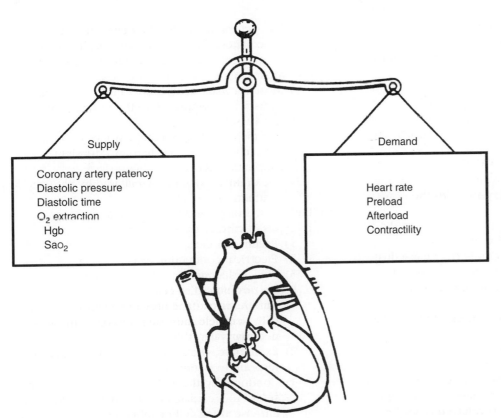

Figure 4-5 Factors that influence myocardial oxygen supply and demand. Hgh, Hemoglobin concentration; Sao$_2$, arterial oxygen saturation. (Reproduced with permission of Edwards Lifesciences, Irvine, CA.)

c) Imbalances between supply and demand cause ischemia; prolonged imbalance causes infarction

c. Coronary arteries and distribution (Figure 4-6)

1) The left coronary artery before bifurcation is referred to as the *left main coronary artery;* the left main coronary artery divides into the left anterior descending artery and the left circumflex artery

a) The left anterior descending coronary artery supplies the following:

i) Anterior left ventricle

ii) Anterior two thirds of the interventricular septum

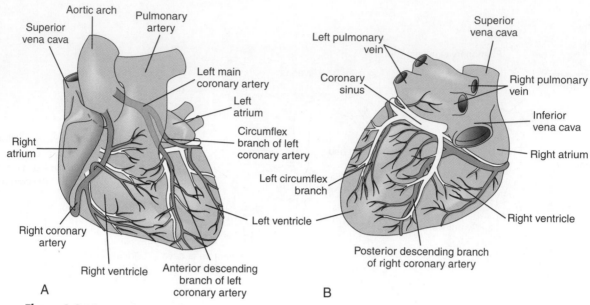

Figure 4-6 The coronary circulation. **A,** Anterior surface. **B,** Posterior surface. (From Hatcheet, R., & Thompson, D. [Eds.] [2002]. *Cardiac nursing: A comprehensive guide.* Edinburgh: Churchill Livingstone.)

iii) Apex of left ventricle
iv) Bundle of His and bundle branches
b) The left circumflex coronary artery supplies the following:
  i) Left atrium
  ii) Sinoatrial node in 45% of hearts
  iii) AV node in 10% of hearts
  iv) The obtuse marginal branch supplies the following:
    (a) Lateral left ventricle
    (b) Posterior left ventricle
2) The right coronary artery supplies the following:
  a) Right atrium
  b) Sinoatrial node in 55% of hearts
  c) Left posterior hemibundle (this has a dual blood supply: the left anterior descending artery and the right coronary artery)
  d) AV node in 90% of hearts
  e) The marginal branch supplies the following:
    i) Lateral right ventricle
    ii) Inferior right ventricle
  f) In hearts in which the right coronary artery is dominant (≈80%), a branch of the right coronary artery that is referred to as the *posterior descending artery* supplies the following:
    i) Anterior right ventricle
    ii) Inferior wall of left ventricle
    iii) Posterior left ventricle
    iv) Posterior third of septum
3) Collateral circulation
  a) This consists of interarterial vessels that connect or anastomose with each other

  b) Factors that foster the development of collateral flow include anemia, hypoxemia, and gradual occlusion (e.g., arteriosclerosis)
d. Coronary veins
  1) Most coronary veins empty into the coronary sinus, which empties into the right atrium
e. Lymph vessels
  1) The main cardiac channel empties into the pretracheal node and then into the right lymphatic duct
  2) The drainage system is facilitated by cardiac contraction
10. Electrophysiology and the conduction system
  a. Types of cardiac cells
    1) Pacemaker cells
    2) Electrical conducting cells
    3) Myocardial muscle cells
  b. Properties of cardiac cells
    1) Automaticity: the ability of the certain cardiac cells to initiate impulses regularly and spontaneously
    2) Excitability: the ability of the cardiac cells to respond to a stimulus
    3) Conductivity: the ability of cardiac cells to respond to a cardiac impulse by transmitting the impulse along cell membranes
    4) Contractility: the ability of the cardiac cells to respond to an impulse by muscle contraction
  c. Conduction system (Figure 4-7)
    1) Sinoatrial node
      a) Functions as the natural pacemaker of the heart because it has the fastest intrinsic rate (i.e., 60–100 beats/minute)
      b) Located in the right atrial wall near the opening of the superior vena cava

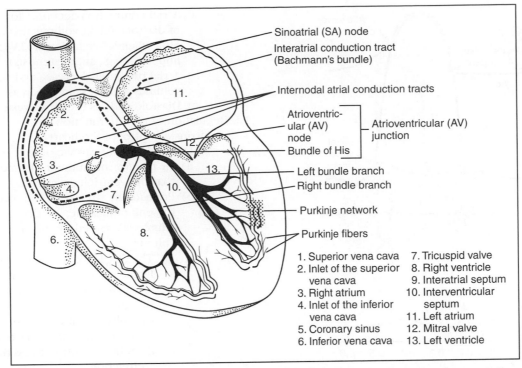

1. Superior vena cava
2. Inlet of the superior vena cava
3. Right atrium
4. Inlet of the inferior vena cava
5. Coronary sinus
6. Inferior vena cava
7. Tricuspid valve
8. Right ventricle
9. Interatrial septum
10. Interventricular septum
11. Left atrium
12. Mitral valve
13. Left ventricle

Figure 4-7 The conduction system. (From Huszar, R. J. [1994]. *Basic dysrhythmias: Interpretation and management* [2nd ed.]. St. Louis: Mosby.)

2) Internodal pathways
3) Bachmann bundle (interatrial pathway): the pathway that takes the impulse from the right atrium to the left atrium
4) AV node
   a) Accounts for the physiologic delay of 0.08 to 0.12 second to allow the atria to completely depolarize, contract, and finish filling the ventricles before the ventricles are stimulated
   b) Contains no pacemaker cells; its primary function is to slow the impulse down
5) AV junction
   a) The tissue that surrounds the AV node and the bundle of His that contains pacemaker cells
   b) Functions as a secondary pacemaker with an intrinsic rate of 40 to 60 beats/minute
6) Bundle of His: first portion of interventricular conduction system
7) Bundle branches
   a) Right bundle branch takes the impulse to the right ventricular (RV) myocardium
   b) Left bundle branch divides into hemibundles; the blockage of either of the two major hemibundles (anterior or posterior) is referred to as a *hemiblock*
8) Purkinje fiber system
   a) Takes the impulse from the bundle branches through the wall of the ventricles to the subendocardial layers

   b) Functions as a final tertiary pacemaker ((i.e., the upper pacemakers fail) at the inherent rate of 20 to 40 beats/minute
11. Cardiac cycle (Figure 4-8)
   a. Systole
      1) Isovolumetric contraction:
         a) Contraction increases pressure in the ventricles, but there is no change in volume because the AV valves are closed and the semilunar valves have not yet opened
         b) Ventricular pressures must exceed the pressure in the respective great vessel to open the semilunar valves
      2) Maximal ejection: when the pressure in the ventricles exceeds the pressure in the great vessels, the semilunar valves open, and blood is rapidly ejected into the great vessels
      3) Reduced ejection: blood is slowly ejected from the ventricles to the great vessels, but when the pressure in the great vessel is greater than the pressure in the ventricles, the semilunar valve closes, and systole ends
   b. Diastole
      1) Isovolumetric relaxation: relaxation occurs and ventricular pressure decreases, but volume does not change because the semilunar valves have closed and the AV valves have not yet opened
      2) Rapid filling:
         a) During this phase, the AV valves open and blood rushes into the ventricles

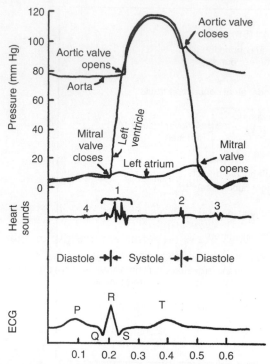

Figure 4-8 Wenger diagram that demonstrates the cardiac cycle and that shows electrocardiographic events, heart sounds, and pressure curves. (From Wenger, N., Hurst, J. W., & McIntyre, M. C. [1980]. *Cardiology for nurses.* St. Louis: McGraw-Hill.)

b) Atrial and ventricular pressures decrease and ventricular volumes increase
3) Reduced filling: atrial and ventricular pressures slowly increase and ventricular volumes increase with the slow filling of the ventricles
4) Atrial contraction (also referred to as the *atrial kick*)

a) Atrial contraction accounts for 15% to 30% of diastolic filling volume; this may be up to 50% when left ventricular (LV) filling is impeded (e.g., mitral stenosis)
b) Atrial pressures decrease and ventricular volumes and pressures increase
c) Diastole ends as the AV valves close
12. Regulation of cardiac function
  a. Intrinsic control of the heart
    1) Determinants of cardiac output (Figure 4-9)
      a) Heart rate: the number of times per minute that the ventricles contract
      b) Preload: the stretch on the myofibrils at the end of diastole; the degree of myofibril stretch is affected by the ventricular volume
        i) The Starling law of the heart and the Frank-Starling mechanism: within physiologic limits, the greater the stretch on the myofibrils, the greater the force of the subsequent contraction; both understretching and overstretching of the myofibrils result in a less-than-optimal contraction
      c) Afterload: the pressure against which the ventricle must pump to open the semilunar valve; this is affected by vascular resistance, ventricular diameter, and the mass and viscosity of the blood
      d) Contractility: the contractile force of the heart independent of preload and afterload
  b. Extrinsic control of the heart
    1) Neurologic control of the heart
      a) Autonomic nervous system
        i) Terms used to describe cardiac effects:
          (a) Chronotropic: effect on heart rate

Figure 4-9 Determinants of cardiac output. (From Price, S. A., & Wilson, L. M. [1996]. *Pathophysiology: Clinical concepts of disease processes* [5th ed.]). St. Louis: Mosby.)

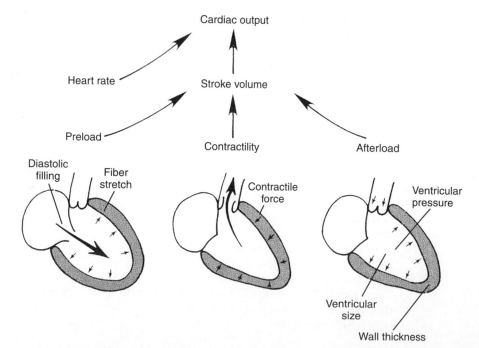

(b) Inotropic: effect on contractility
(c) Dromotropic: effect on conductivity
ii) Sympathetic nervous system (SNS)
(a) This branch is responsible for the "fight or flight" response
(b) The SNS is innervated by physiologic or psychologic stress
(c) It causes positive chronotropic, inotropic, and dromotropic effects
(d) SNS receptors and effects are listed in Table 4-1
(e) Sympathomimetic (also referred to as *adrenergic*) drugs are frequently used to augment these effects, especially after the patient's endogenous supplies are depleted; these drugs vary with regard to their receptor stimulation and the potency of that stimulation (Table 4-2)
b) Parasympathetic (vagal) nervous system
i) This branch maintains the steady state
ii) It causes negative chronotropic, inotropic, and dromotropic effects
iii) Although the cardiovascular effects of the parasympathetic nervous system are generally undesirable in critically ill patients, they may decrease myocardial oxygen consumption by up to 50%
iv) Parasympatholytic (vagolytic) agents (e.g., atropine) block these effects
c) Chemoreceptors
i) Chemoreceptors are located in carotid and aortic bodies
ii) They are sensitive to changes in PaO_2, $PaCO_2$, and pH
iii) Hypoxia, hypercapnia, and acidosis cause changes in the heart rate and the ventilatory rate
d) Baroreceptor reflex
i) Baroreceptors are located in the carotid sinus and the aortic arch
ii) They are sensitive to arterial pressure
iii) Increased BP causes vagal stimulation, which results in a decrease in heart rate and contractility
e) Bainbridge reflex
i) Accelerator receptors are located in the right atrium
ii) These receptors are sensitive to right atrial pressure
iii) Increased right atrial pressure causes an increase in heart rate
f) Respiratory reflex
i) Inspiration decreases intrathoracic pressure, which increases venous return to the right side of the heart, which causes the Bainbridge reflex; when the increased venous return reaches the left side of the heart, LV cardiac output increases, which increases arterial BP and decreases the heart rate through the stimulation of baroreceptors
ii) This process is at least partly responsible for sinus dysrhythmia; an interaction between the respiratory and cardiac centers in the medulla also contributes

TABLE 4-1 Sympathetic Nervous System (Adrenergic) Receptors and Effects

Receptor	Location of Receptor	Effects
α	Vessels	Vasoconstriction of most vessels, especially the arterioles
β₁	Heart	Increase in heart rate (chronotropic effect), contractility (inotropic effect), and conductivity (dromotropic effect)
β₂	Bronchial and vascular smooth muscle	Bronchodilation and vasodilation
Dopaminergic	Renal and mesenteric artery bed	Dilation of renal and mesenteric arteries

From Dennison, R. (2007). *Pass CCRN!* (3rd ed.). St. Louis: Mosby.

TABLE 4-2 Sympathomimetic Agents and Receptor Stimulation

Drug	α	β₁	β₂
Phenylephrine (Neo-Synephrine)	++++	0	0
Norepinephrine (Levophed)	++++	++	0
Epinephrine (Adrenalin)	++++	++++	++
Dopamine (Intropin)	++>5 mcg/kg/min; +++>10 mcg/kg/min	++++<10 mcg/kg/min	+
Dobutamine (Dobutrex)	+	++++	++
Isoproterenol (Isuprel)	0	++++	++++

From Dennison, R. (2007). *Pass CCRN!* (3rd ed.). St. Louis: Mosby.

Vascular system

1. Functions: to supply blood, nutrients, and hormones to tissues and to remove metabolic wastes from tissues
2. Resistance to flow
   a. The Poiseuille formula states that resistance depends on the following:
      1) The length of the vessel
      2) The radius of the vessel
      3) The viscosity of the blood
   b. Blood flow through the body is also influenced by neurologic stimulation that affects vascular tone and features that cause turbulence within the vascular lumen, such as bifurcations or protrusions from the vessel wall into the vessel lumen (e.g., atherosclerosis)
3. Components of the vascular system
   a. Arteries: the delivery system that distributes and regulates the amount of oxygenated blood flow to various tissue beds
      1) Arteries are able to stretch during systole and recoil during diastole
      2) The arterial system is a high-pressure circuit
      3) The layers of the arterial wall consist of the following:
         a) Intima: the thin lining of the endothelium and a small amount of elastic tissue; it decreases resistance to flow and minimizes the chance of platelet aggregation
         b) Media: the smooth muscle and elastic tissue; it changes the lumen diameter as needed
         c) Adventitia: the connective tissue; it strengthens and shapes the vessels
   b. Arterioles
      1) Arterioles are vital to the maintenance of BP and systemic vascular resistance
      2) Arterioles may lead to capillaries, metarterioles, or precapillary sphincters, which control blood flow into the capillary bed

   c. Capillaries: the nutrient beds where the exchange of gases, nutrients, and metabolites take place by the process of diffusion
      1) Capillaries contain no smooth muscle; their diameter depends on changes in precapillary and postcapillary tone
      2) Capillary dynamics are influenced by four pressures (Figure 4-10):
         a) Hydrostatic pressures push
            i) Capillary hydrostatic pressure pushes fluid out of the capillary and into the interstitium
            ii) Interstitial hydrostatic pressure pushes fluid out of the interstitium and into the capillary
         b) Colloidal oncotic pressures pull
            i) Capillary colloidal oncotic pressure pulls and holds fluid in the capillary
            ii) Interstitial colloidal oncotic pressure pulls and holds fluid in the interstitium
         c) Pressures that push fluid out of the capillary dominate at the arterial end; pressures that push fluid back into the capillary dominate at the venous end
         d) Edema is caused by an imbalance in these pressures or by an increase in capillary permeability; the term *third spacing* is used to describe fluid accumulation in any space that is not intravascular or intracellular (e.g., interstitial edema, ascites, pleural effusion, pericardial effusion, into the lumen of the intestine)
            i) HF: peripheral edema is caused by venous congestion and excessive hydrostatic pressure at the venous end
            ii) Protein malnutrition or liver disease: a decrease in plasma proteins decreases capillary colloidal oncotic pressure and allows excessive fluid to leak out of the capillary

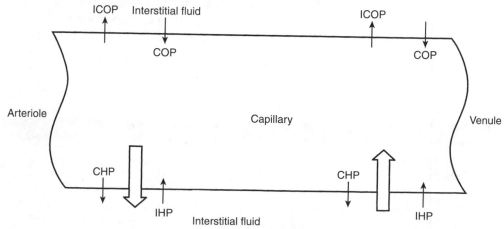

Figure 4-10 Capillary dynamics. Forces out of the capillary dominate at the arteriole end, whereas forces back into the capillary dominate at the venule end. *CHP,* Capillary hydrostatic pressure; *COP,* colloidal oncotic pressure; *ICOP,* interstitial colloidal oncotic pressure; *IHP,* interstitial hydrostatic pressure. (From Dennison, R. D. [2007]. *Pass CCRN!* 3rd ed. St. Louis: Mosby.)

d. Veins: the return system that brings deoxygenated blood back to the heart and lungs
  1) Veins act as a reservoir; the venous system holds 65% to 70% of the total blood volume
  2) The venous pump sends blood back to the right side of the heart; the skeletal muscles contract, compress veins, and propel blood toward the heart
  3) Valves in the veins prevent retrograde blood flow
4. BP
  a. Regulation
    1) Autonomic nervous system
    2) Renin-angiotensin-aldosterone system (Figure 4-11)

a) Renin is secreted by the kidney in response to the following:
  i) Decreased BP that stimulates stretch receptors in juxtaglomerular cells
  ii) SNS stimulation
  iii) Hyponatremia
b) Renin stimulates the conversion of angiotensinogen to angiotensin I
c) Angiotensin I is converted to angiotensin II by angiotensin-converting enzyme (ACE) as the blood travels through the lung
d) Angiotensin II causes vasoconstriction and the secretion of aldosterone

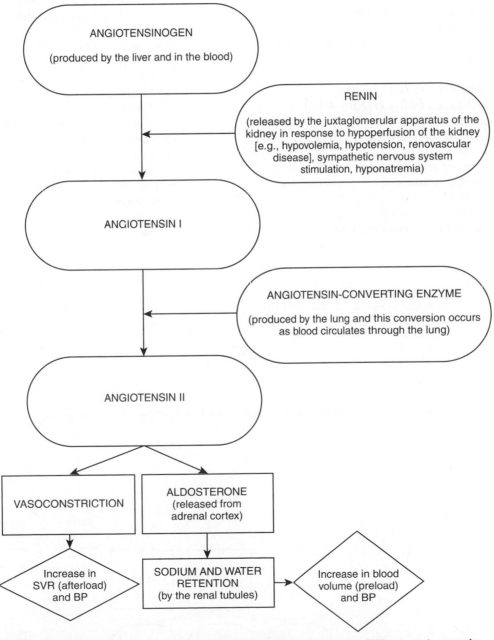

Figure 4-11 Renin-angiotensin-aldosterone system. *BP,* Blood pressure; *SVR,* systemic vascular resistance. (From Dennison, R. D. [2007]. *Pass CCRN!* 3rd ed. St. Louis: Mosby.)

e) Vasoconstriction and sodium and water retention increase BP and decrease renin secretion
    3) Capillary fluid shifts, especially from areas of interstitial space to intravascular space
    4) Local control mechanisms
  b. Factors that affect arterial BP (Figure 4-12)
  c. Pulse pressure: the difference between the systolic and diastolic pressures
    1) Calculated as: Systolic BP − Diastolic BP
    2) Normal is approximately 40 mm Hg
    3) Affected by stroke volume and arterial elastance
  d. Mean arterial pressure: the average pressure in the aorta and its major branches during the cardiac cycle
    1) Calculated by either of the following formulae:
      a) (Systolic BP + [Diastolic BP × 2]) ÷ 3
      b) Diastolic BP + ⅓ Pulse pressure
    2) Normal: 70 to 105 mm Hg
    3) Affected by cardiac output and systemic vascular resistance

Oxygen delivery to tissues (DO_2)/Oxygen consumption by tissues (VO_2) (Figure 4-13)

1. Oxygen delivery to tissues (DO_2)
  a. Product of cardiac output and arterial oxygen content
    1) Cardiac output is a product of heart rate and stroke volume; stroke volume is affected by preload, afterload, and contractility
    2) Arterial oxygen content is a product of hemoglobin and arterial saturation

3) Examples of situations that decrease DO_2
  a) Decrease in SaO_2 (e.g., acute respiratory failure, decrease in inspired oxygen level [e.g., smoke inhalation], decrease in barometric pressure [e.g., high altitudes])
  b) Decrease in hemoglobin (e.g., anemia, hemorrhage)
  c) Decrease in cardiac output (e.g., HF, hypovolemia)
  b. Oxygen consumption by tissues (VO_2)
    1) VO_2: volume of oxygen consumed by the tissues each minute
      a) Determined by comparing the oxygen content in the arterial blood with the oxygen content in the mixed venous blood (e.g., drawn from the distal tip of the PA catheter)
    2) Examples of situations that increase VO_2
      a) Activity (e.g., bathing, repositioning)
      b) Agitation
      c) Shivering
      d) Fever
      e) Increased work of breathing
      f) Severe infection
      g) Burns
    3) Examples of therapeutic methods to decrease VO_2
      a) Hypothermia
      b) Sedation
      c) Analgesia

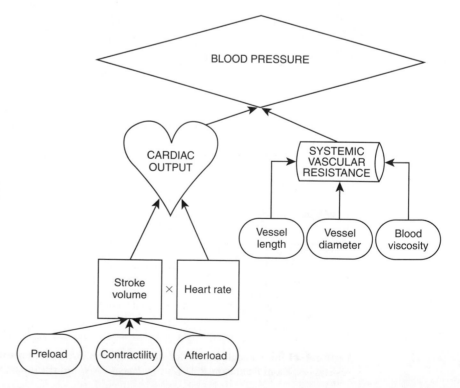

Figure 4-12 Determinants of blood pressure. (From Dennison, R. D. [2007]. *Pass CCRN!* 3rd ed. St. Louis: Mosby.)

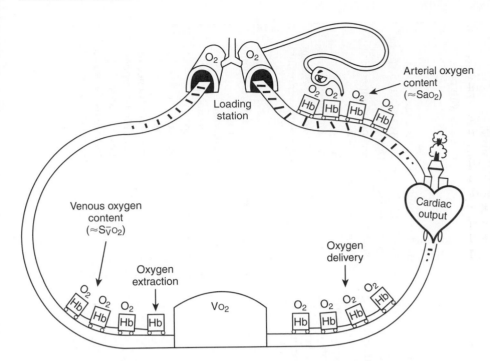

Figure 4-13 A schematic that demonstrates oxygen delivery and oxygen consumption (DO_2/VO_2). (Reproduced with permission of Edwards Lifesciences, Irvine, CA.

c. Serum arterial lactate level
  1) Lactic acidosis is the result of anaerobic metabolism; an elevated serum arterial lactate level indicates a tissue oxygen deficit
  2) Normal serum arterial lactate level: <1 mmol/L

Cardiovascular Assessment

Focused assessment

1. Chief complaint: identifies why the patient is seeking help and the duration of the problem
2. Symptoms related to cardiac disorders
   a. Chest pain: may also be identified as indigestion, burning, discomfort, tightness, or pressure in the mid chest, the epigastrium, or the left arm; Table 4-3 describes the differentiation of chest pain
   1) PQRST format for describing complaint
      a) P
         i) Provocation: what provokes or worsens the pain?
         ii) Palliation: what relieves the pain? (also include what was used but did not relieve the pain)
      b) Q
         i) Quality: what does the pain feel like?
      c) R
         i) Region: where is the pain?
         ii) Radiation: to what area does the pain radiate, if any?
      d) S
         i) Severity: how severe is the pain?
            (a) Pain scale: the most frequently used scale in adults is the 1-to-10 scale, with 1 being negligible and 10 being the worst imaginable

      e) T
         i) Timing: is the pain intermittent or continuous, and what is the relationship of the pain to other events or activities?
   b. Dyspnea
      1) Shortness of breath or "breathlessness"
      2) Exertional dyspnea
      3) Orthopnea: patient is unable to lie flat because of dyspnea
      4) Paroxysmal nocturnal dyspnea: patient awakens with a feeling of suffocation 1 to 2 hours after going to sleep; if accompanied by wheezing, may be called *cardiac asthma*
   c. Cough: cardiac cough usually occurs at night and is precipitated by supine positioning, exertion, or turning to one side
   d. Hemoptysis: may be related to pulmonary edema
   e. Palpitations: unpleasant awareness of the heartbeat when at rest; may be described as skipping, pounding, or thumping sensation; associated with premature beats or other dysrhythmias
   f. Syncope or lightheadedness
   g. Headache: may be related to hypertension
   h. Ascites: may be related to RV failure (RVF)
   i. Abdominal pain: may be related to RVF
   j. Edema or weight gain: frequently related to RVF; also described as involving a bloated feeling, swelling, tightening of clothing, tightening of shoes, and marks left from constricting garments
   k. Fatigue or weakness: may be related to RVF
   l. Nocturia: may be related to HF
   m. Diaphoresis: may be related to SNS stimulation or infection
   n. Unexplained joint pain: may be related to rheumatic fever

TABLE 4-3   Differentiation of Chest Pain

Cause	Provocation	Palliation	Quality	Region/Radiation	Severity	Timing	Associated Signs/Symptoms
Angina pectoris	• Exercise • Exertion • Exposure to cold • Emotional stress • Eating • Smoking	• Rest • Oxygen • Nitroglycerin • Calcium channel blockers (e.g., nifedipine [Procardia])	• Heaviness or pressure • Tightness • Squeezing • Dull ache • Burning • Not always described as pain but as discomfort	• Substernal • May be diffuse and vague • May radiate to arms, neck, jaw, back, and upper abdomen	• Mild to severe	• Gradual or sudden onset • Duration usually 1-4 minutes but may be 5-15 minutes	• Tachycardia, tachypnea • Dyspnea • Nausea, vomiting • Diaphoresis • Weakness • Anxiety • May have ST-T wave changes with pain
Acute myocardial infarction	• No specific precipitator • Lifestyle change and stress • Usually occurs within 3 hours of awakening	• Narcotics • Reperfusion by fibrinolytic or percutaneous coronary intervention (e.g., angioplasty, atherectomy) • No relief with rest and/or nitroglycerin	• As for angina • Heaviness or pressure • May show Levine's sign (clenched fist over sternum)	• As for angina	• No symptoms to severe • Absence of pain is common in patients with diabetes mellitus and in older adults	• Sudden onset • Duration: >30 minutes; usually 1-2 hours	• As for angina • Tachycardia, tachypnea • Dyspnea • Feeling of impending doom • S_4 • ECG changes:T wave inversion, ST segment elevation, eventually Q waves
Dissecting aortic aneurysm	• Peripheral vascular disease • Marfan syndrome • Aortitis • Hypertension and/or hypertensive crisis • Chest trauma	• Narcotics • Surgery • No relief with rest and/or nitroglycerin	• Tearing • Ripping	• Anterior chest • Radiation to shoulders, neck, back, and abdomen	• Severe	• Sudden onset • Worse at onset • Duration: hours to days	• Tachycardia, tachypnea • Dysphagia • Confusion • Diaphoresis • Syncope • Dyspnea • Anxiety • Unilateral absence of pulse; BP differences between sides • Motor/sensory changes • Murmur of aortic regurgitation

Condition	Cause	Quality	Severity	Location	Treatment	Onset/Duration	Signs and Symptoms
Pericarditis	• Myocardial infarction • Cardiac surgery • Trauma • Infections • Uremia • Lupus erythematosus	• Sharp • Stabbing • Knifelike • Worsened by inspiration, coughing, movement, recumbent position	• Mild to severe	• Precordial • Substernal • Radiation to neck, shoulders, arms, and back	• Nonsteroidal anti-inflammatory agents (e.g., ibuprofen [Motrin], indomethacin [Indocin]) • Sitting up and leaning forward	• Sudden onset • Duration: days	• Tachycardia, tachypnea • Fever • Dyspnea • Pericardial friction rub • Leukocytosis • Diffuse concave ST segment
Pulmonary embolism	• Venous stasis (e.g., immobility, pelvic surgery, atrial fibrillation) • Hypercoagulability (e.g., oral contraceptives, malignancy, polycythemia) • Injury to vessel (e.g., IVs, vascular surgery)	• Sharp • Knifelike • Shooting • Deep ache • Pressure • Worsened by deep inspiration or coughing	• Mild to severe	• Substernal or lateral chest • Radiation to shoulder or neck	• Narcotics • High Fowler's position • Splinting of chest	• Sudden onset • Duration: minutes to hours	• Tachycardia, tachypnea • Dyspnea • Pallor or cyanosis • Cough • Anxiety, feeling of impending doom • Sinus tachycardia or atrial dysrhythmias • Accentuated P_2 • Right-sided S_4, possible right-sided S_3 • If RVF: JVD • If pulmonary infarction: pleural friction rub, hemoptysis, fever
Pneumothorax	• Congenital bleb • Emphysematous bullous • Large tidal volumes or PEEP on mechanical ventilator • Chest trauma • Exacerbated by coughing, exertion, or Valsalva maneuver	• Tearing • Sharp • Worsened by breathing	• Mild to severe	• Lateral chest • May radiate to shoulders, back, and arms	• Narcotics • Insertion of chest tube	• Sudden onset • Duration: hours to days	• Tachypnea • Tachycardia • Dyspnea • Anxiety • JVD • Hyperresonance to percussion of affected side • Diminished breath sounds on affected side • Subcutaneous emphysema may be seen • Tracheal deviation may be seen, especially with tension pneumothorax

Continued

TABLE 4-3 Differentiation of Chest Pain—cont'd

Cause	Provocation	Palliation	Quality	Region/Radiation	Severity	Timing	Associated Signs/Symptoms
Pleuropulmonary (e.g., pleurisy)	• Respiratory infection • Aspiration	• Narcotics • Relief with sitting up	• Sharp • Worsened by coughing, inspiration, or movement	• Lateral chest • May radiate to shoulder and neck	• Moderate	• Gradual onset • Duration: days to weeks	• Tachypnea • Tachycardia • Dyspnea • Fever • Productive cough • Pleural friction rub
Gastrointestinal chest pain	• Cold liquids • Food intake, especially spicy foods, acidic foods, or foods high in fat • Alcohol • Caffeine • Stress • Smoking • Exercise	• Sitting up • Antacids • Esophageal spasm (may be relieved by nitroglycerin)	• "Heartburn" • Dull, burning • Squeezing • Worsened by eating or supine position	• Retrosternal or lower substernal • Upper abdomen • Midline • May radiate to left arm, neck, jaw, upper abdomen, back, and shoulder	• Mild to moderate	• Gradual or sudden onset • Duration: minutes to days	• Dyspnea • Diaphoresis • Anxiety • Dysphagia • Eructation • Vomiting
Musculoskeletal chest pain	• Neck or arm strain • Movement • Coughing • Deep breathing • CPR	• Rest • Heat • Nonsteroidal anti-inflammatory agents (e.g., aspirin, ibuprofen [Motrin])	• Soreness • Stabbing or sticking sensation • Tenderness • Worsened with inspiration and movement	• Localized to one side of chest	• Mild to moderate	• Gradual or sudden onset • Duration: weeks	• Tachypnea • Splinting respirations • Localized tenderness over site of pain
Psychosomatic chest pain	• Stress • Fatigue	• Rest • Anxiolytics	• Dull ache • Sharp • Stabbing • Superficial	• Precordium • Localized; frequently on left side • No radiation	• Mild to severe	• Gradual or sudden onset • Duration: minutes to days	• Hyperpnea • Dyspnea • Palpitations • Dry mouth • Dizziness • Tingling of hands, mouth • Fatigue • Frequent sighing

BP, Blood pressure; CPR, cardiopulmonary resuscitation; ECG, electrocardiogram; JVD, jugular venous distention; PEEP, positive end-expiratory pressure; P_2, pulmonic component of second sound; RVF, right ventricular failure; S_3, third heart sound; S_4, fourth heart sound.
From Dennison, R. (2007). *Pass CCRN!* (3rd ed.). St. Louis: Mosby.

o. Intermittent claudication: hip, thigh, or calf pain that occurs with exercise and ceases with rest; indicative of peripheral arterial disease

p. Peripheral skin changes: decrease in hair distribution, skin color changes, skin ulcerations that will not heal, or a thin, shiny appearance of the skin; these may indicate peripheral vascular disease

q. Calf tenderness: may be related to thrombophlebitis; may be accompanied by red, warm skin over the associated vein

r. Varicose veins: dilated and sometimes painful veins

3. History of present illness: use PQRST format
   a. Provocation, palliation
   b. Quality, quantity
   c. Region, radiation
   d. Severity
   e. Timing
   f. Associated symptoms

4. Medical history
   a. Past illnesses
      1) Coronary artery disease (CAD)
         a) Angina
         b) MI
      2) Cerebrovascular disease: transient ischemic attacks or cerebral infarction (i.e., stroke)
      3) Dysrhythmias
      4) Hypertension
      5) Hyperlipidemia
      6) Peripheral vascular disease
      7) Rheumatic fever or rheumatic heart disease
      8) Murmur or known valvular heart disease
      9) Pulmonary disease (e.g., asthma, chronic obstructive pulmonary disease [COPD])
      10) Pulmonary embolism
      11) Connective tissue disorders
      12) Endocrine disorders, especially diabetes mellitus
      13) Kidney disease
      14) Anemia
      15) Bleeding disorders
      16) Substance abuse
      17) Trauma
   b. Past surgical procedures
   c. Allergies and types of reactions
   d. Past diagnostic studies (e.g., stress echocardiogram, cardiac catheterization)

5. Family medical history: strong predictor of cardiac disease

6. Social history
   a. Usual activity level and ability to perform activities of daily living
   b. Stress level and usual coping mechanisms
   c. Recreational habits
   d. Exercise habits
   e. Dietary habits
   f. Caffeine intake
   g. Tobacco use: recorded as pack-years (i.e., the number of packs per day × the number of years that the patient has smoked)
   h. Alcohol use: recorded as alcoholic beverages consumed per month, week, or day
   i. Toxin exposure
   j. Travel

7. Medication history
   a. Prescribed drug, dose, frequency, and time of last dose
   b. Nonprescribed drugs
      1) Over-the-counter drugs, including herbal supplements
      2) Substance abuse (e.g., cocaine, amphetamines)
   c. Patient's understanding of drug actions and side effects
   d. Drugs that potentially cause problems for patients with cardiovascular disease
      1) Sinus or cold remedies: may contain ephedrine and increase BP
      2) Over-the-counter weight-reduction agents: may contain ephedrine
      3) Tricyclic antidepressants: may cause dysrhythmias
      4) Phenytoin (Dilantin): may cause dysrhythmias
      5) Phenothiazines: may cause dysrhythmias or hypotension
      6) Oral contraceptives: may predispose patient to embolus or thrombosis
      7) Doxorubicin (Adriamycin): may cause cardiomyopathy
      8) Lithium (Eskalith): may cause dysrhythmias
      9) Corticosteroids: cause sodium and fluid retention and exacerbate HF
      10) Theophylline preparations: cause tachycardia and may cause dysrhythmias
      11) Cardiac stimulants (e.g., cocaine): cause tachycardia and may cause dysrhythmias and coronary artery spasms
      12) Platelet aggregation inhibitors (e.g., aspirin, clopidogrel [Plavix]) or anticoagulants: may cause bleeding
      13) Erectile dysfunction medicines: may cause significant hypotension, especially when taken with nitrates

Inspection and palpation

1. Vital signs
   a. BP: sitting, lying, and standing
      1) Reduction of up to 15 mm Hg in systolic BP and of up to 5 mm Hg in diastolic BP when standing is normal; a greater reduction indicates orthostatic changes
         a) To assess for orthostatic changes, assist the patient to a standing position, wait 2 to 3 minutes, and then repeat the measurement of BP and heart rate
      2) Variation of up to 15 mm Hg between arms is normal
      3) BP in lower extremities is expected to be 10 mm Hg higher than in the upper extremities

4) Pulse pressure
   a) Narrowed pulse pressure frequently indicates vasoconstriction, which occurs with innervation of the SNS (e.g., hypovolemic shock) or with the use of vasopressors
   b) Widened pulse pressure frequently indicates excessive vasodilation, which occurs with excessive vasodilatory mediator release (e.g., septic shock) or with the use of vasodilators
   b. Heart rate: tachycardia frequently indicates the innervation of the SNS
   c. Respiratory (ventilatory) rate: tachypnea frequently indicates the innervation of the SNS
   d. Temperature: fever may indicate inflammatory or infectious process (e.g., MI, pericarditis, endocarditis)
   e. Height
   f. Weight
2. General survey
   a. Apparent health status: consistency of apparent age and chronologic age
   b. Level of consciousness
   c. Gross deformity
   d. Nutritional status
   e. Stature and posture
   f. Gait
3. Skin and appendages
   a. Color
      1) Pallor: may be an indication of anemia, SNS innervation, or the use of sympathomimetic agents (e.g., phenylephrine [Neo-Synephrine], norepinephrine [Levophed], dopamine [Intropin])
      2) Cyanosis
         a) Peripheral (or cold) cyanosis is seen on the fingertips and toes; it is associated with peripheral hypoperfusion or vasoconstriction
         b) Central (or warm) cyanosis is seen on the lips, tongue, and mucous membranes; it is associated with 5 g of deoxygenated hemoglobin
         c) Among dark-skinned patients, cyanosis appears as an ashen color
      3) Ruddiness: may be related to polycythemia or hypercapnia
   b. Moisture: diaphoresis and dryness
   c. Temperature: cold skin may be related to hypoperfusion
   d. Turgor: decrease in skin turgor, also referred to as *tenting,* is related to interstitial dehydration
   e. Edema
      1) Edema indicates an increase in interstitial fluid of 30% above normal
      2) Note the location of the edema
         a) Facial
            i) Allergies: profound facial edema during anaphylaxis
            ii) Steroids: exogenous (e.g., prednisone) or endogenous (e.g., Cushing syndrome)
            iii) Renal disease (e.g., nephrotic syndrome)
         b) Dependent edema: RVF
         c) Generalized edema (anasarca): end-stage HF, end-stage renal failure, and severe hypoproteinemia
      3) Degree of pitting
         a) Grade 1+ = 0 to ¼ inch
         b) Grade 2+ = ¼ to ½ inch
         c) Grade 3+ = ½ to 1 inch
         d) Grade 4+ = >1 inch
   f. Lesions
      1) Arterial disease may cause ulcers at the toes or at points of trauma
      2) Venous disease may cause ulcers at the sides of the ankles
4. Fingertips and nail beds
   a. Color: bluish nail beds with peripheral cyanosis
   b. Clubbing
      1) The loss of the normal angle between the base of the nail and the skin; clubbing is present if the angle is >180 degrees
      2) Indicative of chronic hypoxia
   c. Splinter hemorrhages
      1) Red to black linear streaks under the nail bed that run from the base to the tip of the nail
      2) May indicate bacterial endocarditis
   d. Osler nodes
      1) Painful, red, subcutaneous nodules on the fingertips
      2) May indicate embolization with infective endocarditis
5. Head and neck
   a. Face
      1) Facial expression
      2) Facial flushing: episodic facial flushing may indicate pheochromocytoma (i.e., tumor of the adrenal medulla that produces large amounts of catecholamines)
   b. Head bobbing up and down with each heartbeat
      1) Referred to as *de Musset sign*
      2) Indicates aortic aneurysm or regurgitation
   c. Eyes
      1) Xanthoma palpebrarum (also called *xanthelasma*)
         a) Benign, fatty, fibrous, yellowish plaque, nodule, or tumor on the eyelids
         b) Associated with hyperlipidemia
      2) Exophthalmos: usually associated with hyperthyroidism but may also be seen in patients with advanced HF with pulmonary hypertension
   d. Ears
      1) Diagonal bilateral earlobe creases (referred to as *McCarty sign*): may indicate CAD if seen in individuals <45 years old
   e. Neck
      1) Jugular vein distention (JVD)
         a) To evaluate JVD (Figure 4-14):
            i) Place the patient in a 45-degree angle
            ii) Identify the sternal angle: appears as a raised notch that is created where the

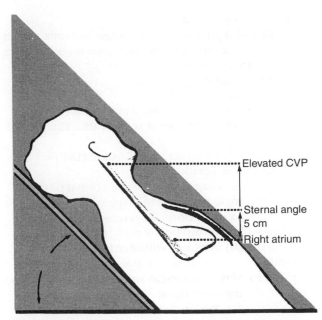

Figure 4-14 Jugular vein distention and an estimation of central venous pressure (CVP). Assess jugular vein distention with the patient at a 45-degree angle. Determine the height of jugular vein distention above the sternal angle. Add 5 cm to this measurement to estimate central venous pressure in centimeters of water pressure. (From Guzzetta, C. E., & Dossey, B. M. [1992]. *Cardiovascular nursing: Holistic practice.* St. Louis: Mosby.)

manubrium and the body of the sternum join; it is also called the *manubriosternal junction* and the *angle of Louis*
   iii) Measure the height of the neck vein distention above the level of the sternal angle
   iv) The normal height of neck vein distention is 1 to 2 cm above the sternal angle
  b) Neck vein distention of >2 cm above the sternal angle is indicative of any of the following:
   i) RVF
   ii) Hypervolemia
   iii) Tension pneumothorax
   iv) Cardiac tamponade

c) To estimate central venous pressure (CVP):
  i) Add 5 cm to the height of neck vein distension
  ii) Normal CVP in centimeters of water: 3 to 8
6. Precordium: inspect and palpate the entire precordium
  a. Point of maximal impulse (PMI) or apical impulse
   1) Frequently visible and usually palpable; may not be palpable in patients with obesity, a muscular chest wall, or an increased anteroposterior diameter
   2) Location: normally at the fifth left intercostal space at the MCL
    a) Displaced to the left in patients with LV hypertrophy
    b) Displaced away from the affected side in patients with tension pneumothorax
   3) Intensity: light tap
    a) HF may cause an increase in the intensity and cause a heave
   4) Size: normal is approximately 1 to 2 cm
    a) The size is more diffuse in patients with ventricular aneurysm
  b. Thrill
   1) Palpable vibration associated with murmur or bruit
   2) Felt where the murmur is heard most loudly or at the location of a bruit
7. Abdomen
  a. Aortic pulsation
   1) Normally visible, especially during expiration
   2) Normally palpable at the midline or slightly to the left of the midline; feel for lateral expansion, which may indicate aneurysm
8. Extremities
  a. Arterial versus venous disease (Table 4-4)
  b. Temperature
   1) Coolness or coldness may indicate decreased blood flow as a result of hypoperfusion or vasoconstriction
   2) Excessive warmth may indicate hyperthyroidism or fever
  c. Peripheral pulses

TABLE 4-4 Comparison of Clinical Indications of Arterial and Venous Peripheral Vascular Disease

	Arterial	Venous
Pain	Excruciating with acute occlusion; intermittent claudication with chronic occlusion	Crampy pain; Homans sign may be present with thrombophlebitis
Pulses	Diminished or absent	Normal but may be difficult to palpate as a result of edema
Color	Pale	Normal or ruddy
Temperature	Cool or cold	Warm
Edema	Absent	Present; may be severe
Skin changes	Thin, shiny, atrophic skin; loss of hair; thickened toenails	Brown pigmentation at ankles
Ulcerations	At toes or points of trauma	At sides of ankles

From Dennison, R. (2007). *Pass CCRN!* (3rd ed.). St. Louis: Mosby.

1) Location (Figure 4-15)
   a) Carotid: palpate only the lower half; never palpate both carotids simultaneously
   b) Brachial
   c) Radial
   d) Ulnar
   e) Femoral
   f) Popliteal
   g) Posterior tibial
   h) Dorsalis pedis
2) Rate and rhythm
3) Amplitude
   a) 0 = not palpable
   b) 1+ = weak and thready, easily obliterated
   c) 2+ = normal, not easily obliterated
   d) 3+ = full and bounding, cannot be obliterated

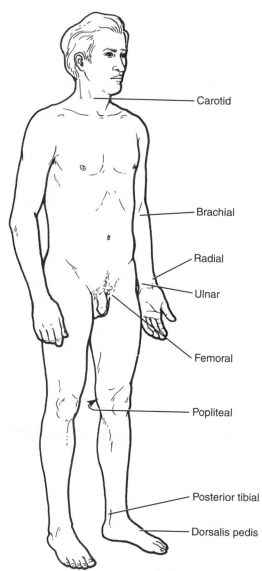

Figure 4-15 The locations of the peripheral pulses. (From Lewis, S. M., Heitkemper, M. M., & Dirksen, S. R. [2007]. *Medical-surgical nursing: Assessment and management of clinical problems* [3rd ed.]. St. Louis: Mosby.)

4) Capillary refill rate
   a) Color should return to blanched area within 3 seconds; delay beyond 3 seconds indicates hypoperfusion
5) Pulse contour
   a) Pulsus alternans
      i) Alternating pulse waves, with every other beat being weaker than the preceding one
      ii) Characteristic of LV failure (LVF)
   b) Pulsus paradoxus
      i) An exaggeration of the normal physiologic response to inspiration
         (a) The normal decrease in BP during inspiration is ≤10 mm Hg
         (b) A drop in BP of ≥10 mm Hg during inspiration is pulsus paradoxus
      ii) May be characteristic of any of the following conditions:
         (a) Pericardial effusion
         (b) Constrictive pericarditis
         (c) Cardiac tamponade
         (d) Severe lung disease
         (e) Advanced HF
         (f) Hemorrhagic shock
d. Homans sign
   1) Identified by dorsiflexion of the foot with the knee slightly bent
   2) Homans sign is present if the patient has pain in the calf with this action
   3) Suggestive of thrombophlebitis, but a negative Homans sign does not rule out the condition
e. Petechiae or ecchymosis
f. Varicose veins
g. Neurovascular assessment
   1) Assess neurovascular status in all of the following situations:
      a) After cardiac catheterization
      b) After percutaneous coronary intervention (PCI) (e.g., angioplasty, atherectomy)
      c) When the patient has a fracture of an extremity (to monitor for compartment syndrome)
      d) When the patient has a circumferential burn of an extremity
   2) Monitor for the clinical indications of acute arterial occlusion: the 6 Ps (Box 4-1)
h. Clinical indications of hypoperfusion: because hypoperfusion is progressive, the earlier that these

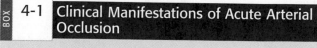

BOX 4-1	**Clinical Manifestations of Acute Arterial Occlusion**

Pain
Pallor
Pulselessness
Paresthesia
Paralysis
Polar (cold)

Adapted from Dennison, R. D. (2007). *Pass CCRN!* (3rd ed.). St. Louis: Mosby.

changes are identified, the more appropriate the management will be and the greater the chances of successfully reversing these changes (Table 4-5)

Auscultation

1. Stethoscope
   a. Earplugs should be snug
   b. Tubing should be no longer than 12 to 15 inches
   c. Chest piece should have both a diaphragm and a bell
      1) Diaphragm
         a) Used for high-pitched sounds (e.g., S_1, S_2, pericardial friction rubs, most murmurs)
         b) Hold firmly against the skin
      2) Bell
         a) Used for low-pitched sounds (e.g., S_3, S_4, murmurs of AV valve stenosis)
         b) Hold tight enough against the skin to create a seal
2. Auscultatory areas (Figure 4-16)
   a. Mitral: Fifth left intercostal space at MCL
   b. Tricuspid: Fifth left intercostal space at left sternal border
   c. Erb's point: Third left intercostal space at left sternal border
   d. Pulmonic: Second left intercostal space at left sternal border
   e. Aortic: Second right intercostal space at right sternal border
3. Heart sounds
   a. S_1
      1) Caused by closure of the AV valves: mitral and tricuspid
      2) Marks the end of diastole and the beginning of systole
      3) Loudest at the apex
      4) Note if the sound is single or split
      5) Note any increase in intensity (e.g., closing snap)
   b. S_2
      1) Caused by closure of the semilunar valves: aortic and pulmonic

2) Marks the end of systole and the beginning of diastole
3) Loudest at the base
4) Note if the sound is single or split
5) Note any increase in intensity
c. Extra heart sounds
   1) S_3
      a) Also called *ventricular gallop*
      b) Dull, low-pitched sound that occurs early during diastole after S_2; may sound like "Ken-tuc-ky" with the "-ky" being the S_3
      c) Caused by a rapid rush of blood into a dilated ventricle; considered abnormal in patients >30 years old
      d) Heard best with bell
         i) Left-sided S_3: heard best at apex
         ii) Right-sided S_3: heard best at sternum
      e) Primarily associated with HF
      f) May also be associated with any of the following:
         i) Fluid overload
         ii) Cardiomyopathy
         iii) Ventricular septal defect or patent ductus arteriosus
         iv) Mitral or tricuspid regurgitation
   2) S_4
      a) Also called *atrial gallop*
      b) Dull, low-pitched sound that occurs late during diastole before S_1; may sound like "Ten-nes-see" with the "Ten-" being the S_4
      c) Caused by the atrial contraction of blood into a noncompliant ventricle; abnormal in adults
      d) Heard best with bell
         i) Left-sided S_4: heard best at apex
         ii) Right-sided S_4: heard best at sternum
      e) Associated with any of the following:
         i) Myocardial ischemia or infarction
         ii) Hypertension
            (a) Systemic: left-sided S_4
            (b) Pulmonary: right-sided S_4
         iii) Ventricular hypertrophy

TABLE 4-5	Clinical Indications of Hypoperfusion		
Normal	**Subclinical Hypoperfusion**	**Clinical Hypoperfusion**	**Shock**
Cardiac index: 2.5–4.0 L/min/m^2	Cardiac index: 2.2–2.5 L/min/m^2	Cardiac index: 2.0–2.2 L/min/m^2	Cardiac index: <2.0 L/min/m^2
• Normal	• No clinical indications of hypoperfusion, although an expert nurse may detect subtle changes in the patient • Hypoperfusion at this stage is detected by invasive hemodynamic monitoring	• Tachycardia • Narrowed pulse pressure • Tachypnea • Cool skin • Oliguria • Diminished bowel sounds • Restlessness leading to confusion	• Dysrhythmias • Hypotension • Tachypnea • Cold, clammy skin • Anuria • Absent bowel sounds • Lethargy leading to coma

From Dennison, R. (2007). *Pass CCRN!* (3rd ed.). St. Louis: Mosby.

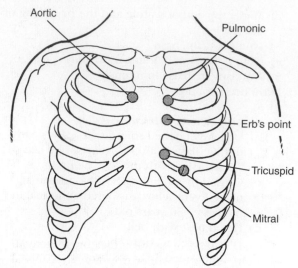

Figure 4-16 Cardiac auscultatory areas. (From Price, S.A., & Wilson, L.M. [1994]. *Pathophysiology: Clinical concepts of disease processes* [4th ed.] St. Louis: Mosby.)

iv) AV blocks

v) Severe aortic or pulmonic stenosis

3) Quadruple rhythm: all four heart sounds heard

4) Summation gallop
   a) All four heart sounds with tachycardia
   b) Merging of S_3 and S_4 causes a louder mid-diastolic sound

5) Pericardial friction rub
   a) High-pitched "to-and-fro" scratchy sound
   b) Heard best at the fourth and fifth intercostal spaces at the lower left sternal blocker with the patient leaning forward
   c) To differentiate between pericardial and pleural friction rubs, ask the patient to hold his or her breath; if the rub persists, it is a pericardial friction rub
   d) Caused by inflammation of the pericardium; commonly heard after MI or cardiac surgery

d. Murmurs

1) Causes of turbulence (referred to as *murmurs* if intracardiac or as *bruits* if extracardiac) (Figure 4-17)
   a) Increased flow across a normal valve (e.g., flow murmur)
      i) May also be called *functional* (as opposed to *structural*); always soft (i.e., not louder than grade II of VI) and systolic (but never holosystolic)
      ii) Caused by any of the following:
         (a) Hyperthermia
         (b) Anemia
         (c) Pregnancy
         (d) Hyperthyroidism
   b) Forward flow through a stenotic valve
   c) Backward flow through a regurgitant (also called *insufficient* or *incompetent*) valve

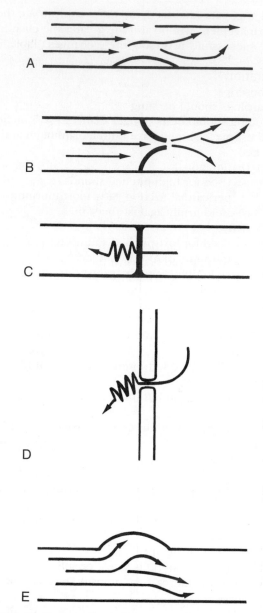

Figure 4-17 Causes of turbulence. **A,** Increased flow across a normal valve. **B,** Forward flow through a stenotic valve. **C,** Backward flow through an incompetent valve. **D,** Flow through a septal defect or an atrioventricular fistula. **E,** Flow into a dilated chamber or a portion of a vessel. (From Thompson, D.A. [1981]. *Cardiovascular assessment.* St. Louis: Mosby.)

   d) Flow through an AV fistula or septal defect
   e) Flow into a dilated chamber or a portion of a vessel

2) Description
   a) Timing: systolic or diastolic
   b) Location: place at which the murmur is loudest
   c) Radiation: direction in which the murmur radiates
   d) Intensity: Levine scale
      i) Grade I of VI: barely audible, difficult to detect
      ii) Grade II of VI: clearly audible but quiet

iii) Grade III of VI: moderately loud, without a thrill
iv) Grade IV of VI: loud, with or without a thrill
v) Grade V of VI: very loud, thrill present, audible with stethoscope partially off of the chest
vi) Grade VI of VI: loudest possible, thrill present, audible with stethoscope off of the chest
e) Configuration
  i) Crescendo: gets louder
  ii) Decrescendo: gets softer
  iii) Crescendo-decrescendo: louder and then softer
  iv) Plateau: even intensity throughout
f) Pitch
  i) High pitched (heard best with diaphragm)
  ii) Low pitched (heard best with bell)
g) Quality: soft, harsh, blowing, musical, rumbling, or rough
4. Vascular sound
  a. Bruit
    1) Turbulent sound
    2) May be heard over carotids, aorta, renals, iliacs, or femorals
    3) Associated with plaque or aneurysm
  b. Doppler pulse
    1) A Doppler stethoscope is used to identify the presence of pulse if the pulse is not palpable; may be used to confirm that the pulse that is being palpated is the patient's and not the nurse's

Diagnostic studies
1. Serum chemistries
  a. Sodium: normal, 136 to 145 mEq/L
  b. Potassium: normal, 3.5 to 5.0 mEq/L
  c. Chloride: normal, 95 to 103 mEq/L
  d. Calcium: normal, 9.0 to 10.5 mg/dl in adults and 8.8 to 10.8 mg/dl in children
  e. Ionized calcium: normal, 4.5 to 5.6 mg/dl in adults and 4.8 to 5.52 mg/dl in children
  f. Phosphorus: normal, 3.0 to 4.5 mg/dl
  g. Magnesium: normal, 1.3 to 2.1 mEq/L in adults, 1.4 to 1.7 mEq/L in children, and 1.4 to 2 mEq/L in infants
  h. Glucose: normal, 65 to 110 mEq/L
  i. Blood urea nitrogen (BUN): normal, 8 to 23 mg/dl
  j. Creatine: normal, 0.6 to 1.1 mg/dl in women and 0.8 to 1.3 mg/dl in men
  k. Enzymes
    1) Total creatine kinase: normal, 55 to 170 U/L in men and 30 to 135 U/L in women
    2) Creatine kinase, myocardial bound: 0% of total creatine kinase
    3) L-lactate dehydrogenase: 90 to 200 U/L
    4) L-lactate dehydrogenase-1: 17% to 25% of total L-lactate dehydrogenase
  l. Muscle proteins (Dennison, 2007)
    1) Myoglobin: normal, <110 ng/ml
    2) Troponin I: normal, 1.5 g/ml
    3) Troponin T: normal, 0.1 g/ml

m. Lipid profile
  1) Cholesterol: normal, 150 to 200 mg/dl
  2) Triglycerides: normal, 40 to 150 mg/dl
  3) Lipoprotein-cholesterol fractionation
    a) High-density lipoprotein: normal, 29 to 77 mg/dl
    b) Low-density lipoprotein: normal, 62 to 130 mg/dl
n. Homocysteine: normal, <15 μmol/L
o. C-reactive protein: normal, <1 mg/dl
p. Brain-type natriuretic peptide: normal, <100 pg/ml
  1) HF
    a) Mild: 100 to 300 pg/ml
    b) Moderate: 300 to 700 pg/ml
    c) Severe: >700 pg/ml
  2) May also be an earlier indicator of acute MI than either CK-MB or troponin I
2. Arterial blood gases (ABGs)
  a. pH: normal, 7.35 to 7.45
  b. $PaCO_2$: normal, 35 to 45 mm Hg
  c. HCO_3: normal, 22 to 26 mM
  d. PaO_2: normal, 80 to 100 mm Hg
  e. SaO_2: >95% (in elderly, >92%)
  f. Arterial lactate: <1 mmol/L
3. Hematology
  a. Hematocrit: normal, 42% to 52% for men and 37% to 47% for women
  b. Hemoglobin: normal, 14 to 18 g/dl for men and 12 to 16 g/dl for females
  c. White blood cells (WBCs): normal, 5800 to 10,800 mm³
  d. Erythrocyte sedimentation rate: normal, ≤15 mm/hour for men and ≤20 mm/hour for women
4. Clotting profile
  a. Prothrombin time: normal 12 to 15 seconds; therapeutic 1.5 to 2.5 times normal
  b. Partial thromboplastin time: normal, 60 to 90 seconds; therapeutic, 1.5 to 2.5 times normal
  c. Activated partial thromboplastin time: normal, 25 to 38 seconds; therapeutic, 1.5 to 2.5 times normal
  d. Activated clotting time: normal, 70 to 120 seconds; therapeutic, 150 to 190 seconds
  e. Thrombin time: normal, 10 to 15 seconds
  f. Bleeding time: normal, 1 to 9.5 minutes
  g. International normalized ratio: normal, <2.0
  h. Platelets: normal, 150,000 to 400,000/mm³
5. Urine
  a. Glucose: normal negative
  b. Ketones: normal negative
  c. Specific gravity: 1.005 to 1.030
  d. Osmolality: normal, 50 to 1200 mOsm/L
6. Other diagnostic studies (Table 4-6)

Hemodynamic Monitoring
General information about hemodynamic monitoring
1. Definition: the monitoring of blood flow, generally with the use of invasive catheters
2. Uses: although invasive monitoring of hemodynamic parameters is not commonplace in most emergency

TABLE 4-6 Cardiovascular Diagnostic Studies

Study	What the Study Evaluates	Comments
Cardiac catheterization and coronary angiography	• Severity of coronary artery stenosis • Cardiac muscle function • Pressures within the heart • Cardiac output and ejection fraction • Blood gas analysis within the heart chambers • Allows for angioplasty, atherectomy, intracoronary stents, or lasers to reduce coronary artery obstruction	• Before test: • Check for allergy to iodine, shellfish, or dye (contrast medium used) • After the test: • Ensure hydration (contrast medium used) • Keep extremity in which catheter was placed immobilized in a straight position for 6–12 hours • Monitor the arterial puncture point for hemorrhage or hematoma • Monitor the neurovascular status of the affected limb • Note complaints of back pain and vital sign changes (may indicate retroperitoneal hemorrhage)
Chest radiography	• Cardiac size and shape • Presence of pulmonary congestion or pleural effusions • Presence of thoracic aneurysm or calcification of the aorta • Position of pulmonary artery and cardiac catheter, pacemaker, and wires	• Inquire about the possibility of pregnancy
Computed tomography	• Left ventricular wall motion • Cardiac tumors • Myocardial infarction • Pericardial effusion • Aortic aneurysm • Aortic dissection	• May be performed with or without contrast medium • If contrast medium is used, check for allergy to iodine, shellfish, or dye; ensure hydration after the procedure
Doppler ultrasonography or duplex ultrasonography	• Vascular disease and degree of occlusion	
Echocardiography • M-mode: single ultrasound beam • Two-dimensional: planar ultrasound beam; wider view of heart and structures • Doppler: addition of Doppler to demonstrate the flow of blood through the heart • Color flow: Doppler blood flow superimposed on a two-dimensional echocardiogram • Stress echocardiography: images before, during, and after exercise or pharmacologic stress • Transesophageal echocardiography: a transducer is placed in the esophagus	• Chamber size and wall thickness • Valve functioning • Papillary muscle functioning • Prosthetic valve functioning • Ventricular wall motion abnormalities • Intracardiac masses • Presence of pericardial fluid • Intracardiac pressures (Doppler) • Ejection fraction and cardiac output (Doppler) • Valve gradients (Doppler) • Intracardiac shunts (Doppler) • Thoracic aneurysm (transesophageal)	• Transesophageal echocardiography is better, particularly if the patient is obese or if the patient has chronic obstructive pulmonary disease, chest wall deformities, chest trauma, or thick chest dressings

TABLE 4-6   Cardiovascular Diagnostic Studies—cont'd

Study	What the Study Evaluates	Comments
Electrocardiography	• Dysrhythmias • Conduction defects, including intraventricular blocks • Electrolyte imbalances • Drug toxicity • Myocardial ischemia, injury, or infarction • Chamber hypertrophy	• List what drugs the patient is receiving on electrocardiography request • Be aware of electrical safety hazards
Electrophysiologic studies	• Dysrhythmias under controlled circumstances • Best therapy for the control of dysrhythmia: drug, required dosage of drug therapy; pacemaker; catheter ablation	• Patients may have near-death experiences during electrophysiologic studies; encourage the expression of fears, concerns, and anxieties • Monitor the puncture site
Holter monitor	• Suspected dysrhythmias over a 24-hour period • Pacemaker function • Silent ischemia	• Instruct the patient regarding the importance of keeping a diary
Magnetic resonance imaging	• Three-dimensional view of the heart • Anatomy and structure of the heart and great vessels, including cardiomyopathy, congenital defects, masses, and aneurysms • Changes in the chemistry of tissues before structural changes occur	• Does not involve radiation or dyes • Cannot be used for patients with any implanted metallic devices, including pacemakers, implantable defibrillators, metallic heart valves, or intracranial aneurysm clips
Signal-averaged electrocardiography	• The presence of late electrical potentials, which may be responsible for malignant ventricular dysrhythmias; may be performed before and after ablation	• The patient must lie still for 10 minutes
Stress electrocardiography	• Persons with a high risk for or who are known to have coronary artery disease or postsurgical patients for ischemia with exercise or pharmacologic agents (e.g., adensoine [Adenocard], dipyridamole [Persantine], dobutamine [Dobutrex]) • Exercise-induced dysrhythmias	• ≥1 mm of transient ST segment depression 80 msec after the J point is suggestive of coronary artery disease • Monitor closely for exercise-induced hypotension or ventricular dysrhythmias
Thallium stress electrocardiography	• Myocardial ischemia during exercise; ischemic areas show a decreased uptake of radioactivity (i.e., cold spots)	• Assure that patient that the amount of radioactive material is minimal

Adapted from Dennison, R. D., (2007). *Pass CCRN!* (3rd ed.). St. Louis: Mosby.

departments, it does occur in many Level 1 trauma centers; questions about hemodynamic monitoring may be seen on the CEN and CFRN examinations

a. Measure hemodynamic parameter pressures and record waveforms
   1) Arterial catheter: systemic arterial BP, including systolic, diastolic, and mean (Figure 4-18)
   2) CVP catheter: CVP measured as a mean (Figure 4-19)
   3) PA catheter
      a) Right atrial pressure (RAP) measured as a mean (Figure 4-20)
      b) PA pressure (PAP) measured as systolic, diastolic, and mean (Figure 4-21)
      c) Pulmonary artery occlusive pressure (PAOP) measured as a mean as an indirect reflection of left atrial pressure (Figure 4-22)
      d) Cardiac output (CO) measured by thermodilution technique
   b. Obtain blood samples from invasive monitoring lines
   c. Provide central venous access for the administration of fluids or drugs
      1) Central venous catheter: usually a triple-lumen catheter
      2) PA catheter
         a) Right atrial (proximal) port

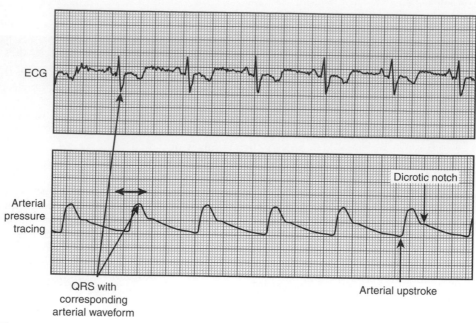

Figure 4-18 Simultaneous electrocardiogram (ECG) and normal arterial pressure tracing. (Modified from Urden, L. D., Stacy, K. M., & Lough, M. E. [2010]. *Critical care nursing: diagnosis and management,* 6th ed. St. Louis: Mosby.

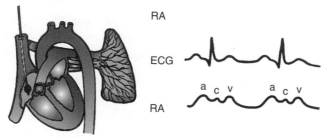

Figure 4-19 Identifying the *a, c,* and *v* waveforms to determine right atrial pressure. (From Urden, L. D., Stacy, K. M., & Lough, M. E. [2010]. *Critical care nursing: diagnosis and management,* 6th ed. St. Louis: Mosby, p. 329.

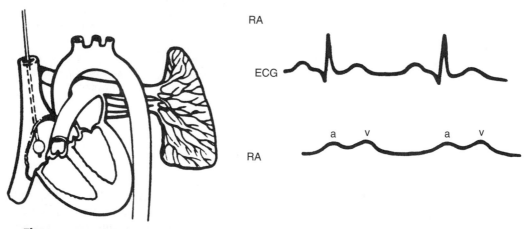

Figure 4-20 Right atrial waveform. (From Sole, M. L., Klein, D. G., & Moseley, M. J. [2009]. *Introduction to critical care nursing,* 5th ed. Philadelphia: W.B. Saunders.)

b) PA (distal) port: heparinized flush solution only to ensure patency; this is not to be used for fluid or drug administration
d. Specialized PA catheters can perform intracardiac pacing, measure SvO_2, measure continuous cardiac output (CCO)

3. Common indications for hemodynamic monitoring:
   a. Shock of any cause
   b. MI, especially with the following:
     1) Acute LVF or RVF
     2) Refractory pain
   c. Acute RVF (e.g., after pulmonary embolism)

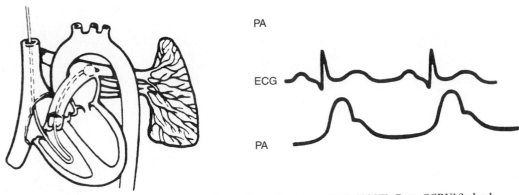

Figure 4-21 Pulmonary artery waveform. (From Dennison, R. D. [2007]. *Pass CCRN!* 3rd ed. St. Louis: Mosby.)

d. Cardiac tamponade
e. The need for the evaluation of fluid status and guided fluid resuscitation (e.g., burns, multiple traumas, complex surgical procedures [especially in patients with preexisting cardiopulmonary disease])
4. Components of a pressure monitoring system (Figure 4-23)
   a. Pascal's law: a change in the pressure of an enclosed incompressible fluid is conveyed undiminished to every part of the fluid and to the surfaces of its container
      1) In essence, this law means that the pressure in a fluid-filled tube (e.g., a pressure monitoring system) will be equal at either end of the tube
   b. Types of monitoring systems
      1) Manometer
         a) Used to measure pressure
         b) Fluid-filled systems attached to water manometers that rise and fall as pressure equalizes within the system
         c) Measured in centimeters of water (cm H_2O)
      2) Fluid system with transducer: intravascular pressure is carried to the transducer by a catheter inserted into the cardiovascular circuit and fluid-filled tubing

a) Transducer: converts the mechanical signal to an electrical signal
b) Monitor
   i) Amplifier: a device that increases the magnitude of the electrical signal and that filters out electrical interference
      (a) Pressure is plotted on the vertical axis
      (b) Time is plotted on the horizontal axis
   ii) Oscilloscope: a device that displays the resultant signal as a pressure waveform and as a numeric value on a meter or a digital display
   iii) Recorder: a device that records the pressure waveform on paper for analysis
3) Fiber-optic monitoring
   a) Used primarily with intracranial pressure monitoring

Hemodynamic parameters (Table 4-7)
1. Arterial and ventricular pressures measured as systolic/diastolic and atrial pressures measured as a mean
2. Systemic arterial BP
   a. Pressure in a systemic artery; reflects systemic arterial BP; changes in BP are the result of either a change in cardiac output or systemic vascular resistance

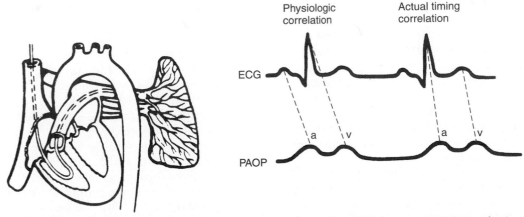

Figure 4-22 Pulmonary artery occlusive pressure waveform. Though the *a* wave correlates physiologically to atrial depolarization and the P wave and the *v* wave correlate physiologically with the QRS complex and ventricular depolarization, tubing and catheter cause a time delay. In actuality, the first wave seen after the QRS complex is the *a* wave, and the first wave seen after the T wave is the *v* wave. (Reproduced with permission of Edwards Lifesciences, Irvine, CA.)

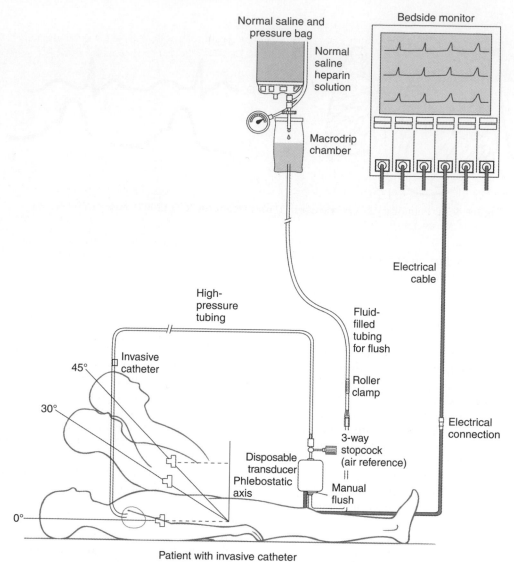

Figure 4-23 Components of a pressure-monitoring system. (From Urden, L. D., Stacy, K. M., & Lough, M. E. [2010]. *Critical care nursing: diagnosis and management* [6th ed.]. St. Louis: Mosby, p. 324.

b. Systolic arterial pressure: maximal pressure with which the blood is ejected from the left ventricle

c. Diastolic arterial pressure: reflects the rapidity of flow of the ejected blood through the arterial system and the vessel's elasticity

1) Diastolic pressure is expected to be higher (and pulse pressure to be narrowed) if there is endogenous catecholamine release or if the patient is receiving sympathomimetic agents (e.g., epinephrine, dopamine [Intropin], norepinephrine [Levophed])

2) Diastolic pressure is expected to be lower (and pulse pressure to be widened) if there are excessive vasodilatory mediators (e.g., septic shock, anaphylactic shock) or if the patient is taking vasodilators

d. Mean arterial pressure (MAP): the average pressure that occurs in the aorta and its major branches during the cardiac cycle; a mean arterial pressure of ≥60 mm Hg is necessary to perfuse the vital organs

1) Formula: (BP systolic + [BP diastolic × 2]) ÷ 3

e. Normal adult pressure values

1) Systolic: 100 to 130 mm Hg

2) Diastolic: 60 to 90 mm Hg

3) Mean: 70 to 105 mm Hg

f. Causes of abnormal pressures (see Table 4-7)

3. Right atrial pressure (RAP)

a. Pressure in the vena cava and the right atrium is reflective of RV end-diastolic pressure

b. Measured through a catheter in the superior vena cava (CVP) or at the proximal port of the PA catheter (RAP)

1) Although these parameters (CVP and RAP) are not the actually the same, they are the same in practicality and are frequently used interchangeably

TABLE **4-7** Causes of Abnormal Hemodynamic Pressures

Parameter	Increased	Decreased
Systemic arterial blood pressure Normal values: • Systolic: 90-140 mm Hg • Diastolic: 60-90 mm Hg • Mean: 70-105 mm Hg	• Increase in systemic vascular resistance (e.g., hypertension, sympathetic nervous system innervation) • Increase in cardiac output (e.g., hyperthyroidism)	• Decrease in systemic vascular resistance (e.g., sepsis, anaphylaxis) • Decrease in cardiac output (e.g., myocardial infarction, tachydysrhythmias)
Right atrial pressure Normal values: • 2-6 mm Hg mean • 3-8 cm H_2O	• Hypervolemia • Tricuspid valve dysfunction: stenosis or regurgitation • Right ventricular failure or infarction • Ventricular septal defect with left-to-right shunt • Pulmonic stenosis • Pulmonary hypertension • Active: hypoxemic pulmonary vasoconstriction (PaO_2 <60 mm Hg) • Pulmonary embolism • Chronic obstructive pulmonary disease • Acute respiratory distress syndrome • Passive: mitral valve dysfunction (stenosis or regurgitation) • Positive pressure ventilation • Constrictive pericarditis • Cardiac tamponade • Mitral valve dysfunction: stenosis or regurgitation • Chronic left ventricular failure (right atrial pressure would be a late indication of left ventricular failure)	• Hypovolemia • Vasodilation • Venous vasodilators (e.g., nitroglycerin, morphine) • Endogenous systemic vasodilation (e.g., septic shock, anaphylactic shock, neurogenic shock)
Pulmonary artery pressure Normal values: • Systolic: 15-30 mm Hg • Diastolic: 5-15 mm Hg • Mean: 10-20 mm Hg	• Hypervolemia • Ventricular septal defect with left-to-right shunt • Pulmonary hypertension • Positive pressure ventilation • Mitral valve dysfunction: stenosis or regurgitation • Constrictive pericarditis • Cardiac tamponade • Left ventricular failure	• Hypovolemia • Excessive vasodilation (e.g., vasodilators, septic shock, anaphylactic shock, neurogenic shock)
Pulmonary artery occlusive pressure Normal values: • 8-12 mm Hg	• Positive pressure ventilation, especially with positive end-expiratory pressure • Hypervolemia • Mitral valve dysfunction: stenosis or regurgitation • Constrictive pericarditis • Cardiac tamponade • Left ventricular failure • Severe aortic stenosis	• Hypovolemia • Excessive vasodilation (e.g., vasodilators, septic shock, anaphylactic shock, neurogenic shock)
Cardiac output and cardiac index Normal values: • Cardiac output: 4-8 L/min • Cardiac index: 2.5-4 L/min	• Sympathetic nervous system innervation (endogenous catecholamines) (e.g., stress, exercise) • Exogenous catecholamines (e.g., epinephrine, isoproterenol [Isuprel], dobutamine [Dobutrex], dopamine [Intropin]) • Other positive inotropes (e.g., digitalis [digoxin {Lanoxin}], amrinone [Inocor]) • Infection or early sepsis • Hyperthyroidism • Anemia	• Decreased contractility (e.g., myocardial infarction, cardiomyopathy, β-blockers) • Increased afterload (e.g., systemic or pulmonary hypertension, aortic or pulmonic stenosis, polycythemia) • Alteration in preload: excessively increased (e.g., hypervolemia, heart failure) or decreased (e.g., hypovolemia, cardiac tamponade, mitral or tricuspid valve disease) • Significantly increased or decreased heart rate (e.g., bradydysrhythmias, tachydysrhythmias)

Adapted from Dennison, R. (2007). *Pass CCRN!* (3rd ed.). St. Louis: Mosby.

continued

TABLE **4-7** Causes of Abnormal Hemodynamic Pressures—cont'd

Parameter	Increased	Decreased
SvO_2 and $ScvO_2$ Normal values: • SvO_2: 60%–80% • $ScvO_2$: 70%–80%	• Increased oxygen supply and delivery • Increased SaO_2 • Increase in cardiac output or cardiac index • Increased hemoglobin • Decreased oxygen demand (e.g., anesthesia, analgesia, muscle paralysis, sedation, hypothermia, sleep) • Decreased oxygen extraction at tissue level • Early sepsis • Cyanide toxicity • Shift of oxyhemoglobin dissociation curve to the left (e.g., alkalosis, hypothermia, decreased levels of 2,3-diphosphoglycerate) • Ventricular septal defect with left-to-right intracardiac shunt (e.g., ventricular septal defect or rupture) • Technical problems • Pulmonary artery catheter in occluded position • Deposits of fibrin on the tip of the catheter	• Decreased oxygen supply and delivery • Decrease in SaO_2 (e.g., decreased FIO_2, continuous positive airway pressure, or positive end-expiratory pressure; suctioning; acute respiratory failure; pulmonary edema) • Decrease in cardiac output or cardiac index (e.g., shock, heart failure, hypovolemia, dysrhythmias, excessive continuous positive airway pressure or positive end-expiratory pressure, negative inotropes, excessive afterload) • Decrease in hemoglobin (e.g., anemia, hemorrhage) or abnormal hemoglobin (e.g., methemoglobinemia, sickle cell anemia) • Increased metabolic needs (e.g., seizures, shivering, restlessness, pain, hyperthermia, increased work of breathing, increased metabolic rate, exertion [e.g., turning, bathing, active range of motion]) • Shift of oxyhemoglobin dissociation curve to the right (e.g., acidosis, hyperthermia)

2) CVP may be measured by a water manometer in cm H_2O pressure or by a transducer in mm Hg pressure
3) RAP from the proximal port of the PA catheter is generally measured by a transducer in mm Hg
   c. Normal pressure value: a mean of 0 to 8 mm Hg (or 3 to 11 cm H_2O)
   d. Trends provide a more reliable measure of a patient's condition than a single value
4. PA pressure (PAP)
   a. Pressure in the PA with the balloon deflated
   b. Measured from the distal tip of the PA catheter with the balloon **deflated**
      1) PA systolic pressure: pressure in the PA during RV systole
      2) PA end-diastolic pressure: pressure in the PA at the end of RV diastole; reflects left atrial pressure in the absence of pulmonary disease
   c. Normal PAP values
      1) Systolic: 15 to 25 mm Hg
      2) Diastolic: 6 to 12 mm Hg

5. Pulmonary artery occlusive pressure (PAOP) (also referred to as *pulmonary capillary wedge pressure* and *PA wedge pressure*)
   a. Pressure in the PA with the balloon **inflated**; reflects pressure from the left atrium in the absence of pulmonary hypertension
   b. Measured from the distal tip of the PA catheter with the balloon inflated; the balloon blocks right heart pressures from the distal tip; left atrial pressure reflects LV end-diastolic pressure and LV preload in the absence of mitral valve disease or left atrial tumor
   c. Normal pressure value: a mean of 4 to 12 mm Hg
6. Mixed venous oxygen saturation (SvO_2)
   a. The oxygen saturation of the blood as it returns to the lung for reoxygenation
      1) Represents the average of the venous oxygen saturations of all organs and tissues
      2) Provides a global perspective of how well the body's demand for oxygen is met by the amount of oxygen supplied
   b. Normal SvO_2: 60% to 80%

7. Central venous oxygen saturation ($ScvO_2$)
   a. The oxygen saturation of the blood in the superior vena cava
      1) Serves as a surrogate for SvO_2 before PA catheterization is performed or when PA catheter placement is not possible (e.g., when admission to a critical care unit is not possible or not yet necessary)
      2) Although the $ScvO_2$ consistently overestimates the SvO_2 (by around 5% to 15%) under shock conditions, there is a close correlation between the two parameters
   b. Measurement
      1) Blood gas analysis of blood drawn from a catheter in the superior vena cava or the right atrium
      2) Fiber-optic oximetric central venous catheter with the tip in the superior vena cava or the right atrium
   c. Normal $ScvO_2$: >70%
      1) Affected by changes in oxygen delivery and/or oxygen consumption
   d. Causes of abnormal parameter as for SvO_2

Measurement, interpretation, and safe use of hemodynamic monitoring for clinical decision making

1. Maximize accuracy, reproducibility, and reliability of measured parameters
   a. The transducer must be leveled and balanced to 0 (i.e., *zeroed*) with each position change of the head of the bed and at least every 12 hours
      1) Level the air-fluid interface of the transducer to the phlebostatic axis at the time of setup, any time that the head of the bed is changed, any time that the transducer and monitoring cable are disconnected, or any time that the accuracy of the pressure readings is questionable
         a) The air-fluid interface (also referred to as the *air reference port*) of the transducer needs to be leveled with the phlebostatic axis to ensure accuracy of measurement; the phlebostatic axis correlates with the right atrium and is at the fourth intercostal space midway between the sternum anterior and the spine posterior
            i) If the transducer is too high, the readings will be too low
            ii) If the transducer is too low, the readings will be too high
         b) Although the patient should be supine, there is no need to put the head of bed flat to take pressure measurements as long as the head of bed is elevated no more than 60 degrees and the air-fluid interface is level with the phlebostatic axis
      2) Balance to 0 at the time of setup, any time that the head of bed is changed, any time that the transducer and monitoring cable are disconnected, or any time that the accuracy of the pressure readings is questionable

   b. Obtain chest radiographs after the insertion of a CVP or PA catheter to ensure the proper positioning of the catheter
   c. Analyze the graphic recording with simultaneous electrocardiography as the most reliable means of measuring hemodynamic pressure at the end of expiration (Figure 4-24)
      1) Pressure readings obtained at the end of expiration minimize the effects of intrathoracic pressure changes because the intrathoracic pressure is closest to atmospheric pressure at the end of expiration
         a) Spontaneously breathing patient: expiration is positive (high point of fluctuation)
         b) Mechanically ventilated patient: expiration is neutral (low point of fluctuation)
         c) Remember: ventilator valley, patient peak
2. Ensure the patency of the catheter by maintaining a flush system
   a. Intermittent flush devices deliver 1 to 5 ml/hour as long as the pressure bag is maintained at 300 mm Hg
   b. Heparin may be used; the usual heparin concentration is 0.5 to 1 unit of heparin/1 ml of flush solution
      1) Heparin is contraindicated in patients with a history of heparin-induced thrombosis and thrombocytopenia (HITT)

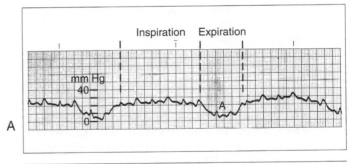

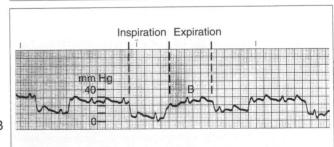

Figure 4-24 Hemodynamic measurements are performed at the end of expiration. **A,** When a patient is receiving positive pressure mechanical ventilation, inspiration is positive and expiration is neutral. Readings should be performed at the valley. Remember: "ventilation, valley." **B,** When a patient is breathing spontaneously, inspiration is negative and expiration is positive. Readings should be performed at the peak. Remember: "patient, peak." (From Schermer, I. [1998]. Physiologic and technical variables affecting hemodynamic measurements. *Critical Care Nurse*, 8[2], 33–40.)

3. Correlate the numeric value of the parameter with the patient's clinical presentation
   a. Hemodynamic parameter changes may precede clinical presentation changes (e.g., subclinical hypoperfusion)
   b. Hemodynamic parameter changes may reflect inaccurate measurements; care must be taken to be consistent among measuring techniques
   c. Note trends of changes in measured parameters over time and in response to therapeutic interventions
   d. Notify the physician of significant changes from the patient's normal values
   e. Use the patient's clinical presentation and hemodynamic parameters to detect physiologic alterations and responses to therapy (Table 4-8)
4. Prevent, detect, and assist with the management of complications of hemodynamic monitoring (Table 4-9)

Electrocardiography
General information
1. The electrocardiograph measures and records the electrical activity of the heart by measuring electrical potential at the skin surface; the electrocardiogram (ECG) is a recording of that activity
2. An ECG is used to detect or demonstrate any of the following:
   a. Rhythm disturbances
   b. Conduction defects
   c. Electrolyte imbalances
   d. Drug effects and toxicity
   e. Chamber enlargement or hypertrophy
   f. Myocardial ischemia, injury, or infarction
3. Electrocardiography paper (Figure 4-25)
   a. Horizontal axis measures time
      1) Each small (1 mm) box is equal to 0.04 second
      2) Each large (5 mm) box is equal to 0.20 second
      3) Small marks at the top of the paper identify 3-second intervals

Rhythm strip analysis
1. Monitoring electrode placement (Figure 4-26)
   a. Lead II: positive at apex; negative under right clavicle; ground usually placed under left clavicle
      1) Advantages
         a) Upright P and QRS waves
         b) Normal appearance
      2) Disadvantage: ectopy and aberrancy look alike
   b. MCL$_1$: positive at fourth intercostal space at RSB; negative under left clavicle; ground usually placed under right clavicle
      1) Advantages
         a) Better differentiation of ectopy from aberrancy
         b) Differentiation of left bundle branch block from right bundle branch block
         c) Differentiation of LV ectopy from RV ectopy

      2) Disadvantages
         a) Diphasic P wave
         b) Negative QRS
   c. MCL$_6$: positive at fifth intercostal space at left midaxillary line has some advantages; may also be used in differentiation of ectopy from aberrancy
2. Components of a single cardiac cycle (Figure 4-27)
   a. P wave
      1) Represents atrial depolarization
      2) First deflection from the isoelectric line
      3) Normal P wave: no more than 2.5 mm tall and no more than 0.11 seconds wide
   b. PR segment
      1) Represents the delay in the AV node
      2) Isoelectric line between the P wave and the QRS complex
   c. PR interval
      1) Represents atrial depolarization and delay in the AV node
      2) Measured from the beginning of the P wave to the beginning of the QRS complex
      3) Normal PR interval: 0.12 to 0.20 second
   d. Q wave: the first negative wave after the P wave but before the R wave
   e. R wave: the first positive wave after the P wave
   f. S wave: the negative wave after the R wave
   g. QRS complex
      1) Represents ventricular depolarization
      2) May have one, two, or all three: Q, R, and S
      3) Measured from the beginning of the first wave of the complex to the end of last wave of the complex
      4) Normal QRS interval: 0.06 to 0.11 second
      5) Normal QRS amplitude: <30 mm in chest leads
   h. ST segment
      1) Represents the time during which the ventricles have completely depolarized and the beginning of repolarization
      2) Located between the QRS complex and the beginning of the T wave
      3) Normally isoelectric at baseline
   i. J point
      1) The angle at which the QRS complex ends and the ST segment begins
      2) The J point deviates from the isoelectric line if the ST segment is elevated or depressed
   j. T wave
      1) Represents ventricular repolarization
      2) Wave after the QRS; may be positive or negative
      3) Normal T wave: <5 mm in limb leads and <10 mm in chest lead
   k. U wave
      1) May represent repolarization of the Purkinje fibers
      2) Small wave after the T wave; often not seen because of its low voltage
      3) Normal U wave: ≤1 mm

TABLE **4-8** Hemodynamic Profiles for Selected Critical Conditions

Condition	Clinical Presentation	Hemodynamic Presentation
Cardiogenic shock	• Tachycardia, hypotension, and tachypnea • S_3 • Crackles • Dyspnea • JVD • Hepatomegaly • Peripheral edema • Oliguria	• CVP, PAP, and PAOP elevated • CO and CI decreased • SaO_2, SvO_2, and $ScvO_2$ decreased
Hypovolemic shock	• Flat neck veins • Tachycardia, hypotension, and tachypnea • Oliguria	• CVP, PAP, and PAOP decreased • CO and CI decreased • SvO_2 and $ScvO_2$ decreased
Anaphylactic shock	• Hypotension and tachypnea • Tachycardia • Angioedema • Warmth, erythema, pruritus, and hives • Wheezing and stridor	• CVP, PAP, and PAOP decreased • CO and CI decreased • SvO_2 and $ScvO_2$ decreased
Neurogenic shock	• Hypotension and tachypnea • Bradycardia • Warm, dry, flushed skin • Hypothermia • Neurologic deficit	• CVP, PAP, and PAOP decreased • CO and CI decreased • SvO_2 and $ScvO_2$ decreased
Septic shock (early and late [e.g., hypovolemic shock])	• Tachycardia, hypotension, and tachypnea • Hyperthermia • Irritability and confusion • Warm, moist, flushed skin	• CVP, PAP, and PAOP decreased • CO and CI increased • SvO_2 and $ScvO_2$ increased as a result of decreased oxygen extraction at the tissues
Pulmonary hypertension (e.g., chronic obstructive pulmonary disease, pulmonary embolism, mitral valve disease, hypoxemia)	• Tachycardia • JVD may occur • Dyspnea	• CVP may be elevated • PAP elevated • SaO_2, SvO_2, and $ScvO_2$ decreased
Cardiac pulmonary edema	• Tachycardia • Dyspnea • Crackles • S_3	• CVP, PAP, and PAOP elevated • SaO_2, SvO_2, and $ScvO_2$ decreased
Noncardiac pulmonary edema (e.g., acute respiratory distress syndrome)	• Dyspnea • Crackles • Evidence of decreased lung compliance (e.g., increased work of breathing if patient is spontaneously breathing, increased peak and plateau pressures if patient is being mechanically ventilated)	• PAP elevated • PAOP normal • SaO_2, SvO_2, and $ScvO_2$ decreased
Cardiac tamponade	• Feeling of fullness in the chest • Tachycardia, hypotension, and tachypnea • Muffled heart sounds • JVD • Electrical alternans	• CVP, PAP, and PAOP elevated • Equalization of intracardiac pressures; all PAP will be elevated within a 5 mm Hg variation • Pulsus paradoxus (i.e., a drop in blood pressure of >10 mm Hg during inspiration) • CO and CI decreased • SvO_2 and $ScvO_2$ decreased
Papillary muscle rupture (e.g., acute mitral regurgitation)	• Tachycardia, hypotension, and tachypnea • Dyspnea • Crackles • S_3 • New holosystolic murmur at apex	• CVP, PAP, and PAOP elevated • SaO_2, SvO_2, and $ScvO_2$ decreased

CI, Cardiac index; *CO,* cardiac output; *CVP,* central venous pressure; *JVD,* jugular vein distention; *PAP,* pulmonary artery pressure; *PAOP,* pulmonary artery occlusive pressure; *SaO2,* arterial oxygen saturation; *ScvO2,* central venous oxygen saturation; *SvO2,* venous oxygen saturation.
Adapted from Dennison, R. (2007). *Pass CCRN!* (3rd ed.). St. Louis: Mosby.

Continued

TABLE 4-8 Hemodynamic Profiles for Selected Critical Conditions—cont'd

Condition	Clinical Presentation	Hemodynamic Presentation
Rupture of ventricular septum	• Tachycardia, hypotension, and tachypnea • New holosystolic murmur at lower left sternal border	• CVP and PAP elevated • Increased SvO_2 and $ScvO_2$
Left ventricular infarction	• Chest pain • S_4 at apex • Characteristic electrocardiogram changes of LVMI	• CVP, PAP, PAOP may be increased
Right ventricular infarction	• Chest pain • S_4 at sternum • JVD • Clear lungs • Characteristic electrocardiogram changes	• CVP may be elevated • PAP and PAOP may be decreased

TABLE 4-9 Management of Hemodynamic Monitoring Complications

Complications	Prevention/Detection/Treatment
Air emboli	• Use the Trendelenburg position for the insertion of deep vein catheters • Place a sterile gloved finger over the needle hub with any disconnection during insertion to prevent air emboli • Aspirate air from the flush solution bag to avoid air embolus with inadvertent emptying of the flush solution bag • Flush all lumens with saline before the insertion of the catheters • Monitor the pressure monitoring system for air bubbles • Use only Luer-Lok connections • Have the patient hold his or her breath during catheter-tubing disconnections (e.g., tubing changes, the removal of deep vein catheters) • If an air embolus is suspected, turn the patient to left side with his or her head down (i.e., Durant maneuver) and administer oxygen
Arterial puncture during venous cannulation	• Hold pressure for at least 5-10 minutes; a longer time may be required for patients who are taking anticoagulants or who have received fibrinolytics
Balloon rupture	• Test the balloon before insertion by inflating the balloon, holding it in a basin of sterile saline, and watching for bubbling • Store catheters away from sunlight and heat • Limit the length of time that the catheter is left in place (ideally <72 hours) • Limit the number of times that the balloon is inflated to only when indicated (balloons are expected to last about 72 inflations); use diastolic pulmonary artery pressure as a reflection of LVEDP in patients without pulmonary hypertension • Do not overinflate the balloon; stop injecting air as soon as the PAOP waveform is seen • Do not aspirate air from the balloon; allow passive deflation to occur, and reattach the empty syringe to the balloon port • This complication is particularly dangerous in right-to-left shunts (i.e., neonates; adults shunt from left to right) • Indications that the balloon has ruptured include the inability to obtain the PAOP waveform and the absence of resistance during inflation • If balloon rupture has occurred, label the balloon lumen accordingly so that others do not continue to try to inflate the balloon; use diastolic pulmonary artery pressure as a reflection of LVEDP in patients without pulmonary hypertension; if a PAOP is required, a new pulmonary artery catheter must be inserted

FIO$_2$, Forced inspiratory oxygen; *LVEDP*, left ventricular end-diastolic pressure; *PAP*, pulmonary artery pressure; *PAOP*, pulmonary artery occlusive pressure; *SaO$_2$*, arterial oxygen saturation.

TABLE 4-9   Management of Hemodynamic Monitoring Complications—cont'd

Complications	Prevention/Detection/Treatment
Clotting and catheter occlusion	• Maintain normal saline drip with an intermittent flush device; heparin may be used according to hospital protocol • Monitor for any change in waveform (e.g., damping)
Dysrhythmias: usually ventricular dysrhythmias or right bundle branch block	• Have emergency equipment (including a transcutaneous pacemaker) available during insertion • Inflate the balloon to capacity (e.g., 1.5 ml) when the catheter is in the right atrium during insertion so that the balloon cushions the catheter tip • Observe the electrocardiography monitor closely during insertion • Ensure that the catheter has been sutured in place to decrease the risk of movement • Assess the PAP waveform for indications that the catheter has flipped back into right ventricle • Request catheter repositioning for catheter fling or right ventricular waveform • If the right ventricular waveform is noted, inflate the balloon to capacity (e.g., 1.5 ml) to cushion the catheter tip • Turn the patient to his or her left side to encourage the distal migration of the catheter back into the pulmonary artery • Deflate the balloon after it has been successfully repositioned in the pulmonary artery • Observe the electrocardiography monitor closely during the removal of the pulmonary artery catheter; the catheter should be removed in one smooth, continuous movement with the balloon deflated
Emboli	• Aspirate (rather than flush) if you suspect a small clot
Exsanguination	• Use only Luer-Lok connections • Maintain alarms in the "on" position; pressure alarms are usually set 10–20 mm Hg above and below the patient's normal values
Fluid overload	• Limit the number of fast flushes • Use 5 ml rather than 10 ml for cardiac outputs when indicated, or use continuous cardiac output, which requires no fluid boluses for the determination of cardiac output • Limit the frequency of cardiac outputs to every 4 hours unless required more often
Hematoma	• Maintain pressure for 5–10 minutes with single-thickness pressure dressings after catheter removal; a longer time may be required for patients who are receiving anticoagulants or fibrinolytics
Hypothermia	• Use room-temperature injectate • Apply blankets and radiant heaters as needed
Infection	• Encourage percutaneous catheter insertion; this results in a much lower incidence of infection than does cutdown • Change the flush solution bag whenever it is empty, every 72–96 hours, or according to hospital protocol • Change the tubing every 72–96 hours or according to hospital protocol • Dress and inspect the site with the use of sterile technique every 72–96 hours or according to hospital protocol • Avoid clear semipermeable dressings for patients with oily skin • Use normal saline rather than 5% dextrose solution for the heparinized flush solution • Flush well after drawing blood samples; do not allow dried blood to stay in stopcock ports or tubing • Limit the number of stopcocks in the pressure-monitoring system • Replace all vented stopcock covers with nonvented "dead end" caps • Use strict sterile technique when handling blood samples and cardiac outputs • Encourage the use of a catheter sleeve over the pulmonary artery catheter to allow for sterile catheter manipulation • Limit the length of time that the catheter is left in place (ideally <72–96 hours) • Monitor for clinical indications of infection at the catheter insertion site: redness, warmth, induration, purulent drainage, and pain • Monitor for clinical indications of catheter sepsis: fever, chills, leukocytosis, positive blood culture, and catheter culture
Microshock	• Recognize that this risk is caused by the elimination of the skin as a protection from microshock in patients with intracardiac catheters • Ensure that all electrical equipment is properly functioning and grounded • Do not touch the patient and a piece of electrical equipment at the same time

Continued

TABLE 4-9	Management of Hemodynamic Monitoring Complications—cont'd	
Complications	**Prevention/Detection/Treatment**
Nerve palsy	• Maintain the limbs in a functional position (e.g., do not keep the wrist hyperextended)
Pneumothorax, hemothorax, or chylothorax during insertion	• Have a chest radiograph taken after central venous catheter cannulation • Assist with the insertion of the chest tube if pneumothorax (air in the pleural space), hemothorax (blood in the pleural space), or chylothorax (lymph fluid in the pleural space) occurs
Pulmonary artery rupture	• Recognize patients who are at high risk: older adult patients; patients with pulmonary hypertension; patients who are receiving anticoagulant, fibrinolytic, or platelet aggregation inhibitor therapy; and hypothermic patients • Inflate the balloon with only enough air to cause the PAOP waveform; do not overinflate the balloon, and limit the inflation time to a maximum of 15 seconds, because both prolonged inflation and excessive balloon volume put too much tension on the vessel wall • Monitor the patient for hemoptysis, dyspnea, and hypotension as indications of pulmonary artery rupture • If rupture of the pulmonary artery does occur, increase the FIO_2, suction the airway, position the patient with the affected lung down, assist with intubation with a double-lumen endotracheal tube, use positive end-expiratory pressure or pulmonary artery catheter balloon inflation for tamponade effect as prescribed, monitor the vital signs and oxygenation levels closely for changes, and prepare the patient for surgery if requested
Pulmonary infarction	• Inflate the balloon only long enough for graphic recording • Continuously monitor PAP so that, if the catheter advances into the PAOP position, it will be noted and the catheter repositioned • Request proximal repositioning if it takes less than 1.25 ml to achieve occluded position, because this indicates that the catheter is positioned too distal and that it may spontaneously occlude the pulmonary arteriole (this is commonly referred to as *spontaneous wedge*) and cause ischemia and infarction • Monitor for chest pain, dyspnea, and decreased SaO_2 as indications of pulmonary infarction
Thrombosis	• Maintain a heparinized normal saline drip with an intermittent flush device; keep the pressure bag at 300 mm Hg • Limit the length of time that the catheter is left in (ideally <72 hours) • Prevent trauma to the intima by performing skillful catheter insertion • To prevent or detect arterial thrombosis with arterial catheters: • Select a site with collateral flow (e.g., radial artery) • Use the smallest catheter feasible (e.g., 20 gauge for radial artery cannulation) • Perform neurovascular assessment hourly to promptly detect acute arterial occlusion • If arterial occlusion occurs, assist with intra-arterial fibrinolytics or embolectomy

From Dennison, R. (2007). *Pass CCRN!* (3rd ed.). St. Louis: Mosby.

I. QT interval
  1) Represents time of ventricular depolarization and repolarization
  2) Measured from first wave of QRS complex to the end of the T wave
  3) Normal QT interval based on heart rate; the slower the heart rate, the longer the normal QT interval; the faster the heart rate, the shorter the normal QT interval
    a) For heart rates between 60 and 100 beats/ minute, the normal QT interval is less than half of the R-R interval
  4) To correct for changes in heart rate (especially for heart rates that are not between 60 and 100 beats/minute), calculate the QT interval corrected for heart rate (QTc)

    a) Formula: QT ÷ The square root of the R-R interval
    b) Normal QTc: 0.32 to 0.44
3. Steps in the analysis of a rhythm strip (Table 4-10)
4. Criteria for basic dysrhythmias and blocks (Table 4-11)
5. ECG changes with electrolyte imbalances
  a. Hypokalemia
    1) If ≤3 mEq/L
      a) Flat T with prominent U wave
      b) T wave and U wave of approximately same amplitude
      c) ST segment flattening, depression, or both
    2) If ≤2.0 mEq/L
      a) U wave taller than T wave
      b) Prolongation of QT interval
      c) ST segment depression

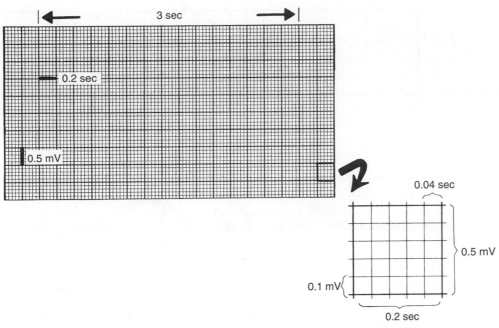

Figure 4-25 Electrocardiogram paper. The horizontal axis represents time, with each small block equal to 0.04 second and each large block equal to 0.20 second, with 3-second intervals marked off at the top of the paper. The vertical axis represents voltage, when standardized, with each small block equal to 0.1 mV and each large block equal to 0.5 mV. (From Kinney, M. R., Packa, D. R., & Dunbar, S. B. [1993]. *AACN's clinical reference for critical-care nursing* [3rd ed.]. St. Louis: Mosby.)

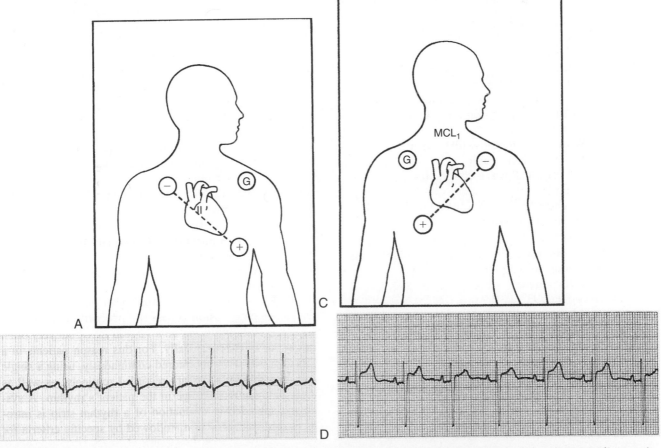

Figure 4-26 Monitoring leads. **A,** Electrode placement for lead II. **B,** Representation of the appearance of the electrocardiogram in lead II. **C,** Electrode placement for MCL₁. **D,** Representation of appearance of electrocardiogram in MCL₁. (From Urden, L. D., Lough, M. E., & Stacy, K. M. [1995]. *Priorities in critical care nursing.a* St. Louis: Mosby.)

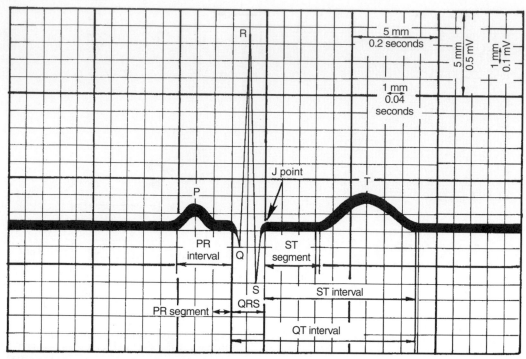

Figure 4-27 Components of a single cardiac cycle. (From Seidel, J. C. [1986]. *The Methodist Hospital: Basic electrocardiography—A modular approach.* St. Louis: Mosby.)

3) If ≤1.0 mEq/L
   a) U wave fuses with T wave
b. Hyperkalemia
  1) If >5.5 mEq/L
    a) Tall, narrow, peaked T waves
    b) QRS complex widens
    c) P wave widens and becomes shallow
  2) If ≥6.5 mEq/L: QRS complex widens more
  3) If ≥8.0 mEq/L
    a) Wide QRS merged with T wave
    b) P wave barely visible
  4) If ≥12 mEq/L: P wave disappears
c. Hypocalcemia
  1) Prolonged QT
  2) Prolonged ST segment
d. Hypercalcemia
  1) Shortened QT
  2) Shortened ST segment
e. Hypomagnesemia
  1) Prolonged QT
  2) Broad, flattened T wave
f. Hypermagnesemia
  1) Prolonged PR and QT
  2) Prolonged QRS

Multiple-lead electrocardiography analysis
1. ECG leads (Figure 4-28)
  a. Limb leads: frontal plane
    1) Lead I: positive at left arm, negative at right arm
    2) Lead II: positive at foot, negative at right arm

    3) Lead III: positive at foot, negative at left arm
    4) Lead aVR: unipolar at right arm
    5) Lead aVL: unipolar at left arm
    6) Lead aVF: unipolar at foot
  b. Chest leads: horizontal plane
    1) Lead V_1: fourth intercostal space at right sternal border
    2) Lead V_2: fourth intercostal at left sternal border
    3) Lead V_3: halfway between V_2 and V_4
    4) Lead V_4: fifth intercostal space at left MCL
    5) Lead V_5: fifth intercostal space at left anterior axillary line
    6) Lead V_6: fifth intercostal space at left midaxillary line
    7) R wave gets taller across the precordium from V_1 to V_6 (this is referred to as the normal progression of the R wave across the precordium); the S wave gets smaller across the precordium (V_1 to V_6)
    8) Conditions associated with poor R-wave progression across the precordium include the following:
      a) Anterior MI
      b) Left bundle branch block
      c) Emphysema
    9) Conditions associated with low voltage across the precordium include the following:
      a) Emphysema
      b) Pericardial effusion
      c) MI
      d) Obesity

TABLE 4-10 Rhythm Strip Analysis

Component	Assessment
Regularity (rhythm)	• Is it regular? • Is it irregular? • Are there any patterns to the irregularity? • Are there any ectopic beats? If so, are they early (premature) or late (escape)? • Is the regularity of the P waves and the QRS complexes the same? (If there is only one P wave for each QRS, only one regularity needs to be recorded.)

Rate	• Methods
	  • Count the dark lines between the P waves or QRS complexes as 300, 150, 100, 75, 60, 50, 43, 38, 33, and 30.
	  • Count the number of QRS complexes in a 6-second strip and multiply by 10.
	  • Use a rate ruler.
	• Are atrial and ventricular rates the same? (If there is only one P wave for each QRS, only one rate needs to be recorded.)

P waves	• Are the P waves regular? • Is there one P wave for every QRS? • Is the P wave in front of the QRS or behind it? • Is the P wave normal and upright in lead II? • Are there more P waves than QRS complexes? • Do all P waves look alike? • Are irregular P waves associated with ectopic beats? If so, are they early (premature) or late (escape)?
PR intervals	• Is the PR interval measurement within the normal range (i.e., 0.12-0.20 second)? • Are all PR intervals constant? • If the PR interval varies, is there a pattern to the changing measurements?
QRS complexes	• Is the QRS measurement within normal limits (i.e., 0.06-0.11 second)? • Are all QRS complexes of equal duration? • Do all QRS complexes look alike? • Are unusual QRS complexes associated with ectopic beats? If so, are they early (premature) or late (escape)?
QT interval	• Is the QT measurement within normal limits (i.e., less than half of the previous R-R interval or 0.32-0.44 second)?
Patient presentation	• Is the patient symptomatic? • Are there clinical indications of hypoperfusion, such as hypotension, syncope, or chest pain?

From Dennison, R. (2007). *Pass CCRN!* (3rd ed.). St. Louis: Mosby.

c. Specialty leads: these leads should be included if there are changes associated with inferior wall injury or infarction so that concurrent posterior or RV infarction is detected
  1) Posterior leads
    a) Lead V7: fifth intercostal space at left posterior axillary line
    b) Lead V8: halfway between V7 and V8
    c) Lead V9: fifth intercostal space next to vertebral column
  2) RV leads
    a) Lead V4R: fifth intercostal space at right MCL
    b) Lead V5R: fifth intercostal space at right anterior axillary line
    c) Lead V6R: fifth intercostal space at right midaxillary line
    d) The standard 12 leads plus V4R, V5R, V6R, V7, V8, and V9 make the 18 leads of an 18-lead ECG

2. Bundle branch blocks (Figure 4-29)
  a. A block of either bundle branch causes a delay in the conduction through the ventricles and a prolongation of the QRS interval; branching (commonly referred to as *rabbit ears*) or slurring of the QRS complex also usually occurs, which indicates that the two ventricles are depolarized out of sync
  b. Left bundle branch block is a bifascicular block (i.e., it involves the loss of both major hemibundles), and it is manifested by the following:
    1) QRS of ≥0.12 seconds
    2) QRS that is positive in V6 and negative in V1
  c. Right bundle branch block is a unifascicular block, and it is manifested by the following:
    1) QRS of ≥0.12 seconds
    2) QRS that is positive in V1 and negative in V6
3. Myocardial ischemia, injury, and infarction
  a. Electrocardiography indicators (Figure 4-30)

4-11   Criteria for Basic Dysrhythmias and Blocks

Rhythm	Rate	Regularity	P Waves	PR Interval	QRS Duration
Normal sinus rhythm	60–100 beats/min	Atrial and ventricular rhythms regular	Normal	0.12–0.20 sec and constant	<0.12 sec
Sinus bradycardia	<60 beats/min	Atrial and ventricular rhythms regular	Normal	0.12–0.20 sec and constant	<0.12 sec
Sinus tachycardia	>100 beats/min (usually 100–160 beats/min)	Atrial and ventricular rhythms regular	Normal	0.12–0.20 sec and constant	<0.12 sec
Sinus dysrhythmias	Usually 60–100 beats/min but may be slower or faster	Atrial and ventricular rhythms regularly irregular; the rate increases with inspiration (so the R-R interval shortens) and decreases with expiration (so the R-R interval lengthens); the difference between the shortest and the longest R-R is <0.12 sec	Normal	0.12–0.20 sec and usually constant; may vary slightly with rate variation	<0.12 sec
Sinus block (sinus exit block)	Dependent on underlying rhythm	Atrial and ventricular rhythms regular with an irregularity; the R-R interval at the block measures an exact multiple of the normal R-R interval	One or more entire cardiac cycle is absent; P wave absent during block	None during block	QRS absent during block
Sinus arrest	Dependent on underlying rhythm	Atrial and ventricular rhythms regular with an irregularity in the form of a pause; the R-R interval at the pause measures more or less than an exact multiple of the normal R-R interval	Indefinite period of time without an entire cardiac cycle; P wave absent during arrest	None during arrest	QRS absent during arrest
Premature atrial contractions	Dependent on underlying rhythm	Dependent on underlying rhythm; premature atrial contractions interrupt the underlying rhythm	P wave of this early beat differs from sinus P; the ectopic P wave is early and may be flattened, notched, or lost in the preceding T wave	Usually 0.12–0.20 sec but may be >0.20 sec	<0.12 sec
Wandering atrial pacemaker	Usually 60–100 beats/min	Atrial and ventricular rhythms usually slightly irregular	P waves look different from beat to beat; there are at least three different-looking P waves	0.12–0.20 sec and may vary	<0.12 sec

Dysrhythmia	Rate	Rhythm	P Wave	PR Interval	QRS Complex
Supraventricular tachycardia*	>160 beats/min; usually 160–250 beats/min	Atrial and ventricular rhythms regular	P waves are impossible to distinguish; may be lost in QRS or the preceding T wave	Cannot measure	<0.12 sec
Atrial tachycardia	150–250 beats/min	Atrial and ventricular rhythms regular	P wave differs from sinus P; may merge with the preceding T wave	0.12–0.20 sec	<0.12 sec
Atrial flutter	Atrial rate approximately 300 beats/min; ventricular rate varies with conduction through the atrioventricular node; a 2:1 atrial flutter has a ventricular rate of approximately 150 beats/min, whereas a 4:1 atrial flutter has a ventricular rate of approximately 75 beats/min	Atrial flutter waves regular; ventricular rhythm (response) usually regular	No true P waves; flutter waves have a characteristic sawtooth appearance	No true P waves	<0.12 sec
Atrial fibrillation	Atrial rate >350 beats/min; ventricular rate varies greatly depending on conduction through the atrioventricular node	Atrial fibrillatory waves irregular; ventricular rhythm irregularly irregular	No true P waves; fibrillatory waves are manifested by a quivering baseline	No true P waves	<0.12 sec
Premature junctional contraction	Dependent on underlying rhythm	Dependent on underlying rhythm; premature junctional contraction interrupts the underlying rhythm	P wave, if visible, will be inverted; may be in front of, in, or after the QRS complex	Can be measured only if P wave is in front of QRS; PR will be <0.12 sec if measurable	<0.12 sec
Junctional escape rhythm	40–60 beats/min	Atrial and ventricular rhythms regular	P wave, if visible, will be inverted; may be in front of, in, or after the QRS complex	Can be measured only if P wave is in front of QRS; PR will be <0.12 sec if measurable	<0.12 sec
Accelerated junctional rhythm	60–100 beats/min	Atrial and ventricular rhythms regular	P wave, if visible, will be inverted; may be in front of, in, or after the QRS complex	Can be measured only if P wave is in front of QRS; PR will be <0.12 sec if measurable	<0.12 sec

*The term *supraventricular tachycardia* refers to any narrow QRS tachycardia with a focus that cannot be clearly identified; the term should only be used when a more definitive diagnosis cannot be made.

Continued

TABLE 4-11   Criteria for Basic Dysrhythmias and Blocks—cont'd

Rhythm	Rate	Regularity	P Waves	PR Interval	QRS Duration
Junctional tachycardia	>100 beats/min; usually 100–180 beats/min	Atrial and ventricular rhythms regular	P wave, if visible, will be inverted; may be in front of, in, or after the QRS complex	Can be measured only if P wave is in front of QRS; PR will be <0.12 sec if measurable	<0.12 sec
First-degree atrioventricular nodal block	Dependent on underlying rhythm	Dependent on underlying rhythm	Normal	>0.20 sec	<0.12 sec
Second-degree atrioventricular nodal block Mobitz I† (Wenckebach)	Atrial rate dependent on underlying rhythm; ventricular rate dependent on the conduction ratio; the atrial rate is higher than the ventricular rate	Atrial rhythm regular, ventricular rhythm irregular (i.e., P-P is regular but R-R is irregular); groupings are identifiable between P waves that were not conducted	P waves normal but some not followed by a QRS	Normal PR interval progressively lengthens until a P wave is not followed by a QRS; entire cycle begins again with a normal PR interval	<0.12 sec
Second-degree atrioventricular nodal block Mobitz II†	Atrial rate dependent on underlying rhythm; ventricular rate dependent on the conduction ratio but usually <60 beats/min; the atrial rate is higher than the ventricular rate	Atrial rhythm regular, ventricular rhythm regular or irregular depending on whether conduction ratio varies or is constant; the P-P is regular, but some R-Rs may be twice the normal rate	P waves normal some not followed by a QRS without a preceding progressive lengthening	Usually 0.12–0.20 sec of conducted P waves but may be longer; constant for each conducted QRS	≥0.12 sec
Third-degree (or complete) atrioventricular block	Atrial rate dependent on underlying rhythm; ventricular rate dependent on the focus of the escape rhythm: 40–60 beats/min if the escape focus is junctional, 20–40 beats/min if the escape focus is ventricular	Atrial rhythm regular, ventricular rhythm usually regular; P-P regular; R-R usually regular	P waves normal but not followed by (or associated with) a QRS	No consistent PR interval; no relationship between the P waves and the QRS complexes	<0.12 sec if escape focus is junctional; ≥0.12 sec if escape focus is ventricular
Left bundle branch block	Dependent on underlying rhythm	Dependent on underlying rhythm	Normal	0.12–0.20 sec as long as no coexisting atrioventricular nodal block	≥0.12 sec; QRS is negative in V_1

	Rate	Rhythm	P Waves	PR Interval	QRS
Right bundle branch block	Dependent on underlying rhythm	Dependent on underlying rhythm	Normal	0.12–0.20 sec as long as no coexisting atrioventricular nodal block	≥0.12 sec; QRS is positive in V_1
Premature ventricular contraction	Dependent on underlying rhythm	Dependent on underlying rhythm; premature ventricular contraction interrupts the underlying rhythm	No associated P waves	No associated P waves; cannot measure PR	≥0.12 sec; QRS of premature ventricular contraction looks different than normal QRS
Monomorphic ventricular tachycardia	100–250 beats/min; ventricular tachycardia is usually ≈150 beats/min; ventricular tachycardia at 200–250 beats/min may be called *ventricular flutter*	Ventricular rhythm usually regular; if dissociated P waves are identifiable, then the atrial rhythm is regular	No associated P waves but may have dissociated P waves scattered throughout the rhythm	No associated P waves; cannot measure PR	≥0.12 sec; QRS of ventricular tachycardia looks different than normal QRS
Polymorphic ventricular tachycardia (torsades de pointes)	150–250 beats/min	Ventricular rhythm may be regular	None	None	≥0.12 sec with a QRS that seems to twist around a center line; there is a gradual alteration in the amplitude and direction of the QRS
Ventricular fibrillation	None	Irregular; chaotic baseline	None	None	None
Idioventricular rhythm	20–40 beats/min	Ventricular rhythm usually regular; no atrial activity	None	None	≥0.12 sec
Accelerated idioventricular rhythm	40–100 beats/min	Ventricular rhythm usually regular; no atrial activity	None	None	≥0.12 sec
Asystole	None	No atrial or ventricular activity	None	None	None

†A 2:1 block is a second-degree block, but it may be either Mobitz type I or type II. The QRS width may be helpful for differentiating between the two: if the QRS is of normal width, it is probably a type I block; if the QRS is ≥0.12 sec, it is probably a type II block.

From Dennison, R. (2007). *Pass CCRN!* (3rd ed.). St. Louis: Mosby.

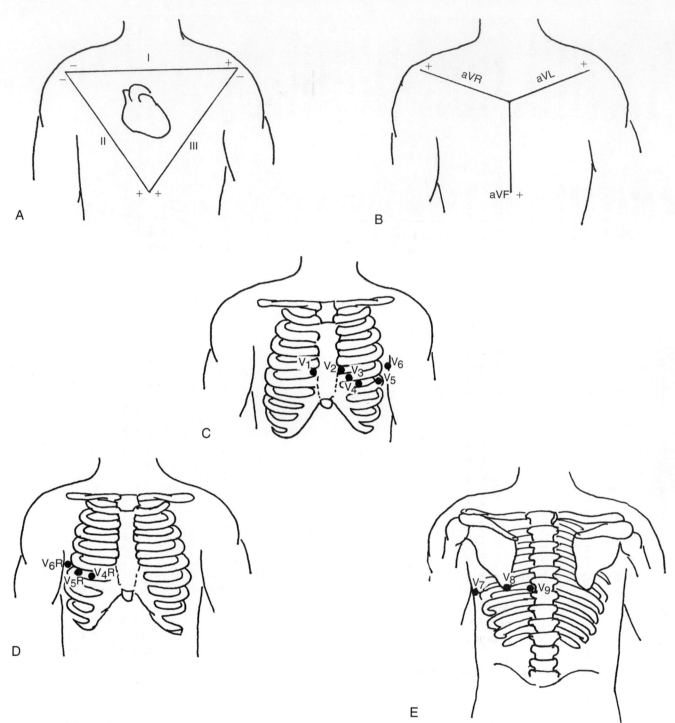

Figure 4-28 Electrocardiogram leads. **A,** Bipolar limb leads: I, II, and III. **B,** Unipolar limb leads: aVR, aVL, and aVE. **C,** Standard chest leads: V_1 to V_6. **D,** Right ventricular leads: V_4R to V_6R. **E,** Posterior leads: V_7 to V_9.

1) Ischemia is manifested by changes in the T waves; these are the earliest changes in the evolution of MI
   a) Indicative change: symmetrically inverted T waves in the leads that face the ischemic area
   b) Reciprocal change: tall T waves in the leads opposite the ischemic area

2) Injury is manifested by ST segment changes; these are intermediate changes in the evolution of MI
   a) Indicative change: ST segment elevation in the leads that face the injured area
   b) Reciprocal change: ST segment depression in the leads opposite the injured area

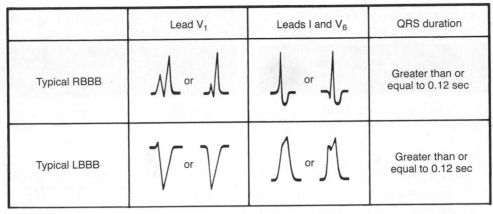

	Lead V₁	Leads I and V₆	QRS duration
Typical RBBB			Greater than or equal to 0.12 sec
Typical LBBB			Greater than or equal to 0.12 sec

Figure 4-29 Bundle branch blocks. *LBBB,* Left bundle branch block; *RBBB,* right bundle branch block. (Modified from Grauer, K. [1992]. *Practical guide to ECG interpretation.* St. Louis: Mosby.)

3) Infarction is manifested by changes in the Q waves; these are the latest changes in the evolution of MI
   a) Indicative change: pathologic Q waves (0.04 second wide or a quarter of the height of the R wave) in the leads that face the necrotic area
   b) Reciprocal change: tall R waves in the leads opposite the necrotic area
   c) Q waves
     i) Normal in many leads; to be pathologic (i.e., indicative of infarction), they must be 0.4 second wide or a quarter of the height of the R wave
     ii) Take up to 24 hours to develop
     iii) Relate to a mass loss of myocardium
     iv) Prevented by successful reperfusion therapies (e.g., fibrinolytics, PCI)
4) Some conditions may make the electrocardiographic diagnosis of MI difficult by changing the morphology of the QRS wave, the ST segment, or the T waves; some examples include the following:
   a) Unstable angina (e.g., Wellens syndrome)

   b) Ventricular pacemakers
   c) Left bundle branch block: the chance of acute MI is more likely if the following are present:
     i) New onset
     ii) ST segment depression of 1 mm in leads V₁ and V₂
     iii) ST segment elevation of >5 mm
   d) Ventricular hypertrophy
   e) Wolff-Parkinson-White syndrome
   f) Pericarditis
   g) Hypothermia
   h) Hemorrhagic stroke
   i) Electrolyte imbalances
b. Location (Table 4-12)
   1) Anterior left ventricle: indicative changes in V₃, V₄, and possibly V₂
   2) Septal: indicative changes in V₁ and V₂
   3) Lateral left ventricle indicative changes in I, aVL, V₅, or V₆
     a) I and aVL are considered high lateral leads
     b) V₅ and V₆ are considered low lateral leads
   4) Inferior left ventricle: indicative changes in II, III, and aVF

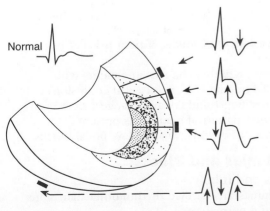

Normal

Ischemia = T wave Inversion

Injury = ST Elevation (at least 2 mm)

Infarction = Pathological Q wave (at least .04 sec or ¼ height of QRS)

Reciprocal Changes = Inverted changes seen in leads opposite

Figure 4-30 Electrocardiogram indicators in ischemia, injury, infarction, and reciprocal changes. (From Harvey, M. [2000]. *Study guide to core curriculum for critical care nursing* [3rd ed.] Philadelphia: Saunders.)

TABLE 4-12 Electrocardiogram Lead Correlations With Myocardial Infarction Locations*

Location	Leads	Coronary Artery Affected
Anterior	(V_2), V_3, and V_4	LAD
Septal	V_1 and V_2	LAD
Anteroseptal	V_1, V_2, V_3, and (V_4)	LAD
Lateral	I, aVL (high lateral), V_5 and V_6 (low lateral)	LCA
Anterolateral	V_3, V_4, V_5, V_6 (may be I and aVL)	LCA
Inferior	II, III, and aVF	RCA
RV	V_4R, V_5R, V_6R; may be transient	RCA
Posterior	V_7, V_8, and V_9 or reciprocal in V_1, V_2, and V_3	RCA, LCA, or both

LAD, Left anterior descending artery; *LCA,* left circumflex artery; *RCA,* right coronary artery.

*Changes may also be seen in leads in parentheses.
From Dennison, R. (2007). *Pass CCRN!* (3rd ed.). St. Louis: Mosby.

TABLE 4-13 Determination of Age of Myocardial Infarction

Description	Electrocardiographic Characteristics	Time From Onset of Pain
Hyperacute	• ST segment elevation • "Tombstone"-shaped T waves or T wave inversion	Minutes to hours
Acute	• ST segment elevation • T wave inversion • Pathologic Q waves	Hours to days
Recent	• T wave inversion • Pathologic Q waves	Weeks to months
Old	• Pathologic Q waves	After several months

From Dennison, R. (2007). *Pass CCRN!* (3rd ed.). St. Louis: Mosby.

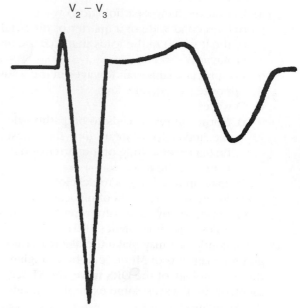

$V_2 - V_3$

Figure 4-31 Wellens syndrome. (From Conover, M. [2003]. *Understanding electrocardiography* [8th ed.] St. Louis: Mosby-Year Book.)

5) Posterior left ventricle
 a) Reciprocal changes in V_1 and V_2
 b) Indicative changes in V_7, V_8, or V_9
  i) V_8 and V_9 are the most significant
 6) RV: indicative changes in V_4R, V_5R, and V_6R; V_4R is the most significant
 c. Determination of age of MI (Table 4-13)
4. Electrocardiographic changes in patients with angina
 a. Variant (also referred to as *Prinzmetal* or *vasospastic*) angina
  1) Angina at rest caused by spasm of the coronary artery or arteries
  2) Manifested by ST segment elevation with pain
 b. Wellens syndrome (Figure 4-31)
  1) Group of signs that are associated with the occlusion of the proximal left anterior descending artery and a high risk of sudden cardiac death in a patient with unstable angina
   a) Symmetric and deeply inverted T waves in V_2 and V_3 that persist even when the patient is pain free
   b) Little or no ST segment elevation
   c) Little or no enzyme elevation
   d) No development of Q waves or loss of precordial R waves
  2) Cardiac catheterization with PCI is indicated
5. Electrocardiographic changes in patients with pericarditis
 a. ST segment normal in V_1 and aVR but all other leads show ST segment elevation
 b. Depression of PR interval in limb leads and left chest leads (V_5 and V_6)
 c. Decrease in QRS voltage if pericardial effusion is present
6. Electrocardiographic changes in patients with myocardial trauma (e.g., myocardial contusion)
 a. Nonspecific ST and T wave changes; there is an infarction pattern if necrosis is present
 b. High risk of dysrhythmias and AV nodal blocks

Dysrhythmias and Blocks
Definitions and rules
1. Dysrhythmias: any cardiac rhythm other than sinus rhythm at a normal rate

2. Block: the failure of an intrinsic impulse to be conducted through the conduction system
3. Premature: a beat that occurs earlier than expected with regard to the underlying rhythm; this is an example of irritability, and treatment is directed toward treating the cause or suppressing the irritability
4. Escape: a beat that occurs later than expected with regard to the underlying rhythm; this is an example of default (i.e., it occurs because upper pacemakers do not initiate a beat), and treatment is directed toward treating the cause or stimulating the upper pacemakers
5. Pacemaker rule: the fastest rate will control the heart
   a. Because the sinus node is the fastest inherent rate, it is usually in control; the underlying rhythm is the sinus rhythm
   b. When irritability occurs, another area will take control away from the sinus node, such as that which occurs with atrial tachycardia, junctional tachycardia, or ventricular tachycardia
   c. When upper pacemakers fail, the pacemaker below with the fastest rate will assume control (e.g., sinus arrest with junctional escape rhythm)
6. Rule of electrical flow: when the impulse is traveling directly toward the positive pole of a lead, the wave will be positive; when the impulse is traveling directly away from the positive pole or directly toward the negative pole of a lead, the wave will be negative

Etiology
1. General
   a. Congenital (e.g., long QT syndrome, accessory pathways, Brugada syndrome)
   b. Myocardial ischemia or infarction
   c. Hypoxemia or hypoxia
   d. Electrolyte imbalance
   e. Acid-base imbalance
   f. SNS stimulation via endogenous catecholamines or sympathomimetic drugs (e.g., epinephrine, isoproterenol [Isuprel], dopamine [Intropin])
   g. Drug effects or toxicity
      1) "Holiday heart" syndrome caused by excessive alcohol consumption; this type of binge drinking may cause acute dysrhythmias (usually a supraventricular tachycardia)
2. Specific to each dysrhythmia (Table 4-14)
3. Pathophysiology: arrhythmogenic mechanisms
   a. Problems with impulse formation
      1) Altered automaticity
         a) Enhanced automaticity
            i) Caused by the following:
               (a) Hypoxia
               (b) Hypercapnia
               (c) Ischemia or infarction
               (d) Hypokalemia or hypocalcemia
               (e) Catecholamines
               (f) Hyperthermia
               (g) Digitalis toxicity
               (h) Stretching of the heart muscle
            ii) Cause of most atrial, junctional, and ventricular ectopic beats and most ventricular tachycardias
         b) Depressed automaticity
            i) Caused by any of the following:
               (a) Vagal stimulation
               (b) Hyperkalemia or hypercalcemia
               (c) Decreased catecholamines
               (d) Hypothermia
               (e) β-blockers
            ii) Cause of bradycardia or blocks
      2) Triggered activity
         a) Early: occurs when the QT is prolonged
            i) Caused by prolongation of repolarization and effective refractory period
            ii) Example: torsades de pointes
         b) Delayed: the result of elevated intracellular calcium
            i) Caused by the following:
               (a) Electrolyte imbalances
               (b) Catecholamines
            ii) Example: tachycardias of digitalis toxicity
   b. Problems with impulse conduction
      1) Reentry: the most common mechanism for tachydysrhythmias
         a) An impulse travels through an area of the myocardium and depolarizes it but then reenters the same area to depolarize it again
         b) Cause of any of the following:
            i) Some ectopy
            ii) Some ventricular tachycardias
            iii) Most supraventricular tachycardias
            iv) Wolff-Parkinson-White tachycardias
      2) Accessory pathways
         a) Wolff-Parkinson-White syndrome
            i) Caused by Kent bundle, which bypasses the AV node
            ii) Cause of the following:
               (a) Short PR, wide QRS wave with slurring of the first portion of the QRS wave (referred to as a delta wave)
               (b) Tachydysrhythmias
         b) Lown-Ganong-Levine syndrome
            i) Caused by the following:
               (a) AV nodal bypass tract
               (b) AV node smaller than normal
               (c) Fibers running through AV node that do not have the built-in delay feature that nodal fibers have
            ii) Causes of the following:
               (a) Short PR with normal QRS wave
               (b) Tachydysrhythmias
         c) Mahaim fibers
            i) Caused by nodoventricular or fasciculoventricular fibers
            ii) Cause of the following:

TABLE 4-14   Basic Dysrhythmia and Block Management

Rhythm	Etiology	Significance	Treatment
General	• Congenital • Myocardial ischemia or MI • Hypoxia • Electrolyte imbalance • Acid-base imbalance • Sympathetic nervous system stimulation • Drug effect or toxicity	• Dependent on patient's clinical presentation • Monitor for clinical manifestations of hypoperfusion	• Treat cause • Correct ischemia if possible • Correct hypoxemia or hypoxia • Correct electrolyte imbalance • Correct acid-base imbalance • Correct drug toxicity • Provide general emergency management for any symptomatic patient • Oxygen • Intravenous access • Multiple-lead electrocardiography if rhythm interpretation is required or if ischemia is suspected
Sinus bradycardia	• Athletic heart • Sleep • Vagal stimulation • Myocardial ischemia or MI • Inferior or posterior MI • Fibrodegenerative changes of the SA node (e.g., sick sinus syndrome) • Increased intracranial pressure • Hypothermia • Hypothyroidism • Cervical or mediastinal tumor • Drug effects: digitalis, β-blockers, calcium-channel blockers, or opiates	• Depends on rate • If too slow, cardiac output decreases • Clinical manifestations of hypoperfusion may include hypotension, syncope, chest pain, and HF • Escape beats (atrial, junctional, or ventricular) may occur	• None if asymptomatic • If clinical manifestations of hypoperfusion occur: • Transcutaneous pacemaker preferred • Atropine may be used as a temporary treatment for patients who do not have myocardial ischemia
Sinus tachycardia	• Stress, fear, anxiety, pain, or anger • Exercise • Hypovolemia or hypervolemia • Shock • Hypoxia • Fever • Anemia • Hyperthyroidism • Inflammatory heart disease • Myocardial ischemia or MI • Anterior MI • Fibrodegenerative changes (e.g., sick sinus syndrome) • HF • Pulmonary embolism • Drug effects: epinephrine, isoproterenol (Isuprel), dopamine (Intropin), atropine, caffeine, nicotine, amphetamines, cocaine, alcohol, or aminophylline	• Usually not significant except in patients with heart disease, in whom it may cause angina, MI, HF, or shock	• Treat cause • Anxiolytics for anxiety • Analgesics for pain • Antipyretics for fever • Fluids for hypovolemia • Treatment of HF • Avoidance of stimulants • Usually does not require other treatment, but the following may also be used: • Sedation or β-blockers may be used to decrease or block the effects of catecholamines
Sinus dysrhythmia	• Normal; variations in sympathetic and parasympathetic stimulation during ventilation • In older patients, may indicate sick sinus syndrome • Digitalis toxicity	• Normal variation • May be seen with digitalis toxicity	• None • Discontinue digitalis if toxicity is the cause

TABLE **4-14**   Basic Dysrhythmia and Block Management—cont'd

Rhythm	Etiology	Significance	Treatment
Sinus block (sinus exit block)	• Fibrodegenerative changes of the sinus node (e.g., sick sinus syndrome) • Ischemia of the SA node (e.g., MI) • Vagal stimulation • Inflammatory heart disease (e.g., myocarditis) • Drug toxicity: digitalis	• Depends on the frequency and duration of the pauses • If the patient loses consciousness (i.e., Stokes-Adams attacks), this is very significant and requires treatment	• Discontinue digitalis if toxicity is the cause • Atropine • Pacemaker if frequent or long pauses or if patient is having Stokes-Adams attacks
Sinus arrest	• Fibrodegenerative changes (e.g., sick sinus syndrome) • Ischemia of the SA node (e.g., MI) • Vagal stimulation • Electrolyte imbalance: potassium or magnesium • Drug toxicity: digitalis	• Depends on the frequency and duration of the pauses • If the patient loses consciousness (i.e., Stokes-Adams attacks), this is very significant and requires treatment	• Discontinue digitalis if toxicity is the cause • Atropine • Pacemaker if frequent or long (>3 sec) pauses or if patient is having Stokes-Adams attacks
Premature atrial contractions	• Increased sympathetic stimulation: stress, fear, anxiety, or pain • Exercise • Inflammatory heart disease (e.g., myocarditis) • Myocardial ischemia • Valvular heart disease (e.g., mitral stenosis, mitral valve prolapse) • HF • Electrolyte imbalance • Hypoxia • Drug effects: caffeine, nicotine, or alcohol • Drug toxicity: digitalis	• Usually benign but may precede atrial tachycardia, flutter, or fibrillation • Considered significant if >6/min	• Treat the cause • Usually no treatment is necessary, but, if frequent, treatment may include digitalis (i.e., digoxin [Lanoxin]), quinidine (Cardioquin), propranolol (Inderal), β-blockers, calcium-channel blockers, or anxiolytics
Wandering atrial pacemaker	• Vagal stimulation • Sinus bradycardia • Drug toxicity: digitalis	• May represent multiple atrial escape beats	• Usually none needed • Discontinue digitalis if toxicity is suspected • Atropine may be used to increase a slow sinus rate
Atrial tachycardia (NOTE: The term *paroxysmal atrial tachycardia* refers to the sudden interruption of the sinus rhythm by a rapid ectopic focus that starts and ends abruptly.)	• Increased sympathetic stimulation: stress, fear, anxiety, or pain • Exercise • Inflammatory heart disease (e.g., myocarditis) • Myocardial ischemia or MI • Hypoxia • Hyperthyroidism • Valvular heart disease (e.g., mitral valve prolapse) • Chronic obstructive pulmonary disease • Wolff-Parkinson-White syndrome • Drug effects: caffeine, nicotine, or alcohol • Drug toxicity: digitalis (frequently paroxysmal atrial tachycardia with block)	• Patient may experience palpitations and clinical manifestations of hypoperfusion (e.g., hypotension, syncope, chest pain, HF) because diastolic filling time and preload are greatly reduced • Myocardial oxygen consumption is increased and myocardial oxygen supply is decreased, so myocardial ischemia may occur or worsen	• Depends on patient's tolerance, the cause, and any history of previous attacks • Discontinue digitalis if toxicity is suspected • Initial treatment: vagal stimulation and adenosine; if the rhythm persists, continue with the following: • Calcium-channel blockers (e.g., diltiazem [Cardizem], verapamil [Calan]) • β-Blockers • Digoxin (if not the cause) • Synchronized cardioversion • NOTE: If the QRS is wide (e.g., associated with Wolff-Parkinson-White syndrome), do not use adenosine, β-blockers, calcium-channel blockers, or digoxin; the preferred agents are amiodarone and procainamide; if Wolff-Parkinson-White syndrome is the cause, ablation is the preferred long-term treatment

Continued

TABLE 4-14 Basic Dysrhythmia and Block Management—cont'd

Rhythm	Etiology	Significance	Treatment
Atrial fibrillation	• HF • Cardiomyopathy • Myocardial ischemia or MI • Anterior MI • Valvular heart disease (e.g., mitral stenosis, mitral regurgitation) • Hyperthyroidism • Inflammatory heart disease (e.g., pericarditis) • Hypertension • Postcardiotomy • Pulmonary hypertension (e.g., chronic obstructive pulmonary disease, pulmonary embolism) • Wolff-Parkinson-White syndrome • Drug effects: alcohol	• No effective atrial contraction, so loss of atrial "kick" • Mural thrombi formation predisposes patient to emboli • Significance varies greatly with regard to rate: may cause clinical manifestations of hypoperfusion (e.g., hypotension, syncope, chest pain, HF)	• Vagal stimulation • Ibutilide (Corvert) or synchronized cardioversion if acute onset • Calcium-channel blockers (e.g., diltiazem [Cardizem], verapamil [Calan]) • β-Blockers • Digoxin (Lanoxin; if not the cause) • If the ventricular response rate is slow, atropine or a pacemaker may be needed • Digitalis (i.e., digoxin [Lanoxin]) should be considered as the cause of a slow ventricular response rate; withhold digitalis if it is the cause • NOTE: If associated with Wolff-Parkinson-White syndrome, do not use β-blockers, calcium-channel blockers, or digoxin (Lanoxin); the preferred agents are amiodarone (Cordarone) and procainamide • Other nonacute considerations: implantable atrial defibrillator, ablation, or maze procedure • Long-term anticoagulation is needed for chronic atrial fibrillation to prevent mural thrombi and the risk for embolic stroke; the desirable international normalized ratio is 2 to 3
Atrial flutter	• HF • Myocardial ischemia or MI • Valvular heart disease • Inflammatory heart disease (e.g., pericarditis) • Hypertension • Postcardiotomy • Pulmonary hypertension (e.g., chronic obstructive pulmonary disease, pulmonary embolism) • Hyperthyroidism • Drug effects: alcohol • Drug toxicity: digitalis	• No effectiveness of atrial contraction • Significance varies greatly depending on rate • If rate is very rapid, may cause clinical manifestations of hypoperfusion (e.g., hypotension, syncope, chest pain, HF) because diastolic filling time and preload are greatly reduced	• The same as for atrial fibrillation • Although adenosine (Adenocard) is not indicated for the treatment of atrial flutter, it may slow the rhythm enough to allow flutter waves to be recognized • Anticoagulation may be prescribed for atrial flutter, but the risk of mural thrombi and stroke are considered lower than that of atrial fibrillation
Premature junctional contractions	• Myocardial ischemia or MI • Inferior MI • HF • Valvular heart disease • Hypoxia • Drug effects: nicotine, caffeine, and alcohol • Drug toxicity: digitalis • Same etiology as premature atrial contractions	• Usually benign but may predispose to junctional tachycardia if frequent	• Usually none necessary, but sedation or β-blockers may be used • Discontinue digitalis if toxicity is the cause

AV, Atrioventricular; *HF,* heart failure; *MI,* myocardial infarction; *SA,* sinoatrial.
Adapted from Dennison, R. (2007). *Pass CCRN!* (3rd ed.). St. Louis: Mosby.

TABLE 4-14   Basic Dysrhythmia and Block Management—cont'd

Rhythm	Etiology	Significance	Treatment
Junctional escape rhythm	• Vagal stimulation • SA block • Complete AV block • Myocardial ischemia or MI • Valvular heart disease • Hypoxia • Postcardiotomy • Drug toxicity: digitalis	• Protects patient from asystole • Do not suppress	• Note that this is not irritability; it is escape, so it should be treated by accelerating the sinus node • Atropine • Pacemaker may be needed • Discontinue digitalis if toxicity is the cause; it is a frequent cause of this rhythm
Accelerated junctional rhythm	• Vagal stimulation • SA block • Complete AV block • Myocardial ischemia or MI • Reperfusion of myocardium • Hypoxia • Inflammatory heart disease (e.g., myocarditis) • Postcardiotomy • Drug toxicity: digitalis	• Protects patient from asystole • Do not suppress	• Treat failure of sinus node • Discontinue digitalis if toxicity is the cause; it is a frequent cause of this rhythm
Junctional tachycardia	• Myocardial ischemia or MI • Reperfusion of myocardium • Inflammatory heart disease • Postcardiotomy • Drug toxicity: digitalis	• Usually stops spontaneously and usually tolerated well	• Treat cause • Discontinue digitalis if toxicity is the cause • Vagal stimulation • Adenosine (Adenocard) • Amiodarone (Cordarone) • β-Blockers or calcium-channel blockers if normal left ventricular function
First-degree AV nodal block	• Normal variation • Myocardial ischemia or MI • Conduction system fibrosis • Inflammatory heart disease (e.g., myocarditis) • Vagal stimulation • Postcardiotomy • Myocardial contusion • Hyperkalemia • Drug toxicity: digitalis, β-blockers, or calcium-channel blockers	• Relatively benign but may progress to second- or third-degree block	• Observe closely for progression of the block • Discontinue digitalis if toxicity is the cause • Drugs or pacemaker not needed unless there is also a sinus bradycardia
Second-degree AV nodal block Mobitz I (Wenckebach)	• Myocardial ischemia or MI • Inferior or posterior MI • Conduction system fibrosis • Inflammatory heart disease • Postcardiotomy • Myocardial contusion • Drug toxicity: digitalis, β-blockers, or calcium-channel blockers	• Block is at AV node • Occurs more often with inferior MI (lesion of the right coronary artery) • Relatively benign: usually transient and does not usually progress to complete heart block	• Does not usually require treatment • Monitor for progression of the block • Discontinue digitalis if toxicity is the cause • Transvenous pacemaker or atropine may be used if the rate is slow and the patient is symptomatic
Second-degree AV nodal block Mobitz II	• Myocardial ischemia or MI • Anterior MI • Hypertension • Valvular heart disease • Conduction system fibrosis • Inflammatory heart disease (e.g., myocarditis) • Postcardiotomy • Myocardial contusion	• Block is at the bundle of His, which accounts for the slight widening of the QRS complex • Occurs more often with anterior MI (lesion of the left anterior descending artery) • Ominous because it often progresses to complete heart block	• Atropine may be used but is not usually helpful • Transcutaneous or transvenous pacemaker

Continued

TABLE **4-14** Basic Dysrhythmia and Block Management—cont'd

Rhythm	Etiology	Significance	Treatment

Third-degree (or complete) AV block	• Myocardial ischemia or MI
	• Conduction system fibrosis
	• Inflammatory heart disease
	• Postcardiotomy
	• Myocardial contusion
	• Hypoxia
	• Electrolyte imbalance: potassium
	• Drug toxicity: digitalis
		• If no escape rhythm is established, the patient has ventricular asystole	• Observe for clinical manifestations of hypoperfusion if inferior MI with junctional escape rhythm
			• Atropine may be used
			• Pacemaker, especially in the presence of the following:
			  • Anterior MI
			  • Inferior MI with ventricular escape rhythm

Left bundle branch block	• Myocardial ischemia or MI • Anterior MI • Fibrodegenerative changes • Postcardiotomy	• Bifascicular block considered more serious than right bundle branch block, especially in the presence of acute MI • Monitor these patients closely during pulmonary artery catheter insertion because trifascicular block may occur	• New left bundle branch block with acute MI may be treated with a prophylactic pacemaker, especially if an AV nodal block is also present
Right bundle branch block	• Myocardial ischemia or MI • Anterior or inferior MI • Fibrodegenerative changes • Postcardiotomy • Pulmonary artery catheter insertion • Acute pulmonary embolus	• None; cardiac output is not affected by delayed ventricular depolarization (i.e., wide QRS)	• Monitor closely for the development of left bundle branch block

Premature ventricular contraction	• Increased sympathetic nervous system stimulation (e.g., endogenous catecholamines, sympathomimetic drugs [e.g., epinephrine, isoproterenol {Isuprel}, dopamine]) {Intropin}
	• Myocardial ischemia or MI
	• Reperfusion of myocardium
	• HF
	• Ventricular aneurysm
	• Cardiomyopathy
	• Hypoxia
	• Acidosis
	• Electrolyte imbalances: potassium, calcium, or magnesium
	• Drug toxicity: digitalis or aminophylline
		• Premature ventricular contractions of most significance may predispose to ventricular tachycardia or ventricular fibrillation:
		  • Frequent (>6/min)
		  • Bigeminal
		  • Multifocal
		  • R-on-T phenomenon
		  • Couplets
		  • Runs of ventricular tachycardia (i.e., three or more premature ventricular contractions in a row)
		• Pulse amplitude of premature ventricular contraction is reduced as a result of decreased filling time
			• Treatment of cause (e.g., oxygen, electrolyte replacement, discontinue digitalis)
			• No treatment required if not significant
			• If frequent or symptomatic: amiodarone (Cordarone), procainamide, lidocaine, and β-blockers

Monomorphic ventricular tachycardia	• Myocardial ischemia or MI • Reperfusion of myocardium • Ventricular aneurysm • Cardiomyopathy • Valvular heart disease • Postcardiotomy • R-on-T premature ventricular contraction • Hypoxia • Acidosis • Electrolyte imbalance: hypokalemia • Drug toxicity: digitalis	• Ominous because it may progress to ventricular fibrillation • Symptoms depend on underlying heart disease, rate, and duration of ventricular tachycardia • May cause angina, HF, or shock	• Treat cause: correct electrolyte imbalance or drug toxicity • Normal left ventricular function: procainamide, amiodarone (Cordarone), lidocaine, or sotalol (Betapace) • Impaired left ventricular function: amiodarone (Cordarone), lidocaine, or cardioversion • If hypotension, chest pain, or pulmonary edema: immediate sedation and cardioversion • If pulseless: treat as ventricular fibrillation (e.g., defibrillation, amiodarone [Cordarone])

TABLE **4-14** Basic Dysrhythmia and Block Management—cont'd

Rhythm	Etiology	Significance	Treatment
Polymorphic ventricular tachycardia (i.e., torsades de pointes if preceded by prolonged QT)	• Class IA antidysrhythmics (e.g., procainamide, quinidine [Cardioquin], disopyramide [Norpace]) • Class III antidysrhythmics (e.g., sotalol [Betapace], amiodarone [Cordarone]) • Tricyclic antidepressants (e.g., amitriptyline [Elavil]) • Phenothiazines (e.g., chlorpromazine [Thorazine]) • Organic insecticides • Electrolyte imbalances: hypomagnesemia, hypocalcemia, or hypokalemia • Congenital long QT syndrome or Brugada syndrome • Marked bradycardia • Hypothermia • Subarachnoid hemorrhage	• No effective perfusion • May go into and out of this rhythm	• Treat cause: treat ischemia or replace electrolytes • Prevent torsades de pointes: monitor the QT interval closely and discontinue any offending drug when the QT prolongs to more than half of the RR interval • Discontinue any offending drugs if characteristic torsades pattern seen • Normal QRS: • Electrolyte replacement • Amiodarone (Cordarone), β-blockers, lidocaine, procainamide, or sotalol (Betapace) • Prolonged QRS (suggests torsades): • Electrolyte replacement (especially magnesium) • Overdrive pacing • Isoproterenol (Isuprel) • Phenytoin (Dilantin) • Lidocaine • Impaired left ventricular function: • Amiodarone (Cordarone) • Lidocaine • Cardioversion
Ventricular fibrillation	• Myocardial ischemia or MI • R-on-T premature ventricular contraction • Electrical shock, including microshock • Brugada syndrome (familial) • Drowning • Hypothermia • Hypoxia • Drug toxicity: digitalis • Dying heart	• Lethal within 4-6 min • No cardiac output • Symptoms include loss of consciousness, pulse, heart sounds, and ventilation; blood pressure changes; and anoxic seizures	• Cardiopulmonary resuscitation until a defibrillator is available and ready and then after defibrillation and between successive defibrillation attempts • Immediate defibrillation (150-200 joules [biphasic energy], 360 joules [monophasic energy]) • Vasopressin or epinephrine • Intubation • Antidysrhythmics: amiodarone or lidocaine • Consideration of therapeutic hypothermia
Idioventricular rhythm	• Vagal stimulation • Failure of higher pacemakers (e.g., ischemia or fibrosis of the conduction system) • Myocardial ischemia or MI • Third-degree AV block • Drug toxicity: digitalis	• Protects the patient from asystole but very unreliable • Do not suppress	• Accelerate higher pacemakers with atropine • Pacemaker • If pulseless: • Cardiopulmonary resuscitation • Epinephrine • Pacemaker • Consider the 6 Hs and the 5 Ts

Continued

TABLE 4-14	Basic Dysrhythmia and Block Management—cont'd		
Rhythm	**Etiology**	**Significance**	**Treatment**
Accelerated idioventricular rhythm	• Failure of higher pacemakers (e.g., ischemia or fibrosis of the conduction system) • Myocardial ischemia or MI • Reperfusion of the myocardium • Drug toxicity: digitalis	• Protects the patient from asystole but very unreliable • Do not suppress	• Accelerate higher pacemakers with atropine • Pacemaker
Asystole	• Vagal stimulation • Myocardial ischemia or MI • Third-degree AV block • Anaphylaxis • Drug overdose • Hypoxia • Acidosis • Shock • Dying heart	• Lethal within 4-6 min • No cardiac output • Symptoms include loss of consciousness, pulse, heart sounds, and ventilation; blood pressure changes; and anoxic seizures	• Cardiopulmonary resuscitation • Epinephrine • Atropine • Pacemaker • Check the rhythm in a second lead to rule out ventricular fibrillation • Consider the 6 Hs and the 5 Ts

(a) Short PR with wide QRS wave
(b) Tachydysrhythmias
3) Aberrant conduction
  a) Aberrant conduction occurs most often in the presence of the following:
    i) Rate is rapid
    ii) Very premature atrial contractions
    iii) There are changes in cycle length (e.g., atrial fibrillation [a QRS wave that ends a short cycle length after a long cycle length is likely to be conducted aberrantly and is referred to as *Ashman phenomenon*])
  b) Because one of the bundle branches (usually the right) is still refractory when a supraventricular impulse reaches it, the impulse must travel down the nonrefractory bundle and across to the other ventricle; this causes a wide QRS wave, which is frequently mistaken for a premature ventricular contraction (PVC) (if a single complex) or ventricular tachycardia (if several complexes in a row)
  c) Unlike ectopy, aberrancy is no more serious than the supraventricular mechanism that caused it (e.g., atrial fibrillation with aberrancy is no more clinically significant than atrial fibrillation)
  d) QRS morphology is the most important criterion for the differentiation between ectopy and aberrancy, but other criteria may also be helpful (Table 4-15); multiple-lead electrocardiography is often helpful to identify P waves and to look at the morphology of the QRS wave
  e) Ectopy is more common than aberrancy; if in doubt, always assume ectopy and treat accordingly

Clinical presentation
1. Anxiety and restlessness
2. Vertigo and syncope
3. Weakness, fatigue, and activity intolerance
4. Palpitations
5. Chest pain
6. Clinical indications of LVF: dyspnea, S_3, and crackles
7. Clinical indications of hypoperfusion (see Table 4-5)
8. Diagnostic
  a. Electrocardiography: multiple-lead ECG
  b. Serum electrolyte levels: may indicate that the cause is an electrolyte imbalance
  c. Drug levels: may indicate that the cause is drug toxicity
  d. ABGs: may indicate that the cause is acidosis or hypoxemia

Collaborative management
1. Continue assessment
  a. Airway, breathing, circulation, and disability (ABCDs)
  b. Vital signs: BP, pulse, respiratory rate, and temperature
  c. Oxygen saturation
  d. Respiratory rate and effort
  e. Cardiac effort and excursion
  f. Clinical indications of hypoperfusion (see Table 4-5)
  g. Pain, discomfort, or dyspnea level
  h. Accurate intake and output
  i. Serum electrolytes
  j. Level of consciousness
  k. Close monitoring for progression of symptoms
2. Provide basic life support (BLS) and advanced cardiac life support (ACLS) as indicated for lethal dysrhythmias
3. Establish and maintain airway, ventilation, and oxygenation
  a. Positioning with the head elevated to 30 to 45 degrees

TABLE 4-15   Differentiation Between Ventricular Ectopy and Aberrancy

Features	Favoring Ventricular Ectopy	Favoring Supraventricular Origin With Aberrancy
Rate	• 130-150 beats/min	• >150 beats/min
Regularity	• Regular	• Irregular (most likely to be atrial fibrillation)
P wave	• None or dissociated (atrioventricular dissociation) • Inverted P wave after QRS (retrograde conduction to atria)	• Premature
QRS width	• >0.14 sec	• 0.12-0.14 sec
QRS morphology	• Initial vector opposite normal beats • Precordial concordance (all QRSs V_1-V_6 positive or all QRSs V_1-V_6 negative) • QRS morphology similar to previously seen premature ventricular complexes	• Initial vector same as normal beats
QRS morphology in V_1 (NOTE: Uppercase letters indicate large waves, and lowercase letters indicate small waves.)	• Monophasic R wave • Rr′ with left peak taller • Biphasic qR interval • Biphasic Rs or rS interval	• Monophasic QS interval • Biphasic rS interval • Triphasic rSR′ or rR′ interval
QRS morphology in V_6 (NOTE: Uppercase letters indicate large waves, and lowercase letters indicate small waves.)	• Monophasic QS interval • Biphasic qR interval • Biphasic rS interval	• Monophasic R wave • Triphasic qRs complex
Fusion beats	• Yes	• No
Compensatory pause after single beat or at end of run	• Yes	• No
Axis	• Indeterminate or left axis deviation of −30 or greater	• Normal or right axis deviation
Patient history	• History of premature ventricular complexes • History of heart disease	• History of premature atrial complexes and atrial fibrillation • History of preexisting bundle branch block
Response to carotid massage	• No effect on ventricular rate	• Often causes at least temporary slowing of ventricular rate
Blood pressure	• Usually very low or absent but may be normal	• Moderately low or normal
Consciousness	• Frequently unconscious but may be conscious	• May complain of lightheadedness
Seizures	• Frequently present but may be absent	• Absent

From Dennison, R. (2007). *Pass CCRN!* (3rd ed.). St. Louis: Mosby.

b. Oxygen by nasal cannula at 2 to 6 L/minute to maintain an SpO$_2$ of 95% unless contraindicated; for patients with COPD, use pulse oximetry to guide oxygen administration to an SpO$_2$ of 90%
c. Endotracheal intubation and mechanical ventilation may be required
4. Maintain adequate circulation and perfusion
   a. Intravenous access with two large-bore catheters for fluid and medication administration
   b. Fluid replacement
     1) Crystalloids: usually 0.9% saline; lactated Ringer solution is contraindicated for patients with liver disease

c. Multiple-lead electrocardiography to help with diagnosis
d. Antidysrhythmic agents as indicated by standing orders or as prescribed
   1) Drugs and treatments of choice for each dysrhythmia (see Table 4-14)
     a) Information about indications, actions, dosage, contraindications, and adverse effects of selected antidysrhythmic agents is included in Appendix E
   2) Close monitoring for adverse effects of antidysrhythmic agents (see Appendix E)

e. Use electrical therapies as indicated
  1) Cardioversion
    a) Uses
      i) Urgent cardioversion is used for tachydys-rhythmias (other than sinus) that are rapid enough to cause hemodynamic compromise or that have not responded to antidysrhythmic drug therapy
      ii) Elective cardioversion is performed for tachydysrhythmias that are reasonably well tolerated hemodynamically but have not responded to antidysrhythmic drug therapy
    b) Contraindications
      i) Tachydysrhythmias that result from digitalis toxicity
      ii) Nonsustained tachydysrhythmias
      iii) Longstanding atrial fibrillation
      iv) Atrial fibrillation with a normal or slow ventricular rate in the absence of AV nodal blocking drugs
      v) Multifocal atrial tachycardia
    c) Method of treatment the same as for defibrillation except in the following situations:
      i) Conscious patients should be sedated with diazepam (Valium), lorazepam (Ativan), or midazolam (Versed)
      ii) Elective procedures should be preceded by at least a 6-hour fast
      iii) Anteroposterior electrode placement is preferable for the cardioversion of atrial fibrillation
      iv) Emergency equipment and drugs must be available
      v) The synchronizer switch should be on so that a charge is delivered only during QRS, thus avoiding the descending limb of the T wave
      vi) Voltage is from 25 to 200 joules

      vii) Antidysrhythmic drug therapy is used after sinus rhythm is restored
    d) Complications: as for defibrillation
  2) Defibrillation: see Cardiopulmonary Arrest
f. Use pacemaker therapies for patients who have problems with impulse formation or conduction
  1) Definition: a pacemaker is an electronic device that delivers an electrical stimulus to the heart to cause the depolarization of the myocardium and to increase or decrease the heart rate
  2) Indications for pacemakers
    a) Sick sinus syndrome with syncope
      i) Symptomatic bradydysrhythmias
      ii) Sinus block or sinus arrest with ventricular asystole
      iii) Alternating tachycardia and bradycardia (called *tachy-brady syndrome*)
    b) Hypersensitive carotid sinus syndrome
    c) AV blocks (Table 4-16)
      i) Second-degree AV block, Mobitz type II
      ii) Third-degree AV block
    d) Bifascicular block with acute MI
    e) Trifascicular block (e.g., bilateral bundle branch block)
    f) Refractory tachydysrhythmias that are unresponsive to drug therapy or cardioversion (referred to as *tachycardia overdrive*); an important treatment modality for torsades de pointes
  3) Components
    a) Pulse generator
      i) Battery
      ii) Circuitry
    b) Leads
      i) Atrial
      ii) Ventricular
    c) Electrodes
      i) Unipolar
        (a) Negative only
        (b) Metal of pulse generator acts as positive

TABLE 4-16   **Indications for Temporary Transvenous Pacemaker in the Presence of Acute Myocardial Infarction**

Degree of Block	Inferior Myocardial Infarction	Anterior Myocardial Infarction
First-degree atrioventricular block	No	No
Second-degree atrioventricular block, type I	No	NA
Second-degree atrioventricular block, type II	NA	Yes
Third-degree atrioventricular block with junctional escape rhythm	No if asymptomatic, Yes if symptomatic	NA
Third-degree atrioventricular block with ventricular escape rhythm	Yes	Yes

NA, Not applicable, because patients with inferior myocardial infarction do not develop type II second-degree block and because patients with anterior myocardial infarction do not develop type I second-degree block or have junctional escape rhythms.
From Dennison, R. (2007). *Pass CCRN!* (3rd ed.). St. Louis: Mosby.

ii) Bipolar
    (a) Positive: proximal; sensing
    (b) Negative: distal; pacing
4) Types of pacemakers
  a) Temporary or permanent
    i) Temporary (external pulse generator): hours to weeks
      (a) Transvenous endocardial (Figure 4-32)
        (i) Pacing leads are inserted percutaneously via the internal jugular or subclavian vein and advanced into the right atria, the right ventricle, or both
      (b) Transcutaneous (Figure 4-33)
        (i) Percutaneous leads are applied to the chest and back; they are used during cardiac arrest until a transvenous pacer can be inserted
  b) Asynchronous versus synchronous
    i) Asynchronous
      (a) Also called *fixed rate*
      (b) The pacemaker delivers a pacing stimulus at a fixed rate, regardless of the heart's intrinsic activity
      (c) Will cause competition with the heart's intrinsic activity; the pacing stimulus may land during the descending limb of the T wave
      (d) Rarely seen today
    ii) Synchronous
      (a) Also called *demand*
      (b) The pacemaker delivers a pacing stimulus only when the heart's

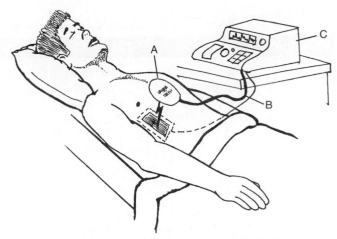

Figure 4-33 Temporary transcutaneous pacing. *A,* Electrode patches (anterior and posterior). *B,* Lead. *C,* Pulse generator. (Drawing by Ann M. Walthall.)

intrinsic pacemaker fails to function at a predetermined rate
      (c) The pacing stimulus will be either inhibited or triggered when the intrinsic activity is seen
5) North American Society of Pacing and Electrophysiology generic codes (Table 4-17) and types of pacemakers (Table 4-18)
  a) Chambers of stimulation
    i) Atrial: AOO and AAI
      (a) Pacing stimulus occurs before the P wave
      (b) Requires an intact AV node
    ii) Ventricular: VOO, VAT, VVI, VVT, and VDD
      (a) Pacing stimulus occurs before the QRS complex
    iii) AV sequential: DOO, DVI, and DDD
      (a) Maintains AV synchrony and the hemodynamic benefit of the atrial kick
      (b) Pacing stimulus before P wave, QRS complex, or both
      (c) Sufficient AV delay is set to allow for atrial depolarization and contraction to complete ventricular filling
    iv) Atriobiventricular (also referred to as *cardiac resynchronization therapy*)
      (a) Used in severe HF in patients with ventricular depolarization asynchrony
      (b) Placement of an LV lead (either placed directly on the left ventricle [epicardial] with a thoracotomy approach or endocardially via the coronary sinus) along with RV and right atrial leads
      (c) An AV delay that is adequate to allow for atrial contraction to contribute optimally to ventricular filling

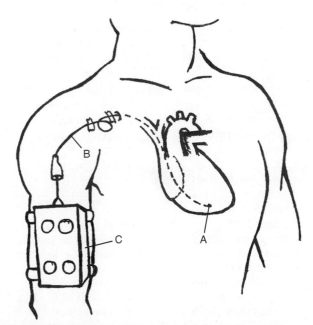

Figure 4-32 Temporary transvenous endocardial pacing. *A,* Electrode. *B,* Lead. *C,* External pulse generator. (Drawing by Ann M. Walthall.)

TABLE **4-17** The NASPE/BPEG Generic (NBG) Pacemaker Code

Position	I	II	III	IV	V
Category	Chamber(s) paced **O** = None **A** = Atrium **V** = Ventricle **D** = Dual (A+V)	Chamber(s) sensed **O** = None **A** = Atrium **V** = Ventricle **D** = Dual (A+V)	Response to sensing **O** = None **T** = Triggered **I** = Inhibited **D** = Dual (T+I)	Programmability, rate modulation **O** = None **P** = Simple Programmable **M** = Multiprogrammable **C** = Communicating **R** = Rate modulation	Antitachyarrhythmia function(s) **O** = None **P** = Pacing (antitachyarrhythmia) **S** = Shock **D** = Dual (P+S)
Manufacturers' designation only	**S** =Single **(A or V)**	**S** =Single **(A or V)**			

NOTE: Positions I through III are used exclusively for antibradyrhythmia function.
From Dennison, R. (2007): *Pass CCRN!* (3rd ed.). St Louis: Mosby, Inc.

TABLE **4-18** Types of Pacemakers

Code	Description	Indications	Advantages	Disadvantages
AOO	Fixed-rate atrial pacer	• Consistently slow sinus rate with intact atrioventricular nodal conduction	• Single lead • Maintains atrioventricular synchrony	• Atrial competition • No protection in case of atrioventricular nodal block
AAI	Demand atrial pacer	• Sick sinus syndrome • Sinus arrest • Sinus bradycardia • Must have intact atrioventricular nodal conduction	• Single lead • Maintains atrioventricular synchrony	• No protection in case of atrioventricular nodal block
VOO	Fixed-rate ventricular pacer	• Complete heart block with slow idioventricular rhythm • Rarely used today	• Single lead • Protection from ventricular asystole	• Ventricular competition with possible stimulation of ventricular dysrhythmias
VAT	Atrial-triggered ventricular pacer	• Complete heart block with intact sinus node	• Synchronized atrioventricular conduction with atrial "kick" optimizes cardiac output • Ventricular rate increases with atrial rate so more exercise responsive	• Two leads • May cause pacemaker-mediated tachycardia: rapid ventricular response in sinus or atrial dysrhythmias
VVI	Demand ventricular pacer	• Sick sinus syndrome • Sinus bradycardia • Sinus arrest • Complete heart block	• Single lead • Simple and reliable • Inexpensive • Protection from ventricular asystole • Little chance of competitive rhythms	• Loss of synchronized atrioventricular conduction and atrial "kick" may reduce cardiac output • Not rate responsive (NOTE: A VVIR is a VVI with rate responsiveness.)

Continued

TABLE **4-18**   Types of Pacemakers—cont'd

Code	Description	Indications	Advantages	Disadvantages
VVT	Pacing stimulus delivered whether needed or not; the stimulus depolarizes the ventricle if there is no intrinsic depolarization; the stimulus lands harmlessly in QRS if intrinsic depolarization is present	• Sick sinus syndrome • Sinus bradycardia • Sinus arrest • Complete heart block	• Single lead • Can evaluate pacer function even if intrinsic activity faster than pacer rate	• Loss of synchronized atrioventricular conduction and atrial "kick" may reduce cardiac output • Not rate responsive • Difficult to evaluate QRS morphology
VDD	Ventricular pacer that can be atrial triggered or inhibited by intrinsic ventricular depolarization	• Sick sinus syndrome • Sinus bradycardia • Sinus arrest • Complete heart block	• Maintains atrioventricular synchrony • If atrial activity is present, pacer functions in atrial triggered mode; if no atrial activity, the device paces the ventricle in demand mode with the inhibition of intrinsic ventricular depolarization	• Two leads • May cause pacemaker-mediated tachycardia • Does not pace the atria, so there may be a loss of atrial contraction if there is no intrinsic atrial activity
DOO	Fixed-rate atrioventricular sequential pacer	• Consistently slow atrial and ventricular rates	• Synchronized atrioventricular conduction with atrial "kick" optimizes cardiac output	• Two leads • Not rate responsive • Atrial and ventricular competition
DVI	Fixed-rate atrial pacer with demand ventricular pacer	• Sick sinus syndrome • Sinus bradycardia • Sinus arrest • Complete heart block	• Synchronized atrioventricular conduction with atrial "kick" optimizes cardiac output	• Two leads • Not rate responsive • Blind to intrinsic atrial activity, so atrial competition and even atrial fibrillation may occur
DDD	Demand atrial and ventricular pacer; ventricular pacing may be atrial triggered or ventricular inhibited	• Sick sinus syndrome • Sinus bradycardia • Sinus arrest • Complete heart block	• Synchronized atrioventricular conduction with atrial "kick" optimizes cardiac output • Near-normal physiologic function	• Two leads • Most expensive • May cause pacemaker-mediated tachycardia • Difficult to troubleshoot • Not used with atrial fibrillation

From Dennison, R. (2007). *Pass CCRN!* (3rd ed.). St. Louis: Mosby.

    (d) The optimal timing of the stimulation of both ventricles; this may be with one ventricle stimulated slightly before the other rather than simultaneously
    (e) May or may not include an implantable cardioverter-defibrillator
  b) Rate-responsive: the heart rate is adjusted according to demands for cardiac output
    i) Heart rate changes are stimulated by changes in muscle activity, minute ventilation, or blood changes in temperature or pH
    ii) Rate-responsive modes: AAIR, VVIR, and DDDR

6) Electrocardiographic evidence of pacing (Figure 4-34)
    a) Spike before paced event
    b) Wide QRS wave if a ventricular pacer is used
    c) Presence of T wave confirms ventricular depolarization
    d) Presence of fusion beats
7) Complications
    a) Infection
    b) Pneumothorax
    c) Myocardial perforation
    d) Hematoma
    e) Frozen shoulder

PACED HEART ACTIVITY

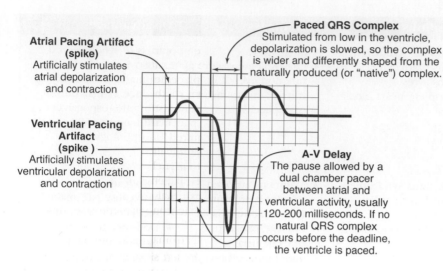

Atrial Pacing Artifact (spike)
Artificially stimulates atrial depolarization and contraction

Paced QRS Complex
Stimulated from low in the ventricle, depolarization is slowed, so the complex is wider and differently shaped from the naturally produced (or "native") complex.

Ventricular Pacing Artifact (spike)
Artificially stimulates ventricular depolarization and contraction

A-V Delay
The pause allowed by a dual chamber pacer between atrial and ventricular activity, usually 120-200 milliseconds. If no natural QRS complex occurs before the deadline, the ventricle is paced.

Figure 4-34 Electrocardiographic evidence of pacing. (From Witherell, C. [1990]. Questions nurses ask about pacemakers. *American Journal of Nursing, 90[12],* 20.)

f) Dysrhythmias
g) Electrical malfunction (Table 4-19)
8) Collaborative management
a) Temporary
   i) Maintain electrical safety
      (a) Ensure the proper grounding of equipment
      (b) Touch side rails before touching patient to discharge static electricity
      (c) Wear rubber gloves when making adjustments
      (d) Avoid sources of electromagnetic interference (e.g., electrocautery, defibrillation, MRI, transcutaneous electrical nerve stimulation units, radiation therapy, lithotripsy)
   ii) Prevent complications
      (a) Cover dial to prevent accidental changes in settings
      (b) Limit the mobility of the affected extremity to prevent accidental catheter dislodgement
      (c) Observe the catheter site for signs of infection
      (d) Assist with the establishment of the pacing threshold and set the milliamperes (mA) slightly above this; it is usually initially set at between 3 and 5 mA, depending on the pacing threshold
      (e) Observe the cardiac monitor for pacemaker malfunction
g. Prepare and care for the patient with an automatic implantable cardioverter-defibrillator
   1) Definition: a cardioverter-defibrillator is an implantable device that provides for the immediate termination of ventricular tachycardia or ventricular fibrillation in patients in

whom these dysrhythmias cannot be pharmacologically or surgically controlled
   2) Tiered therapy (also called *third-generation*) devices have all of the following:
      a) Antitachycardia pacing
      b) Low-energy cardioversion
      c) High-energy defibrillation
      d) Bradycardia backup pacing
   3) Collaborative management
      a) Monitor for dysrhythmias and evaluate the effectiveness of the automatic implantable cardioverter-defibrillator if firing occurs; administer antidysrhythmic agents as prescribed
      b) If cardiopulmonary arrest occurs, do the following:
         i) Obtain emergency equipment and prepare to cardiovert or defibrillate
         ii) Treat the patient as you would any patient who is in cardiopulmonary arrest; do not wait for the device
         iii) Do not place defibrillator paddles within 5 to 10 cm of the generator
         iv) Anteroposterior paddle placement may be more effective
      c) Deactivate the automatic implantable cardioverter-defibrillator with the use of a magnet as requested by the physician
      d) Encourage the patient to express his or her fears and concerns about being shocked; consider referral to support group
5. Treat the cause of the dysrhythmia
   a. Correct ischemia if possible
      1) Coronary artery vasodilators and/or antispasmodics: nitrates, calcium-channel blockers
      2) Fibrinolytics
      3) PCI
   b. Correct hypoxemia and hypoxia

TABLE 4-19 Pacemaker Electrical Malfunctions

Malfunctions	Causes	Interventions
Failure to fire (pace): • Pacemaker does not fire when the need to fire is physiologically indicated • Recognized by pauses longer than the automatic interval and the absence of a pacer spike at the end of the escape interval	• Loose connections • Battery depletion • Lead displacement • Lead fracture • Sensing malfunction (e.g., electromagnetic interference)	• Tighten connections if temporary • Replace battery or pulse generator • Lead repositioning or replacement may be required • Evaluate the patient's own rhythm and the patient's response; if inadequate, administer atropine or apply an external transcutaneous pacemaker; cardiopulmonary resuscitation may be required • May be caused by a sensing malfunction; to identify this, convert the pacemaker to asynchronous by placing a magnet over an implanted pacemaker or by switching to asynchronous on an external pacemaker; if pacer spikes are seen in the asynchronous mode, a sensing malfunction exists • Remove the source of electromagnetic interference
Failure to capture: • Pacemaker fires but depolarization does not occur • Recognized by a spike that is not followed by depolarization (e.g., P wave if atrial pacer l or QRS if ventricular pacer)	• Displacement of lead • Lead fracture • Increased pacing thresholds (e.g., electrolyte imbalance, drug toxicity, acid-base imbalance, ischemia) • Fibrosis or scar tissue at the lead tip • Battery failure • Chamber perforation • Complexes not visible	• Position the patient on the left side or into whatever position he or she was in when the capture was last seen • Increase milliamperes • May require lead repositioning or lead replacement • Replace battery or pulse generator • Check chest radiograph for lead fracture and lead placement • Correct metabolic or electrolyte imbalances • Consider drugs levels and toxicity • Check for diaphragmatic pacing and monitor for cardiac tamponade if catheter perforation is suspected • Change monitoring lead or increase electrocardiogram size (gain) • May require external transcutaneous pacing or cardiopulmonary resuscitation
Failure to sense: • Pacemaker fails to recognize intrinsic activity (e.g., P wave, QRS) • Recognized by pacer spikes that fall closer to the intrinsic beats than to the escape interval; spikes land indiscriminately throughout the cardiac cycle, including potentially on the descending limb of the T wave	• Displacement of lead • Lead fracture • Sensitivity set too low or set on asynchronous • Disconnection of the sensing circuit • Inadequate signal (e.g., low P or QRS voltage) • Battery failure • Increased sensing threshold (e.g., edema or fibrosis at lead tip) • Chamber perforation	• Position patient on the left side or into whatever position he or she was in when the sensing was last seen • Lead repositioning or replacement may be necessary • Make sure that the pacer is not set on asynchronous • Increase sensitivity • Check connections on temporary pacemakers • Administer lidocaine if non-sensed QRSs are premature ventricular contractions • Check the chest radiograph for lead placement or lead fracture • Replace battery or pulse generator • If the patient's own rhythm is adequate, turn the pacer off or turn the heart rate down to minimum • If the patient's own rhythm is inadequate, increase the pacer rate to override the patient's own rhythm
Oversensing: • Pacemaker recognizes extraneous electrical activity or the wrong intrinsic electrical activity as the inhibiting event • Recognized by absence of pacer spikes and failure to fire	• Sensitivity set too high • Electromagnetic interference • Oversensing of P or T waves • Myopotentials • Crosstalk (no ventricular pacing)	• Decrease sensitivity • Remove the electromagnetic interference; ensure that all equipment is properly grounded • Decrease atrial output and ventricular sensitivity and then increase ventricular blanking period • May require external transcutaneous pacing or cardiopulmonary resuscitation

From Dennison, R. (2007). *Pass CCRN!* (3rd ed.). St. Louis: Mosby.

1) Measures to improve SaO_2 (e.g., oxygen, endotracheal intubation, mechanical ventilation, positive end-expiratory pressure)
   2) Measures to improve cardiac output (e.g., inotropes, vasodilators, intra-aortic balloon pumps)
   3) Measures to improve hemoglobin (e.g., blood)
   c. Correct electrolyte imbalances
   1) Replacement of deficient electrolytes
   2) Restriction of excessive electrolyte levels (e.g., electrolyte restriction, diuretics, ion exchange resins, dialysis)
   d. Correct acidosis
   1) Measures to improve oxygen delivery to correct metabolic acidosis caused by lactic acid
   2) Dialysis for patients with renal failure
   3) Hydration and insulin therapy for patients in diabetic ketoacidosis
   4) Improvement of ventilation to correct respiratory acidosis
   e. Eliminate cause of catecholamine release or block effects
   1) Analgesics for pain
   2) Relaxation techniques and anxiolytics for anxiety
   3) β-Blockers for cardioprotection as prescribed

Evaluation

1. Patent airway as well as adequate oxygenation (i.e., normal PaO_2, SpO_2, and SaO_2) and ventilation (i.e., normal $PaCO_2$)
2. Absence of clinical indicators of respiratory distress
3. Absence of clinical indicators of hypoperfusion
4. Alert and oriented with no neurologic deficit
5. Control of chest pain, discomfort, or dyspnea

Typical disposition

1. If evaluation criteria are met: discharge with instructions for follow up
2. If evaluation criteria are not met: admit; may require admission to critical care unit

Cardiopulmonary Arrest

Definition: cardiac arrest followed by ventilatory cessation

Predisposing factors

1. Dysrhythmias
2. Electrical shock
3. Drowning
4. Asphyxiation
5. Trauma
6. Hypothermia
7. Terminal phase of a chronic illness (cardiopulmonary resuscitation [CPR] may not be attempted on these patients in accordance with advanced directives and do-not-resuscitate orders)

Pathophysiology

1. Cardiac arrest stops the delivery of oxygen and the removal of carbon dioxide, thereby causing tissue hypoxia and metabolic (i.e., lactic) acidosis

2. Ventilatory arrest causes hypercapnia, respiratory acidosis, and hypoxemia
3. Eventually the cerebral cortex is irreversibly damaged, and severe neurologic deficit or biologic death occurs

Clinical presentation

1. Loss of consciousness
2. Absence of breathing; agonal breathing may be a precursor to cardiopulmonary arrest
3. Absence of central pulses
4. Absence of auscultated or palpated BP
5. Anoxic seizures may occur
6. Urinary and bowel incontinence may occur
7. Electrocardiography findings
   a. Most commonly ventricular fibrillation
   b. Less commonly ventricular tachycardia
   c. Rarely asystole
   d. Cardiopulmonary arrest with a stable electrical rhythm (referred to as *pulseless electrical activity*)

Collaborative management

1. Continue assessment throughout resuscitation
   a. ABCDs
   b. Vital signs: BP, pulse, respiratory rate, and temperature
   c. Oxygen saturation
   d. Respiratory effort and excursion
   e. Cardiac rate and rhythm
   f. Clinical indications of hypoperfusion (see Table 4-5)
   g. Pain, discomfort, or dyspnea level
   h. Accurate intake and output
   i. Serum electrolytes
   j. Level of consciousness
   k. Close monitoring for the progression of symptoms
2. Initiate CPR (Table 4-20)
3. Provide basic life support (BLS) as recommended by current American Heart Association (AHA) guidelines
   a. Responsiveness: establish unresponsiveness and then call for the resuscitation team
   b. Airway and ventilation
   1) Open airway with the use of the head-tilt/chin-lift maneuver; the jaw-thrust maneuver is used if cervical spine injury is suspected
   2) Evaluate ventilation by looking for the rise and fall of the chest and by listening and feeling for airflow for no more than 10 seconds
      a) If the patient is adequately breathing, position him or her on his or her left side in recovery position
      b) If the patient is not breathing or is breathing inadequately, provide ventilation by delivering 2 breaths (each >1 second) of 500 to 600 ml using any of the following methods:
         i) Mouth-to-mask ventilation
         ii) Manual resuscitation with a bag-valve-mask device secured over the nose and mouth

TABLE 4-20 Primary and Secondary Survey in Cardiopulmonary Arrest

	Primary Survey	Secondary Survey
Focus	Cardiopulmonary resuscitation and defibrillation	Assessment and treatment
A	Open the airway	Use of invasive airways
B	Deliver ventilations	Assess for adequate oxygenation and ventilation
C	Perform chest compressions	Establish intravenous access, diagnose rhythm disturbances, and administer drugs
D	Defibrillate	Diagnosis: search for and treat reversible causes

Source: American Heart Association. *Advanced cardiac life support manual.* Dallas: American Heart Association.

  iii) Manual resuscitation with a bag attached to an endotracheal (ET) tube or a tracheostomy tube if it is already in place
 c) Note that each rescue breath does make the chest rise
  i) If the chest does not rise when the first breath is delivered, perform the head-tilt/chin-lift maneuver again before repeating the attempt to deliver the breath
 d) Maintain a ventilator rate of 10 to 12 breaths/minute in adults and 12 to 20 breaths/minute in infants and children; hyperventilation is associated with poor survival rates
 c. Circulation
  1) Assess for signs of circulation (e.g., adequate breathing, coughing, movement, carotid pulse) for no more than 10 seconds
  2) If there is no pulse, deliver compressions
   a) Place the heel of one hand over the lower half of sternum; place the other hand over the first hand
   b) Compress the sternum at a depth of 1½ to 2 inches in adults and one third to one half the depth of the chest in children and infants at a rate of 100 per minute
    i) New guidelines emphasize that the provider push hard and fast, allowing the chest to completely recoil after each compression
    ii) The compression ratio is 30:2 for CPR that a single lay rescuer provides to adults, children, and infants (excluding newborns); for children and infants, if two health care providers are present, the ratio is 15:2
   c) Do not interrupt chest compressions for 2 minutes (i.e., 5 cycles of 30 compressions to 2 breaths)
    i) Advanced airway interventions (e.g., endotracheal tube, laryngeal mask airway [LAM™], Combitube™) should be performed while compressions are in progress; compressions should be maintained without pauses for ventilation
 d. Coordination of compressions and ventilation

  1) Maintain a ratio of 30 compressions to 2 ventilations for one or two rescuers treating adults
 e. Considerations
  1) CPR that is performed expertly provides only 20% of normal cardiac output, but most of this goes to the upper body, including the heart and brain
  2) Mortality rates increase despite prompt CPR if ACLS is delayed beyond 12 minutes
  3) The resistance of ventricular dysrhythmias to defibrillation occurs over time; prompt defibrillation is critical to survival
4. Provide ACLS as recommended by current AHA guidelines
 a. Use ACLS algorithms to provide assistance with decision making during a cardiopulmonary arrest (Figures 4-35 through 4-40)
 b. Identify and treat the cause of cardiac arrest; this is especially important during the treatment of pulseless electrical activity
  1) The 6 Hs: hypovolemia, hypoxia, hydrogen ion, hyper/hypokalemia, hypoglycemia, and hypothermia
  2) The 5 Ts: toxins, tamponade, tension pneumothorax, thrombosis, and trauma
 c. Electrical therapies to change an abnormal cardiac rhythm to a normal one
  1) Principle: by delivering a shock of sufficient strength, a critical mass of myocardium is depolarized simultaneously, thus allowing for the emergence of a dominant normal rhythm
  2) Precordial thump
   a) Note that the current AHA guidelines provide no recommendation for or against the use of a precordial thump for ACLS providers because there are no prospective studies that evaluate its efficacy
   b) Uses
    i) For witnessed ventricular fibrillation or pulseless ventricular tachycardia only if a defibrillator is not immediately available; do not allow the delivery of a precordial thump in adults to delay defibrillation
    ii) For ventricular tachycardia with a pulse only if a defibrillator and pacemaker are readily available, because deterioration to ventricular fibrillation or asystole may occur

Pulseless VT/VF Algorithm

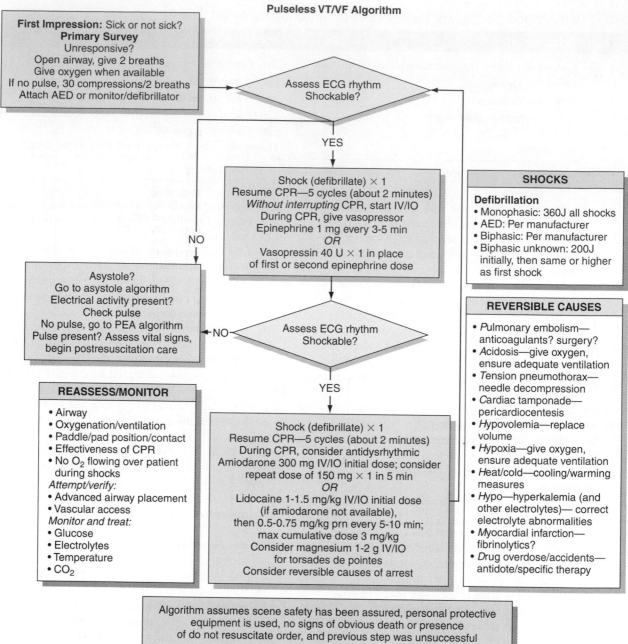

Figure 4-35 Pulseless ventricular tachycardia/ventricular fibrillation algorithm. (From Aehlert, B. [2007]. *ACLS study guide* [3rd ed.]. St. Louis: Mosby.)

iii) For use only early for ventricular dysrhythmias; precordial thump delivers minimal voltage ($\approx$25 joules) so it is only likely to be effective if the duration of the ventricular dysrhythmia is short

c) Method: a solitary thump with the heel of the hand is delivered to the mid sternum from a height of 8 to 12 inches (not recommended for pediatric patients)

3) Defibrillation: defibrillation should be performed for ventricular fibrillation or pulseless ventricular tachycardia within 3 minutes

a) Uses
   i) Pulseless ventricular tachycardia and ventricular fibrillation
   ii) Unstable or refractory ventricular tachycardia with a pulse

b) Method for manual defibrillation
   i) Check the pulse: make sure that the ventricular fibrillation pattern is not merely artifact caused by a loose electrocardiography electrode
   ii) Remove any foil-lined patches from the patient's chest (e.g., nitroglycerin [NTG]

Asystole/Pulseless Electrical Activity Algorithm

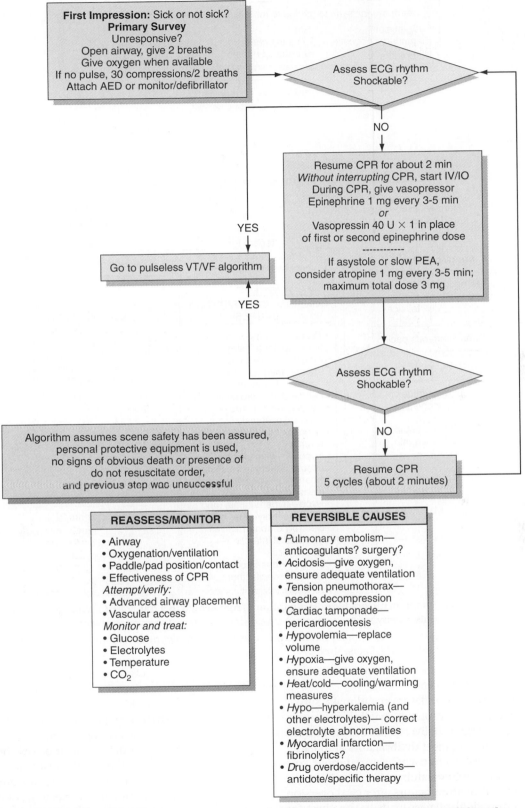

Figure 4-36 Asystole/pulseless electrical activity algorithm. (From Aehlert, B. [2007]. *ACLS study guide* [3rd ed.]. St. Louis: Mosby.)

Symptomatic Bradycardia

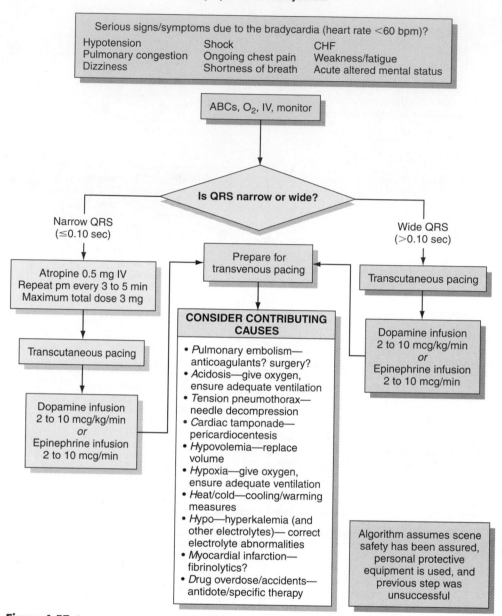

Figure 4-37 Symptomatic bradycardia algorithm. (From Aehlert, B. [2007]. *ACLS study guide* [3rd ed.]. St. Louis: Mosby.)

patches) because they may cause arcing and patient burns

iii) Turn the defibrillator on and make sure that the synchronizer switch is off so that the charge is delivered as soon as buttons are pushed; most defibrillators automatically reset to nonsynchronized mode so you can immediately defibrillate if ventricular fibrillation occurs after cardioversion

iv) Apply defibrillation pads to the chest for paddle placement, or apply conductive jelly to the paddles

(a) Anterior: one paddle is placed to the right of the sternum below the right

clavicle, and the other paddle is placed lateral to the apex in the left midaxillary line

(b) Anteroposterior: the anterior paddle is placed over the apex and the posterior paddle is placed below the right scapula; this paddle placement may be better for obese patients, patients with hyperinflated lungs (e.g., COPD), and for patients with an automatic implantable cardioverter-defibrillator (AICD)

(c) Pacemakers

(i) For patients with permanent pacemakers, the paddles should

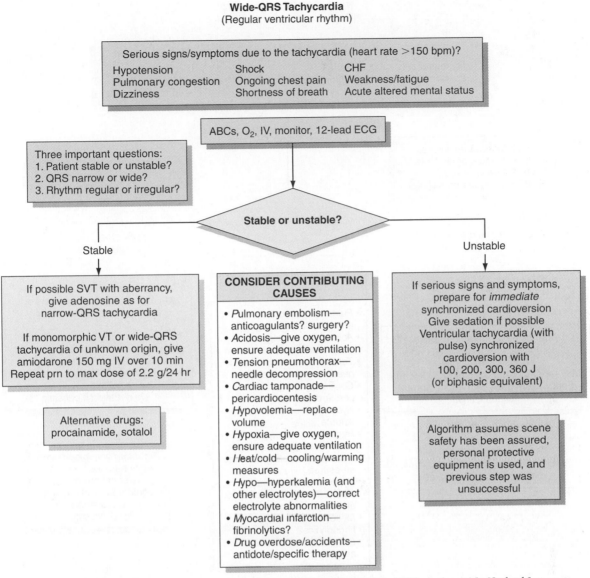

Wide-QRS Tachycardia
(Regular ventricular rhythm)

Serious signs/symptoms due to the tachycardia (heart rate >150 bpm)?

Hypotension	Shock	CHF
Pulmonary congestion	Ongoing chest pain	Weakness/fatigue
Dizziness	Shortness of breath	Acute altered mental status

ABCs, O₂, IV, monitor, 12-lead ECG

Three important questions:
1. Patient stable or unstable?
2. QRS narrow or wide?
3. Rhythm regular or irregular?

Stable or unstable?

Stable

Unstable

If possible SVT with aberrancy, give adenosine as for narrow-QRS tachycardia

If monomorphic VT or wide-QRS tachycardia of unknown origin, give amiodarone 150 mg IV over 10 min Repeat prn to max dose of 2.2 g/24 hr

Alternative drugs: procainamide, sotalol

CONSIDER CONTRIBUTING CAUSES

- *P*ulmonary embolism—anticoagulants? surgery?
- *A*cidosis—give oxygen, ensure adequate ventilation
- *T*ension pneumothorax—needle decompression
- *C*ardiac tamponade—pericardiocentesis
- *H*ypovolemia—replace volume
- *H*ypoxia—give oxygen, ensure adequate ventilation
- *H*eat/cold—cooling/warming measures
- *H*ypo—hyperkalemia (and other electrolytes)—correct electrolyte abnormalities
- *M*yocardial infarction—fibrinolytics?
- *D*rug overdose/accidents—antidote/specific therapy

If serious signs and symptoms, prepare for *immediate* synchronized cardioversion Give sedation if possible Ventricular tachycardia (with pulse) synchronized cardioversion with 100, 200, 300, 360 J (or biphasic equivalent)

Algorithm assumes scene safety has been assured, personal protective equipment is used, and previous step was unsuccessful

Figure 4-38 Wide-QRS tachycardia algorithm. (From Aehlert, B. [2007]. *ACLS study guide* [3rd ed.]. St. Louis: Mosby.)

not be placed within 5 to 10 cm of the pulse generator because this may interfere with the delivery of electricity during defibrillation
  (ii) Turn temporary pacemaker pulse generator off during defibrillation
v) Charge to appropriate voltage for defibrillation
  (a) Biphasic: 100 to 200 joules in adults (see manufacturer instructors for the defibrillator)
  (b) Monophasic: 360 joules in adults
  (c) For pediatric patients, use 2 joules/kg initially, then increase to 4 joules/kg

vi) Apply paddles to defibrillation pads or jellied paddles to chest with the use of firm (≈25 pounds) pressure in the adult patient
vii) For pediatric patients who weigh <10 kg, use infant or small paddles; if the patients weighs >10 kg, use large or adult paddles
viii) Say the word "clear," and ensure that no one is touching the patient or the bed
ix) Press both discharge buttons simultaneously
x) Resume CPR, beginning with chest compressions; note that current guidelines recommend only one shock before resuming CPR
xi) Recheck the rhythm after five cycles of CPR (≈2 minutes)

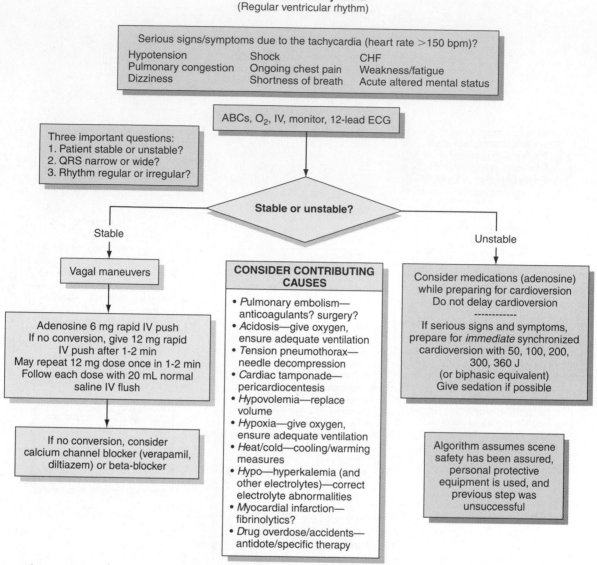

Figure 4-39 Narrow-QRS tachycardia algorithm. (From Aehlert, B. [2007]. *ACLS study guide* [3rd ed.]. St. Louis: Mosby.)

(a) If rhythm and pulse are restored, administer antidysrhythmic drug therapy

(b) If rhythm and pulse are not restored, continue with appropriate algorithm

c) Successful defibrillation is less likely if any of the following are present:
  i) Hypoxia
  ii) Severe acidosis
  iii) Alkalosis
  iv) Electrolyte imbalance
  v) Ischemia
  vi) Long duration of ventricular fibrillation

d) Complications
  i) Dysrhythmias: asystole, bradycardia, AV blocks, or ventricular fibrillation
  ii) Hypotension
  iii) Myocardial damage

  iv) Pulmonary edema
  v) Emboli
  vi) Muscle pain
  vii) Skin burns

4) Temporary pacemaker: for patients who have problems with impulse formation or conduction
  a) Transcutaneous pacemaker
    i) Large surface skin electrodes are applied anteriorly and posteriorly
      (a) Posterior: positive electrode applied between the spine and the left scapula at the level of the heart
      (b) Anterior: negative electrode applied at the left fourth intercostal space at the MCL
    ii) This may be painful for the patient and should be replaced by a transvenous lead as soon as possible

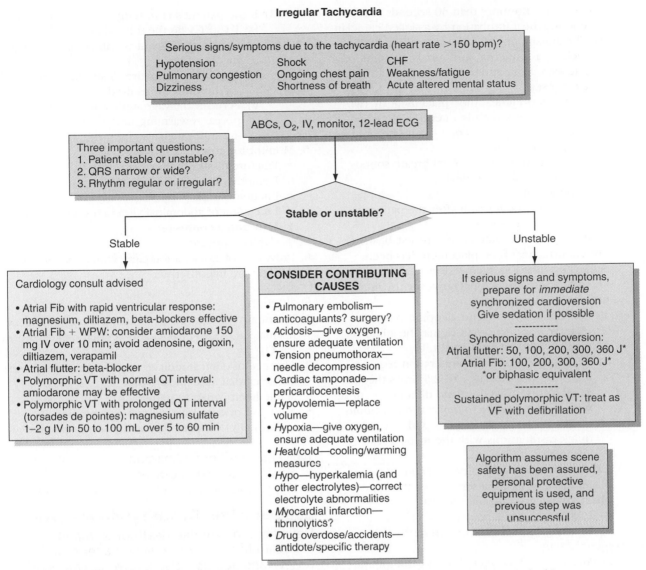

Irregular Tachycardia

Serious signs/symptoms due to the tachycardia (heart rate >150 bpm)?

Hypotension	Shock	CHF
Pulmonary congestion	Ongoing chest pain	Weakness/fatigue
Dizziness	Shortness of breath	Acute altered mental status

ABCs, O₂, IV, monitor, 12-lead ECG

Three important questions:
1. Patient stable or unstable?
2. QRS narrow or wide?
3. Rhythm regular or irregular?

Stable or unstable?

Stable

Unstable

Cardiology consult advised

• Atrial Fib with rapid ventricular response: magnesium, diltiazem, beta-blockers effective
• Atrial Fib + WPW: consider amiodarone 150 mg IV over 10 min; avoid adenosine, digoxin, diltiazem, verapamil
• Atrial flutter: beta-blocker
• Polymorphic VT with normal QT interval: amiodarone may be effective
• Polymorphic VT with prolonged QT interval (torsades de pointes): magnesium sulfate 1–2 g IV in 50 to 100 mL over 5 to 60 min

CONSIDER CONTRIBUTING CAUSES

• *P*ulmonary embolism—anticoagulants? surgery?
• *A*cidosis—give oxygen, ensure adequate ventilation
• *T*ension pneumothorax—needle decompression
• *C*ardiac tamponade—pericardiocentesis
• *H*ypovolemia—replace volume
• *H*ypoxia—give oxygen, ensure adequate ventilation
• *H*eat/cold—cooling/warming measures
• *H*ypo—hyperkalemia (and other electrolytes)—correct electrolyte abnormalities
• *M*yocardial infarction—fibrinolytics?
• *D*rug overdose/accidents—antidote/specific therapy

If serious signs and symptoms, prepare for *immediate* synchronized cardioversion Give sedation if possible
----
Synchronized cardioversion:
Atrial flutter: 50, 100, 200, 300, 360 J*
Atrial Fib: 100, 200, 300, 360 J*
*or biphasic equivalent

Sustained polymorphic VT: treat as VF with defibrillation

Algorithm assumes scene safety has been assured, personal protective equipment is used, and previous step was unsuccessful

Figure 4-40 Irregular tachycardia algorithm. (From Aehlert, B. [2007]. *ACLS study guide* [3rd ed.]. St. Louis: Mosby.)

b) Transvenous pacemaker
   i) The lead is threaded into the apex of the right ventricle via the subclavian or internal jugular vein
d. Intravenous access
   1) Establish the patency of any existing central or peripheral intravenous or heparin lock; if a central venous catheter is in place when the arrest occurs, it should be used to administer drugs during the resuscitation
   2) Antecubital or external jugular veins are preferred if a venous catheter or additional venous catheters must be established
      a) Peak drug concentrations are lower and circulation times are longer when drugs are administered via peripheral sites as compared with central sites
      b) If peripheral venous access is used for resuscitation drugs, administer bolus drugs

rapidly, follow them with 20 ml of saline, and elevate the extremity for 10 to 20 seconds
   3) Central venous cannulation may be performed
      a) The major disadvantage of central venous cannulation during cardiopulmonary arrest is the need to stop CPR
         i) Internal jugular and subclavian sites require the cessation of CPR
         ii) Femoral vein cannulation does not require the cessation of CPR
   4) Distal wrist and hand veins and distal saphenous veins in the legs are the least favorable sites for drug administration during CPR
e. Endotracheal intubation
   1) Attempt as soon as is feasible; however, defibrillation and the administration of epinephrine are the first and second priorities
   2) Hyperventilation with 100% oxygen should precede any intubation attempt

3) Stop CPR for no more than 30 seconds to allow for endotracheal intubation by a skilled clinician
   a) The advantages of endotracheal intubation include a reduction in the risks of vomiting and aspiration and the provision of a relative airway seal
4) Confirm endotracheal tube placement by two methods, one of which is an end tidal carbon dioxide indicator; the second method should be one of the following:
   a) Listening for equal bilateral breath sounds
   b) Esophageal detector device
   c) Capnography
5) Obtain a chest radiograph after the patient is stabilized
6) If an intravenous route cannot be established but endotracheal tube placement has been achieved, some emergency drugs can be given via the endotracheal tube; however, the intravenous route is preferred
   a) Epinephrine, lidocaine, atropine, naloxone (Narcan), and vasopressin may be administered via the endotracheal tube
   b) Endotracheal tube administration requires adjusting the dose to 2 to 2.5 times the usual intravenous dose and diluting the drug with isotonic saline to make a total volume of at least 10 ml; follow this with several quick insufflations with the manual resuscitation bag
7) Two alternative rescue airway techniques are placed orally and are inserted past the hypopharynx but not into the trachea
   a) Laryngeal mask airway (LMA™)
   b) Esophageal-tracheal Combitube™
f. Oxygen therapy
   1) Administer 100% oxygen during cardiopulmonary arrest with a bag-valve-mask device; a reservoir bag or tubing attached to the bag-valve-mask device is required to achieve as high a concentration of oxygen as possible
   2) Remember that there is no contraindication to 100% oxygen during cardiopulmonary arrest
g. Intravenous fluids: normal saline is used to maintain adequate preload and to mix intravenous drug infusions
h. Pharmacologic agents as indicated in algorithms (see Figures 4-35 through 4-40); specific drug information is available in Appendix E
i. Treatment of hypothermia if the patient's body temperature is 86°F to 93°F (30°C to 34°C)
   1). Initial treatment: perform CPR
   a) A single defibrillation attempt for ventricular fibrillation or pulseless ventricular tachycardia and medications are given at longer intervals
   b) Intubate the patient and ventilate with warm humidified oxygen
   c) Obtain intravenous access and administer warmed intravenous saline

2) If the patient's core temperature is less than 86°F (30°C), do the following
   a) Continue CPR but withhold intravenous medications
   b) Continue with warm inspired oxygen and warm intravenous fluids
   c) Peritoneal lavage with warm saline, extracorporeal rewarming, and esophageal rewarming tubes may also be used
5. Monitor for complications of CPR
   a. Fracture of sternum or ribs
   b. Hemothorax
   c. Pneumothorax
   d. Laceration of abdominal viscera (especially the liver)
   e. Myocardial contusion
   f. Cardiac rupture
6. Provide postresuscitation care, which may include therapeutic hypothermia

Evaluation
1. Patent airway as well as adequate oxygenation (i.e., normal PaO_2, SpO_2, SaO_2) and ventilation (i.e., normal $PaCO_2$)
2. Absence of clinical indicators of respiratory distress
3. Stable cardiac rate and rhythm
4. Stable hemodynamic status
5. Alert and oriented with no neurologic deficit
6. Control of chest pain, discomfort, or dyspnea

Typical disposition: admission
1. Admission to critical care unit
2. Preparation for emergent surgery may be required

Sudden Infant Death Syndrome (SIDS)
Definition: the sudden death of an infant <1 year old that is unexplained after examination, review, and autopsy; also known as *crib death* or *cot death*
Predisposing factors: unknown, although there are several theories
1. Brainstem abnormalities
2. Prone sleeping position that causes hypoxia and hypercapnia
3. Abnormal respiratory control and arousal responsiveness
4. Cardiac arrhythmias
5. Metabolic disorders or defects
6. Infections
7. Genetics

Pathophysiology
1. Unknown, although there are characteristic findings noted during postmortem examinations
   a. Frothy discharge from the mouth and nostrils that is occasionally blood tinged
   b. Petechiae may be found on the lungs, heart, and thymus
   c. Pulmonary edema may be present
   d. Markers of hypoxia

Clinical presentation

1. Subjective
   a. Family reports finding infant not breathing
   b. No history of trauma or illness
2. Objective
   a. Apnea
   b. Absence of pulse and BP
3. Diagnostic
   a. Postmortem laboratory tests to rule out other causes
   b. Radiographs to rule out child abuse

Collaborative management

1. Continue assessment throughout resuscitation
   a. ABCDs
   b. Vital signs: BP, pulse, respiratory rate, and temperature
   c. Oxygen saturation
   d. Respiratory effort and excursion
   e. Cardiac rate and rhythm
   f. Level of consciousness
   g. Close monitoring for progression of symptoms
2. Initiate CPR
   a. Basic life support and pediatric life support as appropriate
   b. Family presence: bring the family to the bedside during resuscitation efforts
3. Provide support to the family after resuscitation efforts
   a. Offer to let the family hold the infant
   b. Provide the family with mementos (e.g., lock of hair, footprint)
   c. Reassure the family that it is not their fault
   d. Provide a private area for the family if they would like one
   e. Offer to call the family's religious leader or a representative from pastoral care

Evaluation

1. Appropriate support of family
2. Available resources provided to family

Typical disposition

1. Prepare the family for the autopsy and the release of the body to the funeral home
2. Refer the family to counseling services and support groups
3. Refer the family for genetic counseling and testing if indicated

Coronary Artery Disease/Acute Coronary Syndrome

Definitions

1. CAD: a progressive disease of the coronary arteries that results in their narrowing or obstruction
2. Acute coronary syndrome: a syndrome of acute myocardial ischemia caused by atherosclerotic plaque rupture and thrombus formation; prolonged ischemia can cause necrosis; types include the following:
   a. Non-ST elevation
      1) Prolonged resting chest pain (>20 minutes) within the previous 24 hours without sustained ST segment elevation of >1 mm
         a) Unstable angina: may have ST segment depression
         b) Non-ST elevation MI (NSTEMI): positive creatine kinase, myocardial bound (CK-MB), troponin, or both
      2) Pathophysiology: the partial occlusion of a coronary artery with a platelet-rich thrombus
      3) The goal is to prevent progression to complete occlusion of the coronary artery and resultant ST segment elevation MI
      4) Collaborative management
         a) Close monitoring for progression
         b) Platelet aggregation inhibitors (e.g., aspirin, glycoprotein IIb/IIIa inhibitors) and anticoagulants (e.g., low-molecular-weight heparin [e.g., enoxaparin; Lovenox]) may be used
         c) β-Blockers
         d) Nitrates
         e) PCI
   b. ST elevation
      1) Prolonged resting chest pain (>20 minutes) within the previous 24 hours with ST segment elevation
      2) ST segment elevation MI
         a) Evidence of infarction: ST elevation of >2 mm in leads V_1, V_2, and V_3 and of >1 mm in other leads
         b) Non–Q-wave MI: patient does not develop pathologic Q waves
         c) Q-wave MI: patient does eventually (within 12 to 24 hours) develop pathologic Q waves
      3) Pathophysiology: the complete occlusion of a coronary artery by a thrombus
      4) Goal: restore blood flow
      5) Collaborative management
         a) Aspirin and β-blockers
         b) Reperfusion therapy (e.g., acute PCI, fibrinolytics) followed by therapies to maintain patency (e.g., aspirin, glycoprotein IIb/IIIa inhibitors, anticoagulants)
         c) Nitrates
         d) ACE inhibitors

Predisposing factors: cardiac risk factors increase the incidence of premature CAD

3. Nonmodifiable risk factors
   a. Heredity: when siblings or parents develop CAD before the age of 55 years; several other risk factors also involve a genetic predisposition (e.g., hypertension, hyperlipidemia, diabetes mellitus)
   b. Advancing age: men, >45 years; women, >55 years
   c. Gender: males have twice the risk of premenopausal females; risk increases in women after menopause

4. Modifiable risk factors
   a. Hypertension: BP >140/90 mm Hg
   b. Hyperlipidemia: elevated levels of cholesterol, triglycerides, and low-density lipoproteins or decreased levels of high-density lipoproteins; desirable levels of lipids are as follows:
      1) Cholesterol level <200 mg/dl
      2) Low-density lipoprotein level <100 mg/dl for patients with heart disease or diabetes mellitus; <130 mg/dl for patients with two or more risk factors; <160 mg/dl for patients with only one risk factor
      3) High-density lipoprotein level >40 mg/dl
      4) Triglyceride level <110 mg/dl
   c. Smoking: smoking increases platelet aggregation and fibrinogen levels and may cause vasospasm; elevated carbon monoxide levels decrease the oxygen-carrying capacity of hemoglobin; complete smoking cessation is desired
   d. Diabetes mellitus or glucose intolerance: the control of blood glucose in patients with diabetes mellitus is advocated to control the risk of sequelae, including CAD; the desirable fasting glucose level is <150 mg/dl
   e. Hyperhomocysteinemia: homocysteine level of >14 μmol/L
      1) Homocysteine is an essential sulfur-containing amino acid that is formed during the processing of dietary protein; elevated levels are toxic to the vascular endothelium and increase coagulability
      2) Deficiencies of folate, vitamin B_{12}, and vitamin B_6 have all been implicated in elevated levels of homocysteine; these levels may be successfully reduced with the use of folate, vitamin B_{12}, or pyridoxine therapy
   f. Sedentary lifestyle: exercise is inversely related to cardiovascular mortality; sedentary people also tend to be obese
   g. Stress
      1) Chronic stress promotes the long-term development of CAD
      2) Acute stress increases catecholamine levels, myocardial oxygen consumption, and dysrhythmia potential
   h. Obesity: body weight that is >120% of ideal body weight; ideal body weight is desirable
      1) Obesity also contributes to hypertension, hyperlipidemia, glucose intolerance, and a sedentary lifestyle
      2) Midline fat is of greater risk than hip and thigh fat (i.e., apple shape versus pear shape)
   i. Oral contraceptives increase the risk of MI, especially in smokers; they also may increase BP

Pathophysiology

1. Arteriosclerosis: a group of diseases that are characterized by a thickening and loss of elasticity (calcification) of the arterial walls
2. Atherosclerosis: the most common form of arteriosclerosis
   a. A chronic disease process that is characterized by the buildup of fatty plaque along the subintimal layer of the arteries and that leads to a decrease in the arterial lumen
   b. Progression (Figure 4-41)
      1) Fatty streak: a yellow, smooth lesion of lipid
         a) Injury to the endothelial cells that line the lumen of the artery
            i) The arteries that are the most likely to be affected include the coronary arteries, the aorta, the cerebral arteries, and the arterial bifurcations
         b) The permeability of the endothelial cells to fatty acids and triglycerides increases
         c) Initiation of the inflammatory/immune response
         d) Release of vasoactive peptides; accumulation of macrophages and platelets
      2) Fibrous plaque: a raised, yellow lesion with collagen accumulation
         a) Smooth muscle proliferation occurs

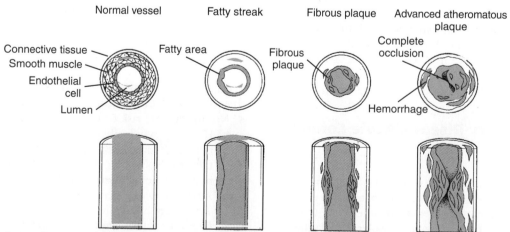

Figure 4-41 Progression of atherosclerosis. (From Urden, L. D., Lough, M. E., & Stacy, K. M. [1998]. *Critical care nursing: Diagnosis and management* [3rd ed.]. St. Louis: Mosby.)

3) Complicated lesion: a calcified lesion with ulceration, rupture, or hemorrhage
   a) Platelet aggregation to the injured arterial endothelium caused by the irregular surface of the intima leads to thrombosis
   b) Decrease in arterial lumen and arterial elasticity
   c) Decreased blood flow distal to the lesion
3. Decreased blood flow and oxygen supply to the myocardium lead to an imbalance between oxygen supply and oxygen demand
   a. Gradual or partial occlusion: ischemia that causes angina
      1) Demand angina is caused by 75% occlusion of the coronary artery lumen; angina at rest is caused by 99% occlusion
   b. Sudden or complete occlusion: necrosis that causes MI
4. Pathologic consequences of atherosclerosis and arteriosclerosis
   a. Angina pectoris
   b. MI
   c. HF
   d. Dysrhythmias caused by ischemia
   e. Sudden death

Collaborative management

1. Continue assessment
   a. ABCDs
   b. Vital signs: BP, pulse, respiratory rate, and temperature
   c. Oxygen saturation
   d. Respiratory effort and excursion
   e. Cardiac rate and rhythm
   f. Discomfort and pain level
   g. Accurate intake and output
   h. Serum electrolytes
   i. Level of consciousness
   j. Close monitoring for the progression of symptoms
2. Establish and maintain airway, oxygenation, and ventilation
   a. Position the patient with the head elevated to 30 to 45 degrees
   b. Oxygen by nasal cannula at 2 to 6 L/minute to maintain an SpO_2 of 95% unless contraindicated; for patients with COPD, use pulse oximetry to guide oxygen administration to an SpO_2 of 90%
3. Maintain adequate circulation and perfusion
   a. Intravenous access if indicated for fluid and medication administration
   b. Antidysrhythmics as prescribed
   c. Platelet aggregation inhibitors, anticoagulants, and fibrinolytics as prescribed
   d. PCI: prepare the patient if required
4. Control chest pain, discomfort, and anxiety
   a. Differentiation of acute chest pain (Figure 4-42)
   b. Coronary vasodilators (e.g., nitroglycerin [NTG; Tridil]) if indicated
   c. Narcotic analgesics if indicated
   d. Antiemetics if indicated
   e. Anxiolytics if indicated
5. Encourage a healthy lifestyle
   a. Well-balanced diet to maintain normal weight
      1) Low in saturated fat and transfatty acids while including monounsaturated fats (e.g., olive oil, canola oil)
      2) High in fiber
         a) Fresh fruit and vegetables
         b) Whole grains
      3) Adequate low-fat proteins
   b. Adequate rest and relaxation
   c. Regular exercise
6. Provide information about the treatment of CAD (as time allows)
   a. Nonpharmacologic and pharmacologic methods to reduce risk factors
   b. Monitoring for the progression of the disease with the use of stress tests and cardiac catheterization as indicated
   c. Treatment of fixed lesions; PCI or coronary artery bypass grafting may be used

Evaluation

1. Patent airway as well as adequate oxygenation (i.e., normal PaO_2, SpO_2, SaO_2) and ventilation (i.e., normal $PaCO_2$)
2. Absence of clinical indicators of respiratory distress
3. Absence of clinical indicators of hypoperfusion
4. Control of pain, discomfort, and dyspnea
5. Alert and oriented with no neurologic deficit

Typical disposition

1. If evaluation criteria met: discharge with instructions for follow up for further cardiac testing and treatment
2. If evaluation criteria not met: admission to step-down unit, critical care unit, or catheterization laboratory for PCI

Angina Pectoris

Definition: transient chest pain associated with myocardial ischemia

Predisposing factors

1. Factors that decrease supply
   a. Arteriosclerosis or atherosclerosis
   b. Coronary artery spasm
   c. Aortitis
   d. Dysrhythmias
   e. Anemia
   f. Shock
2. Factors that increase demand
   a. Hypertension
   b. Aortic valve disease
   c. Tachydysrhythmias
   d. HF
   e. Hyperthyroidism

Ischemic Chest Pain/Discomfort Algorithm

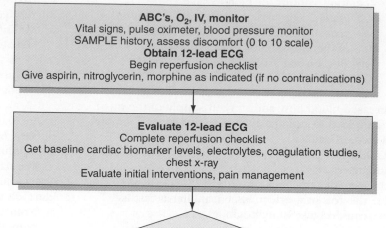

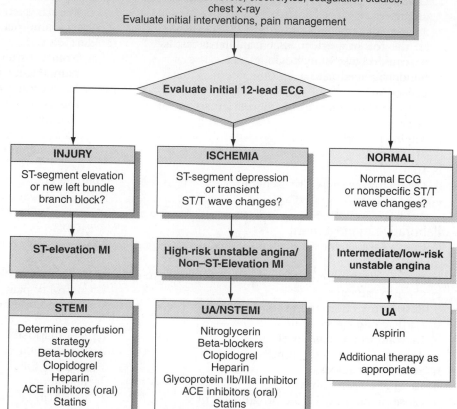

Figure 4-42 Ischemic chest pain/discomfort algorithm. (From Aehlert, B. [2007]. *ACLS study guide* [3rd ed.]. St. Louis: Mosby.)

Pathophysiology

1. There is a temporary imbalance between myocardial oxygen supply and myocardial oxygen demand that causes ischemia
   a. Common precipitating factors: the 5 E's plus smoking
      1) Exercise: volume work (e.g., walking, running)
      2) Exertion: pressure work (e.g., lifting, pushing, Valsalva maneuver)
      3) Emotion: catecholamine release
      4) Eating: shunting of blood to gut
      5) Exposure to cold: vasoconstriction
      6) Smoking
         a) Nicotine increases heart rate and BP
         b) Carbon monoxide decreases the oxygen-carrying capacity of hemoglobin
2. Ischemia leads to anaerobic metabolism and the accumulation of lactic acid, which causes chest pain

Clinical presentation

1. Subjective
   a. Substernal chest discomfort that usually lasts 1 to 4 minutes but that may last up to 15 minutes and that subsides with rest or nitroglycerin (NTG [Tridil])
      1) Discomfort may be described as burning, squeezing, tightness, pressure, heaviness, indigestion, aching, or indigestion
      2) Pain may radiate to shoulders, back, arms, jaw, neck, or epigastrium
      3) Precipitating factors: the 5 E's plus smoking
   b. Dyspnea
   c. Nausea and vomiting
   d. Anxiety
   e. Weakness
2. Objective
   a. Tachycardia
   b. Hypotension or hypertension

c. Tachypnea

d. Levine sign: clenched fist held over sternum

e. Pallor

f. Diaphoresis

g. S_4

3. Diagnostic

a. Cardiac markers (i.e., CK-MB, troponin): negative for cardiac damage

b. Lipid profile: to identify hyperlipidemia as a cardiac risk factor

c. Serum glucose level: to identify diabetes mellitus or glucose intolerance as a risk factor; however, serum glucose is likely to be elevated as a result of stress hormones

d. Complete blood cell count with differential: may show a decrease in hemoglobin as a cause of anemia-induced angina

e. ECG
   1) ST segment depression in unstable angina
   2) ST segment elevation in variant angina
   3) Ventricular dysrhythmias may be present
   4) Pathologic Q waves may be present, thus indicating previous MI

f. Echocardiography: may show segmental wall motion defects

4. Types (Table 4-21)

Collaborative management

1. Continue assessment

   a. ABCDs

   b. Vital signs: BP, pulse, respiratory rate, and temperature

   c. Oxygen saturation

   d. Respiratory effort and excursion

   e. Cardiac rate and rhythm

   f. Chest pain or discomfort

   g. Level of consciousness

   h. Accurate intake and output

   i. Close monitoring for the progression of symptoms

2. Increase oxygen supply to the heart

   a. Oxygen by nasal cannula at 2 to 6 L/minute to maintain an SpO_2 of 95% unless contraindicated; for patients with COPD, use pulse oximetry to guide oxygen administration to an SpO_2 of 90%

   b. Calcium-channel blockers (e.g., nifedipine [Procardia]) or NTG for variant angina

   c. Blood transfusion if angina is caused by anemia

   d. Dysrhythmia management
      1) Tachydysrhythmias decrease the time required for coronary artery filling and may decrease cardiac output

TABLE 4-21 Types of Angina

Type of Angina	Signs and Symptoms
Stable angina	• Unchanging frequency, duration, and severity • Predictable to the patient • ST segment depression may occur during pain
Unstable Angina • De Novo Angina	• Angina of New Onset
• Crescendo angina: angina that has increased in frequency, intensity, or duration • Preinfarction angina: angina of prolonged duration that occurs even at rest	• Associated with the progression of coronary artery disease • Less exertion to cause pain or pain at rest • Greater severity • Longer duration • More difficult to relieve and may not be relieved with nitroglycerin • May have ST segment depression during pain
• Wellens syndrome: critical proximal stenosis of left anterior descending coronary artery	• Associated with critical proximal stenosis of left anterior descending coronary artery • Characteristic electrocardiogram changes that appear even when the patient is pain free • ST segment isoelectric or elevated no more than 1 mm in V_1-V_3 • Symmetric T wave inversion in V_2 and V_3 • No loss of normal R wave progression in V_1-V_3 • No pathologic Q waves • Normal or slightly elevated enzyme levels • Emergency cardiac catheterization is indicated
• Variant angina (also called *Prinzmetal angina* or *vasospastic angina*): angina related to coronary artery spasm	• Associated with coronary artery spasm • Pain occurs at rest • May be caused by tobacco, alcohol, or cocaine • Pain lasts longer than usual anginal pain (i.e., ≥10 min) • ST segment elevation during pain

Adapted from Dennison, R. (2007). *Pass CCRN!* (3rd ed.). St. Louis: Mosby.

2) Bradydysrhythmias increase the time required for coronary artery filling but may decrease cardiac output

   e. Platelet aggregation inhibitors (e.g., aspirin, ticlopidine [Ticlid]); heparin may be prescribed to prevent clotting or to stop the extension of a clot

   f. PCI (Table 4-22): prepare the patient as required

3. Relieve chest pain

   a. NTG

     1) Effects

       a) NTG in doses of <1 mcg/kg/minute is predominantly a venous dilator; it decreases the myocardial workload and myocardial oxygen consumption by decreasing the preload

       b) NTG in doses of >1 mcg/kg/minute is an arterial as well as a venous dilator; it decreases the myocardial workload and myocardial oxygen consumption by decreasing both the afterload and the preload

     2) Route

       a) Usually sublingual tablets or metered-dose spray; one dose every 3 to 5 minutes for up to three doses

       b) Intravenous NTG for unstable angina or for chest pain that is not relieved after three doses of sublingual NTG

     3) Caution: do not give NTG if erectile dysfunction medication has been taken within the last 36 hours because the two medications together can cause severe hypotension and a decreased level of consciousness

   b. Morphine sulfate may be required for unstable angina

4. Decrease oxygen demand

   a. Removal of provoking factors

     1) Cease activity immediately when chest pain occurs

     2) Bed rest during pain; semi-Fowler position is usually the most comfortable for the patient

   b. NTG as prescribed

   c. β-Blockers (e.g., metoprolol [Lopressor]) as prescribed

     1) β-Blockers decrease myocardial workload and myocardial oxygen demand by decreasing heart rate and contractility

     2) β-Blockers are contraindicated in patients with variant angina and ischemia/infarction associated with cocaine; blocking β receptors leaves α receptors unopposed and perpetuates vascular spasm

   d. Control of dysrhythmias: tachydysrhythmias increase myocardial workload and myocardial oxygen consumption

---

TABLE 4-22   Percutaneous Coronary Interventions

Procedures	• *Percutaneous transluminal coronary angioplasty:* the inflation of a balloon-tipped catheter in an area of coronary artery stenosis caused by plaque; the plaque is pushed back against the wall of the vessel and fractured (i.e., controlled trauma)
	• *Coronary artery stent:* the use of a metalcoil that acts as a scaffolding device to support a coronary artery and to maintain patency after percutaneous transluminal coronary angioplasty; previously used only in cases of acute closure; most percutaneous transluminal coronary angioplasty procedures currently include planned stent placements
	• *Coronary atherectomy:* the removal of plaque from a coronary artery with the use of a high-speed diamond-tipped (rotational) or shaving (directional) device
	  • *Directional coronary atherectomy:* a directional device shaves pieces of the atheroma into the catheter tip
	  • *Coronary rotational ablation (Rotablator):* a diamond-coated burr drills through the atheroma and pulverizes the plaque
	  • *Transluminal extraction catheter:* a motorized cutting head shaves the atheroma from the arterial wall and suctions out the pieces
	  • *Excimer laser coronary atherectomy:* the use of a laser to vaporize the atheroma
	  • *AngioJet:* a high-speed saline jet that is most effective for the treatment of thrombus

Indications	• Unstable or chronic angina • Acute or postacute myocardial infarction • Postcoronary artery bypass graft with postoperative angina • Patient must be a surgical candidate in the case of coronary artery dissection
Contraindications	• Left main coronary artery disease (unless there is a patent bypass around this condition, it is referred to as *protected*) • Stenosis of the coronary artery at an orifice • Variant angina • Critical valvular disease
Action	The goal of percutaneous coronary intervention is to reduce the degree of coronary artery stenosis; the intervention is considered successful if the degree of stenosis is reduced to 20%–30% without serious complications.

Adapted from Dennison, R. (2007). *Pass CCRN!* (3rd ed.). St. Louis: Mosby.

e. Control of catecholamine release
   1) Establish and maintain a calm, quiet environment
   2) Keep the patient and his or her family informed
   3) Restrict stimulants
5. Monitor for complications
   a. Progression to MI
   b. Dysrhythmias
   c. Mitral regurgitation caused by ischemia and the dysfunction of papillary muscles
   d. HF

Evaluation
1. Patent airway as well as adequate oxygenation (i.e., normal PaO_2, SpO_2, SaO_2) and ventilation (i.e., normal $PaCO_2$)
2. Absence of clinical indicators of respiratory distress
3. Absence of clinical indicators of hypoperfusion
4. Alert and oriented with no neurologic deficit
5. Control of chest pain, discomfort, or dyspnea

Typical disposition
1. If evaluation criteria met: discharge with instructions for follow up for further cardiac testing and treatment; patient teaching and counseling should include the following:
   a. Identify risk factors and encourage their modification to decelerate arteriosclerotic or atherosclerotic process
   b. Educate the patient regarding the use of NTG tablets or spray
      1) One dose every 3 to 5 minutes for a maximum of three doses; if no relief 5 minutes after first dose, call 911
      2) Do not take NTG within 36 hours of taking erectile dysfunction medications because this may precipitate severe hypotension
2. If evaluation criteria not met: admission to step-down unit, critical care unit, or catheterization laboratory for PCI

Myocardial Infarction
Definition: the death of a portion of the myocardium

Predisposing factors
1. Arteriosclerosis or atherosclerosis
2. Coronary artery thrombosis
3. A combination of these factors: most MIs are caused by atherosclerosis and thrombosis
4. Coronary artery spasm
5. Cocaine induced: excessive SNS stimulation causes tachycardia, hypertension, and arterial vasoconstriction and spasm; coronary artery spasm may cause MI, especially non–Q-wave infarction
6. Other, less-commonly seen causes
   a. Severe prolonged hypotension
   b. Chest trauma (e.g., myocardial contusion)
   c. Trauma to the coronary arteries
   d. Aortic stenosis or insufficiency

e. Thyrotoxicosis
f. Blood dyscrasias
g. Aortic dissection
h. Arteritis
i. Carbon monoxide poisoning

Pathophysiology
1. Atherosclerosis with unstable plaque
2. Plaque rupture may be caused by inflammation or infection
   a. C-reactive protein: a biochemical byproduct that rises rapidly after an inflammatory response; it stimulates the release and expression of inflammatory mediators, and it has been found in atheromatous plaques
3. Platelet aggregation and blood coagulation
4. Coronary artery occlusion
5. Prolonged imbalance between myocardial oxygen supply and demand
6. Inadequate oxygenation causes anaerobic metabolism
7. Anaerobic metabolism causes lactic acidosis
8. Prolonged ischemia causes the electrical and mechanical death of myocardium
9. Contractility and compliance are decreased, thus causing LV dysfunction
10. Ischemia, injury, and acidosis cause electrical irritability; this potentially leads to PVCs, ventricular tachycardia, and ventricular fibrillation
11. Healing takes approximately 2 to 3 months; a firm, white scar is formed, but it does not contract or conduct electrical impulses

Classifications of MIs
1. Non–ST segment elevation MI versus ST segment elevation MI: ST segment indicates actual injury to the myocardium
2. Q wave versus non–Q wave: presence of Q wave correlates to a mass loss of myocardium so that significant loss of myocardium will cause a Q wave while loss of a small area of myocardium will not cause a Q wave
   a. Non–Q-wave infarctions: partial occlusion or early reperfusion
      1) Spontaneous reperfusion: the cessation of spasm or endogenous tissue plasminogen activator
      2) Therapeutic reperfusion: fibrinolytics or PCI
3. Left versus right: Table 4-23 describes the wall of MI along with the coronary artery that is affected, indicative ECG leads, and anticipated complications
4. Factors that affect mortality
   a. Age
   b. LV ejection fraction
   c. Number of occluded vessels
   d. History of MI
   e. Presence of cardiogenic shock: associated with a loss of 40% of LV muscle mass; may be from one MI or several cumulative MIs

TABLE 4-23 Myocardial Infarction Summary

Coronary Artery	Location of Infarct	Indicative Electrocardiogram Leads	Anticipated Complications

Left main coronary artery	Extensive anterior	V₁–V₆	• Sudden cardiac death
			• Dysrhythmias, especially the following:
			  • Sinus tachycardia
			  • Atrial dysrhythmias
			  • Ventricular dysrhythmias
			• Blocks
			  • First-degree atrioventricular block
			  • Second-degree atrioventricular block Mobitz type II
			  • Third-degree atrioventricular block with ventricular escape
			  • Bundle branch block
			• Ventricular rupture
			• Ventricular septal defect
			• Ventricular aneurysm
			• Heart failure
			• Cardiogenic shock

Left anterior descending artery	Septal	V₁ and V₂	• Dysrhythmias, especially the following:
			  • Sinus tachycardia
			  • Atrial fibrillation
			  • Ventricular dysrhythmias
			• Blocks
			  • First-degree atrioventricular block
			  • Second-degree atrioventricular block Mobitz type II
			  • Third-degree atrioventricular block with ventricular escape
			  • Bundle branch block
			• Ventricular septal rupture

	Anterior	V₃ and V₄	• Dysrhythmias, especially the following:
			  • Sinus tachycardia
			  • Atrial fibrillation
			  • Ventricular dysrhythmias
			• Blocks
			  • First-degree atrioventricular block
			  • Second-degree atrioventricular block Mobitz type II
			  • Third-degree atrioventricular block with ventricular escape
			  • Bundle branch block
			• Ventricular aneurysm
			• Heart failure
			• Cardiogenic shock

Left circumflex artery	Lateral	High: I and aVL Low: V₅ and V₆	• Dysrhythmias • Heart failure

Right coronary artery	Inferior	II, III, and aVF	• Dysrhythmias, especially the following:
			  • Sinus bradycardia
			  • Sinus arrest
			  • Junctional rhythms
			  • Ventricular dysrhythmias
			• Blocks
			  • Sinoatrial blocks
			  • First-degree atrioventricular block
			  • Second-degree atrioventricular block Mobitz type I
			  • Third-degree atrioventricular block, usually with atrioventricular junctional escape
			  • Bundle branch block
			• Papillary muscle rupture
			• Heart failure

TABLE 4-23   Myocardial Infarction Summary—cont'd

Coronary Artery	Location of Infarct	Indicative Electrocardiogram Leads	Anticipated Complications

	Posterior	Reciprocal changes in V_1 and V_2; indicative changes in V_7–V_9 (especially V_8 and V_9)	• Dysrhythmias, especially the following:
			  • Sinus bradycardia
			  • Sinus arrest
			  • Junctional rhythms
			  • Ventricular dysrhythmias
			• Blocks
			  • First-degree atrioventricular block
			  • Second-degree atrioventricular block Mobitz type I
			  • Third-degree atrioventricular block, usually with atrioventricular junctional escape
			• Papillary muscle rupture with acute mitral regurgitation

	Right ventricular	V_4R–V_6R (especially V_4R)	• Dysrhythmias, especially the following:
			  • Sinus bradycardia
			  • Sinus arrest
			  • Junctional rhythms
			  • Ventricular dysrhythmias
			• Blocks
			  • First-degree atrioventricular block
			  • Second-degree atrioventricular block Mobitz type I
			  • Third-degree atrioventricular block, usually with atrioventricular junctional escape
			  • Bundle branch block
			• Papillary muscle rupture with acute tricuspid regurgitation
			• Right ventricular failure

From Dennison, R. (2007). *Pass CCRN!* (3rd ed.). St. Louis: Mosby.

f. NOTE: women have twice the mortality of men; this is probably related to the fact that women tend to be older and to have more significant risk factors (e.g., diabetes mellitus, hypertension) when they develop their MIs

Clinical presentation
1. Subjective
   a. Pain: 75% to 85% of all patients with MI have pain
      1) Provocation: emotional or physical stress; may occur at rest
      2) Palliation: not relieved by oxygen, rest, or nitrates; relieved by narcotics or reperfusion (e.g., fibrinolytics, PCI)
      3) Quality
         a) Frequently prescribed as pressure on the chest
         b) May also be described as knife-like, stabbing, burning, or indigestion
         c) May feel like usual anginal pain but more severe
         d) Atypical pain is common among women
         e) If described as tearing or ripping, consider the possibility of a dissecting aortic aneurysm
      4) Region and radiation
         a) The primary location is usually the chest, but it may be epigastric, especially with inferior MI
         b) Radiation is usually to the left arm, the left elbow, the left shoulder, both arms, or the jaw
         c) If pain is radiating to the back, consider the possibility of a dissecting aortic aneurysm
      5) Severity: from vague, slight discomfort to severe pain; it will be more intense than the patient's typical anginal pain
      6) Timing
         a) Most MIs occur within 3 hours of awakening
         b) The pain is continuous from onset, with duration of ≥20 minutes
         c) Pain that comes and goes for as long as several days before the actual MI is referred to as a *stuttering MI pattern;* intermittent pain before continuous pain is *preinfarction angina*
   b. Silent MI: as many as 25% of all patients with MI have no pain
      1) More likely to occur in the older adult or diabetic patient; patients do not have pain with MI after cardiac transplantation because the transplanted heart is denervated
      2) Clues that suggest a possible silent MI: new-onset HF or an acute change in mental status, unexplained abdominal pain, or unexplained dyspnea or fatigue

c. Associated symptoms
   1) Nausea and vomiting: seen more often with inferior or posterior MI
   2) Dyspnea or orthopnea: seen more often with anterior MI
   3) Diaphoresis
   4) Palpitations
   5) Apprehension
2. Objective
   a. Heart rate and rhythm
      1) Tachycardia: seen more often with anterior MI
      2) Bradycardia: seen more often with inferior MI
   b. Normotension, hypotension, and hypertension
      1) Hypertension: seen more often with anterior MI
      2) Hypotension: seen more often with inferior MI
      3) Equality in arms: inequality in arms indicates a possible dissecting thoracic aortic aneurysm
   c. Tachypnea
   d. Elevated temperature: may occur 48 to 72 hours after MI
   e. Levine sign: clenched fist held over sternum
   f. May have JVD: indicative of RVF and commonly seen with RV infarction
   g. May have abnormal PMI: downward and lateral displacement
   h. Heart sound changes
      1) May have diminished heart sounds; this is related to decreased contractility
      2) May have S_4: indicative of LV noncompliance; this is common for the first 24 hours
      3) May have S_3: this is an early sign of LVF
      4) May have pericardial friction rub: this is indicative of pericarditis
      5) Murmurs indicate valve dysfunction
      6) Muffled sounds indicate effusion or cardiac tamponade
   i. May have carotid, aortic, or femoral bruits
   j. May have clinical indications of hypoperfusion (see Table 4-5)
   k. May have clinical indications of HF
      1) LVF (e.g., S_3, crackles, dyspnea) with LV infarction

   2) RVF (e.g., JVD, hepatomegaly, peripheral edema) with RV infarction
3. Diagnostic
   a. Leukocyte count: increased (usually 12,000 to 15,000 mm^3) at 48 to 72 hours
   b. Erythrocyte sedimentation rate: increased at 48 to 72 hours
   c. C-reactive protein: increased with acute MI
   d. Diagnostic studies for cell injury (Table 4-24)
      1) Increased serum enzymes
         a) Creatine kinase: elevation (usually twice the normal level with MI) occurs 4 to 6 hours after MI, peaks 24 hours later, and returns to normal after about 3 days; an early creatine kinase peak is an indication of successful reperfusion
         b) Lactate dehydrogenase (LDH): elevation occurs within 24 hours after MI, peaks at 72 hours, and returns to normal within 2 weeks; may be particularly valuable for the evaluation of patients who delay seeking medical attention for 2 or more days
      2) Positive serum isoenzymes
         a) Creatine kinase: positive CK-MB (>4%) is indicative of MI; this is a highly specific test for MI
            i) Electrophoresis technique: traditional CK-MB; this is not usually diagnostic for 8 to 24 hours after onset of pain
         b) LDH: normally $LDH_2 > LDH_1$; $LDH_1 > LDH_2$ (referred to as *flipped LDH*) is indicative of MI; this does not occur until 48 to 72 hours after the onset of pain
      3) Increased serum muscle proteins
         a) Myoglobin: muscle protein; high sensitivity but low specificity; excellent early negative predictive value
         b) Troponin: contractile protein
            i) Cardiac troponin I: found only in cardiac muscle; more specific but later rise and peak

TABLE 4-24 Laboratory Diagnostic Tests for Acute MI

Test	Normal Values	Time to Rise (After Injury)	Peak (After Injury)	Return to Normal (After Injury)
CK	Men: 55–170 U/L Women: 30–135 U/L	4–6 hours	24 hours	3–4 days
CK-MB	0% of total CK	6–10 hours	12–24 hours	2–3 days
LDH	90–200 IU/L	24–48 hours	72 hours	8–14 days
LDH$_1$	17%–25% of total LDH	8–24 hours	72 hours	8–14 days
Myoglobin	<85 ng/ml	1–4 hours	6–12 hours	1–2 days
Cardiac troponin I	<1.5 ng/ml	3–6 hours	24 hours	5–12 days
Cardiac troponin T	<0.1 ng/ml	3–4 hours	12–48 hours	2–3 weeks

CK, Creatine kinase; *CK-MB,* creatine kinase (myocardial bound); *LDH,* ʟ-lactate dehydrogenase.
Adapted from Dennison, R. (2007). *Pass CCRN!* (3rd ed.). St. Louis: Mosby.

ii) Cardiac troponin T: found in cardiac muscle as well as skeletal muscle; less specific than cardiac troponin I, especially in patients with renal failure, but earlier rise and peak

4. Electrocardiography (ECG)
   a. As a diagnostic tool for acute MI, it is most helpful when things are clearly abnormal
      1) If the initial echocardiogram is nondiagnostic, repeat ECG should be performed every 30 minutes until pain ceases or until the ECG is clearly diagnostic and definitive therapy can be initiated
      2) The typical criteria for prompt reperfusion therapies (e.g., PCI, fibrinolytics) with acute MI include either of the following:
         a) ST segment elevation of >1 mm in at least two contiguous leads
         b) New left bundle branch block
5. Echocardiography
   a. Normal wall motion: strong predictor of nonischemic pain
   b. Reduced wall motion: strong predictor of acute occlusion
   c. May show mechanical complications (e.g., ventricular septal defect, papillary muscle rupture)
6. Chest radiograph: may show cardiomegaly or indications of HF
7. Cardiac catheterization: will likely show coronary artery occlusion; PCI may be performed after diagnosis

Collaborative management

1. Continue assessment
   a. ABCDs
   b. Vital signs: BP, pulse, respiratory rate, and temperature
   c. Oxygen saturation
   d. Respiratory effort and excursion
   e. Cardiac rate and rhythm
   f. Hemodynamic status: indications for invasive hemodynamic monitoring in patients with acute MI include the following:
      1) Persistent chest pain
      2) Persistent tachycardia
      3) Significant hypertension or hypotension
      4) Significant LVF or RVF
      5) Intravenous inotropic or vasoactive agents
      6) New systolic murmur
   g. Discomfort and pain level
   h. Bleeding if receiving fibrinolytics and anticoagulants
   i. Accurate intake and output
   j. Serum electrolytes
   k. Level of consciousness
   l. Close monitoring for the progression of symptoms
      1) S_3 and crackles indicative of LVF
      2) S_3, crackles, and hypotension indicative of cardiogenic shock

2. Manage cardiopulmonary arrest if needed; ventricular fibrillation frequently occurs within 1 hour of infarction
   a. Basic life support (BLS) or ACLS
   b. Intravenous access
   c. Advanced airway management as indicated; rapid-sequence intubation may be required with rapid-sequence premedication
3. Reduce the size of the MI: myocardial salvaging techniques
   a. Treat pain promptly and adequately: this decreases catecholamine release and myocardial oxygen demand
      1) Morphine sulfate: 2 to 4 mg intravenously every 5 minutes until pain is relieved
         a) Actions: decreases preload; decreases catecholamine release via pain relief (which decreases heart rate and afterload); decreases anxiety and restlessness
         b) Cautions: inferior MI; RV MI
      2) NTG (Tridil): may be given prophylactically at 25 to 100 mcg/minute intravenously for 24 to 48 hours
         a) Actions
            i) Decreases preload to decrease myocardial oxygen demand
            ii) Dilates epicardial coronary vessels to increase myocardial oxygen supply
            iii) Augments the analgesic effect of morphine
         b) Caution: may cause reflex tachycardia; β-blockers may be needed
      3) Reperfusion therapies (e.g., fibrinolytics, PCI): these relieve pain by reestablishing blood flow and aerobic metabolism
      4) Intra-aortic balloon pump: may be used for intractable pain because it increases coronary artery perfusion pressure
   b. Increase myocardial oxygen supply
      1) Administer oxygen to maintain an SpO_2 of 95%, which is generally achieved with the use of a nasal cannula and an administration rate of 2 to 6 L/minute
         a) In patients with COPD and chronic hypercapnia, maintain an SpO_2 of approximately 90%
      2) Provide either emergent PCI or fibrinolytics to reestablish the patency of the infarct-related artery within the benchmark time frame
         a) PCI is preferred (especially for older adult patients) if a cardiac catheterization laboratory is available to provide the opening of the infarct-related artery within 60 minutes (i.e., door, data, diagnosis, balloon); if not, fibrinolytics are used and should be administered within 30 minutes (i.e., door, data, diagnosis, drug) (Table 4-25)
         b) Either primary PCI or fibrinolytics are preceded by platelet aggregation inhibitors, anticoagulants, or both

TABLE 4-25 Fibrinolytic Therapy

Actions	• Activates plasminogen to plasmin, which is the active agent that breaks down clots (i.e., it speeds up the normal fibrinolytic process to allow for early reperfusion)
	• Limits cellular necrosis and decreases infarction size
	• Decreases mortality and morbidity
	  • Short term: reestablishes arterial patency
	  • Long term: maintains ejection fraction

Fibrinolytic agents	• Streptokinase (Streptase): rarely used today
	• Recombinant tissue plasminogen activator
	  • Alteplase (Activase): short half-life so administered as a bolus followed by infusion
	  • Tenecteplase (TNKase): longest half-life so administered as a one-time bolus
	• Recombinant plasminogen activator
	  • Reteplase (Retavase): intermediate half-life so administered as two boluses 10 min apart
	• Urokinase (Abbokinase): rarely used with acute myocardial infarction but frequently used to treat peripheral arterial occlusion

Indications	• History that is strongly suggestive of myocardial infarction • ST segment elevation of more than 1 mm in at least two contiguous leads or new left bundle branch block • Pain of <6 hours or still having pain (NOTE: As long as the patient is having pain, salvageable myocardium is assumed, because dead myocardium does not metabolize aerobically or anaerobically and thus neither lactic acid nor pain would be produced.)
Absolute contraindications	• Active internal bleeding • History of hemorrhagic stroke, intracranial neoplasm, atrioventricular malformation, or aneurysm • Intracranial or intraspinal surgery or trauma within 2 months • Known bleeding disorder (e.g., thrombocytopenia, hemophilia) • Suspected aortic aneurysm or acute pericarditis • Systolic blood pressure ≥200 mm Hg, diastolic blood pressure ≥120 mm Hg, or both • Prolonged (i.e., >10 min) or traumatic cardiopulmonary resuscitation • Pregnancy • Streptokinase (Streptase) is contraindicated if the patient has received the drug or had a streptococcal infection within the last 6-9 months; however, tissue plasminogen activator can still be used
Relative contraindications	• Major surgery or trauma within 10 days • Recent gastrointestinal or genitourinary bleeding • Cerebrovascular disease • Oral anticoagulant therapy • Systolic blood pressure ≥180 mm Hg, diastolic blood pressure ≥110 mm Hg, or both • Significant liver dysfunction • Septic thrombophlebitis • Subacute bacterial endocarditis • High likelihood of left heart thrombus (e.g., mitral stenosis with atrial fibrillation, ventricular aneurysm, left atrial myxoma) • Diabetic hemorrhagic retinopathy • Advanced age (>70-75 years) with consideration of physiologic age, severity of concomitant diseases, and mental status • Any condition with which bleeding would be a significant hazard or would be difficult to manage (e.g., recent femoral artery puncture or sheath)

Clinical indications of reperfusion	• Pain cessation
	• ST segment return to baseline
	• Reperfusion dysrhythmias
	  • Sinus bradycardia
	  • Idioventricular rhythm and accelerated idioventricular rhythm
	  • Atrioventricular blocks
	  • Ventricular irritability: premature ventricular contractions, ventricular tachycardia, and ventricular fibrillation
	• Creatine kinase washout: early or markedly elevated creatine kinase peak

TABLE 4-25 Fibrinolytic Therapy—cont'd

Assessment	• Heart rate • Blood pressure • Electrocardiogram rhythm; note reperfusion dysrhythmias • Clinical indications of reperfusion • Bleeding (e.g., puncture points, gums, saliva, sputum, gastric secretions, stools, urine) • Complaints of chest pain, back pain, or headache

Brief summary of nursing management	• Administer adjuvant therapy: tissue plasminogen activator followed by aspirin and heparin (Heparin sodium)
	• Monitor for clinical indications of reperfusion; notify the physician if these are not seen so that emergent percutaneous coronary intervention can be scheduled
	• Avoid punctures: arterial, intravenous, intramuscular, and subcutaneous
	  • Apply pressure until hemostasis is achieved if punctures are required after fibrinolytics have been initiated
	  • Insert multiple (usually two or three) intravenous catheters before the initiation of fibrinolytic therapy; one of these catheters may be used for venous sampling
	• Monitor stools, urine, emesis, sputum, and saliva for blood
	• Monitor for complications

Complications	• Hemorrhage
	  • At site of vascular puncture: 80% incidence
	  • Gastrointestinal or genitourinary bleeding: 15%–20% incidence
	  • Intracranial bleed: 1% incidence
	• Reocclusion: monitor for new pain, ST segment changes, or both
	• Allergic reactions to streptokinase
	  • Monitor for urticaria, fever, bronchospasm, dyspnea, stridor, or dysrhythmias
	  • Administer diphenhydramine (Benadryl), hydrocortisone (Solu-Cortef), or both as prescribed in an attempt to prevent allergic reaction
	• Reperfusion dysrhythmias: usually transient
	  • Administer antidysrhythmics or perform cardioversion or defibrillation as indicated for sustained ventricular tachycardia or ventricular fibrillation (prophylactic antidysrhythmics are no longer recommended with fibrinolytic therapy)
	  • Administer atropine or apply a transcutaneous pacemaker for symptomatic bradycardia or block

Adapted from Dennison, R. (2007). *Pass CCRN!* (3rd ed.). St. Louis: Mosby.

i) Platelet aggregation inhibitors
 (a) Aspirin (160 to 325 mg initially and daily) or other antiplatelet drugs (e.g., clopidogrel [Plavix]) to decrease platelet aggregation and clot extension
 (b) Glycoprotein IIb/IIIa platelet receptor blockers (e.g., abciximab [ReoPro], eptifibatide [Integrilin], tirofiban hydrochloride [Aggrastat])
ii) Anticoagulants
 (a) Indirect thrombin inhibitor
  (i) Unfractionated heparin may be prescribed for 24 to 48 hours to maintain an activated partial thromboplastin time of 45 to 60 seconds: the initial dose should be weight based, with a bolus of 60 units/kg followed by an infusion of 12 units/kg/hour; the infusion is then adjusted with regard to activated partial thromboplastin time results
  (ii) Usual dose of unfractionated heparin

  (iii) Low-molecular-weight heparin (enoxaparin [Lovenox]) given subcutaneously
 (b) Warfarin (Coumadin) is usually prescribed for at least 3 months for patients with any of the following conditions:
  (i) Anterior Q-wave MI
  (ii) HF
  (iii) Severe LV dysfunction
  (iv) Atrial fibrillation
  (v) Previous embolic event
3) Treat anemia if present: maintain a hemoglobin level of >12 g/dl if possible
4) Maintain coronary artery perfusion pressure
 a) Use caution when administering NTG and other vasoactive agents because they may decrease coronary artery perfusion pressure by decreasing the aortic root pressure
 b) Nitroprusside (NTP [Nipride]) is contraindicated during ischemic pain because it may cause coronary artery steal, which shunts blood from ischemic to nonischemic areas and decreases coronary artery

perfusion pressure by decreasing aortic root pressure

5) Control dysrhythmias
   a) Tachydysrhythmias decrease the time required for coronary artery filling and may decrease cardiac output
   b) Bradydysrhythmias increase the time required for coronary artery filling but may decrease cardiac output

c. Decrease myocardial oxygen consumption
   1) Administer β-blockers as prescribed to decrease heart rate and contractility as well as myocardial oxygen consumption
      a) Actions
         i) Decrease the incidence of dysrhythmias and increase the ventricular fibrillation threshold
         ii) Block the effects of catecholamines (i.e., cardioprotection)
         iii) Reduce infarct size and the severity of the HF
      b) Agents: metoprolol (Lopressor) 5 mg intravenously every 2 minutes for three doses is usually given, but atenolol (Tenormin) or esmolol (Brevibloc) may be used
      c) Contraindications
         i) Heart rate <50 beats/minute
         ii) Second- or third-degree AV block
         iii) Systolic BP <100 mm Hg
         iv) HF
         v) Bronchospasm
            (a) No β-blockers should be given to a patient with active bronchospasm
            (b) Cardioselective β-blockers (e.g., metoprolol [Lopressor], esmolol [Brevibloc]) may be given to a patient with a history of bronchospastic lung disease (e.g., asthma), but noncardioselective β-blockers (e.g., propranolol [Inderal]) should not be given
         vi) Cocaine-induced MI
   2) Administer ACE inhibitors (e.g., captopril [Capoten], enalapril [Vasotec]) or angiotensin blockers (e.g., losartan [Cozaar], valsartan [Diovan]) as prescribed to attenuate ventricular remodeling
      a) Action: block the vasoconstriction and the sodium and water retention associated with the activation of the renin-angiotensin-aldosterone system
      b) Indications with acute MI: anterior or large inferior MI or evidence of HF
      c) ACE inhibitors block the conversion of angiotensin I to angiotensin II; angiotensin blockers block angiotensin II and do not block the breakdown of bradykinin, so they are less likely to cause cough
      d) Caution: hypotension
   3) Administer vasodilators as prescribed
      a) Venous vasodilators (usually NTG) to decrease preload
      b) Arterial vasodilators (usually NTP) to decrease afterload
      c) Caution: hypotension may occur; careful titration is necessary to decrease myocardial oxygen consumption and to prevent hypoperfusion

   4) Provide physical and emotional rest
      a) Maintain bed rest
      b) Prevent the Valsalva maneuver: teach the patient to exhale when turning in bed
      c) Explain procedures thoroughly: discuss monitor alarms, equipment, visiting hours, and reasons for procedures
      d) Keep the family informed about the patient's progress and status
      e) Provide for the patient's comfort
         i) Provide prompt pain control: analgesics
         ii) Provide nausea control: antiemetics and mouth care
         iii) Provide for physical comfort: temperature control, lighting, and noise control
      f) Instruct the patient regarding relaxation techniques; encourage the use of these techniques; use calming music, white noise, or nature sounds to help with relaxation
      g) Administer anxiolytics as prescribed: usually diazepam (Valium), lorazepam (Ativan), or alprazolam (Xanax)

d. Collaborative management specific to RV infarctions
   1) Assess for clinical indications of RV MI, especially in the patient with acute inferior MI
      a) ECG changes in V_4R, V_5R, and V_6R
      b) Right-sided S_4
      c) Clinical indications of RVF: JVD, hepatojugular reflux, right-sided S_3, and murmur of tricuspid insufficiency
      d) Minimal to absent pulmonary congestion
   2) Administer therapy specific to RV infarction
      a) Maintain adequate filling volumes
         i) Measure RAP and PA occlusive pressure; patients with significant RV infarction usually require hemodynamic monitoring
         ii) Administer volume: usually in the form of colloids (e.g., dextran, plasma protein fraction, albumin)
         iii) Avoid the use of diuretics and venous vasodilators
      b) Maintain contractility: inotropes (e.g., dobutamine [Dobutrex]) are frequently needed

e. Collaborative management specific to cocaine-induced MI
   1) β-Blockers are contraindicated
   2) Diltiazem (Cardizem) to reduce coronary artery spasm
   3) Diazepam (Valium) to reduce risk of seizures

4. Monitor for complications
   a. Dysrhythmias and conduction system defects
   b. HF
   c. Cardiogenic shock
   d. Papillary muscle dysfunction or rupture

e. Ventricular septal rupture
f. Cardiac rupture
g. Ventricular aneurysm
h. Pericarditis
i. Sudden cardiac death

Evaluation

1. Patent airway as well as adequate oxygenation (i.e., normal PaO_2, SpO_2, SaO_2) and ventilation (i.e., normal $PaCO_2$)
2. Absence of clinical indicators of respiratory distress
3. Absence of clinical indicators of hypoperfusion
4. Alert and oriented with no neurologic deficit
5. Control of chest pain, discomfort, or dyspnea

Typical disposition

1. Admission to critical care unit; preparation for PCI or surgery if indicated
2. Transfer to a another facility if a higher level of services is needed

Heart Failure
Definitions

1. HF: a condition in which one or both ventricles of the heart cannot pump sufficient blood to meet the metabolic needs of the body; it is characterized by one or both of the following:
   a. Clinical indications of intravascular and interstitial volume overload (e.g., dyspnea, crackles, edema)
   b. Clinical indications of tissue hypoperfusion (e.g., fatigue, exercise intolerance)

2. Pulmonary edema
   a. Fluid in the alveoli
   b. Impairs gas exchange and causes hypoxemia by impairing the diffusion between alveoli and the capillaries

Predisposing factors

1. Risk factors
   a. CAD is the primary risk factor, especially if the patient has a history of MI
   b. Congenital heart disease
   c. Valvular heart disease
   d. Hypertension
   e. Diabetes
   f. Obesity
   g. Alcoholism
   h. Smoking
   i. High or low hematocrit level
   j. Sedentary lifestyle
   k. High-fat or high-salt diet
2. Etiologic factors (Table 4-26)
3. Causes of decompensation in a patient with HF
   a. Progression of LV dysfunction
   b. New or worsening ischemia
   c. Hypoxemia
   d. Worsening of anemia
   e. Drugs (e.g., nonsteroidal antiinflammatory drugs, the initiation of β-blocker treatment at too high of a dosage)
   f. Hypertension
   g. New dysrhythmia, particularly atrial fibrillation

TABLE 4-26 Etiologic Factors of Heart Failure

Left Ventricular Failure	Right Ventricular Failure
• Coronary artery disease or left ventricular infarction	• Left ventricular failure
• Cardiomyopathy	• Coronary artery disease or right ventricular infarction
• Hypertension	• Pulmonary hypertension
• Dysrhythmias	• Passive: mitral valve disease
• Volume overload	• Active: hypoxemia or pulmonary embolism
• Valvular disease: mitral or aortic	• Dysrhythmias
• Ventricular septal defect	• Volume overload
• Coarctation of aorta	• Valvular disease: mitral or pulmonic
• Myocarditis	• Ventricular septal defect
• Cardiac tamponade	• Cardiomyopathy
	• Myocardial contusion

Biventricular Failure

Increased Demand	Electrolyte Imbalance
• Thyrotoxicosis	• Hyponatremia
• Anemia	• Hypokalemia
• Pregnancy	• Hypocalcemia
• Systemic infection	• Hypomagnesemia
• Beriberi	• Hypophosphatemia
• Paget disease	

From Dennison, R. (2007). *Pass CCRN!* (3rd ed.). St. Louis: Mosby.

h. Missed or suboptimal medication

i. Dietary indiscretions (e.g., high-salt foods)

j. Alcohol use

Pathophysiology

1. Compensation → decompensation: in the short-term, these mechanisms compensate for a failing heart; in the long-term, however, all of these factors trigger a process of pathologic growth and remodeling

   a. SNS

      1) Increases in heart rate, contractility, and conductivity initially increase cardiac output, thereby leading to dysrhythmias

      2) Vasoconstriction increases preload and afterload, thereby causing an increase in BP and resulting in an increase in myocardial oxygen consumption

   b. Renin-angiotensin-aldosterone system: sodium and water retention and peripheral vasoconstriction increase blood volume and preload

      1) Myocardial oxygen consumption is increased

      2) Pulmonary and peripheral edema may eventually occur

      3) Ventricular dilation and hypertrophy may occur

   c. Hypertrophy: more myofibrils increase cross-bridging; more mitochondria increase the supply of adenosine triphosphate

   d. Interstitial remodeling

      1) Compliance is eventually decreased and diastolic dysfunction results

      2) Force transmission through the ventricular wall is eventually decreased

      3) Ventricular remodeling causes the normal oval shape of the ventricular chamber to become more spherical

2. Classifications of HF

   a. Location: left or right

   b. Onset: acute or chronic

   c. Output state: low output (e.g., MI, cardiomyopathy) or high output (e.g., thyrotoxicosis, anemia)

   d. Type of pumping defect: backward (i.e., high volume and engorgement behind the failing ventricle) versus forward (i.e., low filling volume for the ventricle in front of the failing ventricle)

   e. Relationship to the cardiac cycle: systolic (60% to 70%) or diastolic (30% to 40%)

      1) Systolic dysfunction (pump problem): the inability of the ventricle to shorten against a load; the left ventricle loses its ability to contract normally against progressive increases in afterload

      2) Diastolic dysfunction (filling problem): an impairment in LV filling at near normal or mildly elevated left atrial and ventricular pressures; this is a result of a decrease in ventricular compliance; small changes in volume are associated with a disproportionate increase in pressure

Clinical presentation

1. Subjective

   a. First symptoms are frequently cough, exertional dyspnea, edema, or fatigue

2. Objective (Table 4-27)

3. Diagnostic

   a. Serum electrolyte levels: may reveal or confirm imbalances, especially hypokalemia, hypocalcemia, and hyponatremia

   b. ABGs: may show hypoxemia (especially if pulmonary edema is present) and acid-base imbalances (including lactic acidosis in severe hypoperfusion states)

   c. Drug levels: may reveal abnormal levels of digoxin (Lanoxin) or antidysrhythmic agents

   d. Thyroid profile: may reveal abnormal thyroid function

   e. CBC: may show anemia or leukocytosis

   f. BUN and creatinine levels: may be elevated to detect renal impairment

   g. Brain-type natriuretic peptide

      1) Normal: <100 picograms/ml; levels of >100 picograms/ml indicate HF

      2) Elevated brain-type natriuretic peptide levels correlate with an increased LV end-diastolic pressure and volume

   h. Urine: may show proteinuria or the presence of red blood cells or casts

   i. Chest radiography: shows cardiac enlargement and dilation; may show pulmonary congestion

   j. Echocardiography: shows changes in chamber size, wall thickness, and valve motion

   k. Electrocardiography

      1) May show myocardial ischemia or infarction

      2) May show atrial enlargement or ventricular hypertrophy

Collaborative management

1. Continue assessment

   a. ABCDs

   b. Vital signs: BP, pulse, respiratory rate, and temperature

   c. Oxygen saturation

   d. Respiratory effort and excursion

   e. Cardiac rate and rhythm

   f. Discomfort or pain level

   g. Accurate intake and output

   h. Serum electrolytes

   i. Level of consciousness

   j. Close monitoring for the progression of symptoms

2. Establish and maintain airway, oxygenation, and ventilation

   a. Position the patient with the head elevated to 30 to 45 degrees

   b. Oxygen by nasal cannula at 2 to 6 L/minute to maintain an SpO_2 of 95% unless contraindicated; for patients with COPD, use pulse oximetry to guide oxygen administration to an SpO_2 of 90%

TABLE 4-27 Clinical Indications of Left Ventricular and Right Ventricular Failure

Left Ventricular Failure	Right Ventricular Failure
• Tachypnea, dyspnea, orthopnea, or paroxysmal nocturnal dyspnea	• Jugular venous distention
• Tachycardia	• Hepatojugular reflux
• Left-sided S_3	• Dependent pitting edema
• Displaced point of maximal impulse or heave at apex	• Heave at sternum
• Crackles or wheezes	• Hepatomegaly or splenomegaly
• Cough, frothy sputum, or hemoptysis	• Anorexia, nausea, or vomiting
• Diaphoresis	• Abdominal pain and bloating
• Pulsus alternans	• Ascites
• Oliguria	• Nocturia
• Weakness and fatigue	• Weakness and fatigue
• Mental confusion	• Weight gain
• Murmur of mitral regurgitation	• Murmur of tricuspid regurgitation
• Arterial blood gases: decreased PaO_2 and SaO_2	• Right-sided S_3

• Hemodynamics
  • Elevated PAP and PAOP
	• Hemodynamics
	  • Elevated CVP and RAP

• Abnormal chest radiograph
  • Cardiomegaly
  • Engorged pulmonary vasculature
  • Kerley B lines
  • Pleural effusion
	• Abnormal liver function studies
	  • Alanine aminotransferase
	  • Aspartate aminotransferase
	  • Lactate dehydrogenase

• Electrocardiogram findings
  • Left atrial enlargement
  • Left ventricular hypertrophy
  • Atrial dysrhythmias
	• Electrocardiogram findings
	  • Right atrial enlargement
	  • Right ventricular hypertrophy
	  • Atrial dysrhythmias

From Dennison, R. (2007). *Pass CCRN!* (3rd ed.). St. Louis: Mosby.

c. Noninvasive positive-pressure ventilation may be used to avert intubation
  1) Positive pressure ventilation (also known as *pressure support ventilation*) during inspiration decreases the work of breathing
  2) Continuous positive pressure airway pressure during expiration: increases the driving pressure of oxygen to improve oxygenation; decreases the intrapulmonary shunt by opening collapsed alveoli; decreases surface tension and the work of breathing
d. Intubation and mechanical ventilation may be required; rapid-sequence intubation as indicated
e. Elimination of accumulated fluid: diuretics
f. Treatment of anemia: more than half of patients with HF are anemic, with hemoglobin levels of <12 gm/dl; the treatment of anemia improves cardiac function
3. Maintain adequate circulation and perfusion
  a. Intravenous access with two large-bore catheters for fluid and medication administration
  b. Fluid replacement
    1) Crystalloids: usually 0.9% saline; lactated Ringer solution is contraindicated for patients with liver disease
    2) Red packed cells

  3) Should be given early if significant blood loss is suspected to prevent tissue hypoxia
    a) Replacement of platelets, clotting factors, and calcium should be considered if multiple transfusions are given
c. Measures to reduce myocardial oxygen consumption
  1) Physical and emotional rest
    a) Prevent Valsalva maneuver; teach the patient to exhale when turning in bed
    b) Explain procedures thoroughly: discuss monitor alarms, equipment, visiting hours, and reasons for procedures
    c) Keep the family informed about the patient's progress and status
    d) Provide for physical comfort: temperature control, lighting, and noise control
    e) Instruct the patient regarding relaxation techniques, and encourage their use
    f) Administer anxiolytics as prescribed: usually diazepam (Valium), lorazepam (Ativan), or alprazolam (Xanax)
d. Measures to reduce preload and afterload
  1) Positioning: low Fowler position with legs dependent
  2) Sodium and fluid restrictions acutely
    a) Fluid restriction to <2000 ml/24 hours
    b) Sodium restriction to <2 to 3 g/24 hours

3) Diuretics: usually loop diuretics (e.g., furose-mide [Lasix], bumetanide [Bumex])

4) Venous vasodilators

   a) ACE inhibitors and angiotensin II receptor blockers: decrease preload and afterload

   b) Nesiritide (Natrecor): recombinant form of brain-type natriuretic peptide reduces pre-load and afterload

   c) Nitrates (e.g., NTG): decrease preload

   d) NTP: reduces preload and afterload; particularly helpful for hypertensive patients

5) Dialysis: used if the patient is in renal failure; continuous renal replacement therapy may be initiated

e. Measures to improve contractility

   1) Positive inotropic agents (e.g., dobutamine [Dobutrex])

      a) Indications: temporary treatment of diuretic-refractory decompensation

      b) Agents

         i) Cardiac glycosides (e.g., digoxin [Lanoxin])

         ii) Sympathetic stimulants (e.g., dobutamine [Dobutrex]): especially useful with pulmonary edema if the patient is normotensive

   2) Mechanical cardiac support devices (e.g., ventricular assist devices) if indicated and available

f. Measures to manage dysrhythmias

   1) Atrial

      a) Atrial dysrhythmias frequently resolve with the treatment of HF because atrial stretch and, therefore, atrial irritability, are decreased

      b) Digoxin (Lanoxin): decreases ventricular re-sponse rate by increasing the refractoriness of the AV node

      c) Anticoagulants: used to prevent mural thrombi and embolic events

   2) Ventricular

      a) Antidysrhythmics as prescribed

      b) Correction of electrolyte deficiencies

      c) Cardiac resynchronization therapy: atriobi-ventricular pacing restores synchronous ventricular contraction to optimize LV filling and to improve cardiac output; the patient may already have this type of pacemaker, or it may be planned

4. Monitor for complications

   a. Deep vein thrombosis or pulmonary embolism

   b. Progressive deterioration

   c. Dysrhythmias: common cause of sudden death

   d. Cardiogenic shock

   e. Complications of therapy

      1) Fluid and electrolyte imbalance: hypokalemia, hypocalcemia, and hypomagnesemia as a result of diuretic therapy

      2) Digitalis toxicity

Evaluation

1. Patent airway as well as adequate oxygenation (i.e., normal PaO_2, SpO_2, SaO_2) and ventilation (i.e., normal $PaCO_2$)

2. Absence of clinical indicators of respiratory distress

3. Absence of clinical indicators of hypoperfusion

4. Alert and oriented with no neurologic deficit

5. Control of chest pain, discomfort, or dyspnea

Typical disposition

1. If evaluation criteria met: discharge with instructions for follow up for further cardiac testing and treatment; patient and family teaching should include secondary and contributing causes of HF and preventive measures:

   a. Dietary changes

   b. Smoking cessation

   c. Lipid-lowering agents

   d. Decreased alcohol intake

   e. Weight loss

   f. Antihypertension medication

2. If evaluation criteria not met: admission to step-down unit or critical care unit

Cardiomyopathy

Definition: a disorder that involves the structure and function of the myocardium; the three types are dilated, hypertrophic, and restrictive (Figure 4-43)

Dilated cardiomyopathy

1. Predisposing factors

   a. Idiopathic

   b. Infection, especially viral (e.g., coxsackievirus B, arbovirus)

   c. Toxins (e.g., doxorubicin [Adriamycin], daunorubi-cin [Cerubidine], alcohol, lead, arsenic, cobalt)

   d. Electrolyte, vitamin, or nutrient deficiency

   e. Pregnancy

   f. Neuromuscular disorders (e.g., myasthenia gravis, muscular dystrophy)

   g. Connective tissue disorders (e.g., systemic lupus erythematosus, scleroderma)

   h. Infiltrative disorders (e.g., sarcoidosis, amyloidosis)

   i. Hyperthyroidism

2. Pathophysiology

   a. Damage to myofibrils that causes a decrease in contractility and systolic dysfunction

   b. Preload and afterload increased by the stimulation of the renin-angiotensin-aldosterone system

   c. Gross dilation of the heart that often affects all four chambers

   d. Refractory HF

3. Clinical presentation

   a. Subjective

      1) Fatigue and weakness

      2) Chest pain

      3) Palpitations

      4) Syncope

      5) Symptoms of HF: dyspnea and edema

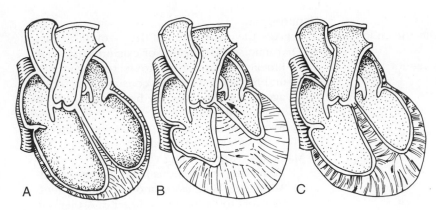

Figure 4-43 Cardiomyopathies. **A,** Dilated. **B,** Hypertrophic. **C,** Restrictive. (From Kinney, M. R., Packa, D. R., & Dunbar, S. B. [1993]. *AACN's clinical reference for critical-care nursing* [3rd ed.]. St. Louis: Mosby.)

b. Objective
  1) Orthostatic BP changes
  2) May have murmurs of tricuspid or mitral regurgitation
  3) Signs of biventricular failure
    a) LVF: S_3, crackles, and PMI displaced laterally
    b) RVF: JVD, peripheral edema, and hepatomegaly
c. Diagnostic
  1) Chest radiography: cardiomegaly, pulmonary congestion, and possibly pleural effusion
  2) Electrocardiography: biventricular hypertrophy, biatrial enlargement, dysrhythmias (i.e., atrial fibrillation is common), and blocks; bundle branch block may be seen
  3) Echocardiography: decreased ventricular wall motion, decreased ejection fraction, enlarged chamber size, and abnormal wall motion
  4) Cardiac catheterization: elevated intracardiac pressures and mitral or tricuspid regurgitation

Hypertrophic cardiomyopathy (previously called *idiopathic hypertrophic subaortic stenosis* [IHSS])
1. Predisposing factors
  a. Idiopathic
  b. Heredity: genetically transmitted autosomal-dominant trait
  c. Neuromuscular disorders
  d. Hypoparathyroidism
2. Pathophysiology
  a. Hypertrophy of the heart muscle, including the ventricular septum and the ventricular free wall
  b. Rigid, noncompliant ventricles that will not stretch to fill, thereby causing diastolic dysfunction with a decrease in preload and cardiac output
  c. Mitral regurgitation caused by papillary muscles and mitral valve pulled out of alignment
  d. With severe hypertrophy, LV outflow tract obstruction occurs, especially when contractility is increased by an increase in circulating catecholamines
  e. Decrease in blood flow to coronary arteries (angina) and brain (syncope)
  f. Sudden cardiac death may result

3. Clinical presentation
  a. Subjective
    1) Dyspnea, orthopnea, and paroxysmal nocturnal dyspnea (PND)
    2) Chest pain
    3) Palpitations
    4) Syncope
  b. Objective
    1) PMI displaced laterally
    2) Crackles
    3) S_4
    4) Murmurs
      a) Subaortic stenosis: systolic ejection murmur that is loudest along the left sternal border; it increases with the Valsalva maneuver and decreases with a squatting position
      b) Mitral regurgitation: holosystolic blowing murmur that is loudest at the apex and that radiates to the axilla
  c. Diagnostic
    1) Chest radiography: left atrial dilation, cardiomegaly, and pulmonary congestion
    2) Electrocardiography: left atrial enlargement and LV hypertrophy, ST and T wave abnormalities, dysrhythmias (i.e., atrial fibrillation, ventricular dysrhythmias), and blocks; left anterior hemiblock is frequently seen
    3) Echocardiography: left atrial enlargement; increased thickness of the LV free wall and the interventricular septum that causes a narrowing of the LV outflow tract; abnormal wall motion, especially of the septum; mitral regurgitation is possible
    4) Cardiac catheterization: elevated left ventricular end diastolic pressure (LVEDP); mitral regurgitation may be evident

Restrictive cardiomyopathy
1. Predisposing factors
  a. Idiopathic
  b. Infiltrative disorders (e.g., sarcoidosis, amyloidosis)
  c. Endomyocardial fibrosis
  d. Glycogen deposition
  e. Radiation
  f. Lymphoma
  g. Connective tissue disorders (e.g., scleroderma)

2. Pathophysiology
   a. Fibrous tissue infiltrates the myocardium, the endocardium, and the subendocardium
   b. The heart becomes noncompliant and cannot stretch, fill, or contract well
   c. Decreased preload and contractility
   d. Decreased cardiac output
   e. HF
3. Clinical presentation
   a. Subjective
      1) Chest pain
      2) Fatigue and weakness
      3) Dyspnea, orthopnea, and PND
   b. Objective
      1) Signs of RVF: JVD, hepatomegaly, peripheral edema, and right-sided S_3
      2) May also have signs of LVF: left-sided S_3 and crackles
   c. Diagnostic
      1) Chest radiography: cardiomegaly, pulmonary congestion, and possibly pleural effusion
      2) Electrocardiography: low QRS voltage; AV blocks are common
      3) Echocardiography: atrial enlargement; enlarged ventricular outside dimension but small ventricular chamber; pericardial effusion may be evident
      4) Cardiac catheterization: elevated intracardiac pressures

Collaborative management

1. Continue assessment
   a. ABCDs
   b. Vital signs: BP, pulse, respiratory rate, and temperature
   c. Oxygen saturation
   d. Cardiac rate and rhythm
   e. Respiratory rate and effort
   f. Level of consciousness
   g. Accurate intake and output
   h. Discomfort or pain level
   i. Close monitoring for the progression of symptoms
2. Dilated
   a. Provide care as for HF
   b. Decrease myocardial oxygen consumption
   c. Monitor for complications
      1) Dysrhythmias
         a) Atrial fibrillation: digoxin (Lanoxin)
         b) Ventricular dysrhythmias: antidysrhythmic agents (e.g., amiodarone [Cordarone]) and automatic implantable cardioverter-defibrillators
      2) Systemic emboli: anticoagulation is frequently prescribed, especially for patients with ejection fractions of <30%
   d. Assist with the preparation of the patient for mitral valve replacement or cardiac transplantation as requested

3. Hypertrophic
   a. Prevent the obstruction of the LV outflow tract
      1) Administer β-blockers or calcium-channel blockers as prescribed to decrease contractility and myocardial oxygen consumption; these agents also decrease the heart rate to improve ventricular filling
      2) Avoid inotropic agents, which would increase outflow tract obstruction
   b. Maintain adequate filling volumes
      1) Administer intravenous fluids as prescribed
      2) Administer β-blockers and calcium-channel blockers to decrease the heart rate, thereby allowing more time for filling
      3) Use caution with or avoid drugs that decrease preload, such as venous vasodilators and diuretics
   c. Monitor for complications
      1) Dysrhythmias
         a) Atrial: digoxin (Lanoxin) is not used because it may increase outflow tract obstruction; diltiazem (Cardizem) or verapamil (Calan) may be used
         b) Ventricular: antidysrhythmics (e.g., amiodarone [Cordarone])
      2) Systemic emboli: anticoagulants are frequently prescribed, especially for patients with ejection fractions of <30%
   d. Assist with the preparation of the patient for percutaneous transluminal septal myocardial ablation, ventricular septal myectomy, dual-chamber pacemaker, or cardiac transplantation as requested
4. Restrictive
   a. Treat the cause: may include steroids
   b. Provide care as for HF
   c. Monitor for complications
      1) Dysrhythmias
         a) Atrial fibrillation: digoxin
         b) Ventricular dysrhythmias: antidysrhythmic agents (e.g., amiodarone [Cordarone])
      2) AV blocks: pacemaker may be needed
      3) Systemic emboli: anticoagulants are frequently prescribed, especially for patients with ejection fractions of <30%
   d. Assist with the preparation of the patient for cardiac transplantation as requested

Evaluation

1. Patent airway as well as adequate oxygenation (i.e., normal PaO_2, SpO_2, SaO_2) and ventilation (i.e., normal $PaCO_2$)
2. Absence of clinical indicators of respiratory distress
3. Absence of clinical indicators of hypoperfusion
4. Alert and oriented with no neurologic deficit
5. Control of chest pain, discomfort, or dyspnea

Typical disposition

1. If evaluation criteria met: discharge with instructions for follow up for further cardiac testing and treatment

2. If evaluation criteria not met: admission to step-down unit or critical care unit

Pericarditis

Definition: an inflammatory process that involves the visceral or parietal pericardium

Predisposing factors

1. Idiopathic: most common cause
2. MI
   a. Acute: usually occurs within 7 days; related to inflammation and the healing process
   b. Subacute (referred to as *Dressler syndrome*): occurs later (usually 2 weeks or more); thought to be an autoimmune response
3. Trauma
4. Connective tissue diseases (e.g., systemic lupus erythematosus)
5. Infection: viral or bacterial (e.g., tuberculosis)
6. Malignancy
7. Dissecting thoracic aortic aneurysms
8. Radiation therapy
9. Uremia
10. Myxedema
11. Drugs: procainamide, hydralazine (Apresoline), phenytoin (Dilantin), and penicillin

Pathophysiology

1. Inflammation of the layers of the pericardium occurs
2. Increased capillary permeability as a result of inflammation may cause fluid to leak into the pericardial space; cardiac tamponade is possible
   a. As little as 50 to 100 ml may cause cardiac tamponade if the fluid accumulation is acute and rapid (e.g., trauma, postcardiotomy)
   b. As much as 2 L may not cause cardiac tamponade if the fluid accumulation is chronic and slow (e.g., uremia with pleural effusion)
3. If scarring, thickening, and fibrosis of the pericardium occurs, constrictive pericarditis develops
4. Either constrictive pericarditis or cardiac tamponade decreases the diastolic filling of the heart and causes systemic or pulmonary venous congestion, decreased cardiac output, and cardiac index, thereby leading to shock

Clinical presentation

1. Subjective
   a. Precordial or left pleuritic chest pain
      1) Persistent sharp or stabbing pain, pleuritic pain, or dull ache
      2) Radiates to the left shoulder, the neck, the arms, or the abdomen
      3) Aggravated by inspiration, cough, and supine positioning
      4) Relieved by sitting up or leaning forward
   b. Hoarseness, dysphagia, and dyspnea occur if pericardial effusion compresses adjacent structures

c. Cough
d. Hemoptysis
2. Objective
   a. Tachypnea
   b. Tachycardia
   c. Fever and malaise
   d. Heart sound changes
      1) Pericardial friction rub (this is a hallmark sign, but it is frequently absent)
      2) Muffled heart sounds if pericardial effusion or cardiac tamponade occur
3. Diagnostic
   a. WBC: increased
   b. Sedimentation rate: increased
   c. C-reactive protein: increased
   d. CK-MB and troponin: negative
   e. Antinuclear antibodies: positive if caused by connective tissue disease
   f. Blood cultures: positive if caused by infection
   g. Chest radiography
      1) Pericardial effusion causes "water bottle" silhouette
      2) Pleural effusion and pulmonary infiltrates may be seen
   h. Electrocardiography
      1) Diffuse concave ST elevation in all leads except aVL, aVR, and V_1; upright T waves flattened; no Q waves
      2) PR segment depression
      3) Low voltage if pericardial effusion
      4) Dysrhythmias: atrial fibrillation, atrial flutter, premature atrial contractions, and paroxysmal atrial tachycardia
   i. Echocardiography
      1) Pericardial effusion may be seen
      2) If constrictive pericarditis: pericardial thickening or calcification
   j. Computerized tomography or magnetic resonance imaging: pericardial effusion; thickened or calcified pericardium in constrictive pericarditis

Collaborative management

1. Continue assessment
   a. ABCDs
   b. Vital signs: BP, pulse, respiratory rate, and temperature
   c. Oxygen saturation
   d. Respiratory effort and excursion
   e. Cardiac rate and rhythm
   f. Discomfort and pain level
   g. Level of consciousness
   h. Accurate intake and output
   i. Close monitoring for the progression of symptoms
2. Maintain airway, oxygenation, and ventilation
   a. Elevate the head of the bed to 30 to 45 degrees; an overbed table may be helpful for the patient to lean on

b. Oxygen by nasal cannula at 2 to 6 L/minute to maintain an SpO_2 of 95% unless contraindicated; for patients with COPD, use pulse oximetry to guide oxygen administration to an SpO_2 of 90%

3. Control pain and discomfort
   a. Nonsteroidal antiinflammatory agents
   b. Steroids may be prescribed if no response to nonsteroidal antiinflammatory agents or if effusion present
   c. Narcotic analgesics if necessary
4. Administer drugs and therapies for the treatment of the cause
   a. Antibiotics if bacterial
   b. Steroids if connective tissue disorders
   c. Thyroid hormone replacement for myxedema
   d. Withdrawal of suspect drugs
5. Discontinue anticoagulants as ordered
   a. If anticoagulants must be continued, heparin will be used because it is much easier to reverse than warfarin (Coumadin)
   b. If anticoagulants are not discontinued, monitor the patient closely for clinical indications of cardiac tamponade
6. Monitor for complications
   a. Dysrhythmias
   b. Constrictive pericarditis
   c. Cardiac tamponade
   d. HF

Evaluation

1. Patent airway as well as adequate oxygenation (i.e., normal PaO_2, SpO_2, SaO_2) and ventilation (i.e., normal $PaCO_2$)
2. Absence of clinical indicators of respiratory distress
3. Absence of clinical indicators of hypoperfusion
4. Alert and oriented with no neurologic deficit
5. Control of chest pain, discomfort, or dyspnea

Typical disposition

1. If evaluation criteria met: discharge with instructions for follow up for further cardiac testing and treatment
2. If evaluation criteria not met or if the cause is unclear: admission to step-down unit, critical care unit, or catheterization laboratory for pericardiocentesis
   a. Pericardiocentesis and biopsy are indicated if the cause is unclear, if purulent pericarditis is suspected, or if cardiac tamponade occurs

Myocarditis

Definition: an inflammation of the myocardium

Predisposing factors

1. Viral infections (e.g., coxsackievirus A and B [most common cause])
2. Bacterial infections (e.g., diphtheria, staphylococcal infections)
3. Parasitic infections (e.g., toxoplasmosis)
4. Helminthic infections (e.g., trichinosis)
5. Fungal infections (e.g., *Candida, Aspergillus*); usually seen in patients with immunosuppression

6. Hypersensitivity reactions (e.g., rheumatic fever)
7. Radiation therapy of the chest
8. Chronic alcoholism

Pathophysiology

1. Three stages
   a. Stage 1: viral infection triggers the immune response, which should attenuate viral proliferation
   b. Stage 2: autoimmunity
      1) If the immune system does not downregulate after viral proliferation is controlled, autoimmune disease occurs
      2) T cells target the patient's own tissue
      3) Cytokine activation and cross-reacting antibodies may further accelerate the process
   c. Stage 3: dilated cardiomyopathy may occur
      1) This is caused by direct effect of coxsackie viral protease, by cytokines such as tumor necrosis factor activating proteinases, and by the effect of viruses on the myocyte
      2) Ventricular dilation and remodeling occur
      3) Progressive HF develops, which may cause death or necessitate cardiac transplantation
2. Damage to the myocardium may be diffuse to focal
   a. Diffuse injury frequently causes HF
   b. Focal injury may cause the necrosis of portions of the conduction system and result in conduction blocks

Clinical presentation

1. Subjective
   a. Chest soreness, burning, or pressure: increased by inspiration and supine positioning
   b. Easily fatigued
   c. Syncope
   d. Clinical indications of upper respiratory or gastrointestinal viral infection
   e. Sudden unexplained dyspnea, orthopnea, or PND
2. Objective
   a. Fever
   b. Crackles
   c. Heart sound changes
      1) Distant heart sounds
      2) S_3 and S_4
      3) Murmur of mitral regurgitation may be heard
      4) Pericardial friction rub may be heard
3. Diagnostic
   a. WBC: increased
   b. CK-MB and troponin: may be increased
   c. Sedimentation rate: increased
   d. Chest radiography
      1) Cardiomegaly
      2) Pleural or pericardial effusion
      3) Pulmonary congestion
   e. Electrocardiography
      1) Diffuse ST segment and T wave abnormalities
      2) Low voltage
      3) Left axis deviation

4) Dysrhythmias: supraventricular or ventricular

5) Blocks: AV or bundle branch blocks

Collaborative management

1. Continue assessment
   a. ABCDs
   b. Vital signs: BP, pulse, respiratory rate, and temperature
   c. Respiratory effort and excursion
   d. Oxygen saturation
   e. Cardiac rate and rhythm
   f. Discomfort or pain level
   g. Level of consciousness
   h. Accurate intake and output
   i. Close monitoring for the progression of symptoms
2. Maintain airway, oxygenation, and ventilation
   a. Elevate the head of the bed to 30 to 45 degrees; an overbed table may be helpful for the patient to lean on
   b. Oxygen by nasal cannula at 2 to 6 L/minute to maintain an SpO_2 of 95% unless contraindicated; for patients with COPD, use pulse oximetry to guide oxygen administration to an SpO_2 of 90%
   c. Suction as needed
   d. Intubation and mechanical ventilation may be required
3. Maintain adequate circulation and perfusion
   a. Intravenous access for fluid and medication administration
   b. Fluid replacement if required; usually 0.9% saline
4. Administer drug therapies for the treatment of the cause
   a. Antibiotics for bacterial infections
   b. Amphotericin B (Abelcet) for fungal infections
   c. Corticosteroids for connective tissue diseases (this contraindicated for early infectious viral myocarditis because these drugs may enhance myocardial damage by increasing tissue necrosis and viral replication and thus should not be used)
5. Monitor for complications
   a. Dilated cardiomyopathy
   b. Dysrhythmias
   c. Blocks: a temporary or permanent pacemaker is frequently required
   d. Pericarditis: monitor closely for clinical indications of cardiac tamponade
   e. Systemic emboli: anticoagulants may be prescribed; if so, monitor closely for clinical indications of cardiac tamponade

Evaluation

1. Patent airway as well as adequate oxygenation (i.e., normal PaO_2, SpO_2, SaO_2) and ventilation (i.e., normal $PaCO_2$)
2. Absence of clinical indicators of respiratory distress
3. Absence of clinical indicators of hypoperfusion
4. Alert and oriented with no neurologic deficit
5. Control of chest pain, discomfort, or dyspnea

Typical disposition: admission

Infective Endocarditis

Definition: an inflammation of the endocardium that usually occurs in the membranous lining of the heart valves but that also may involve cardiac prostheses

Predisposing factors

1. Congenital or acquired valvular heart disease
   a. Septal defects
   b. Bicuspid aortic valve
   c. Mitral valve prolapse (with murmur)
   d. Rheumatic heart disease
   e. Degenerative heart disease
   f. History of endocarditis
2. Cardiac surgery: especially valve repair or replacement
3. Invasive tests or monitoring
4. Skin, bone, or pulmonary infections
5. Poor oral hygiene
6. Dental procedures
7. Intravenous drug use
8. Long-term venous access devices
9. Body piercing
10. Immunosuppressed state (e.g., acquired immunodeficiency virus, cancer, diabetes mellitus, burns, hepatitis, immunosuppressive drugs or steroids)

Causative agents

1. Bacteria
   a. *Staphylococcus aureus*
   b. *Streptococcus viridans*
   c. Group A nonhemolytic streptococcus
   d. *Streptococcus pneumoniae* (pneumococcus)
   e. *Staphylococcus epidermidis*
   f. *Streptococcus faecalis* (enterococci)
   g. *Pseudomonas aeruginosa*
   h. *Enterococcus*
   i. *Aspergillus fumigatus*
   j. *Haemophilus*
   k. *Serratia marcescens*
   l. *Candida albicans*
2. Viruses (e.g., coxsackievirus, adenovirus)

Pathophysiology

1. May be described as acute or subacute
   a. Acute infective endocarditis
      1) Typically a fulminant systemic illness of brief duration
      2) Most frequently occurs with normal valves and causes severe damage to the valves
      3) Organism is usually *Staphylococcus aureus*
   b. Subacute endocarditis
      1) Manifests initially as a flu-like illness that progresses slowly
      2) Most frequently associated with already damaged valves (e.g., rheumatic heart disease, mitral valve prolapse)
      3) Outcome is usually good with adequate treatment
      4) Organism is usually *Streptococcus viridans*

2. May affect right-sided or left-sided valves
   a. Left-sided valves are affected most often, with the aortic valve being affected twice as often as the mitral valve
   b. Right-sided valves are affected more often in intravenous drug users
3. Bacteria and blood products adhere to structural irregularities in the cardiac valves
4. Lesions form as a result of the colonization of bacteria
   a. These lesions, called *vegetations,* contain bacteria, red blood cells, platelets, fibrin, collagen, and necrotic tissue
5. Valvular tissue is damaged by the vegetations
6. Valve becomes incompetent and may later scar to become stenotic
7. Other problems include allergic vasculitis and the embolization of vegetations and bacteria

Clinical presentation

1. Subjective
   a. Infectious symptoms (e.g., fever, chills, diaphoresis, malaise, weakness, anorexia, myalgias, arthralgias, headache, weight loss)
   b. Pleuritic chest pain
   c. Abdominal pain
   d. Back pain
   e. May have symptoms of HF: dyspnea, orthopnea, and PND
   f. Cough and hemoptysis
   g. Medical history
      1) Predisposing factors
      2) Recent valve surgery in a patient who had a dental procedure without prophylactic antibiotics
2. Objective
   a. Fever
   b. Heart sound changes: new or changed murmur
   c. Confusion or delirium
   d. Signs of embolic or allergic vasculitis
      1) Splinter hemorrhages of the nail beds (these are thought result from an immune response or emboli)
      2) Petechiae: conjunctiva, chest, abdomen, and oral mucosa
      3) Roth spots: round white lesions on the retina
      4) Janeway lesions: flat, painless erythematous lesions on the palms, the soles of the feet, and the extremities
      5) Osler nodes: painful nodules on the fingers and toes
      6) Clinical indications of embolic stroke (e.g., hemiparesis, hemiplegia, aphasia, ataxia)
   e. May have signs of HF: S_3, crackles, JVD, hepatomegaly, splenomegaly, and peripheral edema
3. Diagnostic
   a. WBC: increased
   b. RBC: decreased
   c. Hemoglobin: decreased

   d. Sedimentation rate: elevated
   e. Blood cultures: persistently positive
   f. Urine: microscopic hematuria, proteinuria
   g. Chest radiography
      1) If tricuspid or pulmonic valve
         a) Multiple bilateral infiltrates, primarily in the lower lobes
         b) Infiltrates
      2) If mitral or aortic valve
         a) Cardiomegaly
         b) Pulmonary congestion
   h. Electrocardiography
      1) Dysrhythmias
         a) Atrial: supraventricular tachydysrhythmias, including paroxysmal atrial tachycardia (PAT), atrial fibrillation, and atrial flutter
         b) Ventricular: premature ventricular contractions (PVCs)
      2) Blocks: AV blocks or bundle branch blocks
   i. Echocardiography: transesophageal is more sensitive and specific than transthoracic

Collaborative management

1. Continue assessment
   a. ABCDs
   b. Vital signs: BP, pulse, respiratory rate, and temperature
   c. Oxygen saturation
   d. Respiratory effort and excursion
   e. Cardiac rate and rhythm
   f. Discomfort or pain level
   g. Level of consciousness
   h. Accurate intake and output
   i. Close monitoring for the progression of symptoms
2. Maintain airway, oxygenation, and ventilation
   a. Elevate the head of the bed to 30 to 45 degrees; an overbed table may be helpful for the patient to lean on
   b. Oxygen by nasal cannula at 2 to 6 L/minute to maintain an SpO_2 of 95% unless contraindicated; for patients with COPD, use pulse oximetry to guide oxygen administration to an SpO_2 of 90%
3. Maintain adequate circulation and perfusion
   a. Intravenous access for fluid and medication administration
   b. Fluid replacement if required; usually 0.9% saline
4. Decrease myocardial oxygen consumption
   a. Bed rest and activity restrictions until fever and cardiac symptoms subside
   b. Treatment of fever (this is controversial, because pyrogens are helpful for mobilizing the immune system)
      1) Antipyretics (e.g., acetaminophen [Tylenol])
      2) Cooling blankets may be used, but shivering should be avoided because of its effect on oxygen consumption
5. Control and treat infection
   a. Blood cultures
   b. Antibiotics as prescribed; antibiotic therapy for endocarditis is usually for 4 to 8 weeks' duration

6. Monitor for complications
   a. HF, cardiogenic shock, and pulmonary edema may occur as a result of valve perforation or dehiscence, ruptured chordae tendineae, or valvular obstruction by vegetation
   b. Extension of the infection with abscess or fistula formation or purulent pericardial effusion
      1) Septic emboli
      2) Perivalvular abscess
   c. Neurologic complications: stroke-like systems
   d. Systemic emboli
   e. Bacterial or mycotic aneurysm (this is a localized abnormal expansion of a vessel as a result of the destruction of a part or all of the vessel wall from the growth of bacteria or fungi): may be intracranial, intrathoracic, abdominal, or peripheral
   f. Dysrhythmias or blocks
   g. Septic shock

Evaluation

1. Patent airway as well as adequate oxygenation (i.e., normal PaO_2, SpO_2, SaO_2) and ventilation (i.e., normal $PaCO_2$)
2. Absence of clinical indicators of respiratory distress
3. Absence of clinical indicators of hypoperfusion
4. Alert and oriented with no neurologic deficit
5. Control of chest pain, discomfort, or dyspnea
6. Afebrile

Typical disposition: admission

1. Patient may go from the emergency department to surgery for valve repair or replacement if indicated
2. Instruct patients with valvular disease or valve replacement about the prevention of endocarditis
   a. People with valvular heart disease should receive prophylactic antibiotics before intrusive procedures (e.g., dental procedures, cardiac catheterization)
   b. Good hygiene—especially oral—may also help to prevent endocarditis, especially in susceptible persons

Hypertensive Crises

Definitions

1. Hypertension: an elevation in BP above 140/90 mm Hg in an adult patient
2. Hypertensive crisis: a rapid rise in BP that occurs when the BP elevation is severe enough to cause the threat of immediate vascular necrosis and end-organ damage; note that the defining characteristics are how rapidly the BP rises and the resulting end-organ effects rather than the absolute BP
3. Hypertensive emergency: an acute elevation of BP that is associated with acute and ongoing organ damage to the kidneys, brain, heart, eyes, or vascular system
   a. There is no absolute BP level, but the BP is usually >240/140 mm Hg
   b. The BP must be lowered within minutes to a few hours to reduce potential complications of new or progressive end-organ damage
   c. The condition requires immediate hospitalization in a critical care unit and intravenous antihypertensive agents

Predisposing factors

1. Primary
   a. Untreated or inadequately treated essential (idiopathic) hypertension
      1) Risk factors: family history; black race; obesity; hyperlipidemia; diabetes or glucose intolerance; tobacco use; excessive alcohol intake; high fat diet, high-sodium diet, or both; stress; sedentary lifestyle; aging; and oral contraceptives
      2) Poor compliance is frequently a factor in hypertensive crisis; factors that are closely related to poor compliance include a lack of symptoms (i.e., the silent killer), the side effects of pharmacologic agents, and the costs of pharmacologic agents
2. Secondary
   a. Renal disease
      1) Increased renin-angiotensin levels
         a) Renin-secreting tumors
         b) Renovascular disease
      2) Acute glomerulonephritis
      3) Chronic pyelonephritis
   b. Eclampsia or preeclampsia of pregnancy
   c. Central nervous system injuries
      1) Head injury
      2) Spinal cord injury: autonomic dysreflexia is hypertension with bradycardia that occurs in patients with spinal cord injury at T6 or above in response to noxious stimuli
   d. Burns
   e. Drug side effects: oral contraceptives, steroids, cocaine, amphetamines, methamphetamine, and decongestants

Pathophysiology

1. Hypertension produces changes in the arterioles and decreases in blood flow to vital organs
   a. Severe hypertension causes necrosis of the intima and media of the arteries
   b. Systolic hypertension is now considered to more contributory to LV hypertrophy, LVF, and stroke than diastolic hypertension
2. Organ ischemia occurs from platelet aggregation, intravascular coagulation, arteriolar spasm, and edema
3. Target organs most likely to be damaged by hypertensive crises
   a. Heart: hypertensive disease, LV hypertrophy, LVF, angina, and MI
   b. Kidney: decreased renal perfusion, proteinuria, and renal failure
   c. Retina: hemorrhages and blindness
   d. Brain: hypertensive encephalopathy

Clinical presentation

1. Subjective
   a. History of hypertension common (Table 4-28)
   b. Significant elevation of BP above normal
2. Objective
   a. Significant elevation of BP above normal
   b. Epistaxis may occur
3. Evidence of end-organ involvement
   a. Cardiovascular involvement may be present
      1) Chest pain
      2) Signs of LV hypertrophy: PMI displaced to the left, S_4, ECG indicators of LV hypertrophy (i.e., deep S in V_1 and V_2 and tall R in V_5 and V_6)
      3) Signs of LVF and pulmonary edema: dyspnea, orthopnea, LV heave, S_3, and crackles
      4) Carotid and abdominal bruits are common
   b. Renal involvement may be present
      1) Nocturia
      2) Pressure-related diuresis
      3) Hematuria
      4) Elevated BUN and creatinine levels
   c. Retinal involvement may be present
      1) Visual disturbances (e.g., blurred vision, reduced visual acuity, photophobia, temporary loss of vision)
      2) Funduscopic changes: arteriolar narrowing, hemorrhages, exudates, and papilledema
   d. Neurologic involvement may be present, especially with hypertensive encephalopathy
      1) Occipital or anterior headache, especially in the morning; may be severe
      2) Nausea and vomiting
      3) Seizures
      4) Altered mental status: irritability, confusion, and agitation that progress to lethargy and coma
      5) Focal neurologic signs (e.g., cranial nerve palsy, sensory or motor deficits, aphasia, positive Babinski reflex)
4. Diagnostic
   a. Potassium: hypokalemia occurs with primary hyperaldosteronism
   b. BUN and creatinine levels may be elevated, thus indicating renal involvement
   c. Lipid profile to evaluate additional cardiac risk
   d. Aldosterone may be elevated
   e. Urine: hematuria or proteinuria may be present
   f. Chest radiography
      1) Cardiomegaly may be present
      2) Widening of the mediastinum suggests dissecting thoracic aortic aneurysm
   g. Electrocardiography: may show left atrial enlargement or LV hypertrophy
   h. Computed tomography of brain: may show cerebral edema or hemorrhage

Collaborative management

1. Continue assessment
   a. ABCDs
   b. Vital signs: BP, pulse, respiratory rate, and temperature
   c. Oxygen saturation
   d. Respiratory effort and excursion
   e. Cardiac rate and rhythm
   f. BP every 5 minutes until stable
   g. Discomfort or pain level
   h. Level of consciousness
   i. Accurate intake and output
   j. Close monitoring for the progression of symptoms
2. Maintain airway, oxygenation, and ventilation
   a. Elevate the head of the bed to 30 to 45 degrees; an overbed table may be helpful for the patient to lean on
   b. Oxygen by nasal cannula at 2 to 6 L/minute to maintain an SpO_2 of 95% unless contraindicated; for patients with COPD, use pulse oximetry to guide oxygen administration to an SpO_2 of 90%
   c. Airway maintenance: oropharyngeal or nasopharyngeal airway or endotracheal intubation may be required, especially if an altered level of consciousness or pulmonary edema is present
   d. Ventilation: mechanical ventilation may be required, especially if neurologic impairment or pulmonary edema is present
3. Maintain adequate circulation and perfusion
   a. Intravenous access for fluid and medication administration

TABLE 4-28 New Classification of Blood Pressure Levels According to the Seventh Report of the Joint National Committee on Prevention, Detection, Evaluation, and Treatment of High Blood Pressure

Category	Systolic (mm Hg)	and/or	Diastolic (mm Hg)
Optimal	<120	and	<80
Normal	<130	and	<85
Stage 1 hypertension	140–159	or	90–99
Stage 2 hypertension	≥160	or	≥100

Adapted from Bakris, G. (2003). The implications of JNC 7 for antihypertensive treatment protocols. Retrieved May 9, 2010, from www.medscape.com/viewprogram/2513_pnt

b. Measures to decrease myocardial oxygen consumption
   1) Activity restriction initially
   2) Sodium restriction to less than 2 g/24 hours
   3) Smoking cessation
   4) Physical comfort: temperature control, lighting, and noise control
   5) Anxiolytics as prescribed: usually diazepam (Valium), lorazepam (Ativan), or alprazolam (Xanax)
4. Decrease BP gradually
   a. Reduction of mean arterial pressure by no more than 20% to 25% during the first 2 hours because BP that is decreased too aggressively may cause neurologic damage by significantly decreasing cerebral perfusion pressure
      1) If neurologic changes occur, BP reduction should be slowed or temporarily stopped
   b. Antihypertensive agents
      1) Vasodilators
         a) Nitroprusside (Nipride): usually the first-line agent for hypertensive emergency because of its rapid onset and short duration of effect
         b) NTG: particularly helpful for patients with acute coronary syndrome or HF
         c) Hydralazine (Apresoline)
            i) Use with caution because this drug may cause severe, prolonged, and uncontrolled hypotension
            ii) Medication of choice for eclampsia
         d) Nicardipine (Cardene)
            i) Intravenous vascular calcium-channel blocker
            ii) Contraindicated with HF
      2) Sympathetic blockers
         a) α-Blockers block vasoconstriction
            i) Phentolamine (Regitine): especially helpful if hypertension is caused by autonomic dysreflexia because bradycardia contraindicates β-blockers
         b) β-Blockers block the reflex tachycardia associated with vasodilators
            i) Esmolol (Brevibloc): rapid-acting, cardioselective β-blocker
            ii) Contraindicated with HF, heart block, and hypertension caused by stimulants (e.g., cocaine)
            iii) Propranolol (Inderal) preferred over esmolol for hypertension in patients with aortic dissection (ENA, 2007)
         c) α- and β-blockers: block both vasoconstriction and tachycardia
            i) Labetalol (Normodyne): α-blocker and noncardioselective β-blocker
               (a) Contraindicated with HF, asthma, and heart block
      3) ACE inhibitors
         a) Enalapril (Vasotec): only intravenous ACE inhibitor; particularly helpful with HF

   4) Diuretics: usually loop diuretics (e.g., furosemide [Lasix], bumetanide [Bumex])
5. Monitor for complications
   a. Cerebral infarction
   b. MI
   c. HF or pulmonary edema
   d. Dissection of aorta
   e. Renal failure

Evaluation
1. Patent airway as well as adequate oxygenation (i.e., normal PaO_2, SpO_2, SaO_2) and ventilation (i.e., normal $PaCO_2$)
2. Absence of clinical indicators of respiratory distress
3. Absence of clinical indicators of hypoperfusion
4. Alert and oriented with no neurologic deficit
5. Control of chest pain, discomfort, or dyspnea

Typical disposition
1. If evaluation criteria met and this was not a true hypertensive crisis: discharge with instructions for follow-up
   a. Provide patient and family instruction and counseling regarding nonpharmacologic and pharmacologic BP management
2. If evaluation criteria not met: admission to step-down unit or critical care unit

Acute Arterial Occlusion
Definition: acute complete occlusion of an artery by thrombosis in the presence of an already narrowed artery, embolism, or trauma

Predisposing factors
1. Arterial embolization
   a. Atrial fibrillation
   b. Valvular heart disease
   c. HF
   d. Ventricular aneurysm
   e. Bacterial endocarditis
2. Injury to the arterial wall
   a. Vascular trauma
   b. Arterial punctures
   c. Postcardiac catheterization, PCI, and vascular surgery
3. Compression of artery with swelling
   a. Fracture (i.e., compartment syndrome)
   b. Circumferential burn

Pathophysiology
1. Occlusion of an artery
2. Ischemia occurs
3. Vasoactive factors (e.g., serotonin) may be released; this causes vasospasm and the worsening of the ischemia
4. Ischemia progresses to necrosis if it is not promptly resolved

Clinical presentation
1. Neurovascular status: evaluate the 6 Ps
   a. Pain: usually severe and sudden but may be muscle soreness or tenderness

b. Pallor: cyanosis or petechiae may also be noted
c. Pulselessness
d. Paresis or paralysis; rigor may be noted late
e. Paresthesia or anesthesia
f. Polar: cool or cold below the level of the injury
2. Objective
    a. Muscle tenderness and cool with palpation
    b. Muscle rigor with prolonged ischemia
    c. Petechiae are seen with microemboli
    d. Doppler stethoscope indicates diminished or absent blood flow
3. Diagnostics
    a. Complete blood cell count and coagulation studies: to detect anemia or clotting abnormalities
    b. Doppler flow studies: diminished or absent blood flow
    c. Ankle-brachial index: a comparison of ankle and brachial systolic BP obtained with a Doppler stethoscope; a value of <0.30 is not compatible with limb viability
    d. Diagnostic study: angiography indicates arterial occlusion

Collaborative management

1. Continue assessment
    a. ABCDs
    b. Vital signs: BP, pulse, respiratory rate, and temperature
    c. Oxygen saturation
    d. Respiratory effort and excursion
    e. Cardiac rate and rhythm
    f. Discomfort and pain level
    g. Level of consciousness
    h. Neurovascular status: the 6 Ps
    i. Accurate intake and output
    j. Close monitoring for the progression of symptoms
2. Maintain airway, oxygenation, and ventilation
    a. Elevate the head of the bed to 30 to 45 degrees
    b. Oxygen by nasal cannula at 2 to 6 L/minute to maintain an SpO_2 of 95% unless contraindicated; for patients with COPD, use pulse oximetry to guide oxygen administration to an SpO_2 of 90%
3. Maintain adequate circulation and perfusion
    a. Intravenous access in the unaffected limb for fluid and medication administration
    b. Proper positioning of the limb: keep the extremity straight, warm, and dependent
        1) Bed rest
        2) Elevate the head of the bed to facilitate flow to the ischemic limb
        3) Do not elevate the extremity
        4) Do not apply heat to the ischemic area
    c. Notify the physician immediately of perfusion deficit; prepare the patient for an angiogram
    d. Procedures to reestablish the patency of artery
        1) Intra-arterial fibrinolytics (e.g., urokinase [Abbokinase], recombinant tissue plasminogen activator [rt-PA]) followed by anticoagulants
        2) Preparation for percutaneous endovascular or surgical procedures if indicated

4. Control pain and discomfort
    a. Narcotic analgesics
    b. Anxiolytics
5. Monitor for complications
    a. Reocclusion
    b. Infection

Evaluation

1. Patent airway as well as adequate oxygenation (i.e., normal PaO_2, SpO_2, SaO_2) and ventilation (i.e., normal $PaCO_2$)
2. Absence of clinical indicators of respiratory distress
3. Absence of clinical indicators of hypoperfusion
4. Absence of neurovascular compromise
5. Alert and oriented with no neurologic deficit
6. Control of chest pain or discomfort

Typical disposition: admission to critical care unit, to radiology for intervention procedure, or to surgery

Acute Aortic Aneurysm

Definition: a permanent localized dilation of the aorta with an increase of ≥1.5× the normal diameter

Predisposing factors

1. Hypertension
2. Degenerative changes caused by aging; familial predisposition
3. Congenital weakness of the aorta
4. Pregnancy: especially during the third trimester
5. Coarctation of the aorta
6. Syphilis
7. Severe systemic infection (e.g., bacterial aneurysm)
8. Marfan syndrome
9. Trauma: especially blunt trauma with acceleration-deceleration injury

Pathophysiology

1. Elastin provides elasticity of the vessel wall, and collagen is responsible for mechanical strength; abnormal proteolytic enzyme activity causes increased synthesis and the degradation of elastin and collagen
2. Elastin destruction may be the triggering event for aneurysm formation followed by the weakening of the collagen, which allows the dilation of the aorta to occur
3. An expanding hematoma compresses or occludes the arteries that branch off of the aorta and may compress structures
4. Hematoma formation in the medial layer causes longitudinal separation of the layers of the aorta (dissection)
5. The resultant thin-walled channel can easily rupture and hemorrhage into mediastinal, pleural, or abdominal cavities
6. Pain moves from the site of origin to other sites as the dissection extends

Clinical presentation

1. Subjective
   a. Usually asymptomatic until dissection or rupture occurs
   b. If pain is present, it is described as sharp, knife-like, tearing, or ripping
   c. Medical history
2. Objective
   a. Normal to high BP; hypotension suggests cardiac tamponade or aortic rupture
   b. Pulsatile mass
   c. Increased aortic diameter on palpation
   d. Bruit over the aorta
3. Specifically the ascending thoracic aorta
   a. May be asymptomatic
   b. Dyspnea
   c. Chest pain
   d. Clinical indications of aortic regurgitation: diastolic murmur, LVF, and widened pulse pressure
4. Specifically the aortic arch
   a. Dyspnea
   b. Stridor
   c. Cough
   d. JVD
   e. Hoarseness
   f. Weak voice
5. Specifically the descending thoracic arch
   a. Dull chest pain and upper back pain
   b. Hoarseness
6. Dissecting thoracic aortic aneurysm
   a. Sudden, sharp, tearing or ripping pain in the chest that radiates to the shoulders, neck, or back
   b. Hypotension
   c. Dyspnea
   d. Syncope
   e. Leg weakness and transient paralysis
   f. May have BP and pulse difference between the arms or between the arms and legs
   g. May have clinical indications of thrombotic stroke
   h. May have clinical indications of cardiac tamponade (see the Cardiac Tamponade section)
7. Specifically abdominal aortic aneurysm
   a. Dull abdominal and back pain
   b. Nausea and vomiting
   c. Abdominal bloating
   d. Pulsation in abdomen
8. Specifically ruptured abdominal aortic aneurysm
   a. Severe, sudden, dull, continuous abdominal pain that radiates to the low back, hips, and scrotum; this is unaffected by movement
   b. Feeling of abdominal fullness
   c. Nausea and vomiting
   d. Syncope and shock
   e. Pulsation in abdomen: periumbilical area
9. Diagnostic
   a. Hemoglobin and hematocrit may be decreased
   b. Chest radiography
      1) Mediastinal widening
      2) Widening of aortic silhouette
      3) Aortic calcification
      4) Left pleural effusion
   c. Electrocardiography
      1) May show LV hypertrophy
      2) May show nonspecific ST-T wave changes
      3) Absence of ECG indicators of MI
   d. Transesophageal echocardiography: may show aortic root dilation and an intimal flap that divides the true and false lumen in dissection
   e. Aortography: diameter, size, and location of aneurysm
   f. Computed tomography scanning and magnetic resonance imaging: presence and location of aneurysm
   g. Ultrasound: presence, size, shape, and location of aneurysm
   h. Flat plate of abdomen: outline of aneurysm

Collaborative management

1. Continue assessment
   a. ABCDs
   b. Vital signs: BP, pulse, respiratory rate, and temperature
   c. Oxygen saturation
   d. Respiratory effort and excursion
   e. Cardiac rate and rhythm
   f. Hemodynamic status
   g. Discomfort and pain level
   h. Level of consciousness
   i. Neurovascular status: the 6 Ps
   j. Accurate intake and output
   k. Close monitoring for the progression of symptoms
2. Maintain airway, breathing, and circulations
   a. Oxygen by nasal cannula at 2 to 6 L/minute to maintain an SpO_2 of 95% unless contraindicated; for patients with COPD, use pulse oximetry to guide oxygen administration to an SpO_2 of 90%
   b. Intubation and mechanical ventilation may be necessary
3. Maintain adequate circulation and perfusion
   a. Intravenous access with two large-bore catheters
   b. Normal saline or lactated Ringer solution by rapid infusion until blood is available; colloids (e.g., albumin, dextran) may also be used
   c. Control of mean arterial pressure at approximately 70 mm Hg if dissection occurs or if patient is hypertensive;
      1) Nitroprusside [Nitropres]: may be used with propranolol (Inderal)
      2) Labetalol (Normodyne)
   d. Measures to decrease tissue oxygen requirements
      1) Activity restriction
      2) Physical comfort: temperature control, lighting, and noise control
      3) Anxiolytics as prescribed: usually diazepam (Valium), lorazepam (Ativan), or alprazolam (Xanax)

4) Assist with the preparation of the patient for procedures or surgical repair as indicated
4. Control pain and discomfort
   a. Nonsteroidal antiinflammatory agents
   b. Narcotic analgesics are required for rupture or dissection, but use extreme caution if the patient is hypotensive
   c. Anxiolytics
5. Monitor for complications
   a. Hemorrhage
   b. Hypovolemic shock
   c. Death

Evaluation

1. Patent airway as well as adequate oxygenation (i.e., normal PaO_2, SpO_2, SaO_2) and ventilation (i.e., normal $PaCO_2$)
2. Absence of clinical indicators of respiratory distress
3. Absence of clinical indicators of hypoperfusion
4. Absence of neurovascular compromise
5. Alert and oriented with no neurologic deficit
6. Control of chest pain or discomfort

Typical disposition: admission to critical care unit or to surgery for surgical repair

Peripheral Arterial Disease

Definition: the partial or total occlusion of an artery by atherosclerosis or arteriosclerosis obliterans

Predisposing factors

1. Arteriosclerosis or atherosclerosis (the same risk factors as referred to in the discussion of CAD)
   a. Atherosclerosis: most common cause
   b. Arteriosclerosis: significant cause in older patients
2. Hypertension
3. Arteritis
4. Raynaud disease: vasospasm of the fingers and toes in response to cold or emotional stress
5. Thromboangiitis obliterans (i.e., Buerger disease): the inflammation and blockage of the small and medium-sized arteries of the extremities

Pathophysiology

1. Most significant occlusion usually occurs at bifurcations
2. Damage to intima with progressive deterioration and thrombus formation
3. Partial or complete occlusion
   a. Stage 1: pathologic changes within the artery but no clinical symptoms
   b. Stage 2: intermittent claudication; 75% occlusion
   c. Stage 3: pain at rest; ≈90% to 95% occlusion
   d. Stage 4: necrosis; ≈99% to 100% occlusion

Clinical presentation

1. History of other arteriosclerotic or atherosclerotic disease (e.g., CAD) or risk factors for arteriosclerotic or atherosclerotic disease (e.g., smoking, hypertension, hyperlipidemia)

2. Occlusive disease of the terminal aorta and iliac arteries
   a. Subjective
      1) Intermittent claudication in thigh and hip: pain increases with exercise and decreases with rest
      2) Impotence
   b. Objective
      1) Coolness of the lower extremities
      2) Hair loss over the lower extremities
      3) Decreased or absent iliac and femoral pulses
      4) Bruit or thrill over the iliac area
3. Occlusive disease of the femoral and popliteal arteries
   a. Subjective
      1) Intermittent claudication in the lower leg that progresses to pain at rest
      2) Decreased sensation or paresthesia of the lower extremities
   b. Objective
      1) Coolness of the lower extremities
      2) Hair loss over the lower extremities
      3) Pallor or mottling of the lower extremities
      4) Nonhealing ulcers on the toes or points of trauma
      5) Decreased motor strength in the lower extremities
      6) Decreased or absent femoral and popliteal pulses
      7) Bruit or thrill over the femoral or popliteal area
4. Diagnostic
   a. Arteriography: shows partial or complete arterial occlusion
   b. Doppler and duplex ultrasonography shows partial to complete vascular occlusion
   c. Antinuclear antibody testing: positive with Sjögren syndrome, scleroderma, Raynaud disease, rheumatoid arthritis, and other autoimmune conditions

Collaborative management

1. Continue assessment
   a. ABCDs
   b. Vital signs: BP, pulse, respiratory rate, and temperature
   c. Oxygen saturation
   d. Respiratory effort and excursion
   e. Cardiac rate and rhythm
   f. Discomfort and pain level
   g. Level of consciousness
   h. Neurovascular status: the 6 Ps
   i. Accurate intake and output
   j. Close monitoring for the progression of symptoms
2. Maintain airway, oxygenation, and ventilation
   a. Elevate the head of the bed to 30 to 45 degrees; an overbed table may be helpful for the patient to lean on
   b. Oxygen by nasal cannula at 2 to 6 L/minute to maintain an SpO_2 of 95% unless contraindicated; for patients with COPD, use pulse oximetry to guide oxygen administration to an SpO_2 of 90%
3. Maintain adequate circulation and perfusion
   a. Intravenous access for fluid and medication administration

b. Intravenous fluids: usually 0.9% saline
c. Measures to decrease peripheral oxygen requirements
   1) Activity cessation when pain occurs
   2) Bed rest during acute occlusion
   3) Limb at the level of the heart: do not elevate the ischemic extremity
   4) Maintenance of normothermia
   5) Prevention of trauma
d. Measures to reestablish blood flow
   1) Pharmacologic agents to reestablish blood flow: fibrinolytics (e.g., urokinase [Abbokinase], streptokinase [Streptase], rt-PA [Activase])
   2) Preparation of the patient
     a) Percutaneous procedures aimed at decreasing occlusion (e.g., catheter embolectomy, percutaneous balloon angioplasty)
     b) Surgery
4. Control pain and discomfort
  a. Nonsteroidal antiinflammatory agents
  b. Narcotic analgesics
  c. Anxiolytics
5. Monitor for complications
  a. Infection
  b. Limb necrosis

Evaluation
1. Patent airway as well as adequate oxygenation (i.e., normal PaO_2, SpO_2, SaO_2) and ventilation (i.e., normal $PaCO_2$)
2. Absence of clinical indicators of respiratory distress
3. Absence of clinical indicators of hypoperfusion
4. Absence of neurovascular compromise
5. Alert and oriented with no neurologic deficit
6. Control of chest pain or discomfort

Typical disposition
1. If evaluation criteria met: discharge with instructions for follow-up for further vascular testing and treatment
2. If evaluation criteria not met: admission to step-down unit, to critical care unit, to cardiac catheterization laboratory for percutaneous endovascular procedure, or to surgery for vascular bypass

Peripheral Venous Thrombosis
Definition: the occlusion of a vein by a blood clot
Predisposing factors (Virchow triad)
1. Hypercoagulability
  a. Malignancy: especially of the breast, the lung, the pancreas, the gastrointestinal tract, or the genitourinary tract
  b. Estrogen, especially in smokers
   1) Oral contraceptives
   2) Postmenopausal hormone replacement therapy
  c. Dehydration and hemoconcentration
  d. Fever

e. Sickle-cell anemia
f. Pregnancy and postpartum period
g. Polycythemia vera
h. Abrupt discontinuance of anticoagulants
i. Sepsis
2. Alterations in the vessel wall
  a. Trauma
  b. Intravenous drug use
  c. Aging
  d. Vasculitis
  e. Varicose veins
  f. Diabetes mellitus
  g. Atherosclerosis
  h. Inflammatory process
3. Venous stasis
  a. Prolonged bed rest or immobilization
  b. Obesity
  c. Advanced age
  d. Burns
  e. Pregnancy
  f. Postpartum period
  g. HF
  h. MI
  i. Bacterial endocarditis
  j. Recent surgery, especially of the legs, pelvis, or abdomen
  k. Thrombus formation in heart (e.g., atrial fibrillation)
  l. Cardioversion

Pathophysiology
1. More than 90% of thrombi develop in the deep veins of the lower extremities; superficial thrombophlebitis poses little risk unless the associated clot extends into the major deep veins; this would be suggested by swelling of the leg
2. Thrombus formation enhances platelet adhesiveness and causes a release of scrotonin (vasoconstrictor)
3. Factors that contribute to the dislodgment of the thrombi
  a. Intravascular pressure changes
   1) Sudden standing (e.g., initial ambulation)
   2) Valsalva maneuver (e.g., coughing, sneezing, vomiting)
   3) Fluid challenges
   4) Massaging of the legs
  b. Natural mechanism of clot dissolution: 7 to 10 days after the clot develops

Clinical presentation
1. Subjective
  a. History of predisposing factors (e.g., Virchow triad)
  b. Pain: aching, localized pain with movement; tenderness with palpation
2. Objective
  a. Unilateral edema, erythema, warmth, and dilated collateral veins on the affected extremity
  b. Positive Homans sign: pain in the calf with dorsiflexion of the foot with the knee slightly bent

1) The presence of this sign is suggestive of but not definitive for venous thrombosis
2) The absence of this sign does not rule out venous thrombosis
  c. Low-grade fever
3. Diagnostic
  a. Positive D-dimer
  b. Venography and Doppler ultrasonography show occlusion
  c. Impedance plethysmography shows occlusion

Collaborative management

1. Continue assessment
  a. ABCDs
  b. Vital signs: BP, pulse, respiratory rate, and temperature
  c. Oxygen saturation
  d. Respiratory effort and excursion
  e. Cardiac rate and rhythm
  f. Discomfort and pain level
  g. Level of consciousness
  h. Neurovascular assessment
  i. Close monitoring for the progression of symptoms
2. Maintain airway, oxygenation, and ventilation
  a. Elevate the head of the bed to 30 to 45 degrees
  b. Oxygen by nasal cannula at 2 to 6 L/minute to maintain an SpO_2 of 95% unless contraindicated; for patients with COPD, use pulse oximetry to guide oxygen administration to an SpO_2 of 90%
3. Prevention of progression or dislodgement of clot
  a. Elevation of affected extremity
  b. Warm compresses
  c. Compression stockings
  d. Low-molecular-weight heparin
    1) Enoxaparin (Lovenox): 30 mg every 12 hours
    2) Dalteparin sodium (Fragmin): 2,500 IU daily
  e. Instruction regarding the avoidance of Valsalva maneuver
  f. Avoid leg massage
  g. Hydrate with oral or intravenous fluids
4. Monitor for complications
  a. Pulmonary embolism
  b. Post phlebitis syndrome

Evaluation

1. Patent airway as well as adequate oxygenation (i.e., normal PaO_2, SpO_2, SaO_2) and ventilation (i.e., normal $PaCO_2$)
2. Absence of clinical indicators of respiratory distress
3. Absence of clinical indicators of hypoperfusion
4. Alert and oriented with no neurologic deficit
5. Control of chest pain, discomfort, or dyspnea

Typical disposition

1. If evaluation criteria met: discharge with instructions for follow up and subcutaneous low-molecular-weight heparin, warm compresses, and compression stockings
2. If evaluation criteria not met: admission to step-down unit or to critical care unit for evaluation for the presence of pulmonary embolism

Blunt Cardiac Injury (also known as *myocardial contusion*)

Definition: a transient or permanent myocardial dysfunction caused by blunt trauma to the heart; may include myocardial necrosis without CAD

Predisposing factors

1. Usually acceleration-deceleration injury sustained during a motor vehicle collision; the sternum may hit the steering wheel or the dashboard; injury may also be caused by the shoulder strap of the seatbelt
2. Other vehicular collisions: motorcycle collisions, automobile–pedestrian collisions
3. Kicking of the chest by a large animal
4. Assault with a blunt instrument
5. Industrial crush injury
6. Explosion
7. Vigorous CPR
8. Projectile objects (e.g., baseballs, hockey pucks)

Pathophysiology

1. The heart is compressed between the sternum and the spine
2. Red blood cells extravasate around the myocardial fibers (i.e., bruising of the myocardium)
3. Subpericardial and subendocardial myocardial fibers become edematous and may fragment; necrosis may even occur in severe cases
4. The atria and the right ventricle are the primary sites of injury because of their anterior position
5. Decreased RV contractility causes an increase in the RV end-diastolic volume and a decrease in the RV ejection fraction (i.e., the backward failure of the right ventricle)
6. This decrease in the RV ejection fraction decreases preload to the left ventricle (i.e., forward failure of the left ventricle)
7. The dilation of the right ventricle shifts the interventricular septum to the left, thus compromising LV compliance
8. An increase in pulmonary vascular resistance (PVR) is frequently seen, which increases RV afterload and further decreases RV ejection fraction
9. Damage to the cardiac valves may occur (especially mitral and aortic) because LV pressures are higher
10. In addition to the effect of blunt trauma on myocardial contractility, sudden cardiac death may occur as a result of a blunt, nonpenetrating blow to the precordium or the left lateral chest during the electrically vulnerable period of the cardiac cycle, thereby causing fatal ventricular dysrhythmias; this sudden cardiac death is referred to as *commotio cordis*

Clinical presentation

1. Subjective
   a. May be asymptomatic
   b. History of events and mechanism of injury
   c. Treatment before arrival
   d. Precordial angina-like chest pain
      1) Frequently increases with inspiration, cough, and movement
      2) Unresponsive to NTG but frequently responsive to oxygen, anti-inflammatory agents, and narcotics
   e. Dyspnea
   f. Palpitations
2. Objective
   a. Tachycardia and tachypnea
   b. Hypotension may occur
   c. Ecchymosis may be present on the anterior chest
   d. Chest wall tenderness with palpation
   e. Clinical indications of RVF: JVD, peripheral edema, and hepatomegaly
   f. Clinical indications of LVF less likely: S_3 and crackles
   g. Cardiac arrest as a result of fatal ventricular dysrhythmias may occur
3. Diagnostic
   a. Serum: CK-MB and cardiac troponin may be positive depending on the severity of the injury
   b. Electrocardiography with RV leads
      1) ST segment changes, T wave inversion; Q waves may be seen if injury is severe or if a coronary artery is lacerated or thromboses
      2) Dysrhythmias
         a) Atrial dysrhythmias: premature atrial contractions (PACs), atrial fibrillation, and atrial flutter
         b) Ventricular dysrhythmias: PVCs, ventricular tachycardia, and ventricular fibrillation
         c) Blocks: AV blocks and right bundle branch blocks
   c. Echocardiography
      1) Decreased regional wall motion (especially RV)
      2) Decreased RV ejection fraction
      3) May show complications (e.g., apical thrombi, pericardial effusion, cardiac tamponade)

Collaborative management

1. Continue assessment
   a. ABCDs
   b. Vital signs: BP, pulse, respiratory rate, and temperature
   c. Oxygen saturation
   d. Respiratory effort and excursion
   e. Cardiac rate and rhythm
   f. Hemodynamic status
   g. Discomfort and pain level
   h. Level of consciousness
   i. Accurate intake and output
   j. Close monitoring for the progression of symptoms
2. Maintain airway, oxygenation, and ventilation
   a. Elevation of the head of the bed to 30 to 45 degrees
   b. Oxygen by nasal cannula at 2 to 6 L/minute to maintain an SpO_2 of 95% unless contraindicated; for patients with COPD, use pulse oximetry to guide oxygen administration to an SpO_2 of 90%
3. Maintain adequate circulation and perfusion
   a. Intravenous access for fluid and medication administration
   b. Measures to decrease myocardial oxygen demand
      1) Oxygen by nasal cannula at 2 to 6 L/minute to maintain an SpO_2 of 95% unless contraindicated; for patients with COPD, use pulse oximetry to guide oxygen administration to an SpO_2 of 90%
      2) Bed rest
      3) Anxiolytics as prescribed and indicated
   c. Measures to ensure adequate RV contractility, LV filling, and cardiac output
      1) Intravenous isotonic fluids as prescribed to ensure adequate LV filling; avoid venous vasodilators and diuretics
      2) Inotropes (e.g., dobutamine [Dobutrex]) as prescribed to improve RV contractility
   d. Treatment of dysrhythmias
      1) Atrial: digitalis (i.e., digoxin [Lanoxin]) and cardioversion
      2) Ventricular: usually amiodarone (Cordarone)
      3) Blocks: temporary pacemaker; a permanent pacemaker may be necessary
4. Control pain and discomfort
   a. Nonsteroidal antiinflammatory agents
   b. Narcotic analgesics in doses that are adequate to allow the patient to deep breathe and cough as indicated
   c. Anxiolytics
5. Monitor for complications
   a. Ventricular rupture
   b. Cardiac tamponade
   c. Coronary artery thrombosis
   d. Valve rupture
   e. Conduction defects
   f. HF
   g. Ventricular aneurysm
   h. Cardiogenic shock: monitor for clinical manifestations of hypoperfusion
   i. Systemic emboli

Evaluation

1. Patent airway as well as adequate oxygenation (i.e., normal PaO_2, SpO_2, SaO_2) and ventilation (i.e., normal $PaCO_2$)
2. Absence of clinical indicators of respiratory distress
3. Absence of clinical indicators of hypoperfusion
4. Alert and oriented with no neurologic deficit
5. Control of chest pain, discomfort, or dyspnea

Typical disposition: admission to step-down unit or critical care unit

Penetrating Cardiac Trauma
Definition: the puncture of the heart with a sharp object or rib

Predisposing factors
1. Violence (e.g., knife wound, gunshot wound, ice pick)
2. Industrial accident (e.g., scaffolding)
3. Motorcycle collision (e.g., handlebar impalement)
4. Sports injury
5. Explosion
6. Crush injury

Pathophysiology
1. Puncture of the heart (usually the right ventricle) with a sharp object or rib
2. Loss of blood into the pericardial space or into the mediastinum
3. Cardiac tamponade or shock may occur

Clinical presentation
1. Subjective
   a. Chest pain
   b. History of events and occurrence
   c. Mechanism of injury
   d. Treatment before arrival
   e. Medical history
2. Objective
   a. Visible wound; object that is causing penetration may be seen
   b. Bleeding from chest
   c. Hypotension
   d. Clinical indications of hypoperfusion
   e. Clinical indications of cardiac tamponade
3. Diagnostic
   a. hemoglobin and hematocrit levels decreased

Collaborative management
1. Continue assessment
   a. ABCDs
   b. Vital signs: BP, pulse, respiratory rate, and temperature
   c. Oxygen saturation
   d. Respiratory effort and excursion
   e. Cardiac rate and rhythm
   f. Hemodynamic status
   g. Discomfort and pain level
   h. Level of consciousness
   i. Accurate intake and output
   j. Close monitoring for the progression of symptoms
2. Maintain airway, oxygenation, and ventilation
   a. Airway, oxygenation, and circulation support with the use of BLS and ACLS if needed
   b. 100% oxygen by face mask; intubate and mechanically ventilate as indicated
3. Maintain adequate circulation and perfusion
   a. Intravenous access with two large-bore catheters for fluid and medication administration
   b. Circulating volume replacement
      1) Normal saline or lactated Ringer solution by rapid infusion until blood is available; colloids (e.g., albumin, hetastarch, dextran) may also be used
      2) Blood and blood products
   c. Control of hemorrhage
      1) Stabilization of object(s) with intravenous bags or dressings; do not remove an impaled object
      2) Application of pressure to the site if the object has been removed and there is a bleeding wound
      3) Application of pressure around the site if the object has not already been removed and there is bleeding around the wound
      4) Assistance with the insertion of a chest tube for hemothorax or pneumothorax
      5) Assistance with pericardiocentesis for cardiac tamponade
   d. Preparation of the patient for exploratory thoracotomy
4. Control pain and discomfort
   a. Nonsteroidal antiinflammatory agents
   b. Narcotic analgesics in doses that are adequate to allow patient to deep breathe and cough as indicated
   c. Anxiolytics
5. Monitor for complications
   a. Hemorrhagic shock
   b. Cardiac tamponade
   c. Hemothorax
   d. Pneumothorax

Evaluation
1. Patent airway as well as adequate oxygenation (i.e., normal PaO_2, SpO_2, SaO_2) and ventilation (i.e., normal $PaCO_2$)
2. Absence of clinical indicators of respiratory distress
3. Absence of clinical indicators of hypoperfusion
4. Alert and oriented with no neurologic deficit
5. Control of chest pain, discomfort, or dyspnea

Typical disposition: admission to surgery

Great Vessel Injury
Definition: condition in which fluid (blood, effusion fluid, or pus) in the pericardial space compromises cardiac filling and cardiac output

Predisposing factors
1. Acceleration-deceleration injury (e.g., motor vehicle collision)
2. Compression injury
3. Penetrating trauma

Pathophysiology: the disruption of major vessel integrity causes a loss of effective circulating blood volume, which leads to shock

Clinical presentation
1. Subjective
   a. History of events and mechanism of injury

b. Treatment before arrival

c. Pain that frequently radiates to back or consistent back pain

d. Dyspnea

e. Dysphagia or hoarseness

f. Sensory or motor changes in the lower extremities

2. Objective
   a. Tachycardia
   b. BP changes
      1) Hypertension or hypotension
      2) Difference between the left and right arms
      3) Difference (greater than the patient's normal difference) between the upper and lower extremities
   c. Tracheal shift
   d. Clinical indications of hypoperfusion
   e. Harsh systolic murmur may be audible along the precordium

3. Diagnostic
   a. Serum: hemoglobin and hematocrit levels decreased
   b. ECG: may show dysrhythmias or ST-T wave changes that are indicative of ischemia
   c. Chest radiograph
      1) Mediastinal widening
      2) Loss of aortic knob shadow
   d. Transesophageal echocardiography or spiral computed tomography scanning
   e. Aortogram: will show extravasation of dye

Collaborative management

1. Continue assessment
   a. ABCDs
   b. Vital signs: BP, pulse, respiratory rate, and temperature
   c. Oxygen saturation
   d. Respiratory effort and excursion
   e. Cardiac rate and rhythm
   f. Discomfort and pain level
   g. Level of consciousness
   h. Accurate intake and output
   i. Close monitoring for the progression of symptoms

2. Manage cardiopulmonary arrest if needed: manage airway, oxygenation, and circulation with the use of BLS and ACLS if needed

3. Maintain airway, oxygenation, and ventilation
   a. Airway, oxygenation, and circulation with the use of BLS and ACLS if needed
   b. 100% oxygen by nonrebreathing mask; intubate and mechanically ventilate as indicated

4. Maintain adequate circulation and perfusion
   a. Intravenous access with two large-bore catheters for fluid and medication administration
   b. Circulating volume replacement
      1) Normal saline or lactated Ringer solution by rapid infusion until blood is available; colloids (e.g., albumin, hetastarch, dextran) may also be used
      2) Blood and blood products
   c. Control of hemorrhage

1) Antihypertensives may be needed to keep the mean arterial pressure <90 mm Hg

2) Preparation of the patient for exploratory thoracotomy as soon as possible; it is not possible to truly stabilize these patients except in the operating room with vascular repair

5. Control pain and discomfort
   a. Narcotic analgesics in doses that are adequate to allow the patient to deep breathe and cough as indicated
   b. Anxiolytics

6. Monitor for complications
   a. Hemorrhagic shock
   b. Cardiac tamponade
   c. Hemothorax
   d. False aneurysm

Evaluation

1. Patent airway as well as adequate oxygenation (i.e., normal PaO_2, SpO_2, SaO_2) and ventilation (i.e., normal $PaCO_2$)
2. Absence of clinical indicators of respiratory distress
3. Absence of clinical indicators of hypoperfusion
4. Alert and oriented with no neurologic deficit
5. Control of chest pain, discomfort, or dyspnea

Typical disposition: admission to surgery

Cardiac Tamponade

Definition: condition in which fluid (blood, effusion fluid, or pus) in the pericardial space compromises cardiac filling and cardiac output

1. Tamponade is not dependent on the amount of fluid in the pericardial space but rather on the presence of the hemodynamic consequences of pericardial fluid

Predisposing factors

1. Blunt or penetrating injury of the heart
2. Post MI
   a. Pericarditis, especially in the anticoagulated patient
   b. Cardiac rupture
3. Iatrogenic causes: perforation of the myocardium by transvenous pacemaker wires, invasive catheters, intracardiac injection, or cardiac needle biopsy
4. Transmyocardial revascularization
5. After CPR or electrical cardioversion
6. Fibrinolytic or anticoagulant therapy
7. Rupture of the great vessels
8. Dissecting aortic aneurysms
9. Malignancy or radiation therapy
10. Connective tissue disease: rheumatoid arthritis, systemic lupus erythematosus, or scleroderma
11. Metabolic disease: renal failure, hepatic failure, or myxedema
12. Inflammation: pericarditis
13. Infection: viral; bacterial; fungal
14. Drugs: procainamide, hydralazine (Apresoline), minoxidil (Loniten), phenytoin (Dilantin), daunorubicin (Cerubidine), methyldopa (Aldomet), sulfasalazine

(Azulfidine), isoniazid (INH), methysergide (Sansert), sargramostim (Leukine), and tetracycline derivatives

Pathophysiology

1. The accumulation of fluid or blood in the pericardial space
   a. The pericardial space normally contains <50 ml of fluid
   b. If the fluid accumulates rapidly (e.g., cardiac trauma, cardiac surgery), a relatively small volume ($\approx$100 ml to 200 ml) may cause cardiac tamponade
   c. If the fluid accumulates slowly (e.g., uremia, myxedema), a large volume may be accommodated before hemodynamic consequences related to poor cardiac filling occur
2. When intrapericardial pressure is very high and approaches atrial pressures and ventricular diastolic pressure, the transmural cardiac pressure falls, which leads to the inability of the heart to fill
3. End-diastolic volume (preload) decreases
4. Contractility decreases
5. Stroke volume decreases
6. Cardiac output decreases
7. LVF, RVF, and shock

Clinical presentation

1. Subjective
   a. History of events or occurrence
   b. Precordial fullness or pain
   c. Dyspnea that is improved when sitting upright
   d. Anxiety or feeling of impending doom
   e. Medical history
2. Objective
   a. Tachycardia is usually an early sign, but, as the impairment in ventricular filling progresses, the patient may be pulseless (i.e., pulseless electrical activity)
   b. Hypotension and narrowed pulse pressure
   c. Increased JVD: may not be seen if the patient is hypotensive
   d. Absent PMI
   e. Dullness to percussion below the left scapula (i.e., Ewart sign)
   f. Pulsus paradoxus: a systolic pressure decrease of $\geq$10 mm Hg with inspiration
   g. Beck triad: hypotension, distended neck veins, and muffled heart sounds
3. Diagnostic
   a. Complete blood cell count with differential: to assess for anemia
   b. Type and cross-matching: in preparation for the need for blood
   c. Chest radiograph
      1) Widened mediastinum
      2) Enlarged heart (i.e., water-bottle silhouette)
   d. Electrocardiography
      1) Diffuse ST segment elevation across the precordial leads
      2) Decrease in the amplitude of the QRS or electrical alternans (i.e., alternating tall and small QRSs) across the precordial leads
      3) Bradycardia may indicate impending pulseless electrical activity
      4) Ventricular dysrhythmias
   e. Echocardiogram: two-dimensional or transesophageal
      1) Echo-free space will be evident between the pericardium and epicardium
   f. FAST: focused assessment with sonography
   g. Fluoroscopy of chest: may be used during pericardiocentesis

Collaborative management

1. Continue assessment
   a. ABCDs
   b. Vital signs: BP, pulse, respiratory rate, and temperature
   c. Oxygen saturation
   d. Respiratory effort and excursion
   e. Cardiac rate and rhythm
   f. Discomfort and pain level
   g. Level of consciousness
   h. Accurate intake and output
   i. Close monitoring for the progression of symptoms
2. Maintain airway, oxygenation, and ventilation
   a. Airway, oxygenation, and circulation support with the use of BLS and ACLS if needed
   b. 100% oxygen by face mask; intubate and mechanically ventilate as indicated
3. Maintain adequate circulation and perfusion
   a. Intravenous access with two large-bore catheters for fluid and medication administration
   b. Circulating volume replacement
      1) Normal saline or lactated Ringer's solution by rapid infusion until blood is available; colloids (e.g., albumin, hetastarch, dextran) may also be used
      2) Blood and blood products
   c. Inotropes (e.g., dobutamine [Dobutrex]) as prescribed
   d. Atropine or transcutaneous pacing may be necessary for bradycardia
   e. Pericardiocentesis for emergency cardiac tamponade (Figure 4-44)
      1) Place patient in semi-Fowler position; the subxiphoid and left parasternal approaches are most commonly used
      2) Apply ECG electrodes
      3) Have echocardiography technician available to assist with two-dimensional echocardiography guidance if possible; fluoroscopy may also be used
      4) Have emergency equipment available, including a transcutaneous pacemaker
      5) Assist with the administration of local anesthetic and sedation

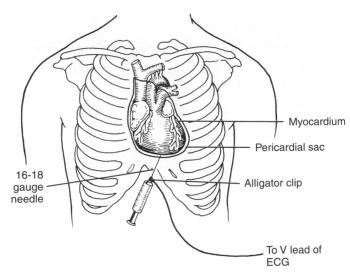

16-18 gauge needle

Myocardium

Pericardial sac

Alligator clip

To V lead of ECG

Figure 4-44 Pericardiocentesis. *ECG,* Electrocardiogram. (From Dennison, R. D. [2007]. *Pass CCRN!* [3rd ed.]. St. Louis: Mosby.)

6) Assist with the slow aspiration of the fluid and with sending it to the laboratory department for analysis
7) Monitor for complications during the procedure
   a) Laceration of coronary artery or conduction system
   b) Myocardial perforation
   c) Pneumothorax
   d) Dysrhythmias
   e) Hypotension (usually reflexogenic)

f. Surgical intervention as indicated; pericardiocentesis may not resolve the tamponade if effusion is posterior; surgical drainage may be indicated
4. Administer drugs or therapies related to the cause
   a. Protamine (protamine sulfate) or vitamin K if the patient is taking anticoagulants
   b. Dialysis for patients with renal failure
   c. Antibiotics if purulent effusion is present
   d. Thyroid hormone replacement for myxedema
   e. Corticosteroids may be prescribed for drug-related pericardial effusions, uremia, and pericarditis
5. Control pain and discomfort
   a. Narcotic analgesics in doses that are adequate to allow the patient to deep breathe and cough as indicated
   b. Anxiolytics
6. Monitor for complications
   a. HF
   b. Cardiac arrest

Evaluation
1. Patent airway as well as adequate oxygenation (i.e., normal PaO_2, SpO_2, SaO_2) and ventilation (i.e., normal $PaCO_2$)
2. Absence of clinical indicators of respiratory distress
3. Absence of clinical indicators of hypoperfusion
4. Alert and oriented with no neurologic deficit
5. Control of chest pain, discomfort, or dyspnea

Typical disposition: admission; may go from emergency department to surgery

LEARNING ACTIVITIES

1. DIRECTIONS: Identify the coronary artery that usually supplies the following structures as LAD (left anterior descending artery), LCA (left circumflex artery), or RCA (right coronary artery).

Structure	Coronary Artery
Anterior left ventricle	
Atrioventricular node	
Bundle branches	
Inferior left ventricle	
Lateral left ventricle	
Left atrium	
Posterior left ventricle	
Right atrium	
Right ventricle	
Sinoatrial node	
Septum	

2. DIRECTIONS: Match the dysrhythmia with the appropriate characteristic.

____ 1. Normal sinus rhythm
____ 2. Sinus bradycardia
____ 3. Sinus tachycardia
____ 4. Premature atrial contraction
____ 5. Atrial fibrillation
____ 6. Atrial flutter
____ 7. Supraventricular tachycardia
____ 8. Premature junctional contraction
____ 9. Junctional escape rhythm
____ 10. Accelerated junctional rhythm
____ 11. Junctional tachycardia
____ 12. Premature ventricular complex
____ 13. Accelerated idioventricular rhythm
____ 14. Ventricular tachycardia
____ 15. Ventricular fibrillation
____ 16. Asystole
____ 17. First-degree atrioventricular block
____ 18. Second-degree atrioventricular block, type 1
____ 19. Second-degree atrioventricular block, type 2
____ 20. Third-degree atrioventricular block

a. PR interval >0.20 second
b. Early P wave that looks different from other P waves followed by a normal QRS
c. Sawtooth waves on baseline, no clearly identifiable P waves, and a normal QRS
d. QRS is early and ≥0.12 second, with a T wave in the opposite direction of the QRS
e. Regular rhythm, normal P waves, normal QRS complexes, and a rate of <60 beats/minute
f. Quivering baseline with irregularly occurring QRSs
g. QRS complex is early, with inverted P wave immediately (<0.12 second) before the QRS, during the QRS, or immediately after the QRS
h. Regular rhythm with rate of 40 to 60 beats/minute with a normal QRS and an inverted P wave immediately (<0.12 second) before the QRS, during the QRS, or immediately after the QRS
i. Flat line, with no QRS complexes
j. Regular rhythm, normal P waves, normal QRS complexes, and a rate of >100 beats/minute
k. Regular rhythm, normal P waves, normal QRS complexes, and a rate of 60 to 100 beats/minute
l. Progressive PR lengthening until a P wave is not followed by a QRS
m. Regular rhythm with rate of 60 to 100 beats/minute with a narrow QRS with an inverted P wave immediately (<0.12 second) before the QRS, during the QRS, or immediately after the QRS
n. Wide QRS (≥0.12 second) rhythm with rate of 40 to 100 beats/minute
o. Regular rhythm with rate of >100 beats/minute with a narrow QRS and an inverted P wave immediately (<0.12 second) before the QRS, during the QRS, or immediately after the QRS
p. Regular rhythm with a rate of 150 to 250 beats/minute without clearly discernible P waves with a narrow QRS
q. P wave not followed by QRS without the preceding progression of the PR interval
r. No relationship between P waves and QRS complexes; escape rhythm established by the atrioventricular junction or ventricle
s. Irregular baseline and the absence of QRS complexes
t. Wide QRS (≥0.12 second) rhythm with a rate of >100/minute

3. DIRECTIONS: Analyze the following electrocardiogram rhythm strips. All strips represent 6-second intervals.

a.

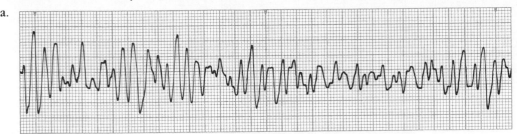

Interpretation _____

b.

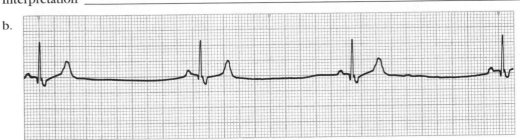

Interpretation _____

c.

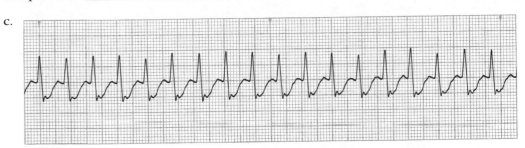

Interpretation _____

d.

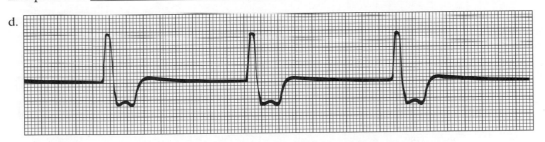

Interpretation _____

e.

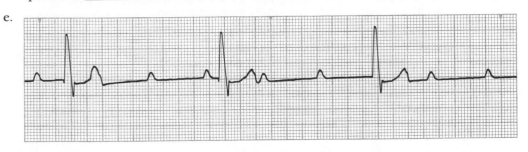

Interpretation _____

f.

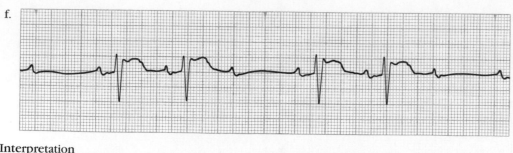

Interpretation _____

g.

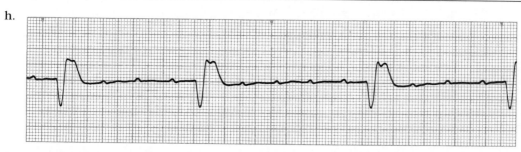

Interpretation _____

h.

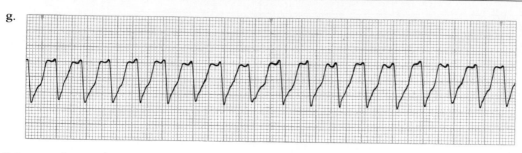

Interpretation _____

i.

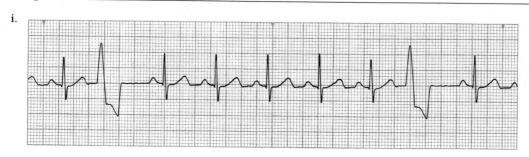

Interpretation _____

4. DIRECTIONS: Complete the table by identifying which cardiac wall the following lead groupings evaluate and corresponding types of myocardial infarction. Identify the coronary artery as LAD (left anterior descending artery), LCA (left circumflex artery), or RCA (right coronary artery).

Cardiac Wall	Lead Grouping	Artery
Anterior		
Septal		
Anteroseptal		
Lateral		
Anterolateral		
Inferior		
Right ventricular		
Posterior		

5. DIRECTIONS: Analyze the following 12-lead electrocardiograms from patients with acute chest pain for indications of myocardial infarction. Identify the location and age of the myocardial infarction if present.

a.

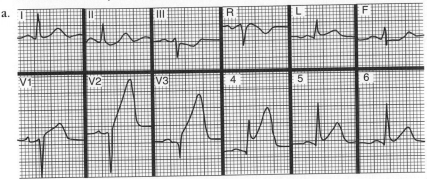

Interpretation _____

b.

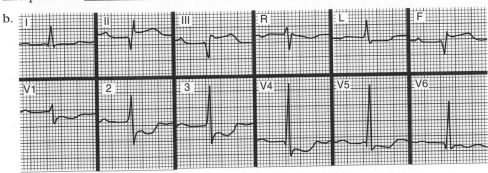

Interpretation _____

6. DIRECTIONS: Match the dysrhythmia with the most appropriate treatment summary

____ 1. Ventricular fibrillation
____ 2. Stable monomorphic ventricular tachycardia
____ 3. Asystole
____ 4. Symptomatic bradycardia
____ 5. Pulseless electrical activity
____ 6. Stable supraventricular tachycardia
____ 7. Acute-onset atrial fibrillation
____ 8. Pulseless ventricular tachycardia
____ 9. Junctional tachycardia
____ 10. Sinus tachycardia
____ 11. Torsades de pointes

a. Cardiopulmonary resuscitation, intubation, transcutaneous pacing, epinephrine, and atropine
b. Treatment of the cause followed by β-blockers or sedatives
c. Ibutilide, calcium-channel blockers, β-blockers, amiodarone (Cordarone), sedation, and cardioversion
d. Amiodarone (Cordarone) or lidocaine and β-blockers or calcium-channel blockers; do not cardiovert
e. Magnesium, overdrive pacing, and isoproterenol
f. Defibrillation, cardiopulmonary resuscitation, vasopressin or epinephrine, intubation, and amiodarone (Cordarone) or lidocaine
g. Amiodarone (Cordarone) or lidocaine followed by synchronized cardioversion
h. Atropine, transcutaneous pacing, or both
i. Cardiopulmonary resuscitation, intubation, assessment for possible causes, epinephrine, and atropine
j. Vagal maneuvers and adenosine, (Adenocard) calcium-channel blockers, β-blockers, and digoxin (Lanoxin)

7. DIRECTIONS: Match the following treatments for acute myocardial infarction with the rationales for their use. More than one rationale may apply.

____ 1. Fibrinolytics
____ 2. Percutaneous interventional procedures such as angioplasty and atherectomy
____ 3. Angiotensin-converting enzyme inhibitors
____ 4. Nitroglycerin
____ 5. Calcium-channel blockers
____ 6. β-Blockers
____ 7. Aspirin
____ 8. Heparin

a. Increases myocardial oxygen supply by reestablishing the patency of the infarct-related artery
b. Decreases myocardial oxygen demand by blocking the effects of catecholamines
c. Increases myocardial oxygen supply by reducing spasm
d. Decreases myocardial oxygen demand by reducing preload
e. Prevents the extension of a clot by decreasing platelet aggregation
f. Prevents the extension of a clot by preventing the conversion of prothrombin to thrombin
g. Prevents ventricular dilation and the adverse remodeling of the myocardium
h. Used for secondary prevention after myocardial infarction

8. DIRECTIONS: Complete the following crossword puzzle related to cardiovascular emergencies.

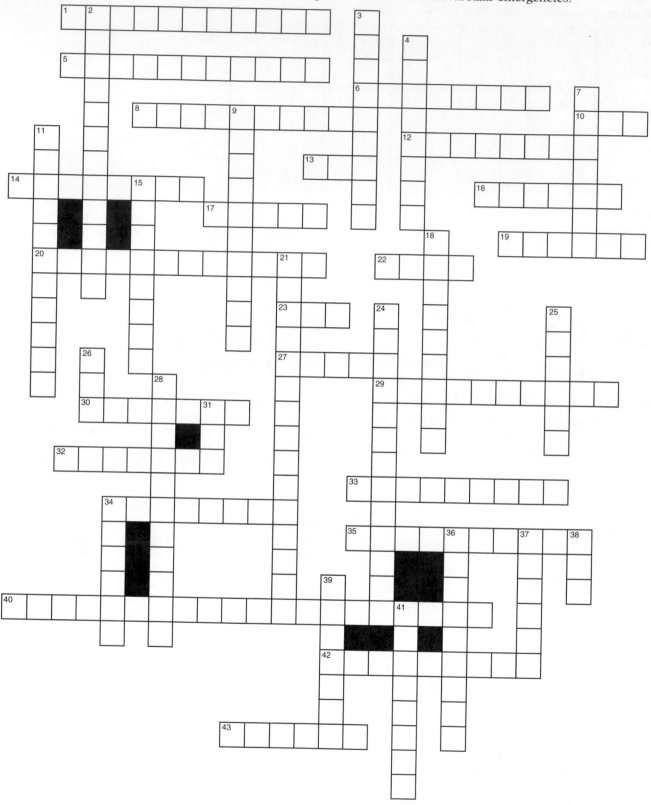

ACROSS

1. Percutaneous interventional procedure that opens an occluded artery with the use of a shaving device
5. Percutaneous interventional procedure that opens an occluded artery with the use of balloon dilation
6. A cardiac muscle protein that is measured when diagnosing myocardial infarction
8. A calcium-channel blocker that is used to treat coronary artery spasm
10. A platelet aggregation inhibitor (abbrev)
12. The indicative leads for this cardiac wall are V_3 and V_4

13. The preferred method of reperfusion for acute myocardial infarction (abbrev)
14. The analgesic of choice for acute myocardial infarction
16. The indicative leads for this cardiac wall are V_1 and V_2
17. This device is used during percutaneous interventional procedures to prevent closure
19. A new holosystolic murmur at the lower sternum, an increase in SvO_2, and shock indicate the rupture of the _____
20. The most common complication of myocardial infarction

22. The device that is used to decrease afterload and to increase myocardial perfusion during cardiogenic shock (abbrev)
23. Good cholesterol (abbrev)
27. This coronary artery supplies the right artery, the right ventricle, and the inferior wall of the left ventricle
29. Angiotensin-converting enzyme inhibitors are used after myocardial infarction to prevent this
30. The indicative leads for this cardiac wall are I and aVL, V_5 and V_6, or all of these
32. This syndrome is caused by proximal left anterior descending disease and causes T wave inversion

33. This muscle protein is sensitive but not specific for myocardial infarction
34. The indicative leads for this cardiac wall are II, III, and aVF
35. This cardioselective β-blocker is often used for the treatment of acute myocardial infarction
40. This risk factor for coronary artery disease is treated with folic acid
42. This is a tissue plasminogen activator with a short half-life that must be given as a bolus followed by an infusion
43. Patients with diabetes are more likely to have this type of myocardial infarction

DOWN

2. This is a tissue plasminogen activator that has a longer half-life and that is administered as a single bolus
3. The indicative leads for this cardiac wall are V_8 and V_9
4. The internal mammary is now referred to as the internal _____
7. The type of angina caused by spasm
9. The inotropic agent that is most likely to be used for the treatment of cardiogenic shock with myocardial infarction

11. An oral platelet aggregation inhibitor that is frequently used after a percutaneous interventional procedure
15. This is demonstrated on an electrocardiogram by T wave inversion
18. This glycoprotein IIb/IIIa inhibitor is frequently used after a percutaneous interventional procedure (generic)
21. The most likely cause of acute myocardial infarction
24. This nitrate is used for the treatment of acute chest pain

25. This is a major cause for a delay in seeking assistance for chest pain
26. Bad cholesterol (abbrev)
28. This is evidenced by the cessation of pain, the return of the ST segment to baseline, and dysrhythmias
31. A general term used for undifferentiated chest pain (abbrev)
34. This is evidenced on an electrocardiogram by ST segment elevation
36. The rupture of the _____ muscle causes acute mitral regurgitation

37. This sign is a clenched fist over the sternum
38. S_3, dypsnea, and crackles indicate this complication of acute myocardial infarction (abbrev)
39. This anticoagulant is used to prevent the extension of a clot or reocclusion
41. This activity is likely to decrease body weight, blood pressure, lipids, and stress

9. DIRECTIONS: Match the physical findings from the following with the appropriate pathologic conditions. More than one physical finding may be listed for each pathologic condition.

____ 1. Right ventricular failure
____ 2. Left ventricular failure
____ 3. Left ventricular myocardial infarction
____ 4. Pulmonary embolism
____ 5. Cardiac tamponade
____ 6. Valvular dysfunction
____ 7. Pericarditis
____ 8. Endocarditis
____ 9. Hyperlipidemia
____ 10. Chronic arterial insufficiency
____ 11. Chronic venous insufficiency

a. Jugular vein distention
b. Displaced point of maximal impact
c. S_3 at apex
d. S_3 at sternum
e. S_4 at apex
f. S_4 at sternum
g. Murmur
h. Pericardial friction rub
i. Muffled heart sounds
j. Splinter hemorrhages
k. Intermittent claudication
l. Xanthelasma
m. Peripheral edema
n. Peripheral pallor
o. Peripheral rubor
p. Fever
q. Crackles in lung bases
r. Corneal arcus
s. Hepatomegaly
t. Pulsus paradoxus

10. DIRECTIONS: Identify the following signs, symptoms, causes, or treatments as being associated with pericarditis, myocarditis, or endocarditis. You may identify more than one type of cardiomyopathy for each feature.

Feature	Pericarditis	Myocarditis	Endocarditis
Associated with myocardial infarction			
May cause cardiomyopathy			
Causes splinter hemorrhages and petechiae			
Treated with anti-inflammatory drugs			
Sudden onset of heart failure			
Causes pericardial friction rub			
Valve replacement may be necessary			
Usually associated with viral infection			
Associated with cardiac surgery			
Definitive diagnosis requires biopsy			
May cause systemic emboli			
Monitor closely for cardiac tamponade			
Causes murmur			
Associated with uremia			
Associated with ST segment elevation			
Treated with antimicrobials			
Increased incidence among patients with rheumatic heart disease			

11. DIRECTIONS: Match the chest trauma with the appropriate treatment or assessment finding.

____ 1. Myocardial contusion
____ 2. Penetrating chest trauma
____ 3. Great vessel tear
____ 4. Cardiac tamponade

a. Dysphagia and hoarseness
b. May cause tamponade
c. Blood pressure differences between upper and lower extremities
d. Can be caused by a rib
e. May be associated with false aneurysm
f. May have the same electrocardiogram findings as myocardial infarction
g. Decreased hemoglobin and hematocrit levels
h. Hypotension, muffled heart sounds, and jugular vein distention

LEARNING ACTIVITIES ANSWERS

1.

Structure	Coronary Artery
Anterior left ventricle	LAD
Atrioventricular node	Most commonly the RCA; less commonly the LCA
Bundle branches	LAD
Inferior left ventricle	RCA
Lateral left ventricle	LCA
Left atrium	LCA
Posterior left ventricle	Most commonly the RCA; less commonly the LCA
Right atrium	RCA
Right ventricle	RCA
Sinoatrial node	Most commonly the RCA; less commonly the LCA
Septum	LAD

2.

k   1. Normal sinus rhythm
e   2. Sinus bradycardia
j   3. Sinus tachycardia
b   4. Premature atrial contraction
f   5. Atrial fibrillation
c   6. Atrial flutter
p   7. Supraventricular tachycardia
g   8. Premature junctional contraction
h   9. Junctional escape rhythm
m 10. Accelerated junctional rhythm
o 11. Junctional tachycardia
d 12. Premature ventricular complex
n 13. Accelerated idioventricular rhythm
t 14. Ventricular tachycardia
s 15. Ventricular fibrillation
i 16. Asystole
a 17. First-degree atrioventricular block
l 18. Second-degree atrioventricular block, type 1
q 19. Second-degree atrioventricular block, type 2
r 20. Third-degree atrioventricular block

3.

a. Ventricular fibrillation
b. Sinus bradycardia with wide QRS (bundle branch block should be assessed for on a 12-lead electrocardiogram)
c. Supraventricular tachycardia; this is a regular narrow QRS tachycardia with no discernible P waves; the P waves could be hidden in the QRS or T wave, so there is no way to identify where above the ventricle the rhythm originates; however, the rate of 180 beats/minute suggests an atrial origin
d. Idioventricular (escape) rhythm
e. Underlying rhythm is sinus rhythm (atrial rate is 90 beats/minute); there is a third-degree atrioventricular block with a ventricular escape rhythm (ventricular rate is 35 beats/minute)
f. Underlying rhythm is sinus rhythm (atrial rate is 80 beats/minute); there is a second-degree Mobitz I (Wenckebach) atrioventricular block present; the conduction ratio is 3:2, and the ventricular rate is 40 to 50 beats/minute
g. Ventricular tachycardia (monomorphic)
h. Underlying rhythm is sinus tachycardia (atrial rate is 145 beats/minute); there is a second-degree Mobitz II block present; the conduction ratio is variable, but the PR interval of the conducted P wave is consistent
i. Sinus rhythm with two unifocal premature ventricular complexes

4.

Cardiac Wall	Lead Grouping	Artery
Anterior	$(V_2), V_3, V_4$	LAD
Septal	V_1, V_2	LAD
Anteroseptal	$V_1, V_2, V_3, (V_4)$	LAD
Lateral	I, aVL (high lateral), V_5, V_6 (low lateral)	LCA
Anterolateral	V_3, V_4, V_5, V_6, (I, aVL)	LCA
Inferior	II, III, aVF	RCA
Right ventricular	V_4R, V_5R, V_6R may be transient	RCA
Posterior	V_7, V_8, V_9 or reciprocal in V_1, V_2, V_3	RCA, LCA, or both

5.

a. ST segment elevation is noted from V_1 through V_6. Pathologic Q waves are noted in V_2 and V_3. There is a small R wave in V_1, so the negative wave in that lead in an S wave. This electrocardiogram shows evidence of hyperacute anterior myocardial infarction with injury that extends to the septal and lateral walls.

b. ST segment elevation and pathologic Q waves are noted in II, III, and aVF, which is indicative of acute inferior myocardial infarction. Reciprocal changes in the V leads (ST segment depression from V_1 through V_5) also suggest posterior wall involvement.

6.

1. f
2. g
3. a
4. h
5. i
6. j
7. c
8. f
9. d
10. b
11. e

7.

1. a
2. a
3. g
4. d, c
5. c
6. b
7. e
8. e, f

8.

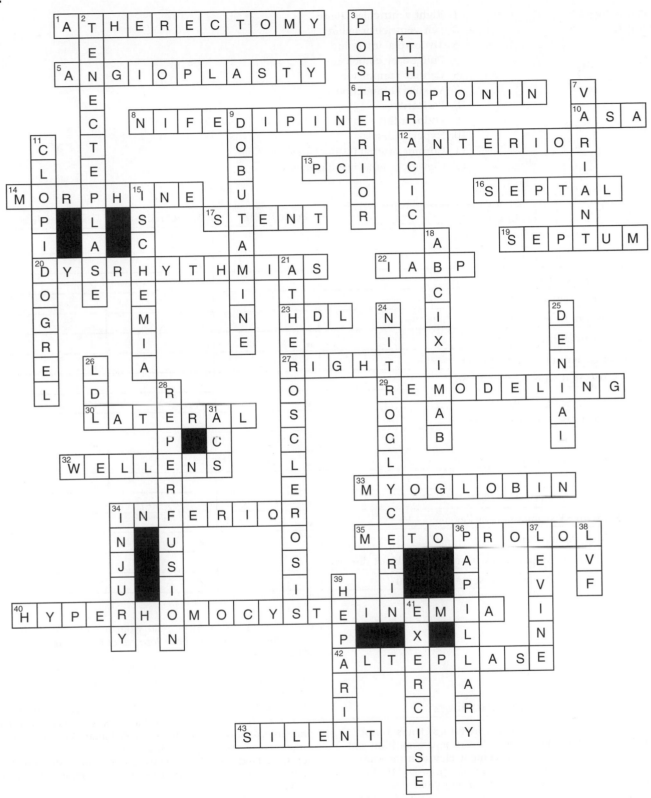

9.

a, b, d, g, m, s	1. Right ventricular failure
b, c, g, q	2. Left ventricular failure
e	3. Myocardial infarction
f, q	4. Pulmonary embolism
a, e, i, t	5. Cardiac tamponade
g	7. Valvular dysfunction
h, p	8. Pericarditis
g, j, p	9. Endocarditis
l, r	10. Hyperlipidemia
k, n	11. Chronic arterial insufficiency
m, o	12. Chronic venous insufficiency

10.

Feature	Pericarditis	Myocarditis	Endocarditis
Associated with myocardial infarction	✓		
May cause cardiomyopathy		✓	
Causes splinter hemorrhages, petechiae			✓
Treated with anti-inflammatory drugs	✓		
Sudden onset of heart failure		✓	
Causes pericardial friction rub	✓		
Valve replacement may be necessary			✓
Usually associated with viral infection		✓	
Associated with cardiac surgery	✓		✓
Definitive diagnosis requires biopsy		✓	
May cause systemic emboli		✓	✓
Monitor closely for cardiac tamponade	✓		
Causes murmur			✓
Associated with uremia	✓		
Associated with ST segment elevation	✓		
Treated with antimicrobials		✓	✓
Increased incidence in patients with rheumatic heart disease		✓	✓
May be treated with therapeutic septal infarction		✓	

11.

1. f
2. b, d, g
3. a, c, e, g
4. h

References and Suggested Readings

Aehlert, B. (2007). ACLS study guide (3rd ed.). St. Louis: Mosby.

Aghababian, R. (2004). Emergency department evaluation and treatment of patients with ST-segment elevation myocardial infarction. *Critical Pathways in Cardiology, 3(3),* 110–113.

Akhondi, H. & Rahimi, A. R. (2002). *Haemophilus aphrophilus* endocarditis after tongue piercing. *Emerging Infectious Disease, 8(8),* 2002 August. Retrieved November 4, 2008, from http://www.cdc.gov/ncidod/EID/vol8no8/01-0458.

American Heart Association. (2006). *Advanced cardiac life support manual.* Dallas, TX: American Heart Association.

Bakris, G. (2003). The implications of JNC 7 for antihypertensive treatment protocols. Retrieved May 9, 2010, from www.medscape.com/viewprogram/2513_pnt.

Baxter, G. L. (2008). A 58-year-old woman with stress-induced cardiomyopathy (Takotsubo). *Journal of Emergency Nursing, 34(2),* 134–136.

Buttaro, T. M., Trybulski, J., Bailey, P. P., & Sandberg-Cook, J. (2003). *Primary care: A collaborative practice.* St. Louis: Mosby.

Dennison, R. D. (2007). Pass CCRN! (3rd ed.). St. Louis: Mosby.

Calder, S. (2008). Clinical pearls and pitfalls of electrocardiogram interpretation in acute myocardial infarction. *Journal of Emergency Nursing, 34(4),* 324–329.

Casey, C. & Emde, K. (2008). Displaced fractured sternum following blunt chest trauma. *Journal of Emergency Nursing, 34(1),* 83–85.

Castellano, G., Affuso, F., Di Conza, P., & Fazio, S. (2008). Myocarditis and dilated cardiomyopathy: Possible connections and treatments. *Journal of Cardiovascular Medicine, 9(7),* 666–671.

Chng, Y., & Kosowsky, J. (2004). A triage algorithm for the rapid clinical assessment and management of emergency department patients presenting with chest pain. *Critical Pathways in Cardiology: A Journal of Evidence-Based Medicine, 3(3),* 154–157.

Constantine, E., & Linakis, J. (2005). The assessment and management of hypertensive emergencies and urgencies in children. *Pediatric Emergency Care, 21(6)*, 391–396.

Conway, G. (2006). Case management for heart failure in the emergency department. *Critical Pathways in Cardiology, 5(1)*, 25–28.

Cottrell, D. B., & Mack, K. (2008). Atrial fibrillation: An emergency nurse's rapid response. *Journal of Emergency Nursing, 34(3)*, 207–210.

Darovic, G. O. (2002). *Hemodynamic monitoring: Invasive and noninvasive clinical application* (3rd ed.). Philadelphia: W. B. Saunders.

Darovic, G. O., & Franklin, C. M. (2004). *Handbook of hemodynamic monitoring* (2nd ed.). St. Louis: W. B. Saunders.

Decker, C. J., Amin, A., Jones, P., Maddox, T. M., Ramesh, P., & Spertus, J. A. (2006). Risk factor management post-MI: Adherence and outcomes. *Circulation, 113(21)*, e802.

Dennison, R. D. (2007). *Pass CCRN!* (3rd ed.). St. Louis: Mosby.

Domino, F. J. (2008). *The 5-minute clinical consultant* (16th ed.). Philadelphia: Lippincott, Williams, & Wilkins.

Eggers, K., Lagerqvist, B., Venge, P., Wallentin, L., & Lindahl, B. (2007). Persistent cardiac troponin I elevation in stabilized patients after an episode of acute coronary syndrome predicts long-term mortality. *Circulation, 116(17)*, 1907–1914.

Emergency Nurses Association. (2007). *Emergency nursing core curriculum* (6th ed). Philadelphia: Saunders.

Emergency Nurses Association. (2005). *Sheehy's manual of emergency care* (6th ed.). St Louis: Mosby.

Fultz, J., & Sturt, P. A. (2005). *Mosby's emergency nursing reference* (3rd ed.). St. Louis: Mosby.

Gardetto, N., & Carroll, K. (2007). Management strategies to meet the core heart failure measures for acute decompensated heart failure: A nursing perspective. *Critical Care Nursing Quarterly, 30(4)*, 307–320.

Imazio, M., Trinchero, R., & Shabetai, R. (2007). Pathogenesis, management, and prevention of recurrent pericarditis. *Journal of Cardiovascular Medicine, 8(6)*, 404–410.

Jarvis, C. (2008). *Physical examination and health assessment* (5th ed.). St. Louis: Saunders.

Kemmerer, D. A. (2008). Devious digoxin: A case review. *Journal of Emergency Nursing, 34(5)*, 487–489.

Mayo Clinic. (2009). Wolff-Parkinson-White syndrome. Retrieved December 1, 2008, from http://www.mayoclinic.com/health/wolff-parkinson-white-syndrome/DS00923.

McCowan, C. (2007). Hypertensive emergencies. Retrieved November 4, 2008, from http://www.emedicine.com/emerg/TOPIC267

Medina, D. L., Sumter, D., George, J., Rushenberg, J., & Leonard, C. (2007). Reducing door-to-balloon times in acute myocardial infarction. *Journal of Emergency Nursing, 33(4)*, 336–341.

Mosley, M. (2004). Glycoprotein IIb IIIa inhibitors in ACS with PCI: Little prospective data. *Emergency Medicine News, 26(8)*, 4, 43.

Novotny, A. (2006). Chest pain screening area within a busy emergency department: Lakeland Regional Medical Center's 6-month experience. *Journal of Emergency Nursing, 32(4)*, 304–309.

Pickman, D., & Drew, B. J. (2008). QT/QTc interval monitoring in the emergency department. *Journal of Emergency Nursing, 34(5)*, 428–434.

Pearlman, M. K., Tanabe, M. B., Mycyk, D. N., & Stone, D. B. (2008). Evaluating disparities in door-to-EKG time for patients with noncardiac chest pain. *Journal of Emergency Nursing, 34(5)*, 414–418.

Price, S. A., & Wilson, L. M. (2003). *Pathophysiology: Clinical concepts of disease process* (6th ed.). St. Louis: Mosby.

Proehl, J. A. (2004). *Emergency nursing procedures* (3rd ed.). St. Louis: Saunders.

Roppolo, L. P., Davis, D., Kelly, S. P., & Rosen, P. (2007). *Emergency medicine handbook: Critical concepts for clinical practice.* St. Louis: Mosby.

Schulenburg, M. (2007). Management of hypertensive emergencies: Implications for the critical care nurse. *Critical Care Nursing Quarterly, 30(2)*, 86–93.

Spangler, S. (2008). Pericarditis, acute. Retrieved November 3, 2008, from http://www.emedicine.com/med/topic1781.htm.

Stephens, E. (2007). Peripheral vascular disease. Retrieved November 3, 2008, from http://www.emedicine.com/emerg/topic862.htm.

Stern, S. (2002). Angina pectoris without chest pain: Clinical implications of silent ischemia. *Circulation, 106(15)*, 1906–1908.

Zimmerman, P. G., & Herr, R. (2006). *Triage nursing secrets.* St. Louis: Mosby.

CHAPTER 5

Respiratory Emergencies

Introduction

Constitutes 12% (18 items) of the CEN examination
The focus is on respiratory conditions commonly
encountered in an emergency department setting
The continuum of age needs to be considered
from infancy to older adulthood

Age-Related Considerations

Neonates, infants, and children
1. The head of a neonate or infant is large and naturally
   flexed in a supine position
   a. Extension of head may cause tracheal extubation
   b. Flexion of head may lead to mainstem intubation
2. Infants under 6 months of age are obligate nose
   breathers (Emergency Nurses Association [ENA],
   2007); keep nares clear of secretions
3. Infants have relatively less oxygen (O_2) reserve due to
   greater O_2 consumption, so hypoxemia occurs
   relatively more rapidly
4. Airway resistance in infants is 15 times greater than
   in adults (ENA, 2007)
5. The larynx is high and anterior; vocal cords have
   lower attachments
6. The smallest portion of airway is at the cricoid in
   infants and children younger than 10 years of age;
   this is why a cuff on an endotracheal (ET) tube is not
   necessary in patients younger than 10 years
7. The tongue is large and therefore the most common
   cause of airway obstruction in children
8. The chest wall is pliable, contributing to sternal
   retractions
9. Accessory muscles of inspiration tire quickly because
   of limited glycogen reserve (ENA, 2007)

Older adults
1. Decreased diffusion capacity decreases normal PaO_2;
   may estimate expected normal PaO_2 by subtracting
   one half of the patient's age in years from 105
2. Elastase breaks down elastic tissue (i.e., lung) over time,
   causing senile emphysema; decreased alveolar surface
   area, and loss of supporting tissue for peripheral airways,
   resulting in decreased ability of the lungs to return to
   their original position (i.e., decreased elastance) and increased residual volume and functional residual capacity
3. Compliance of the chest wall diminishes, thereby
   increasing work of breathing; tidal volume decreases
   and respiratory rate increases

4. Respiratory muscle strength decreases with aging
   and is correlated to nutritional status
5. There is a decreased sensitivity of the respiratory
   centers to hypoxemia or hypercapnia resulting in a
   diminished ventilatory response when illness occurs
   (e.g., heart failure, infection) (ENA, 2007)
6. Diminished physical activity may decrease awareness of disease and delay diagnosis and treatment
7. Older adults may report dyspnea as "breathlessness"
   (ENA, 2007)
8. The presenting symptom of myocardial infarction
   (MI) in older adults is frequently dyspnea
9. Anemia is common in older adults and may be a
   cause of dyspnea and hypoxia
10. Diminished pulmonary defense mechanisms and
    immunosenescence predispose older adults to
    respiratory infections; pneumonia is the leading
    cause of death among older adults (ENA, 2007) and
    is sometimes referred to as the "old man's friend"

Selected Concepts in Anatomy and Physiology

General information
1. The pulmonary system consists of lungs, conducting air passages, muscles of ventilation, central
   nervous system control, thoracic cage, and alveoli
   (Figure 5-1)
2. Functions of the pulmonary system include the
   following:
   a. Allows interchange of gases between the
      atmosphere and the bloodstream
   b. Assists in maintenance of acid-base balance
   c. Contributes to phonation (making sounds and
      speaking)
   d. Acts as a reservoir for blood for the left atrium and
      ventricle
   e. Assists in metabolism

Functional anatomy
1. Conducting airways: nose to terminal bronchioles
   a. Conduct airflow toward gas exchange units; no gas
      exchange occurs in these airways
      1) Consists of branching tubes with diminishing
         diameter
      2) Accounts for ≈2 ml/kg of inspired tidal
         volume (this volume is referred to as
         anatomical deadspace)

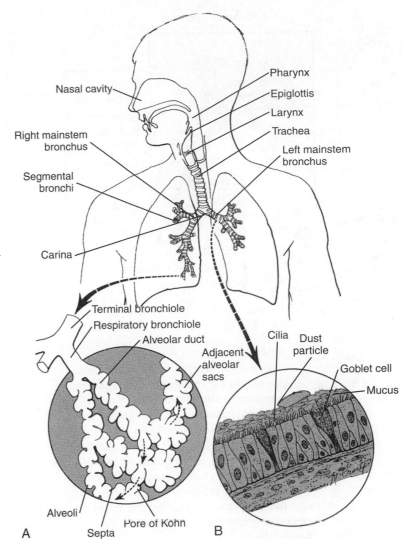

Figure 5-1 The respiratory system. **A,** Acinus. **B,** Mucociliary escalator. (From Price, S., & Wilson, L. M. [1997]. *Pathophysiology: Clinical concepts of disease processes* [5th ed.]. St. Louis: Mosby.)

b. Upper airway (Figure 5-2): nose or mouth to external opening of vocal cords; serves as a passageway for food and inspired gas
   1) Mouth: not as effective as the nose in conditioning the inspired air
   2) Nose
      a) Structure
         i) Mucous membrane lining contains cilia and mucus-producing cells
         ii) Rich supply of blood vessels lies under the mucous membranes to provide warmth
         iii) Skeletal rigidity maintains patency during inspiration
         iv) Turbinates increase surface area
         v) Four sinuses surround and drain into the nasal cavity: frontal, maxillary, ethmoid, sphenoid
         vi) Septum divides the nose into two fossae
      b) Functions
         i) Warm inspired gas to body temperature
         ii) Protects the lower airway from foreign material; filters inspired air of particles 5 microns (μm) or larger
         iii) Prevents inspiration of potentially dangerous environmental gases
         iv) Assists in production of sound in phonation
         v) Provides sense of olfaction: sniffing directs air toward the olfactory area located in the superior turbinate
      c) More resistance (two to three times) than the mouth; this is rationale for why dyspneic patients are more likely to breathe through their mouth
   3) Pharynx: posterior nasal cavity to esophagus
      a) Structure
         i) Nasopharynx: between posterior nasal cavity to soft palate; contains the pharyngeal tonsils and eustachian tubes
            (a) Pharyngeal tonsils (also called adenoids): dense concentration of lymphatic tissue; guards entryway into respiratory and gastrointestinal tracts

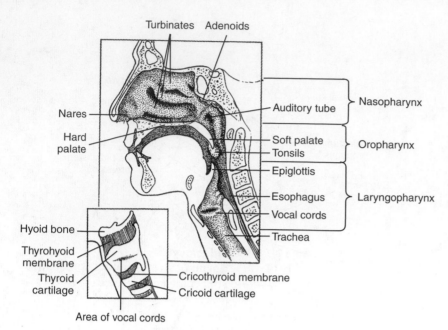

Turbinates   Adenoids

Nares

Hard
palate

Hyoid bone

Thyrohyoid
membrane

Thyroid
cartilage

Area of vocal cords

Auditory tube — Nasopharynx

Soft palate
Tonsils — Oropharynx

Epiglottis

Esophagus
Vocal cords — Laryngopharynx

Trachea

Cricothyroid membrane
Cricoid cartilage

Figure 5-2 The upper airway (lateral view). (From Luce, J. M. & Pierson, D. J. [1998]. *Critical care medicine.* Philadelphia: W.B. Saunders.)

(b) Eustachian tubes: connection between nasopharynx and middle ears; opens during swallowing to equalize pressure in the middle ear

ii) Oropharynx: between the soft palate and base of tongue

(a) Contains palatine and lingual tonsils

(b) Center of the gag reflex: controlled by cranial nerves IX (glossopharyngeal) and X (vagus)

iii) Laryngopharynx (also called the hypopharynx): from base of tongue to the epiglottis

(a) Functions

(i) Swallowing

(ii) Protection because the area is rich in lymphatic tissue

4) Larynx: upper portion of the trachea; connects the laryngopharynx with the trachea

a) Structure: consists of thyroid cartilage, vocal cords, cricoid cartilage

i) Epiglottis: flexible cartilage attached to the thyroid cartilage, overhangs the larynx like a lid; prevents food from entering the larynx and trachea during swallowing

ii) Thyroid cartilage: largest laryngeal cartilage

(a) Contains the vocal cords

(b) Also referred to as the Adam's apple

iii) Vocal folds: two pairs of membranes that protrude into the lumen of the larynx; controlled by recurrent laryngeal nerve, a branch of the vagus nerve

(a) True vocal cords: form a triangular opening leading to the trachea

(i) Change shape and vibrate in response to contraction of muscles in the larynx to result in phonation

(b) Glottis: passage through the vocal cords

iv) Cricothyroid membrane: avascular structure that connects the thyroid and cricoid cartilage; cricothyrotomy, an emergency opening of the airway, is performed here

v) Cricoid cartilage: complete ring located below the thyroid cartilage

b. Functions: allows speech, prevents aspiration, and allows for cough reflex and Valsalva maneuver

c. Lower airway (Figure 5-3): below larynx; conducts air to the gas exchange surface

1) Structure

a) Trachea: first portion of tracheobronchial tree

i) The esophagus and trachea share a common wall; erosion through this wall (tracheoesophageal fistula) may be caused by an overinflated ET tube or tracheostomy tube cuff

b) Carina: bifurcation of trachea into left and right mainstem bronchi

i) The carina is rich in parasympathetic nervous system fibers and cough receptors

ii) Suctioning may stimulate the carina and cause bradycardia and hypotension

c) Bronchi

i) Right mainstem bronchus is almost straight (25 degrees) off trachea and larger in diameter than the left (40 to 60 degrees); aspiration of liquid or food, foreign bodies, suction catheter, and ET tube go to right preferentially

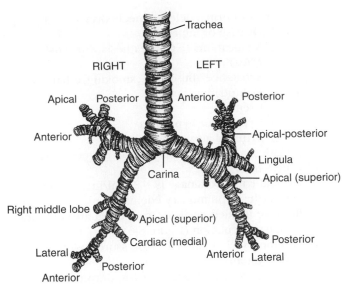

Figure 5-3 The lower airway. (Modified from Frownfelter, D. L. [ed.]. [1978]. *Chest physical therapy and pulmonary rehabilitation.* Chicago: Mosby.)

    ii) Conducting airways branch from mainstem bronchi branch → lobar bronchi; from lobar bronchi branch → segmental bronchi; from segmental bronchi branch → subsegmental bronchi and so on

    iii) Bronchi are supported by cartilage and smooth muscle

    iv) Mast cells lie just beneath the bronchial epithelium near the smooth muscle and blood vessels

  2) Function

    a) The lower airway conducts, warms, cleanses, and humidifies air

    b) The bronchi are responsible for most of total airway resistance in a healthy person

    c) Mast cells secrete histamine and other mediators of the inflammatory process when stimulated by antigen-antibody response

  3) Terminal bronchioles

    a) Structure: 1 mm in diameter; fibrous, elastic smooth muscle; no cartilage, mucous glands, or cilia

    b) Function

      i) Terminal bronchioles are particularly sensitive to carbon dioxide (CO_2) and dilate in response to increased CO_2 levels

      ii) Bronchospasm may significantly narrow the lumen and increase airway resistance

2. Lung

  a. Lobes separated by fissures

    1) Right: three lobes

    2) Left: two lobes

  b. Segments

    1) Right: 10 segments

    2) Left: 8 segments

  c. Subsegments

  d. Lobules

    1) Primary functional units of lung

    2) Consists of terminal bronchiole, alveolar ducts, alveolar sacs, alveoli, pulmonary circulation

  e. Gas exchange units (Figure 5-4):

    1) Acinus: the terminal respiratory unit distal to the terminal bronchioles

      a) Respiratory bronchioles

      b) Alveolar ducts

      c) Alveolar sacs

      d) Alveoli

    2) Lined with alveolar epithelium: the site of diffusion of O_2 and CO_2 between inspired air and blood

    3) Cells

      a) Type I pneumocytes

      b) Type II pneumocytes: produce, store, and secrete surfactant, a lipoprotein that lines the inner aspect of the alveolus

        i) Surfactant decreases surface tension of the fluid lining the alveoli and prevents alveolar collapse at the end of expiration, especially at low volumes

        ii) A deficiency of surfactant causes alveolar collapse, poorly compliant lungs, and alveolar edema

        iii) The half-life of surfactant is only 14 hours; injury to these cells quickly results in massive atelectasis

  f. Alveolar-capillary membrane

    1) Structure

      a) Lines respiratory bronchioles to alveoli

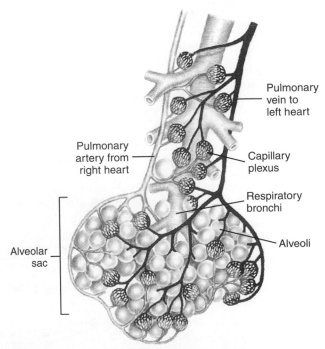

Figure 5-4 The acinus. (From Wilson, S. F. & Thompson, V. M. [1990]. *Mosby's clinical nursing series: Respiratory disorders.* St. Louis: Mosby.)

b) Diffusion pathway (Figure 5-5): gases travel through the pathway from alveolus to blood (O_2) or blood to alveolus (CO_2)
   i) Alveolar epithelium
   ii) Epithelial basement membrane
   iii) Interstitial space
   iv) Capillary basement membrane
   v) Capillary endothelium

2) Function: immense surface area and thinness of membrane allow for rapid gas exchange by diffusion

g. Defense mechanisms
  1) Upper airway
    a) Nasal cilia: filters particles
    b) Sneeze: reaction to irritation in the nose
    c) Cough: reaction to irritation in the upper airway distal to the nose
    d) Mucociliary escalator: combination of mucus and cilia, which filters particles not filtered by nasal cilia (smaller than 5 mm—are trapped in mucus and then propelled upward by the pulsatile motion of the cilia)
    e) Lymphatics: contains lymphocytes
  2) Lower airway
    a) Cough: especially at level of carina
    b) Mucociliary escalator
    c) Lymphatics
  3) Alveoli
    a) Immune system
    b) Lymphatics
    c) Alveolar macrophages: mononuclear phagocytes that engulf and remove bacteria and other foreign substances

4) Loss of normal defense mechanisms
    a) Disease or injury
    b) Medications (e.g., anesthesia, corticosteroids)
    c) Substance abuse (e.g., smoking, ethanol)
    d) Malnutrition
    e) Uremia
    f) Hypoxia or hyperoxia
    g) Artificial airways

3. Lymphatics: remove interstitial fluid to keep lung free of excess fluid
  a. Normal lymph drainage is ≈20 ml/hr; may be 200 ml/hr in pulmonary edema
  b. Remove inhaled particles from distal areas of lung

4. Pulmonary circulation (Figure 5-6)
  a. Pulmonary circulation: low pressure, low resistance system
   1) Lungs receive the full cardiac output (≈5 L/min)
   2) Right ventricle → main pulmonary artery → left and right pulmonary arteries → arterioles → capillaries that spread over the surface of the alveoli → red blood cells (RBCs) move through in single file to allow the diffusion of gases and the attachment of O_2 to hemoglobin (Hgb)
   3) Veins move out of lung toward pleura
    a) Numerous veins gradually form four pulmonary veins that empty into the left atrium
    b) The venous system serves as an immense reservoir of blood for the left atrium and left ventricle
   4) Mean pressure in pulmonary artery: 10 to 20 mm Hg

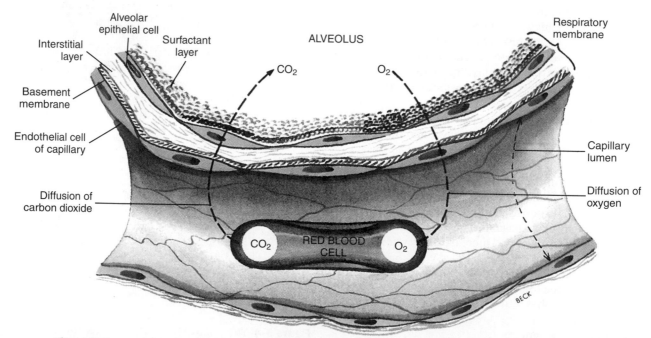

Figure 5-5 The diffusion pathway. (From Lewis, S. M. & Collier, I. [1992]. *Medical-surgical nursing* [3rd ed.] St. Louis: Mosby.)

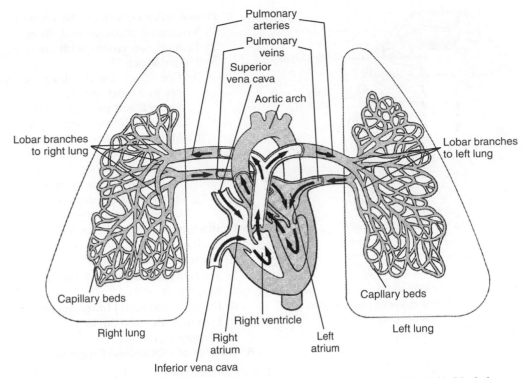

Figure 5-6 The pulmonary circulation. (From Wilson, S. F. & Thompson, V. M. [1990]. *Mosby's clinical nursing series: Respiratory disorders.* St. Louis: Mosby.)

a) Pulmonary hypertension (pulmonary artery pressure >20 mm Hg)
  i) Primary pulmonary hypertension: idiopathic
  ii) Secondary pulmonary hypertension
    (a) Passive pulmonary hypertension: result of back pressure
      (i) Mitral stenosis
      (ii) Left ventricular failure
    (b) Active pulmonary hypertension
      (i) Constriction of the pulmonary circulation is caused by decreased alveolar O_2 concentration (called hypoxemic pulmonary hypertension), acidosis, or endogenous agents such as epinephrine; norepinephrine; angiotensin II
      (ii) Obstruction in pulmonary circuit: pulmonary embolus
  b) Dilation of the pulmonary circulation caused by:
    i) O_2
    ii) Pulmonary vasodilators (e.g., isoproterenol [Isuprel], aminophylline, epoprostenol [Flolan], bosentan [Tracleer], nitric oxide)
b. Bronchial circulation
  1) This system consists of the nutrient and O_2 circulation for the tracheobronchial tree down to terminal bronchioles, visceral pleura, interstitial and connective tissue, some arteries and veins, lymph nodes, nerves within the thoracic cavity
  2) Gas exchange units are supplied with nutrients and O_2 by the pulmonary circulation
  3) Bronchial venous blood enters the pulmonary veins, causing some desaturation of the oxygenated blood in the pulmonary vein; this venous blood and the blood from the thebesian veins cause the normal physiologic shunt of 3% to 5%
5. Thoracic cage (Figure 5-7)
  a. Muscular walls reinforced by bones
    1) Sternum anterior: three connected flat bones
      a) Manubrium
      b) Body
      c) Xiphoid
    2) Spine posterior: 12 pairs of ribs attached to the vertebrae
    3) Ribs anterior, lateral, and posterior
      a) Seven pairs of ribs (true ribs) attached to sternum
      b) Five pairs of ribs attached to the rib above it
    4) Clavicles superior
    5) Diaphragm: inferior border of the thoracic cage
  b. Properties
    1) Rigid to protect the lungs
    2) Resilient to allow expansion and reduction of lung volume that occurs during ventilation
  c. Contents
    1) Heart
    2) Lungs
    3) Esophagus
    4) Great vessels

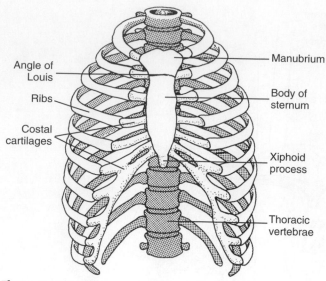

Angle of
Louis

Ribs

Costal
cartilages

Manubrium

Body of
sternum

Xiphoid
process

Thoracic
vertebrae

Figure 5-7 The thoracic cage. (From Scanlan, C. L., Spearman, C. B., & Sheldon, R. L. [Eds.]. [1990]. *Egan's fundamentals of respiratory care* [6th ed.]. St. Louis: Mosby.)

     5) Liver
     6) Spleen
6. Pleural cavities (Figure 5-8)
  a. Each lung hangs in its own pleural cavity attached only at the hilum; the hilum is where the two mainstem bronchi branch and where the pulmonary vessels enter and leave the thoracic space
  b. Pleural cavities are independent of one another

  c. Pleural linings consist of two layers
    1) Visceral: contiguous with lung
    2) Parietal: contiguous with chest wall
    3) Pleural space
      a) Contains a few milliliters of serous fluid acting as a lubricant and adhesive between the visceral and parietal pleura as they slide along each other with each ventilatory cycle
      b) Maintains a negative intrapleural pressure of ≈ -5 mm Hg below atmospheric pressure; pressure becomes more negative (-10 mm Hg) during inspiration; loss of this negative intrapleural pressure causes the lung to collapse (e.g., pneumothorax)
7. Mediastinum: center of thoracic cavity; contains the following:
  a. Heart and great vessels
  b. Trachea and mainstem bronchi
  c. Esophagus
  d. Phrenic, vagus, and other nerves
  e. Lymph nodes and ducts
  f. Thymus gland
8. Muscles of ventilation (Figure 5-9)
  a. Inspiratory
    1) Diaphragm
      a) Innervation occurs via phrenic nerves (C3 to C5)
      b) The diaphragm consists of two hemidiaphragms connected by a central membranous tendon; this tendon is contiguous with the fibrous pericardium
      c) Contraction flattens the diaphragm

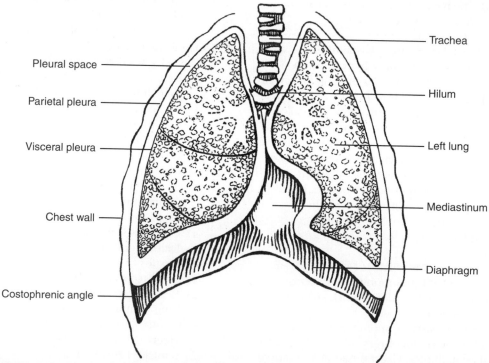

Pleural space

Parietal pleura

Visceral pleura

Chest wall

Costophrenic angle

Trachea

Hilum

Left lung

Mediastinum

Diaphragm

Figure 5-8 Internal structures of the thorax, including pleural cavities. (From Dettenmeier, P. [1992]. *Pulmonary nursing care.* St. Louis: Mosby.)

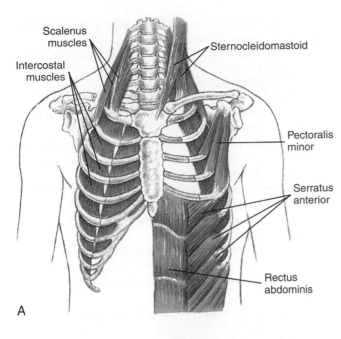

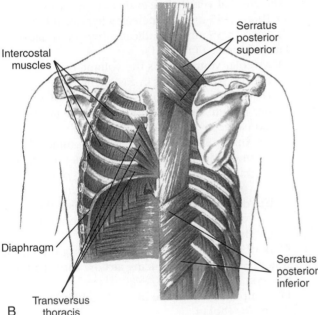

Figure 5-9 Muscles of ventilation. **A,** Anterior. **B,** Posterior. (From Urden, L. D., Stacy, K. M., & Lough, M. E. [2007]. *Critical care nursing: Diagnosis and management* [6th ed.]. St. Louis: Mosby.)

i) Increases size of thorax superior-inferior
ii) Normally accounts for 70% of tidal volume during quiet breathing
d) Relaxation makes the diaphragm dome shaped and decreases the volume of the thoracic cavity
2) External intercostals
a) Innervation occurs from T1 to T12
b) Contraction raises the ribs, increasing the size of thorax anteroposteriorly

3) Accessory muscles of inspiration
a) Scalene: enlarges the upper rib cage
i) Located in the neck; stretch from the first cervical vertebrae to the first and second ribs
b) Sternocleidomastoid: elevates the sternum to increase the anteroposterior (AP) and transverse diameter of the chest
i) Located in the neck; stretch from the manubrium and clavicle to the mastoid process and occipital bone
c) Not used in normal resting ventilation but used during exercise and in respiratory distress; also used in the inspiratory phase of sneeze or cough
b. Expiratory
1) Expiration is normally passive
a) It occurs when diaphragm and external intercostals relax and return to resting position
b) The natural tendency of the lungs is to collapse as they are made of elastic tissue; elastance is the quality of the lungs to recoil after inspiration
2) Accessory muscles of expiration: internal oblique, external oblique, rectus abdominis, internal intercostal, and transverse abdominis
a) Depress the lower ribs and pull down the anterior portion of the lower chest
b) Increase pressure in abdominal cavity and compress the abdominal viscera up against the diaphragm
c) Used when increased levels of ventilation are needed
d) Important in forceful expiration, coughing, and sneezing
9. Neuroanatomy
a. Medulla: central chemoreceptors sensitive to cerebrospinal fluid (CSF) pH ($\uparrow$Pa$_{CO_2}$ → acidosis)
1) Primary control of ventilation is by these central chemoreceptors and Pa$_{CO_2}$ and pH levels
2) They respond to minimal changes in Pa$_{CO_2}$ very quickly
3) Adjustment of alveolar ventilation occurs
a) Increase in Pa$_{CO_2}$ causes an increase in the rate and depth of ventilation
b) Decrease in Pa$_{CO_2}$ causes a decrease in the rate and depths of ventilation
b. Arterial chemoreceptors in aortic arch and carotid bodies: sensitive to pH, Pa$_{O_2}$
1) These peripheral chemoreceptors and Pa$_{O_2}$ levels provide secondary control of ventilation
2) They will not respond to Pa$_{CO_2}$ levels until a 10 mm Hg change is seen
3) They respond when Pa$_{O_2}$ falls below ≈60 mm Hg; particularly important in patients with chronically elevated levels of Pa$_{CO_2}$
c. Pontine: control rhythmic ventilation
1) Apneustic center stimulates inspiratory center
2) Pneumotaxic center inhibits inspiratory activity

d. Alveolar stretch receptors: inhibit further inspiration preventing overdistention of alveoli; may cause bronchodilation, tachycardia, vasodilation

e. Proprioceptors in muscles and tendons: increase ventilation in response to body movements

f. Baroreceptors in aortic arch and carotid bodies: increase in blood pressure inhibits ventilation

g. Juxtacapillary receptors (also called pulmonary J receptors): stimulated by increase in interstitial fluid volume; may cause laryngeal constriction, hypotension, bradycardia, mucous production, dyspnea

h. Chest wall pain receptors
   1) Lung parenchyma does not have pain receptors
   2) Parietal pleura do have pain receptors; transmit impulses via intercostal nerves and thoracic ganglia

i. Irritant receptors: stimulated by pulmonary edema, chemical or mechanical irritation; may cause bronchospasm, cough, mucus production

j. Modifying influences: drugs; brain trauma, edema, or increased intracranial pressure; chronic hypercapnia

Physiology

1. Ventilation: movement of air between atmosphere and alveoli and distribution of air within the lungs to maintain appropriate concentrations of O_2 and CO_2 in the alveoli
   a. Process (Figure 5-10)
      1) Inspiration (inhalation): the movement of atmospheric air into the alveoli

   a) Message from medulla travels down phrenic nerve to diaphragm
   b) Diaphragm and external intercostals contract
   c) Size of thorax increases
   d) Lungs are stretched and intrapulmonary pressure is decreased to less than atmospheric pressure (-1 cm H_2O)
   e) Air movement into lungs to equalize the difference between atmospheric and alveolar pressure

   2) Expiration (exhalation): movement of air from alveoli to the atmosphere
      a) Relaxation of diaphragm and external intercostals
      b) Recoil of lungs to their resting size and a concomitant increase in alveolar pressure above atmospheric pressure ($+1$ cm H_2O)
      c) Air movement out of lungs to equalize the pressure difference

   b. Efficiency of ventilation: evaluated by Pa_{CO_2}
      1) Pa_{CO_2} >45 mm Hg indicates hypoventilation
      2) Pa_{CO_2} <35 mm Hg indicates hyperventilation

   c. Lung volumes (Table 5-1)
      1) Alveolar ventilation is the volume of air per minute participating in gas exchange
      2) Deadspace ventilation is the volume of air per minute that does not participate in gas exchange
         a) Anatomical deadspace is the volume of air in conducting airways and does not participate in gas exchange; $\approx$2 ml/kg of tidal volume
         b) Alveolar (pathologic) deadspace is the volume of air in contact with nonperfused alveoli

   d. Work of breathing = work of deforming the elastic system + work of producing airflow through the airways
      1) Compliance: measure of expandability of lungs and/or thorax
      2) Airway resistance: pressure differential required to produce a unit flow change; affected by airway caliber and length

2. Perfusion: movement of blood through the pulmonary capillaries
   a. Pulmonary vasculature: resistance varies to accommodate the blood flow that it receives
   b. Distribution of perfusion
      1) Related to gravity and intra-alveolar pressures
      2) Hypoxemic pulmonary vasoconstriction
         a) Localized
            i) Protective mechanism which decreases blood flow to an area of poor ventilation so that blood can be shunted to areas of better ventilation
            ii) Stimulated by decreased alveolar O_2 levels

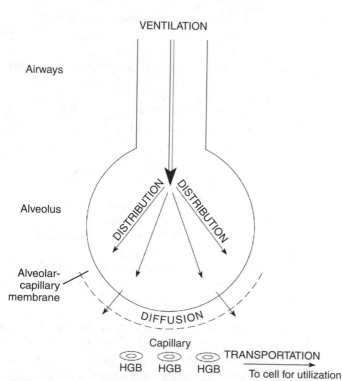

Figure 5-10 Respiratory process: ventilation, distribution, diffusion, transportation, and cellular utilization. HGB, hemoglobin. (Drawing by Ann M. Walthall.)

Image labels: VENTILATION; Airways; Alveolus; Alveolar-capillary membrane; DISTRIBUTION; DISTRIBUTION; DIFFUSION; Capillary; HGB HGB HGB; TRANSPORTATION; To cell for utilization

TABLE 5-1 Lung Volumes

Volume	Definition	Normal
Tidal volume (V_T)	Volume of air moved in and out of the lungs with each normal breath	7 ml/kg or ≈500 ml
Inspiratory reserve volume (IRV)	Volume of air that can be maximally inspired above the normal inspiratory level	3000 ml
Expiratory reserve volume (ERV)	Volume of air that can be maximally exhaled beyond the normal expiratory level	1000 ml
Residual volume (RV)	Volume of air remaining in the lungs at the end of a maximal expiration	1000 ml
Inspiratory capacity (IC)	V_T + IRC; volume of air that can be maximally inspired from a normal expiratory level	3500 ml
Functional residual capacity (FRC)	RV + ERV; volume of air remaining in the lungs at the end of normal expiration	2000 ml
Vital capacity (VC)	V_T + IRC + ERV; volume of air that can be maximally expired after a maximal inspiration	4500 ml
Total lung capacity (TLC)	V_T + IRC + ERV + RV; volume of air that the lungs can hold with maximal inspiration	5500–6000 ml
Respiratory rate or frequency (*f*)	Number of breaths per minute	12–20
Minute ventilation (M_E)	$V_T \times f$; volume of air expired per minute	5–10 liters
Deadspace (VF_D)	$V_D/V_T = Paco_2 - Peco_2/Paco_2$ $Paco_2$ (arterial); $Peco_2$ (exhaled) volume or percentage of the V_T that does not participate in gas exchange; includes the volume of air in the conducting pathways (anatomical deadspace) plus the volume of alveolar air that is not involved in gas exchange due to pathology (alveolar deadspace)	V_D/V_T ratio is normally <0.4; V_D/V_T >0.6 usually indication for mechanical ventilation
Alveolar ventilation (V_A)	$V_T - V_D$; volume of tidal air that is involved in alveolar gas exchange	350 ml
Forced vital capacity (FVC)	Volume of air in a forceful maximal expiration	Normally the same as VC: 4500 ml
Forced expiratory volume (FEV)	Volume of air exhaled in a given time period; FEV_1: volume of air exhaled in 1 second; FEV_3: volume of air exhaled in 3 seconds	FEV_1: >75% of VC FEV_3: >95% of VC

From Dennison, R. D. (2007). *Pass CCRN!* (3rd ed.). St. Louis: Mosby.

b) Generalized
  i) If all alveoli have low O_2 levels as occurs with alveolar hypoventilation, hypoxemic pulmonary vasoconstriction may be distributed over the lungs
  ii) Increases pulmonary vascular resistance (PVR) and pulmonary artery pressure (PAP)
  iii) Right ventricular hypertrophy and failure (cor pulmonale) may result
    (a) Chronic cor pulmonale: chronic conditions such as chronic obstructive pulmonary disease (COPD)
    (b) Acute cor pulmonale: acute conditions such as pulmonary embolism
c. Ventilation/perfusion ($\dot{V}/\dot{Q}$)
  1) Normal $\dot{V}/\dot{Q}$
    a) Alveolar minute ventilation equals ≈4 L/min
    b) Normal cardiac output (100% goes to lungs) equals ≈5 L/min
    c) Normal $\dot{V}/\dot{Q}$ ratio equals 0.8

2) Pathologic mismatch
  a) Deadspace: $\dot{V}$ greater than $\dot{Q}$
    i) $\dot{V}/\dot{Q}$ ratio will be >0.8 when ventilation is greater than perfusion (e.g., high $\dot{V}/\dot{Q}$ ratio)
    ii) Examples include pulmonary embolism, shock, and decrease in perfusion to the lung caused by excessive tidal volume or positive end-expiratory pressure (PEEP)
  b) Shunt: $\dot{Q}$ greater than $\dot{V}$
    i) $\dot{V}/\dot{Q}$ ratio will be <0.8 when perfusion is greater ventilation (e.g., low $\dot{V}/\dot{Q}$ ratio)
    ii) Examples include atelectasis, acute respiratory distress syndrome (ARDS), and pneumonia
3) Positional mismatch
  a) Greatest ventilation in superior areas
  b) Greatest perfusion in inferior areas
  c) This is rationale for "good lung down" in unilateral lung conditions

i) Improves ventilation to the "bad lung" (e.g., atelectasis, pneumonia, pneumothorax) and optimizes perfusion to the "good lung"

3. Distribution: movement of inspired air into lobes, segments, lobules
4. Diffusion: movement of gases between the alveoli, plasma, and RBCs
   a. Gases diffuse from areas of higher concentration to areas of lower concentration regardless of medium until concentration is the same throughout the chamber
   b. Determinants of diffusion
      1) Surface area available for gas transfer: negatively affected by pulmonary resection (e.g., lobectomy or pneumonectomy), emphysema, or pneumothorax
      2) Thickness of the alveolar-capillary membrane: negatively affected by pulmonary edema or fibrosis
      3) Diffusion coefficient of gas
         a) CO_2 20 times more diffusible than O_2
            i) Diffusion problems cause hypoxemia but they do not cause hypercapnia
            ii) Hypercapnia indicates hypoventilation (e.g., respiratory muscle fatigue)
      4) Driving pressure
         a) Fraction of the gas × barometric pressure
         b) Negatively affected by low inspired fraction of O_2 (e.g., smoke inhalation) or low barometric pressure (e.g., high altitudes)
         c) Positively affected by higher than normal fraction of inspired O_2 (F_{IO_2}) (e.g., supplemental O_2) or higher than normal barometric pressure (e.g., hyperbaric O_2 chamber)
            i) Continuous positive airway pressure (CPAP) and PEEP increase the driving pressure of O_2 by keeping the pressure above zero throughout the entire ventilatory cycle
5. Transport of gases in blood: movement of O_2 and CO_2 through the circulatory system; O_2 moving from the alveolus to the tissues to be utilized and CO_2 moving from the tissues to the alveolus for exhalation
   a. O_2
      1) Mode of transport
         a) Hgb: 97% of O_2 is combined with Hgb; represented by the Sa_{O_2}
            i) One molecule of Hgb can carry four molecules of O_2
            ii) The amount of O_2 that the Hgb actually carries depends on the affinity of the Hgb for O_2; there is normally more affinity at the lung level and less affinity at the tissue level due to the Bohr effect, which controls the reaction between Hgb and O_2 and CO_2

iii) Ability of Hgb to deliver O_2 to the tissues is negatively affected by:
   (a) Anemia
   (b) Abnormal Hgb (e.g., methemoglobinemia, carboxyhemoglobin, or Hgb S [sickle cell])
b) Plasma: 3% of O_2 is dissolved in the plasma; represented by the Pa_{O_2}
2) Oxyhemoglobin dissociation curve: shows the relationship between Pa_{O_2} and Hgb saturation (Figure 5-11)
   a) Critical point: Pa_{O_2} 60 mm Hg
      i) Pa_{O_2} >60: horizontal limb of curve; increase in Pa_{O_2} >60 results in minimal increases in O_2 saturation
      ii) Pa_{O_2} <60: vertical limb of curve; decrease in Pa_{O_2} <60 mm Hg results in dramatic decreases in O_2 saturation
   b) Correlation between Pa_{O_2} and Sa_{O_2} with a normal curve (Table 5-2)
   c) Shifting of the oxyhemoglobin dissociation curve
      i) Shifting of the oxyhemoglobin dissociation curve to the left
         (a) Affinity of Hgb for O_2 is increased, therefore Hgb is more saturated for a given Pa_{O_2} and less O_2 is unloaded for a given Pa_{O_2}
         (b) This means that it is easier to pick up O_2 at the lung level but more difficult to drop off O_2 at the tissue level

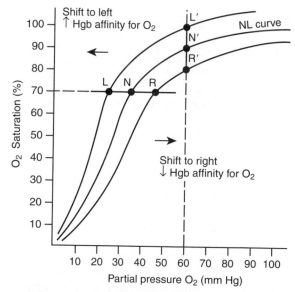

Figure 5-11 Oxyhemoglobin dissociation curve. Normal curve (N) optimizes pickup of O_2 at the lung and drop-off of O_2 at the tissue level; left shift (L) increases the affinity between O_2 and hemoglobin (Hgb), which optimizes pickup of O_2 at the lung level but impairs drop-off of O_2 at the tissue level; right shift (R) decreases affinity between O_2 and Hgb, which impairs pickup of O_2 at the lung level but optimizes drop-off of O_2 at the tissue level. (From Dettenmeier, P. [1992]. *Pulmonary nursing care.* St. Louis: Mosby.)

TABLE 5-2   Correlation Between Pao_2 and Sao_2

Pao_2 (in mm Hg)	Sao_2 (in %)
100	98
90	97
80	95
70	93
60	90
50	85
40	75
30	57
27	50

From Dennison, R. D. (2007). *Pass CCRN!* (3rd ed.). St. Louis: Mosby.

      (c) Factors that shift the oxyhemoglobin dissociation curve to the left: alkalemia, hypothermia, hypocapnia, decreased 2,3-diphosphoglycerate (2,3-DPG)

    ii) Shifting of the oxyhemoglobin dissociation curve to the right

      (a) Affinity of Hgb for O_2 is decreased, therefore Hgb is less saturated for a given Pao_2 and more O_2 is unloaded for a given Pao_2

      (b) This means that it is more difficult to pick up O_2 at the lung level but easier to drop off O_2 at the tissue level

      (c) Factors that shift the oxyhemoglobin dissociation curve to the right: acidemia, hyperthermia, hypercapnia, increased 2,3-DPG

b. CO_2: most transported as bicarbonate

  1) Carbonic acid and water in the presence of carbonic anhydrase form bicarbonate in the erythrocyte

  2) Five percent is dissolved in plasma ($Paco_2$)

  3) Five percent is combined with Hgb as carbaminohemoglobin; CO_2 attaches to Hgb at a different bonding site than O_2

6. O_2 delivery to the tissue

  a. O_2 delivery (Do_2): volume of O_2 delivered to the tissues by the left ventricle each minute; affected by the following:

    1) Cardiac ouput

    2) Sao_2

    3) Hgb

  b. O_2 consumption ($\dot{V}o_2$): volume of O_2 consumed by the tissues each minute; affected by the following:

    1) Increased O_2 consumption

      a) Increased work of breathing

      b) Hyperthermia

      c) Trauma

      d) Infection

      e) Anxiety

      f) Hyperthyroidism

      g) Muscle tremors or seizures

    2) Decreased O_2 consumption

      a) Hypothermia

      b) Sedation

      c) Neuromuscular blockade

      d) Anesthesia

      e) Hypothyroidism

      f) Inactivity

7. Cellular respiration: utilization of O_2 by the cell

  a. Estimated by the amount of CO_2 produced and the O_2 consumed

  b. O_2 is utilized by the mitochondria in the production of cellular energy; O_2 deficit may result in lethal cell injury if prolonged

Pulmonary Assessment

Primary and secondary assessment (see Chapter 2)
Focused assessment

1. Chief complaint: why the patient is seeking help and duration of the problem; possible symptoms related to pulmonary disorders that may be identified as chief complaint may include any of the following:

  a. Dyspnea or shortness of breath

    1) Onset

    2) Duration

    3) Frequency

    4) Timing: time of day; weather or season; activity; eating; talking; deep breathing

    5) Position (e.g., orthopnea)

    6) Severity: effect on ability to perform activities of daily living (ADLs)

    7) Palliation: what is effective in relieving dyspnea

    8) Accompanying symptoms

      a) Cough

      b) Chest pain

      c) Wheezing

  b. Cough

    1) Onset

    2) Duration

    3) Frequency

    4) Timing: time of day, weather or season, activity, eating, talking, deep breathing

    5) Position

    6) Pattern: regular or occasional

    7) Sputum production

      a) Duration

      b) Frequency

      c) Amount: use household measurements (e.g., teaspoons, tablespoons, shot glass, paper cup, iced tea glass)

      d) Color

      e) Consistency

      f) Odor

      g) Hemoptysis

        i) May be related to tuberculosis, lung cancer, bronchiectasis, pneumonia, pulmonary embolism

ii) Character
    (a) Grossly bloody
    (b) Blood-tinged
    (c) Blood-streaked
    (d) Hematest positive
iii) Differentiation from hematemesis
    (a) Hemoptysis: frothy, alkaline, accompanied by sputum
    (b) Hematemesis: nonfrothy, acidic, dark red or brown, accompanied by food particles
    (c) Usual treatment (e.g., expectorants, cough drops, a cigarette)

8) Accompanying symptoms
  a) Sputum production
  b) Hemoptysis
  c) Chest pain
  d) Wheezing
  e) Dyspnea

9) Medication history: may be side effect of angiotensin-converting enzyme (ACE) inhibitors (e.g., captopril [Capoten], enalapril [Vasotec])

c. Chest pain
  1) P
    a) Provocation: pulmonary pain is frequently provoked by trauma, coughing, deep breathing, or movement
    b) Palliation: pulmonary pain may be relieved by sitting upright or by narcotics
  2) Q
    a) Quality: pulmonary pain is most frequently sharp and increased by coughing, inspiration, movement
  3) R
    a) Region: pulmonary pain is usually located at lateral chest
    b) Radiation: pulmonary pain may radiate to shoulder, neck
  4) S
    a) Severity: pulmonary pain is usually moderate but may be severe
  5) T
    a) Timing
      i) Onset: pulmonary pain onset is usually gradual
      ii) Duration: pulmonary pain duration is usually days to weeks

d. Wheezing
  1) Onset
  2) Duration
  3) Timing: time of day, weather or season, activity, eating, talking, deep breathing; position
  4) Identified triggers (e.g., dust, pollen, propellants)
  5) Usual treatment

e. Nasal or sinus problems
  1) Epistaxis
  2) Nasal stuffiness
  3) Postnasal drip
  4) Sinus pain

f. Hoarseness: chronic hoarseness may be related to cancer of larynx
g. Ascites: may be related to cor pulmonale
h. Abdominal pain: may be related to cor pulmonale
i. Edema or weight gain: may be related to cor pulmonale
j. Fatigue or weakness: may be related to cor pulmonale
k. Fever: may be related to pulmonary infections
l. Night sweats: may be related to tuberculosis
m. Anorexia: may be related cor pulmonale, dyspnea, or drug side effects (e.g., xanthine bronchodilators)
n. Weight loss: may be related to dyspnea, fatigue (preventing food preparation), or hypermetabolism
o. Sleep disturbances: may be related to dyspnea or coughing

2. History of present illness; use PQRST
  a. Associated symptoms
  b. Specific to chest trauma
    1) Blunt trauma leaves the body surface intact
    2) Penetrating trauma disrupts the body surface
    3) Etiology
      a) Motor vehicle or motorcycle collision
      b) Vehicle/pedestrian collision
      c) Fall
      d) Assault
      e) Explosion
      f) Projectiles: bullet, knives, impalement
    4) Mechanisms of injury
      a) Blunt chest trauma
        i) Rapid acceleration/deceleration: shearing force causes stretching of tissue, organs, blood vessels with resultant tearing, leaking, or rupture
        ii) Direct impact: object striking chest or chest striking object causes rib, sternal, or scapular fractures, injury to the heart or lung parenchyma
        iii) Compression: force of rapid deceleration as tissues hit a fixed object such as the sternum or rib cage causes concussion, contusion, bleeding, rupture of an organ
      b) Penetrating chest trauma
        i) Penetration of lung, heart, great vessel, or diaphragm causes bleeding and may cause loss of intactness of an organ or vessel

3. Past medical history
  a. Current or past illnesses
    1) Recurrent respiratory infections
    2) Asthma
    3) COPD
      a) Possible components
        i) Chronic bronchitis: dominant reported symptoms are coughing with sputum production
        ii) Emphysema: dominant reported symptom is dyspnea

iii) Patients with COPD often also have asthma: dominant reported symptom is wheezing

4) Tuberculosis
5) Lung cancer
6) Pulmonary fibrosis: frequently related to occupational lung disease
7) Pulmonary embolism
8) Chest trauma (e.g., pneumothorax, flail segment)
9) Connective tissue disorders (e.g., lupus)
10) Fungal disease (e.g., histoplasmosis)
11) Granulomatous diseases (e.g., sarcoidosis)
12) Immunosuppression
13) Recent aspiration
14) Cardiovascular disease

b. Substance abuse: alcohol, tobacco, drugs
c. Past surgical procedures (e.g., thoracotomy)
d. Recent travel out of the country
e. Past diagnostic studies (e.g., allergy testing, pulmonary function test, chest radiograph)

4. Family medical history
5. Social history
   a. Usual activity level and ability to perform ADLs
   b. Stress level and usual coping mechanisms
   c. Work environment
      1) Occupation
      2) Environmental hazards: pulmonary irritants, allergens
      3) Use of protective devices
   d. Home environment
      1) Allergens: pets, plants, trees, molds, dust
      2) Type of heating: gas heat is drying
      3) Use of air conditioner and/or humidifier
   e. Exercise and recreational habits: exposure to inhalants and allergens
   f. Tobacco use: present and past
      1) Type of tobacco, duration and amount
         a) Cigarettes: record as pack-years (number of packs per day times the number of years patient has been smoking)
         b) Chewing or rubbing tobacco: type and amount per day
         c) Marijuana: joints per day
      2) Efforts to quit
      3) Second-hand smoke exposure
   g. Fluid intake
   h. Dietary habits: pulmonary symptoms during meals
6. Medication history
   a. Prescribed drug, dose, frequency, time of last dose
   b. Nonprescribed drugs
      1) Over-the-counter drugs, including herbs
         a) St. John's Wort can worsen asthma symptoms if taken with aminophylline or amitriptyline (Elavil)
         b) Guarana can increase the likelihood of side effects if taken with respiratory medications because it contains theophylline

c) Ginseng reduces the effectiveness of β-blockers
d) Licorice elimination is reduced if taken with corticosteroids
e) Blue cohosh and *Lobelia* may increase the side effects of nicotine patches
f) Ma huang can increase toxicity of methylxanthines in asthmatic patients
      2) Substance abuse
   c. Medication allergies and type of reaction (e.g., cough may be side effect of ACE inhibitors)
   d. Patient's understanding of drug actions and side effects; knowledge of how to use and clean inhaler if prescribed
7. Immunization status

General Survey

1. Vital signs
   a. Blood pressure
   b. Heart rate
   c. Respiratory rate, rhythm, and depth; note pursed-lip breathing, which may be used in times of dyspnea
   d. Temperature
2. Apparent health status: compare apparent age relative to chronologic age
3. Level of consciousness: note restlessness and/or confusion, which may indicate hypoxia
4. Increased work of breathing: note use of accessory muscles
5. Speech pattern: note pausing mid sentence to take a breath indicates problem
6. Nutritional status
7. Gait
8. Position: tripod (sitting up leaning forward) indicates respiratory distress

Inspection and palpation

1. Skin and mucous membranes
   a. Color
      1) Pallor: may indicate anemia
      2) Rubor: may indicate hypercapnia or polycythemia
      3) Cyanosis
         a) Peripheral cyanosis: noted on peripheral areas and associated with hypoperfusion or vasoconstriction
         b) Central cyanosis: noted on lips and mucous membranes and associated with deoxygenated Hgb
      4) Cherry-red: may indicate carbon monoxide (CO) intoxication
2. Thoracic scars indicating previous surgery or trauma
3. Petechiae: may indicate blood dyscrasias, liver disease, fat embolism
4. Edema: may be associated with cor pulmonale
5. Nailbeds

a. Color: note cyanosis
b. Clubbing: indicates chronic decrease in O_2 supply to tissues (e.g., restrictive lung diseases, cyanotic heart disease)
6. Tracheal position
  a. Normal: midline
  b. Deviation
    1) Local causes: hematoma or goiter
    2) Mediastinal shift toward affected side: spontaneous pneumothorax, atelectasis, pneumonectomy
    3) Mediastinal shift away from affected side: tension pneumothorax, large pleural effusion, hemothorax
7. Lymph nodes: enlarged with inflammatory response or malignancy
8. Jugular neck vein distention: may indicate any of the following:
  a. Right ventricular failure (e.g., cor pulmonale)
  b. Tension pneumothorax
  c. Cardiac tamponade
  d. Superior vena cava syndrome
9. Accessory muscle use: indicates respiratory distress
10. Thorax
  a. Normal contour
    1) Slope of ribs: ribs are normally at 45-degree angle to vertebrae
    2) Costal angle: normally <90 degrees
    3) AP diameter: normally one half of lateral diameter so that normal ratio of AP to lateral diameter is 1:2
    4) Symmetrical
  b. Abnormal contour
    1) Pectus excavatum (funnel chest)
      a) Sternum pushed inward
      b) May cause hypoventilation, restrictive lung disease
    2) Pectus carinatum (pigeon chest)
      a) Sternum pushed outward
      b) May cause hypoventilation, restrictive lung disease
    3) Scoliosis
      a) S curvature to spine
      b) May cause hypoventilation, restrictive lung disease
    4) Kyphosis (hunchback)
      a) Frequently occurs with aging due to osteoporosis
      b) May cause hypoventilation, restrictive lung disease
    5) Increased AP diameter: indicates obstructive lung disease
  c. Intercostal spaces
    1) Retraction of interspaces during inspiration
      a) Tracheal obstruction
      b) Asthma
    2) Bulging of interspaces during expiration
      a) Asthma
      b) Tension pneumothorax
      c) Pleural effusion

  d. Chest movement
    1) Respiratory excursion: symmetrical, $\approx$3 to 6 cm during normal breathing
    2) Impaired movement
      a) Thoracic pain with splinting
      b) Restrictive lung disease
    3) Asymmetrical expansion
      a) Massive pleural effusion
      b) Pneumonia
      c) Pneumothorax
      d) Right mainstem intubation (no movement on left)
      e) Flail chest
  e. Inspiration-to-expiration (I:E) ratio
    1) Normally 1:2 with expiration lasting twice as long as inspiration
    2) Obstructive lung diseases causes prolonged expiratory time with ratios $\geq$1:3
  f. Respiratory rate and rhythm (Table 5-3)
  g. Chest wall
    1) Point of maximal impulse
      a) Normally palpated at fifth left intercostals space (LICS) at medial collateral ligament (MCL)
      b) Frequently shifted medially in patients with chronic lung disease and pulmonary hypertension due to right ventricular hypertrophy
    2) Tenderness may be caused by any of the following:
      a) Fracture
      b) Tumor
      c) Costochondritis
    3) Fremitus
      a) Vocal fremitus: evaluate by asking the patient to say "99" while palpating the thorax with ball of hand
        i) Decreased vocal fremitus is frequently noted in bronchial obstruction, pleural effusion, pneumothorax, emphysema, and with thick chest wall
        ii) Increased vocal fremitus is frequently noted in pneumonia, tumor, pulmonary fibrosis, pulmonary infarction, over large airways, and with thin chest wall
    4) Subcutaneous emphysema
      a) Air in tissues under the skin
      b) May indicate esophageal or airway injury
      c) May be noted around stab wound or chest tube
11. Abdominal muscles
  a. Infants and children breathe abdominally
  b. Patients with obstructive lung disease use their abdominal muscles as accessory muscles to help push the air out of the lungs
12. Clinical indications of respiratory distress (Box 5-1)
13. Clinical indications of hypoxemia/hypoxia
  a. Hypoxemia (decreased O_2 in the blood): noted by PaO_2 <80 mm Hg and SaO_2 <95% on arterial blood gases (ABGs) or pulse oximetry (i.e., SpO_2)

TABLE **5-3** Respiratory Rhythms

Rhythm	Description	Possible causes
Eupnea	Adult rate: 12–20 breaths/min and normal depth of ventilation; regular with occasional sigh Pediatric: 16 to 40/min depending on age Infants: 30 to 60/min	• Normal
Bradypnea	Slow (<10 breaths/min), regular ventilation	• Depression of respiratory center with opium, alcohol, or tumor • Sleep • Increased intracranial pressure • Hypercapnia (i.e., CO_2 narcosis) • Metabolic alkalosis
Tachypnea	Rapid (>24 breaths/min) ventilation; depth may be normal or decreased	• Restrictive lung disease • Pneumonia • Pleurisy • Chest pain • Fear and/or anxiety • Respiratory insufficiency
Hypopnea	Shallow ventilation, normal rate	• Deep sleep • Heart failure • Shock • Meningitis • Central nervous system depression • Coma
Hyperpnea	Deep ventilation; rate may be normal or increased	• Exercise • Hypoxia • Fever • Hepatic coma • Midbrain or pons lesions • Acid-base imbalance • Salicylate overdosage
Cheyne-Stokes	Increasing and decreasing rate and depth of ventilation followed by apnea lasting 20–60 seconds	• Increased intracranial pressure • Heart failure • Renal failure • Meningitis • Cerebral hemisphere damage • Drug overdosage
Kussmaul	Deep, gasping, rapid (usually >35 breaths/min) ventilation	• Metabolic acidosis (e.g., diabetic ketoacidosis; renal failure) • Peritonitis
Apneustic	Prolonged gasping inspiration followed by short inefficient expiration	• Lesion of pons
Biot's	Periods of apnea alternating with a series of breaths of equal depth; breathing may be slow and deep or rapid and shallow	• Meningitis • Encephalitis • Head trauma • Increased intracranial pressure
Ataxic	Lack of any pattern to ventilation	• Brain stem lesion
Obstructive	I:E ratio of ≥1:4	• Asthma • Emphysema • Chronic bronchitis
Apnea	Cessation of ventilation for >15 seconds	• Central nervous system damage • Sleep apnea

From Dennison, R. D. (2007). *Pass CCRN!* (3rd ed.). St. Louis: Mosby.

5-1 Clinical Indications of Respiratory Distress

Pursed-lip breathing
Tripod positioning
Speaking only one or two words between breaths
Cough
Use of accessory muscles
Intercostal retractions

From Dennison, R. D. (2007). *Pass CCRN!* (3rd ed.). St. Louis: Mosby.

  b. Hypoxia (decreased O_2 in the tissues): noted by clinical indications of hypoxia (Box 5-2) and increased serum lactate level
14. Clinical indications of hypercapnia (increased CO_2 in the blood): noted by increased $Paco_2$ on ABGs and clinical indications of hypercapnia (Box 5-3)

Percussion
1. Description of percussion tones (Table 5-4)
2. Thorax
   a. Percussion tones normally heard
      1) Lung: resonance
      2) Diaphragm: flat
      3) Heart: dull
   b. Abnormal percussion tones over thorax
      1) Hyperresonant: asthma, emphysema, pneumothorax
      2) Dull: atelectasis, pneumonia, tumor
      3) Flat: pleural effusion

5-2 Clinical Indications of Hypoxia

Restlessness → confusion → lethargy → coma
Tachycardia → dysrhythmias
Tachypnea
Dyspnea
Use of accessory muscles
Mild hypertension (early) → hypotension (late)
Cyanosis may be present (depending on hemoglobin level)

From Dennison, R. D. (2007). *Pass CCRN!* (3rd ed.). St. Louis: Mosby.

5-3 Clinical Indications of Hypercapnia

Headache
Irritability
Confusion
Inability to concentrate → somnolence → coma
Bradypnea
Tachycardia → dysrhythmias
Hypotension
Facial rubor (plethora)

From Dennison, R. D. (2007). *Pass CCRN!* (3rd ed.). St. Louis: Mosby.

  c. Diaphragmatic excursion
     1) Evaluated by percussing the position of the diaphragm at expiration and then during full inspiration
     2) Normal diaphragmatic excursion is 3 to 5 cm
     3) May be decreased by the following:
        a) Increased intrathoracic volume: emphysema
        b) Increased intra-abdominal volume and pressure
           i) Ascites
           ii) Hepatomegaly
           iii) Pregnancy
           iv) Gaseous abdominal distention
        c) Decreased chest excursion and tidal volume: thoracic or abdominal pain
        d) Phrenic nerve injury
3. Abdomen
   a. Liver
      1) Normal liver span in the right MCL is 6 to 12 cm
      2) Hepatomegaly (liver span >12 cm in left MCL) may be seen in cor pulmonale

Auscultation
1. Method of lung auscultation
   a. Use diaphragm
   b. Ask patient to take deep breaths through his or her mouth
   c. Listen to at least one full breath at each location
   d. Compare symmetrical areas
2. Breath sounds
   a. Intensity
      1) Increased
         a) Hyperventilation
         b) Anything that decreases the distance between the lung and your stethoscope (e.g., thin chest wall)
      2) Decreased
         a) Hypoventilation
            i) Emphysema
            ii) Thoracic pain
            iii) Restrictive lung lungs (e.g., atelectasis, pulmonary fibrosis)
         b) Anything that increases the distance between the lung and your stethoscope
            i) Muscular or obese chest
            ii) Pneumothorax (may be diminished or absent)
            iii) Hemothorax (may be diminished or absent)
            iv) Pleural effusion
      3) Absent
         a) Severe bronchospasm
         b) Massive atelectasis
         c) Pneumonectomy
         d) Pneumothorax
         e) Hemothorax
         f) Malpositioned ET tube (absent breath sounds over left lung)

TABLE 5-4 Percussion Tones

Tone	Intensity	Pitch	Duration	Quality	Normal Location
Tympanic	Loud	High	Medium	Drumlike	Stomach, bowel
Hyperresonant	Loud	Low	Long	Booming	Hyperinflated lungs
Resonant	Medium	Low	Long	Hollow	Normal lung
Dull	Soft	High	Medium	Thudlike	Liver, spleen, heart
Flat	Soft	High	Short	Extreme dullness	Muscle, bone

From Dennison, R. D. (2007). *Pass CCRN!* (3rd ed.). St. Louis: Mosby.

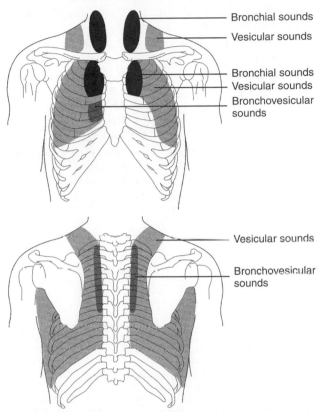

Figure 5-12 Quality of breath sounds: normal locations. (From Barkauskas, V. H., Baumann, L., and Darling-Fischer, C. S. [2002]. *Health and physical assessment* [3rd ed.]. St. Louis: Mosby.)

b. Quality
   1) Descriptions and normal locations (Figure 5-12, Table 5-5)
   2) Implications
     a) Bronchial in areas other than normal location: consolidation (e.g., atelectasis, pneumonia, tumor)

     b) Bronchovesicular in areas other than normal location: partial consolidation, partial aeration

     c) Adventitious sounds (Table 5-6): pathologic extra sounds that may be heard at points in the ventilatory cycle or throughout the ventilatory cycle

     d) Voice sounds: abnormal and indicative of consolidation

   1) Bronchophony: increase in clarity of voice sounds
     a) Ask patient to say "99"
     b) Voice sounds are normally muffled
     c) If voice sounds are clear over a particular area, bronchophony is present

   2) Egophony: "e" to "a" conversion of voice sounds
     a) Ask patient to say "e"
     b) Muffled "e" should be heard over normal lung
     c) If "a" is heard over a particular area, egophony is present

   3) Whispered pectoriloquy: increase in clarity of whispered sounds
     a) Ask the patient to whisper "99"
     b) Whispered sounds are normally muffled
     c) If whispered sounds are clear over a particular area, whispered pectoriloquy is present

Bedside assessment of pulmonary function

1. Spirometry: measured with Wright respirometer
   a. Tidal volume (V_T)
     1) Amount of air moved in and out each breath
     2) Normal: 7 ml/kg
       a) V_T <5 ml/kg indicates need for artificial airway and/or mechanical ventilation
       b) V_T >5 ml/kg indicates that the patient can be weaned and/or extubated

TABLE 5-5 Normal Breath Sounds

Quality	I:E Ratio	Intensity	Pitch	Quality	Normal Location
Bronchial	I < E	Loud	High	Hollow	Trachea
Bronchovesicular	I = E	Medium	Medium	Breezy	Mainstem bronchi
Vesicular	I > E	Soft	Low	Swishy	Peripheral lung

From Dennison, R. D. (2007). *Pass CCRN!* (3rd ed.). St. Louis: Mosby.

TABLE **5-6** Breath Sounds: Adventitious Sounds

Sound	Alternative Terms	Phase	Description	Cause
• Stridor	• Croupy	• Inspiratory	• High-pitched whistle audible without a stethoscope	• Upper airway obstruction • Epiglottitis • Foreign body • Laryngospasm • Laryngeal edema
• Crackles	• Rales	• Inspiratory	• Discontinuous crackling sound; similar to rubbing hair between fingers	• Pulmonary edema • Atelectasis • Pulmonary fibrosis
• Rhonchi	• Gurgles, sonorous rhonchi	• Expiratory	• Continuous gurgling sound	• Fluid or mucus in airways
• Wheezes	• Whistles; sibilant rhonchi	• Inspiratory or expiratory	• High-pitched whistling sound	• Decrease in airway lumen • Bronchospasm • Mucus plug • Tumor
• Pleural friction rub		• Inspiratory and expiratory	• Grating or scratching sound	• Pulmonary infarction • Pleurisy • Tuberculosis • Lung cancer

From Dennison, R. D. (2007). *Pass CCRN!* (3rd ed.). St. Louis: Mosby.

b. Vital capacity (V_C)
   1) Maximal amount of air that can be exhaled after a maximal inspiration
   2) Normal: 15 ml/kg
      a) V_C <10 ml/kg indicates need for artificial airway and/or mechanical ventilation
      b) V_C >10 ml/kg indicates that the patient can be weaned and/or extubated
2. Ventilatory mechanics
   a. Peak expiratory flow rate (PEFR): used to make serial measurements of lung function in patients with asthma
3. Capnography (i.e., end-tidal CO_2 monitoring)
   a. Continuous noninvasive method for evaluating the adequacy of CO_2 exchange in the lungs; assesses $Paco_2$ indirectly by detecting the level of CO_2 in the exhaled air
      1) Measurement of expired CO_2 tension displaying the CO_2 waveform from breath to breath (Figure 5-13)
      2) Normal value: the $Petco_2$ is usually 1 to 5 mm Hg below the $Paco_2$
         a) Increased $Petco_2$ assumes hypoventilation
         b) Decreased $Petco_2$ assumes hyperventilation
      3) Implication: changes in $Petco_2$ indicates that the patient requires prompt assessment and ABGs for analysis
   b. Colormetric CO_2: inexpensive and disposable indicators initially used to confirm ET placement in the emergency department (ED)

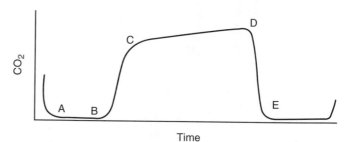

Figure 5-13 Typical normal CO_2 waveform. **A–B,** Exhalation of CO_2–free gas from deadspace. **B–C,** Combination of deadspace and alveolar gases. **C–D,** Exhalation of mostly alveolar gas. **D,** Exhalation of CO_2 at maximal point (end-tidal point). **D–E,** Inspiration begins and CO_2 concentration rapidly falls to baseline or zero. (From St. John, R. E. [2004]. Airway management. *Critical Care Nurse, 24*[2], 93–96.)

4. Pulse oximetry (Spo_2): continuous noninvasive monitoring of arterial O_2 saturation
   a. Indications
      1) Assessment of adequacy of oxygenation (does not adequately evaluate ventilation because $Paco_2$ increases with hypoventilation but Pao_2 and O_2 saturation do not decrease until much later)
   b. Description
      1) Sensor with light source is placed on the fingertip, toe, bridge of nose, forehead, or earlobe; care must be taken to use the appropriate sensor for the location

2) The amount of arterial Hgb saturated with O_2 is determined by beams of light passed through the tissue

c. Values
   1) Normal value: >95%
   2) Abnormal value: <95% with moderate to severe hypoxemia should be suspected if <90%; causes of decreased SpO_2 include the following:
      a) Decrease in SaO_2 and PaO_2
      b) Decrease in cardiac output
d. Limitations
   1) Inadequate pulsations may result from the following:
      a) Significant hypotension
      b) Vasopressor use
      c) Severe hypothermia
      d) Arterial compression
   2) Tends to overestimate SaO_2 by 2% to 5%; accuracy of SpO_2 <70% is questionable; the lower the SaO_2, the greater is the difference between it and the SpO_2
   3) Does not accurately reflect O_2 tissue delivery in patients with anemia or abnormal Hgb values
      a) Carboxyhemoglobin
         i) Results in overestimation of O_2 saturation reading because Hgb is saturated but with CO
         ii) Smokers may have elevated carboxyhemoglobin levels
      b) Methemoglobin
         i) Results in overestimation of SaO_2
         ii) Methemoglobin is a form of Hgb that cannot carry O_2
         iii) May be related to the administration of nitroglycerin, nitroprusside, sulfonamides, local anesthetics
      c) Hgb S: sickle cell anemia
   4) Other variables may impair accuracy
      a) Increased bilirubin (>20 mg%): results in inaccurately low readings
      b) Ambient light: may affect accuracy
      c) Motion artifact: may affect accuracy
      d) Edema: may result in inaccurately low readings
      e) Nail polish: blue, green, gold, black, or brown nail polish should be removed
      f) Pierced earlobe: results in inaccurate reading
e. Implication: changes in SpO_2 indicate that the patient requires prompt assessment and arterial blood gases ABGs for analysis

Diagnostic Studies

1. Serum chemistries
   a. Sodium: normal 136 to 145 mEq/L
   b. Potassium: normal 3.5 to 5.0 mEq/L
   c. Chloride: normal 95 to 103 mEq/L
   d. Total calcium: normal
      1) Adults: 9.0 to 10.5 mg/dl
      2) Children: 8.8 to 10.8 mg/dl
   e. Ionized calcium: normal
      1) Adults: 4.5 to 5.6 mg/dl
      2) Children: 4.8 to 5.52
   f. Phosphorus: normal 3.0 to 4.5 mg/dl
   g. Magnesium: normal
      1) Adults: 1.3 to 2.1 mEq/L
      2) Children: 1.4 to 1.7 mEq/L
      3) Infants 1.4 to 2 mEq/L
   h. Fasting glucose: 65 to 110 mEq/L
   i. Blood urea nitrogen: normal 8 to 23 mg/dl
   j. Creatinine: normal 0.6 to 1.1 mg/dl for females; 0.8 to 1.3 mg/dl for males
   k. Lactate dehydrogenase: 110 to 250 milliunits/ml
   l. Serum toxicology level: to rule out cause of increase or decreased respirations
   m. Serum alcohol level: elevation causes respiratory depression and possible aspiration
2. ABGs
   a. pH: normal 7.35 to 7.45
   b. $PaCO_2$: normal 35 to 45 mm Hg
   c. HCO_3^-: normal 22 to 26 mM
   d. PaO_2: normal 80 to 100 mm Hg
   e. SaO_2: >95% (older adults >92%)
3. Hematology
   a. Hct: normal 42% to 52% for males; 37% to 47% for females
   b. Hgb: normal 14 to 18 g/dl for males; 12 to 16 g/dl for females
   c. WBCs: normal 4.8 to 10.8 mm^3
   d. D-dimer: positive if level >500 ng/ml
4. Sputum analysis:
   a. Characteristics: color, odor, viscosity, presence of blood
   b. Culture and sensitivity tests: identify infecting organism and effective antibiotic agent
   c. Gram stain: differentiates between gram-negative or gram-positive bacteria
   d. Acid-fast stain: determines presence of acid-fast bacilli (tuberculosis)
   e. Cytology studies: determines presence of malignant cells
5. Urine
   a. Urine toxicology level: to rule out cause of increase or decreased respirations
   b. Urine pregnancy in all women of child-bearing age
6. Other diagnostic studies (Table 5-7)

Acid-Base Balance and Arterial Blood Gas Interpretation

Physiology review

1. Acid: a substance that can give up a H^+ ion; acids are produced by the body as a result of cellular metabolism
   a. Volatile (e.g., carbonic acid)
      1) Exhalable
      2) Results from aerobic metabolism of glucose
      3) Eliminated by the lungs
   b. Nonvolatile (also called fixed) (e.g., sulfuric, phosphoric, uric)

TABLE **5-7** Pulmonary Diagnostic Studies

Study	Evaluates	Comments
Chest radiograph	• Detects lung pathology (e.g., pneumonia, pulmonary edema, atelectasis, tuberculosis, etc) • Determines size and location of lung lesions and tumors • Verifies placement of endotracheal tube, central venous catheters, chest tubes	• Noninvasive test with minimal radiation exposure • Inquire about possibility of pregnancy • Posteroanterior (PA) and lateral films are done most commonly but in critical care areas anteroposterior (AP) portable films are frequently necessary due to inability to transport patient • Lateral decubitus films aid in identification of pleural effusion
Laryngoscopy, bronchoscopy, mediastinoscopy	• Obtain cytology specimen or biopsy • Identify tumors, obstructions, secretions, foreign bodies in tracheobronchial tree • Locate a bleeding site • May be used therapeutically to remove secretions, foreign bodies, other contaminants	• Patient is sedated prior to the procedure, usually with a benzodiazepine (e.g., diazepam [Valium], midazolam [Versed]) • Monitor the patient for subcutaneous emphysema after study; indicates tracheal or bronchial tear • Monitor for hemoptysis; some blood in sputum is normal after biopsy but frank hemoptysis requires immediate attention
Magnetic resonance imaging (MRI)	• Distinguishes tumors from other structures (e.g., tumor, pleural thickening, fibrosis)	• Noninvasive test • Contraindicated for patients with pacemakers or implanted metallic devices
Pulmonary angiography	• Detects changes in lung tissue (e.g., masses) • Diagnoses abnormalities in pulmonary vasculature include thrombi and emboli • Identifies congenital abnormalities of the circulation	• Invasive test • Inquire about possibility of pregnancy • Contrast media injected into pulmonary artery: ensure adequate hydration after study • Monitor arterial puncture point for hematoma or hemorrhage
Pulmonary function studies (See Table 5-1 for lung volumes and parameters with normal values.) Spirometry: volumes and capacities	• Measure lung volumes, capacities, and flow rates • Identify features of restrictive or obstructive lung disease • Evaluate responsiveness to bronchodilator therapy • Aid in evaluation of surgical risk • Document a disability or cause of dyspnea	• Noninvasive study • Frequently repeated after bronchodilator therapy
Thoracentesis (may include pleural biopsy)	• Obtain pleural fluid and/or tissue specimen • May be used therapeutically to remove pleural fluid	• Monitor patient for indications of pneumothorax • Monitor for leakage from puncture point
Thoracic computed tomography (CT)	• Defines lesions, masses, cavities, or shadows seen on a normal chest radiograph • Evaluates tracheal or bronchial narrowing • Aids in planning radiation therapy	• Radiographs taken at different angles
Ultrasonography	• Evaluates pleural disease • Visualizes diaphragm and detects disease around diaphragm (e.g., subphrenic hematoma or abscess)	• Noninvasive test
Ventilation scan Lung perfusion scan Ventilation/perfusion ($\dot{V}/\dot{Q}$) scan	• Diagnoses ventilation and/or perfusion abnormalities including emphysema, pulmonary emboli	• Invasive test: radioisotope inspired and injected intravascularly • Inquire about possibility of pregnancy • Nuclear scan study: assure patient that amount of radioactive material is minimal

Adapted from Dennison, R. D. (2007). *Pass CCRN!* (3rd ed.). St. Louis: Mosby.

1) Nonexhalable and cannot be converted into a gas
2) Results from aerobic metabolism of protein and fat and the anaerobic metabolism of glucose
3) Eliminated by the kidney
c. Elimination or neutralization necessary
2. Acidemia: the condition of the blood with pH <7.35
3. Acidosis: the process that causes the acidemia
4. Base: a substance that can accept a H^+ (the primary base in the body is bicarbonate)
5. Alkalemia: the condition of the blood with pH >7.45
6. Alkalosis: the process that causes the alkalemia
7. pH
   a. Indirect measurement of hydrogen ion concentration
   b. Reflection of the balance between carbonic acid (acid regulated by the lungs) and bicarbonate (base regulated by the kidneys)
   c. Inversely proportional to H^+ concentration
      1) Increase in H^+ concentration: lower pH, more acid
      2) Decrease in H^+ concentration: higher pH, more base
   d. Must be maintained within a narrow range to allow functioning of enzymatic systems in the body; pH <6.8 or >7.8 is incompatible with life

Acid-base regulation

1. Chemical buffers
   a. Weak acid and strong base
   b. Immediate response when a change in acid-base status occurs by combining with excess acid or base
   c. Buffer systems
      1) Bicarbonate–carbonic acid buffer system
         a) The most important buffer system
         b) Bicarbonate is generated by the kidney and aids in the elimination of H^+
      2) Phosphate system: aids in excretion of H^+ by the kidney
      3) Ammonium: H^+ is added to ammonia (NH_3) in the renal tubule to form ammonium (NH_4); allows greater excretion of H^+ by the kidney
      4) Hgb and other proteins: aids in buffering extracellular fluid
2. Respiratory system
   a. Regulates the excretion or retention of carbonic acid
      1) If pH decreases, the rate and depth of ventilation increase
      2) If pH increases, the rate and depth of ventilation decrease
   b. Responds within minutes: fast but weak
3. Renal system
   a. Regulates the excretion or retention of bicarbonate and the excretion of hydrogen and nonvolatile acids
      1) If pH decreases, the kidney retains bicarbonate
      2) If pH increases, the kidney excretes bicarbonate
   b. Responds within 48 hours: slow but powerful

Acid-base imbalances (Table 5-8)

1. Acidemia: pH <7.35
   a. Acidosis: the process causing acidemia
      1) Caused by acid gain
         a) If acid is volatile (reflected by increase in $Paco_2$): respiratory acidosis
         b) If acid is nonvolatile (reflected by decrease in HCO_3^-): metabolic acidosis
      2) Caused by base loss or metabolic acid gain (reflected by decrease in HCO_3^-): metabolic acidosis
      3) Anion gap is used to differentiate between metabolic acid gain or base loss as cause of metabolic acidosis
         a) Calculated: $Na^+ - (Cl^- + CO_2^-)$
         b) Normal: 10-14
         c) If anion gap is normal (between 10-14): metabolic acidosis is due to a base loss
         d) If anion gap is increased (>14): metabolic acidosis is due to acid gain
2. Alkalemia: pH >7.45
   a. Alkalosis: the process causing alkalemia
      1) Caused by acid loss
         a) If acid is volatile (reflected by decrease in $Paco_2$): respiratory alkalosis
         b) If acid is nonvolatile (reflected by increase in HCO_3^-): metabolic alkalosis
      2) Caused by base gain or metabolic acid loss (reflected by increase in HCO_3^-): metabolic alkalosis
3. Compensation
   a. Respiratory acidosis
      1) The kidneys reabsorb more bicarbonate or excrete more H^+
      2) The bicarbonate and base excess levels increase
      3) This change will be slow and may take as long as 2 to 3 days
   b. Respiratory alkalosis
      1) The kidneys excrete more bicarbonate
      2) The bicarbonate and base excess levels decrease

TABLE 5-8	**Acid-Base Imbalances**		
Imbalance	Ph	Primary Change	Compensatory Change
Respiratory acidosis	<7.35	↑ $Paco_2$	↑ HCO_3^-
Metabolic acidosis	<7.35	↓ HCO_3^-	↓ $Paco_2$
Respiratory alkalosis	>7.45	↓ $Paco_2$	↓ HCO_3^-
Metabolic alkalosis	>7.45	↑ HCO_3^-	↑ $Paco_2$

↑, Increased; ↓, decreased.

3) This change will be slow and may take as long as 2 to 3 days
  a) Because respiratory alkalosis is almost always a short-term process (e.g., hyperventilation), compensation for respiratory alkalosis is rarely seen because it takes too long and the problem would be resolved
c. Metabolic acidosis
  1) The lungs increase the rate and depth of ventilation
  2) The $Paco_2$ level decreases
  3) This change will be rapid, usually within minutes to hours
d. Metabolic alkalosis
  1) The lungs decrease the rate and depth of ventilation
  2) The $Paco_2$ level increases
  3) This change will be rapid, usually within minutes to hours
e. Correction versus compensation
  1) Correction may be a physiologic process or the result of appropriate therapeutic measures; correction is achieved when there the pH is normal and both indicators ($Paco_2$, HCO_3^-) are normal
  2) Compensation is a physiologic process; the pH is normal and both indicators are abnormal
    a. Partial compensation: pH is still abnormal but the secondary parameter is outside normal range in the direction to move the pH toward normal
    b. Full compensation: pH is normal and the secondary parameter is outside normal range in the direction to move the pH toward normal
4. Mixed disorders (Table 5-9)
  a. More than one disorder may coexist
  b. The degree of respiratory component versus metabolic component can be calculated utilizing these formulas
    1) As the $Paco_2$ changes by 10 mm Hg (from normal of 40), it is associated with a change in pH of 0.8 in the opposite direction
    2) As the pH changes by 0.15 (from normal of 7.40), it is associated with a change in base of 10 mEq in the same direction
  c. Compensation cannot exist in mixed disorders because each system is independently abnormal and cannot help the other

Analysis of arterial blood gases

1. Purposes of ABGs
  a. Evaluate ventilation: $Paco_2$
  b. Evaluate acid-base status: pH; to determine the cause of the acid-base imbalance, determine which parameter is abnormal
    1) Respiratory: $Paco_2$
    2) Metabolic: HCO_3^-
  c. Evaluate oxygenation: Pao_2

TABLE 5-9 Mixed Acid-Base Disorders	
Mixed Disorder	**Clinical Example**
Mixed acidosis	Cardiac and respiratory arrest
Mixed alkalosis	Compensated respiratory acidosis (e.g., COPD) being excessively mechanically ventilated
Respiratory acidosis and metabolic alkalosis	Patient with COPD on diuretics
Respiratory alkalosis and metabolic acidosis	Hepatic and renal failure

2. Parameters and normal values (Box 5-4)
  a. pH: negative logarithm of hydrogen ion concentration in arterial blood
    1) Normal pH is 7.35 to 7.45
    2) Levels <7.35 indicate an acidosis
    3) Levels >7.45 indicate an alkalosis
  b. $Paco_2$: partial pressure of CO_2 in arterial blood
    1) Normal $Paco_2$ is 35 to 45 mm Hg
    2) Levels <35 indicate a respiratory alkalosis or respiratory compensation for a metabolic acidosis
    3) Levels >45 indicate a respiratory acidosis or respiratory compensation for a metabolic alkalosis
  c. HCO_3^-: bicarbonate ion level in arterial blood
    1) Normal HCO_3^- is 22 to 26 mEq/L
    2) Levels <22 indicate a metabolic acidosis or metabolic compensation for respiratory alkalosis
    3) Levels >26 indicate a metabolic alkalosis or metabolic compensation for respiratory acidosis
  d. Base excess (BE): difference between acid and base levels in arterial blood
    1) Normal BE is +2 to −2
    2) Levels <−2 (actually a base deficit) indicate a metabolic acidosis or metabolic compensation for respiratory alkalosis
    3) Levels >+2 indicate a metabolic alkalosis or metabolic compensation for respiratory acidosis
  e. Pao_2: partial pressure of O_2 in arterial blood
    1) Normal Pao_2 is 80 to 100 mm Hg
    2) Levels >100 indicate hyperoxemia
    3) Levels <80 indicate mild hypoxemia
    4) Levels <60 indicate moderate hypoxemia
    5) Levels <40 indicate severe hypoxemia

BOX 5-4 Normal Arterial Blood Gas Values	
pH	7.35-7.45
$Paco_2$	35-45 mm Hg
HCO_3^-	22-26 mEq/L
Pao_2	80-100 mm Hg

f. Sao$_2$: saturation of Hgb by O$_2$
  1) Normal Sao$_2$ is $\geq$95%
  2) Levels <95% indicate mild desaturation of Hgb
  3) Levels <90% indicate moderate desaturation of Hgb
  4) Levels <75% indicate severe desaturation of Hgb
3. Steps in analysis
  a. Is pH acidotic, alkalotic, or normal?
  b. Which parameter is abnormal?
    1) Paco$_2$: respiratory
    2) HCO$_3^-$: metabolic
  c. If the pH is normal, is it leaning? If so, consider compensation
    1) Compensation causes a leaning pH: the pH leans toward the initial disorder
      a) The body never overcompensates; a normal nonleaning pH with two abnormal indicators (Paco$_2$, HCO$_3^-$) suggests a mixed disorder (e.g., one alkalotic process + one acidotic process)
    2) For compensation to be occurring, one parameter change must help the other
      a) Full compensation: normal pH with both indicators abnormal
      b) Partial compensation
        i) pH is still abnormal
        ii) Both indicators (Paco$_2$, HCO$_3^-$) are abnormal with the secondary indicator moving in the direction to help normalize the pH
  d. Assess oxygenation
    1) Pao$_2$ <80 mm Hg is hypoxemia
    2) Pao$_2$ <60 mm Hg on room air is usually an indication for O$_2$ administration
    3) Acceptable Pao$_2$ should be adjusted for age; one method is to subtract 1 mm Hg for each year >60 years from 80 mm Hg; this gives acceptable Pao$_2$ on room air for a patient of that age
4. Technical problems that may affect accuracy of arterial blood gas values
  a. Too much heparin: decrease in Paco$_2$, decrease in HCO$_3^-$, increase in base excess
  b. Air bubble: increase in pH, decrease in Paco$_2$, increase in Pao$_2$
  c. Not chilled immediately: decrease in pH, decrease in Pao$_2$, increase in Paco$_2$
  d. Inadequate discard volume when drawing from catheter with flush solution: decreased Paco$_2$

Discussion of acid-base imbalances (Table 5-10)

Airway Management
Etiology of airway obstruction
1. Upper airway
  a. Relaxation of tongue against hypopharynx: primary cause of obstruction in unconscious patient
  b. Foreign body aspiration
    1) Aspiration of food: primary cause of obstruction in conscious patient
    2) Vomitus
    3) Dentures
  c. Tumor
  d. Hematoma
  e. Laryngeal spasm, edema
  f. Vocal cord paralysis
  g. Infection (e.g., epiglottis)
  h. Trauma (e.g., fractured trachea)
2. Lower airway
  a. Foreign bodies
  b. Secretions
  c. Hemorrhage
  d. Pneumonia
  e. Space-occupying lesions, tumors
  f. Bronchospasm

Clinical presentation of airway obstruction
1. Partial obstruction
  a. Presence of air movement
  b. Restlessness, agitation, anxiety
  c. Respiratory distress: intercostal retractions; use of accessory muscles
  d. Cyanosis
  e. Coughing
  f. Altered speech
  g. Inspiratory sounds: snoring; stridor
  h. Breath sound changes: wheezes; rhonchi
2. Complete obstruction
  a. Lack of air movement
  b. Extreme anxiety in conscious patient
  c. Respiratory distress: intercostal retractions; use of accessory muscles
  d. Cyanosis
  e. Inability to speak, cough, or produce any sound
  f. Universal sign of choking: patient clutches throat with hand
  g. Unconsciousness within seconds

Collaborative management of airway obstruction and/or respiratory distress
1. Evaluate patency of the airway: look, listen, feel for airflow
2. Maintain optimal airway and thoracic position
  a. Use head-tilt, chin lift (also called sniffing) position for optimal airway position
    1) True hyperextension should be avoided
    2) Contraindicated if cervical spine fracture possible (instead use jaw thrust)
  b. Position head of bed for optimal chest excursion: semi-Fowler's to high Fowler's position if no spinal trauma is suspected
3. Remove any obstruction
  a. Inspect the mouth for blood, teeth, loose dentures, food, or anything else that may cause obstruction
  b. Remove any visible obstruction

TABLE 5-10 Discussion of Acid-Base Imbalances

Imbalance	Etiology	Clinical Presentation	Collaborative Mgt

Respiratory acidosis: pH low; $Paco_2$ high	• Hypoventilation
	• Airway obstruction
	• CNS depression from drugs, injury, or disease
	• Chest wall injury (e.g., flail chest)
	• Obstructive lung disease (e.g., chronic bronchitis, emphysema, late asthma)
	• Restrictive lung disease (e.g., kyphoscoliosis, obesity hypoventilation syndrome)
	• O_2–induced hypoventilation in patients with chronic hypercapnia
	• Neuromuscular abnormality (e.g., Guillain-Barré syndrome, myasthenia gravis, multiple sclerosis)
	• Atelectasis, pneumonia
	• Pulmonary edema
	• Respiratory arrest
		• Initially
		  • Sympathetic nervous system stimulation symptoms (e.g., tachycardia, tachypnea, diaphoresis)
		• Later
		  • Bradypnea
		  • Hypotension
		  • Dysrhythmias
		  • Confusion
		  • Headache
		  • Blurred vision
		  • Flushed face (plethora)
		  • Somnolence leading to coma
		  • (These late symptoms are also referred to as CO_2 *narcosis*)
			• Increase ventilation and treat cause
			• Maintain patent airway
			• Position for optimal ventilation
			• Implement bronchial hygiene measures
			• Administer drug therapy (e.g., bronchodilators, mucolytics, antibiotics)
			• Mechanical ventilation may be necessary
			• If patient is already on mechanical ventilation:
			  • Increase rate
			  • Increase tidal volume

Respiratory alkalosis: pH high; $Paco_2$ low	• Hyperventilation
	• Anxiety or hysteria
	• Thoracic pain
	• Early asthma
	• Pneumothorax
	• Pulmonary embolus
	• Early salicylate intoxication
	• Hyperthyroidism
	• Hepatic failure
	• Fever
	• Gram-negative septicemia
	• CNS infection or injury
	• Excessive mechanical ventilation
		• Tachycardia
		• Palpitations
		• Dry mouth
		• Anxiety
		• Profuse perspiration
		• Paresthesia around mouth and extremities
		• Dizziness, vertigo, syncope
		• Increased muscle irritability, twitching
		• Tetany
		• Inability to concentrate
		• Seizures
		• Coma
			• Decrease ventilation and treat cause
			• Provide reassurance and maintain a calm attitude
			• Administer sedatives (frequently given intravenously)
			• Ask patient to breathe into and out of a paper bag or use a rebreathing mask
			• If patient is already on mechanical ventilation:
			  • Decrease rate
			  • Decrease tidal volume
			  • Change from assist-control to IMV
			  • Consider sedation
			  • Consider addition of deadspace tubing

Metabolic acidosis: pH low; HCO_3^- low	• Acid gain (increased anion gap)
	  • Tissue hypoxia (e.g., shock [lactic acidosis])
	  • Ketoacidosis (diabetic ketoacidosis or starvation)
	  • Renal failure
	  • Drugs and toxins (e.g., salicylates; methanol, ethylene glycol)
	• Bicarbonate loss (normal anion gap)
	  • Bile drainage
	  • Pancreatic fistula
	  • Diarrhea
	  • Acetazolamide (Diamox) therapy
		• Nausea, vomiting, abdominal discomfort
		• Weakness
		• Tremors
		• Malaise
		• Headache
		• Tachypnea progressing to Kussmaul's
		• Hypotension
		• Dysrhythmias
		• Confusion
		• Lethargy → coma
			• Treat cause as appropriate
			• Improve oxygenation and/or perfusion (lactic acidosis)
			  • Give insulin (DKA)
			  • Dialysis (renal failure)
			  • Antidiarrheals (diarrhea)
			• Administer buffer
			  • Bicarbonate IV or orally for pH ≤7.0

TABLE

5-10   Discussion of Acid-Base Imbalances—cont'd

Imbalance	Etiology	Clinical Presentation	Collaborative Mgt

Metabolic alkalosis: pH high; HCO_3^- high	• Acid loss
	  • Nasogastric suction or severe vomiting
	  • Potassium-wasting diuretic therapy
	  • Steroid therapy
	  • Cushing's disease
	  • Hyperaldosteronism
	  • Hepatic disease
	  • Hypokalemia, hypochloremia
	• Bicarbonate gain
	  • Dosing with bicarbonate
	  • Excess infusion of lactated Ringer's solution
		• Bradypnea
		• Nausea, vomiting, diarrhea
		• Paresthesia around mouth and extremities
		• Confusion
		• Dizziness
		• Increased muscle irritability
		• Tetany
		• Seizures
		• Coma
			• Treat cause
			• Antiemetic
			• Electrolyte replacement: potassium and/or chloride
			• Discontinuance of sodium bicarbonate or lactated Ringer's solution
			• Administer carbonic anhydrase inhibitor:
			  • Acetazolamide (Diamox)
			• Administer buffer:
			  • Arginine monohydrochloride
			  • Ammonium chloride
			  • Weak HCl acid solution

From Dennison, R. D. (2007). *Pass CCRN!* (3rd ed.). St. Louis: Mosby.

1) Fingers are used to remove visible foreign bodies; blind sweeps are not recommended due to concern that the obstruction may be pushed deeper into the airway
2) Magill forceps may be used but care must be taken to prevent pushing the obstruction deeper into the airway

c. Use abdominal thrusts (also referred to as Heimlich maneuver): subxiphoid thrusts to relieve upper airway obstruction
1) Alternate five abdominal thrusts with attempts to ventilate in unconscious patient
2) Avoid abdominal thrusts (use chest thrusts) in any of the following situations:
   a) Patient is too obese for you to get your arms around them
   b) Patient has had recent abdominal surgery
   c) Patient is pregnant
   d) Place in recovery position: side-lying on left side
4. Encourage deep breathing: sustained inspiratory effort to increase air in the alveoli and prevent atelectasis
5. Remove secretions as required
   a. Cough: forceful expiration to dislodge and remove secretions from the tracheobronchial tree
   b. Suctioning of oropharynx: removal of secretions from the oropharynx with a suction catheter and negative pressure
   c. Suctioning of tracheobronchial tree: removal of secretions from the tracheobronchial tree through the use of a suction catheter and negative pressure
      1) If the patient has a tracheostomy or ET tube
         a) Suction only if indicated and limit number of passes to minimum required
         b) Use a suction catheter with the outer diameter of the catheter no more than one-half the inner diameter of the ET tube

c) Use sterile technique if suctioning is performed through ET tube or tracheostomy; aseptic technique is used if suctioning nasotracheally
   i) Two gloves should be used
   ii) Goggles should be worn to protect the nurse's eyes if open suction system is used
d) Explain procedure to the patient; protect the patient's eyes
e) Provide hyperoxygenation (100% O_2) before and after suctioning
f) Advance the catheter only 1 cm past the length of the ET tube to avoid mucosal trauma
g) Apply suction as the catheter is withdrawn
h) Limit suctioning to 10 seconds; hyperoxygenate for 30 seconds between passes
i) Avoid excessive negative pressure; keep pressure ≤ 100 mm Hg
j) Liquefy secretions with humidification and hydration; the use of saline lavage is not helpful and may be harmful and is not indicated
k) Monitor of complications
   i) Hypoxemia
   ii) Dysrhythmias
   iii) Hypertension
   iv) Intracranial hypertension
   v) Tracheal trauma
l) Stop suctioning if there is a change in heart rate, ECG rhythm, or drop in SpO_2
m) Assess breath sounds after suctioning to evaluate effectiveness
2) For nasotracheal suctioning
   a) Preoxygenate with a nonrebreathing mask first

b) Place patient in "sniffing" position while sitting up or place towel roll between shoulders if supine

c) Lubricate catheter with water-soluble lubricant prior to insertion

d) Prevent injury to the nasal mucosa
   i) Placement of a nasopharyngeal airway may be done to prevent injury to the nasal mucosa if frequent suctioning is required
   ii) Endotracheal intubation or tracheostomy may also be required if frequent suctioning is required

e) Ask the patient to cough and advance the catheter during that time since the glottis is open; if the patient cannot follow commands, advance the catheter during inspiration

f) Note indications that the catheter is in the trachea
   i) Patient becomes anxious
   ii) Patient cannot speak

g) Complete suctioning as for a patient with an ET or tracheostomy tube

6. Chest physiotherapy (chest PT)
   a. Used to promote bronchial hygiene and improve breathing efficiency
   b. Postural drainage (PD): positioning of the patient to use gravity to drain secretions from peripheral areas into the major bronchi or trachea so that they can be coughed and expectorated or suctioned to prevent respiratory complications
   c. Percussion: clapping the chest with cupped hands to mechanically dislodge secretions from the bronchial walls into the major bronchi or trachea so that they can be coughed and expectorated or suctioned
   d. Vibration: vibration during expiration of areas of the chest with either an open hand or a vibrating device to loosen secretions from the bronchial walls into the major bronchi or trachea so that they can be coughed and expectorated or suctioned

7. If patient is boarding or staying in the ED for an extended period, turn the patient at least every 2 hours unless contraindicated; consider "good lung down" principle for patients with unilateral lung conditions

8. Use artificial airways safely and appropriately
   a. Indications for emergency airway management
      1) Apnea
      2) Upper airway obstruction
      3) Need for airway protection (e.g., vomiting, bleeding, altered mental status)
      4) Acute respiratory failure or impending respiratory failure
   b. General principles
      1) Provide humidification because natural humidification mechanisms are bypassed

2) Use aseptic technique with upper airway artificial airways; use sterile technique with lower airway artificial airways

3) Suction as indicated; because ET tubes splint the epiglottis open, effective coughing is impaired

4) Provide method of communication if appropriate; this is the most significant stressor experienced by intubated patients

c. Summary of artificial airways (Table 5-11)
   1) Upper airway artificial airways (Figure 5-14)
      a) Oropharyngeal airway
      b) Nasopharyngeal airway
      c) Cricothyrotomy
   2) Lower airway artificial airways
      a) Esophageal-tracheal combitube (Figure 5-15)
      b) Laryngeal mask airway (LMA) (Figure 5-16)
      c) ET tube (Figure 5-17)
         i) Nasotracheal tube
         ii) Orotracheal tube
      d) Tracheostomy (see Figure 5-17)

d. ET intubation
   1) Indications
      a) Inability of conscious patient to ventilate adequately
      b) Inability to ventilate unconscious patient with bag-valve-mask (BVM)
      c) Inability to control secretions and maintain airway
      d) Loss of protective reflexes (i.e., cough or gag)
   2) Insertion of ET tube
      a) Collect supplies and select tube size
         i) Tube
            (a) Size
               (i) Females usually 7.5 to 8.0
               (ii) Males usually 8.0 to 8.5
               (iii) Pediatric formula for ET tube size is (age/4) + 4 for uncuffed tubes and (age/4) + 3 for cuffed tubes
            (b) It is important to have tubes of different sizes available—one larger and one smaller than anticipated
         ii) Equipment to insert and secure tube: laryngoscope with straight (Miller) and curved (MacIntosh) blades with working lights, stylet, lubricant, syringe, tape, or device to stabilize tube
         iii) Suction equipment including suction catheter and Yankauer suction device
      b) Monitor ECG and SpO_2 during intubation
      c) Hyperoxygenate with 100% O_2 for at least 2 minutes
      d) Place patient in head tilt-chin lift position (unless cervical spine injury is suspected; then use jaw thrust and maintain inline cervical immobilization)

TABLE 5-11   Summary of Artificial Airways

Type of Airway	Advantages	Disadvantages	Miscellaneous
Oropharyngeal airway	• Easy to insert • Inexpensive • Effectively holds tongue away from pharynx	• Improper insertion technique can push tongue back and occlude airway • Easily dislodged • Poorly tolerated by conscious patients as it may stimulate gag reflex • Causes increased oral secretions • Contraindicated in patients with trauma to lower face, recent oral surgery, loose or avulsed teeth	• Determine appropriate size: with flange at teeth, end of airway should not extend beyond the angle of the jaw • Large adult: usually 100 mm (size 5) • Medium adult: usually 90 mm (size 4) • Small adult: usually 80 mm (size 3) • Insert by holding tongue down with tongue blade and sliding into place; alternative method: insert upside down and turn over when into pharynx; take care not to traumatize palate • Do not use as a bite block; likely to cause vomiting and potential aspiration in conscious patients • Remove, wash, and give mouth care every 4 hours; check mucous membranes for ulcerations
Nasopharyngeal airway (also called a *nasal trumpet*)	• Easy to insert • Inexpensive • Effectively holds tongue away from pharynx • May be used in conscious or unconscious patients • Prevents trauma to nasal mucosa during nasotracheal suctioning • May be inserted when mouth cannot be opened (e.g., during seizures, jaw fractures)	• May cause nosebleeds, pressure necrosis, or sinus infection • Kinks and clogs easily • Contraindicated in patients predisposed to nosebleeds, nasal obstruction, bleeding disorder, sepsis and in patients with basal skull fracture • Not used in infants and small children because the small size required does not permit enough air flow for adequate ventilation	• Determine appropriate size: 1 inch longer than nose to earlobe; lumen smaller than naris • Large adult: usually 8–9 internal diameter • Medium adult: usually 7–8 internal diameter • Small adult: usually 6–7 internal diameter • Insert with bevel against septum • Use viscous lidocaine (Xylocaine) as a lubricant for insertion to decrease discomfort • Do not use in patients receiving anticoagulants • Provide humidification of inspired air • Confirm placement by visualizing the tip of the airway next to the uvula • Rotate naris to naris every 8 hours • Limit the duration of use to reduce risk of sinus infection
Esophageal-tracheal combitube	• Allows ventilation whether the tube is inserted into the trachea or the esophagus • Reduces risk of aspiration over mask ventilation • Permits easier placement over endotracheal tube because visualization of the vocal cords is not necessary • Provides comparable ventilation and oxygenation to that achieved with an endotracheal tube	• Incorrect identification of the position of the distal lumen may result in absence of ventilation • May cause esophageal trauma • Cannot mechanically ventilate the patient with a combitube • Not used in children	• Use of an end-tidal CO_2 or esophageal detector device is recommended to confirm placement as either being in the trachea or esophagus

From Dennison, R. D. (2007). *Pass CCRN!* (3rd ed.). St. Louis: Mosby.

Continued

TABLE 5-11 Summary of Artificial Airways—cont'd

Type of Airway	Advantages	Disadvantages	Miscellaneous
Laryngeal mask airway (LMA)	• Permits easier placement than endotracheal tube because visualization of the vocal cords is not necessary • Provides comparable ventilation and oxygenation to that achieved with an endotracheal tube • Allows placement when there is a possibility of unstable neck injury or when appropriate positioning of the patient for tracheal intubation is impossible • Reduces risk of aspiration over mask ventilation • Permits coughing and speech	• Small proportion of patients cannot be ventilated with an LMA so an alternative strategy is needed • Cannot prevent aspiration because it does not separate the gastrointestinal tract from the respiratory tract • May cause laryngospasm, bronchospasm • May be difficult to ventilate patients who require high airway pressures to attain adequate tidal volumes	• If lubrication is required, only the posterior aspect of the airway should be lubricated • If used for mechanical ventilation, an audible air leak may occur

Endotracheal tube (general)	• Provides relatively sealed airway for mechanical ventilation, prevention of aspiration
	• Permits easy suctioning
	• Prevents gastric distention with air during CPRl
		• Requires skilled personnel for insertion
		• Splints epiglottis opens and prevents effective cough
		• Causes loss of physiologic PEEP because epiglottis is splinted open; patient should receive 3-5 cm PEEP to reestablish physiologic PEEP
		• May kink and clog
		• Causes aphonia
		• May cause laryngeal or tracheal damage
		• Contraindicated in patients with laryngeal obstruction caused by tumor, infection, or vocal cord paralysis
			• Determine appropriate size
			  • Females: usually 7.5-8.0 internal diameter
			  • Males: usually 8.0-8.5 internal diameter
			  • Tube may need to be 0.5-1.0 smaller if to be inserted nasally
			• Provide humidification of inspired air
			• Mark tube at corner of mouth or at naris to assess any movement
			• Use minimal occlusive volume or minimal leak volume for cuff inflation; insure that cuff pressure does not exceed 18 mm Hg (if pressure >18 mm Hg required to achieve seal, tube is too small and needs to be replaced with larger tube)
			• Confirm placement by chest radiograph: tip of tube should be 3-5 cm above carina
			• Provide mouth care every 4 hours; observe oral or nasal mucosa for signs of ulcerations or necrosis
			• Position to prevent kinking; use mechanical ventilator's support arms to support ventilator tubing

TABLE 5-11   Summary of Artificial Airways—cont'd

Type of Airway	Advantages	Disadvantages	Miscellaneous
Specific to oral endotracheal tube	• Easier insertion than nasal intubation • Permits larger tube than nasal intubation	• Less stable, less comfortable than nasal tube • May stimulate gag reflex • May be bitten or chewed • May cause necrosis at corner of mouth • Increases oral secretions; makes mouth care more difficult • Contraindicated in patients with acute unstable cervical spine injury due to need for neck extension (blind nasotracheal intubation may be attempted in these patients)	• Avoid unnecessary manipulation of tube
Specific to nasal endotracheal tube	• More comfortable for patient than oral endotracheal tube • Permits good oral hygiene • Cannot be bitten or chewed	• More difficult insertion than oral intubation • May cause pressure necrosis or sinus infection • Requires smaller size • Contraindicated in patients with nasal obstruction, fractured nose, sinusitis, bleeding disorder, basal skull fracture	• Monitor for clinical indications of sinus infection: fever; increased pharyngeal drainage; halitosis; leukocytosis; sinus pain or headache
Cricothyrotomy	• Provides immediate airway access, especially helpful if complete upper airway obstruction	• May cause bleeding • Only temporary; very small opening if established with large needle; larger if airway opened with scalpel and small tracheostomy tube used	• Provide humidification of inspired air • Use large bore over-the-needle catheter; adaptor required to attach to manual resuscitation bag • Physician may use scalpel and insert small tracheostomy tube • Monitor for bleeding, subcutaneous emphysema
Tracheostomy	• Provides long-term airway access • Minimizes risk of vocal cord damage from an endotracheal tube during long-term airway maintenance • Decreases deadspace and decreases work of breathing • Provides a relative seal to prevent aspiration • Allows the patient to eat, swallow • Allows easier suctioning • Permits Valsalva maneuver and effective cough • Is more comfortable for patient • Is less likely to be dislodged than endotracheal tube • Bypasses upper airway obstruction	• May require surgery but may be performed done percutaneously • Causes aphonia • May cause false passage anterior to trachea in patients with thick necks • May cause erosion of innominate artery with tip of tube or low stoma • Causes scar • May cause tracheocutaneous or tracheoesophageal fistula	• Usually considered if artificial airway is required longer than 2-3 weeks • Determine appropriate size: usually 5-6 • Requires humidification of inspired air • Preferred if airway obstruction (e.g., tumor or laryngeal edema or spasm) • Provide tracheostomy care that includes cleaning stoma and tube every 8 hours with saline; keep stoma dry (if 4 × 4 pads are used, change often if secretions present) • Keep obturator, extra tracheostomy tube, and tracheal spreader at bedside

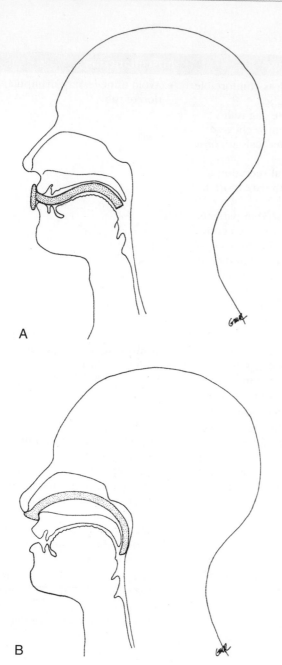

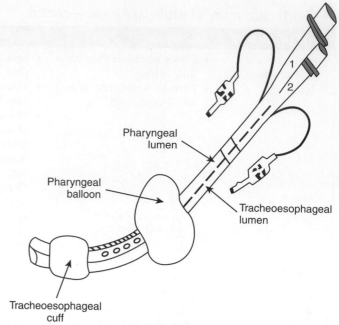

Figure 5-15 Esophageal-tracheal combitube. (From Urtubia, R. N., Aguila, M., & Cumsille, M. [2000]. Combitube: A study for proper use. *Anesthesia and Analgesia, 90*[4], 958–962.)

Figure 5-14 Upper airway artificial airways. **A,** Oropharyngeal airway. **B,** Nasopharyngeal airway. (From Sheehy, S. [1992]. *Emergency nursing: Principles and practice* [3rd ed.]. St. Louis: Mosby.)

e) Ensure patient safety
  i) Intubation should be performed by the most qualified person available who has been trained in ET intubation and frequently performs the procedure (usually physician, nurse practitioner, nurse anesthetist, or respiratory therapist)
  ii) Intubation attempt should be no longer than 30 seconds; if unable to intubate, attempts should be ceased and the patient should again be hyperoxygenated before trying again

f) Confirm placement of ET tube
  i) Feel air movement through tube
  ii) Assess bilateral chest excursion
  iii) Auscultate bilateral breath sounds; if breath sounds are audible on the right but not on the left, right mainstem intubation has occurred; pull the tube back slightly and then recheck breath sounds
  iv) Use a capnometer to confirm consistent exhalation of CO_2
  v) Auscultate over epigastrium: air movement should not be audible in adults but may be in pediatrics due to thin wall chest so not reliable in children
  (vi) Confirm tube positioning by chest radiograph; distal tip of tube should be 2 cm above the carina

g) Inflate the cuff using the either minimal occlusive volume or minimal leak volume
  i) Minimal occlusive volume
    (a) Listen over trachea with stethoscope
    (b) Inflate cuff until no air leak is audible during the inspiratory cycle of the ventilator
  ii) Minimal leak volume
    (a) Listen over trachea with stethoscope
    (b) Inflate cuff until no air leak is audible during the inspiratory cycle of the ventilator
    (c) Remove 0.1 cm of air or until a minimal leak is audible during the inspiratory cycle of the ventilator

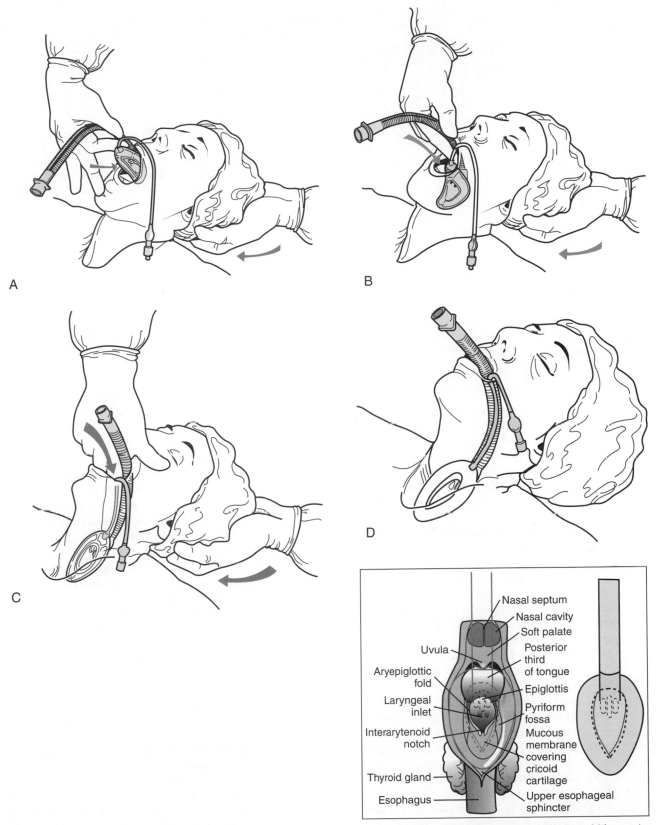

Figure 5-16 Laryngeal mask airway (LMA). **A,** LMA is an adjunctive airway that consists of a tube with a cuffed masklike projection at distal end. **B,** LMA is introduced through mouth into pharynx. **C,** Once LMA is in position, a clear, secure airway is present. **D** (anatomic detail), during insertion, LMA is advanced until resistance is felt as distal portion of tube locates in hypopharynx. Cuff then is inflated. This seals larynx and leaves distal opening of tube just above glottis, providing a clear, secure airway. (From European Resuscitation Council. [2000]. Part 6: Advanced cardiovascular life support. Section 3: Adjuncts for oxygenation, ventilation, and airway control. *Resuscitation, 46*[1–3], 115–125.)

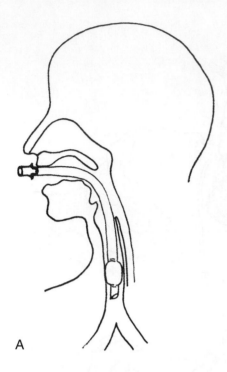

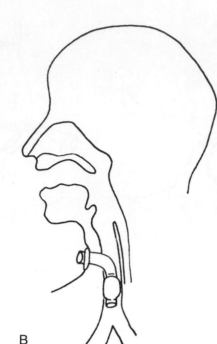

Figure 5-17 Lower airway artificial airways. **A,** Endotracheal tube. **B,** Tracheostomy tube. (From Phipps, W. J., et al. [1995]. *Medical-surgical nursing: Concepts and clinical practice* [5th ed.]. St. Louis: Mosby.)

h) Tape tube in place
 i) Secure tape to minimize pressure areas on the face; tape with tension to both sides to avoid excessive pressure on corner of mouth if oral tube
 ii) If a commercial stabilization device is used, assess lips and oral mucosa frequently for evidence of excessive pressure
i) Note the depth marking on the side of the tube; usually at 19 to 23 cm for an average adult
j) Attach O_2 deliver system or mechanical ventilator

3) Rapid sequence intubation (RSI): use of pharmacologic agents for sedation and paralysis to secure an airway in the most rapid way possible
a) Preparation: 5 to 10 minutes prior
 i) Confirm that intubation equipment is functional
 ii) Establish intravenous (IV) access
 iii) Prepare medications and determine sequence of administration: lidocaine, opioids, atropine, defasciculating agents (LOAD)
 iv) Assess if there are possible contraindications to RSI medications
 v) Monitor SpO_2, ECG rhythm, and blood pressure throughout procedures
b) Preoxygenation: 5 minutes prior
 i) Administer 100% O_2 via a nonrebreather mask to washout nitrogen
 ii) Assist ventilation with BVM system only if needed to obtain O_2 saturation >90% (use cricoid pressure)

c) Pretreatment: 3 minutes prior
 i) Administer IV medications:
  (a) Lidocaine: to decrease intracranial pressure
  (b) Opiate: to sedate
  (c) Atropine: for bradycardia
  (d) Defasciculating agent: small dose of defasciculating paralytic to prevent muscle fasciculations (involuntary muscle contraction)
d) Paralytic agent: Just prior to procedure
 i) Administer short-acting neuromuscular blocking agent (e.g., succinylcholine, vecuronium)
 ii) BVM ventilate patient
e) Placement: 30 to 45 seconds after paralytic agent
 i) Apply cricoid pressure (Sellick maneuver) to prevent regurgitation of gastric contents
 ii) Maintain pressure throughout intubation sequence until the position of the ET tube is verified
 iii) Visualization of ET tube going through the cords
 iv) Inflate cuff
f) Placement verification
 i) Confirm tube placement by colormetric $ETCO_2$ device
 ii) Symmetrical rise and fall of chest
 iii) Auscultation breath sounds: listen over each lateral lung field, the left axilla, and the left supraclavicular region for good breath sounds, and no air movement should occur over the stomach

g) Post intubation
   i) Secure ET tube
   ii) Place on mechanical ventilation
   iii) Administer analgesic and sedative agents as prescribed for comfort
   iv) Obtain a chest radiograph for verification of placement
4) Prevention of unplanned extubation
   a) Identify patients at high risk for unplanned extubation: restless, confused, anxious
   b) Explain to the patient the purpose of the ET tube, that it temporarily prevents the patient from speaking; explain the hazards of self-extubation
   c) Secure the ET tube with tape around head or with a commercially available stabilization device
   d) Note the size of the ET tube and the position of the tube at the teeth
   e) Restrain the patient's hands as necessary (need physician order)
   f) Ensure support of ventilator tubing to decrease tension on the ET tube
   g) Ensure that appropriate equipment is available at the bedside: bag-valve-mask, replacement ET tube, suction equipment
   h) Treatment of unplanned extubation
      i) Assess patency of airway, respiratory rate, SpO_2, breath sounds, neurologic status
      ii) Administer O_2 with BVM if the patient requires ventilatory assistance or by mask or cannula if the patient is breathing spontaneously
      iii) Notify the physician and assemble equipment for emergency reintubation
5) Assessment of sudden decrease in oxygenation in the intubated patient: Think DOPE
   a) Displaced tube
   b) Obstructed tube
   c) Pneumothorax
   d) Equipment problem (e.g., O_2 empty, disconnected from ventilator)
6) Complications of ET intubation
   a) Trauma: damage to teeth, mucous membranes, perforation or laceration of pharynx, larynx, trachea
   b) Aspiration
   c) Laryngospasm, bronchospasm
   d) Esophageal mainstem intubation
   e) Hypoxia, anoxia: prolonged attempts

O_2 Therapy

Definitions
1. Hypoxemia: decrease in arterial blood O_2 tension
   a. Diagnosis by ABGs
   b. Decrease in PaO_2 and SaO_2
      1) Mild hypoxemia: PaO_2 <80 mm Hg ($\approx SaO_2$ 95%)
      2) Moderate (significant) hypoxemia: PaO_2 <60 mm Hg ($\approx SaO_2$ 90%)
      3) Severe hypoxemia: PaO_2 <40 mm Hg ($\approx SaO_2$ 75%)
2. Hypoxia: decrease in tissue oxygenation
   a. Diagnosis by clinical indications (see Box 5-2)
   b. Affected by PaO_2 and SaO_2, Hgb, patency of vessels, cellular demand

Factors indicating need for O_2 therapy
1. Hypoxemia
   a. Low inspired O_2 concentration (e.g., high altitudes)
   b. Hypoventilation (e.g., asthma)
   c. $\dot{V}/\dot{Q}$ mismatching (e.g., pulmonary embolism)
   d. Shunt (e.g., acute respiratory distress syndrome)
   e. Diffusion abnormalities (e.g., pulmonary fibrosis)
2. Hypoxia
   a. Hypoxemic hypoxia: secondary to a gas exchange problem (e.g., ventilation-perfusion mismatch, shunt, diffusion abnormalities)
   b. Hypemic hypoxia: secondary to reduced O_2-carrying capacity of the blood (e.g., anemia, CO poisoning, methemoglobinemia)
   c. Stagnant hypoxia: secondary to a reduced blood flow in the body or a reduction in cardiac output (e.g., shock)
   d. Histotoxic hypoxia: secondary to the inability of the cells to utilize O_2 (e.g., cyanide poisoning)

Pathophysiology of hypoxia
1. Decrease in PaO_2 initially stimulates the sympathetic nervous system (SNS)
2. O_2 extraction at tissue level increases
3. As PaO_2 becomes critically low, tissue oxygenation becomes inadequate and hypoxia occurs
4. Nutrient metabolism changes from aerobic to anaerobic, which results in 20 times less ATP than aerobic metabolism and lactic acid as a waste product
5. Acidosis and decreased cellular energy results

Clinical presentation of hypoxia
1. Evidence of altered perfusion
   a. Tachycardia
   b. Hypotension
   c. Changes in skin color and temperature
2. Evidence of anaerobic metabolism: lactic acidosis
3. Evidence of organ dysfunction
   a. Cerebral: altered sensorium
   b. Myocardial: decreased cardiac output; dysrhythmias
   c. Renal: decreased urine output
4. Parameters of O_2 delivery
   a. PaO_2, SaO_2, SpO_2
   b. Hgb, Hct
   c. Cardiac output, cardiac index

Indications for O_2 therapy
1. Significant hypoxemia: PaO_2 <60 mm Hg; SaO_2 or SpO_2 <90%
2. Suspected hypoxemia (e.g., asthma, pulmonary embolism, aspiration, drug overdose, seizure or postictal state, pneumothorax, trauma)

3. Increased myocardial workload (e.g., heart failure, hypertensive crisis, MI)
4. Decreased cardiac output (e.g., shock, hypotension, cardiopulmonary arrest)
5. Increased O_2 demand (e.g., sepsis, increased ventilatory work)
6. Decreased O_2 carrying capacity (e.g., CO or cyanide poisoning, methemoglobinemia, sickle cell disease, anemia)
7. Prior to procedures that may cause hypoxemia (e.g., suctioning, during and after anesthesia, transportation of unstable patient, bronchoscopy)

Principles of O_2 therapy

1. Airway is always the first priority; O_2 is useless without an adequate airway
2. O_2 is a potent drug that is administered as prescribed; may be prescribed as flow rate, O_2 concentration (expressed as a %), or fraction of inspired O_2 (FIO_2) (expressed as a decimal)
3. The objective is to improve tissue oxygenation
   a. Maintain Pao_2 at least 60 mm Hg and Sao_2 at 90%; serial serum lactate levels are also helpful in monitoring progression or improvement of hypoxia and degree of anaerobic metabolism
   b. Determine the effectiveness of O_2 therapy: determined by pathology
      1) O_2 therapy is ineffective for shunt; alveoli must be opened (also referred to as alveolar recruitment) to get the O_2 to the alveolar-capillary membrane; PEEP is required in these cases
4. If high concentrations are necessary, limit duration to prevent O_2 toxicity
   a. Exact concentration of inspired O_2 should be measured with O_2 analyzer
5. Safety guidelines
   a. Keep O_2 source at least 10 feet from open flame
   b. Do not allow smoking in a room with supplemental O_2
   c. Do not use electrical appliances within 5 feet of O_2 source
   d) Do not use petroleum-based products around O_2 source; use only water-soluble lubricants, creams
   e) Turn the O_2 off when not in use
   f) Secure the O_2 tanks to prevent accidental dropping; keep O_2 source away from heat or direct sunlight

High-flow versus low-flow O_2 delivery systems

1. Low-flow O_2 delivery systems
   a. Do not provide total inspired gas; remainder of patient's inspiratory volume is met by patient breathing varying amounts of room air
   b. FIO_2 dependent on rate and depth of ventilation and fit of device
   c. Low flow does not necessarily mean low FIO_2
   d. Devices
      1) Nasal cannula
      2) Reservoir systems
         a) Simple face mask

   b) Partial rebreathing mask
   c) Nonrebreathing mask
2. High-flow O_2 delivery systems
   a. Provide the entire inspired gas by high flow of gas or entrainment of room air
   b. Provide a predictable FIO_2
   c. Does not necessarily mean high FIO_2
   d. Devices
      1) Venturi mask
      2) T-piece: may be high or low flow depending on flow rate
      3) Trach collar: may be high or low flow depending on flow rate
      4) Mechanical ventilator
O_2 delivery systems (Table 5-12)

Hazards of O_2 therapy

1. Oxygen-induced hypoventilation
2. Oxygen toxicity
   a. Cause: a concentration that is too high for too long a period (hours to days)
   b. Clinical indications
      1) Early
         a) Substernal chest pain that increases with deep breathing
         b) Dry cough and tracheal irritation
         c) Dyspnea
         d) Upper airway changes (e.g., nasal stuffiness, sore throat, eye and ear discomfort)
         e) Anorexia, nausea, vomiting
         f) Fatigue, lethargy, malaise
         g) Restlessness
      2) Late
         a) Changes on chest films: atelectasis, patches of pneumonia
         b) Progressive ventilatory difficulty: decreased vital capacity; decreased compliance; hypercapnia
         c) Increased intrapulmonary shunt: increasing A-a gradient and decreased Pao_2/FIO_2 ratio; hypoxemia
            i) The A-a gradient is a measure of the difference between the alveolar and arterial concentration of O_2; it is used in diagnosing the source of hypoxemia
   c. Prevention
      1) Use the lowest FIO_2 possible to maintain a Pao_2 of at least 60 mm Hg (Sao_2 90%)

Hyperbaric oxygenation

1. Definition: administration of high concentration (usually 100%) O_2 under greatly increased pressure (usually 2 to 3 atmospheres [atm])
2. Indications: CO or cyanide poisoning; air embolism; radiation therapy; gas gangrene; burns; nonhealing wounds, necrotizing fasciitis, decompression illness, osteomyelitis, intracranial abscess
3. Complications: O_2 toxicity; absorptive atelectasis; acute respiratory distress syndrome, bleeding and edema of eustachian tubes, rupture of tympanic membrane

Selected Concepts in Mechanical Ventilation

Indications for mechanical ventilation

1. Acute ventilatory failure with respiratory acidosis not relieved by ordinary methods
2. Hypoxemia despite maximum O_2 therapy
3. Relief of hypoxemia causes increased CO_2 retention
4. Apnea: consideration needs to be given to the reversibility of the situation (i.e., not indicated to prolong a terminal condition)

TABLE 5-12 Summary of Oxygen Delivery Systems

System	Advantages	Disadvantages	Miscellaneous
Nasal cannula 1-6 L/min delivers 24%-44% O_2 (3% increase with each liter)	• Safe and simple • Comfortable • Effective for low O_2 concentration • Allows eating and talking • Inexpensive	• Contraindicated in nasal obstruction • May cause drying and irritation of nasal mucosa • Variable concentrations of O_2 depending on tidal volume, ventilatory rate, flow rate, and nasal patency	• Ensure that flow rates do not exceed 6 l/min • Provide humidification if flow rates exceed 4 L/min • Use gauze pads under cannula at tops of ears to prevent pressure ulceration
Simple face mask 5-10 L/min delivers 40%-60% O_2 (ENA, 2005)	• Delivers high O_2 concentration • Does not dry mucous membranes of nose and mouth • Can be used in patients with nasal obstruction	• Hot, confining, uncomfortable • Tight seal necessary • Frequently poorly tolerated in dyspneic patient • Interferes with eating and talking • May cause CO_2 retention if flow rate is <6 L/min • Variable concentrations of O_2 depending on tidal volume, ventilatory rate, and flow rate • Cannot deliver <40% • Potential for O_2 toxicity • Impractical for long-term therapy	• Place pads between mask and bony facial parts • Wash and dry face every 4 hours • Clean mask every 8 hours • Ensure flow rate of at least 5 L/min • Watch for signs of O_2 toxicity
Partial rebreathing mask 8-12 L/min delivers 50%-80% (ENA, 2005)	• Delivers high O_2 concentrations • Does not dry mucous membranes	• As for face mask • May cause CO_2 retention if reservoir bag is allowed to collapse	• Ensure that bag not totally deflate during inhalation (increase flow rate) • Keep mask snug • Watch for signs of O_2 toxicity
Nonrebreathing mask 6-12 L/min delivers 60%-90%	• As for other masks • One-way valves prevent rebreathing of CO_2 and increases O_2 concentrations	• As for other masks except does not cause CO_2 retention	• As for partial rebreathing mask • Watch for signs of O_2 toxicity
Face tent (face shield)	• Large, soft plastic bucket fits around child's entire face and lower jaw • Easy access for suctioning both nose and mouth • O_2 can be provided warm, cooled, or humidified	• Cannot provide O_2 concentrations >40% even with high flow rate	• As for other masks • Watch for signs of O_2 toxicity
Blow-by	• Less stressful for child; caregiver can hold child in lap and direct O_2 toward child's face	• Variable delivery depending on technique • Cannot provide >40% O_2	• Allows for "alternative" delivery: may attach tubing to toys or "sippy" cups

Adapted from Dennison, R. D. (2007). *Pass CCRN!* (3rd ed.). St. Louis: Mosby and Emergency Nurses Association. (2005). *Sheehy's manual of emergency care* (6th ed.). St. Louis: Mosby.

Continued

TABLE **5-12** Summary of Oxygen Delivery Systems—cont'd

System	Advantages	Disadvantages	Miscellaneous
Venturi mask 2–12 L/min delivers 24%–50% ENA, 2005)	• Delivers accurate O_2 concentration depending on flow rate and diluter jet inserted despite changes in patient's respiratory pattern • O_2 concentration can be changed • Does not dry mucous membranes	• FIO_2 can be lowered if mask does not fit snugly, if tubing is kinked, if O_2 intake ports are blocked, or if less than recommended liter flow is used • Hot, confining, uncomfortable • Tight seal necessary • Frequently poorly tolerated in dyspneic patient • Interferes with eating and talking	• Watch for signs of O_2 toxicity • As for other masks
Pocket mask 10 L/min delivers 50% (ENA, 2005)	• Avoid direct mouth to mouth contact • O_2 source can be added • In children can produce a good tidal volume	• Rescuer fatigue	• Watch for good seal
Bag-valve-mask Room air delivers 21%; 12 L/min delivers 40%–90% (ENA, 2005)	• Can use quickly • Can increase O_2 concentration easily • Can feel lung compliance • Can be used on apneic or breathing patient	• Increased air into stomach • Difficulty obtaining and maintaining a good seal	• Maintain tight seal
O_2–powered breathing device 100 L/min delivers 100% (ENA, 2005)	• High O_2 flow • Provide positive pressure • Improvement in lung inflation	• Gastric distention • Requires O_2 source • Not recommended for children unless special adapter available	
Trach collar 21%–70% 10 L or to provide visible mist	• Does not pull on tracheostomy • Elastic ties allow movement of mask away from tracheostomy without removing it	• O_2 diluted by room air • Increased likelihood of infection and skin irritation around stoma because of high humidity • Condensation can collect in the tubing and drain into patient's airway especially during turning	• Ensure that O_2 be warmed and humidified • Empty condensation from tubing frequently; empty into water trap or container for appropriate discard; do not empty water back into humidifier
T-piece or tube Flow rate set at 2.5 times patient's minute ventilation to deliver 21%–100%	• Delivers variable concentrations • Less moisture around tracheostomy than with tracheostomy collar	• May cause CO_2 retention at low flow rates • Weight of T-piece can pull on tracheostomy tube • Condensation can collect in the tubing and drain into patient's airway especially during turning	• Requires heated nebulizer • Use extension on open side to act as a reservoir and increase O_2 concentration as prescribed • Empty condensation from tubing frequently • Check ABGs frequently • Watch for signs of O_2 toxicity
Mechanical ventilation 21%–100%	• Delivers predictable, constant concentrations of O_2 • Supports ventilation as well as oxygenation • Addition of positive end-expiratory pressure (PEEP) augments the driving pressure of O_2; this aids in the achievement of acceptable Po_2 levels at lower O_2 concentrations	• Requires skilled personnel • Requires electricity and backup power generator (plug into red outlet) • Condensation can collect in the tubing and drain into patient's airway, especially during turning	• Requires heated humidifier • Empty condensation from tubing frequently • Check ABGs frequently • Watch for signs of O_2 toxicity

Commonly used mechanical ventilator parameters

1. Mode refers to how the machine senses or signals the initiation of inspiration; Table 5-13 describes ventilator modes frequently used in an emergency department setting
2. Tidal volume: 5 to 10 ml/kg
3. Respiratory rate: usually 8 to 16 breathes/min for adults
4. FIO_2
   a. Initially 1.0 (i.e., 100%) for 20 minutes, especially if cardiac arrest
   b. Adjusted so that Pao_2 is 60 mm Hg
   c. Use lowest FIO_2 that achieves desired Pao_2
   d. PEEP may be added to maintain acceptable Pao_2 with lower FIO_2 to reduce the risk of O_2 toxicity
5. PEEP
   a. Definition: maintenance of pressure above atmospheric at airway opening at end-expiration
      1) Physiologic: 3 to 5 cm
      2) Therapeutic: >5 cm
      3) Best (or optimal) PEEP: provides Sao_2 of at least 90% without compromising cardiac output

TABLE 5-13   **Ventilator Modes**

Mode	Description	Comments
Control	• Preset tidal volume and rate; the ventilator delivers the tidal volume at the rate set on the ventilators	• Patient must be apneic or paralyzed or they "fight" the ventilator • Guarantees ventilation with a specific minute ventilation • Allows ventilatory muscle rest
Assist/control (also called assisted mandatory ventilation)	• Preset tidal volume, minimum rate (control rate), and inspiratory effort required to "trigger" the ventilator to cycle to assist breaths (sensitivity); the ventilator delivers the control breaths of the specified tidal volume and responds by cycling additionally if the patient's inspiratory effort (negative pressure) is adequate	• More comfortable than control mode • Less work of breathing for patient than spontaneous breathing or IMV • Allows ventilatory muscle rest • Risk for hyperventilation because each assisted breath is delivered at same tidal volume as mandatory breaths; sedation may be necessary
Synchronized intermittent mandatory ventilation (SIMV)	• Preset tidal volume and minimum rate; the patient may take additional breaths between the mandatory breaths • Mandatory breaths are synchronized so that they do not occur during the patient's ventilatory efforts	• Less potential for hyperventilation because patient-initiated breaths are at the tidal volume determined by the patient • More work of breathing for patient than assist/control because patient-initiated breaths are not assisted • Less need for sedation than assist/control or control modes • Does not decrease cardiac output as much as assist/control or control modes • Frequently used for weaning
Pressure support ventilation (PSV)	• Preset inspiratory support pressure level; when the patient initiates a breath, this positive pressure flows to assist the patient's spontaneous breaths; tidal volume and rate are patient controlled	• Low level (5–10 cm H_2O) helps to eliminate the increased work of breathing associated with an endotracheal tube; higher levels help to augment the patient's own intrinsic tidal volume • Lessens work of breathing but also allows use of respiratory muscles to lessen muscular atrophy • Lower mean airway pressures than volume ventilation • May be used with IMV or alone; if used alone, patient must be spontaneously breathing • There is no preset ventilatory rate and apnea occurs if the patient does not initiate a breath; newer models provide a volume ventilation backup (called volume-assured pressure support ventilation [VAPSV])

From Dennison, R. D. (2007). *Pass CCRN!* (3rd ed.). St. Louis: Mosby.

b. Physiologic effects of PEEP
  1) Decreases surface tension and work of breathing
  2) Reduces shunt by opening alveoli that are collapsed (i.e., alveolar recruitment) and keeping alveoli open that are open
  3) Increases the driving pressure of O_2 to allow achievement of a better Pao_2 at the same Fio_2 or achievement of the same Pao_2 at a lower Fio_2; decreases risk of O_2 toxicity
c. Common uses of PEEP
  1) ARDS (also referred to as noncardiac pulmonary edema)
  2) Cardiac pulmonary edema
  3) Acute respiratory failure with persistent hypoxemia
d. Contraindications/cautions of PEEP
  1) Untreated hypovolemia and hypotensive states: the decrease in venous return causes by PEEP can accentuate hypotension
  2) COPD: increased risk of barotrauma in patients with COPD
e. Adverse effects of PEEP
  1) Increased risk of barotrauma
  2) Increased need for patient sedation

Noninvasive Positive Pressure Ventilation (NPPV)

Description: positive pressure ventilation (usually CPAP or BiPAP) of a nonintubated spontaneously breathing patient, may be administered via a face or nasal mask or an ET tube and may be delivered via a mechanical ventilator or specialized NIPPV machine

1. CPAP: maintenance of positive pressure during spontaneous ventilation
2. BiPAP: combination of pressure support ventilation (I-PAP) and continuous positive airway pressure (E-PAP)

Indications

1. Acute respiratory failure; frequently used as an interim treatment to prevent the need for intubation, especially in patients with COPD
2. Severe respiratory distress in a patient opposed to intubation
3. Pulmonary edema
4. Sleep apnea

Advantages over traditional mechanical ventilation

1. Avoidance of intubation and complications of intubation
2. Improved patient comfort
3. Lower incidence of nosocomial pneumonia
4. Lower sedation requirements
5. No loss of speech

Contraindications

1. Absolute
  a. Hemodynamic instability
  b. Problems with airway patency (e.g., copious secretions)
  c. Risk for aspiration
  d. Altered level of consciousness (i.e., patients without airway protective reflexes)
2. Relative
  a. Uncooperative patient
  b. Morbid obesity
  c. Unstable angina or acute MI
  d. Inability to fit mask

Complications

1. Discomfort related to mask; can lead to facial skin breakdown
2. Nasal congestion
3. Conjunctivitis
4. Gastric distention, vomiting, aspiration
5. Pneumothorax
6. Restlessness and agitation, especially in claustrophobic patients

Specific Respiratory Emergencies

Acute respiratory failure

Definitions

1. Acute respiratory failure: failure of the respiratory system to provide for the exchange of O_2 and CO_2 between the environment and tissues in quantities sufficient to sustain life
2. COPD with acute exacerbation: acute process in a patient with a chronic condition; usually caused by respiratory infection
  a. COPD: a disease state characterized by the presence of airflow obstruction due to chronic bronchitis or emphysema; the airflow obstruction is progressive, may be accompanied by airway hyperactivity, and may be partially reversible (American Thoracic Society)
    1) Chronic bronchitis: defined clinically by excessive mucus secretion in the bronchi (also known as the blue bloaters)
    2) Emphysema: defined pathophysiologically by enlargement of the air spaces distal to the terminal bronchioles with destruction of alveolar walls (Also known as the pink puffers)
  b. Acute exacerbation of COPD: worsening dyspnea, increase in sputum volume, and increase in sputum purulence

Precipitating factors

1. COPD with acute exacerbation
2. Pneumonia
3. Chest trauma
4. Pulmonary edema
5. Pulmonary fibrosis
6. Pleural effusion
7. Pneumothorax
8. Asthma
9. Atelectasis
10. Aspiration pneumonitis
11. Acute respiratory distress syndrome
12. Smoke inhalation

13. Pulmonary embolism: thrombotic, fat, air, amniotic
14. Status asthmaticus
15. Central nervous system (CNS)-depressant drugs such as opiates, sedatives/hypnotics
16. Neuromuscular blocking drugs such as muscle paralytics, aminoglycosides, organophosphate poisoning
17. Neurologic conditions such as head trauma, poliomyelitis, amyotrophic lateral sclerosis, spinal cord injury, Guillain-Barré syndrome, myasthenia gravis, multiple sclerosis, muscular dystrophy
18. Morbid obesity
19. Sleep apnea
20. Tracheal obstruction
21. Epiglottis
22. Cystic fibrosis
23. Drowning

Pathophysiology
1. Impairment in ventilation and/or diffusion of O_2
2. Hypercapnia and/or hypoxemia

Clinical presentation
1. Subjective
   a. History of precipitating factor
   b. Clinical indications of respiratory distress (see Box 5-1)
   c. Clinical indications of hypoxia (see Box 5-2)
   d. Clinical indications of hypercapnia (see Box 5-3)
2. Objective
   a. Clinical indications of respiratory distress see Box 5-1)
   b. Hypoxemia: decrease in SpO_2, SaO_2, PaO_2
   c. Clinical indications of hypoxia (see Box 5-2)
   d. Clinical indications of hypercapnia (see Box 5-3)
3. Diagnostic
   a. Arterial blood gas changes
      1) PaO_2 <50 to 60 mm Hg
      2) $PaCO_2$ >50 mm Hg with pH <7.30
   b. Chest radiograph: may identify cause

Collaborative management
1. Continue assessment
   a. ABCDs
   b. O_2 saturation
   c. Vital signs: blood pressure, pulse, respiratory rate, and temperature
   d. Respiratory effort and excursion
   e. Cardiac rate and rhythm
   f. Pain, discomfort, or dyspnea level
   g. Accurate intake and output
   h. Serum electrolytes
   i Level of consciousness
   j. Close monitoring for progression of symptoms
2. Treat the cause
3. Establish and maintain airway
   a. Positioning for optimal ventilation
      1) Head of bed to 30 to 45 degrees
      2) Overbed table for patient to lean on

3) "Good lung down" if unilateral lung condition exists
b. Bronchial hygiene and chest physiotherapy as indicated
   1) Inspiratory maneuvers: deep breathing; incentive spirometry
   2) Analgesics in doses adequate to allow patient to deep breathe and cough as indicated
   3) Encouragement of the patient to cough if rhonchi are audible; suctioning if the patient is unable to clear airways
   4) Postural drainage, percussion, vibration may be necessary
   5) Bronchoscopy may be necessary if airway clearance techniques are inadequate
   6) Intubation and mechanical ventilation may be necessary if $PaCO_2$ continues to rise and acidosis develops
c. Intubation and mechanical ventilation may be necessary if $PaCO_2$ continues to rise and acidosis develops
d. O_2 as indicated for hypoxemia
   1) Nasal cannula or mask; masks are contraindicated in hypercapnic patients as the high concentration of O_2 provided by these delivery systems would likely eliminate the hypoxic drive
   2) Flow rate or O_2 concentration to keep SpO_2 ≈95% unless contraindicated; in patients with chronic hypercapnia, adjust flow rate or O_2 concentration to keep SpO_2 ≈90%
   3) Intubation and mechanical ventilation may be necessary if $PaCO_2$ continues to rise and acidosis develops
e. Pharmacologic therapies
   1) Bronchodilators may be indicated
      a) β_2-Adrenergic agonists (these agents are preferred over non–respiratory-selective β stimulants like epinephrine and isoproterenol because they cause fewer cardiovascular side effects)
         (i) Terbutaline (Brethine)
         (ii) Albuterol (Proventil)
         (iii) Isoetharine HCl (Bronkosol)
         (iv) Metaproterenol (Alupent)
      b) Parasympatholytics (e.g., ipratropium [Atrovent])
      c) Xanthines (e.g., aminophylline, theophylline)
      d) Magnesium
   2) Expectorants (e.g., guaifenesin [Robitussin], potassium iodide [SSKI]) may be used but hydration is most important
   3) Mucolytics (e.g., acetylcysteine [Mucomyst]) may be used to decrease the tenacity of the mucus; frequently causes bronchospasm so given with a bronchodilator

4) Sedatives: generally avoided unless patient is very agitated
5) Antitussives: avoid use of antitussives unless nonproductive cough is causing patient fatigue
f. Quiet, restful environment
4. Optimize O_2 delivery and decrease O_2 consumption
   a. Improvement of O_2 delivery to the tissues (Do_2)
      1) Sao_2: O_2, PEEP as required
      2) Cardiac output: fluid administration, inotropic agents, intra-aortic balloon pump, vasoactive agents, etc. as required
      3) Hgb: packed RBCs as required
   b. Treatment of fever (controversial because pyrogens helpful in mobilizing the immune system)
      1) Antipyretics (e.g., acetaminophen [Tylenol])
      2) Cooling blankets may be used but shivering should be avoided due to effect on O_2 consumption
5. Maintain adequate hydration but prevent overhydration
   a. IV access for fluid and medication administration
   b. Fluids usually D_5NS
6. Treat infection (if present) and prevent sepsis
   a. Antimicrobials as indicated: empirically or specific to cultured microorganism
   b. Bronchial hygiene techniques
   c. Antipyretics and cooling methods to reduce fever
7. Monitor for/prevent complications
   a) Dysrhythmias
   b) Pulmonary infections
   c) Acid-base imbalance
      1) Respiratory acidosis
      2) Respiratory alkalosis occurs in patients with chronic hypercapnia when $Paco_2$ is normalized rather than the pH due to long-term renal retention of bicarbonate
   d) Electrolyte imbalance
   e) Thromboembolism
   f) Gastrointestinal complications: abdominal distention; ileus; ulcer; hemorrhage
   g) Renal failure
   h) Sepsis; septic shock

Evaluation
1. Patent airway, adequate oxygenation (i.e., normal Pao_2, Spo_2, Sao_2) and ventilation (i.e., normal $Paco_2$)
2. Absence of clinical indications of respiratory distress
3. Absence of clinical indicators of hypoperfusion
4. Absence of clinical indications of infection/sepsis
5. Alert and oriented with no neurologic deficit
6. Control of pain, discomfort, or dyspnea
7. Absence of clinical indications of bleeding
8. Alert and oriented with no neurologic deficit

Typical disposition
1. If evaluation criteria met: discharge with instructions
2. If evaluation criteria not met: admission to progressive care unit or critical care unit

Acute Respiratory Distress Syndrome
Definitions
1. Acute lung injury
   a. A syndrome of lung inflammation and increased alveolar-capillary permeability characterized by hypoxemia resistant to O_2 therapy
   b. The less severe end of the spectrum of the pulmonary component of systemic inflammatory response syndrome (SIRS)
2. Acute respiratory distress syndrome
   a. A syndrome of acute respiratory failure characterized by noncardiac pulmonary edema and manifested by refractory hypoxemia caused by intrapulmonary shunt
   b. May be considered the severe end of the spectrum of the pulmonary component of SIRS

Predisposing factors
1. Direct injury
   a. Chest trauma: pulmonary contusion
   b. Drowning
   c. Hypervolemia, pulmonary edema
   d. Inhalation: smoke, chemicals
   e. Pneumonia: viral, bacterial, or fungal
   f. Pulmonary embolism: particularly fat or amniotic fluid
   g. Radiation
2. Indirect injury
   a. Sepsis: most likely cause
   b. Shock or prolonged hypotension
   c. Multisystem trauma, especially multiple fractures
   d. Burns
   e. Toxemia of pregnancy
   f. Acute pancreatitis
   g. Diabetic ketoacidosis
   h. CNS injury
   i. Massive blood transfusion
   j. Drug overdosage: heroin, methadone, barbiturates, aspirin, thiazide diuretics, tricyclic antidepressants

Pathophysiology
1. Acute lung injury reduces normal perfusion to the lungs causing platelet aggregation and stimulation of the inflammatory-immune system and release of various mediators that activate or stimulate neutrophils, macrophages, and other cells to release toxic substances that cause microvascular injury
2. Damage to alveolar-capillary membrane and increase in capillary permeability
3. Capillary leak allows proteins and fluids to spill into the interstitium and alveolar spaces; pulmonary lymphatic drainage capacity is overwhelmed and alveolar flooding occurs

4. Pulmonary edema results and causes interference with O_2 diffusion and inactivation of surfactant; damage to type II pneumocytes results in decreased production of surfactant
5. Massive atelectasis causes extensive intrapulmonary shunting and profound hypoxemia
6. Vasoconstrictive mediators cause increased pulmonary vasoconstriction and pulmonary hypertension
7. Decrease in lung compliance and increasing alveolar deadspace
8. Interstitial collagen deposition causes pulmonary fibrosis

Clinical presentation

1. Subjective
   a. History of recent injury or toxic inhalation
   b. Dyspnea
   c. Fatigue
2. Objective
   a. Tachypnea
   b. Tachycardia
   c. Clinical indications of respiratory distress (see Box 5-1)
   d. Clinical indications of hypoxemia (see Box 5-2)
   e. Cyanosis may be evident
   f. Breath sound changes: crackles
3. Phases of ARDS (Table 5-14)
4. Diagnostic
   a. CBC with differential: may have high WBC count
   b. Blood cultures: sepsis is the most common cause
   c. ABGs: refractory hypoxemia (hypoxemia despite high concentration of O_2); PaO_2 <55 mm Hg despite FIO_2 ≥0.5 for 24 hours
   d. Chest radiograph
      1) May be normal initially
      2) Bilateral diffuse interstitial and alveolar infiltrates
      3) Ground-glass appearance
      4) "White-out" due to massive atelectasis
      5) Heart size is normal (one factor that differentiates ARDS from cardiac pulmonary edema)
   e. Computed tomography (CT) of chest
      1) Gravity-dependent infiltrates
      2) Lack of homogeneity of infiltrates

Collaborative management

1. Continue assessment
   a. ABCDs
   b. Vital signs: blood pressure, pulse, respiratory rate, and temperature
   c. O_2 saturation
   d. Respiratory effort and excursion
   e. Cardiac rate and rhythm
   f. Pain and Discomfort level
   g. Level of consciousness
   h. Accurate intake and output
   i. Close monitoring for progression of symptoms

TABLE 5-14 Phases of ARDS

Parameter	Phase I	Phase II	Phase III	Phase IV
Heart rate	Tachycardia	Tachycardia	Tachycardia	Bradycardia
Tidal volume/minute ventilation	Increased	Increased	Normal or decreased	Decreased
$PaCO_2$	Decreased	Decreased	Normal or increased	Increased
Acid-base	Respiratory alkalosis	Respiratory alkalosis	Metabolic (and possibly respiratory) acidosis	Respiratory and metabolic acidosis
PaO_2 on room air	Normal	Normal or slightly decreased (≈60 mm Hg)	Significantly decreased (≈ 40 mm Hg)	Severely decreased (≈ 25 mm Hg)
Shunt	<6%	10%	20%	>30%
Compliance	Normal	Slightly decreased	Moderately decreased	Severely decreased
Pulmonary clinical manifestations	Dyspnea	Dyspnea; fatigue; retractions	Dyspnea; fatigue; retractions; cyanosis	Dyspnea; fatigue (may have had respiratory arrest); cyanosis; rusty sputum
Breath sounds	Clear	Fine crackles	Coarse crackles and/or wheezes	Crackles, rhonchi, and/or wheezes
Chest radiograph	Normal	Patchy infiltrates usually in dependent areas	Diffuse infiltrates	Consolidation
Other signs/ symptoms	Tachycardia	Tachycardia	Tachycardia; dysrhythmias; decreasing sensorium	Bradycardia; dysrhythmias; hypotension; decreasing sensorium

From Dennison, R. D. (2007). *Pass CCRN!* (3rd ed.). St. Louis: Mosby.

2. Maintain airway, oxygenation, and ventilation
   a. Positioning for optimal ventilation
      1) Head of bed to 30 to 45 degrees with overbed table for patient to lean on; prone positioning is frequently used as ARDS progresses
   b. O_2 as indicated
      1) May require high concentrations (up to 100%) with nonrebreathing mask prior to intubation and mechanical ventilation
      2) FIO_2 should be maintained as the lowest level possible to achieve an acceptable oxygenation (e.g., PaO_2 60 mm Hg; SaO_2 90%) to prevent O_2 toxicity; positive pressure (CPAP or PEEP) will increase driving pressure allowing the use of a lower FIO_2 to maintain the acceptable O_2 level
   c. Adequate ventilation
      1) NPPV (e.g., PSV, BiPAP) with face mask may be used prior to need for intubation
      2) Endotracheal intubation: indicated to deliver mechanical ventilation and PEEP when FIO_2 >0.50 is required to maintain acceptable oxygenation or as patient fatigues
      3) Mechanical ventilation to maintain adequate ventilation and oxygenation; tidal volume at 4 to 8 ml/kg of ideal body weight (IBW)
   d. Reduction of intra-alveolar fluid
      1) Avoidance of overhydration as may occur in fluid resuscitation of trauma patients
      2) Diuretics as prescribed
      3) CPAP or PEEP to increase intra-alveolar pressure and aid in prevention of further fluid sequestration into the alveoli
3. Maintain adequate circulation and perfusion
   a. IV access for fluid and medication administration
   b. Cautious IV fluid (usually 0.9% saline) administration because fluid overload contributes to excess intra-alveolar fluid
4. Optimize O_2 delivery and decrease O_2 consumption
   a. Improvement of O_2 delivery to the tissues (DO_2)
      1) SaO_2: O_2, PEEP as required
      2) Cardiac output: fluid administration, inotropic agents, intra-aortic balloon pump, vasoactive agents, etc. as required
      3) Hgb: packed RBCs as required
   b. Treatment of fever (controversial because pyrogens helpful in mobilizing the immune system)
      1) Antipyretics (e.g., acetaminophen [Tylenol])
      2) Cooling blankets may be used but shivering should be avoided due to effect on O_2 consumption
5. Treat the cause of ARDS; for example:
   a. Antimicrobials for infection
   b. Treatment of pulmonary embolism
   c. Treatment of shock states

6. Monitor for/prevent complications
   a. Acute respiratory failure
   b. Secondary infections: nosocomial pneumonia
   c. Sepsis
   d. Shock
   e. Multiple organ dysfunction syndrome (MODS)
   f. Dysrhythmias
   g. Gastrointestinal hemorrhage
   h. Heart failure
   i. Renal failure
   j. Residual lung damage; pulmonary fibrosis

Evaluation
1. Patent airway, adequate oxygenation (i.e., normal PaO_2, SpO_2, SaO_2) and ventilation (i.e., normal $PaCO_2$)
2. Absence of clinical indications of respiratory distress
3. Absence of clinical indicators of hypoperfusion
4. Absence of clinical indications of infection/sepsis
5. Alert and oriented with no neurologic deficit
6. Control of pain, discomfort, or dyspnea

Typical disposition: admission to the critical care unit
Asthma
Definition
1. Asthma: a recurrent, reversible airway disease characterized by episodic wheezing, chronicity, hyperresponsiveness of airways to a variety of stimuli, and largely reversible obstruction of airways
   a. Mild intermittent
      1) Symptoms 1 to 2 days per week
      2) Brief exacerbations
      3) Nocturnal symptoms less than three times per month
      4) FEV_1 or PEFR at least 80%
      5) PEFR or FEV_1 variability <20%
   b) Mild persistent
      1) Symptoms more than twice per week but less than once per day
      2) Exacerbations may affect activity and sleep
      3) Nocturnal symptoms two to four times per month
      4) FEV_1 or PEFR at least 80%
      5) PEFR or FEV_1 variability 20% to 30%
   c) Moderate persistent
      1) Symptoms daily
      2) Exacerbations may affect activity and sleep
      3) Nocturnal symptoms more than five times a month
      4) Daily use of inhaled short-acting β_2-agonist
      5) FEV_1 or PEFR 60% to 80% predicted
      6) PEFR or FEV_1 variability >30%
   d) Severe persistent
      1) Symptoms daily
      2) Frequent exacerbations
      3) Frequent nocturnal symptoms
      4) Limitation of physical activities
      5) FEV_1 or PEFR <60% predicted
      6) PEFR or FEV_1 variability >30%

2. Status asthmaticus: exacerbation of acute asthma characterized by severe airflow obstruction that is not relieved after 24 hours of maximal doses of traditional therapy

Predisposing factors

1. Extrinsic: when a specific allergy can be related to the attack
   a. Dust and dust mites
   b. Animal dander, feathers
   c. Pollen
   d. Mold
   e. Preservatives (e.g., bisulfites)
   f. Food such as nuts, legumes (e.g., peanuts), chocolate, eggs, shellfish, food additives
2. Intrinsic: when the attack is seemingly unrelated to a specific allergen
   a. Infection, such as bacterial or viral pneumonia, bronchitis, or sinusitis
   b. Stress
   c. Exercise
   d. Gastroesophageal reflux disease (GERD)
   e. Aspiration
   f. Fear, anger, crying, laughing
   g. Menstrual cycle
   h. Smoke
   i. Propellants
   j. Air pollution
   k. Changes in inspired air such as cold or hot air, very high or very low humidity
   l. Alcohol
      1) Medications such as aspirin, nonsteroidal anti-inflammatory drugs (NSAIDs), β-blockers

Pathophysiology

1. Triggers
   a. Extrinsic triggers cause IgE to be released; IgE stimulates the mast cells in the pulmonary submucosa to release histamine and slow-reacting substance of anaphylaxis (SRS-A)
      1) Histamine attaches to the receptor sites in the large bronchi causing swelling and inflammation
      2) SRS-A, composed of three types of leukotrienes, causes inflammation and edema of the smooth muscle of the smaller bronchi and release of prostaglandins, which enhance the effects of histamine
      3) Inflammation causes epithelial damage and airway smooth muscle hyperresponsiveness
   b. Intrinsic triggers affect the balance between sympathetic and parasympathetic branches of the autonomic nervous system
2. Airway narrowing, caused by inflammation and bronchoconstriction, is greatest during expiration
   a. Work of breathing is increased and fatigue occurs impairing ventilation
   b. Air trapping causes hyperinflation of alveoli
3. Mucus further narrows the airway lumen
   a. Increased amount of thick, tenacious mucus is caused by increased number of goblet cells, excessive secretion of mucus caused by histamine, dehydration related to increased insensible water loss via respiratory tract during tachypnea
   b. Excessive mucus in smaller airways causes $\dot{V}/\dot{Q}$ mismatching and shunt
4. Acute respiratory failure with hypoxemia and respiratory acidosis eventually occurs if the attack is not promptly reversed

Clinical presentation

1. Subjective
   a. History of a slow, progressive worsening of airflow obstruction over the course of several days or weeks; history may include recent upper respiratory tract infection (URI) or exposure to allergen or environmental factors
   b. Dyspnea
   c. Chest tightness
   d. Fatigue
2. Objective
   a. Tachycardia
   b. Tachypnea
   c. Inability to speak in full sentences due to dyspnea
   d. Cough with thick tenacious sputum production
   e. Use of accessory muscles and intercostal retractions
   f. Prolonged expiratory phase (I: E ratio >1:3)
   g. Diaphoresis
   h. PEFR <80% of patient's personal or predicted best
   i. Clinical indications of dehydration: poor skin turgor, dry mucous membranes, increased specific gravity of urine
   j. Breath sound changes: rhonchi, wheezing
   k. Indications of potential imminent respiratory arrest
      1) Change in consciousness: drowsiness or confusion
      2) Paradoxical thoracoabdominal movement
      3) Absence of rhonchi and wheezes may occur in critical stages; indication of absence of airflow
      4) Bradycardia
      5) Pulsus paradoxus >15 mm Hg
3. Diagnostic
   a. WBCs increased if respiratory infection
   b. HCT increased due to dehydration
   c. Electrolytes: potassium and/or magnesium may be low during an acute attack
   d. ABGs (Table 5-15)
   e. Sputum culture: positive if infection present
   f. Chest radiograph
      1) Normal or hyperinflated lungs with flattened diaphragms
      2) Helpful to rule out other causes of respiratory distress

TABLE 5-15 Asthma: ABG Analysis				
Stage	**Pao$_2$**	**Paco$_2$**	**pH**	**Acid-Base Imbalance**
I	Normal	Decreased	Increased	Respiratory alkalosis
II	Decreased	Decreased	Increased	Respiratory alkalosis
				Mild to moderate hypoxemia
III	Very low	Normal	Normal	Significant hypoxemia
IV	Extremely low	Elevated	Decreased	Respiratory acidosis
				Critical hypoxemia

From Dennison, R. D. (2007). *Pass CCRN!* (3 ed.). St. Louis: Mosby.

Collaborative management

1. Continue assessment
   a. ABCDs
   b. Vital signs: blood pressure, pulse, respiratory rate, and temperature
   c. O$_2$ saturation
   d. Respiratory effort and excursion
   e. PEFR after each treatment
   f. Cardiac rate and rhythm
   g. Pain, discomfort, or dyspnea level
   h. Accurate intake and output
   i. Level of consciousness
   j. Close monitoring for progression of symptoms
2. Assess predisposing factors; eliminate and/or treat cause
   a. Antibiotics to promptly treat infection
   b. Avoidance of exposure to pulmonary irritants and pollutants
   c. Avoidance of drugs or foods that may trigger an attack
3. Establish and maintain airway, oxygenation, and ventilation
   a. Elevation of head of bed to 30 to 45 degrees; over-bed table may be helpful for patient to lean on
   b. O$_2$ by nasal cannula at 2 to 6 L/min to maintain Spo$_2$ of 95% unless contraindicated; for patients with COPD, use pulse oximetry to guide O$_2$ administration to Spo$_2$ of 90%
   c. Bronchial hygiene and chest physiotherapy as indicated
      1) Inspiratory maneuvers: deep breathing; incentive spirometry
      2) Encouragement of the patient to cough if rhonchi are audible; suctioning if the patient is unable to clear airways
      3) Postural drainage, percussion, vibration may be necessary
   d. Noninvasive ventilatory methods (CPAP, BiPAP) by mask may be used in an attempt to avert intubation and mechanical ventilation
   e. Intubation and mechanical ventilation may be necessary as patient fatigues, Paco$_2$ increases, and acidosis develops
      1) Use of RSI for intubation
      2) Assist-control mode is used to allow respiratory muscle rest and recovery

f. Pharmacologic therapies
   1) Bronchodilators to relax bronchial smooth muscle
      a) Leukotriene inhibitors/leukotriene receptor antagonists (e.g., zafirlukast [Accolate], zileuton [Zyflo], montelukast sodium [Singulair]) may have been used as a preventative agent; they are not helpful for treatment of acute bronchospasm
      b) β$_2$-Stimulants
         (i) Action: stimulate β$_2$-receptors to cause smooth muscle relaxation, bronchodilation, improved airflow
         (ii) Agents
            (a) Long-acting (e.g., salmeterol [Serevent]) by metered-dose inhaler will likely have usually been used long-term by the patient with a diagnosis of asthma
            (b) Short-acting β$_2$-agonists (e.g., metaproterenol [Alupent, Metaprel], albuterol [Proventil, Ventolin], pirbuterol [Maxair], bitolterol [Tornalate], terbutaline [Brethaire], epinephrine)
         (iii) Administration
            (a) Metered-dose inhaler is usually used and may be as effective as nebulizers when used with a spacing device
            (b) Nebulizer is frequently used if the PEFR is <50% of the patient's personal best; the β-agonist is administer by nebulizer every 20 minutes or continuously for 1 hour
         (iv) Monitor closely for adverse effects such as significant tachycardia, dysrhythmias, hypertension, headache, tremor, anxiety, hypokalemia
      c) Anticholinergics (e.g., ipratropium bromide [Atrovent]) may be used in severe attacks to augment the effects of β$_2$-agonists
         (i) Action: block parasympathetic stimulation (making sympathetic stimulation dominant) to cause smooth muscle

relaxation; may be especially helpful for asthma stimulated by an intrinsic trigger

(ii) Administered as a metered-dose inhaler or nebulizer; may be administered as a combination agent with β-agonist (e.g., ipratropium bromide and albuterol sulfate [Combivent])

d) Xanthines (e.g., theophylline, aminophylline) may be given intravenously for refractory attack

  (i) Actions

 (a) Smooth muscle relaxation causing bronchodilation though less effective than nebulized β-agonists; also more adverse effects than β-agonists

 (b) Immune-modulating effects including inhibition of T-lymphocytes and other inflammatory cells and inhibition of cytokine release

  (ii) Administration orally for long-term therapy but usually by IV infusion in acute asthma

  (iii) Monitor closely for indications of theophylline toxicity

 (a) Gastrointestinal: anorexia; nausea, vomiting

 (b) Cardiac: dysrhythmias

 (c) Neurologic: restlessness; seizures

e) Magnesium: used in acutely ill asthmatic patients with severe exacerbation

  (i) Actions: smooth muscle relaxation

  (ii) Administered as intravenous infusion: usual dose is 1 to 2 g over 20 minutes

  (iii) Contraindicated in hypotension or renal failure

  (iv) Monitor blood pressure during infusion; note and report significant hypotension or loss of deep tendon reflexes

2) Corticosteroids to reduce inflammation

a) Actions

  (i) Decrease mucosal swelling and release of histamine by the mast cells

  (ii) Potentiates bronchodilators

b) Administration

  (i) Patient has usually administered steroids (e.g., beclomethasone [Vanceril, Beclovent], flunisolide [AeroBid], triamcinolone [Azmacort], fluticasone [Flovent]) via metered-dose inhaler prior to hospitalization

  (ii) Steroids may be initially administered intravenously (e.g., methylprednisolone [Solu-Medrol]) or orally (prednisone [Deltasone] and prednisolone [Pediapred]) in status asthmaticus

(iii) Expectorants (e.g., guaifenesin [Robitussin], potassium iodide [SSKI]) may be used but hydration is most important; water is the best expectorant

(iv) Mucolytics (e.g., acetylcysteine [Mucomyst]) are generally contraindicated because of the adverse effect of bronchospasm

(v) Sedatives: generally avoided unless patient is very agitated

(vi) Antitussives: avoid use of antitussives

(vii) Heliox as prescribed (controversial in acute asthma)

 (a) Helium is a light gas that decreases work of breathing when it replaces nitrogen in the inspired air; O_2 percentage is prescribed and helium replaces nitrogen to make up the remainder (e.g., 80% helium/20% O_2, 70% helium/30% O_2, 60% helium/40% O_2)

 (b) Actions: decreases airway resistance and work of breathing; decreases hypercapnia and need for intubation and mechanical ventilation

 (c) Administration by face mask or mechanical ventilator

g. Maintain bronchial hygiene

1) Abdominal (i.e., deep) breathing

2) Effective coughing

3) Suctioning only if coughing is ineffective

4) Maintain adequate circulation

a) IV access for fluid and medication administration

b) Rehydration: significant insensible fluid loss occurs with tachypnea

  (i) Oral fluids: noncaffeinated

  (ii) IV fluids: usually 0.9% saline

5) Monitor for/prevent complications

a) Acute respiratory failure

b) Barotrauma (e.g., pneumothorax)

c) Pneumonia

d) Dysrhythmias

e) Hypovolemia

Evaluation

1. Patent airway, adequate oxygenation (i.e., normal Pao_2, Spo_2, Sao_2) and ventilation (i.e., normal $Paco_2$)
2. Absence of clinical indications of respiratory distress
3. Absence of clinical indicators of hypoperfusion
4. Absence of clinical indications of infection/sepsis
5. Alert and oriented with no neurologic deficit
6. Control of pain, discomfort, or dyspnea

Typical disposition

1. If evaluation criteria met: discharge with instructions
   a. Instruction and counseling regarding lifestyle modification and need for pharmacologic therapy

b. Recognition and avoidance of triggers; allergy testing and desensitization may be needed

c. Increased fluid intake

d. Follow-up appointment with the primary care provider

e. Return to ED for increased shortness of breath, worsening PEFR (in patients who have a spirometer), fever, worse coughingv

2. If evaluation criteria not met: admission to progressive care unit or critical care unit

Acute Bronchitis
Definition: acute: inflammation of the trachea, bronchi, and bronchioles, usually viral in nature (Carolan & Callahan, 2006)
Predisposing factors
1. Asthma
2. Environmental allergens
3. Exposure to cigarette smoking
4. Inhalation of toxic substances: chemical fumes, sulfur dioxide, nitrogen dioxide, ammonia
5. Immunosuppressed
6. Viral infection
   a. Adenovirus
   b. Influenza
   c. Parainfluenza
   d. Respiratory syncytial virus (RSV)
   e. Rhinovirus
   f. Coxsackievirus
   g. Herpes simplex virus

Pathophysiology
1. Transient inflammatory changes occur, causing an inflammatory response
2. Bronchial edema and mucus formation occur, leading to symptoms of airway obstruction

Clinical presentation
1. Subjective
   a. History of URI or exposure to smoke or other irritant
   b. Dyspnea
2. Objective
   a. Low-grade fever
   b. Dry cough initially, then turned productive
   c. Breath sound changes
      1) Wheezes especially with forced expiration
      2) Rhonchi that clear with coughing
   d. Lymphadenopathy
   e. Prolonged expiratory phase
   f. Jugular venous distention (JVD) secondary to cor pulmonale with chronic bronchitis
3. Diagnostic
   a. CBC with differential: increased WBCs if infection
   b. Peak flow spirometry decreased with airway obstruction
   c. Chest radiograph: to rule out other causes

Collaborative management
1. Continue assessment
   a. ABCDs

b. Vital signs: blood pressure, pulse, respiratory rate, and temperature

c. O_2 saturation

d. Respiratory effort and excursion

e. Cardiac rate and rhythm

f. Pain, discomfort, or dyspnea level

g. Accurate intake and output

h. Level of consciousness

i. Close monitoring for progression of symptoms

2. Maintain airway, oxygenation, and ventilation
   a. Elevation of head of bed to 30 to 45 degrees; overbed table may be helpful for patient to lean on
   b. O_2 by nasal cannula at 2 to 6 L/min to maintain Spo_2 of 95% unless contraindicated; for patients with COPD, use pulse oximetry to guide O_2 administration to Spo_2 of 90%
   c. Pharmacologic therapies
      1) Corticosteroids: to reduce inflammation as prescribed
      2) Bronchodilators: may help patients with evidence of airflow obstruction
      3) Guaifenesin (Mucinex): may be helpful in reducing ineffective cough in adults
      4) Antihistamines and dextromethorphan (Delsym): not effective in children and may cause adverse effects
   d. Maintain bronchial hygiene
      1) Abdominal (i.e., deep) breathing
      2) Effective coughing
      3) Suctioning only if coughing is ineffective
      4) Chest physical therapy may be prescribed
3. Maintain adequate circulation and perfusion
   a. IV access for fluid and medication administration
   b. Hydration
      1) Oral fluids: noncaffeinated
      2) IV fluids: usually 0.9% saline
4. Treat infection (if present) and prevent sepsis
   a. Antimicrobials as indicated: empirically or specific to cultured microorganism
   b. Antivirals if indicated; influenza vaccination
   c. Bronchial hygiene techniques
   d. Antipyretics and cooling methods to reduce fever
5. Control pain, discomfort, and anxiety
   a. NSAIDs and/or narcotic analgesics in doses that will allow patient to deep breathe and cough may be indicated
   b. Anxiolytics may be indicated
6. Monitor for/prevent complications
   a. Acute respiratory failure
   b. Pneumonia

Evaluation
1. Patent airway, adequate oxygenation (i.e., normal Pao_2, Spo_2, Sao_2) and ventilation (i.e., normal $Paco_2$)
2. Absence of clinical indications of respiratory distress
3. Absence of clinical indications of infection/sepsis

4. Absence of clinical indicators of hypoperfusion
5. Alert and oriented with no neurologic deficit
6. Control of pain, discomfort, or dyspnea

Typical disposition

1. If evaluation criteria met: discharge with instructions
   a. Rest
   b. Use of antibiotics, bronchodilators, antipyretics
   c. Adequate hydration
   d. Avoidance of smoking
   e. Return for increased shortness of breath, high temperature, or change in sputum
   f. Follow up with primary care provider or specialist as directed
2. If evaluation criteria not met: admission to progressive care unit or critical care unit

Aspiration of a Foreign Body
Definition: aspiration of a foreign body into the airway
Predisposing factors

1. Age
   a. Foreign body aspiration occurs more commonly in children younger than 9 years and in older adults
   b. Laryngeal foreign body is common in children younger than 6 years
2. Developmental disability
3. Lapses in supervision
4. Eating too quickly

Pathophysiology

1. Foreign objects can obstruct any part of the airway, disrupting ventilation and oxygenation
   a. Mainstem bronchi or distal trachea near the carina and esophagus are common sites
2. Foreign objects can also become lodged in the esophagus

Clinical presentation

1. Subjective
   a. May or may not report history of aspiration
   b. Dyspnea
   c. Sense of impending doom
2. Objective
   a. Sudden onset of choking and severe coughing
   b. Clinical indications of respiratory distress (see Box 5-1)
   c. Complete airway obstruction: severe respiratory distress, inability to speak or cough, clutching at neck
   d. Partial airway obstruction: sudden onset of coughing, difficulty in breathing, wheezing, or stridor
3. Diagnostic
   a. Chest radiograph: inspiratory and expiratory posteroanterior (PA) and lateral
   b. Neck: AP and lateral imaging of the soft tissues
   c. Indirect laryngoscopy: to visualize and possibly retrieve cause of obstruction

Collaborative management

1. Continue assessment
   a. ABCDs
   b. Vital signs: blood pressure, pulse, respiratory rate, and temperature
   c. O_2 saturation
   d. Respiratory effort and excursion
   e. Cardiac rate and rhythm
   f. Pain, discomfort, or dyspnea level
   g. Level of consciousness
   h. Accurate intake and output
   i. Close monitoring for progression of symptoms
2. Establish and maintain airway, oxygenation, and ventilation
   a. Suction and intubation equipment at bedside
   b. O_2 by nasal cannula at 2 to 6 L/min to maintain SpO_2 of 95% unless contraindicated; for patients with COPD, use pulse oximetry to guide O_2 administration to SpO_2 of 90%
   c. Removal of foreign body
      1) If conscious: elevation of head of bed to 30 to 45 degrees; coughing should be encouraged if the patient can still move air
      2) If unconscious and breathing: abdominal thrusts
      3) If unconscious and not breathing: assist with direct laryngoscopy, removal, and possible intubation
      4) If unable to remove in ED or if lodged in trachea or bronchus, prepare patient for surgery
3. Maintain adequate circulation and perfusion
   a. IV access for fluid and medication administration
   b. Hydration
      1) Oral fluids: noncaffeinated
      2) IV fluids: usually 0.9% saline
4. Control pain, discomfort, and anxiety
   a. NSAIDs and/or narcotic analgesics in doses that will allow patient to deep breathe and cough may be indicated
   b. Anxiolytics may be indicated
5. Monitor for/prevent complications
   a. Cardiopulmonary arrest
   b. Hemoptysis
   c. Bronchial stricture
   d. Pneumonia

Evaluation

1. Patent airway, adequate oxygenation (i.e., normal PaO_2, SpO_2, SaO_2) and ventilation (i.e., normal $PaCO_2$)
2. Absence of clinical indications of respiratory distress
3. Absence of clinical indications of infection/sepsis
4. Absence of clinical indicators of hypoperfusion
5. Alert and oriented with no neurologic deficit
6. Control of pain, discomfort, or dyspnea

Typical disposition

1. If evaluation criteria met: discharge with instructions

a. Rest
b. Pediatric patients: education on prevention for parents (e.g., age-appropriate toys, list of most frequent foreign bodies)
c. Adults: education on prevention (e.g., cut food into small pieces, chew food thoroughly)
2. If evaluation criteria not met: admission to progressive care unit or critical care unit
a. If unable to remove foreign body in the ED, surgery to remove foreign body may be required

Aspiration
Definition
1. Aspiration lung disorder: lung injury related to the inhalation of gastric contents, oropharyngeal secretions, food, or other foreign material into the tracheobronchial tree
2. Aspiration pneumonitis: chemical injury of the lung caused by aspiration of gastric contents, oropharyngeal secretions, or exogenous liquids
3. Aspiration pneumonia: lung infection caused by aspiration of material colonized with bacteria

Predisposing factors
1. Altered consciousness and/or gag reflex
a. Sedation
b. Anesthesia especially emergency surgery when the patient has eaten recently
c. CNS disorders (e.g., cerebral hemorrhage, seizures, neuromuscular diseases)
2. Drug or alcohol intoxication
3. Altered anatomy
a. ET tube keeps the epiglottis splinted open
b. Nasogastric or orogastric tube can cause incompetence of the gastroesophageal sphincter
c. Gastrointestinal tamponade (e.g., Sengstaken-Blakemore tube)
d. Facial, neck, or oral trauma
4 Esophageal abnormalities (e.g., tracheoesophageal fistula)
5. Gastroesophageal reflux
6. Decreased gastrointestinal motility (e.g., diabetic gastroparesis)
7. Gastrointestinal hemorrhage
8. Vomiting
9. Intestinal obstruction (e.g., ileus, tumor, volvulus)
10. Drugs that decrease gastroesophageal sphincter tone: anticholinergics (e.g., atropine), adrenergics (e.g., dopamine), nitrates, caffeine, calcium channel blockers (e.g., nifedipine [Procardia]), estrogen

Pathophysiology
1. Oropharyngeal secretions are most commonly aspirated
2. Aspiration of large particles can obstruct major airways, cause asphyxia, and potentially death
3. Aspiration of smaller particles causes segmental atelectasis and subacute inflammatory pulmonary reaction with extensive hemorrhage

a. Clear acidic liquid causes chemical burn and destruction of the type II pneumocytes; frequently referred to as aspiration pneumonitis
b. Clear nonacidic liquid causes reflex airway closure, pulmonary edema, surfactant changes; contaminated material may cause massive infection
c. Aspiration of material colonized with bacteria potentially causes severe lung infections (e.g., pneumonia, lung abscess)
4. Aspiration into the right lung is more common than into the left lung due to the straighter angle of the right mainstem bronchus

Clinical presentation
1. Subjective
a. May have history of witnessed vomiting, aspiration
b. Dyspnea
c. Chest pain: pleuritic in nature
d. Anxiety
2. Objective
a. Tachycardia
b. Tachypnea
c. Fever
d. Clinical indications of respiratory distress (see Box 5-1)
e. Productive cough or suctioned material
1) Foul-smelling sputum
2) Food, stomach contents may be seen in secretions suctioned from lungs
a) Note: aspirated tube feedings will test positive for glucose
3) Pink, frothy sputum may occur with acidic aspiration
f. Breath sound changes
1) Stridor if obstruction of the upper airway occurs
2) Diminished breath sounds
3) Adventitious sounds: crackles; rhonchi; wheezing
g. Clinical indications of hypoxemia/hypoxia (see Box 5-2)
3. Diagnostic
a. CBC: increased WBCs
b. ABGs
1) Pao_2 and Sao_2: decreased
2) $Paco_2$ may be normal, decreased, or increased depending on ventilation pattern (i.e., low with hyperventilation)
c. Tracheal aspirate: visualization or analysis to determine if aspiration has occurred
d. Sputum: presence of polymorphonuclear leukocytes
e. Chest radiograph: may have bilateral patchy infiltrates, atelectasis, pulmonary edema

Collaborative management
1. Continue assessment
a. ABCDs
b. Vital signs: blood pressure, pulse, respiratory rate, and temperature

c. O_2 saturation

d. Respiratory effort and excursion

e. Cardiac rate and rhythm

f. Pain, discomfort, or dyspnea level

g. Level of consciousness

h. Accurate intake and output

i. Close monitoring for progression of symptoms

2. Establish and maintain airway, oxygenation, and ventilation

a. Positioning of the stretcher in a slight Trendelenburg position with the patient in a right lateral decubitus position

b. Suctioning of the airway immediately providing adequate oxygenation during suctioning

1) Endotracheal intubation may be necessary

2) Bronchoscopy for removal of large particles may be necessary

c. O_2 by nasal cannula at 2 to 6 L/min to maintain Spo_2 of 95% unless contraindicated; for patients with COPD, use pulse oximetry to guide O_2 administration to Spo_2 of 90%

1) CPAP or PEEP may be necessary to maintain adequate oxygenation

d. Intubation and mechanical ventilation may be necessary as patient fatigues, $Paco_2$ increases, and acidosis develops

e. Bronchodilators as prescribed

f. Corticosteroids may be prescribed but controversial

g. Bronchial hygiene techniques

3. Maintain adequate circulation

a. IV access for fluid and medication administration

b. Hydration

1) Oral fluids: noncaffeinated

2) IV fluids: usually 0.9% saline

4. Control pain, discomfort, and anxiety

a. NSAIDs and/or narcotic analgesics in doses that will allow patient to deep breathe and cough may be indicated

b. Anxiolytics may be indicated

5. Treat infection (if present) and prevent sepsis

a. Antimicrobials as indicated: empirically or specific to cultured microorganism

b. Bronchial hygiene techniques

c. Antipyretics and cooling methods to reduce fever

6. Prevent aspiration of gastric contents

a. Appropriate positioning to reduce risk of aspiration and reduce volume of aspiration should vomiting occur; place unconscious patient in side-lying position

b. ET intubation may be necessary to protect the airway

7. Monitor for/prevent complications

a. Acute respiratory failure

b. ARDS

c. Pneumonia

d. Lung abscess

Evaluation

1. Patent airway, adequate oxygenation (i.e., normal Pao_2, Spo_2, Sao_2) and ventilation (i.e., normal $Paco_2$)

2. Absence of clinical indications of respiratory distress

3. Absence of clinical indicators of hypoperfusion

4. Absence of clinical indications of infection/sepsis

5. Alert and oriented with no neurologic deficit

6. Control of pain, discomfort, or dyspnea

Typical disposition: admission; critical care unit admission may be required
Bronchiolitis/respiratory syncytial virus
Description

1. Bronchiolitis is an infection of the lower respiratory tract that leads to an inflammatory response and obstruction of the lower airways

2 RSV is a contagious respiratory virus that infects the lungs and breathing passages

a. RSV is the most common cause of bronchiolitis in infants 12 months and younger

b. The Centers for Disease Control and Prevention (CDC) estimates that most children will be infected with RSV by age 2 years

c. Usually seen during the fall, winter, and early spring

d. Infants usually contagious 3 to 8 days but can be contagious up to 4 weeks (CDC, 2008)

e. Symptoms in adults <5 days and similar to those of URI

Precipitating factors

1. Contact with multiple children (e.g., day care, school, health care workers)

2. Immunosuppression

3. Males more likely to develop severe infections

4. Exposure to tobacco smoke

5. Children under 2 are primarily affected, particularly the following

a. Premature or chronically ill children

b. Infants 2 to 6 months of age

c. Bottle-fed infant (breast-fed babies receive immune benefits from their mother)

d. Child with underlying heart-lung condition

Pathophysiology

1. Bronchiolitis

a. Virus attaches itself to epithelial cells in the nasopharynx or through the eyes

b. The virus is attracted to a protein in the epithelial cells of the respiratory tract

c. Immune response leads to increased secretions

1) Increased mucus can lead to mucus plugging

2) Tissue necrosis and sloughing of dead cells increase the mucus production

3) Copious secretions obstruct the bronchioles and even the bronchi

4) Eventually distal lung tissue collapses due to the inflammatory changes

d. The virus spreads to the lower respiratory tract by fusing with uninfected cells

e. Increased airway resistance, atelectasis, $\dot{V}/\dot{Q}$ mismatching, and hypoxemia

1. RSV
   a. Spread via droplets, which become airborne with sneezing and coughing and can hang around briefly in the air
      1) RSV can survive on hard surfaces for several hours; shorter life span on soft surfaces (e.g., tissue, hands)
   b. Droplets come in contact when the host inhales or makes contact via the nose, mouth, or eyes of host
   c. Transmission can also occur by direct or indirect contact with nasal or oral secretions from an infected individual
   d. Limited to the upper respiratory tract with symptoms similar to the common cold
   e. In infants, if it moves to the lower respiratory tract, they can develop bronchiolitis or pneumonia

Clinical presentation

1. Subjective
   a. History of URI symptoms, prematurity, respiratory or cardiac problem
   b. Parent reports fussy child or infant
   c. Dyspnea
   d. Decreased appetite or poor feeding
2. Objective
   a. Tachypnea, tachycardia
   b. Increased work of breathing: nasal flaring, retractions, grunting
   c. Infant and young child may be lethargic
   d. Breath sound changes: wheezes, crackles
   e. Cough, may be productive
   f. Fever
   g. Clinical indications of dehydration; infants with depressed fontanels
3. Specific to RSV: runny nose, sneezing, decreased appetite and activity, yellow-green conjunctival/nasal drainage
4. Diagnostic
   a. CBC: WBCs usually normal
   b. Chest radiograph
      1) Hyperinflation
      2) Atelectasis, patchy infiltrates
      3) Used to rule out other causes
   c. Nasal swab or nasal washing: positive for RSV
   d. Viral cultures: positive

Collaborative management

1. Continue assessment
   a. ABCDs
   b. Vital signs: blood pressure, pulse, respiratory rate, and temperature
   c. O_2 saturation
   d. Respiratory effort and excursion
   e. Cardiac rate and rhythm
   f. Pain, discomfort, or dyspnea level
   g. Level of consciousness
   h. Accurate intake and output
   i. Close monitoring for progression of symptoms
2. Establish and maintain airway, oxygenation, and ventilation
   a. Head of bed to 30 to 45 degrees
   b. Suction as required
   c. O_2 by nasal cannula at 2 to 6 L/min to maintain SpO_2 of 95% unless contraindicated; for patients with COPD, use pulse oximetry to guide O_2 administration to SpO_2 of 90%
      1) Blow-by O_2 may be used for infants
   d. Anticholinergics (e.g., ipratropium bromide [Atrovent]): relax smooth muscle of the bronchi (large airways)
   e. Corticosteroids: little use unless history of asthma
   f. Guaifenesin (Mucinex) may be helpful in reducing ineffective cough in adults
   g. Antihistamines and dextromethorphan (Delsym) not effective in children and may cause adverse effects
3. Maintain adequate circulation
   a. IV access for fluid and medication administration may be indicated
   b. Hydration
      1) Oral fluids: noncaffeinated
      2) IV fluids may be required: usually 0.9% saline
4. Control pain, discomfort, and anxiety
   a. NSAIDs and/or narcotic analgesics in doses that will allow patient to deep breathe and cough may be indicated
   b. Anxiolytics may be indicated
5. Treat infection and prevent sepsis
   a. Antimicrobials as indicated: empirically or specific to cultured microorganism
   b. Antivirals (e.g., ribavirin [Virazole]) if viral
      1) Inhibit viral replication
      2) Given by aerosolization and small-particle aerosol generator
   c. Bronchial hygiene techniques
   d. Antipyretics and cooling methods to reduce fever
6. Monitor for/prevent complications
   a. Acute respiratory failure
   b. Acute respiratory distress syndrome
   c. Pneumonia
   d. Lung abscess

Evaluation

1. Patent airway, adequate oxygenation (i.e., normal PaO_2, SpO_2, SaO_2) and ventilation (i.e., normal $PaCO_2$)
2. Absence of clinical indications of respiratory distress, especially episodes of apnea
3. Absence of clinical indicators of hypoperfusion
4. Absence of clinical indications of infection/sepsis
5. Alert and oriented with no neurologic deficit
6. Control of pain, discomfort, or dyspnea

Typical disposition

1. If evaluation criteria met: discharge with instructions
   a. Rest and increase fluid intake
   b. Infants: small frequent feedings

c. Medications as prescribed (may include nebulizer)
d. Follow up with primary care provider within 24 hours
e. Return to the ED for worsening respiratory status
2. If evaluation criteria not met or patient is immuno-suppressed: admission to progressive care unit or critical care unit

Chronic Obstructive Pulmonary Disease
Definition
1. Chronic bronchitis: daily productive cough >3 months per year for 2 years
2. Emphysema: permanent abnormal enlargement of air spaces distal to terminal bronchioles
3. Patients frequently have both and may also have asthma

Pathophysiology
1. Inhalation of a noxious product (e.g., cigarette smoke) produces an inflammatory response
2. Macrophages and leukocytes increase in number and begin releasing inflammatory mediators
3. These mediators damage lung tissue, leading to infiltration by neutrophils, which release their own inflammatory mediators
4. Results in destruction of elastic tissue of alveolar membranes, distention of air spaces, "air trapping" in emphysema
5. Hypertrophy of goblet cells causes increased production of thick mucus, leading to chronic cough in chronic bronchitis
6. Small airways eventually remodel from the continuous cycle of injury and healing, which leads to fibrosis
7. Eventually lung tissue is damaged, causing a loss of elastic attachments that connect the airways; results in small airway collapse
8. Air enters the airways easily but becomes trapped, leading to lung hyperinflation and a change in the shape of the chest to barrel-shaped

Predisposing factors
1. Found almost exclusively in smokers
2. Genetic type of emphysema (i.e., α_1-antitrypsin deficiency)
3. Chronic inhalation of respiratory irritants: chemicals, dust, fumes, air pollution
4. Advancing age
   a. Peak onset 40 to 44 years for chronic bronchitis
   b. Peak onset 50 to 75 years for emphysema

Clinical presentation
1. Clinical presentation of chronic bronchitis and emphysema is summarized in Table 5-16
2. Subjective
   a. Dyspnea, orthopnea
   b. Chest tightness
   c. Fatigue
3. Objective
   a. Cyanosis
   b. Cough; may be productive
   c. Pursed lip breathing
   d. Breath sound changes
      1) Decreased intensity in emphysema
      2) Rhonchi and wheezes in chronic bronchitis
   e. Clinical indications of respiratory distress (see Box 5-1)
   f. Clinical indications of hypoxemia/hypoxia (see Box 5-2)
   g. Clinical indications of hypercapnia (see Box 5-3)
4. Diagnostic
   a. CBC
      1) Polycythemia: from chronic hypoxemia; more likely in chronic bronchitis
      2) Eosinophilia: especially with asthma
      3) WBCs: may be increased
   b. Brain natriuretic peptide (BNP): may be helpful in differentiating between COPD and heart failure
   c. ABGs: hypoxemia and hypercapnia
   d. Chest radiograph
      1) Hyperinflation with increased retrosternal air spaces
      2) Flattened diaphragm
      3) Heart shadow appears long and narrow
   e. Sputum for Gram stain (stain that determines whether gram positive or gram negative) and culture and sensitivity tests
      1) Mucoid sputum seen with stable chronic bronchitis
      2) Purulent sputum with exacerbation

Collaborative management
1. Continue assessment
   a. ABCDs
   b. Vital signs: blood pressure, pulse, respiratory rate, and temperature
   c. O_2 saturation
   d. Respiratory effort and excursion
   e. Cardiac rate and rhythm
   f. Pain, discomfort, or dyspnea level
   g. Level of consciousness
   h. Accurate intake and output
   i. Close monitoring for progression of symptoms
2. Establish and maintain airway, oxygenation, and ventilation
   a. Elevation of head of bed to 30 to 45 degrees; overbed table may be helpful for patient to lean on
   b. Suction as needed
   c. Intubation may be required
   d. Provide O_2 to keep Sao_2 (or Spo_2) around 90% to 92%
      1) Because patients with COPD are frequently hypercapnic, their primary stimulus to breathe is stimulation of secondary chemoreceptors sensitive to low blood O_2 levels; therefore, the blood

TABLE 5-16   Summary of the Clinical Presentations of Chronic Bronchitis and Emphysema

	Chronic Bronchitis Predominates	Emphysema Predominates
Predominant pathophysiology	Chronic inflammation and hypertrophy of goblet cells	Destruction of alveolar walls, enlarged alveoli with resultant decrease in surface area for transfer of gases
Predominant sign(s)	Blue: polycythemia causes cyanosis because >5 mg/dl of hemoglobin desaturated Bloater: hypoxia also causes pulmonary vasoconstriction and pulmonary hypertension and right-sided heart failure (i.e., cor pulmonale)	Pink: maintain fairly normal O_2 level until late in disease Puffer: tachypneic; may use pursed lip breathing and assume tripod position
Predominant symptom	Cough	Dyspnea
Age	Earlier onset of disease: 40–50 years of age	Later onset of disease: 50–75 years
Body shape	Usually obese or stocky	Thin body structure with barrel chest; causes of weight loss include: Increased calorie consumption from increased work of breathing Dyspnea limiting ability to eat comfortably
Predominant ABG characteristic	Elevated $Paco_2$ and decreased Pao_2 and Sao_2	Normal $Paco_2$, and Pao_2 and Sao_2 only mildly decreased until late in course
Laboratory	Elevated hemoglobin (caused by stimulation of erythropoietin in response to hypoxemia)	
Response to bronchodilators evaluated during pulmonary function tests	Some, especially if coexisting asthma	None unless coexisting asthma
Chest radiograph	Shows cardiac enlargement	Shows a flattened diaphragm with lung hyperinflation

Adapted from Hoyt, K. S., & Selfridge-Thomas, J. (Eds.). (2007). *Emergency nursing core curriculum* (6th ed.). St. Louis: Elsevier Saunders.

O_2 levels need to be low enough to continue to stimulate them to breathe but not so low that the tissues are hypoxic
  a) If the Sao_2 is normal (95% to 99%), the respiratory drive is lost
  b) If the Sao_2 is <90%, tissue hypoxia occurs
  c) Sao_2 of 90% to 92% is desirable in these patients to avoid both of these risks
e. CPAP or BiPAP by mask may be used in an attempt to avoid intubation and mechanical ventilation
f. Intubation and mechanical ventilation as indicated
  1) If $Paco_2$ continues to rise and acidosis develops
  2) The goal of mechanical ventilation is to normalize the pH, not necessarily the $Paco_2$

  3) Mode may be pressure support, assist-control, or intermittent mandatory ventilation
g. Heliox may be used in combination with O_2 because it is lighter than nitrogen and decreases the work of breathing
h. Bronchial hygiene and chest physiotherapy as indicated
  1) Inspiratory maneuvers: deep breathing; incentive spirometry
  2) Analgesics in doses adequate to allow patient to deep breathe and cough as indicated
  3) Encouragement of the patient to cough if rhonchi are audible; suctioning if the patient is unable to clear airways
  4) Postural drainage, percussion, vibration may be necessary

i. Pharmacologic agents
    1) Bronchodilators: usually β_2-adrenergic agents and/or anticholinergic agents
    2) Mucolytics
    3) Corticosteroids
    4) Antibiotics if infection present
    5) Drugs to aid in nicotine withdrawal if patient is still a smoker
       a) Nicotine patch
       b) Antidepressants: bupropion (Wellbutrin) and nortriptyline (Pamelor, Aventyl)

3. Maintain adequate circulation
   a. IV access for fluid and medication administration may be indicated
   b. Hydration
     1) Oral fluids: noncaffeinated
     2) IV fluids may be required: usually 0.9% saline

4. Control pain, discomfort, and anxiety
   a. NSAIDs and/or narcotic analgesics in doses that will allow patient to deep breathe and cough may be indicated
   b. Anxiolytics may be indicated

5. Treat infection (if present) and prevent sepsis
   a. Antimicrobials as indicated: empirically or specific to cultured microorganism
   b. Bronchial hygiene techniques
   c. Antipyretics and cooling methods to reduce fever

6. Monitor for/prevent complications
   a. Acute respiratory failure
   b. Pulmonary hypertension and cor pulmonale
   c. Thromboembolism; pulmonary embolism
   d. Peptic ulcer
   e. Pneumonia: *Haemophilus influenzae* and *Streptococcus pneumoniae* most likely related to acute exacerbations of COPD
   f. Sepsis

Evaluation

1. Patent airway, adequate oxygenation (i.e., normal Pao_2, Spo_2, Sao_2) and ventilation (i.e., normal $Paco_2$)
2. Absence of clinical indications of respiratory distress
3. Absence of clinical indicators of hypoperfusion
4. Absence of clinical indications of infection/sepsis
5. Alert and oriented with no neurologic deficit
6. Control of pain, discomfort, or dyspnea

Typical disposition

1. If evaluation criteria met: discharge with instructions
2. If evaluation criteria not met: admission to progressive care unit or critical care unit, especially if mechanical ventilation required

Pneumonia
Definitions

1. Pneumonia: inflammatory process of the lung parenchyma, including alveolar spaces and interstitial tissue, produced by an infectious agent

2. Community-acquired pneumonia: pneumonia: pneumonia not acquired in a hospital or a long-term care facility; causative agent is viral in 90% of the cases (ENA, 2007)
3. Hospital-acquired pneumonia (HAP): acute pneumonia that develops after 48 hours of hospitalization; also referred to as nosocomial pneumonia; assumption of a more virulent organism which are often resistant to multiple antibiotics
4. Nursing home–acquired pneumonia (NHAP): pneumonia that occurs in a resident of a nursing home or long-term care facility
   a. Pneumonia is one of the most common infectious diseases in chronic care facilities and a significant cause of mortality and morbidity among residents of nursing homes and long-term care facilities
   b. Similar to pneumonias that occurs in other settings, with the exception that many older adults have subtle signs with little to no change in vital signs

Predisposing factors

1. History of smoking
2. Advanced age
3. Periodontal disease
4. Upper respiratory infection or influenza
5. Altered level of consciousness
6. Chronic illness: diabetes, cardiac or pulmonary disease, malignancy
7. Malnutrition: alcoholism, substance abuse, eating disorder, poverty
8. Immunosuppression
9. Chronic immobility

Pathophysiology

1. Causative agents are inhaled or aspirated
   a. Bacteria
     1) *S. pneumoniae:* (most common)
     2) *H. influenzae*
     3) *Mycobacterium pneumoniae*
     4) *Staphylococcus aureus*
     5) *Klebsiella pneumonia*
     6) *Pseudomonas aeruginosa*
   b. Viruses
     1) Adenovirus
     2) Hantavirus
     3) Influenza types A and B
     4) RSV
   c. Fungi
     1) *Histoplasma capsulatum*
     2) *Coccidioides immitis*
     3) *Candida* sp.
     4) *Aspergillus* sp.
   d. Parasites (e.g., *Pneumocystis jiroveci* [previously known as *Pneomosystis carinii*])
   e. Mycoplasma: *Mycoplasma pneumoniae*

2. Alveoli become inflamed and edematous
3. Alveolar spaces fill with exudate and consolidate
4. Alveoli are not ventilated but they are perfused: $\dot{V}/\dot{Q}$ mismatch; shunt

5. Diffusion of O_2 obstructed causing hypoxemia and hypercapnia
6. Stimulation of goblet cells increase mucus, which causes increased airway resistance and increased work of breathing
7. Acute respiratory failure

Clinical presentation
1. Subjective
   a. Frequently begins with cold or flulike symptoms; infectious symptoms: chills, fever, malaise, tachycardia, headache, myalgia
   b. Chest pain: frequently pleuritic-type pain
   c. Confusion: especially in older adults; a change in behavior may be the only presenting symptom
   d. Older adults and children may complain of abdominal pain
   e. Infants present with history of poor feeding, vomiting
2. Objective
   a. Tachycardia
   b. Tachypnea
   c. Fever and diaphoresis; infants and older adults may be normothermic or hypothermic
   d. Productive cough; sputum mucoid, rusty, blood, or purulent; may have foul odor
   e. Cyanosis may be seen
   f. Clinical indications of respiratory distress (see Box 5-1)
   g. Clinical indications of hypoxemia/hypoxia (see Box 5-2)
   h. Increased tactile fremitus
   i. Clinical indications of dehydration particularly in infants: poor skin turgor; dry mucous membranes; increased specific gravity of urine
   j. Dullness to percussion over areas of consolidation
   k. Breath sounds changes: diminished; bronchial breath sounds; crackles and/or rhonchi; rub may be audible
   l. Voice sounds: egophony; bronchophony
3. Diagnostic
   a. WBCs: increased
   b. ABGs: decreased Pao_2; $Paco_2$ may be increased, decreased, or normal depending on ventilation
   c. Blood culture: to identify microorganism; drawn twice at least 15 minutes apart and prior to antibiotic administration
   d. Sputum
      1) Gram stain
      2) Acid-fast stain: differential stain that distinguishes organisms with waxy cell walls that can resist decolorization; used to rule out tuberculosis
      3) Culture and sensitivity tests to identify specific organism if bacterial; sensitivity test is done if culture is positive to determine to what the organism is susceptible
   e. Chest radiograph
      1) Initially normal, then progresses to diffuse alveolar infiltrate

2) Localization and pattern
   a) Bronchopneumonia: inflammation of the bronchioles and alveoli
   b) Interstitial pneumonia: inflammation of the tissue around alveoli
   c) Alveolar pneumonia: inflammation of the alveoli; usually caused by a virus
   d) Necrotizing pneumonia: necrosis of a portion of lung tissue
3) Viral pneumonias cause diffuse changes
4) Pleural effusion may indicate empyema

Collaborative management
1. Continue assessment
   a. ABCDs
   b. Vital signs: blood pressure, pulse, respiratory rate, and temperature
   c. O_2 saturation
   d. Respiratory effort and excursion
   e. Cardiac rate and rhythm
   f. Pain, discomfort, or dyspnea level
   g. Level of consciousness
   h. Accurate intake and output
   i. Close monitoring for progression of symptoms
2. Establish and maintain airway, oxygenation, and ventilation
   a. Elevation of head of bed to 30 to 45 degrees; over-bed table may be helpful for patient to lean on
   b. Suction as needed
   c. Intubation may be required
   d. O_2 by nasal cannula at 2 to 6 L/min to maintain Spo_2 of 95% unless contraindicated; for patients with COPD, use pulse oximetry to guide O_2 administration to Spo_2 of 90%
   e. CPAP or BiPAP by mask may be used in an attempt to avoid intubation and mechanical ventilation
   f. Intubation and mechanical ventilation as indicated
      1) If $Paco_2$ continues to rise and acidosis develops
      2) The goal of mechanical ventilation is to normalize the pH, not necessaaryy the $Paco_2$
   g. Mechanical ventilation may be required; pressure support, assist-control, or intermittent mandatory ventilation may be used
3. Treat infection and prevent sepsis
   a. Antibiotics for bacterial cause
      1) *S. pneumoniae:* macrolides (azithromycin [Zithromax]), doxycycline (Vibramycin), fluoroquinolones (levofloxacin [Levaquin])
      2) *Staphylococcus aureus:* fluoroquinolones (levofloxacin [Levaquin]), vancomycin (Vancocin)
      3) *Klebsiella pneumoniae:* third-generation cephalosporins and aminoglycosides
      4) *Pseudomonas aeruginosa:* cefepime (Maxipime), meropenem (Merrem), piperacillin (Zosyn), ciprofloxacin (Cipro)

5) *H. influenzae:* macrolides (azithromycin [Zithromax]), second- or third-generation cephalosporins

b. Antivirals for viral cause: amantadine (Symmetrel), zanamivir (Relenza), oseltamivir (Tamiflu)

c. Bronchial hygiene techniques

d. Antipyretics and cooling methods to reduce fever

4. Maintain bronchial hygiene and provide chest physiotherapy as indicated

a. Inspiratory maneuvers: deep breathing; incentive spirometry

b. Humidified air and/or O_2

c. Encouragement to cough or suctioning if the patient is unable to clear airways

d. Postural drainage, percussion, vibration if necessary

e. Bronchodilators as prescribed

f. Expectorants (e.g., guaifenesin [Robitussin], potassium iodide [SSKI]) may be used but hydration is most important; water is the best expectorant

g. Mucolytics (e.g., acetylcysteine [Mucomyst]) may be used to decrease the tenacity of the mucus

h. Sedatives: generally avoided unless patient is very agitated or on mechanical ventilation

i. Antitussives: avoid use of antitussives unless the cough is nonproductive and causing fatigue

j. Preparation of the patient for bronchoscopy as requested: may be necessary if airway clearance techniques are inadequate

5. Maintain adequate circulation

a. IV access for fluid and medication administration may be indicated

b. Hydration

1) Oral fluids: noncaffeinated

2) IV fluids may be required: usually 0.9% saline

6. Control pain, discomfort, and anxiety

a. NSAIDs and/or narcotic analgesics in doses that will allow patient to deep breathe and cough may be indicated

b. Anxiolytics may be indicated

7. Monitor for/prevent complications

a. Acute respiratory failure

b. Pleural effusion

c. Empyema

d.) Lung abscess

e. Septic shock

Evaluation

1. Patent airway, adequate oxygenation (i.e., normal PaO_2, SpO_2, SaO_2) and ventilation (i.e., normal $PaCO_2$)

2. Absence of clinical indications of respiratory distress

3. Absence of clinical indicators of hypoperfusion

4. Absence of clinical indications of infection/sepsis

5. Alert and oriented with no neurologic deficit

6. Control of pain, discomfort, or dyspnea

Typical disposition

1. If evaluation criteria met: discharge with instructions

2. If evaluation criteria not met: admission to progressive care unit or critical care unit especially if mechanical ventilation required or sepsis

Hyperventilation Syndrome (HVS)
Definition: manifestation of rapid and/or deep breathing causing hypocapnia and respiratory alkalosis
Predisposing factors

1. Anxiety

2. Salicylate poisoning

3. Early asthma

4. Drug or alcohol abuse

Pathophysiology

1. Rapid breathing (tachypnea) or deep breathing (hyperpnea) causes excessive loss of CO_2 and carbonic acid leading to respiratory alkalosis

2. Alkalosis cause vasoconstriction

3. Alkalosis increases the binding between plasma proteins and calcium, reducing serum ionized calcium level and causing tetany

4. Hyperventilation and its results lead to anxiety, perpetuating the hyperventilation

5. Patients with chronic HVS have overinflated lungs due to their breathing mechanics (they tend to breath with their upper thorax instead of with the diaphragm, as do most people), so any need to increase lung volume (i.e., taking a deep breath) can be perceived as dyspnea

Clinical presentation

1. Subjective

a. May have history of panic attacks

b. Dyspnea, "air hunger"

c. Tingling of the lips, hands, feet

d. Dizziness

e. Chest discomfort

f. Headache

2. Objective

a. Tachypnea or hyperpnea

b. Diaphoresis

c. Restless and agitated

d. Clinical indications of decrease in ionized calcium: Carpopedal spasms, Chvostek and Trousseau signs; may have seizures

3. Diagnostic

a. ABGs: hypocapnia, respiratory alkalosis with normal PaO_2, SaO_2

1) The normal O_2 levels help to differentiate this syndrome from other causes of hyperventilation such as pulmonary embolism

b. Toxicology screen: to rule out drug cause

c. D-dimer: negative rules out pulmonary embolism

d. ECG: changes include prolonged QT interval, ST-segment changes, and T-wave elevation or depression

e. Chest radiograph: to rule out other causes

Collaborative management

1. Continue assessment
   a. ABCDs
   b. Vital signs: blood pressure, pulse, respiratory rate, and temperature
   c. O_2 saturation
   d. Respiratory effort and excursion
   e. Cardiac rate and rhythm
   f. Pain, discomfort, or dyspnea level
   g. Level of consciousness
   h. Accurate intake and output
   i. Close monitoring for progression of symptoms
2. Establish and maintain airway, oxygenation, and ventilation
   a. Elevation of head of bed to 30 to 45 degrees; overbed table may be helpful for patient to lean on
   b. Calm, reassuring environment
   c. Diaphragmatic breathing: encourage the use of the diaphragm when breathing, which provides distraction and a sense of control over breathing, which leads to a decrease in respiratory rate
   d. Physically compressing the upper thorax while the patient exhales maximally helps decrease the lung hyperinflation
   e. Partial rebreathing bag with 21% O_2 may be used; having the patient breathe into a paper bag is usually ineffective because they often cannot cooperate with this treatment
   f. Anxiolytics as prescribed to decrease stress and anxiety
3. Control pain, discomfort, and anxiety
   a. NSAIDs and/or narcotic analgesics in doses that will allow patient to deep breathe and cough may be indicated
   b. Anxiolytics may be indicated
4. Monitor for/prevent complications
   a. Cerebral ischemia
   b. Seizures

Evaluation

1. Patent airway, adequate oxygenation (i.e., normal Pao_2, Spo_2, Sao_2), and ventilation (i.e., normal $Paco_2$)
2. Absence of clinical indications of respiratory distress
3. Absence of clinical indicators of hypoperfusion
4. Absence of clinical indications of infection/sepsis
5. Alert and oriented with no neurologic deficit
6. Control of pain, discomfort, or dyspnea

Typical disposition: discharge with instructions

1. Instructions on diaphragmatic breathing
2. May receive a referral to a psychologist/psychiatrist

Inhalation Injury
Definition

a. Lung damage caused by inhalation of noxious material: smoke, toxic combustion byproducts, superheated air or steam, or other noxious fumes

2. Inhalation injuries account for the majority of deaths in fires

Precipitating factors

1. Patient in an enclosed space when fire or explosion occurs
2. Industrial accidents involving steam or gasses

Pathophysiology

1. Three pathophysiologic processes
   a. Asphyxiation: toxic gases (e.g., CO and cyanide) displace environmental O_2 so inspired O_2 concentration decreases to <21%
      1) CO is a colorless, odorless, tasteless gas produced by combustion of organic material
         a) CO binds with Hgb at 200 to 250 times the affinity of O_2, so Hgb is unavailable to transport O_2, leading to cellular hypoxia
         b) Clinical significance increases with the patient's carboxyhemoglobin level
         c) Smokers or those exposed to automobile exhaust will have higher baseline CO levels
      2) Cyanide is produced by burning synthetic materials
         a) Leads to asphyxiation by interfering with mitochondrial oxidative phosphorylation and cellular respiration
         b) The resulting anaerobic metabolism produces lactic acid
   b. Thermal injury: caused by the inhalation of superheated air/steam
      1) Laryngospasm limits the thermal injury to the upper airway in most cases
      2) Inhalation of steam can produce both upper and lower airway injuries, however; most injuries below the glottis are from inhalation of chemical by products
      3) Heat in the airways produces redness, edema, blisters, and charring that can cause airway obstruction
   c. Smoke and soot
      1) Inhaling smoke damages respiratory epithelial cells, destroys cilia, and leads to pulmonary edema
      2) The size of the soot particles and the location where they are deposited in the respiratory tract influence the degree of damage
      3) Soot particles are acidic and can form free radicals, which further damage mucosal surfaces and alveoli, leading to a massive inflammatory response

Clinical presentation

1. Subjective
   a. History consistent with inhalation injury
   b. Pain or irritation in upper airways
   c. Burning chest pain or throat pain
2. Objective
   a. Tachycardia
   b. Tachypnea
   c. Hypotension

d. Clinical indications of respiratory distress (see Box 5-1)

e. Stridor

f. Cough

g. Hoarseness: indicates edema and may indicate impending airway obstruction

h. Change in level of consciousness: restlessness, agitation, lethargy

i. Singed facial hairs

j. Soot in nose or mouth, carbonaceous sputum

3. Specific for potential asphyxiation

  a. CO

    1) Headache (common)

    2) Nausea, vomiting

    3) Dizziness

    4) Chest pain

    5) Seizures

    6) Cherry red skin and mucous membranes

    7) Dysrhythmias: changes indicative of ischemia or infarction (ST-segment changes, T-wave changes)

  b. Cyanide (Leybell, Hoffman, Baud, & Borron, 2006)

    1) Dramatic onset

    2) Vertigo, dizziness

    3) Abdominal pain, nausea, vomiting

    4) Cherry red skin color

    5) Bitter almond smell

    6) Bright red retinal arteries

4. Specific for potential thermal injury: oral pharyngeal burns or blisters

5. Diagnostic

  a. ABGs: hypoxemia, respiratory and/or metabolic acidosis

  b. Blood urea nitrogen, creatinine: to evaluate renal function

  c. Electrolytes: to calculate anion gap

  d. Toxicology screen (both serum and urine): to identify possible toxin

  e. Carboxyhemoglobin level: >10% suggests inhalation injury

  f. Urinalysis for myoglobin as an indication of rhabdomyolysis

  g. Methemoglobin level

    1) <2% of total Hgb is normal

    2) 40% of total Hgb is critical

  h. Chest radiograph: may be inconclusive unless pulmonary edema or other problems develop

Collaborative management

1. Continue assessment

  a. ABCDs

  b. Vital signs: blood pressure, pulse, respiratory rate, and temperature

  c. O$_2$ saturation

  d. Respiratory effort and excursion

  e. Cardiac rate and rhythm

  f. Pain, discomfort, or dyspnea level

  g. Level of consciousness

  h. Accurate intake and output

  i. Close monitoring for progression of symptoms

2. Establish and maintain airway, oxygenation, and ventilation

  a. O$_2$ by nasal cannula at 2 to 6 L/min to maintain Spo$_2$ of 95%

    1) Humidification required

    2) If CO: 100% O$_2$ by nonrebreathing mask; hyperbaric oxygenation may be required depending on CO levels

  b. Coughing should be encouraged to expel mucus, soot if patient is capable of effective coughing

  c. Elective intubation may be performed if the patient has airway edema before the airway becomes obstructed; cricothyrotomy may be necessary

  d. Mechanical ventilation with PEEP may be needed to maintain alveolar ventilation

  e. Pharmacologic agents

    1) Racemic epinephrine for upper airway obstruction

    2) Bronchodilators for lower airway obstruction

3. Maintain adequate circulation

  a. IV access for fluid and medication administration may be indicated

  b. Hydration

    1) Oral fluids: noncaffeinated

    2) IV fluids may be required: usually 0.9% saline

4. Treat cyanide poisoning if present

  a. Cyanide antidote kit contains amyl nitrate pearls for inhalation, sodium nitrite and sodium thiosulfate for IV administration

    1) Amyl nitrate and sodium nitrite induces methemoglobin

    2) Methemoglobin does not combine with O$_2$ but will attract cyanide molecules

    3) Thiosulfate combines with cyanide to produce thiocyanate, which is excreted by the kidneys

    4) Hydroxocobalamin given if antidote kit not available; combines with cyanide to form cyanocobalamin (vitamin B$_{12}$), which is also excreted via the kidneys

    5) Control of pain, discomfort, and anxiety

      a) NSAIDs and/or narcotic analgesics in doses that will allow patient to deep breathe and cough may be indicated

      b) Anxiolytics may be indicated

5. Detect and treat rhabdomyolysis

  a. Foley catheter and monitoring of urine output for myoglobinuria: urine is tea colored

  b. Usually treated with IV saline and mannitol to flush this heavy pigment through the renal tubules along with sodium bicarbonate IV to alkaline the urine

6. Monitor for/prevent complications

  a. Laryngospasm and airway obstruction

  b. Respiratory arrest

  c. Acute renal failure caused by rhabdomyolysis

Evaluation

1. Patent airway, adequate oxygenation (i.e., normal Pao_2, Spo_2, Sao_2) and ventilation (i.e., normal $Paco_2$)
2. Absence of clinical indications of respiratory distress
3. Absence of clinical indicators of hypoperfusion
4. Absence of clinical indications of infection/sepsis
5. Alert and oriented with no neurologic deficit
6. Control of pain, discomfort, or dyspnea

Typical disposition

1. If evaluation criteria met: discharge with instructions
2. If evaluation criteria not met: admission to progressive care unit or critical care unit
   a. If inhalation injury or cyanide toxicity, admission to the critical care unit

Submersion injuries
Definition: hypoxic event that occurs from submersion in a fluid
Precipitating factors

1. Overestimation of swimming capability
2. Alcohol or drug intoxication
3. Seizure
4. Spinal cord or head injury
5. Myocardial infarction
6. Dysrhythmia
7. Hypoglycemia
8. Air embolus (e.g., scuba diving)
9. Attempted suicide, homicide, or child abuse
10. Developmental: improper supervision around swimming pools, standing buckets of water, etc; residential swimming pools and bathtubs are common sites for pediatric drowning

Pathophysiology

1. Submersion
   a. Breath holding
   b. Sudden, involuntary gasping results in aspiration and possible swallowing of the fluid
2. Factors to be considered
   a. Temperature of water
      1) Water has a thermal conductive property that is 32 times that of air, so the body temperature rapidly changes toward the temperature of the water
      2) Cold water (temperature of $<20°C$)
         a) Survival rates are greater than for warm water because of the following:
            (i) Hypothermic mechanism: reduction of cerebral metabolic rate reduces cerebral O_2 requirements
            (ii) Diving reflex: decreases the heart rate and shunts blood to the brain and heart; probably less of a factor in adults but is a significant reflex in children
         b) Adverse effects
            (i) May cause fatal dysrhythmias
            (ii) May increase blood viscosity and slow circulation of blood through the coronary and cerebral arteries
            (iii) Perpetuates hypoxia by shifting the oxyhemoglobin dissociation curve to the left, which increases the affinity between Hgb and O_2 and decreases O_2 unloading at the tissue level
            (iv) May cause hyperventilation, hypocapnia, disorientation, and possible loss of consciousness leading to drowning
   b. Quantity of water
      1) Dry: aspiration does not occur but the patient becomes hypoxic from laryngospasm or breath holding
      2) Wet: aspiration of water or gastric contents into lungs occurs
         a) Aspiration of at least 22 ml/kg of fluid is required to cause significant changes in electrolytes and aspiration of at least 11 ml/kg is required to cause changes in blood volume; only $\approx15\%$ of drowning victims ever aspirate that much fluid
         b) Aspiration of acidic gastric contents may cause pneumonitis and acute respiratory distress syndrome; aspiration of solid gastric contents may cause airway obstruction or contribute to intrapulmonary shunt
   c. Type of water: freshwater or saltwater; presence of contaminants
      1) If the patient does aspirate significant amounts of fluid into their lungs, the following physiologic changes occur
         a) Saltwater (hypertonic)
            (i) Fluid is drawn from the vascular space and interstitium into the alveoli
            (ii) This leads to hemoconcentration, pulmonary edema, intrapulmonary shunt, and hypoxemia
            (iii) Hypernatremia, hyperchloremia, and hypermagnesemia occur
         b) Freshwater (hypotonic)
            (i) Hemodilution, hypervolemia, and acute hemolysis along with damage to the type II pneumocytes occur
            (ii) This leads to a decrease in surfactant, resultant alveolar collapse and atelectasis, intrapulmonary shunt, and hypoxemia
            (iii) Seizures may occur due to dilutional hyponatremia
      2) Particulate matter: sand, algae, weeds, mud, chloride, or bacteria
         a) Lung infection and even pulmonary fibrosis may occur
         b) Saltwater is considered twice as lethal as freshwater per unit volume because of the degree of impurity

3. Pulmonary consequences
   a. Aspiration causes laryngospasm, which causes asphyxia and loss of consciousness
   b. Glottic relaxation usually follows, which leads to additional aspiration of water into the lungs
   c. Aspirated fluid causes an inflammatory reaction in the alveolar-capillary membrane
   d. Pulmonary edema occurs as interstitial fluid moves into the alveolus
   e. This dilutes and inactivates the surfactant and causes atelectasis
   f. Hypoxic vasoconstriction occurs and pulmonary hypertension occurs
   g. $\dot{V}/\dot{Q}$ mismatch, intrapulmonary shunt, increased pathologic deadspace, and decreased pulmonary compliance occur
   h. Atelectasis, pneumonitis, and eventually ARDS occur
4. Cardiovascular consequences: hypothermia, hypoxemia, and acidosis may cause fatal dysrhythmias
5. Neurologic consequences
   a. Hypoxemia, hypercapnia, and decreased cerebral perfusion pressure cause cerebral hypoxia and intracranial hypertension
   b. Permanent brain injury occurs as the period of cerebral hypoxia and anoxia continues
   c. Freshwater drowning may cause hyponatremia and seizures
6. Renal consequences: hypoxia, hypoperfusion, myoglobinuria, and hemoglobinuria may lead to acute tubular necrosis and intrarenal renal failure
   a. Myoglobinuria may occur secondary to muscle trauma
   b. Hemoglobinuria may occur secondary to hemolysis as occurs after the aspiration of significant amounts of freshwater

Clinical presentation

1. Subjective
   a. History of submersion (mechanism of injury)
   b. History of contributing event (e.g., alcohol or drug intoxication, MI, spinal cord injury)
   c. Dyspnea
   d. Substernal burning and/or pleuritic chest pain
2. Objective
   a. Dysrhythmias or cardiopulmonary arrest
   b. Tachycardia, hypotension
   c. Tachypnea, possibly apnea
   d. Clinical indications of respiratory distress (see Box 5-1)
   e. Cough: may have pink, frothy sputum
   f. Cyanosis may be evident
   g. Chest dullness to percussion
   h. Breath sound changes: crackles; rhonchi; wheezes
   i. Abdominal distention may be present due to swallowing large volumes of water
   j. Change in level of conscious with signs of cerebral anoxia may be evident

   k. Paralysis may be evident if there is a spinal cord injury
   l. Hyporeflexia or seizures may occur related to hyponatremia in freshwater near-drowning
   m. Oliguria, proteinuria, and elevated blood urea nitrogen may be seen if acute tubular necrosis develops
   n. Brownish (tea-colored) urine may be seen if myoglobinuria is present; reddish (port wine–colored) urine may be seen if hemoglobinuria is present
   o. Temperature may be increased or decreased
      1) May be hypothermic related to exposure in cold water
      2) May have fever related to pulmonary infection
   p. Signs of trauma may be evident
   q. Clinical indications of hypoxemia/hypoxia (see Box 5-2)
3. Diagnostic
   a. Sodium, chloride, potassium, and magnesium may be decreased in freshwater near-drowning and increased in saltwater near-drowning
   b. Potassium may be increased if any of the following occurs:
      1) Freshwater near-drowning with significant hemolysis
      2) Hypothermia
      3) Renal failure
   c. Hct: may be increased in saltwater drowning and decreased in freshwater drowning
   d. Hgb: may be decreased along with later potassium and bilirubin increase if significant hemolysis occurs (must have aspiration of at least 11 ml/kg of freshwater)
   e. WBCs
      1) May be increased due to pulmonary infection
      2) May be decreased in hypothermia due to cells being sequestered in the liver and spleen
   f. ABGs
      1) Respiratory acidosis progressing to respiratory and metabolic acidosis
      2) Hypoxemia
   g. Toxicology screen: to identify any drugs and alcohol
   h. Urine
      1) May show hemoglobinuria
      2) May show myoglobinuria
   i. ECG: may show dysrhythmias
      1) Bradycardia to asystole
      2) Ventricular fibrillation
   j. Chest radiograph
      1) May show diffuse indistinct, nodular infiltrates
      2) May show atelectasis, pneumonia, pulmonary edema, and/or ARDS
   k) Spine radiographs: may be indicated to rule out spinal fracture

l. Electroencephalogram (EEG): may indicate seizure activity

m. CT of head: may indicate head injury

n. Other diagnostic studies depending on possible suspected medical cause

o. Orlowski score: two or fewer of the following variables is associated with a >90% chance of a good outcome; three or more of the following variables is associated with <5% chance of normal recovery (Orlowski, 1987)

1) Age 3 years or younger
2) Submersion time >5 minutes
3) No resuscitative efforts for >10 minutes after rescue
4) Comatose on admission to the ED
5) Arterial pH <7.10

Collaborative management

1. Continue assessment
   a. ABCDs
   b. Vital signs: blood pressure, pulse, respiratory rate, and temperature
   c. O_2 saturation
   d. Respiratory effort and excursion
   e. Cardiac rate and rhythm
   f. Pain, discomfort, or dyspnea level
   g. Level of consciousness
   h. Accurate intake and output
   i. Close monitoring for progression of symptoms

2. Manage cardiopulmonary arrest if needed; establish and maintain airway, ventilation, and oxygenation
   a. BCLS and/or ACLS; resuscitation efforts should not be ceased until the patient has a normal body temperature and continues to fail to respond
   b. Initially use 100% O_2; decrease O_2 levels if possible and still maintain Sao_2 at least 95%
   c. Intubation and mechanical ventilation; PEEP increases intra-alveolar pressure and decreases the pulmonary edema
   d. Bronchodilators
   e. Bronchoscopy may be performed for removal of aspirated foreign solid material

3. Maintain adequate circulation, electrolytes, and renal function
   a. IV access for fluid and medication administration may be indicated
   b. IV fluid prescription will be determined by the patient's sodium level
      1) 0.9% Saline if patient's sodium level is normal
      2) If the patient aspirated significant amounts of saltwater, the serum sodium may be significantly elevated and 0.45% saline may be prescribed
      3) If patient aspirated significant amounts of freshwater, the serum sodium may significantly decreased and 3% saline may be prescribed to prevent neurologic complications such as seizures

c. Fluids and diuretics (e.g., mannitol [Osmitrol]) along with sodium bicarbonate as prescribed for myoglobinuria, hemoglobinuria

4. Restore normal body temperature
   a. Monitoring of core body temperature via rectal probe or Foley catheter with thermistor
   b. Dysrhythmia monitoring
   c. Warming if hypothermic
      1) Use central warming techniques (e.g., IV fluids warmed to 37°C, humidified O_2 warmed to 40°C, gastric lavage, peritoneal lavage, and/or enemas at 37°C) initially
      2) Use surface warming techniques (e.g., warm blankets, radiant heat lamps) after core body temperature is at least 32°C
      3) Monitor for afterdrop (hypotension due to rewarming causing peripheral vasodilation and the shifting of acidotic blood back into the central circulation)
      4) Monitor skin perfusion

5. Treat infection (if present) and prevent sepsis
   a. Antimicrobials as indicated: empirically or specific to cultured microorganism
   b. Bronchial hygiene techniques
   c. Antipyretics and cooling methods to reduce fever

6. Prevent aspiration: orogastric or nasogastric tube to decompress the stomach and prevent vomiting and aspiration

7. Monitor for/prevent complications
   a. Cardiopulmonary arrest
   b. Dysrhythmia
   c. ARDS
   d. Seizures
   e. Fluid and electrolyte imbalances
   f. Renal failure
   g. Cerebral ischemia and damage
   h. Sepsis

Evaluation

1. Patent airway, adequate oxygenation (i.e., normal Pao_2, Spo_2, Sao_2) and ventilation (i.e., normal $Paco_2$)
2. Absence of clinical indications of respiratory distress
3. Absence of clinical indicators of hypoperfusion
4. Absence of clinical indications of infection/sepsis
5. Alert and oriented with no neurologic deficit
6. Control of pain, discomfort, or dyspnea

Typical disposition

1. If evaluation criteria met: admit for 23-hour observation
2. If evaluation criteria not met: admission to critical care unit

Pulmonary Embolism (PE)

Definition: obstruction of blood flow to one or more arteries of the lung by a thrombus lodged in a pulmonary vessel; includes fat, air, amniotic fluid, tumor, and foreign body emboli

1. Massive: more than 50% occlusion of pulmonary blood flow; caused by occlusion of a lobar artery or larger artery

2. Submassive: <50% occlusion of pulmonary blood flow

Predisposing factors

1. Virchow's triad: hypercoagulability, damage to the vascular endothelium, venous stasis (described in the Peripheral Venous Thrombosis section of Chapter 4)
2. For fat embolism
   a. Long bone fractures, pelvic fracture, multiple fractures
   b. Orthopedic surgery with intramedullary manipulation
   c. Trauma to adipose tissue or liver
   d. Osteomyelitis
   e. Sickle cell crisis
   f. Burns
   g. Acute pancreatitis
   h. Liposuction
3. For air embolism
   a. Recent surgical procedure
   b. Insertion of central venous catheter or accidental removal of central venous catheter
   c. Hemodialysis
   d. Endoscopy
   e. Rapid ascend from deep sea diving

Pathophysiology

1. More than 90% of thrombi develop in the deep veins of the lower extremities
2. Thrombus formation enhances platelet adhesiveness and causes release of serotonin (vasoconstrictor)
3. Factors contributing to dislodgment of the thrombi include sudden standing (e.g., initial ambulation), Valsalva maneuver (e.g., coughing, sneezing, vomiting), fluid challenges, and massaging legs
4. Consequences: development of a clot that moves to the pulmonary vessels, where it stops when it becomes too large to move through
   a. Ventilation continues but perfusion is decreased: $\dot{V}/\dot{Q}$ mismatch; increased alveolar deadspace
   b. No gas exchange takes place so there is decreased alveolar CO_2, which causes bronchoconstriction and alveolar shrinking so that less inspired air goes into nonperfused alveoli and more inspired air goes into perfused alveoli
   c. Cessation of blood flow damages type II pneumocytes and leads to a decrease in surfactant
   d. Loss of surfactant causes atelectasis, interstitial fluid movement into the alveolus, and decreased lung compliance
   e. Increased airway resistance and decreased lung compliance increases work of breathing
   f. Pulmonary infarction can occur, causing hemorrhage, consolidation, and necrosis
   g. Systemic hypotension and cardiac arrest may occur

5. Fat emboli: fat globules enter bloodstream
   a. More likely to develop 1 to 3 days or up to 1 week after injury
   b. Fat globules enter the bloodstream and form emboli
   c. Presence of fat emboli in the bloodstream causes interactions with platelets and free fatty acids along with release of vasoactive substances
   d. Cerebral ischemia
6. Air emboli: activation of the clotting cascade and interruption of circulation

Clinical presentation

1. If thrombotic embolism
   a. Subjective
      1) Small embolus: may be asymptomatic
      2) Anxiety
      3) Dyspnea
      4) Chest pain
      5) Palpitations
      6) Feeling of impending doom (if massive PE)
      7) Light headed, weakness
      8) Syncope (massive PE)
      9) If pulmonary infarction develops (hours to days after embolism), the patient will also have pleuritic chest pain
   b. Objective
      1) Tachycardia
      2) Hypotension; may present as pulseless electrical activity (PEA)
      3) Tachypnea
      4) Restlessness
      5) Cough
      6) Cyanosis may be evident in massive PEA
      7) Breath sound changes: crackles, rales
      8) Clinical indications of respiratory distress (see Box 5-1)
      9) Clinical indications of hypoxemia/hypoxia (see Box 5-2)
   c. Diagnostics
      1) D-dimer: high sensitivity but low specificity; 99% negative predictive value; indeterminate $\dot{V}/\dot{Q}$ and a positive D-dimer are indications for pulmonary angiogram
      2) ABGs
         a) Decreased Pao_2, Sao_2, Svo_2; Pao_2 <50 mm Hg in a patient with previously normal ABGs indicates >50% obstruction of the pulmonary tree and that pulmonary hypertension is present
         b) Decreased $Paco_2$
         c) Respiratory alkalosis initially; may have metabolic acidosis if severe hypoxemia; respiratory acidosis may develop with significant atelectasis or fatigue
      3) ECG
         a) Dysrhythmias
            (i) Sinus tachycardia
            (ii) Atrial dysrhythmias, especially atrial fibrillation are common

(iii) Ventricular dysrhythmias may occur in hypoxemia
- b) Blocks: new right bundle branch block may be seen
- c) Tall, peaked P waves in lead II (P-pulmonale)
  - (i) Echocardiogram: rule out cardiac tamponade, dissection of the aorta, acute MI
- 5) Chest radiograph
  - a) Initially normal
  - b) After 24 hours: small infiltrates may be seen secondary to atelectasis; elevated hemidiaphragm on affected side; decreased pulmonary vascularity
    - (i) May show Westermark sign: dilation of pulmonary vessels proximal to the PE along with collapse of vessels distal to the PE
  - c) If pulmonary infarction: infiltrates and pleural effusion may be seen
- 6) $\dot{V}/\dot{Q}$ scan: shows perfusion defect with normal ventilation
- 7) Spiral (helical) CT: easier study to obtain than a $\dot{V}/\dot{Q}$ scan or pulmonary angiogram
- 8) Pulmonary angiography: shows cutoff of a vessel or a filling defect within 24 to 72 hours
- d. Magnetic resonance angiography: allows high-resolution angiography during a single breath

2. If fat embolism: may have no symptoms for 12 to 48 hours
  - a. Subjective
    1) Restlessness, agitation, irritability, confusion
    2) Dyspnea
    3) Delirium
  - b. Objective
    1) Tachypnea
    2) Tachycardia
    3) Fever
    4) Petechiae on conjunctivae, anterior chest, neck, axilla
    5) Breath sound changes: stridor, wheezes, crackles
    6) Lethargy, coma
    7) Seizures
    8) Clinical indications of respiratory distress (see Box 5-1)
    9) Clinical indications of hypoxemia/hypoxia (see Box 5-2)
  - c. Diagnostic
    1) Elevated lipase
    2) Elevated triglycerides
    3) Increased free fatty acids
    4) Elevated sedimentation rate
    5) Decreased Hgb, Hct
    6) Thrombocytopenia
    7) Elevated fibrin split products

8) ABGs
  - a) Decreased Pa_{O_2}, Sa_{O_2}
  - b) Increased Pa_{CO_2}
  - c) Respiratory acidosis; may have metabolic acidosis if severe hypoxemia
9) Chest radiograph: diffuse extensive interstitial and alveolar infiltrates
10) Urinalysis: fat globules in the urine
11) Sputum: fat globules in the sputum

3. If air embolism
  - a. Subjective
    1) Feeling of impending doom
    2) Lightheadedness
    3) Weakness
    4) Nausea
    5) Chest pain
    6) Dyspnea
    7) Palpitations
    8) Confusion
  - b. Objective
    1) Tachypnea
    2) Tachycardia
    3) Hypotension
    4) Churning noise ("mill wheel murmur") may be audible;
    5) Clinical indications of respiratory distress (see Box 5-1)
    6) Clinical indications of hypoxemia/hypoxia (see Box 5-2)
    7) Clinical indications of pulmonary edema: S_3, crackles
    8) Seizures
  - c. Diagnostic
    1) ABGs
      - a) Decreased Pa_{O_2}, Sa_{O_2}
      - b) Increased Pa_{CO_2}
      - c) Respiratory acidosis; may have metabolic acidosis if severe hypoxemia
    2) Chest radiograph: may show evidence of right ventricular failure and/or pulmonary edema
    3) $\dot{V}/\dot{Q}$ scan: similar to PE but may resolve within 24 hours
    4) Echocardiography: shows air in right ventricle, right ventricular dilation, and/or pulmonary hypertension

Collaborative management

1. Continue assessment
  - a. ABCDs
  - b. Vital signs: blood pressure, pulse, respiratory rate, and temperature
  - c. O_2 saturation
  - d. Respiratory effort and excursion
  - e. Cardiac rate and rhythm
  - f. Pain, discomfort, or dyspnea level
  - g. Level of consciousness
  - h. Accurate intake and output
  - i. Close monitoring for progression of symptoms

2. Establish and maintain airway, ventilation, and oxygenation
   a. Elevation of head of bed to 30 to 45 degrees; overbed table may be helpful for patient to lean on
   b. O_2 to maintain SpO_2 of 95% unless contraindicated
      1) Although nasal cannula may be adequate in small PEs, 100% O_2 by nonrebreathing mask is frequently necessary in patients with moderate to massive PE
      2) In patients with COPD, use pulse oximetry to guide O_2 administration to SpO_2 of 90%
   c. Intubation and mechanical ventilation may be necessary
      1) The primary initial problem in PE is diffusion due to the perfusion defect; the patient is generally ventilating adequately initially (frequently even excessively as evidenced by a low $PaCO_2$) but may require intubation and mechanical ventilation as respiratory muscle fatigue occurs
3. Maintain adequate circulation
   a. IV access for fluid and medication administration may be indicated
   b. Hydration: IV fluids may be required: usually 0.9% saline
4. Reestablish pulmonary perfusion and reduce pulmonary hypertension
   a. Baseline clotting profile
   b. Fibrinolytic (i.e., alteplase [Activase]): to cause clot lysis
      1) Indications in PE
         a) Refractory hypoxemia
         b) Acute right ventricular failure
         c) Hemodynamic instability
      2) Contraindications/precautions as for MI
   c. Anticoagulants: to prevent extension of the clot and reocclusion
      1) Unfractionated heparin: weight-dosed and then titrated
      2) Low-molecular-weight heparin (LMWH) (e.g., enoxaparin [Lovenox]): may be prescribed subcutaneously in stable patients
   d. Warfarin (Coumadin): usually prescribed for 6 months after PE
   e. Catheter embolectomy
   f. Surgical embolectomy
5. Control pain, discomfort, and anxiety
   a. NSAIDs and/or narcotic analgesics in doses that will allow patient to deep breathe and cough may be indicated
   b. Anxiolytics may be indicated
6. Specific to air embolism
   a. Left lateral decubitus position with head down (referred to as Durant maneuver) if air embolism suspected
   b. O_2 via 100% nonrebreathing mask; hyperbaric O_2 is indicated for arterial emboli and deterioration
   c. Anticoagulants may be administered

7. Specific to fat embolism
   a. Steroids may be prescribed
   b. IV fluids and osmotic diuretic (e.g., mannitol)
8. Monitor for/prevent complications
   a. Pulmonary infarction
   b. Cerebral infarction
   c. Myocardial infarction
   d. Right ventricular failure
   e. Dysrhythmias or block
   f. Pulmonary abscess
   g. ARDS
   h. Disseminated intravascular coagulation
   i. Shock

Evaluation

1. Patent airway, adequate oxygenation (i.e., normal PaO_2, SpO_2, SaO_2) and ventilation (i.e., normal $PaCO_2$)
2. Absence of clinical indications of respiratory distress
3. Absence of clinical indicators of hypoperfusion
4. Absence of clinical indications of infection/sepsis
5. Alert and oriented with no neurologic deficit
6. Control of pain, discomfort, or dyspnea

Typical disposition

1. Admission; may require admission to critical care unit

Pleural Effusion
Definition: abnormal collection of fluid in the pleural space
Precipitating factors

1. Transudate: hydrothorax
   a. Heart failure
   b. Malignancy
   c. Pulmonary embolism
   d. Renal failure
   e. Liver failure
   f. Tuberculosis
   g. Pancreatitis
   h. Myxedema
2. Exudate: empyema
   a. Pneumonia
   b. Pulmonary infarction
   c. Malignancies
   d. Rheumatoid arthritis
   e. Lupus erythematosus
3. Blood: hemothorax
   a. Chest trauma
   b. Malignancy
   c. Rupture of a great vessel
4. Chyle (i.e., a milky fluid found in lymph fluid from the gastrointestinal tract): chylothorax
   a. Trauma
   b. Inflammation
   c. Malignancy

Pathophysiology

1. Normally <15 ml of fluid in the pleural space that functions as a lubricant between the parietal and visceral pleura

a. The pleural fluid is formed by capillaries lining the parietal pleura and is absorbed by capillaries in the visceral pleura and by the lymphatic system; any disruption in either secretion or reabsorption of the fluid has the potential to cause an effusion

2. Several factors can contribute to increasing amounts of fluid in the pleural space (Black & Hawks, 2009; Selfridge-Thomas & Hoyt, 2007)
   a. Increased capillary pressure: seen in heart failure
   b. Decreased capillary oncotic pressure: seen in liver and renal failure
   c. Increase in capillary permeability: seen in inflammatory conditions
   d. Impairment in lymphatic drainage of the pleura
3. The end result is decreased lung capacity as the fluid increases and lung expansion is inhibited, causing dyspnea

Clinical presentation

1. Subjective
   a. Chest pain, pleuritic pain
   b. Dyspnea
2. Objective
   a. Tachycardia
   b. Tachypnea
   c. Cough: hemoptysis
   d. Fever
   e. Percussion: dullness on the affected side; increased fremitus above effusion and absent over it
   f. Breath sound changes: decreased or absent breath sounds on the affected side
   g. Pleural friction rub
      1) To distinguish from pericardial friction rub, have the patient hold his or her breath; if the rub continues without the patient breathing, it is pericardial rather than pleural
3. Diagnostic
   a. CBC with differential: may have increased WBCs
   b. ECG: to rule out MI
   c. Chest radiograph: lateral decubitus preferred for detecting smaller effusions
   d. CT chest and spiral to identify effusion
   e. Ultrasound: to identify area for thoracentesis if planned

Collaborative management

1. Continue assessment
   a. ABCDs
   b. Vital signs: blood pressure, pulse, respiratory rate, and temperature
   c. O_2 saturation
   d. Respiratory effort and excursion
   e. Cardiac rate and rhythm
   f. Pain, discomfort, or dyspnea level
   g. Level of consciousness
   h. Accurate intake and output
   i. Close monitoring for progression of symptoms
2. Establish and maintain airway, oxygenation, and ventilation
   a. Elevation of head of bed to 30 to 45 degrees; over-bed table may be helpful for patient to lean on

b. O_2 by nasal cannula at 2 to 6 L/min to maintain SpO_2 of 95% unless contraindicated; for patients with COPD, use pulse oximetry to guide O_2 administration to SpO_2 of 90%
   c. Thoracentesis or chest tube insertion if effusion is large; surgical repair of chest trauma may be required in hemothorax
3. Maintain adequate circulation
   a. IV access for fluid and medication administration may be indicated
   b. Hydration
      1) Oral fluids: noncaffeinated
      2) IV fluids may be required: usually 0.9% saline
4. Treat infection (in empyema) and prevent sepsis
   a. Antimicrobials as indicated: empirically or specific to cultured microorganism
   b. Antipyretics and cooling methods to reduce fever
5. Control pain, discomfort, and anxiety
   a. NSAIDs and/or narcotic analgesics in doses that will allow patient to deep breathe and cough may be indicated
   b. Anxiolytics may be indicated
6. Monitor for/prevent complications
   a. Atelectasis
   b. Sepsis if empyema
   c. Shock if hemothorax
   d. Pneumothorax as a complication of thoracentesis

Evaluation

1. Patent airway, adequate oxygenation (i.e., normal PaO_2, SpO_2, SaO_2) and ventilation (i.e., normal $PaCO_2$)
2. Absence of clinical indications of respiratory distress
3. Absence of clinical indicators of hypoperfusion
4. Absence of clinical indications of infection/sepsis
5. Alert and oriented with no neurologic deficit
6. Control of pain, discomfort, or dyspnea

Typical disposition

1. If evaluation criteria met: discharge with instructions following thoracentesis
2. If evaluation criteria not met: admission to progressive care unit or critical care unit
   a. If hemothorax, admission to surgery will likely be required

Croup

Definition: laryngeal or tracheal obstruction characterized by a harsh barking cough, inspiratory stridor, hoarse voice; also known as acute viral laryngotracheobronchitis (LTB)
Predisposing factors
1. Pharyngitis
2. Parainfluenza
3. Upper respiratory infection
   a. Usually affects pediatrics 6 months to 6 years of age, although can be seen in adults
   b. More common in winter months
   c. Parainfluenza virus types 1 and 2 are the primary cause

d. Other causative viruses include: RSV, adenovirus, rhinovirus, diphtheria, *M. pneumoniae*

Pathophysiology

1. Transmission occurs via respiratory droplets
2. The virus enters by the nasopharynx and then spreads to the larynx and trachea
3. Virus sheds by budding (i.e., cells break off or split from parent viral cell to form new viral cells)
4. An inflammatory exudate forms along with erythema and edema of the trachea and the larynx including the vocal cords

Clinical presentation

1. Subjective
   a. History of upper respiratory infection for 1 to 2 days with symptoms of cough, sore throat, drooling, and fever; symptoms worse at night
   b. Fatigue
2. Objective
   a. Tachycardia
   b. Tachypnea
   c. Fever usually <102.2°F (ENA, 2007)
   d. Harsh barking (croupy) cough
   e. Drooling
   f. Erythremic pharynx
   g. Inspiratory and expiratory stridor
   h. Breath sounds normal or diminished
   i. Sternal retractions in severe cases
3. Diagnostic
   a. CBC with differential: usually normal or WBCs increased
   b. ABGs: hypoxemia with severe causes
   c. Neck radiograph
      1) Frontal view: steeple sign (i.e., subglottic narrowing, funneling of tracheal lumen)
      2) Lateral neck view: to rule out epiglottitis
   d. Laryngoscopy: erythema of trachea, larynx

Collaborative management

1. Continue assessment
   a. ABCDs
   b. Vital signs: blood pressure, pulse, respiratory rate, and temperature
   c. O_2 saturation
   d. Respiratory effort and excursion
   e. Cardiac rate and rhythm
   f. Pain, discomfort, or dyspnea level
   g. Level of consciousness
   h. Accurate intake and output
   i. Close monitoring for progression of symptoms
2. Establish and maintain airway, oxygenation, and ventilation
   a. Calm, quiet environment
   b. Cool humidified O_2
   c. Pharmacologic therapies to decrease laryngeal edema
      1) Racemic epinephrine nebulizer: dilates larynx and decreases edema but may have a rebound effect in 60 to 90 minutes

2) Corticosteroids (e.g., dexamethasone [Decadron]) intramuscular or IV injection or nebulizer: reduces inflammation but use controversial
      3) Avoidance of sedatives, opiates, expectorants, bronchodilators, antihistamines
   d. RSI and intubation along with mechanical ventilation may be required
3. Maintain adequate circulation
   a. IV access for fluid and medication administration may be indicated
   b. Hydration
      1) Oral fluids: noncaffeinated
      2) IV fluids may be required: usually 0.9% saline
4. Monitor for/prevent complications
   a. Severe airway obstruction
   b. Acute respiratory failure
   c. Pneumomediastinum
   d. Tracheitis
   e. Laryngotracheopneumonitis

Evaluation

1. Patent airway, adequate oxygenation (i.e., normal Pao_2, Spo_2, Sao_2) and ventilation (i.e., normal $Paco_2$)
2. Absence of clinical indications of respiratory distress, especially no retractions or stridor
3. Absence of clinical indicators of hypoperfusion/ sepsis
4. Improvement in clinical indications of infection (e.g., decrease in fever)
5. Absence of clinical indications of dehydration
6. Alert and oriented with no neurologic deficit
7. Control of pain, discomfort, or dyspnea

Typical disposition

1. If evaluation criteria met: discharge with instructions
   a. Use cool humidified air
   b. Increase fluid intake
2. If evaluation criteria not met: admission to progressive care unit or critical care unit

Epiglottitis

Definition: inflammation and upper airway obstruction caused by a rapidly spreading bacterial infection of the epiglottis and the supraglottic tissues surrounding the epiglottis; includes the aryepiglottic folds, arytenoid soft tissue, and, occasionally, the uvula

Predisposing factors

1. Upper airway infection
2. Immunocompromise
3. Smoking increases risk in adults
4. Caustic or corrosive agents
5. Thermal injury from hot liquids

Pathophysiology

1. Usually caused by infection
   a. Most likely causative organisms
      1) *H. influenzae*: most likely organism in adults who did not receive H. flu vaccine
      2) β-Hemolytic streptococci

3) *S. aureus*
4) *K. pneumoniae*
5) Fungi

   b. Rapid onset of high fever and upper airway obstruction in children but may be more benign onset in adults with just severe sore throat

2. Inflammation and swelling between the base of the tongue and the epiglottis causes the throat structures to push the epiglottis backward
3. Complete blockage of the airway may occur as inflammation and swelling continue
4. Suffocation and death may occur

Clinical presentation

1. Subjective
   a. Parent report of irritability, being fussy
   b. Dyspnea
   c. Anxiety, apprehension
   d. Sore throat, dysphagia
   e. Odynophagia: pain with swallowing and eating
2. Objective
   a. Tripod position with neck extended common in pediatrics
   b. Clinical indications of respiratory distress, air hunger
   c. Stridor
   d. Hoarse or muffled voice
   e. Drooling
   f. Cough
   g. High fever >101.5°F
   h. Stridor (late finding)
   i. Toxic appearance
3. Diagnostic
   a. CBC: elevated WBCs
   b. Throat and blood cultures: positive for causative organism
   c. Lateral neck radiograph: thumbprint sign (i.e., enlarged epiglottis)
   d. Nasopharyngoscopy: direct visualization using fiberoptics shows inflamed epiglottis

Collaborative management

1. Continue assessment
   a. ABCDs
   b. Vital signs: blood pressure, pulse, respiratory rate, and temperature
   c. O_2 saturation
   d. Respiratory effort and excursion
   e. Cardiac rate and rhythm
   f. Pain, discomfort, or dyspnea level
   g. Level of consciousness
   h. Accurate intake and output
   i. Close monitoring for progression of symptoms
1. Establish and maintain airway, oxygenation, and ventilation
   a. Calm, quiet environment
   b. Cool humidified O_2
   c. Avoidance of vigorous examination of posterior pharynx because this may initiate laryngeal obstruction (Fleisher, Ludwig, & Henretig, 2006)

   d. Pharmacologic therapies to decrease airway edema
      1) Racemic epinephrine nebulizer: dilates airway and decreases edema but may have a rebound effect in 60 to 90 minutes
      2) Corticosteroids (e.g., dexamethasone [Decadron]) intramuscular or IV injection or nebulizer: reduces inflammation but use controversial
      3) Heliox: helium–O_2 mixture may be used to allow air passage through narrowed airway
      4) Avoidance of sedatives, opiates, expectorants, bronchodilators, antihistamines
   e. Emergent airway management
      1) Intubation
         a) Awake intubation with sedative such as ketamine (Ketalar) is recommended; muscle paralysis should be avoided (Walls, 2004)
         b) Should be performed by the most experienced person, preferably in the operating room
      2) Cricothyroidotomy, needle cricothyrotomy, or tracheostomy may be necessary
      3) Maintain adequate circulation
         a) IV access for fluid and medication administration may be indicated
         b) Hydration
            (i) Oral fluids: noncaffeinated
            (ii) IV fluids may be required: usually 0.9% saline
      4) Control pain, discomfort, and anxiety
         a) NSAIDs and/or narcotic analgesics in doses that will allow patient to deep breathe and cough may be indicated
         b) Anxiolytics may be indicated
      5) Treat infection (if present) and prevent sepsis
         a) Antimicrobials as indicated: empirically or specific to cultured microorganism
         b) Antipyretics and cooling methods to reduce fever
      6) Monitor for/prevent complications
         a) Upper airway obstruction and respiratory arrest
         b) Postobstructive pulmonary edema

Evaluation

1. Patent airway, adequate oxygenation (i.e., normal Pao_2, Spo_2, Sao_2) and ventilation (i.e., normal $Paco_2$)
2. Absence of clinical indications of respiratory distress
3. Absence of clinical indicators of hypoperfusion
4. Absence of clinical indications of infection/sepsis
5. Alert and oriented with no neurologic deficit
6. Control of pain, discomfort, or dyspnea

Typical disposition: admission to progressive care unit or critical care unit

1. Consultation with ENT specialist

Chest Trauma Emergencies
General Information
Types of trauma
1. Blunt trauma leaves the body surface intact
2. Penetrating trauma disrupts the body surface
3. Perforating trauma leaves both entrance and exit wounds as an object passes through the body

Etiology
1. Motor vehicle collision
2. Motorcycle collision
3. Vehicle/pedestrian collision
4. Fall
5. Assault
6. Explosion
7. Projectiles: bullet, knives, impalement

Mechanisms of injury
1. Blunt chest trauma
   a. Rapid acceleration/deceleration: shearing force causes stretching of tissue, organs, blood vessels with resultant tearing, leaking, or rupture
   b. Direct impact: object striking chest or chest striking object causes rib, sternal, or scapular fractures, injury to the heart or lung parenchyma
   c. Compression: force of rapid deceleration as tissues hit a fixed object such as the sternum or rib cage causes concussion, contusion, bleeding, or rupture of an organ
2. Penetrating chest trauma
   a. Penetration of lung, heart, great vessel, or diaphragm causes bleeding and may cause loss of intactness of an organ or vessel

Pulmonary contusion
Definition: damage to the lung parenchyma that results in localized edema and hemorrhage
Predisposing factors
1. High-velocity blunt trauma dispersed across the chest; pulmonary contusion occurs in ≈75% of blunt trauma patients
2. Crush injuries
3. Chest compressions during cardiopulmonary resuscitation
4. Frequently associated with other chest injuries (e.g., flail chest)

Pathophysiology
1. Blunt trauma causes deceleration injury to chest wall and compression of thoracic cavity
2. Diminished thoracic size compresses lung tissue resulting in capillary rupture and subsequent hemorrhage
3. Initial hemorrhage from bruising, pulmonary tears, and lacerations leads to interstitial and alveolar edema
4. Interstitial edema and inflammation causes $\dot{V}/\dot{Q}$ mismatch
5. Atelectasis develops
6. Hemothorax rated to severe pulmonary lacerations

7. Pulmonary contusion may accompany flail chest and may be masked by the obvious ventilation difficulties seen in flail chest

Clinical presentation (may be delayed 12 to 48 hours)
1. Subjective
   a. History of events leading from injury to symptoms
   b. Anxiety, restlessness
   c. Dyspnea
   d. Chest tenderness or pain
2. Objective
   a. Tachycardia
   b. Tachypnea
   c. Increased work of breathing: use of accessory muscles; tripod position, sternal or intercostal retractions
   d. Cough: nonproductive
   e. Ecchymosis or discoloration at injury site
   f. Palpation of chest: crepitus or deformity if rib fractures
   g. Subcutaneous emphysema: suggests concurrent pneumothorax or upper airway injury
   h. Percussion: dullness on affected side
   i. Breath sounds: diffuse crackles, wheezes
2. Diagnostic
   a. ABGs
      1) Decreased Pao_2
      2) $Paco_2$ may be normal or decreased depending on ventilation pattern (e.g., may be low due to hyperventilation)
   b. Chest radiograph: initially normal
      1) In 12 to 48 hours: patchy, poorly defined areas of increased parenchymal density reflecting intra-alveolar hemorrhage
      2) If severe, extensive areas of increased parenchymal density within one or both lungs
      3) To differentiate ARDS from pulmonary contusion
         a) Pulmonary contusion is usually localized and occurs near the site of external trauma
         b) ARDS causes diffuse bilateral changes
   c. CT assesses damage to pulmonary parenchyma and pleural cavity

Collaborative management
1. Continue assessment
   a. ABCDs
   b. Vital signs: blood pressure, pulse, respiratory rate, and temperature
   c. O_2 saturation
   d. Respiratory effort and excursion
   e. Cardiac rate and rhythm
   f. Pain, discomfort, or dyspnea level
   g. Level of consciousness
   h. Accurate intake and output
   i. Close monitoring for progression of symptoms
2. Establish and maintain airway, oxygenation, and ventilation

a. Positioning
1) Elevation of head of bed to 30 to 45 degrees; overbed table may be helpful for patient to lean on
2) Good lung down when in side-lying position
b. Airway with cervical spine precautions (e.g., jaw thrust) as indicated; intubation may be required
c. O_2 by nasal cannula at 2 to 6 L/min to maintain SpO_2 of 95% unless contraindicated; for patients with COPD, use pulse oximetry to guide O_2 administration to SpO_2 of 90%
3. Maintain adequate circulation
a. IV access for fluid and medication administration may be indicated
b. Hydration
1) Oral fluids: noncaffeinated
2) IV fluids may be required: usually 0.9% saline
4. Control pain and discomfort
a. NSAIDs and/or narcotic analgesics in doses that will allow patient to deep breathe and cough may be indicated
b. Anxiolytics
5. Monitor for/prevent complications
a. Pneumonia: very common complication
b. ARDS
c. Pulmonary edema
d. Pulmonary embolism
e. Lung abscess

Evaluation
1. Patent airway, adequate oxygenation (i.e., normal PaO_2, SpO_2, SaO_2) and ventilation (i.e., normal $PaCO_2$)
2. Absence of clinical indications of respiratory distress
3. Absence of clinical indicators of hypoperfusion
4. Absence of clinical indications of infection/sepsis
5. Alert and oriented with no neurologic deficit
6. Control of pain, discomfort, or dyspnea

Typical disposition
1. If evaluation criteria met: discharge with instructions and to return if respiratory distress develops
2. If evaluation criteria not met: admission to progressive care unit or critical care unit

Pneumothorax
Definition: air in pleural space causing a loss of negative pressure, which causes causing partial or total collapse of the lung (Figure 5-18)
Predisposing factors
1. Primary: related to congenital bleb (common in endomorphic males, age 20 to 40 years)
2. Secondary
a. Emphysematous bullous
b. Tuberculosis
c. Lung cancer
3. Traumatic
a. Blunt trauma caused by motor vehicle collision, falls, blows to chest, blast injuries

b. Cardiopulmonary resuscitation
c. Positive pressure mechanical ventilator
4. Iatrogenic causes: central venous catheterization via subclavian or low jugular vein puncture; intracardiac injection; thoracentesis; positive pressure ventilation

Types of pneumothorax and pathophysiology
1. Simple pneumothorax
a. Unilateral collection of air in the pleural space
b. Can be spontaneous or from trauma
c. No pressure or hemothorax in conjunction with the disease
2. Spontaneous pneumothorax
a. Occurs abruptly with no obvious trauma
b. Subpleural blebs at lung apices rupture directly into pleural space
3. Secondary pneumothorax
a. Occurs in patients with underlying pulmonary disease
b. Overdistention and rupture of an alveolus with dissection of air into the pleural space
4. Closed pneumothorax
a. Disruption of normal negative intrapleural pressure
1) Lung laceration by rib fracture or needle
2) Compression of the lung at the height of inspiration when alveolar pressure is high
3) Rupture of weak alveolus, bleb, or bullous
b. Lung collapse
c. Decreased surface area for exchange of gases
d. Acute respiratory failure
5. Open pneumothorax
a. Communication between the intrathoracic space and the atmosphere results in equilibrium between intrathoracic and atmospheric pressures
b. Air movement in and out of opening in chest wall
c. If opening in chest wall is smaller than the diameter of the trachea, patient may tolerate condition well
d. If opening is larger, more air enters pleural space than enters lungs through trachea
e. During inspiration, the affected lung collapses resulting in ineffective gas exchange
f. May cause tension pneumothorax
6. Tension pneumothorax
a. Air rushes into, but not out of, the pleural space
b. Disruption of negative intrapleural pressure; creation of a positive pressure in the pleural space
c. Ipsilateral lung collapses
d. If tear does not seal, a one-way valve effect may be produced, allowing air to enter during inspiration but not to escape during exhalation
e. Increasing positive intrapleural pressure may cause mediastinal shift leading to compression of the contralateral lung, thoracic aorta, vena cava, and heart

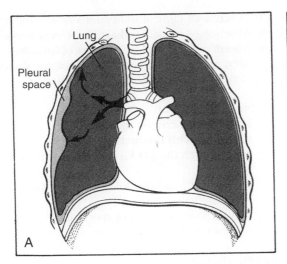
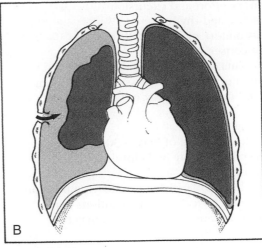
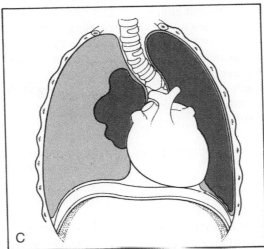

Figure 5-18 Pneumothorax. **A,** Closed. **B,** Open. **C,** Tension. (From Wilson, S. F. & Thompson, J. M. [1990]. *Respiratory disorders.* St. Louis: Mosby–Year Book.)

f. Decreased right ventricular filling, decreased cardiac output

g. Acute respiratory failure and shock may occur

Clinical presentation

1. Subjective
   a. History of injury or onset of symptoms
   b. Dyspnea
   c. Chest pain: sudden, sharp, may be referred to corresponding shoulder, across chest, or abdomen
   d. Feeling of impending doom with tension pneumothorax
2. Objective
   a. Tachycardia
   b. Tachypnea
   c. Cough: dry, nonproductive
   d. Asymmetrical chest excursion with limited motion of affected hemithorax
   e. Subcutaneous emphysema
   f. Decreased fremitus on affected side
   g. Hyperresonance to percussion on affected side
   h. Diminished to absent breath sounds on affected side

   i. Positive Hamman sign: crunching, bubbling, or crackling sound heard with each heartbeat, which indicates pneumomediastinum
3. Diagnostic
   a. ABGs: decreased Pa_{O_2}; increased Pa_{CO_2}
   b. Chest radiograph
      1) Air in pleural space and lung collapse on affected side
      2) Absence of lung marking
      3) Widening of the intercostal spaces on the affected side and mediastinal shift toward unaffected side in tension pneumothorax (late)
   c. CT of chest: to detect small or anterior pneumothorax, which may be missed on chest radiograph

Collaborative management

1. Continue assessment
   a. ABCDs
   b. Vital signs: blood pressure, pulse, respiratory rate, and temperature
   c. O_2 saturation

d. Respiratory effort and excursion

e. Cardiac rate and rhythm

f. Pain, discomfort, or dyspnea level

g. Level of consciousness

h. Accurate intake and output

i. Close monitoring for progression of symptoms

2. Establish and maintain airway, oxygenation, and ventilation

  a. Positioning

    1) Elevation of head of bed to 30 to 45 degrees; overbed table may be helpful for patient to lean on

    2) Good lung down when in side-lying position

  b. Airway with cervical spine precautions (e.g., jaw thrust) as indicated; intubation may be required

  c. O_2 by nasal cannula at 2 to 6 L/min to maintain SpO_2 of 95% unless contraindicated; for patients with COPD, use pulse oximetry to guide O_2 administration to SpO_2 of 90%

  d. Assistance with procedures as indicated

    1) If patient is in immediate distress from tension pneumothorax: immediate needle decompression during primary assessment followed by insertion of chest tube

    2) Chest tube placement

      a) Inserted into fourth to fifth intercostal space at midaxillary line

      b) Connected to a Heimlich flutter valve or chest drainage system

      c) Close open pneumothorax with a Vaseline gauze dressing taped on three sides so that air can escape during expiration; if a tension pneumothorax develops after application of the dressing, remove it to relieve tension and then reapply dressing

      d) Surgical intervention may be needed

3. Maintain adequate circulation

  a. IV access for fluid and medication administration may be indicated

  b. Hydration

    1) Oral fluids: noncaffeinated

    2) IV fluids may be required: usually 0.9% saline

4. Control pain, discomfort, and anxiety

  a. NSAIDs and/or narcotic analgesics in doses that will allow patient to deep breathe and cough may be indicated

  b. Anxiolytics may be indicated

5. Administer tetanus immunization as indicated

6. Monitor for/prevent complications

  a. Atelectasis

  b. Pneumonia, abscess

  c. Tension pneumothorax may result from open pneumothorax

  d. Mediastinal shift, damage to great vessels, and shock

  e. Cardiopulmonary arrest

Evaluation

1. Patent airway, adequate oxygenation (i.e., normal PaO_2, SpO_2, SaO_2) and ventilation (i.e., normal $PaCO_2$)

2. Absence of clinical indications of respiratory distress

3. Absence of clinical indicators of hypoperfusion

4. Absence of clinical indications of infection/sepsis

5. Alert and oriented with no neurologic deficit

6. Control of pain, discomfort, or dyspnea

Typical disposition

1. If evaluation criteria met (e.g., small pneumothorax): discharge with instructions

  a. Return to the ED for increased pain or shortness of breath

  b. Follow up as scheduled with primary care or specialist

2. If evaluation criteria not met: admission to progressive care unit or critical care unit

Hemothorax

Definition: accumulation of blood in pleural space causing compression and collapse of the lung; usually the result of injury to the chest wall vessels (e.g., intercostals or internal mammary) or great vessels

Precipitating factors

1. Blunt or penetrating trauma to chest wall, lung tissue, or mediastinum; often associated with rib fractures or flail chest

2. Pleural or pulmonary neoplasm

3. Anticoagulant therapy

4. Iatrogenic causes: subclavian vein puncture (e.g., insertion of deep vein catheter), lung biopsy

Pathophysiology

1. Hemorrhage into pleural space compresses and collapses lung

2. Bleeding into the pleural space can occur with virtually any disruption of the tissues of the chest wall and pleura or the intrathoracic structures

3. Ventilation and oxygenation are impaired by the space-occupying effect of a large accumulation of blood within the pleural space

4. A massive hemothorax (≥ 1500 ml) can lead to mediastinal shifting, decreased venous return, decreased cardiac output, and hypotension

5. Hemorrhage may lead to shock

Clinical presentation

1. Subjective

  a. History of trauma

  b. Pain that increases with breathing

  c. Dyspnea

2. Objective

  a. Tachycardia

  b. Tachypnea

  c. Asymmetrical chest wall movement with limited excursion on affected side

  d. Chest ecchymosis

  e. Chest wall deformity

  f. Dullness to percussion on affected side

  g. Breath sound changes: diminished or absent on affected side

h. May have clinical indications of shock if 1000 ml loss

3. Diagnostic
   a. CBC with differential: decreased Hgb and Hct
   b. ABGs: decreased Pao_2, increased $Paco_2$
   c. Cervical spine radiograph: to detect cervical injury
   d. Chest radiograph
      1) Air-fluid level in pleural space and lung compression
      2) Blunting of costophrenic angle if >250 ml
      3) Hazy appearance over the lower chest

Collaborative management

1. Continue assessment
   a. ABCDs
   b. O_2 saturation
   c. Respiratory rate and effort
   d. Cardiac rate and rhythm
   e. Discomfort and pain level
   f. Level of consciousness
   g. Accurate intake and output
   h. Close monitoring for progression of symptoms
2. Establish and maintain airway, oxygenation, and ventilation
   a. Positioning
      1) Elevation of head of bed to 30 to 45 degrees if tolerated; if blood pressure decreases or heart rate increases, lower the head of the bed
      2) Good lung down when in side-lying position
   b. Airway with cervical spine precautions (e.g., jaw thrust) as indicated; intubation may be required
   c. O_2 by nasal cannula at 2-6 L/min to maintain Spo_2 of 95% unless contraindicated, for patients with COPD, use pulse oximetry to guide O_2 administration to Spo_2 of 90%
   d. Procedures as indicated
      1) Chest tube with chest drainage system may be adequate treatment if bleeding is self-limiting
      2) If drainage >than 1,000 ml of blood after placement of chest tube or more than 250 ml/hour for more than 3-4 hours, thoracotomy may be indicated
      3) Autotransfusion as indicated: transfusion of patient's blood that has been collected via the chest drainage system and filtered
3. Maintain adequate circulation
   a. IV access for fluid and medication administration may be indicated
   b. Type and crossmatch; blood administration may be required
   c. IV fluids: usually 0.9% saline
   d. Avoidance of overhydration which may contribute to ARDS
4. Control pain, discomfort, and anxiety
   a. NSAIDs and/or narcotic analgesics in doses that will allow patient to deep breathe and cough may be indicated
   b. Anxiolytics may be indicated
5. Administer tetanus immunization as indicated

6. Monitor for indications of other injuries
   a. Fracture of the first or second rib requires extreme force and underlying organs can be damaged
   b. Splenic injury may accompany left lower rib fractures
   c. Hepatic injury may accompany right lower rib fractures
7. Monitor for/prevent complications
   a. Atelectasis
   b. Pneumonia, abscess
   c. Tension pneumothorax may result from open pneumothorax
   d. Mediastinal shift, damage to great vessels, and shock
   e. Cardiopulmonary arrest

Evaluation

1. Patent airway, adequate oxygenation (i.e., normal Pao_2, Spo_2, Sao_2) and ventilation (i.e., normal $Paco_2$)
2. Absence of clinical indications of respiratory distress
3. Absence of clinical indicators of hypoperfusion
4. Absence of clinical indications of infection/sepsis
5. Alert and oriented with no neurologic deficit
6. Control of pain, discomfort, or dyspnea

Typical disposition: admission

1. May require critical care unit admission
2. May require direct admission to surgery from the ED

Rib fracture/sternal fracture/flail chest
Definitions

1. Rib fracture: break in the bony continuity of the ribs
2. Sternal fracture: break in the bony continuity of the sternum
3. Flail chest: instability of chest wall as a result of multiple rib or sternal fractures causing paradoxical movement of the chest wall during ventilation
   a. Two or more ribs broken in two or more places
   b. Fractured sternum
   c. Sternotomy that has not healed

Precipitating factors

1. Blunt trauma from motor vehicle crash, assault
2. Relatively minor trauma in patients with the following:
   a. Osteoporosis
   b. Total sternectomy
   c. Multiple myeloma

Pathophysiology

1. Rib fracture
   a. Fracture of the first and second rib is rare and requires extreme force so suspect underlying injury to great vessel, lungs, and spine
   b. Left lower rib fractures suspect spleen injuries
   c. Right lower rib fractures suspect hepatic injury
   d. The thorax is more cartilaginous in children so rib fracture is less common but an indication of concurrent thoracic or abdominal injuries if they are present

e. Older adult patients are more likely to have complications because they are likely to have senile emphysema and concurrent cardiopulmonary disease

2. Sternal fracture
   a. Tremendous force (i.e., impact with steering wheel) required to cause sternal fracture
      1) This force may also cause myocardial contusion or cardiac tamponade
   b. Most common location is the junction of the manubrium and body of the sternum

3. Flail chest (Figure 5-19)
   a. Fractured segment is free of the bony thorax and moves independently in response to intrathoracic pressure
      1) During inspiration, atmospheric pressure exceeds intrathoracic pressure on affected side causing chest wall to move inward
      2) On expiration, intrathoracic pressure exceeds atmospheric causing chest wall to move outward until the thorax contracts

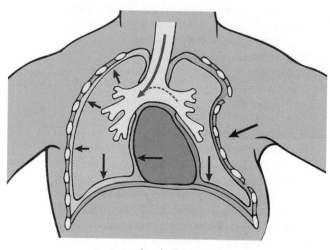

Inspiration

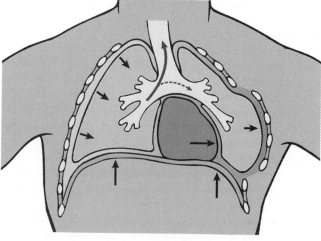

Expiration

Figure 5-19 Flail chest produces paradoxical chest excursion. On inspiration, the flail section sinks in. On expiration, the flail section bulges outward.

b. The bellows effect of the thorax is lost, intrapleural pressure is less negative than normal
c. Ventilation is diminished; tidal volume is decreased causing hypercapnia and resultant hypoxemia; atelectasis may occur
d. Increased work of breathing causes fatigue
e. Note related injuries: pulmonary contusion frequently accompanies flail chest; pneumothorax, pleural effusion may also be present

Clinical presentation

1. Subjective
   a. History of injury
   b. Dyspnea
   c. Excruciating pain with inspiration, coughing, and movement
2. Objective
   a. Tachycardia
   b. Tachypnea
   c. Ecchymosis over thorax
   d. Paradoxical movement of flail segment in flail chest
   e. Subcutaneous emphysema with pneumothorax or laryngeal injury
   f. Tenderness and crepitus or deformity with palpation
   g. Breath sound changes: diminished breath sounds on affected side
   h. Clinical indications of hypoxia (see Box 5-2)
3. Diagnostic
   a. ABGs: decreased Pao_2, increased $Paco_2$
   b. ECG: to assess for indications of myocardial contusion if sternal fracture
   c. Echocardiography: to assess for cardiac tamponade if sternal fracture
   d. Chest radiograph: rib and/or sternal fractures
   e. CT of chest: shows fractures

Collaborative management

1. Continue assessment
   a. ABCDs
   b. Vital signs: blood pressure, pulse, respiratory rate, and temperature
   c. O_2 saturation
   d. Respiratory effort and excursion
   e. Cardiac rate and rhythm
   f. Pain, discomfort, or dyspnea level
   g. Level of consciousness
   h. Accurate intake and output
   i. Close monitoring for progression of symptoms
2. Establish and maintain airway, oxygenation, and ventilation
   a. Airway with cervical spine precautions (e.g., jaw thrust) as indicated; intubation may be required
   b. O_2 by nasal cannula at 2-6 L/min to maintain Spo_2 of 95% unless contraindicated; for patients with COPD, use pulse oximetry to guide O_2 administration to Spo_2 of 90%

c. Positioning on affected side if cervical spine fracture has been ruled out

d. Stabilization of fracture
   1) Stabilization of flail segment with hand or tape (temporary); avoid binding or constricting chest excursion
   2) Internal fixation with plates and screws may be required for multiple rib fractures or massive flail chest
   3) Surgical reduction of displaced sternal fracture
   e) Deep breathing and incentive spirometry to prevent atelectasis

3. Maintain adequate circulation
   a. IV access for fluid and medication administration
   b. Hydration:
      1) IV fluids: usually 0.9% saline
      2) Avoidance of overhydration because the patient may have associated pulmonary contusion and at risk for ARDS

4. Control pain, discomfort, and anxiety
   a. NSAIDs and/or narcotic analgesics in doses that will allow patient to deep breathe and cough may be indicated
   b. Anxiolytics may be indicated

5. Administer tetanus immunization as indicated

6. Monitor for/prevent complications
   a. Atelectasis
   b. Pneumonia
   c. Acute respiratory failure
   d. Myocardial infarction (in sternal fracture)
   e. Cardiac tamponade (in sternal fracture)

Evaluation

1. Patent airway, adequate oxygenation (i.e., normal PaO_2, SpO_2, SaO_2) and ventilation (i.e., normal $PaCO_2$)
2. Absence of clinical indications of respiratory distress
3. Absence of clinical indications of infection/sepsis
4. Stable hemodynamic status
5. Alert and oriented with no neurologic deficit
6. Control of pain and discomfort

Typical disposition

1. If evaluation criteria met: discharge with prescription for analgesics and follow-up
2. If evaluation criteria not met: admission to progressive care unit or critical care unit (especially is flail chest or sternal fracture)

Diaphragmatic Rupture

Definition: a sudden, dramatic increase in abdominal or thoracic pressure causes a tear in the diaphragm

Predisposing factors: injury below nipple line, in flanks, or lateral chest wall

1. Blunt trauma: MVC, assault, fall against a immobile object
2. Penetrating injury (e.g., gunshot or stab wound)
3. Often associated with other injuries

Pathophysiology

1. The intrathoracic pressure is negative while the intra-abdominal pressure is positive
2. Rupture of the diaphragm allowing the movement of abdominal contents into the thorax
   a. More common on the left side because the left hemidiaphragm is weaker than the right and the right hemidiaphragm is somewhat protected by the liver
   b. Penetrating trauma may cause a perforation in the diaphragm
3. The size of the rupture determines the extent to which the organs migrate upward: the stomach and/ or loops of intestine may enter the chest and compromise lung expansion
   a. Abdominal contents compress the lung on the affected side and may even cause mediastinal shift
   b. The decrease in the effectiveness of the diaphragm causes ineffective ventilatory excursion
4. Ventilation problems are most evident if the left hemidiaphragm is affected since when the right hemidiaphragm is affected, the liver is fixed and cannot move upward into the thorax

Clinical presentation

1. Subjective
   a. History of traumatic event; may be concurrent with hemothorax, pneumothorax, or intra-abdominal hemorrhage
   b. Pain in shoulder, chest or abdomen
      1) Kehr sign: pain radiates to left shoulder
   c. Dyspnea
   d. Dysphagia
   e. Nausea, eructation
2. Objective
   a. Obvious injury to chest, abdomen
   b. Ecchymosis
   c. Tachypnea, tachycardia, hypotension
   d. Palpation: crepitus or deformity
   e. Heart sounds: shifting to opposite side of the injury
   f. Breath sound changes: diminished or absent breath sounds on affected side
   g. Bowel sounds audible in chest over the affected side
   h. If chest tubes are placed for another condition, may see fecal matter or undigested food in the chest drainage system
3. Diagnostic
   a. Chest radiograph
      1) Normal if no abdominal contents displaced in chest
      2) May have unilateral elevation of hemidiaphragm
      3) May have hollow or solid mass above the diaphragm (the stomach) that may be visible
      4) May have mediastinal shift away from affected side
      5) May place nasogastric tube prior to radiography and tube will be seen in the chest

b. CT of the chest and abdomen
1) Confirms rupture of the diaphragm and any movement of abdominal contents into the thorax
2) Focused assessment sonography trauma (FAST): indicates whether intra-abdominal fluid present

Collaborative management

1. Continue assessment
   a. ABCDs
   b. Vital signs: blood pressure, pulse, respiratory rate, and temperature
   c. O_2 saturation
   d. Respiratory effort and excursion
   e. Cardiac rate and rhythm
   f. Pain, discomfort, or dyspnea level
   g. Level of consciousness
   h. Accurate intake and output
   i. Close monitoring for progression of symptoms
2. Establish and maintain airway, oxygenation, and ventilation
   a. Airway with cervical spine precautions (e.g., jaw thrust) as indicated; intubation may be required
   b. O_2 by nasal cannula at 2 to 6 L/min to maintain SpO_2 of 95% unless contraindicated; for patients with COPD, use pulse oximetry to guide O_2 administration to SpO_2 of 90%
   c. Elevation of head of bed to 30 to 45 degrees; over-bed table may be helpful for patient to lean on
   d. Surgical repair to pull the abdominal organs back into the abdomen and repair the diaphragm
   e. Deep breathing and incentive spirometry to prevent atelectasis
3. Maintain adequate circulation
   a. IV access for fluid and medication administration
   b. Hydration
      1) IV fluids: usually 0.9% saline
      2) Avoidance of overhydration because the patient may have associated pulmonary contusion and at risk for ARDS
4. Control pain, discomfort, and anxiety
   a. NSAIDs and/or narcotic analgesics in doses that will allow patient to deep breathe and cough may be indicated
   b. Anxiolytics may be indicated
5. Treat infection (if present) and prevent sepsis
   a. Antimicrobials as indicated: empirically or specific to cultured microorganism
   b. Antipyretics and cooling methods to reduce fever
6. Assist/perform procedures
   a. Conscious sedation may be done prior to procedures
   b. Chest tube and drainage system as required for pneumothorax
   c. Nasogastric tube placement to decompress the stomach
   d. Foley catheter to monitor urine output

7. Administer tetanus immunization as indicated
8. Monitor for/prevent complications
   a. Atelectasis
   b. Bowel strangulation
   c. Sepsis
   d. Shock

Evaluation

1. Patent airway, adequate oxygenation (i.e., normal PaO_2, SpO_2, SaO_2) and ventilation (i.e., normal $PaCO_2$)
2. Absence of clinical indications of respiratory distress
3. Absence of clinical indicators of hypoperfusion
4. Absence of clinical indications of infection/sepsis
5. Alert and oriented with no neurologic deficit
6. Control of pain, discomfort, or dyspnea

Typical disposition: admission; prepare patient for surgical repair

Tracheobronchial Injury

Definition: disruption in the integrity of the tracheobronchial tree; usually occurs at the proximal trachea or near the carina

Predisposing factors

1. Blunt trauma (e.g., motor vehicle crashes, clothesline injury): most common cause resulting in a partial or complete tear of the tracheal or bronchial wall
2. Deceleration injuries: can cause shearing forces between the fixed carina or proximal bronchus
3. Rapid anteroposterior compression of the chest: can cause lateral traction on the lungs resulting in a tearing of the bronchus from the fixed carina
   a. Rupture can occur from an abrupt increase in pressure against a closed glottis
4. Compression of the trachea between the sternum and spinal column
5. Penetrating trauma

Pathophysiology

1. Injury causes a tear of the bronchial tree
2. Ineffective ventilation as inspired air escapes into the thoracic cavity and does not reach the lungs
3. Swelling can cause airway obstruction
4. Severity of symptoms related to the level of the injury, degree of injury, and airflow changes that occur

Clinical presentation

1. Subjective
   a. History of trauma; injury to may go unrecognized for 3 to 4 days
   b. Pain that increases with breathing and swallowing
   c. Dyspnea
2. Objective
   a. Tachycardia
   b. Tachypnea
   c. Clinical indications of respiratory distress (see Box 5-1)
      1) Sitting up and leaning forward
      2) Use of inspiratory accessory muscles in neck and shoulders

d. Hoarse voice

e. May have stridor

f. Hemoptysis

g. Chest contusion, ecchymosis, or wound

h. Altered level of consciousness

i. Subcutaneous emphysema palpated in the chest, face, neck, and /or suprasternal area

j. Breath sound changes: decreased or absent on the affected side

k. Hamman sign: mediastinal crunch associated with pneumomediastinum

l. Persistent air leak from chest tube

3. Diagnostic

a. ABGs: may show hypoxemia

b. Radiography

1) Soft tissue lateral neck films

2) Chest: pneumomediastinum below the carina

c. Bronchoscopy: direct visualization of injury

Collaborative management

1. Continue assessment

a. ABCDs

b. Vital signs: blood pressure, pulse, respiratory rate, and temperature

c. O_2 saturation

d. Respiratory effort and excursion

e. Cardiac rate and rhythm

f. Pain, discomfort, or dyspnea level

g. Level of consciousness

h. Accurate intake and output

i. Close monitoring for progression of symptoms

2. Establish and maintain airway, oxygenation, and ventilation

a. Once tracheobronchial injury confirmed, prepare for rapid-sequence intubation and intubate even if no evidence of respiratory compromise

1) Placement of ET tube below the level of injury

2) Cricothyrotomy or emergent tracheostomy may be required

b. O_2 by nasal cannula at 2 to 6 L/min to maintain Spo_2 of 95% unless contraindicated; for patients with COPD, use pulse oximetry to guide O_2 administration to Spo_2 of 90%

c. Elevation of head of bed to 30 to 45 degrees

d. Open chest wounds should be covered; remove if clinical indications of tension pneumothorax occur

e. Thoracotomy for surgical repair

f. Deep breathing and incentive spirometry to prevent atelectasis

3. Maintain adequate circulation

a. IV access for fluid and medication administration

b. Hydration

1) IV fluids: usually 0.9% saline

2) Warming of fluids, especially if patient is hypothermic

4. Control pain, discomfort, and anxiety

a. NSAIDs and/or narcotic analgesics in doses that will allow patient to deep breathe and cough may be indicated

b. Anxiolytics may be indicated

5. Assist/perform procedures

a. Conscious sedation may be done prior to procedures

b. Chest tube and drainage system as required for pneumothorax

c. Nasogastric tube placement to decompress the stomach

d. Foley catheter to monitor urine output

6. Administer tetanus immunization as indicated

7. Monitor for/prevent complications

a. Airway obstruction

b. Acute respiratory failure

c. Shock

Evaluation

1. Patent airway, adequate oxygenation (i.e., normal Pao_2, Spo_2, Sao_2) and ventilation (i.e., normal $Paco_2$)

2. Absence of clinical indications of respiratory distress

3. Absence of clinical indicators of hypoperfusion

4. Absence of clinical indications of infection/sepsis

5. Alert and oriented with no neurologic deficit

6. Control of pain, discomfort, or dyspnea

Typical disposition: admission; prepare patient for surgical repair

LEARNING ACTIVITIES

1. DIRECTIONS: Complete the following crossword puzzle related to respiratory emergencies.

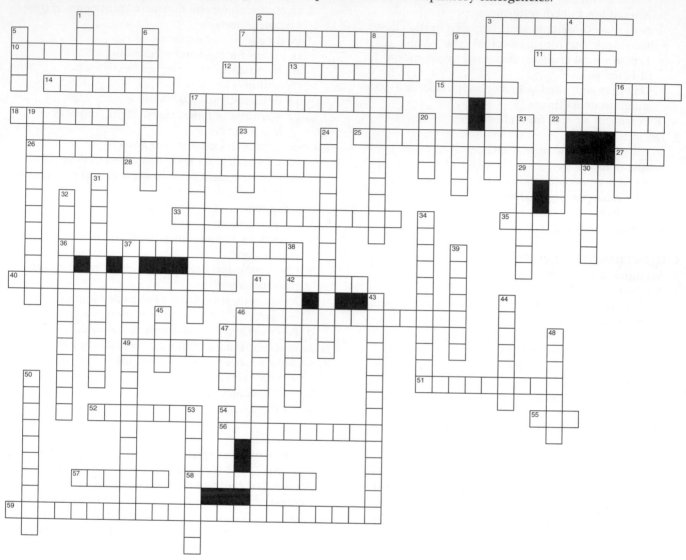

ACROSS

3. A β_2-stimulant that is administered orally or by inhalation

7. A surgical procedure to create an opening in the trachea

10. The ability of the lungs to snap back to their original position; decreased in COPD

11. The combination of pressure support ventilation and CPAP

12. The most likely cause of this syndrome is anxiety (abbreviation)

13. This triad describes factors that contribute to clotting, DVT, and, potentially, PE (possessive)

14. A risk of high concentrations of O_2 is O_2 _____

15. A forceful expiration to expel mucus from the lungs

16. An expiratory maneuver used in a spontaneously breathing patient to decrease shunt and increase the driving pressure of O_2 (abbreviation)

17. This type of airway should not be used in conscious patients because it would trigger the gag reflex

18. A type of O_2 mask which ensures a desired O_2 concentration

22. This sign is associated with pneumomediastinum (possessive)

25. A β_2-stimulant that may be given orally, subcutaneously, or by inhalation (generic)

26. This reflex is protective and most likely to occur in children and when submersion is in cold water

27. A mechanical ventilation mode that allows the patient to breath between the mandatory breaths (abbreviation)

28. This type of O_2 mask delivers the highest O_2 concentration

29. The smallest portion of a child's airway

33. This results from lysis of RBCs that may occur in freshwater drowning
35. This virus is the most common cause of bronchiolitis (abbreviation)
36. This group of drugs includes β_2-adrenergic agents, anticholinergic agents, xanthines, and magnesium
40. This type of airway may be used in conscious patients to hold the tongue away from the hypopharynx

42. This condition may be confused with epiglottis
46. A function normally performed by the upper airway that must be included in the care of a patient with an artificial airway
49. Hyperventilation causes an imbalance of this electrolyte
51. The component of COPD characterized by significant dyspnea, especially with exertion

52. This type of O_2 delivery system is comfortable for patients but provides up to only 40% O_2 concentration
55. This type of embolism may occur with deep sea diving
56. Avoidance of vigorous examination of the posterior pharynx may cause airway obstruction in this condition
57. This type of asthma is when the attack has lasted 24 hours even with maximal therapy

58. _____ drainage is a method of bronchial hygiene that uses gravity to drain secretions into the upper airway so that they can be coughed out
59. This condition is characterized by a Pao_2 <50 to 60 mm Hg and/or $Paco_2$ >50 mm Hg with pH <7.30 (three words)

DOWN

1. This type of embolism is associated with petechiae and confusion
2. This condition is characterized by decreased lung compliance, intrapulmonary shunt, and refractory hypoxemia (abbreviation)
3. Group of drugs that should be administered to allow a patient to breathe deeply after thoracotomy
4. This condition is characterized by pus in the pleural space
5. One method of ensuring that cuff pressure is not excessive is the minimal _____ technique
6. A machine that pushes air into the lungs to inflate them
8. A diagnostic study to obtain fluid from the pleural space for analysis
9. A complication of mechanical ventilation; risk is increased when large tidal volumes or peep are used
16. This toxic gas is produced by burning synthetic materials

17. Sao_2, Hgb, and cardiac output all affect this parameter (two words)
19. This type of airway provides a relative seal to allow mechanical ventilation without the surgical risks of tracheostomy
20. A device attached to an ET tube or tracheostomy that provides a relative seal for mechanical ventilation and airway protection
21. A method of airway clearance that uses tapping with cupped hands to loosen secretions
22. A gas that may be used in place of nitrogen in inspired air for patients with increased airway resistance
23. An expiratory maneuver used in a mechanically ventilated patient to decrease shunt and increase the driving pressure of O_2 (abbreviation)
24. This toxic gas is produced by combustion of organic material (2 words)
30. Indicated when Sao_2 is <90%

31. Xanthine bronchodilator; also dilates pulmonary vasculature (generic)
32. This occurs from muscle destruction and may cause acute renal failure
34. Intubated patients identify their major stressor as the inability to _____
37. The component of COPD characterized by cough with mucus production (two words)
38. A method of airway clearance used if the patient cannot effectively cough; used only when indicated
39. Placing a patient with an air embolism in a left lateral decubitus position with his head down is referred to as _____ maneuver (possessive)
41. The less severe end of the spectrum of the pulmonary component of SIRS (three words)
43. A drug that breaks down the disulfide bonds in mucus (generic)
44. Testing sputum for _____ _ is a common method to check for aspiration of enteral feeding

45. The most common cause of epiglottis in adults (abbreviation)
47. Type of heparin that may be administered subcutaneously to prevent deep vein thrombosis and pulmonary embolism (abbreviation)
48. A drug used to prevent extension or recurrence of a clot in patients with pulmonary embolism (generic)
50. The change in volume for a given change in pressure or expansibility of the lung; decreased in ARDS
53. A drug used in patients with pulmonary embolism with acute right ventricular failure or refractory hypoxemia to break down the clot (generic)
54. This sign is pain referred to the left shoulder that may occur in diaphragmatic rupture (possessive)

2. DIRECTIONS: Identify whether the following factors cause a shift of the oxyhemoglobin curve to the left or right.

	Left	Right
Increased 2,3-DPG		
Hypothermia		
Hypercapnia		
Hyperthermia		
Acidosis		
Decreased 2,3-DPG		
Hypocapnia		
Alkalosis		
Hypophosphatemia		
Massive blood transfusion		

3. DIRECTIONS: Identify the primary breath sound change that occurs in the following conditions.

Condition	Breath Sound Change or Changes
Emphysema	
Atelectasis	
Pneumonia	
Chronic bronchitis	
Pneumothorax	
Pulmonary fibrosis	
Asthma	
Pulmonary edema	
Pleurisy	
Hemothorax	
Pleural effusion	
Pulmonary embolism	

4. DIRECTIONS: Analyze the following arterial blood gases. Identify any acid-base imbalance, any partial or total compensation, and the presence of hypoxemia. Assume all patients to be younger than 60 years.

	pH	$Paco_2$	HCO_3^-	Pao_2	Answer
1.	7.30	54	26	64	
2.	7.48	30	24	96	
3.	7.30	40	18	85	
4.	7.50	40	33	92	
5.	7.35	54	30	55	
6.	7.21	60	20	48	
7.	7.54	25	30	95	

5. DIRECTIONS: Match the O_2 delivery system with the O_2 concentration range that it can deliver. Choices may be used more than once.

___1. Nasal cannula	a. 21% to 100%
___2. Simple face mask	b. 24% to 40%
___3. Partial rebreathing mask	c. 24% to 44%
___4. Nonrebreathing mask	d. 35% to 60%
___5. Venturi mask	e. 40% to 60%
	f. 60% to 80%

6. DIRECTIONS: Identify the type of artificial airway in each of the following situations. More than one may be listed.

Problem	Preferred Artificial Airway
Tongue against hypopharynx	
Need for frequent nasotracheal suctioning	
Inability to open mouth (e.g., seizure)	
Facial or jaw fracture	
Complete upper airway obstruction when endotracheal intubation is impossible (e.g., laryngeal edema or spasm, tracheal fracture)	
Need for sealed airway (e.g., mechanical ventilation or potential for aspiration)	
Need for long-term lower airway access and sealed airway	

7. DIRECTIONS: List at least five age-related differences important to know when working with respiratory emergencies.

Pediatric	Older Adult
a.	f.
b.	g.
c.	h.
d.	i.
e.	j.

8. DIRECTIONS: Match the sentence on the left with the type of ventilation listed on the right. Types of ventilation may be used more than once.

_____1. uses a mask that fits over the nose, or over both nose and mouth. _____2. is more costly than other types of ventilation. _____3. Facial trauma is a contraindication for. _____4. may be the most effective type of NIV. _____5. should be used with the claustrophobic patient. _____6. is contraindicated in respiratory arrest. _____7. can be used with PEEP. _____8. provides support for both inspiration and expiration. _____9. does not directly provide respiratory assistance. _____10. is the choice intervention in patients with a need for assistance to protect their airway. _____11. may decrease sedation requirements.	a. Invasive ventilation b. BiPAP c. CPAP d. Noninvasive ventilation

9. DIRECTIONS: List five pulmonary and five nonpulmonary causes for acute respiratory distress syndrome (ARDS).

Pulmonary	Nonpulmonary
a.	f.
b.	g.
c.	h.
d.	I.
e.	j.

10. DIRECTIONS: Match the pathophysiology to the treatment of ARDS. Choices may be used more than once.

____ 1. Pulmonary hypertension	a. PEEP
____ 2. Intrapulmonary shunt	b. Fluid restriction and diuretics
____ 3. Diffusion defect	c. High concentrations of O_2
____ 4. Pulmonary edema	
____ 5. Ventilation/perfusion ($\dot{V}/\dot{Q}$) mismatch	

11. DIRECTIONS: Match the pathology to the treatment in pulmonary embolism. More than one choice may be used.

____ 1. Pulmonary hypertension	a. Embolectomy
____ 2. Occlusion of pulmonary blood supply	b. Heparin
____ 3. Low levels of antithrombin III	c. Tissue plasminogen activator (tPA)

12. DIRECTIONS: Match the clinical presentation to the type of chest trauma.

____ 1. Chest pain, dyspnea, diminished breath sounds on affected side, hyperresonance to percussion, tracheal shift away from affected side	a. Pulmonary contusion
____ 2. Chest pain, dyspnea, diminished breath sounds on affected side, hyperresonance to percussion, tracheal shift toward affected side	b. Flail chest
____ 3. Ecchymosis at site of impact, chest tenderness, dyspnea, hemoptysis	c. Simple pneumothorax
____ 4. Epigastric pain, dyspnea, dysphagia, bowel sounds audible over affected side of chest	d. Hemothorax
____ 5. Chest pain, dyspnea, diminished breath sounds on affected side, dullness to percussion	e. Tension pneumothorax
____ 6. Chest tenderness, dyspnea, paradoxical chest movement	f. Diaphragmatic rupture

LEARNING ACTIVITIES ANSWERS

1.

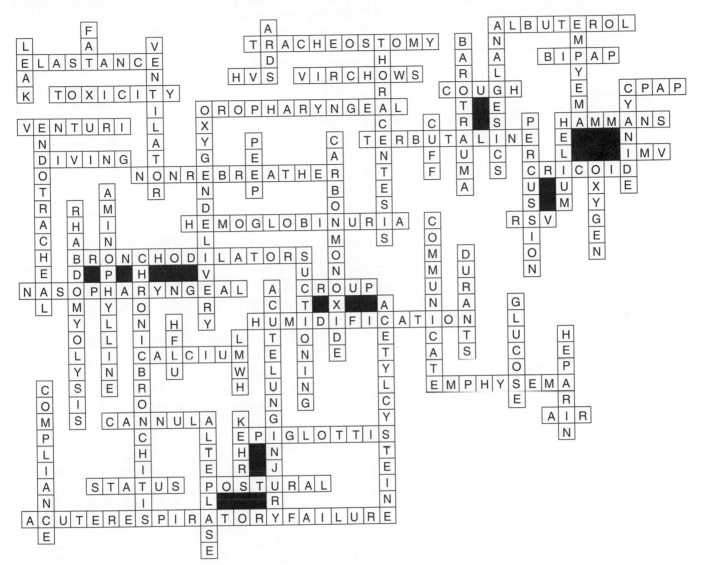

2.

	Left	Right
Increased 2,3-DPG		X
Hypothermia	X	
Hypercapnia		X
Hyperthermia		X
Acidosis		X
Decreased 2,3-DPG	X	
Hypocapnia	X	
Alkalosis	X	
Hypophosphatemia	X	
Massive blood transfusion	X	

3.

Condition	Breath Sound Change or Changes
Emphysema	Diminished breath sounds
Atelectasis	Diminished breath sounds Bronchial or bronchovesicular breath sounds Crackles
Pneumonia	Diminished breath sounds Bronchial or bronchovesicular breath sounds
Chronic bronchitis	Rhonchi Wheezes may also be present
Pneumothorax	Diminished or absent breath sounds
Pulmonary fibrosis	Diminished breath sounds Crackles
Asthma	Wheezes Rhonchi
Pulmonary edema	Crackles Wheezes (referred to as *cardiac asthma*) may be present
Pleurisy	Pleural friction rub
Hemothorax	Diminished or absent breath sounds
Pleural effusion	Diminished breath sounds
Pulmonary embolism	Crackles Pleural friction rub if pulmonary infarction develops

4.

	pH	$Paco_2$	HCO_3^-	Pao_2	Answer
1.	7.30	54	26	64	Respiratory acidosis with mild hypoxemia
2.	7.48	30	24	96	Respiratory alkalosis
3.	7.30	40	18	85	Metabolic acidosis
4.	7.50	40	33	92	Metabolic alkalosis
5.	7.35	54	30	55	Compensated respiratory acidosis with moderate hypoxemia
6.	7.21	60	20	48	Mixed disorder: respiratory and metabolic acidosis with critical hypoxemia
7.	7.54	25	30	95	Mixed disorder: respiratory alkalosis and metabolic alkalosis

5.

1. c
2. e
3. d
4. f
5. b

6.

Problem	Preferred Artificial Airway
Tongue against hypopharynx	Oropharyngeal or nasopharyngeal
Need for frequent nasotracheal suctioning	Nasopharyngeal
Inability to open mouth (e.g., seizure)	Nasopharyngeal
Facial or jaw fracture	Nasopharyngeal or nasotracheal tube
Complete upper airway obstruction when endotracheal intubation is impossible (e.g., laryngeal edema or spasm, tracheal fracture)	Cricothyrotomy or tracheostomy
Need for sealed airway (e.g., mechanical ventilation or potential for aspiration)	Endotracheal tube or tracheostomy LMA but less protection from aspiration
Need for long-term lower airway access and sealed airway	Tracheostomy

7.

Pediatric	Older Adult
Airway resistance in infants is 15 times greater than in adults	Dilatation of alveoli, enlargement of airspaces, decrease in exchange surface area and loss of supporting tissue for peripheral airways result in decreased static elastic recoil of the lung, and increased residual volume and functional residual capacity
Larynx high and anterior; vocal cords have lower attachments	
Smallest portion of airway is at the cricoid (patient younger than 10 years)	Compliance of the chest wall diminishes, thereby increasing work of breathing
Infants under 6 months of age are obligate nose breathers; keep nares clear of secretions	Respiratory muscle strength also decreases with aging and strongly correlated with nutritional status
Tongue is large the most common cause of airway obstruction in children	Ventilation perfusion ($\dot{V}/\dot{Q}$) ratio increases with aging causing a low $\dot{V}/\dot{Q}$ zone as a result of premature closing of dependent airways
Young infants have relatively less O_2 reserve (greater O_2 consumption), so hypoxemia occurs relatively more rapidly	
Infant head is relatively larger and naturally flexed in supine position	Carbon monoxide transfer decreases with age due to loss of surface area
Extension of head may cause tracheal extubation	Decreased sensitivity of respiratory centers to hypoxia or hypercapnia results in a diminished ventilatory response when illness present (e.g., heart failure, infection)
Flexion of head may lead to mainstem intubation	
Pliable chest wall: compensate with use of accessory muscles	Decreased perception of bronchoconstriction along with diminished physical activity may decrease awareness of disease and delay diagnosis and treatment
Accessory muscles of inspiration tire quickly because of less reserve glycogen	
Diaphragm is the main muscle used for inspiration; therefore, injury or restriction of the diaphragm can compromise respiratory status	May report shortness of air or dyspnea as "breathlessness" (ENA, 2005)
Mediastinum thinner and more mobile	Pneumonia is leading cause of death in older adults (ENA, 2007)

8.

1.	d
2.	a
3.	d
4.	b
5.	a
6.	d
7.	a
8.	b
9.	c
10.	a
11.	d

9.

Pulmonary	Nonpulmonary
Chest trauma: pulmonary contusion	Sepsis (No. 1 cause)
Near-drowning	Shock or prolonged hypotension
Hypervolemia, pulmonary edema	Septic shock
Inhalation of toxic gases and vapors	Hypovolemic shock
Smoke	Anaphylactic shock
Chemicals	Cardiogenic shock
O_2 toxicity	Neurogenic shock
Pneumonia: viral, bacterial, or fungal	Multisystem trauma
Aspiration pneumonitis	Burns
Radiation pneumonitis	Cardiopulmonary bypass
Pulmonary embolism: thrombotic; air; fat; amniotic fluid	Disseminated intravascular coagulation (DIC)
Radiation	Toxemia of pregnancy
Drugs: bleomycin	Acute pancreatitis
	Diabetic coma
	Head injury
	Drug overdose: heroin; methadone; barbiturates; aspirin; thiazide diuretics
	Multiple blood transfusions

10.

1. c
2. a
3. a, c
4. a, b
5. a, b, c

11.

1. a, c
2. a, c
3. b

12.

1. e
2. c
3. a
4. f
5. d
6. b

References and Selected Readings

Bowman, J. G. (2006, December). Epiglottitis, adults. Retrieved March 22, 2009, from http://emedicine.medscape.com/article/763612–overview.

Buttaro, T. M., Trybulski, J., Bailey, P. P., & Sandberg-Cook, J. (2003). *Primary care: A collaborative practice*. St. Louis: Mosby.

Carolan, P. L., & Callahan, C. (2006, October). Bronchitis, acute and chronic. Retrieved March 11, 2009, from http://emedicine.medscape.com/article/1001332-overview.

Centers for Disease Control and Prevention Website. (2008). Respiratory syncytial virus (RSV) overview. Retrieved March 18, 2008, from http://www.cdc.gov/RSV/.

Conrad, S. (2005). Respiratory distress syndrome, adult. Retrieved March 18, 2009, from http://emedicine.medscape.com/article/808260-overview.

Coyne, E. (2007). Adult epiglottitis. *Advanced Emergency Nursing Journal, 29(1),* 52–57.

Dennison, R. D. (2007). *Pass CCRN!* (3rd ed.). St. Louis: Mosby.

Domino, F. J. (2008). *The 5-minute clinical consultant* (16th ed.). Philadelphia: Lippincott Williams and Wilkins.

Emergency Nurses Association. (2007). *Emergency nursing core curriculum* (6th ed.). Philadelphia: WB Saunders.

Emergency Nurses Association. (2005). *Sheehy's manual of emergency care* (6th ed.). St Louis: Mosby.

Felter, R., & Waldrop, R. (2009, January). Pediatrics, epiglottitis. Retrieved March 22, 2009, from http://emedicine.medscape.com/article/801369-overview.

Fleisher, G. R., Ludwig, S., & Henretig, F. M. (2006). *Textbook of pediatric emergency medicine*. Philadelphia: Lippincott Williams and Wilkins.

Fultz, J., & Sturt, P. (2005). *Mosby's emergency nursing reference* (3rd ed.). St. Louis: Mosby.

Gardner, J. (2008, April). Viral croup in children. *Nursing, 38(4),* 57–58.

Jarvis, C. (2008). *Physical examination and health assessment* (5th ed.). St. Louis: Saunders.

Karras, D. J. (2003, February). Managing community-acquired pneumonia in the ED. *Emergency Medicine News, 25(1)*, 17.

Keough, V., & Pudelek, B. (2001, May). Blunt chest trauma: Review of selected pulmonary injuries focusing on pulmonary contusion. *AACN Clinical Issues: Advanced Practice in Acute and Critical Care, 12(2)*, 270–281.

Kerns, B., & Rosh, A. J. (2008). Hyperventilation syndrome. *eMedicine*. Retrieved March 18, 2008, from http://emedicine.medscape.com/article/807277-overview.

Lafferty, K., & Kulkarni, R. (2008, October). Tracheal intubation, rapid sequence intubation. Retrieved March 8, 2009, from http://emedicine.medscape.com/article/80222-overview.

Lutfiyya, M., Henley, E., & Chang, L. F. (2006). Diagnosis and treatment of community acquired pneumonia. Retrieved March 17, 2009, from http://www.a-afp.org/afp/20060201/442.html.

Mancini, M. (2008, October). Hemothorax. Retrieved March 22, 2009, from http://emedicine.medscape.com/article/425518-overview.

Mandanas, R. (2007). Pneumonia, fungal. Retrieved March 17, 2009, from http://emedicine.medscape.com/article/300341-overview.

Mayo Clinic Website. (2007). ARDS. Retrieved March 18, 2009, from http://mayoclinic.com/health/ards/DS00944.

McClintick, C. M. (2008). Open pneumothorax resulting from blunt thoracic trauma: A case report. *Journal of Trauma Nursing, 15(2)*, 72–76.

Orlowski, J. P. (1987). Drowning, near-drowning, and ice-water submersions. *Pediatric Clinics of North America, 3(4)*, 75–92.

Price, S., & Wilson, L. M. (2003). *Pathophysiology: Clinical concepts of disease process* (6th ed.). St. Louis: Mosby.

Proehl, J. (2004). *Emergency nursing procedures* (3rd ed.). St. Louis: Saunders.

Roppolo, L. P., Davis, D., Kelly, S. P., & Rosen, P. (2007). *Emergency medicine handbook: Critical concepts for clinical practice*. St. Louis: Mosby.

Scolnik, D., Coates, L., Stephens, D., Da Silva, Z., Lavine, E., & Schuh, S. (2006). Controlled delivery of high versus low humidity versus mist Therapy for croup in emergency departments: A randomized controlled trial. *Journal of the American Medical Association*, 295(11):1274–1280.

St. John, R. E. (2004). Airway management. *Critical Care Nurse, 24(2)*, 93–96.

Verive, M., & Fiore, M. (2007). Near drowning. Retrieved March 20, 2009, from http://emedicine.medscape.com/article/908677-overview.

Walls, R. W. (2004). *Manual of emergency airway management*. Philadelphia: Lippincott Williams and Wilkins.

Introduction to the Neurologic Emergencies Chapter

This content constitutes 10% (15 items) of the CEN examination

The focus is on neurovascular conditions that are commonly encountered in an emergency department setting

The continuum of age needs to be considered from infancy through older adulthood

Age-Related Considerations

Neonates, infants, and children

1. Infants normally have a flexion posture; floppy is abnormal
2. The Babinski reflex is normal in children <2 years old
3. The heads of infants and small children have prominent occiputs that cause flexion of the neck when the child is laid supine
4. The skulls of these patients are more pliable and thin and less likely to absorb trauma through fracturing
5. Heads in this age group are disproportionately large as compared with body size, thus making these patients more prone to head injury
6. In infants, the anterior fontanelle closes between 9 and 18 months of age; the posterior fontanelle closes by 2 months of age
7. Opisthotonos positioning: if the neck is hyperextended, infants may stiffen up the extremities
8. Symptoms of meningeal irritation in infants include a shrill cry, irritability, and poor feeding
9. It may be necessary to pad the area under the child's torso to the pelvis to keep the cervical spine in neutral alignment

Older adults

1. Cerebral atrophy, weakness of bridging vessels, adherent dura, and more fragile cerebral vasculature make the older adult prone to subdural hematomas
2. Dentures can cause airway obstruction in patients with altered levels of consciousness
3. Reflex time and senses gradually decrease with age:
   a. Movement
   b. Touch and pain perception
   c. Hearing
   d. Visual acuity and depth perception

4. Older adults are less likely to report symptoms related to their decrease in senses
5. Spinal column abnormalities (e.g., kyphosis, lordosis) frequently make cervical spine immobilization more difficult for these patients
6. Degenerative joint disease and osteoporosis make spinal fractures more common
7. The most common type of fall in the older population is a same-level fall (e.g., in the bathroom), which may be perceived as minor even when serious injury has occurred

Selected Concepts in Anatomy and Physiology

General information about the neurologic system

1. Functions of the neurologic system
   a. Receiving stimuli from the internal and external environment over sensory pathways
   b. Communicating information between the body periphery and the central nervous system
   c. Processing information received at reflex or conscious levels to determine appropriate responses
   d. Transmitting information over motor pathways to the organs responsible for responding to the stimuli
2. Components of the neurologic system
   a. Central nervous system (CNS)
      1) Brain
      2) Spinal cord
   b. Peripheral nervous system
      1) Cranial nerves
      2) Spinal nerves
      3) Peripheral nerves
   c. Autonomic nervous system
      1) Sympathetic nervous system (SNS)
      2) Parasympathetic nervous system (PNS)

Microscopic anatomy and physiology

1. Nerve cells
   a. Neuroglia (also called *glial cells*)
      1) Neuroglia are more numerous than neurons; 85% of the cells in the CNS are neuroglia
      2) These cells provide support, nourishment, and protection to the neurons
      3) Most tumors of the CNS are neuroglial because neuroglia are mitotic and can replicate themselves

4) Types: microglia, oligodendroglia, astrocytes, and ependyma

b. Neurons (Figure 6-1)
 1) Transmit nerve impulses
 2) 10 billion in CNS; most are in the cerebral cortex
 3) Cannot regenerate in the CNS; can regenerate in the peripheral nervous system by growing within the myelin if the cell body is intact
 4) Components
  a) Cell body (soma)
   i) Nucleus: controls the metabolic processes of the cell
   ii) Cytoplasm: contains organelles to carry out metabolic functions
  b) Axons
   i) Conduct impulses away from the cell body to other neurons or to end organs
   ii) One axon per neuron
   iii) May be myelinated or unmyelinated
  c) Dendrites
   i) Conduct impulses toward the cell body, which receives nerve impulses from the axons of other neurons
   ii) May be more than one dendrite per neuron
  d) Neurofibrils: thin, thread-like fibers that form a network in the cytoplasm
  e) Nissl bodies
   i) Specialize in protein synthesis with RNA
   ii) Maintain and regenerate neuronal processes
  f) Myelin sheath
   i) On some neurons, the axons are covered with myelin (a white lipid substance) between the nodes of Ranvier
   ii) Myelin acts as insulation to speed the conduction of impulses down the axon sheath
   iii) It accounts for the white color found in parts of the brain and spinal cord
   iv) It is made by oligodendroglia in the CNS and by Schwann cells in the peripheral nervous system

g) Nodes of Ranvier
 i) Constrictions that occur periodically along the axon where it is not covered by myelin
 ii) Allows for the rapid conduction of impulses by saltatory conduction (i.e., node to node)
h) Neurilemma
 i) The outer coating of the neurons in the peripheral nervous system
 ii) Provides for peripheral nerve regeneration
 iii) Synaptic knobs: contain vesicles that store neurotransmitter substances
5) Categorization
 a) Direction of impulse formation
  i) Afferent sensory neurons transmit impulses to the spinal cord or brain
  ii) Efferent motor neurons transmit impulses away from the brain or spinal cord
  iii) Remember: SAME (*Sensory Afferent, Motor Efferent*)
  iv) Interneurons transmit impulses from sensory neurons to motor neurons
 b) Number of processes
  i) Unipolar neurons have one process coming from the cell body; it bifurcates into an axon and a dendrite
  ii) Bipolar neurons have two processes (one axon and one dendrite) coming from the cell body
  iii) Multipolar neurons have one axon and more than one dendrite
 c) Location
  i) Upper motor neurons originate above the brainstem
  ii) Lower motor neurons originate below the brainstem

2. Neurophysiology
 a. Impulse transmission
  1) Initiated by a stimulus: chemical, electrical, mechanical, or thermal

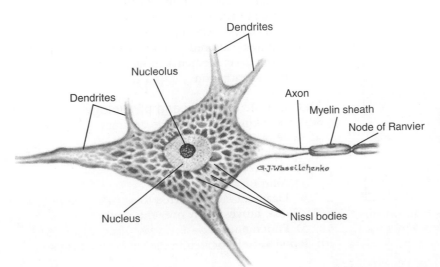

Figure 6-1 The neuron. (From Long, B. C., Phipps, W. J., & Cassmeyer, V. L. [1993]. *Medical-surgical nursing: A nursing process approach* [3rd ed.]. St. Louis: Mosby.)

2) Change in permeability of the cell membrane caused by sodium
3) Depolarization of the cell caused by sodium influx; results in the initiation of an action potential
4) Repolarization and return to normal resting polarized (ready) state occurs
5) Synaptic transmission (Figure 6-2)
   a) Unidirectional conduction of an impulse from one neuron to the next
   b) As the impulse nears the end of the axon, a release of neurotransmitter from the synaptic vesicles occurs
   c) Diffusion of neurotransmitter across the synaptic gap changes the permeability of the cell membrane of the adjoining cell
   d) The impulse then continues to its end organ or cell
   b. Refractory periods
   1) Absolute: period of time when the nerve cannot be stimulated again
   2) Relative: period of time when the nerve can only be stimulated by a strong impulse
3. Cerebral metabolism
   a. Oxygen requirements
   1) The brain comprises 2% of the body weight but receives 20% of the cardiac output and uses 20% of the oxygen delivered
   2) The brain, especially the cerebral cortex, is very susceptible to changes in oxygen delivery; the brainstem is the area that is most resistant to hypoxic damage
   3) Anoxia causes brain edema and neuron death
   b. Nutrient requirements
   1) The brain has high metabolic energy needs
   2) Glucose is the main source of cellular energy (i.e., adenosine triphosphate [ATP])

   a) When triggered by the SNS, gluconeogenesis is a very important process, because it causes the conversion of protein and fat to glucose; the brain does not require insulin to use glucose
   b) Hypoglycemia is associated with neurologic symptoms
      i) Confusion usually occurs if the blood glucose level is <50 to 70 mg/dl
      ii) Coma occurs if the blood glucose level is <20 mg/dl
   c) Although hyperglycemia does not cause direct neurologic effects, the osmotic effect may cause serum hyperosmolality and brain dehydration (e.g., hyperglycemic hyperosmolar nonketotic coma)
   3) Vitamins
      a) Thiamine (B_1) is important in the Krebs cycle; a deficiency of B_1 causes Wernicke encephalopathy
      b) Vitamin B_{12} is important for the spinal cord and the peripheral nervous system; a deficiency of B_{12} causes pernicious anemia and the gradual deterioration of the CNS and the peripheral nerves
      c) Pyridoxine (B_6) is a coenzyme that participates in many enzymatic reactions in the CNS; a deficiency of B_6 causes neuropathy and seizures
      d) Niacin ((i.e., nicotinic acid) is needed for the synthesis of coenzymes; a deficiency of niacin causes pellagra
4. Blood-brain barrier
   a. This is not a true structure but rather refers to the special permeability characteristics of brain capillaries and the choroid plexus
   b. Functions
   1) It acts to limit the transfer of certain substances into the extracellular fluid (ECF) or the cerebrospinal fluid (CSF) of brain
   2) It prevents toxic substances from readily entering the extracellular space of the nervous system; it may also hinder the effective use of certain drug therapies for the treatment of neurologic system problems
   3) It may be altered by trauma, the induction of some toxic elements, intracranial tumors, and brain irradiation

C. Macroscopic anatomy and physiology
1. Scalp: the skin that covers the cranium
   a. Made of five layers
   1) **Skin:** thicker than anywhere else on the body
   2) **Cutaneous** tissue
   3) **Adipose** tissue
   4) **Ligament** layer referred to as *galea aponeurotica;* moves freely over the skull
   5) **Pericranium**
   b. Blood vessels located in the subcutaneous tissue

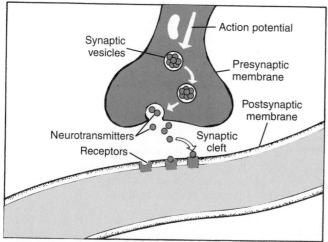

Figure 6-2 Synaptic transmission. (From Chipps, E. M., Clanin, N. J., & Campbell, V. G. [1992]. *Neurologic disorders: Mosby's clinical nursing series.* St. Louis: Mosby.)

1) The scalp is very vascular
2) Blood vessels here do not contract well when injured
3) Scalp laceration can result in significant blood loss

2. Skull (Figure 6-3): the bony structure of the head that consists of the cranium and the skeleton of the face
   a. The skull is composed of an inner table and an outer table that are separated by cancellous (spongy) bone; this structure allows for maximum strength and minimal weight
   b. The cranium is a body vault that holds and protects the brain from external forces; its volume capacity is approximately 1500 ml
   c. The cranium consists of eight bones
      1) Frontal: one
      2) Parietal: two
      3) Temporal: two
      4) Occipital: one
      5) Ethmoid: one
      6) Sphenoid: one
   d. The sphenoid bone divides the interior of the skull into three fossae (Figure 6-4)
      1) Anterior fossa: contains the frontal lobes
      2) Middle fossa: contains the temporal, parietal, and occipital lobes
      3) Posterior fossa: contains the cerebellum
   e. The foramen magnum is a large oval-shaped opening at the base of the skull; this is the location of the connection of the brain and spinal cord

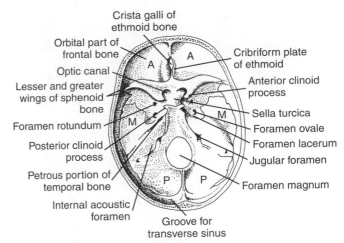

A = Anterior cranial fossa
M = Middle cranial fossa
P = Posterior cranial fossa

Figure 6-4 Bones that form the floor of the cranial cavity and the three fossae formed by these bones. (From Kinney, M. R., Packa, D. R., & Dunbar, S. B. [1998]. *AACN's clinical reference for critical-care nursing* [4th ed.]. St. Louis: Mosby.)

3. Meninges (Figure 6-5): the protective coverings of the brain and the spinal cord
   a. Pia mater: the innermost layer of the brain and spinal cord; the blood vessels of the pia mater form the choroid plexus
   b. Arachnoid mater: the middle layer of the meninges

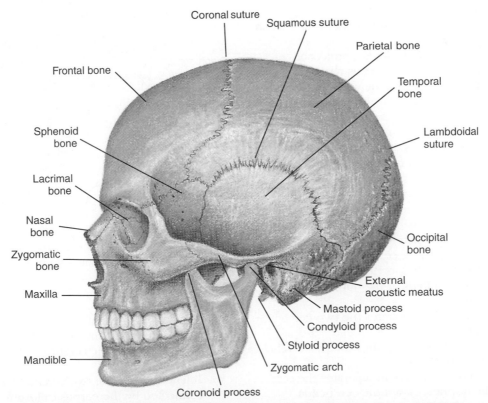

Figure 6-3 Lateral view of the skull. (From Chipps, E. M., Clanin, N. J., & Campbell, V. G. [1992]. *Neurologic disorders: Mosby's clinical nursing series.* St. Louis: Mosby.)

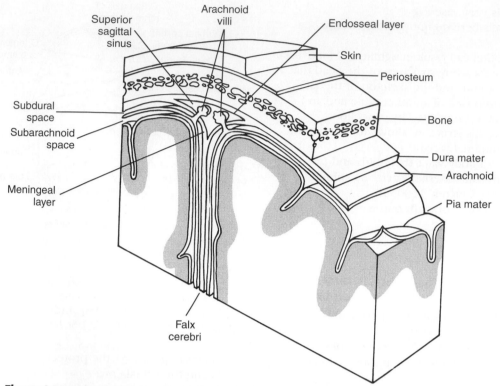

Figure 6-5 Coronal section of the skull and brain that shows the relationship of the meninges. (From Barker, E. [1994]. *Neuroscience nursing.* St. Louis: Mosby.)

1) The subarachnoid space is between the arachnoid mater and the pia mater
   a) Contains the larger blood vessels of the brain
   b) Contains CSF
   c) Contains arachnoid villi (i.e., projections of arachnoid mater that serve as channels for the absorption of CSF into the venous system)
c. Dura mater: the outermost layer of the meninges
  1) Meningeal arteries and venous sinuses lie within clefts formed by the separation of the inner and outer layers of dura
  2) The epidural space is between the skull and the dura mater
   a) Only a potential space
   b) Site of epidural hemorrhage or hematoma
  3) The subdural space is between the dura mater and the arachnoid mater
   a) Only a potential space
   b) Site of subdural hemorrhage or hematoma
  4) There are several folds of the dura mater (Figure 6-6)
   a) The falx cerebri separates the two cerebral hemispheres
   b) The falx cerebelli separates the two cerebellar hemispheres
   c) The tentorium cerebelli separates the cerebral hemispheres from the cerebellum
   d) The diaphragma sellae canopies the sella turcica (where the pituitary gland is located) and encloses the pituitary gland

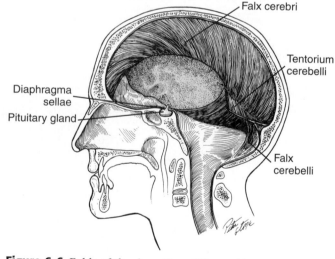

Figure 6-6 Folds of the dura. (From Kinney, M. R., Packa, D. R., & Dunbar, S. B. [1998]. *AACN's clinical reference for critical-care nursing* [4th ed.]. St. Louis: Mosby.)

4. Brain (Figure 6-7)
  a. General information
   1) Weighs approximately 1.5 kg
   2) Divided into the cerebrum, the brainstem, and the cerebellum
  b. Telencephalon: the two cerebral hemispheres connected by the corpus callosum
   1) Cerebral cortical areas and functions (Table 6-1 and Figure 6-8)
    a) Lobes

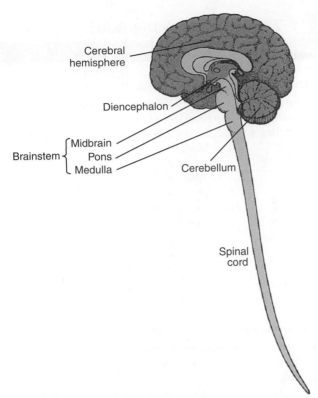

Figure 6-7 Major divisions of the central nervous system. (From Lewis, S. M., & Collier, I. C. [1992]. *Medical-surgical nursing* [3rd ed.] St. Louis: Mosby.)

6-1   Cerebral Cortical Areas and Functions

Cerebral Cortical Area	Functions
Frontal lobe	• Personality • Behavior: ethical, moral, and social • Intellectual functions • Conscious thought • Abstract thinking • Judgment and foresight • Short-term memory • Voluntary motor function • Motor speech (Broca area in dominant hemisphere)
Parietal lobe	• Localization of sensory information to the body surface • Sensory integration and discrimination • Object recognition • Position sense • Body awareness and image
Temporal lobe	• Emotion • Long-term memory • Processing of olfactory, gustatory, and auditory input • Sensory speech (Wernicke area in dominant hemisphere)
Occipital lobe	• Processing of visual input

From Dennison, R. D. (2007). *Pass CCRN!* (3rd ed.). St. Louis: Mosby.

i) Frontal
ii) Parietal
iii) Temporal
iv) Occipital
b) Cerebral hemispheres
  i) Each hemisphere of the brain receives sensory information from the opposite side of the body and controls the skeletal muscles of the opposite side
  ii) Each hemisphere has specialization
    (a) The left cerebral hemisphere is specialized for analysis, problem solving, language, mathematics, abstract reasoning, and the interpretation of symbols
    (b) The right cerebral hemisphere is specialized for visuospatial patterns, nonverbal communication, music, and artistic ability
  iii) Hemispheric dominance
    (a) Ninety percent of right-handed people are left-hemisphere dominant
    (b) Sixty percent of left-handed people are right-hemisphere dominant

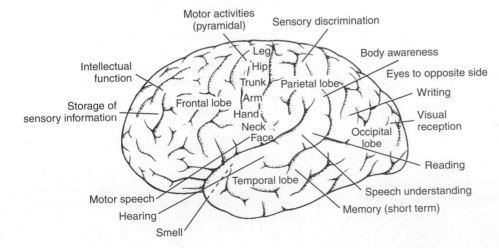

Figure 6-8 Functional areas of the cerebral cortex. (From Kinney, M. R., Packa, D. R., & Dunbar, S. B. [1998]. *AACN's clinical reference for critical-care nursing* [4th ed.]. St. Louis: Mosby.)

(c) Language centers are located in the dominant hemisphere; lesions in the dominant hemisphere frequently cause aphasia
  c) Corpus callosum: the path for fibers to cross from one cerebral hemisphere to the other
  d) Basal ganglia
    i) Regulates and controls motor integration
    ii) Influences posture
    iii) Allows fine voluntary movements
  c. Diencephalon
    1) Thalamus: relays incoming messages to appropriate areas of the brain
    2) Hypothalamus
      a) Temperature regulation
      b) Regulation of food and water intake
      c) Sleep patterns
      d) Autonomic responses
      e) Control of hormonal secretion of pituitary gland
    3) Limbic system
      a) Self-preservation behaviors, including aggression
      b) Basic drives (e.g., food, sex)
      c) Affective aspect of emotional behavior
      d) Some aspects of memory
  d. Brainstem
    1) Functions
      a) Relays messages between the brain and the lower levels of the nervous system
      b) Is the origin of all cranial nerves except the first and second
    2) Divisions
      a) Mesencephalon (midbrain)
        i) Location of reticular activating system, which is responsible for arousal from sleep, wakefulness, and the focusing of attention
      b) Pons
        i) Connects the cerebral cortex and the cerebellum
        ii) Contains respiratory centers
      c) Medulla oblongata
        i) Connects the motor and sensory tracts of the spinal cord to the medulla
        ii) Contains cardiac and respiratory centers
  e. Cerebellum
    1) Coordinates muscle movement with sensory input
    2) Controls balance
    3) Influences muscle tone in relation to equilibrium
    4) Affects locomotion and posture
    5) Controls nonstereotyped movements
    6) Synchronizes muscle action
5. Cerebral circulation (Table 6-2)
  a. The brain receives 20% of cardiac output
  b. Arterial system (Figures 6-9 and 6-10)
    1) External carotid system: arises from common carotid arteries

TABLE 6-2	Cerebral Artery Distribution	
Artery	**Areas**
Anterior Circulation: Internal Carotid System	
• Anterior cerebral arteries	• Superior surface of the frontal and parietal lobes • Medial surface of the cerebral hemispheres • Basal ganglia • Corpus callosum • Hypothalamus
• Middle cerebral arteries	• Lateral surfaces of the frontal, parietal, and temporal lobes • Superior surface of the temporal lobe • Subcortical structures (e.g., thalamus, hypothalamus, basal ganglia) • Precentral (motor) gyri • Postcentral (sensory) gyri
Posterior Circulation: Vertebrobasilar System	
• Basilar artery	• Most of the brainstem • Cerebellum
• Posterior cerebral arteries	• Thalamus • Medial portion of the occipital lobe • Inferior portion of the temporal lobe • Vestibular organs • Cochlear apparatus

From Dennison, R. D. (2007). *Pass CCRN!* (3rd ed.). St. Louis: Mosby.

  a) Occipital arteries: supply the posterior fossa
  b) Temporal arteries: supply the temporal area
  c) Maxillary arteries: form the middle meningeal arteries
  d) Meningeal arteries: branches of external carotid arteries that supply the dura mater; the internal carotid and vertebral arteries supply the pia and arachnoid maters
    2) Anterior circulation: internal carotid system
      a) Arises from common carotid arteries
      b) Accounts for 80% of cerebral perfusion
    3) Posterior circulation: vertebrobasilar system
      a) Arises from subclavian arteries and joins at lower border of pons to form basilar artery
    4) Circle of Willis
      a) Formed by internal carotids and vertebral arteries
      b) Permits collateral circulation if one of the carotid or vertebral arteries becomes occluded; many people have an incomplete circle of Willis, which prevents this collateral flow when injury or occlusion occurs
      c) Prone to aneurysmal formation as a result of multiple bifurcations
  c. Cerebral blood flow
    1) Brings oxygen and nutrients to the brain tissue for cellular energy production; waste products are removed from the blood

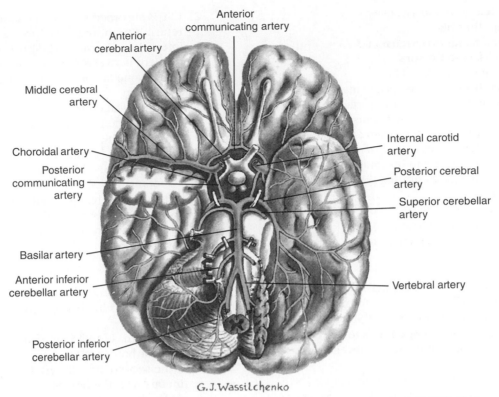

Figure 6-9 Arterial system of the brain. (From Urden, L., Stacy, K., & Lough, M. [2002]. *Thelan's critical care nursing: Diagnosis and management* [4th ed.]. St. Louis: Mosby.)

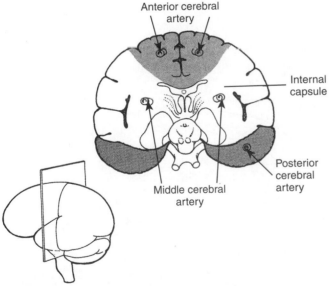

Figure 6-10 Distribution of the arterial blood supply. (From Urden, L., Stacy, K., & Lough, M. [2002]. *Thelan's critical care nursing: Diagnosis and management* [4th ed.]. St. Louis: Mosby.)

2) Cerebral blood flow varies with changes in cerebral perfusion pressure (CPP) and the diameter of the cerebrovascular bed
3) CPP = Mean arterial pressure (MAP) – Mean intracranial pressure (ICP)
   a) Changes in MAP or ICP will affect CPP

b) Normal MAP is 70 to 105 mm Hg
c) Normal ICP is 1 to 15 mm Hg
d) Normal CPP is 70 to 100 mm Hg
   i) CPP of <50 mm Hg is associated with impaired neuronal functioning
4) Autoregulation is the ability of the brain to alter the diameter of the arterioles to maintain cerebral blood flow at a constant level despite changes in CPP
   a) When ICP approaches MAP, CPP decreases to the point where autoregulation is impaired and cerebral blood flow decreases
   b) Limits on autoregulation occur when the CPP is between 50 and 150 mm Hg
      i) CPP of <50 mm Hg causes hypoperfusion (e.g., cardiopulmonary arrest, shock), which results in anoxic encephalopathy
      ii) CPP of >150 mm Hg causes hyperperfusion (e.g., hypertensive crisis), which results in brain edema and hypertensive encephalopathy
5) Factors that can increase cerebral blood flow
   a) Hypercapnia
   b) Hypoxemia
   c) Decreased blood viscosity
   d) Hyperthermia
   e) Drugs: vasodilators
6) Factors that can decrease cerebral blood flow
   a) Hypocapnia
   b) Hyperoxemia

c) Increased blood viscosity
d) Hypothermia
e) Intracranial hypertension
f) Drugs: vasopressors
d. Venous system (Figure 6-11)
  1) The cerebrum has external veins that lie in the subarachnoid space on the surfaces of the hemispheres and internal veins that drain the central core of the cerebrum and that lie beneath the corpus callosum
  2) Both the external and internal venous systems empty into venous sinuses that lie between the dural layers
  3) The internal jugular veins collect blood from the dural venous sinuses
6. CSF: cushions brain and spinal cord
  a. Characteristics
    1) Functions
      a) Cushions brain and spinal cord
      b) Allows for compensation for changes in ICP; the displacement of CSF out of the cranial cavity compensates for increases in intracranial volume to prevent increases in ICP
    2) Pressure: normally 80 to 180 mm H_2O, measured at the lumbar level, with patient in a side-lying position
  b. CSF production and reabsorption
    1) CSF is a transudate of plasma that is formed by the choroid plexus in the ventricles

  2) CSF is absorbed by the arachnoid villi, which return it to the systemic circulation via the internal jugular veins; the hydrostatic pressure gradient between the CSF and the venous sinus is one factor that determines CSF absorption
  c. CSF communication system within the brain
    1) Ventricles: hollow spaces that are lined with ependyma; they contain specialized epithelium called *choroid plexus* that produces CSF
    2) Pathway of CSF circulation: lateral ventricles → foramen of Monro → third ventricle → aqueduct of Sylvius → fourth ventricle → cisterns and subarachnoid space, where arachnoid villi reabsorb CSF into the systemic circulation
7. Spine and spinal cord
  a. Structure
    1) Vertebral column: composed of 7 cervical, 12 thoracic, 5 lumbar, 5 sacral, and 4 coccygeal vertebrae
    2) Spinal cord: 42 to 45 cm that extends from the superior border of the atlas to the upper border of the second lumbar vertebrae (L2); it is continuous with the brainstem
      a) Meninges: pia mater, arachnoid mater, and dura mater
      b) Central canal: opening in the center of the spinal cord that contains CSF; it communicates with the fourth ventricle

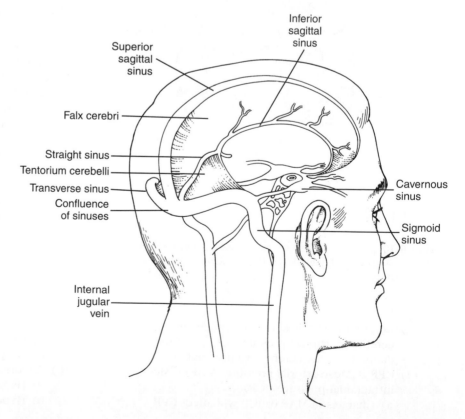

Figure 6-11 Venous system of the brain that shows the major dural venous sinuses and their connection to the internal jugular veins. (From Barker, E. [1994]. *Neuroscience nursing.* St. Louis: Mosby.)

c) Central gray horns that form an "H" shape: they primarily contain cell bodies (Figure 6-12)
  i) The anterior (or ventral) horn of gray matter contains cell bodies of efferent or motor fibers
  ii) The posterior (or dorsal) horn of gray matter contains cell bodies of afferent or sensory fibers
  iii) The lateral horns of gray matter contain the preganglionic fibers of the autonomic nervous system
d) Columns of white matter that are fiber tracts surround the gray matter: they primarily contain myelinated axons
  i) Spinal tracts are named by column, origin, and termination (e.g., the lateral corticospinal tract is located in the lateral column, originates in the cortex, and terminates in the spine; it is therefore a descending tract [i.e., cortex to spine])
3) Upper and lower motor neurons
  a) Upper motor neurons: located in the cerebral cortex and the brainstem
    i) Cell bodies lie in the motor area of the cerebral cortex
    ii) Axons pass through the spinal cord to synapse with the lower motor neurons
    iii) Damage to upper motor neurons causes spastic paralysis and hyperactive reflexes
  b) Lower motor neurons: located in the spinal cord
    i) Cell bodies lie in the anterior horn of gray matter in the spinal cord

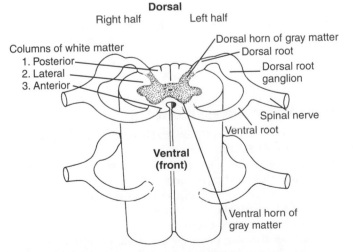

Figure 6-12 Segment of the thoracic spinal cord in cross section. (From Kinney, M. R., Packa, D. R., & Dunbar, S. B. [1998]. *AACN's clinical reference for critical-care nursing* [4th ed.]. St. Louis: Mosby.)

ii) Axons directly innervate striated muscle fibers
iii) Damage to lower motor neurons causes flaccid paralysis and areflexia
b. Function
  1) Mediates the reflex arc
    a) An involuntary response to a stimulus (e.g., touching a hot stove causes the reflex withdrawal of the hand)
    b) Does not go beyond the spinal cord to the brain and does not require cerebral interpretation
  2) Serves as the communicating pathway between the brain and the peripheral nervous system
8. Peripheral nervous system
  a. Spinal segments that consist of 31 pairs of spinal nerves: 8 cervical (C1 through C8), 12 thoracic (T1 through T12), 5 lumbar (L1 through L5), 5 sacral (S1 through S5), and 1 coccygeal
    1) Fibers of the spinal nerve
      a) Motor fibers
        i) Originate in the anterior gray column of the spinal cord
        ii) Form the ventral root of the spinal nerve and pass to the skeletal muscles
      b) Sensory fibers
        i) Originate in the spinal ganglia of the dorsal roots
        ii) Peripheral branches distribute to visceral and somatic structures as mediators of sensory impulses to the CNS
    2) Dermatomes: each spinal nerve innervates a specific portion of the skin identified as the dermatome for that spinal nerve (Figure 6-13 and Table 6-3)
    3) Spinal nerves form various nerve plexuses that innervate the skin and muscles throughout the body
  b. Cranial nerves (Figure 6-14 and Table 6-4) consist of 12 pairs of nerves that carry impulses to and from the brain
9. Autonomic nervous system: controls the activities of the viscera at an unconscious level
  a. Structure
    1) Consists of two neuron chains that carry information from the CNS to the peripheral effector organs
    2) Neurotransmitters form a chemical bridge in the transmission of a nerve impulse
      a) Sympathetic branch: epinephrine and norepinephrine
      b) Parasympathetic branch: acetylcholine
  b. Function
    1) Controls activities of the viscera at an unconscious level
    2) Consists of two parallel systems that regulate visceral organs by acting in opposing manners (Table 6-5)

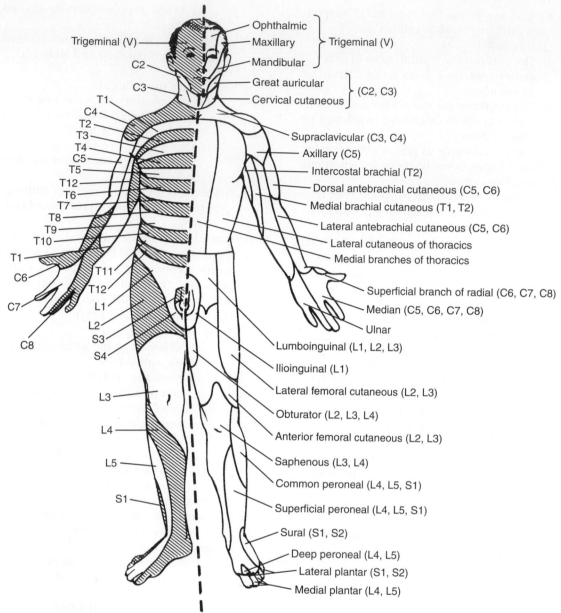

Figure 6-13 Left, Dermatome distribution. **Right,** Peripheral distribution of the cutaneous nerves. (From Long, B. C., Phipps, W. J., & Cassmeyer, V. L. [1993]. *Medical-surgical nursing: A nursing process approach* [3rd ed.]. St. Louis: Mosby.)

a) Sympathetic branch (also called *adrenergic*)
   i) Dominates in crisis situations and is frequently referred to as the "fight-or-flight" system
   ii) Innervated by physiologic or psychologic stressors
   iii) Promotes activities that prepare the body for crisis situations
b) Parasympathetic branch (also called *cholinergic*)
   i) Dominates in moments of calm or "steady state"
   ii) Promotes activities that restore the body's energy sources

Neurologic Assessment
Primary and secondary assessment (see Chapter 2)
Focused assessment
1. Chief complaint: why the patient is seeking help and the duration of the problem
2. Symptoms related to neurologic problems
   a. Head or spinal cord trauma
      1) Sequence of events
      2) Mechanism of injury and time of injury
      3) Treatment before arrival
   b. Change in consciousness (e.g., difficulty staying awake)
   c. Headache

TABLE 6-3	Relationship of Spinal Cord Segments to Peripheral Nerves, Muscles, and Functional Abilities		
Spinal Cord Segment	**Peripheral Nerves**	**Muscles**	**Functional Ability**
C3–C5	• Phrenic nerve	• Diaphragm	• Diaphragmatic chest excursion
C5	• Spinal accessory nerve	• Trapezius	• Shoulder shrug
C5–C6	• Axillary nerve • Musculocutaneous nerve • Radial nerve	• Deltoid • Biceps • Brachioradialis	• Arm elevation • Forearm flexion
C6–C8	• Radial nerve	• Triceps • Extensor carpi radialis and ulnaris • Flexor carpi radialis and ulnaris	• Forearm extension • Wrist extension • Wrist flexion
C8 and T1	• Median nerve • Ulnar nerve	• Adductor pollicis • Dorsal interossei	• Hand grip • Finger spreading
T1–T12	• Thoracic and lumbosacral branches	• Intercostals • Rectus abdominis and obliques	• Intercostal chest excursion • Rotation at waist
L1–L3	• Femoral nerve	• Iliopsoas • Quadriceps	• Hip flexion • Knee extension
L2–L4	• Deep peroneal nerve • Sciatic nerve	• Extensor hallucis and digitorum • Biceps femoris and hamstrings	• Foot dorsiflexion • Knee flexion
L5–S2	• Inferior gluteal nerve • Tibial nerve	• Gluteus maximus • Gastrocnemius	• Hip extension • Plantar flexion

From Dennison, R. D. (2007). *Pass CCRN!* (3rd ed.). St. Louis: Mosby.

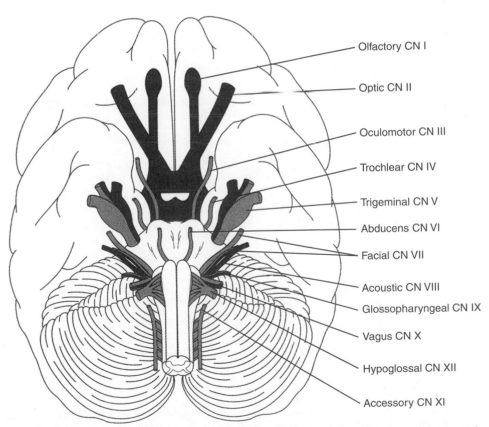

Olfactory CN I
Optic CN II
Oculomotor CN III
Trochlear CN IV
Trigeminal CN V
Abducens CN VI
Facial CN VII
Acoustic CN VIII
Glossopharyngeal CN IX
Vagus CN X
Hypoglossal CN XII
Accessory CN XI

Figure 6-14 Diagram of the base of the skull that shows the entrance or exit of the cranial nerves. CN, Cranial nerve. (From Barkauskas, V. H., et al. [1994]. *Health and physical assessment.* St. Louis: Mosby.)

TABLE 6-4   Cranial Nerve Summary

Number	Name	Memory Jogger: Name	Memory Jogger: Motor/Sensory/Both	Functions
I	Olfactory	On	Some	Sensory • Smell
II	Optic	Old	Say	Sensory • Vision
III	Oculomotor	Olympus	Marry	Motor • Upward and lateral eye movement • Pupillary constriction • Eyelid elevation
IV	Trochlear	Towering	Money	Motor • Downward and medial eye movement
V	Trigeminal	Tops	But	Sensory • Sensation of the scalp and face • Sensation of the cornea of the eye Motor • Temporal and masseter muscles
VI	Abducens	A	My	Motor • Lateral eye movement
VII	Facial	Fin	Brother	Sensory • Taste on the anterior two thirds of the tongue Motor • Muscles of facial expression • Eyelid closure • Lacrimal and salivary glands
VIII	Acoustic	And	Says	Sensory • Hearing • Equilibrium and balance
IX	Glossopharyngeal	German	Bad	Sensory • Taste on the posterior third of the tongue • Pharynx Motor • Parotid gland
X	Vagus	Viewed	Business	Sensory • Pharynx, larynx, and neck Motor • Palate, larynx, and pharynx • Swallowing • Cardiac muscle • Secretory glands of the pancreas and the gastrointestinal tract
XI	Spinal accessory	Some	Marry	Motor • Shoulder and neck movement • Sternocleidomastoid and trapezius muscles
XII	Hypoglossal	Hops	Money	Motor • Tongue

From Dennison, R. D. (2007). *Pass CCRN!* (3rd ed.). St. Louis: Mosby.

TABLE 6-5 Autonomic Nervous System: Sympathetic and Parasympathetic Branch Function

	Sympathetic (Adrenergic)	Parasympathetic (Cholinergic)
Eyes	• Pupils dilate	• Pupils constrict
Heart	• Heart rate increased • Contractility increased • Coronary arteries dilate	• Heart rate decreased • Contractility decreased • No effect on coronary arteries
Lungs	• Bronchodilation	• Bronchoconstriction
Liver	• Glycogenolysis and lipolysis	• Glycogenesis
Gastrointestinal system	• Salivary flow decreased • Gastric mobility and secretion decreased • Intestinal motility decreased	• Salivary flow increased • Gastric mobility and secretion increased • Intestinal motility increased
Urinary bladder	• Bladder relaxed • Sphincter closed	• Bladder contracted • Sphincter open
Adrenal gland	• Secretes epinephrine and norepinephrine	• No effect
Skin	• Piloerection (i.e., goose pimples) • Increased perspiration	• No effect

From Dennison, R. D. (2007). *Pass CCRN!* (3rd ed.). St. Louis: Mosby.

1) Focal or generalized
2) Unilateral or bilateral
3) With or without fever
   a) Headache with fever: infectious process (e.g., meningitis, encephalitis)
   b) Headache without fever: intracerebral hemorrhage or tumor
4) Time of day: early morning headache is suggestive of tumor
d. Seizures
  1) New onset
  2) Increased frequency if patient has a history of seizure disorder
e. Visual changes
  1) Loss of a portion of the visual field
  2) Diplopia: double vision
  3) Photophobia: light sensitivity (may be experienced with increased ICP or meningitis)
  4) Nystagmus: involuntary movements of the eyes
f. Impaired speech
  1) Dysarthria: difficulty articulating words
  2) Aphasia: inability to use or understand language (spoken or written)
g. Change in mood (e.g., depression, euphoria, emotional lability)
h. Change in thought processes (e.g., hallucinations, delusions, illusions, paranoia) and cognition
i. Change in behavior (e.g., hygiene habits, inappropriate laughter)
j. Change in motor function (e.g., tremors, paresis, paralysis)
k. Change in gait
l. Dizziness, syncope, or vertigo
m. Change in sensory function (e.g., pain, paresthesia, anesthesia)
n. Memory changes
o. Swallowing difficulties
p. Difficulty with activities of daily living

3. History of present illness: determine PQRST
4. Medical history
  a. Congenital disorders (e.g., spina bifida, cerebral palsy, Down syndrome)
  b. Childhood diseases: poliomyelitis
  c. Epilepsy
  d. Trauma: head or spinal cord involvement
  e. Infectious neurologic conditions (e.g., encephalitis, meningitis)
  f. Neuromuscular disease
    1) Multiple sclerosis
    2) Myasthenia gravis
    3) Amyotrophic lateral sclerosis
    4) Parkinson disease
  g. Alzheimer disease
  h. Cancer
  i. Cardiovascular disease
  j. Cerebrovascular disease
  k. Diabetes mellitus
  l. Renal insufficiency or failure
  m. Pulmonary embolism
  n. Impairment of vision: eyeglasses, contact lenses, or prosthesis
  o. Impairment of hearing: hearing aid
5. Family history of neurologic disease
6. Social history
  a. Occupation: exposure to toxins (e.g., solvents, pesticides)
  b. Stress level and usual coping mechanisms
  c. Recreational and exercise habits
  d. Caffeine intake
  e. Tobacco use: recorded as pack-years (i.e., the number of packs per day multiplied by the number of years of smoking)
  f. Alcohol and drug use or abuse
  g. Toxin exposure
  h. Travel
  i. Handedness: left or right

7. Medication history
   a. Prescribed drug, dose, frequency, and time of last dose
   b. Nonprescribed drugs
      1) Over-the-counter remedies, including herbal compounds
      2) Substance abuse
   c. Patient understanding of drug actions and side effects
   d. Drugs frequently used for neurologic problems
      1) Tranquilizers
      2) Sedatives
      3) Aspirin
      4) Anticonvulsants
      5) Antihypertensives
      6) Platelet aggregation inhibitors
   e. Drugs that may cause neurologic problems
      1) Tranquilizers
      2) Sedatives
      3) Aspirin
      4) Anticoagulants
      5) Alcohol

Inspection and palpation

1. Vital signs
   a. Hypotension
      1) Hemorrhage
         a) Because the cranium is an inexpansible vault, intracranial hemorrhage cannot result in hypotension, because herniation would result before significant hypotension
         b) Consider other sources of bleeding (e.g., lacerated liver, ruptured spleen, thoracic trauma)
      2) General neurologic deterioration
   b. Hypertension
      1) Systolic hypertension may be seen as a component of the Cushing triad, which is a late sign of intracranial hypertension
      2) May indicate a change in arterial resistance; associated with vessel occlusion (e.g., stroke)
   c. Pulse pressure: difference between systolic and diastolic pressures
      1) Normal: 30 to 40 mm Hg
      2) Increased pulse pressure is a component of the Cushing triad
2. Pulse
   a. Sinus bradycardia: a component of the Cushing triad
   b. Sinus tachycardia
      1) Hypoxia
      2) Hemorrhage
      3) General neurologic deterioration
   c. Atrial dysrhythmias (e.g., atrial fibrillation, atrial flutter) may be an etiologic factor in ischemic stroke
3. Ventilatory rate and rhythm (Table 6-6)
4. Temperature
   a. Decreased (subnormal)

   1) Shock
   2) Drug overdose
   3) Metabolic coma (e.g., myxedema coma)
   4) Terminal stages of neurologic disease
   b. Increased
      1) Infection
      2) Subarachnoid hemorrhage
      3) Seizures
      4) Restlessness
      5) Injury to the hypothalamus

General appearance

1. Apparent health status: consistency of apparent age and chronologic age
2. General behavior
   a. Demeanor
   b. Affect: facial expressions and body language
   c. Mood: euphoria, anger, depression, or suicidal thoughts
3. Posture: gestures, fidgeting, restlessness, tremor, or rigidity
4. Gait: ataxia (i.e., uncoordinated movements of the body)
5. Obvious physical defects
   a. Hemiparalysis
   b. Facial asymmetry
   c. Ptosis
   d. Tremor
   e. Mass response: decorticate or decerebrate posturing

Mental status and cognition

1. Level of consciousness: the most sensitive clinical indicator of a change in neurologic status
   a. Consciousness is a state of awareness: of the self, the environment, and one's responses to the environment
      1) Arousal
         a) Measure of being awake
         b) Function of the reticular activating system in the midbrain
      2) Awareness
         a) Involves interpreting sensory input and giving an appropriate response
         b) Requires both the reticular activating system and the cerebral hemispheres to be intact
   b. Evaluate the degree of stimulus required to obtain a response
      1) Verbal stimulus: speak the patient's name at normal voice volume
      2) Tactile stimulus: touch or shake the patient
      3) Painful stimulus: use only if the other methods are unsuccessful; avoid trauma and bruising that can be caused by pinching
         a) Techniques to elicit a pain response
            i) Central: brain responds
               (a) Pressure to the trapezius muscle: squeeze the large muscle mass

TABLE 6-6   Ventilatory Rhythms

Rhythm	Description	Diagram	Significance
Eupnea	Regular rhythm at normal rate		• Normal
Bradypnea	Regular rhythm with a rate of <12 breaths/min		• Central nervous system depression as a result of injury, disease, or drugs
Cheyne-Stokes	Increasing rate and depth of ventilation followed by decreasing rate and depth of ventilation and then apnea		• Bilateral lesions of the cerebral hemispheres • Lesion of the basal ganglia • Cerebellar lesion • Lesion of the upper brainstem • Metabolic conditions
Central nervous system hyperventilation	Sustained increased rate and depth of ventilation		• Lesions of the lower midbrain or the upper pons • May be secondary to transtentorial herniation
Apneustic	Periods of apnea with full inspiration		• Lesions of the mid to lower pons
Cluster	3-4 breaths of identical rate and depth followed by apnea, and the sequence is then repeated		• Lesions of the lower pons or the upper medulla
Ataxic	No pattern to ventilation; completely irregular with mostly apnea		• Lesions of the medulla

From Dennison, R. D. (2007). *Pass CCRN!* (3rd ed.). St. Louis: Mosby.

between the thumb and the index finger; do not pinch the skin

(b) Pressure to the Achilles tendon: squeeze the large muscle mass between the thumb and the index finger; do not pinch the skin

(c) Sternal rub: rub the sternum gently with the knuckle

ii) Peripheral: spine responds

(a) Nail bed pressure: apply pressure to the nail bed with the flat surface of a pen or pencil

c. Glasgow Coma Scale (Table 6-7)
1) Method to standardize the observation of responsiveness in patients
2) The best or highest response is recorded; E (eye), M (motor), or V (verbal)
3) Note if certain responses cannot be evaluated because of any of the following:
   a) Endotracheal intubation or tracheostomy
   b) Aphasia
   c) Eyes swollen shut
   d) May have to make other adaptations for children older than infants
   e) Considerations for intoxicated patients
      i) Best verbal response may be affected by the inebriated patient's confusion, use of inappropriate words, or even incomprehensible mumbling and sounds

ii) Best motor response may also be affected by alcohol, which can cause a loss of motor function and coordination
4) Parameters
   a) Minimum: 3
   b) Maximum (normal): 15
   c) Clinically significant:
      i) Change of 2 points or more
      ii) A score of ≤8 indicates severe brain dysfunction and the need for airway protection via an endotracheal tube with mechanical ventilation

d. National Institutes of Health Stroke Scale (Table 6-8)
1) Used to assess the severity of presenting signs and symptoms
2) Score of ≥22 indicates severe neurologic deficit
3) Baseline assessment is completed at admission; repeat assessments 2 hours after treatment, 24 hours after the onset of symptoms, 7 to 10 days after the onset of symptoms, and 3 months after the onset of symptoms

2. Cognitive function
a. Orientation: patient may be alert but confused
   1) Orientation to time
      a) Ability to give today's date
      b) Ability to state the year
   2) Orientation to place

TABLE 6-7   Glasgow Coma Scale

Parameter	Adult Response	Infant Response	Score
Eye opening	Spontaneous	Spontaneous	4
	To speech	To speech	3
	To pain	To pain	2
	None	None	1
Best motor response	Obeys commands	Spontaneous movement	6
	Localizes pain	Withdraws from touch	5
	Withdraws from pain	Withdraws from pain	4
	Abnormal flexion (decorticate posturing)	Abnormal flexion (decorticate posturing)	3
	Abnormal extension (decerebrate posturing)	Abnormal extension (decerebrate posturing)	2
	None	None	1
Best verbal response	Oriented	Coos or babbles	5
	Confused	Irritable cry	4
	Inappropriate	Cries only to pain	3
	Incomprehensible	Moans to pain	2
	None	None	1

From Dennison, R. D. (2007). *Pass CCRN!* (3rd ed.). St. Louis: Mosby.

a) Ability to identify surroundings (e.g., "Where are you now?")
b) Ability to state address
3) Orientation to person
a) Ability to identify self by name
b) Recognition of friends and family
4) Orientation to situation: ability to identify why he or she is in the hospital (e.g., "Why are you here?")
b. Memory
1) "How old are you?"
2) Remote memory: "When is your birthday?"
3) Recent memory: "What did you have for breakfast?"
c. Short-term recall: can the patient repeat three or four words after 3 to 5 minutes?
d. General knowledge: can the patient answer a question about current events?
e. Attention span: is the patient able to focus on a subject?
f. Thought content: note evidence of illusions, hallucinations, delusions, or paranoia
g. Calculation skills: can the patient count backward from 20 to 1?
h. Judgment: "Why are you here?"; "What would you do if there was a fire in the wastebasket?"
i. Abstraction: ask the patient to spell the word *world* backward
3. Speech and language
a. Note speech, sentence structure, and appropriate use of words; speech should be fluent with the expression of connected thoughts
b. If the patient cannot use or understand verbal communication:
1) Can he or she understand or use gestures?

2) Can he or she understand written language or write messages?
c. Identify the presence of speech disorders
1) Dysphonia: difficulty producing sound
2) Dysarthria: difficulty with articulation
3) Dysprosody: lack of inflection while talking
4) Aphasia: impaired understanding or expression of verbal or written language
a) Receptive (sensory) aphasia: lesion in Wernicke area in the temporal area
b) Expressive (motor) aphasia: lesion in Broca area in the frontal area
c) Global: both

Motor function

1. Muscle size
a. Symmetry
b. Atrophy or hypertrophy
2. Symmetric movement and strength of extremities
a. Movement: spontaneous and symmetric
b. Muscle strength (Table 6-9)
1) Arm strength
a) Test flexor and extensor muscle groups by evaluating strength against resistance
b) Pronator drift
i) Detection: have patient hold arms out in front of himself or herself with palms up and eyes closed
ii) Normal: patient should be able to hold the arms even for at least 20 seconds
iii) Abnormal: the weak arm begins to drift and pronate (i.e., palm turns downward)
2) Leg strength
a) Test flexor and extensor muscle groups by evaluating strength against resistance

TABLE 6-8 National Institutes of Health Stroke Scale

Item/Domain	Response	Score
1A: Level of consciousness	Alert and keenly responsive	0
	Obeys commands and answers or responds to minor stimulation	1
	Responds only to repeated stimulation or painful stimulation (excludes reflex response)	2
	Responds only with reflex motor response or totally unresponsive	3
1B: Orientation Ask the month and the patient's age; response must be exactly right	Answers both questions correctly	0
	Answers one question correctly or unable to speak as a result of any reason other than aphasia or coma	1
	Answers neither question correctly or too stuporous or aphasic to answer	2
1C: Response to commands Ask the patient to open and close the eyes and then grip and release the nonparetic hand	Performs both tasks correctly	0
	Performs one task correctly	1
	Performs neither task correctly	2
2: Gaze Only horizontal movements tested	Normal	0
	Partial gaze palsy	1
	Forced deviation or total gaze paresis not overcome by oculocephalic maneuver	2
3: Visual field Tested by confrontation	No visual loss	0
	Partial hemianopia	1
	Complete hemianopia	2
	Bilateral hemianopia (blind from any cause, including cortical blindness)	3
4: Facial movement Encourage the patient to smile and close the eyes, or check the grimace symmetry	Normal symmetric movement	0
	Minor paralysis (flattened nasolabial fold, asymmetry when smiling)	1
	Partial paralysis (total or near-total lower face paralysis)	2
	Complete paralysis (absence of facial movement of the upper and lower face)	3
5A: Left arm motor function Extend the left arm with the palm down at 90 degrees (sitting) or 45 degrees (supine)	No drift; holds position for full 10 seconds	0
	Drifts down before 10 seconds but does not hit the bed or other support	1
	Some effort against gravity but cannot get up to 90 degrees (or 45 degrees if supine)	2
	No effort against gravity, limb falls	3
	No movement	4
5B: Right arm motor function Extend the right arm with the palm down at 90 degrees (sitting) or 45 degrees (supine)	No drift; holds position for full 10 seconds	0
	Drifts down before 10 seconds but does not hit the bed or other support	1
	Some effort against gravity but cannot get up to 90 degrees (or 45 degrees if supine)	2
	No effort against gravity, limb falls	3
	No movement	4
6A: Left leg motor function Extend the left leg and flex at the hip to 30 degrees	No drift; holds position for full 5 seconds	0
	Drifts down before 5 seconds but does not hit the bed or other support	1
	Some effort against gravity	2
	No effort against gravity, limb falls	3
	No movement	4
6B: Right leg motor function Extend the right leg and flex at the hip to 30 degrees	No drift; holds position for full 5 seconds	0
	Drifts down before 5 seconds but does not hit the bed or other support	1
	Some effort against gravity	2
	No effort against gravity, limb falls	3
	No movement	4

Continued

TABLE 6-8   National Institutes of Health Stroke Scale—cont'd

Item/Domain	Response	Score
7: Limb ataxia Finger/nose and heel/shin performed on both sides; not ataxia if patient is hemiplegic or unable to comprehend; ataxia must be out of proportion to any weakness present	Absent Present in one limb Present in two limbs	0 1 2
8: Sensory	Normal Pinprick less sharp or dull on affected side Severe to total sensory loss; patient unaware of being touched	0 1 2
9: Best language Name items and read short sentences	No aphasia Some loss of fluency or comprehension Severe aphasia: fragmentary communication, listener carries burden of communication Mute, global aphasia; no usable speech or auditory comprehension	0 1 2 3
10: Dysarthria If not obviously present, have the patient read	Normal Slurs some words So slurred as to be unintelligible or mute	0 1 2
11: Extinction/inattention	No abnormality Inattention to any sensory modality or extinction to bilateral simultaneous stimulation in one sensory modality Profound hemi-inattention or hemi-inattention to more than one modality; does not recognize own hand	0 1 2

From National Institutes of Health (2009). NIH stroke scale. Retrieved May 16, 2010 at http://stroke.nih.gov/documents/NIH_Stroke_Scale_Booklet.pdf

TABLE 6-9   Muscle Strength Grading Scale

Grade	Description
0/5	No movement or muscle contraction
1/5	Trace; no movement but evidence of muscle contraction
2/5	Not greater than gravity; movement with gravity eliminated
3/5	Greater than gravity; movement against gravity
4/5	Slight weakness; movement against some resistance
5/5	Normal; movement against full resistance

From Dennison, R. D. (2007). *Pass CCRN!* (3rd ed.). St. Louis: Mosby.

b) Ask the patient to raise the legs one at a time to 30 degrees off of the bed from the supine position and to hold them in place for a count to 5; observe for drift
3. Muscle tone
   a. Flaccidity: no resistance to passive movement
     1) Generally associated with lower motor neuron lesions; may also occur early with upper motor neuron lesions
   b. Hypotonia: little resistance to passive movement
   c. Hypertonia: increased muscle resistance to passive movement

   d. Rigidity: increased muscle resistance to passive movement of a stiff (i.e., rigid) limb that is uniform through both flexion and extension
   e. Spasticity: gradual increase in tone that causes increased resistance until tone is suddenly reduced
     1) Clonus (i.e., the continued rhythmic contraction of a muscle after the stimulus has been applied) may be evident
     2) Spastic paralysis: a chronic condition in which muscles are affected by persistent spasms and exaggerated tendon reflexes because of damage to motor nerves of the CNS
4. Coordination
   a. Point-to-point movements
     1) Finger–nose test: ask the patient to touch his or her nose with a finger with the eyes closed
     2) Heel–knee test: ask the patient to run the heel of one foot down the opposite leg from the knee to the foot
   b. Rapid, rhythmic, alternating movements
     1) Pronation–supination test: ask the patient to rapidly pronate and supinate one of his or her hands
5. Gait
   a. Tandem gait: patient asked to walk heel to toe in a straight line
     1) Normal: walk heel to toe without difficulty
     2) Abnormal: loss of balance indicates cerebellar dysfunction

6. Involuntary movements
   a. Posturing may occur spontaneously or in response to pain in comatose patients; may also be considered a mass response
      1) Abnormal flexion (Figure 6-15)
         a) Decorticate posturing: arms are flexed toward the body while legs are extended
         b) Indicates cerebral lesion
      2) Abnormal extension (see Figure 6-15)
         a) Decerebrate posturing: arms are extended, wrists are externally rotated, and legs are extended
         b) Indicates midbrain or brainstem lesion
      3) Opisthotonos: extension of arms and legs with arching of the back and neck (may indicate brainstem injury)
      4) Flaccid posture: entire body is flaccid, even with painful stimulation
   b. Tremor
      1) Resting: Parkinson disease
      2) Intentional: cerebellar disease
      3) Flapping: metabolic encephalopathy (e.g., hepatic or renal failure)
      4) Physiologic: stress induced
      5) Senile: age induced
   c. Seizure: describe
      1) Preceding events: aura
      2) Initial cry or sound
      3) Onset
         a) Initial body movements
         b) Deviation of head and eyes
         c) Chewing and salivation
         d) Posture of body
         e) Sensory changes
      4) Tonic and clonic phases
         a) Progression of movements of the body
         b) Skin color and airway
         c) Pupillary changes
         d) Incontinence
         e) Duration of each phase
      5) Level of consciousness during seizure
      6) Postictal phase
         a) Duration
         b) General behavior
         c) Memory of events
         d) Orientation
         e) Pupillary changes
         f) Headache
         g) Aphasia
         h) Injuries
      7) Duration of entire seizure
      8) Medications given and response
      9) Findings obtained with diagnostic studies
         a) Serum electrolytes
         b) Diagnostic imaging (e.g., computed tomography [CT], magnetic resonance imaging [MRI])
         c) Electroencephalography (EEG)

Sensory function

1. Ability to perceive sensation
   a. Superficial sensation
      1) Light touch: wisp of cotton on skin
      2) Superficial pain: light pinprick on skin (use a sterile needle and discard it appropriately after testing)
      3) Skin temperature: hot and cold test tubes on skin (this test is rarely performed)
   b. Deep sensation
      1) Vibration: vibration of tuning fork on bony surface
      2) Position sense: position of great toe or thumb with eyes closed
      3) Deep pain: pressure on Achilles tendon, calf muscles, or upper arm muscles
   c. Ability to recognize objects through the special senses
      1) Agnosia: the inability to recognize objects through the special senses: may be visual, auditory, or tactile or relate to body parts and their relationships
   d. Distribution of sensory loss
      1) Entire side of body: parietal or thalamic lesion
      2) Dermatomal (Table 6-10; see Figure 6-13)
         a) Dermatome: the skin area supplied by the sensory fibers of a single spinal nerve
      3) Peripheral nerve distribution (see Figure 6-13)
   e. Degrees of sensory loss
      1) Anesthesia: loss of sensation
      2) Dysesthesia: impaired sensation
      3) Hyperesthesia: increased sensation

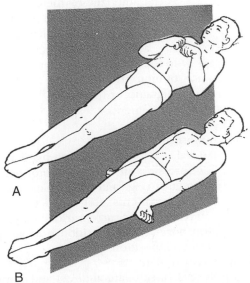

Figure 6-15 A, Abnormal flexion (decorticate) posturing. **B,** Abnormal extension (decerebrate) posturing. (From Urden, L., Stacy, K., & Lough, M. [2002]. *Thelan's critical care nursing: Diagnosis and management* [4th ed.]. St. Louis: Mosby.)

TABLE 6-10   Dermatomal Levels for Bedside Assessment

Anatomic Location	Spinal Level
Front of neck	C3
Thumb	C6
Ring and little finger	C8
Nipple line	T4
Umbilicus	T10
Groin crease	L1
Knee	L3
Anterior ankle and foot	L5
Lateral foot and heel	S1
Genitalia	S3-S4

From Dennison, R. D. (2007). *Pass CCRN!* (3rd ed.). St. Louis: Mosby.

4) Hypesthesia: decreased sensation
5) Paresthesia: burning or tingling sensation

Cranial nerve function

1. Olfactory (I)
   a. Test: the patient's ability to identify familiar odors (e.g., coffee, cloves, tobacco, alcohol) is tested; each nostril is tested separately with the eyes closed; this test is rarely performed in acute care
   b. Normal: able to identify familiar odors
   c. Abnormal: unable to identify familiar odors; referred to as *anosmia*
2. Optic (II)
   a. Visual acuity: test with the use of the following:
      1) Snellen chart: have the patient read lines at 20 feet from the chart or use the pocket Snellen card held 14 inches away from the patient
         a) Record the number on the lowest line that the patient can read with 50% accuracy
         b) Test the patient with glasses or contact lenses
      2) If the patient cannot see well enough to read the Snellen chart, ask the patient how many fingers you are holding up
      3) If the patient cannot see well enough to tell you how many fingers you are holding up, assess whether he or she blinks in response to a visual threat
   b. Visual fields
      1) Test by confrontation: compare the patient's visual field with the examiner's visual field with the eye on the same side covered
      2) Note a loss of vision or of a portion of the visual field
3. Oculomotor (III), trochlear (IV), and abducens (VI)
   a. Eyelids: the elevation of the eyelids is controlled by cranial nerve III; ptosis may indicate cranial nerve III injury
   b. Pupil size

1) Normal: 2 to 6 mm
2) Abnormal: clinically significant change is a change of >1 mm
   a) Pinpoint and nonreactive
      i) Pontine lesion
      ii) Medication effect
         (a) Opiates (e.g., morphine)
         (b) Miotics (e.g., pilocarpine)
   b) Midsize (2 to 6 mm) and nonreactive: midbrain lesion
   c) Unilateral large (>6 mm) and nonreactive (may be referred to as *blown pupil* or *Hutchinsonian pupil*): pressure on the oculomotor nerve on the same side
   d) Bilateral large (>6 mm) and nonreactive
      i) Brainstem lesion
      ii) Medication effect
         (a) Parasympatholytics (e.g., atropine)
         (b) Sympathomimetic (e.g., epinephrine)
c. Pupil equality
   1) Normal: equal
   2) Abnormal: unequal (referred to as *anisocoria*)
      a) Normal variation: 15% to 20% of the population has unequal pupils (usually of difference of ≤1 mm)
      b) Abnormal: difference of >1 mm or change from baseline
      c) Injury effects
         i) Injury to parasympathetic fibers of the oculomotor nerve: ipsilateral (same side) pupil dilation
         ii) Injury to sympathetic fibers of the oculomotor nerves (e.g., Horner syndrome: ipsilateral pupil constriction)
            (a) Horner syndrome: a rare interruption of the sympathetic nerve fibers that is characterized by the classic triad of miosis (i.e., constricted pupil), partial ptosis, and loss of hemifacial sweating (i.e., anhidrosis); results from injury to the sympathetic fibers as a result of injury to the carotid artery, stroke, migraine, or tumor
   3) Shape
      a) Normal: round
      b) Abnormal
         i) Oval: may precede dilated pupil as a sign of pressure on the oculomotor nerve
         ii) Irregular (e.g., a keyhole shape may be seen in patients after cataract removal as a result of concurrent iridectomy)
   4) Position: normal is midposition; note any deviation from midposition
   5) Reactivity to light
      a) Normal: brisk bilateral direct and consensual reaction to light
      b) Abnormal: sluggish or absent reaction
   6) Accommodation
      a) Test: ask the patient to focus on a distant object and accommodate as the object moves closer

  b) Pupils dilate when focusing on a far object
  c) Pupils constrict when focusing on a near object
  d. Extraocular movements
   1) Test: ask the patient to keep the head straight and to follow your finger with his or her eyes; move your finger in the direction of the six cardinal positions of gaze (Figure 6-16)
   2) Normal: both eyes move conjugately in the direction of your finger
   3) Abnormal: one or both eyes do not move to follow your finger; this is indicative of cranial nerve injury or isolated muscular dysfunction
  e. Abnormal eye movements
   1) Nystagmus: jerky eye movement that oscillates the eye back and forth quickly; may be seen with lesions of the vestibular system or the brainstem
   2) Disconjugate eye movement: may indicate damage to the brainstem
   3) Conjugate eye movement: may indicate cerebral hemispheric damage
4. Trigeminal (V)
  a. Sensory branch
   1) Test
    a) Three branches (i.e., ophthalmic, maxillary, and mandibular) are tested on both sides with a wisp of cotton (light touch) and pinprick (superficial pain)
     i) Normal: detects touch and pain
     ii) Abnormal: no detection of touch or pain
    b) Corneal blink reflex
     i) Detection: cornea touched with a wisp of cotton
     ii) Normal: bilateral blink; indicates intactness of trigeminal (V) and facial (VII) cranial nerves
     iii) Abnormal: decreased or absent blink; may indicate cranial nerve V injury; note that contact lens wearers may have a diminished corneal blink reflex
  b. Motor branch
   1) Test: the face is inspected for muscle atrophy or tremor; the masseter muscle is palpated while the patient clenches his or her teeth, and the

temporal muscles are palpated as the patient squeezes his or her eyes closed
   2) Normal: symmetry of muscle strength with no atrophy or tremor
   3) Abnormal: asymmetry of muscle strength; may indicate cranial nerve V injury
5. Facial (VII)
  a. Motor branch
   1) Test: symmetry of facial expressions noted while patient raises eyebrows, frowns, smiles, and closes eyelids tightly
   2) Abnormal: asymmetry of facial expression; loss of nasolabial fold or eye remaining open; indicates cranial nerve VII injury (Bell's palsy)
  b. Sensory branch
   1) Test: ability to taste sour and bitter on posterior tongue; rarely performed in acute care
   2) Normal: ability to taste
   3) Abnormal: inability to taste; indicates cranial nerve VII injury
6. Acoustic (VIII)
  a. Cochlear branch: hearing acuity
   1) Whisper test
    a) Have the patient turn away and then have the examiner whisper to see if the patient can hear what is whispered
    b) Test each ear separately
    c) This test differentiates between hearing and lip reading
   2) Weber test
    a) A tuning fork is placed at the midline vertex of the skull
    b) Normal: patient hears equally on both sides
    c) Abnormal: patient indicates difference between the two ears; will hear the sound better with the "good" ear
   3) Rinne test
    a) Test: a tuning fork is placed on the mastoid; when the patient can no longer hear the sound by the bone, the tuning fork is moved to in front of the ear
    b) Normal: air conduction is greater than bone conduction, so the patient should still be able to hear the sound when the tuning fork is moved in front of the ear
    c) Abnormal: inability to hear the sound by air conduction after the cessation of the sound by bone conduction; diminished air conduction is associated with middle ear infection or disease
  b. Vestibular branch
   1) Not tested directly; problems may be detected by symptoms such as nystagmus, vertigo, nausea, vomiting, pallor, sweating, and hypotension
   2) Reflexes: vestibular branch of cranial nerve VIII and connections with cranial nerves III and VI provide information regarding the integrity of the brainstem
    a) Oculocephalic reflex (also called *doll's eyes reflex*) (Figure 6-17)

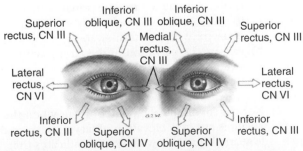

Figure 6-16 The six cardinal positions of gaze. CN, Cranial nerve. (From Seidel, H. M., et al. [1991]. *Mosby's guide to physical examination* [2nd ed.]. St. Louis: Mosby.)

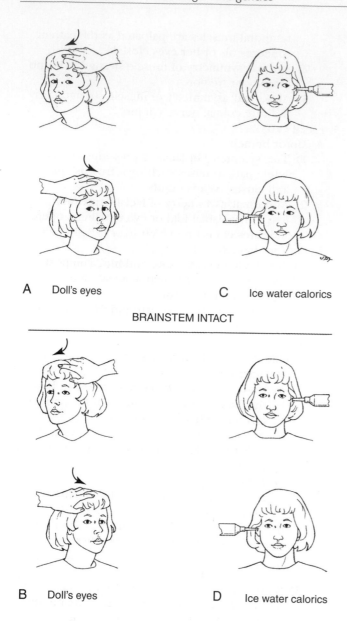

A   Doll's eyes

C   Ice water calorics

BRAINSTEM INTACT

B   Doll's eyes

D   Ice water calorics

BRAINSTEM NOT INTACT

Figure 6-17 A, Oculocephalic (doll's eyes) reflex with normal response: the eyes move in the direction opposite from the direction in which the head is turned. **B,** Oculocephalic (doll's eyes) reflex with abnormal response: the eyes move in the same direction that the head is being turned or stay midline. **C,** Oculovestibular (caloric) reflex with normal response: nystagmus is present, and there may be conjugate movement toward the irrigated ear. **D,** Oculovestibular (caloric) reflex with abnormal response: no nystagmus or disconjugate movement of the eyes. (From Beare, P. G., & Myers, J. L. [1994]. *Principles and practice of adult health nursing* [2nd ed.]. St. Louis: Mosby.)

i) Prerequisites: the cervical spine has been radiologically cleared, and the patient is unconscious; the examiner can hold the patient's eyes open so that eye movement can be observed

ii) Test: head rotated side to side

iii) Normal: eyes move in the opposite direction of the head; this indicates the presence of the doll's eyes reflex (i.e., like the eyes of an expensive china doll); it indicates a supratentorial cause for the coma

iv) Abnormal: eyes stay midline or turn to the same direction as the head (i.e., absence of doll's eyes reflex); this indicates compression in the midbrain-pontine area

b) Oculovestibular reflex (also called *caloric testing;* see Figure 6-17)

i) Prerequisites: must have an intact tympanic membrane and the absence of a basal skull fracture

ii) Test

(a) Elevation of the head of the bed 30 degrees

(b) Injection of 20 to 50 ml of iced water into the ear canal and against the tympanic membrane

iii) Normal: nystagmus with deviation toward the irrigated ear

iv) Abnormal

(a) No eye movement

(b) Disconjugate eye movement

7. Glossopharyngeal (IX) and vagus (X)

a. Phonation

1) Test: patient is asked to say "ah"

2) Normal: bilateral elevation of the palate

3) Abnormal: no elevation of the palate on one side

b. Speech

1) Test: speech is assessed, and any hoarseness is detected

2) Normal: voice is clear with the ability to change volume and pitch

3) Abnormal: hoarseness is present; this indicates damage to the laryngeal branch of cranial nerve X

c. Taste

1) Test: ability to taste sour and bitter on posterior tongue; rarely performed in acute care

2) Normal: ability to taste

3) Abnormal: inability to taste sour or bitter

d. Swallowing

1) Test

a) Hold the patient's tongue down with a tongue blade and touch each side of the pharynx with a cotton swab

b) Palpate the elevation of the larynx with swallow

c) If the patient is conscious, give a sip of water

2) Normal: involuntary swallow or gag when the palate is stroked, elevation of larynx with swallow, and effective swallow; this indicates the intactness of cranial nerves IX and X

3) Abnormal

a) No swallow or gag; do not give fluids, position patient on his or her side, and have suction equipment available

b) Cough on water swallow: request evaluation by a speech and language pathologist

e. Gag

1) Test: palate stroked with a tongue blade; note that this test should not be performed within 2 hours after eating

2) Normal: involuntary gag; this indicates the intactness of cranial nerves IX and X

3) Abnormal: no gag; do not give this patient fluids, position him or her on his or her side, and have suction equipment available

f. Cough

1) Test: touch the hypopharynx with a suction catheter

2) Normal: involuntary cough; this indicates the intactness of the reflexes of cranial nerves IX and X

3) Abnormal: no cough

8. Spinal accessory (XI)

a. Test: Sternocleidomastoid and trapezius muscles inspected for size and symmetry

1) Patient is asked to shrug his or her shoulders as you push down with your hands on the shoulders

2) Patient is asked to turn his or her head to each side against resistance

b. Normal: symmetry; adequate muscle strength

c. Abnormal: asymmetry; poor muscle strength

9. Hypoglossal (XII)

a. Tongue inspected for atrophy, fasciculations, and alignment

b. Tongue strength tested with your index finger when the patient pushes his or her tongue against the cheek

1) Normal: no atrophy or fasciculations; midline alignment when tongue protrudes; normal strength

2) Abnormal: atrophy and fasciculations; deviation from midline; decreased strength

Reflexes

1. Deep tendon reflexes (also called *muscle-stretch reflexes*)

a. Test: tendon tapped with a reflex hammer

b. Normal: contraction of the muscle and a jerk of the affected limb

c. Abnormal

1) Hyporeflexia: less-than-normal contraction

a) May be seen in patients with hypocalcemia, hyperphosphatemia, hypomagnesemia, or lower motor neuron lesions

2) Hyperreflexia: more-than-normal contraction; may be associated with clonus

a) May be seen in patients with hypercalcemia, hypophosphatemia, hypermagnesemia, or upper motor neuron lesions

d. Grading scale (Table 6-11)

e. Locations and spinal levels

TABLE 6-11	Grading Scale for Deep Tendon Reflexes	
Grade	**Description**
0	Absent
1+	Diminished
2+	Normal
3+	More brisk than average but may be normal
4+	Hyperactive with clonus

From Dennison, R. D. (2007). *Pass CCRN!* (3rd ed.). St. Louis: Mosby.

1) Jaw: cranial nerve V (trigeminal)

2) Biceps: elbow flexion; C5 and C6

3) Brachioradialis: wrist extension; C5 and C6

4) Triceps: elbow extension; C7 and C8

5) Patellar: knee extension; L2 and L4

6) Achilles: foot extension; S1 and S2

2. Superficial reflexes

a. Abdominal reflexes

1) Test: abdomen stroked toward umbilicus with the blunt end of a cotton-tipped applicator

2) Normal: umbilicus moves toward the quadrant that is stroked

3) Abnormal: no response; indicates a lesion at T7 through T9 for the upper abdomen or at T11 or T12 for the lower abdomen

b. Cremasteric reflex

1) Test: inner thigh stroked

2) Normal: testis on stimulated side elevates

3) Abnormal: no response; indicates lesion at L1 or L2

c. Plantar reflex

1) Test: sole of the foot stroked with a blunt instrument (Figure 6-18)

2) Normal: toes curl downward

3) Abnormal (Babinski reflex): extension of great toe and fanning of other toes; indicates upper motor neuron lesion

3. Pathologic reflexes

a. Babinski reflex (described previously)

b. Grasp

1) Test: something (frequently a finger) placed in the patient's hand

2) Normal: releases grasp on command

3) Abnormal: will not release grasp on command; infantile reflex: indicates diffuse cerebral dysfunction

c. Sucking

1) Test: corner of the patient's mouth touched

2) Normal: no response

3) Abnormal: patient purses lips and starts to suck; infantile reflex: indicates diffuse cerebral dysfunction

d. Glabellar

1) Test: patient's forehead tapped

2) Normal: no response

3) Abnormal: patient repeatedly blinks; indicates diffuse cerebral dysfunction

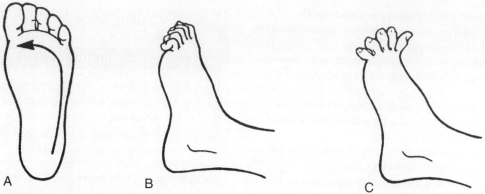

Figure 6-18 Babinski reflex. **A,** Method of stroking the sole of the foot. **B,** Normal response (absence of Babinski reflex). **C,** Abnormal response (presence of Babinski reflex).

Miscellaneous

1. Clinical indications of neurologic trauma
   a. Scalp: tears or swelling
   b. Head and face
      1) Face, maxilla, and mandible should be palpated for fractures
      2) Battle sign: bruising of the mastoid (behind ear); indicative of basal skull fracture (Figure 6-19)
   c. Eyes
      1) Orbits should be palpated; note complaints of pain
      2) Visual acuity should be evaluated if corneal burn or trauma present
      3) Raccoon eyes: bruising around eyes indicative of basal skull fracture (see Figure 6-19)
   d. Nose
      1) Nose should be palpated; note complaints of pain
      2) Note CSF leak: may be seen with basal skull fracture; referred to as *rhinorrhea*
         a) Halo test: CSF leaves a "halo" on 4 × 4s or linens; this term refers to blood settling in the middle with lighter-colored concentric rings around the blood (see Figure 6-19)
   e. Ears
      1) Note edema or trauma to the external ear or the ear canal
      2) Note blood in the external ear canal or behind the eardrum; seen with basal skull fracture
      3) Note CSF leak from ear; seen with basal skull fracture; referred to as *otorrhea*
   f. Injury to teeth, tongue, gums, or mucosa
      1) Malocclusion: inability of teeth to fit together normally when mouth is closed or inability to close mouth
   g. Alteration in consciousness
   h. Clinical indications of intracranial hypertension (see Intracranial Hypertension section)
2. Clinical indications of meningeal irritation
   a. Nuchal rigidity: indicative of meningeal irritation (e.g., infection, hemorrhage)
   b. Brudzinski sign (Figure 6-20)
      1) Prerequisite: cervical spine must be radiologically cleared

      2) Detection: chin brought toward chest and head moved forward
      3) Normal: absence of neck pain; absence of involuntary adduction and flexion of knees toward body
      4) Abnormal: neck pain and involuntary adduction and flexion of legs with attempts to flex the neck; indicates irritation of the meninges by infection or blood
   c. Kernig sign (see Figure 6-20)
      1) Detection: patient is placed on his or her back and assisted to flex the thigh toward the chest until the hip is at 90-degree angle; the leg is then extended at the knee
      2) Normal: ability to fully extend leg without pain
      3) Abnormal: inability to fully extend leg when thigh is flexed toward abdomen; neck pain may also occur; this indicates irritation of the meninges by infection or blood

Intracranial pressure monitoring

1. Purposes
   a. Diagnosing intracranial hypertension
   b. Allowing for the drainage of CSF to maintain pressure
   c. Observing for effects of medical or nursing management
   d. Predicting outcomes: patients who sustain an ICP of >50 mm Hg for >20 minutes have a very poor prognosis
2. Indications
   a. Glasgow Coma Scale score of 8 or less
   b. Severe head trauma
   c. Intracerebral masses
   d. Subarachnoid hemorrhage
   e. Intracerebral hemorrhage (e.g., massive stroke)
   f. Infectious processes (e.g., encephalitis, meningitis)
   g. Encephalopathy
   h. Hydrocephalus
   i. ICP monitoring should be used if deep sedation, paralysis, or barbiturate coma is being used, because the level of consciousness as an assessment parameter is eliminated

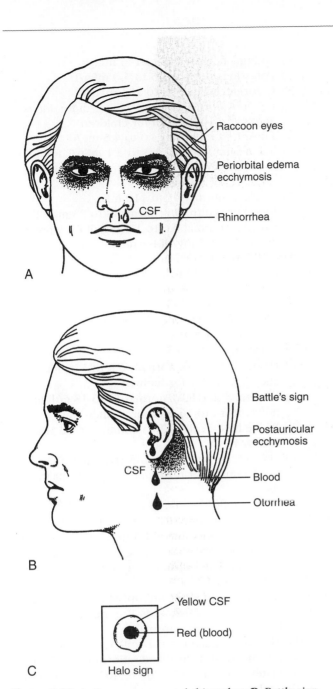

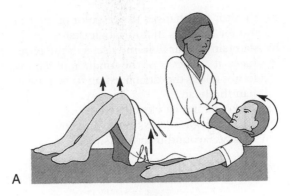

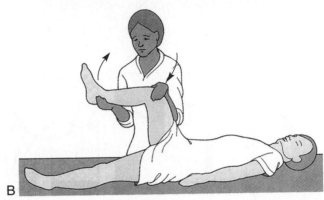

Figure 6-20 **A,** Brudzinski sign. **B,** Kernig sign. (From Barker, E. [1994]. *Neuroscience nursing*. St. Louis: Mosby.)

Figure 6-19 **A,** Raccoon eyes and rhinorrhea. **B,** Battle sign with otorrhea. **C,** Halo sign. *CSF,* Cerebrospinal fluid. (From Barker, E. [1994]. *Neuroscience nursing*. St. Louis: Mosby.)

j. Shunt dysfunction
  1) An intraventricular catheter may be used to relieve increased ICP that is caused by hydrocephalus
  2) Cerebral ventricular shunts are siphoning devices that are placed within cerebral ventricles and peripheral cavities (e.g., ventricular atrium, peritoneal cavity)
  3) Shunt complications
    a) All shunts are subject to kinking, developing plugs, being pulled apart, or infection
    b) Symptoms of malfunction
      i) Mental status: decreased alertness, decreased intellectual functioning, or behavior changes

      ii) Eye changes: alterations in visual acuity or inability to look up
      iii) Incontinence, gait changes, or increased motor tone
      iv) Infants: tense fontanels, shrill cry, flaccidity, of loss of appetite
    c) Symptoms of infection
      i) Fever
      ii) Meningeal sign
      iii) Altered level of consciousness
3. General information
  a. There are several types of ICP measuring devices (Figure 6-21 and Table 6-12)
    1) The insertion of all of these devices occurs either during craniotomy or through a small burr hole made with a twist drill with the use of strict aseptic technique
    2) Systems with a transducer need to be level at the foremen of Monro
  b. ICP values
    1) Normal: <15 mm Hg
    2) Slightly elevated: 16 to 20 mm Hg
    3) Moderately elevated: 21 to 40 mm Hg
    4) Severely elevated: >40 mm Hg
  c. Prevent, detect, and treat complications of ICP monitoring
    1) Infection (e.g., bacterial meningitis, bacterial ventriculitis)
    2) Intracerebral hemorrhage or hematoma

a) Monitor for changes in the color of the CSF and for changes in neurologic status
b) Maintain the air-fluid meniscus of the transducer at the level of the foramen of Monro; do not allow the drainage bag to be lower than the head
3) CSF leak: maintain a closed system
4) Dislodgement or occlusion of catheter
5) CSF leakage around insertion site

Diagnostic studies
1. Serum
   a. Chemistries (Emergency Nurses Association, 2005, 2007)

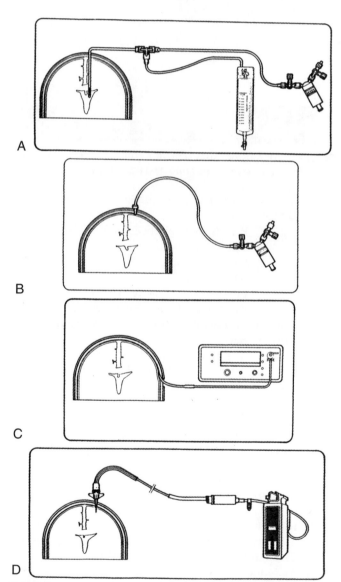

Figure 6-21 Devices for the measurement of intracranial pressure. **A,** Intraventricular catheter and system. **B,** Subarachnoid screw or bolt and system. **C,** Epidural transducer and system. **D,** Intraparenchymal transducer and system. (From Urden, L., Stacy, K., & Lough, M. [2002]. *Thelan's critical care nursing: Diagnosis and management* [4th ed.]. St. Louis: Mosby.)

1) Sodium: normal 136 to 145 mEq/L
2) Potassium: normal 3.5 to 5.0 mEq/L
3) Chloride: normal 95 to 103 mEq/L
4) Calcium: normal 9.0 to 10.5 mg/dl for adults and 8.8 to 10.8 mg/dl for children
5) Phosphorus: normal 3.0 to 4.5 mg/dl
6) Magnesium: normal 1.3 to 2.1 mEq/L for adults, 1.4 to 1.7 mEq/L for children, and 1.4 to 2 mEq/L for infants
7) Glucose: normal 65 to 110 mEq/L
8) Blood urea nitrogen: normal 8 to 23 mg/dl
9) Creatine: normal 0.6 to 1.1 mg/dl for women and 0.8 to 1.3 mg/dl for men
   b. Arterial blood gases
1) pH: normal 7.35 to 7.45
2) $PaCO_2$: normal 35 to 45 mm Hg
3) HCO_3: normal 22 to 26 mM
4) PaO_2: normal 80 to 100 mm Hg
5) SaO_2: normal >95%
   c. Hematology
1) Hematocrit (Hct): normal 42% to 52% for men and 37% to 47% for women
2) Hemoglobin (Hgb): normal 14 to 18 g/dl for men and 12 to 16 g/dl for women
3) White blood cell (WBC) count: normal 5800 to 10,800 mm^3
4) Erythrocyte sedimentation rate: normal up to 15 mm/hr for males; up to 20 mm/hr for females
   d. Clotting profile
1) Prothrombin time (PT): normal 12 to 15 seconds; the therapeutic time is 1.5 to 2.5 times normal
2) Partial thromboplastin time (PTT): normal 60 to 90 seconds; the therapeutic time is 1.5 to 2.5 times normal
3) Activated partial thromboplastin time (aPTT): normal 25 to 38 seconds; the therapeutic time is 1.5 to 2.5 times normal
4) Bleeding time: normal 1 to 9.5 minutes
5) International normalized ratio: normal <2.0
6) Platelets: normal 150,000 to 400,000/mm^3
   e. Toxicology
1) Alcohol: normal 0 mg/dl
2) Dilantin: therapeutic, 10 to 20 mcg/ml
2. CSF analysis
   a. Properties
1) Colorless: cloudy indicates infection
2) Specific gravity: normal 1.007
3) pH: normal 7.35
4) Glucose: normal 60% of serum glucose value; decreased in patients with bacterial meningitis
   b. Protein: elevated in patients with meningitis
3. Other diagnostic studies (Table 6-13)

Intracranial Hypertension (Also known as *increased ICP [↑ICP]*)
Definition: a rise in the pressures within the brain
1. If ICP exceeds MAP, blood flow to the brain will stop

TABLE 6-12 Intracranial Pressure Measuring Devices

Device	Location	Accuracy	Comments
Intraventricular catheter	Usually the lateral ventricle of the nondominant hemisphere is used	Excellent	• Preferred because most accurate and reliable, low cost, and provides opportunity to drain cerebrospinal fluid for specimen or treatment of intracranial hypertension • May be difficult to insert, especially if ventricles are small or displaced • Therapeutic or diagnostic removal of cerebrospinal fluid possible • Provides access for the determination of the volume–pressure relationship • Fluid-filled system used if an intraventricular catheter is placed
Subarachnoid bolt	Subarachnoid space	Fair, but unreliable at high intracranial pressures	• Easy to insert; especially useful if ventricles are small • Inexpensive • Does not penetrate brain • Requires intact skull • Bolt can become occluded with clots or tissue and may require irrigation • Needs to be recalibrated frequently • Unable to drain cerebrospinal fluid • Fluid-filled system used
Intraparenchymal transducer	1 cm into brain tissue	Excellent	• Easy to insert • Unable to drain cerebrospinal fluid or to test volume–pressure response • Catheter is relatively fragile; avoid sharp kinks or pulls • Head position has no effect on pressure reading • Cannot be rezeroed after it is in place • Risk of intracerebral bleeding and infection

From Dennison, R. D. (2007). *Pass CCRN!* (3rd ed.). St. Louis: Mosby.

Predisposing factors

1. Mass lesion
   a. Hematoma (e.g., epidural, subdural, subarachnoid, intracerebral)
   b. Neoplasm
   c. Abscess
   d. Head injury or trauma
2. Cerebral edema: most common cause of intracranial hypertension
   a. Cytotoxic edema: intracellular swelling of neurons and glial cells; it is caused by any of the following:
      1) Hypo-osmolality (e.g., low serum osmolality and sodium)
      2) Hypoxia, which decreases adenosine triphosphate production, which impairs the sodium–potassium pump
      3) Cardiac arrest, which causes anoxic encephalopathy
   b. Vasogenic edema: increase in ECF caused by the breakdown of the blood–brain barrier or by increased vascular permeability and the leakage of plasma protein; it is caused by any of the following:
      1) Trauma (e.g., contusion)
      2) Tumors
      3) Hemorrhage
      4) Abscesses
      5) Surgical trauma (e.g., craniotomy)
3. Cerebrovascular alterations
   a. Venous outflow obstruction caused by decreased venous return from the head (e.g., tight tracheostomy ties or cervical collar, neck flexion, increased intrathoracic pressure)
   b. Increase in CPP (e.g., hypertensive encephalopathy)
   c. Vasodilation (e.g., hypercapnia, acidosis, hyperthermia, vasodilating drugs)
4. Increase in CSF volume (i.e., hydrocephalus)
   a. Communicating hydrocephalus (e.g., subarachnoid hemorrhage, meningitis)
   b. Noncommunicating hydrocephalus (e.g., tumor, surgical, or traumatic edema, hemorrhage or infarction obstructing outflow of CSF)

Pathophysiology

1. Intracranial volumes (Figure 6-22)
   a. Brain tissue: approximately 80-88%
      1) Note: older adults and alcohol or drug abusers may have cerebral atrophy; traction on bridging vessels increases the risk of intracranial bleeding; hemorrhage or hematoma may be very large before symptomatic
   b. Circulating blood: approximately 2-10%
   c. Cerebrospinal fluid: approximately 10%

TABLE

6-13   Neurologic Diagnostic Studies

Study	Purposes	Comments

Angiography	• Visualizes extracranial and intracranial vasculature
	• Identifies aneurysm, arteriovenous malformation, vasospasm, and vascular tumors
	• Detects arterial occlusion and allows for the delivery of intra-arterial therapy to restore blood flow
		• May cause local hematoma, vasospasm, vessel occlusion, allergic reaction to contrast media, and transient or permanent neurologic dysfunction
		• Before the test:
		  • Patient should receive nothing by mouth
		  • Provide sedation before the study as prescribed
		  • Check for allergy to iodine or seafood
		  • Evaluate renal function
		• After the test:
		  • Ensure hydration (contrast medium used)
		  • Maintain bed rest for 8–12 hours
		  • Monitor arterial puncture point for bleeding
		  • Monitor neurovascular status of affected limb
		  • Monitor for indications of systemic emboli
		  • Reevaluate renal function

Computed tomography (CT)	• Views intracranial structures: size, shape, location, and shifts • Differentiates among tumors, hemorrhage, and infarction • Identifies hydrocephalus, brain edema, infectious processes, trauma, aneurysm, hematoma, arteriovenous malformation, brain atrophy, and subacute and old brain infarction	• Patient must be cooperative • Contrast media may be used; possible after a noncontrast computed tomography scan • Check for allergies to iodine or seafood before study • Patient should receive nothing by mouth before study • Sedation may be given • Monitor for signs of an allergic reaction • Encourage fluids • Evaluate renal function when contrast media used
Electroencephalography (EEG)	• Differentiates epilepsy from mass lesion • Detects the focus of seizure activity • Evaluates the electrical function of the brain, which may be abnormal in the presence of cerebrovascular alterations • May be used for the designation of brain death	• Stimulants, anticonvulsants, tranquilizers, and antidepressants may be withheld for 24–48 hours before the study
Lumbar puncture (LP)	• Obtains cerebrospinal fluid for analysis • Measures cerebrospinal fluid opening pressure; this is roughly equivalent to intracranial pressure for most patients if performed with the patient in a recumbent position and if no blockage is present	• Patient must be cooperative • Contraindicated for patients with intracranial hypertension, because herniation may occur • Contraindicated for patients with bleeding disorders and for patients who are receiving anticoagulants • Patient kept flat for 4–8 hours after the procedure to prevent headache • May cause headache, low back pain, meningitis, abscess, cerebrospinal fluid leak, or puncture of the spinal cord

TABLE 6-13   Neurologic Diagnostic Studies—cont'd

Study	Purposes	Comments
Magnetic resonance angiography (MRA) and magnetic resonance imaging (MRI)	• As for computed tomography • Visualizes tissue state (diffusion and perfusion) so that early ischemic changes are apparent (computed tomography cannot visualize most early changes) • Identifies vascular lesions, tissue abnormalities, hemorrhage, infarction, epileptic foci, and multiple sclerosis • Identifies the patency of large veins and venous sinuses • Identifies brainstem abnormalities • Identifies the type, location, and extent of brain injury	• Patient must be cooperative • Contraindicated for patients with any implanted metallic device, including pacemakers • Tends to overestimate the degree of stenosis
Skull radiography	• Detects skull fractures, facial fractures, tumors, bone erosion, cranial anomalies, air–fluid levels in the sinuses, abnormal intracranial calcifications, and radiopaque foreign bodies	• Linear and basal fractures are frequently missed by routine radiography • Contraindicated for pregnant patients • Usually not performed for patients with head trauma because computed tomography is a better diagnostic tool in these cases
Spinal cord arteriography	• Differentiates among spinal arteriovenous malformation, angioma, tumor, and ischemia	• As for skull radiography • May cause the thrombosis of the spinal vessels or an allergic reaction to the contrast agent
Spinal radiography	• Detects vertebral dislocation or fracture, degenerative disease, tumor, bone erosion, and calcification • Identifies structural spinal deficits and rules out associated cervical spine injuries	• Care must be taken to prevent fracture displacement and spinal cord injury • C1–C2 view best obtained via an open mouth; C6–C7 view best obtained with the arms pulled down

From Dennison, R. D. (2007). *Pass CCRN!* (3rd ed.). St. Louis: Mosby.

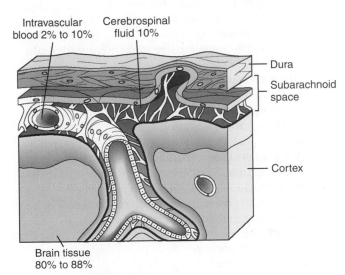

Figure 6-22 Intracranial volumes.

2. Intracranial pressure: the pressure exerted by brain tissue, blood, and cerebrospinal fluid against the inside of the skull; normal ICP is <15 mm Hg with only slight fluctuation under normal circumstances
3. Monro-Kellie hypothesis
    a. The cranium is an inexpansible vault
    b. Inside the cranium is a closed system with three fluctuating volumes
        1) Compensation is the ability of the cranium's contents to change or rearrange; compensation is more effective when volume increase is slower
        2) If the volume of one of the constituents of the intracranial cavity increases, a reciprocal decrease in volume of one or both of the others will occur
            a) Displacement of CSF from the cranium to the lumbar cistern
            b) Increased CSF reabsorption
            c) Compression of low pressure venous system; blood is shunted to venous sinuses
    c. As successive units of any of the three volumes are added to the cranium, a critical point is reached at

which each additional unit of volume added increases ICP dramatically and herniation occurs

   1) There is a volume–pressure relationship; when the critical point is reached, herniation syndromes occur (Figure 6-23 and Table 6-14)

4. Compliance
   a. The ability of the brain to tolerate increases in volume without a corresponding increase in pressure
   b. Compliance is poor: a small increase in volume causes a large increase in pressure

5. CPP
   a. Pressure at which brain tissue is perfused; used to estimate adequacy of cerebral blood flow
   b. Calculated by subtracting ICP from MAP
      1) MAP − ICP = CPP
   c. Normal CPP: 60 to 100 mm Hg; a CPP of >60 mm Hg is considered a minimum desirable CPP for patients with brain injuries
      1) Autoregulation (i.e., the intrinsic ability of the cerebral blood vessels to dilate or constrict in response to changes in the brain's environment) fails if CPP is <50 mm Hg or >150 mm Hg
   d. Increased ICP and decreased CPP decrease cerebral blood flow; the brain receives less oxygen and nutrients, which eventually causes neuronal death

6. Decompensation: the brain loses its ability to compensate
   a. Pressure on cerebral vessels slows blood flow to the brain
   b. Diminished circulation produces ischemia and an accumulation of carbon dioxide and lactic acid
   c. Hypoxia and hypercapnia trigger vasodilation, which increases blood volume and brain edema
   d. Brain edema increases ICP further
   e. The compression of cerebral vessels occurs and causes further ischemia
   f. Eventually, the cerebral circulation stops, and brain death occurs

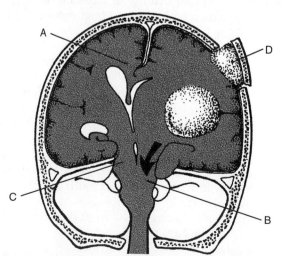

Figure 6-23 Supratentorial herniation. **A,** Cingulate. **B,** Uncal. **C,** Central. **D,** Transcalvarial. (From Thelan, L. A., Urden, L. D., Lough, M. E., & Stacy, K. M. [1998]. *Critical care nursing: Diagnosis and management* [3rd ed.]. St. Louis: Mosby.)

Clinical presentation

1. Subjective
   a. History of traumatic event
   b. Family may report a change in personality
   c. May have headache, nausea, vomiting, or difficulty concentrating

2. Objective
   a. Vital sign changes
      1) Cushing triad: late sign that indicates probable herniation
         a) Increased systolic blood pressure
         b) Widening pulse pressure as a result of diastolic blood pressure being normal or decreased along with increased systolic blood pressure
         c) Bradycardia
      2) Respiratory pattern changes dependent on location of injury (see Table 6-6)
      3) Temperature: central hyperthermia may occur late in patients with intracranial hypertension as a result of pressure on the thermoregulatory center in the hypothalamus
   b. Change in level of consciousness
      1) Early: yawning, restlessness, or confusion
      2) Late: diminishing level of consciousness or posturing
         a) Children: high-pitched cry or agitation
   c. Pupil changes
      1) Early
         a) Ipsilateral pupil changes
            i) Changes in size and shape (i.e., oval)
            ii) Sluggish reaction to light
         b) Conjugate eye deviation
      2) Late
         a) Ipsilateral pupil changes
            i) Dilated and nonreactive to light
            ii) Ptosis
            iii) Disconjugate eye movement with brainstem lesions
   d. Motor changes: contralateral
      1) Caused by compression or pressure on the corticospinal tracts
      2) Early: paresis and plegia
      3) Late: posturing
   e. Parinaud syndrome: paralysis of the upward gaze
   f. Vomiting may occur, especially with lesions below the tentorium
   g. Reflexes: decrease in or absence of reflexes (e.g., cough, gag, and corneal reflexes)
   h. Speech alterations: dysphasia, aphasia, and dysarthria
   i. Seizures may occur
   j. Specific to infants
      1) Bulging fontanels
      2) High-pitched cry
      3) "Setting sun" sign: looks like eyes are sinking into lower lids and there is visible sclera above the irises
      4) Persistent vomiting

TABLE 6-14   Herniation Syndromes

Type of Herniation	Description	Symptomatology	Comments
Cingulate (or subfalcine) herniation	An expanding lesion of one hemisphere that shifts laterally and forces the cingulate gyrus under the falx cerebri; the compression of vessels causes brain edema, ischemia, and intracranial hypertension	• No specific clinical manifestations • May have an altered level of consciousness or plegia • Cheyne-Stokes ventilatory pattern may be seen	• Not life threatening but a sign of brain decompensation • If condition not controlled, uncal or central herniation will occur
Uncal herniation	An expanding lesion in the middle fossa or the temporal lobe that causes a lateral displacement that pushes the uncus of the temporal lobe over the edge of the tentorium; the uncus may be lacerated by the sharp edge of the tentorium	• First symptom is unilateral (ipsilateral) pupil dilation with sluggish reaction to light: fixed, dilated pupils • Decreased level of consciousness • Ventilatory pattern change • Contralateral hemiplegia that progresses to posturing	• Most common herniation syndrome • Life threatening when hemorrhage or brainstem compression occurs
Central (or transtentorial) herniation	Expanding lesions of the frontal, parietal, or occipital lobes or severe generalized edema causes the downward displacement of the basal ganglia and the diencephalon through the tentorial notch, thereby causing pressure on the midbrain	• First symptom is a change in the level of consciousness • Small, reactive pupils become fixed, dilated pupils • Ventilatory pattern changes: apnea • Decorticate posturing becomes flaccidity	• May be preceded by cingulate or uncal herniation • Life threatening
Transcalvarial herniation	Extrusion of brain tissue through the cranium	• No specific clinical manifestations	• May occur through an opening from a skull fracture, a craniotomy site, or a burr hole • Risk of infection
Downward cerebellar (or tonsillar) herniation	An expanding lesion of the cerebellum exerts downward pressure, thereby sending the cerebellar tonsils through the foramen magnum; compression and displacement of the medulla oblongata occurs	• Coma • Flaccid paralysis • Respiratory and cardiac arrest occur	• May be a complication of lumbar puncture in presence of high intracranial pressure • Causes death

From Dennison, R. D. (2007). *Pass CCRN!* (3rd ed.). St. Louis: Mosby.

3. Diagnostic studies
   a. ABGs to evaluate ventilation and oxygenation
   b. CT may show cause of intracranial hypertension or intracerebral shifts
      1) Note that lumbar puncture (LP) is contraindicated; it may cause downward cerebellar herniation with medullary herniation and death
   c. Cerebral angiography: may show cause of intracranial hypertension
   d. Skull radiography: may show cause of intracranial hypertension or shift of pineal gland or sella turcica; rarely performed
   e. Shunt series for child with ventriculoperitoneal shunt
   f. ECG
      1) May show prolonged QT interval
      2) Dysrhythmias: especially with subarachnoid hemorrhage

Collaborative management

1. Continue assessment
   a. ABCDs
   b. Vital signs: blood pressure, pulse, respiratory rate, and temperature
   c. Level of consciousness, pupils, and motor function

d. Clinical indications of intracranial hypertension; invasive ICP monitoring may be used
e. Oxygen saturation
f. Respiratory effort and excursion
g. Cardiac rate and rhythm
h. Accurate intake and output
i. Close monitoring for the progression of symptoms
2. Maintain airway, oxygenation, and ventilation
  a. Positioning: do not tilt or hyperextend the head to maintain an open airway until the spine has been radiologically cleared; use the jaw-thrust technique
  b. Artificial airways as indicated
    1) Oral or nasopharyngeal airway to hold the tongue away from the hypopharynx in patients with altered consciousness
      a) Do not use a nasopharyngeal airway or nasal suctioning if a facial or skull fracture is present
      b) Do not use oral airways in conscious patients because these airways stimulate the gag reflex
    2) Endotracheal intubation if required
      a) Use rapid-sequence intubation premedications
      b) The blind method for intubation may be required if the spine has not been radiologically cleared
  c. Prevention of aspiration
    1) Position the patient on his or her side if the spine has been cleared
    2) Suction only as necessary and limit the duration of suctioning to 10 seconds
    3) Hyperoxygenate with 100% oxygen before and after suctioning
    4) Do not suction by nose if there is evidence of head or facial trauma
  d. Oxygen by nasal cannula at 2 to 6 L/minute if required to maintain an SpO_2 level of 95% unless contraindicated; for patients with chronic obstructive pulmonary disease, use pulse oximetry to guide oxygen administration to an SpO_2 level of 90%
  e. Mechanical ventilation may be necessary
    1) Recognize that positive pressure mechanical ventilation will increase ICP; the use of lower tidal volumes and PEEP may minimize this effect
3. Maintain MAP, CPP, and cerebral blood flow
  a. Identification and control of bleeding from chest, abdomen, pelvis, extremities, and scalp
  b. IV access with two large-bore catheters for fluid and medication administration
  c. Intravenous fluids as prescribed: avoid hypotonic fluids (e.g., dextrose 5% solution [D_5W]), which may contribute to brain edema
  d. Vasopressors as required for patients in neurogenic shock
4. Prevent and monitor for clinical indications; treat intracranial hypertension

a. Recognize factors that increase ICP (Box 6-1); prevent as many of these factors as possible; space activities that increase ICP that cannot be eliminated
b. Adequate venous drainage from head
  1) Positioning
    a) Raise head of bed to promote venous drainage from the brain (avoid if blood pressure decreases when the head of the bed is elevated)
    b) Maintain head and neck in straight alignment to prevent the compression of jugular veins
  2) Avoidance of compression of jugular veins that may be caused by cervical collars or tracheostomy ties that are too tight
  3) Instruction to the patient to avoid straining, bending, and sneezing
  4) Antiemetics as required
c. If there is evidence of intracranial hypertension, therapy should be aimed at reducing the volume of one of the three components of ICP:

BOX 6-1 Causes of Intracranial Pressure Elevations

Ventilation and oxygenation problems
- Airway obstruction
- Hypercapnia
- Hypoxia
- Suctioning without hyperoxygenation
- Deep breathing

Position changes
- Prone position
- Trendelenburg position
- Extreme hip flexion (>90 degrees)

Decreased venous return from head
- Neck flexion, hyperextension, or rotation
- Tight tracheostomy ties or cervical collars
- Increased intrathoracic pressure
- Positive pressure mechanical ventilation
- PEEP
- Valsalva maneuver
- Straining at stool
- Vomiting
- Coughing
- Suctioning
- Isometric exercise

Increased metabolic rate
- Hyperthermia
- Seizure activity
- Rapid eye movement sleep

Stress
- Disturbing conversation
- Noise
- Bright lights
- Pain or noxious stimuli

From Dennison, R. D. (2007). *Pass CCRN!* (3rd ed.). St. Louis: Mosby.

1) CSF: drain CSF if there is an intraventricular catheter present
2) Blood volume: hyperventilation may be used in dire circumstances, because alkalosis causes vasoconstriction, which will decrease intracranial volume and pressure (note that this vasoconstriction will decrease cerebral blood flow and that it may cause cerebral ischemia, so it is only used in extreme situations [e.g., herniation])
3) Brain mass
   a) Osmotic diuretics (e.g., mannitol [Osmitrol]) as prescribed to reduce cerebral edema
   b) Fluid restrictions
   c) Corticosteroids as prescribed
5. Decrease the metabolic requirements of the brain
   a. Prophylactic anticonvulsants as prescribed
   b. Normothermia (<38°C); therapeutic hypothermia (≈33°C) may be used to further lower metabolic and oxygen requirements
      1) Antipyretics
      2) Cooling measures
   c. Sedatives, muscle paralytics, and barbiturates as prescribed
   d. Calm, quiet environment
      1) Prevent loud noises and disturbing conversations
      2) Explain procedures thoroughly; talk to the patient even if there is no apparent awareness
      3) Encourage the family to touch the patient and to speak to him or her encouragingly; a high percentage of patients remember things that were said or read to them while they were "unconscious"
6. Monitor for complications
   a. Herniation
   b. Brain death

Evaluation

1. Patent airway, adequate oxygenation (i.e., normal PaO_2, SpO_2, SaO_2) and ventilation (i.e., normal $PaCO_2$)
2. Absence of clinical indications of respiratory distress
3. Absence of clinical indications of hypoperfusion
4. Absence of clinical indications of infection or sepsis
5. Alert and oriented with no neurologic deficit

Typical disposition: admission to critical care unit; surgery may be required

Traumatic Brain Injury

Definition: an injury that occurs as a result of a blow or jolt to the head or that is caused by a penetrating head injury that disrupts the normal function of the brain; also called *head injury*; may range from mild to severe

1. Primary injury: the injury that occurs as a result of the initial trauma; this can be local or diffuse

a. The Glasgow Coma Scale score is used to define severity within 48 hours of injury
   1) Mild: 13 to 15
   2) Moderate: 9 to 12
   3) Severe: 3 to 8
b. Types of primary injuries
   1) Concussion: a brief alteration in the level of consciousness caused by the movement of the brain within the cranial vault; this results in a brief interruption of the reticular activating system, which causes a brief loss of awareness
   2) Contusion: a bruise on the surface of the brain
   3) Skull fractures (see Skull Fractures section)
   4) Contrecoup injuries: the impact occurs on one side, which causes the brain to move and hit the opposite side of the skull, thus injuring the opposite side of the brain
   5) Diffuse axonal injuries: characterized by extensive generalized damage to the white matter in of the brain
   6) Intracranial hemorrhages
   7) Penetrating head injuries: these occur when an object penetrates the cranial vault and causes damage to the scalp, skull, vessels, and brain tissue
2. Secondary injury: this occurs as an indirect result of the primary injury (e.g., cerebral edema, ischemia, hemorrhage, hematoma)

Predisposing factors

1. Blunt or penetrating trauma; risk is decreased by the use of helmets, airbags, and seatbelts; risk is increased with the ingestion of alcohol or drugs
   a. Motor vehicle collision
   b. Falls
   c. Violence: assault; gunshot or knife wound
   d. Sports-related accidents (e.g., boxing, football)
   e. Industrial accidents

Pathophysiology

1. Focal injury: large enough that it can be identified macroscopically (e.g., skull fracture, hematoma, hemorrhage, contusion, edema with shifting of tissue)
   a. Trauma causes the brain to strike the internal surfaces of the skull and the orbital roof, thereby resulting in bruising and petechial hemorrhages
   b. Laceration of the brain may occur
   c. Areas of infarction and necrosis may occur as a result of vascular injury, which may lead to the oozing of blood into the injured area
   d. Subpial and intracerebral extravasation of blood may occur
   e. Hemorrhage and edema may act as intracranial masses and cause intracranial hypertension
   f. Injury may be at the site of impact (coup), on the opposite side (contrecoup), or both
2. Diffuse injury: diffuse microscopic damage
   a. Widespread axonal disruption throughout the cerebral hemispheres
   b. Anatomic interruption of neuronal pathways

3. Secondary injury (remember that the actual physical damage that occurs at the time of injury cannot be changed, so optimal outcomes are dependent on avoiding or minimizing secondary injury to the brain caused by these systemic or intracranial causes); brain ischemia is the most important cause of secondary brain injury
   a. Systemic causes
      1) Hypotension
      2) Hypoxia
      3) Anemia
      4) Hyperthermia
      5) Hypercapnia or hypocapnia
      6) Electrolyte imbalance
      7) Hyperglycemia or hypoglycemia
      8) Acid-base imbalance
      9) Systemic inflammatory response syndrome
   b. Intracranial causes
      1) Intracranial hypertension
      2) Mass lesions
      3) Brain edema
      4) Vasospasm
      5) Hydrocephalus
      6) Infection
      7) Seizures

Clinical presentation

1. Concussion
   a. Subjective
      1) History of precipitating event
      2) Report of immediate brief period of unconsciousness
      3) Memory loss
      4) Headache or scalp tenderness or pain
      5) Dizziness
      6) Visual changes
      7) Nausea and vomiting
   b. Objective
      1) Confusion, restlessness, or irritability
      2) Disorientation or a "blank" look
      3) Seizures may occur
      4) Specific to infants
         a) Bulging fontanel may be noted
         b) If retinal hemorrhages are noted, abuse possible
   c. Diagnostic
      1) CT of the head is recommended for any focal neurologic signs (e.g., Glasgow Coma Score of <15, seizures)
      2) Cervical spine film for suspected injury
2. Contusion
   a. Subjective
      1) History of precipitating event
      2) Report of altered level of consciousness of >6 hours
      3) Memory loss
   b. Objective
      1) Change in level of consciousness or behavior for several hours
      2) Motor or sensory dysfunction

      3) Cranial nerve dysfunction
      4) Focal neurologic signs (e.g., hemiparesis, hemiplegia)
      5) Seizures may occur
   c. Diagnostic
      1) Serum: to rule out causes of injury
         a) CBC with differential
         b) Blood chemistries
         c) Coagulation profile
         d) Blood alcohol level
      2) Radiology
         a) CT of the head (may initially be normal)
         b) Consider MRI
         c) Consider cervical spine films if warranted by mechanism of injury
      3) Urine: toxicology screen
3. Diffuse axonal injury
   a. Subjective
      1) History of precipitating event
   b. Objective
      1) Immediate loss of consciousness that takes >6 hours to resolve (if it resolves at all)
      2) Retrograde amnesia, confusion, and possible behavioral changes upon awakening
      3) May have purposeful movements, withdrawal from pain, or restlessness
      4) May show signs of brainstem disruption
         a) Loss of brainstem reflexes (e.g., gag)
         b) Hypertension or hyperthermia
         c) Posturing (i.e., decorticate or decerebrate)
   c. Diagnostic
      1) Serum: to rule out cause of injury
      2) Radiology
         a) CT of the head (may initially be normal)
         b) Consider MRI
         c) Cervical spine films
4. Penetrating injuries
   a. Subjective
      1) Mechanism of injury: high versus low velocity
   b. Objective
      1) Altered level of consciousness
      2) Open wounds or bleeding
      3) Clinical indications of hypoperfusion may be present, depending on blood loss and neurologic impairment
      4) Character of gunshot wound: gauge, bullet type, and distance
   c. Diagnostics
      1) CT of the head
      2) MRI of the head: contraindicated if penetrating object is metallic

Collaborative management

1. Continue assessment
   a. ABCDs
   b. Vital signs: blood pressure, pulse, respiratory rate, and temperature

c. Oxygen saturation

d. Respiratory effort and excursion

e. Cardiac rate and rhythm

f. Level of consciousness, pupils, and motor function

g. Clinical indications of intracranial hypertension; invasive ICP monitoring may be used

h. Pain and discomfort level

i. Accurate intake and output

j. Close monitoring for the progression of symptoms

2. Maintain airway, oxygenation, and ventilation

a. Positioning: do not tilt or hyperextend the head to maintain an open airway until the spine has been radiologically cleared; use the jaw-thrust technique

b. Artificial airways as indicated

1) Oral or nasopharyngeal airway to hold the tongue away from the hypopharynx for patients with altered level of consciousness

a) Do not use a nasopharyngeal airway or nasal suctioning if a facial or skull fracture is present

b) Do not use oral airways in conscious patients because these airways stimulate the gag reflex

2) Endotracheal intubation if required

a) Rapid-sequence intubation premedications

b) The blind method for intubation may be required if the spine has not been radiologically cleared

c. Prevention of aspiration

1) Position the patient on his or her side if the spine has been radiologically cleared

2) Suction only as necessary, and limit the duration of suctioning to 10 seconds

3) Hyperoxygenate with 100% oxygen before and after suctioning

4) Do not suction by nose if there is evidence of head or facial trauma

d. Oxygen by nasal cannula at 2 to 6 L/minute if required to maintain an SpO_2 level of 95% unless contraindicated; for patients with chronic obstructive pulmonary disease, use pulse oximetry to guide oxygen administration to an SpO_2 level of 90%

e. Mechanical ventilation may be necessary

1) Recognize that positive pressure mechanical ventilation will increase ICP; the use of lower tidal volumes and PEEP may minimize this effect

3. Maintain MAP, CPP, and cerebral blood flow

a. Identification and control of bleeding from the chest, abdomen, pelvis, extremities, and scalp

b. IV access with two large-bore catheters for fluid and medication administration

c. Intravenous fluids as prescribed: avoid hypotonic fluids (e.g., D_5W), which may contribute to brain edema

d. Vasopressors required for neurogenic shock

4. Prevent, monitor, and treat clinical indications of intracranial hypertension (see Intracranial Hypertension section)

5. Prepare the patient for procedures as indicated

a. Nothing by mouth

b. Nasogastric tube for low suction

c. Foley catheter

d. Surgery for penetrating objects: stabilize the objects in place until they can be removed during surgery

6. Monitor for complications

a. Secondary brain injury (e.g., cerebral edema, ischemia)

b. Intracerebral hematoma or hemorrhage

c. Subarachnoid hemorrhage with contusion

d. Fluid and electrolyte imbalance

e. Antidiuretic hormone (ADH) imbalance: diabetes insipidus (DI) or syndrome of inappropriate antidiuretic hormone (SIADH)

Evaluation

1. Patent airway, adequate oxygenation (i.e., normal PaO_2, SpO_2, SaO_2) and ventilation (i.e., normal $PaCO_2$)

2. Absence of clinical indications of respiratory distress

3. Absence of clinical indications of hypoperfusion

4. Absence of clinical indications of infection or sepsis

5. Alert and oriented with no neurologic deficit

6. Absence of clinical indications of bleeding

Typical disposition

1. If evaluation criteria met: discharge with instructions

a. Concussion and contusion

1) Instructions to return if increased headache, nausea, vomiting, confusion, or other signs of increased ICP occur

2) May need to wake patient every 2 to 4 hours and assess orientation at home

3) Follow up with primary care physician or specialist as directed

2. If evaluation criteria not met: admission

a. If a patient with a contusion or a concussion has an altered level of consciousness, skull fracture, or severe vomiting, then he or she should be admitted

b. If the patient has diffuse axonal injury, admit him or her to a critical care unit

Skull Fractures

Definition: a disruption in the bony integrity of the skull

1. Several different types

a. Linear: simple fracture, single line, or crack

b. Linear stellate: multiple linear fractures that radiate from the site of impact

c. Diastatic: involves a separation of the bones at a suture line or a marked separation of a bone fragment

d. Comminuted: fragmentation of the bone into many pieces

e. Depressed: inward depression of bone fragments

f. Basal: fracture in the skull base or fossa (anterior, middle, or posterior)

Predisposing factors

1. Motor vehicle collision
2. Falls
3. Violence (e.g., assault, gunshot wound, knife wound)
4. Sports-related accidents (e.g., boxing, football)
5. Industrial accidents

Pathophysiology (Figure 6-24)

1. Linear fractures; these account for 80% of skull fractures
   a. Fractures with no displacement of bone
   b. May interrupt major vascular channels
      1) Linear fractures of the temporal and parietal bones may tear the middle meningeal artery and lead to epidural hematoma
      2) Linear fractures of the occipital bone may tear the occipital artery and lead to epidural hematoma
2. Depressed fractures
   a. Fractures that depress the outer table of the skull
   b. May cause brain laceration
   c. May cause intracranial hematoma
3. Basal fractures
   a. Fractures of the base of the skull
   b. May cause injury to one or more cranial nerves or cause tearing of the dura with CSF leak

Clinical presentation

1. Subjective
   a. History of precipitating event or condition
   b. Headache
   c. Nausea and vomiting
   d. Scalp tenderness
2. Objective
   a. Altered level of consciousness with focal neurologic deficits (e.g., hemiparesis, hemiplegia)
   b. Swelling or ecchymosis on the scalp
   c. Scalp laceration
   d. Deformity or crepitus with palpation

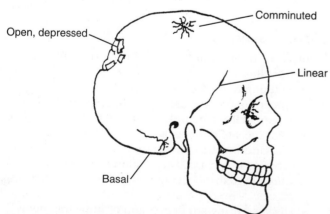

Figure 6-24 Types of skull fractures. (From Barker, E. [1994]. *Neuroscience nursing.* St. Louis: Mosby.)

   e. Seizures
   f. Specific to basal skull fracture
      1) Anterior fossa
         a) May have rhinorrhea; usually lasts 2 to 3 days
         b) May have bilateral ecchymotic eyes (referred to as *raccoon eyes*); takes 3 to 4 hours after injury occurs to develop
         c) May have injury to cranial nerve I (olfactory), which may cause anosmia
         d) May have facial fractures
      2) Middle fossa
         a) May have otorrhea or rhinorrhea
         b) May have CSF or blood behind the tympanic membrane if the tympanic membrane remains intact; may cause hearing deficit
         c) May have ecchymosis over the mastoid bone (referred to as *Battle sign*); takes 4 to 6 hours after the injury occurs to develop
         d) May have cranial nerve injuries
      3) Posterior fossa
         a) May have epidural hematoma, which may result in signs of intracranial hypertension
         b) May have cerebellar, brainstem, or cranial nerve signs (e.g., visual changes, tinnitus, facial paralysis, conjugate eye deviation)
3. Diagnostic
   a. Skull radiography
      1) Linear or depressed skull fractures may be seen on plain films
      2) Basal skull fracture is difficult to confirm with radiography; pneumocephalus, opacity of the mastoid or sphenoid sinus, or an air-fluid level in one of the sinuses may be seen
   b. CT or MRI may visualize depressed fractures

Collaborative management

1. Continue assessment
   a. ABCDs
   b. Vital signs: blood pressure, pulse, respiratory rate, and temperature
   c. Oxygen saturation
   d. Respiratory effort and excursion
   e. Cardiac rate and rhythm
   f. Level of consciousness, pupils, and motor function
   g. Clinical indications of intracranial hypertension
   h. Pain and discomfort level
   i. Accurate intake and output
   j. Close monitoring for the progression of symptoms
2. Maintain airway, oxygenation, and ventilation
   a. Positioning: do not tilt or hyperextend the head to maintain an open airway until the spine has been radiologically cleared; use the jaw-thrust technique
   b. Artificial airways as indicated

1) Oral or nasopharyngeal airway to hold the tongue away from the hypopharynx for patients with an altered level of consciousness
   a) Do not use nasopharyngeal airway or nasal suctioning if a facial or skull fracture is present
   b) Do not use oral airways in conscious patients because these airways stimulate the gag reflex
2) Endotracheal intubation if required; use rapid-sequence intubation premedications
   c. Prevention of aspiration
   1) Position the patient on his or her side if the spine has been radiologically cleared
   2) Suction only as necessary, and limit the duration of suctioning to 10 seconds
   3) Hyperoxygenate with 100% oxygen before and after suctioning
   4) Do not suction by nose if there is evidence of head or facial trauma
   d. Oxygen by nasal cannula at 2 to 6 L/minute if required to maintain an SpO_2 level of 95% unless contraindicated; for patients with chronic obstructive pulmonary disease, use pulse oximetry to guide oxygen administration to an SpO_2 level of 90%
   e. Mechanical ventilation may be necessary
   1) Recognize that positive-pressure mechanical ventilation will increase ICP; the use of lower tidal volumes and PEEP may minimize this effect
3. Maintain MAP, CPP, and cerebral blood flow
   a. Identification and control of bleeding from the chest, abdomen, pelvis, extremities, and scalp; direct pressure as indicated
   b. Intravenous access with two large-bore catheters for fluid and medication administration
   c. IV fluids as prescribed: avoid hypotonic fluids (e.g., D_5W), which may contribute to brain edema
   d. Vasopressors required for patients in neurogenic shock
4. Prevent, monitor, and treat clinical indications of intracranial hypertension (see Intracranial Hypertension section)
   a. Treatment of rhinorrhea or otorrhea, if present:
   1) Do not obstruct flow: use mustache dressing
   2) Elevate head of bed 30 degrees
   3) Avert further tearing of the dura by discouraging sneezing, blowing the nose, and the Valsalva maneuver
      a) Instruct the patient to cough with the mouth open and to exhale when turning (rather than holding the breath)
   4) Do not insert anything into the patient's nose if a CSF leak is suspected
   b. Protection of the part of the brain underneath the cranial defect by not positioning the patient on the side of the injury

5. Control pain and discomfort
   a. Nonsteroidal antiinflammatory drugs
   b. Narcotic analgesics
   c. Anxiolytics
6. Prepare the patient for procedures and assist as indicated
   a. Cleansing of abrasions and lacerations
   b. Preparation for surgery as indicated
7. Monitor for complications
   a. Epidural hematoma
   b. Injury to internal carotid artery at foreman
   c. Intracerebral hemorrhage or contusion
   d. CSF leakage
   e. CNS infection (e.g., meningitis, encephalitis)

Evaluation

1. Patent airway, adequate oxygenation (i.e., normal PaO_2, SpO_2, SaO_2) and ventilation (i.e., normal $PaCO_2$)
2. Absence of clinical indications of respiratory distress
3. Absence of clinical indications of hypoperfusion
4. Absence of clinical indications of infection or sepsis
5. Alert and oriented with no neurologic deficit
6. Control of pain or discomfort
7. Absence of clinical indications of bleeding
8. Alert and oriented with no neurologic deficit

Typical disposition

1. If evaluation criteria met: discharge with instructions
   a. Linear skull fracture with other injuries
2. If evaluation criteria not met: admission to progressive care unit or critical care unit
   a. Depressed skull fracture with scalp laceration: surgery for debridement and repair

Intracranial Hematomas

Definitions

1. Subdural hematoma: a collection of blood in the subdural space
   a. May be classified as acute, subacute, or chronic on the basis of how rapidly signs and symptoms become apparent
2. Epidural hematoma: a collection of blood between the skull and the dura mater
3. Intracerebral hematoma: bleeding directly into the brain tissue either at the site of the original injury or at points distant to the injury

Predisposing factors

1. Trauma
2. Subdural hematoma
   a. May occur spontaneously, particularly if the patient has a coagulation disorder or is taking anticoagulants
   b. May occur in the absence of trauma in older adults and alcoholics
3. Epidural hematoma: often associated with linear skull fractures that cross major vascular channels

Pathophysiology (Figure 6-25)

1. Subdural hematoma
   a. Usually venous bleeding; arterial origin is rare
   b. Blood accumulates below the dura mater
   c. Classifications
      1) Acute: onset within 48 hours after injury
      2) Subacute: onset within 2 weeks after injury
      3) Chronic: may occur weeks to months after injury
         a) Fibroblasts accumulate around the hematoma and encapsulate it
         b) Hemolysis of the clot liberates plasma proteins; this causes the encapsulated area to have a high osmotic pressure
         c) This causes an influx of water and a swelling of the mass
2. Epidural hematoma
   a. Usually arterial bleeding; associated with the tearing of arteries from skull fractures
      1) Linear fractures of the temporal and parietal bones may tear the middle meningeal artery and lead to epidural hematoma
      2) Linear fractures of the occipital bone may tear the occipital artery and lead to epidural hematoma
   b. Blood accumulates above the dura mater
3. Intracerebral hematoma: hematoma into the brain mass itself: may be the result of bleeding caused by missile injury (e.g., gunshot wound, knife wound) or a severe acceleration–deceleration force that causes bleeding into the deep cerebral tissues

Clinical presentation

1. Subdural
   a. Subjective
      1) History of precipitating event or condition
      2) Headache
      3) Increasing irritability that progresses to confusion and then decreased level of consciousness
   b. Objective
      1) Decreased level of consciousness
      2) Ipsilateral oculomotor paralysis
      3) Contralateral hemiparesis or hemiplegia
2. Epidural
   a. Subjective
      1) History of precipitating event or condition
      2) Report of short period of unconsciousness followed by a lucid interval and then rapid deteri-

oration; the lucid interval may be absent if the initial blow is significant
      3) Headache
   b. Objective
      1) Lucid interval followed by decreasing level of consciousness
      2) Ipsilateral oculomotor paralysis
      3) Contralateral hemiparesis or hemiplegia
3. Intracerebral
   a. Subjective
      1) History of precipitating event or condition
   b. Objective
      1) Varies with the area of the brain involved, the size of the hematoma, and the rate of blood accumulation
      2) May or may not show clinical indications of intracranial hypertension
4. Diagnostic
   a. Skull and cervical spine radiography: may reveal associated skull or spine fractures
   b. LP: contraindicated by intracranial hypertension
   c. CT: will show an area of increased density; may also show a midline shift
   d. MRI: shows hematoma
   e. Cerebral angiogram (rarely performed): may reveal an avascular area with the displacement or stretching of vessels

Collaborative management

1. Continue assessment
   a. ABCDs
   b. Vital signs: blood pressure, pulse, respiratory rate, and temperature
   c. Oxygen saturation
   d. Respiratory effort and excursion
   e. Cardiac rate and rhythm
   f. Level of consciousness, pupils, and motor function
   g. Clinical indications of intracranial hypertension; invasive ICP monitoring may be used
   h. Pain and discomfort level
   i. Accurate intake and output
   j. Close monitoring for the progression of symptoms
2. Maintain airway, oxygenation, and ventilation
   a. Positioning: do not tilt or hyperextend the head to maintain an open airway until the spine has been radiologically cleared; use the jaw-thrust technique

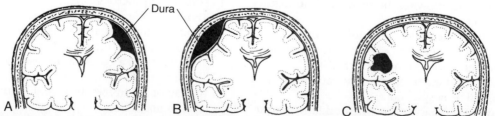

Figure 6-25 Types of hematomas. **A,** Subdural. **B,** Epidural. **C,** Intracerebral. (From Chipps, E. M., Clanin, N. J., & Campbell, V. G. [1992]. *Neurologic disorders: Mosby's clinical nursing series.* St. Louis: Mosby.)

b. Artificial airways as indicated
   1) Oral or nasopharyngeal airway to hold the tongue away from the hypopharynx in patients with altered consciousness
     a) Do not use a nasopharyngeal airway or nasal suctioning if a facial or skull fracture is present
     b) Do not use oral airways in conscious patients because these airways stimulate the gag reflex
   2) Endotracheal intubation if required
     a) Rapid-sequence intubation premedications
     b) The blind method for intubation may be required if the spine has not been radiologically cleared
c. Prevention of aspiration
   1) Position the patient on his or her side if the spine has been radiologically cleared
   2) Suction only as necessary, and limit the duration of suctioning to 10 seconds
   3) Hyperoxygenate with 100% oxygen before and after suctioning
   4) Do not suction by nose if there is evidence of head or facial trauma
d. Oxygen by nasal cannula at 2 to 6 L/minute if required to maintain an SpO_2 level of 95% unless contraindicated; for patients with chronic obstructive pulmonary disease, use pulse oximetry to guide oxygen administration to an SpO_2 level of 90%
e. Mechanical ventilation may be necessary
   1) Recognize that positive pressure mechanical ventilation will increase ICP; the use of lower tidal volumes and PEEP may minimize this effect
3. Maintain MAP, CPP, and cerebral blood flow
  a. IV access with two large-bore catheters for fluid and medication administration
  b. Intravenous fluids as prescribed: avoid hypotonic fluids (e.g., D_5W), which may contribute to brain edema
4. Prevent, monitor, and treat clinical indications of intracranial hypertension (see Intracranial Hypertension section)
  a. Osmotic diuretics are generally not used because the tamponade effect of the hematoma helps to stop the bleeding
  b. Preparation for surgery: note that mortality increases if surgery is delayed
   1) Epidural and subdural hematomas: usually treated with a burr hole and clot evacuation though small hematomas may be observed through serial computed tomography scans to verify the gradual reabsorption of the hematomas
   2) Intracranial hematoma (ICH): surgery is indicated if the ICH is large or if there is a deteriorating neurologic status
  c. Anticonvulsants prophylactically or therapeutically as prescribed

5. Monitor for complications
  a. Intracranial hypertension
  b. Hydrocephalus
  c. CNS infection
  d. Fluid and electrolyte imbalance: DI or SIADH
  e. Seizures

Evaluation
1. Patent airway, adequate oxygenation (i.e., normal PaO_2, SpO_2, SaO_2) and ventilation (i.e., normal $PaCO_2$)
2. Absence of clinical indications of respiratory distress
3. Absence of clinical indications of hypoperfusion
4. Alert and oriented with no neurologic deficit
5. Absence of clinical indications of infection or sepsis
6. Control of pain or discomfort
7. Absence of clinical indications of bleeding

Typical disposition: admission
1. Usually to critical care unit
2. May go directly to surgery

Hemorrhagic Stroke
Definitions
1. Hemorrhagic stroke: a neurologic deficit caused by the interruption of blood flow to the brain as a result of vessel rupture
2. Intraparenchymal hemorrhage: bleeding into the parenchyma of the brain
3. Subarachnoid hemorrhage: bleeding into the subarachnoid space caused by an aneurysm or an arteriovenous malformation
  a. Cerebral aneurysm: a weakened, bulging area on an intracranial blood vessel; these aneurysms account for the majority of subarachnoid hemorrhages
  b. Arteriovenous malformation: a tangle of abnormal arteries and veins; arteries feed directly into veins without a capillary bed

Predisposing factors
1. Intraparenchymal hemorrhage
  a. Trauma
  b. Hypertensive rupture of a cerebral vessel
  c. May also be caused by vascular intracerebral tumor, fibrinolytics, anticoagulants, bleeding disorders, or the spontaneous hemorrhagic conversion of an ischemic infarct
2. Subarachnoid hemorrhage
  a. Most cerebral aneurysms are small (2–6 mm) and saccular, and they most frequently occur at bifurcations in the circle of Willis
   1) Saccular (berry) aneurysms: usually congenital defects
   2) Fusiform aneurysms: result from atherosclerosis
   3) Mycotic aneurysms: result from necrotic vasculitis and septic emboli (rare)
   4) Traumatic aneurysms: result from skull fractures that disrupt a vessel (very rare)
  b. Arteriovenous malformation: congenital

Pathophysiology

1. Intraparenchymal hemorrhage causes pressure on the cerebral tissues and nerves and may lead to a loss of function and the death of neurons
2. Aneurysm
   a. Two contributing factors
      1) Congenital weakness
      2) Stress (e.g., hypertension)
   b. The aneurysm may act as a mass lesion if it is intact and large
   c. Weakness of an artery and high pressure lead to hemorrhage; 90% of ruptured aneurysms are associated with hypertension
   d. A clot initially forms in and around a rupture site and temporarily inhibits continuing hemorrhage; increases in ICP and pressure from local tissues may stop bleeding
   e. Blood leakage into the subarachnoid space and that comes in contact with the meninges causes meningeal irritation
   f. Cerebral vascular spasm often occurs and contributes to ischemia or infarction
   g. Communicating hydrocephalus can develop as a result of the obstruction of CSF outflow through the arachnoid villi
   h. As the clot around the aneurysm is broken down by the body's natural fibrinolytic processes, rebleeding may occur
3. Arteriovenous malformation
   a. This condition steals blood from other areas because it involves an area of low resistance that causes the ischemia of surrounding tissue
   b. Hemorrhage may occur

Clinical presentation

1. Subjective
   a. Intraparynchymal hemorrhage: may report a precipitating traumatic event
   b. Aneurysm:
      1) May report atypical headache that occurs days or weeks prior to rupture (i.e., warning leak phenomenon)
      2) Sudden and severe headache
         a) Described as "the worst headache of my life"
         b) Pain radiates to the neck and back
      3) Generalized, transient weakness
      4) Ptosis, diplopia, or blurred vision
      5) Nausea and vomiting
   c. Arteriovenous malformation
      1) May report hearing a constant swishing sound in the head with each heartbeat
      2) Dizziness or syncope
2. Objective
   a. Restlessness that progresses to an altered level of consciousness
      1) Loss of consciousness is common with hemorrhage from aneurysm
      2) Loss of consciousness is uncommon with hemorrhage from arteriovenous malformation

   b. If hemorrhage into ventricles
      1) Nuchal rigidity
      2) Photophobia
      3) Kernig sign or Brudzinski sign
      4) Hyperthermia
   c. Seizures
   d. Aphasia may occur
   e. Motor or sensory defects may occur
3. Diagnostic
   a. Serum
      1) Hyponatremia may be present as a result of SIADH or cerebral salt wasting
      2) Prothrombin and partial thromboplastin times may be abnormal
   b. CT: identifies the extent of intraparenchymal or subarachnoid hemorrhage and detects the presence of hydrocephalus
   c. LP: performed only if computed tomography is nondiagnostic and if there are no clinical indications of intracranial hypertension
   d. ECG
      1) Subarachnoid hemorrhage: flat, peaked, or inverted T wave; prominent U wave; prolonged QT; dysrhythmias (particularly torsades de pointes) are common
   e. Transcranial Doppler: helps with the diagnosis of vasospasm
   f. MRI or MRA: may show small aneurysms, intracranial hypertension, intraventricular blood, or vasospasm
   g. Cerebral arteriogram: will illustrate size, shape, and location of aneurysm; may show vasospasm

Collaborative management

1. Continue assessment
   a. ABCDs
   b. Vital signs: blood pressure, pulse, respiratory rate, and temperature
   c. Oxygen saturation
   d. Respiratory effort and excursion
   e. Cardiac rate and rhythm
   f. Level of consciousness, pupils, and motor function
   g. Clinical indications of intracranial hypertension; invasive ICP monitoring may be used
   h. Pain and discomfort level
   i. Accurate intake and output
   j. Close monitoring for the progression of symptoms
2. Maintain airway, oxygenation, and ventilation
   a. Positioning: head of bed elevated 30 degrees; place patient in a side-lying position if he or she has nausea or vomiting
   b. Artificial airways as indicated
      1) Oral or nasopharyngeal airway to hold the tongue away from the hypopharynx for patients with altered consciousness
         a) Do not use oral airways in conscious patients because these airways stimulate the gag reflex

2) Endotracheal intubation if required; use rapid-sequence intubation premedications

c. Prevention of aspiration

1) Position the patient on his or her side

2) Suction only as necessary, and limit the duration of suctioning to 10 seconds

3) Hyperoxygenate with 100% oxygen before and after suctioning

d. Oxygen by nasal cannula at 2 to 6 L/minute if required to maintain an SpO_2 level of 95% unless contraindicated; for patients with chronic obstructive pulmonary disease, use pulse oximetry to guide oxygen administration to an SpO_2 level of 90%

e. Mechanical ventilation may be necessary

1) Recognize that positive pressure mechanical ventilation will increase ICP; the use of lower tidal volumes and PEEP may minimize this effect

3. Maintain MAP, CPP, and cerebral blood flow

a. Identification and control of bleeding from the chest, abdomen, pelvis, extremities, and scalp

b. IV access with two large-bore catheters for fluid and medication administration

c. Intravenous fluids as prescribed: avoid hypotonic fluids (e.g., D_5W), which may contribute to brain edema

d. Pharmacologic agents to maintain blood pressure within 10% of prehemorrhage levels; hypotension is associated with hypoperfusion, and hypertension is associated with rebleeding

1) α- and β-blockers (e.g., labetalol [Normodyne]) or vasodilators (e.g., hydralazine [Apresoline])

2) Vasopressors (e.g., phenylephrine [Neo-Synephrine]) for hypotension

e. Calcium-channel blockers to prevent or reduce vasospasm

4. Prevent, monitor, and treat clinical indications of intracranial hypertension (see Intracranial Hypertension section)

5. Decrease environmental stimuli; these interventions may be referred to as *aneurysm precautions:*

a. Provide a quiet, dimly lit, private room

b. Enforce bed rest with the head of the bed elevated 15 to 30 degrees

c. Instruct the patient regarding how to avoid the Valsalva maneuver (e.g., cough with the mouth open, exhale when turning in bed, use stool softeners)

d. Instruct visitors that the patient should not be upset in any way; limit the number of visitors and the duration of visits

e. Do not perform any rectal procedures (e.g., rectal temperatures, enemas)

f. Provide sedation (usually phenobarbital [Luminal]) if the patient is restless

g. Treat fever with acetaminophen (Tylenol)

6. Control pain and discomfort: use narcotic analgesics for headache but avoid oversedation that would impair assessment

7. Prepare the patient for interventional neuroradiology procedures or surgery as indicated

8. Monitor for complications

a. Vasospasm (with aneurysms)

b. Rebleeding

c. Brain edema and intracranial hypertension

d. Hydrocephalus: may require ventriculoperitoneal shunt

e. Fluid and electrolyte imbalance: DI or SIADH

f. Seizures

g. Dysrhythmias (e.g., torsades de pointes)

Evaluation

1. Patent airway, adequate oxygenation (i.e., normal PaO_2, SpO_2, SaO_2) and ventilation (i.e., normal $PaCO_2$)

2. Absence of clinical indications of respiratory distress

3. Absence of clinical indications of hypoperfusion

4. Absence of clinical indications of infection or sepsis

5. Alert and oriented with no neurologic deficit

6. Control of pain or discomfort

Typical disposition: admission to critical care unit

Ischemic Stroke

Definitions

1. Stroke: an infarction of the central nervous system tissue (Adams et al., 2008)

a. Ischemic stroke: the sudden death of brain cells in a localized area as a result of inadequate blood flow

2. Transient ischemic attack: a transient episode of neurologic dysfunction caused by focal brain, spinal cord, or retinal ischemia without infarction (Adams et al., 2008)

Predisposing factors

1. Risk factors include the following:

a. Family history

b. Hypertension

c. Smoking

d. Diabetes mellitus

e. Valvular heart disease

f. Coronary artery disease

g. Heart failure

h. Hyperlipidemia

i. Obesity

j. Sedentary lifestyle

k. Drugs

1) Alcohol, especially heavy episodic consumption

2) Stimulants (e.g., cocaine, phenylpropanolamine)

3) Oral contraceptives

l. Dysrhythmias, especially atrial fibrillation

m. Hypercoagulability

2. Thrombosis
   a. Intracranial arteriosclerosis
   b. Extracranial (i.e., carotid) atherosclerosis
   c. Hypertension
   d. Hypercoagulability (e.g., polycythemia)
3. Embolism
   a. Mural thrombi
      1) Dysrhythmia (e.g., atrial fibrillation)
      2) Ventricular aneurysm
   b. Carotid artery atherosclerosis
   c. Bacterial endocarditis
   d. Valvular heart disease
   e. Prosthetic cardiac valves

Pathophysiology

1. Occlusive vascular disease (thrombosis or embolus) causes a decreased level of oxygen to reach the brain tissue, which causes ischemia and leads to infarction
2. Brain edema develops slowly, usually over the first 72 hours; brain edema and persistent ischemia cause progressive damage to the penumbra (i.e., the ischemic brain tissue that surrounds the infarction)

Clinical presentation

1. Subjective
   a. May report a history of risk factors or transient ischemic attack
   b. Sudden onset of signs and symptoms
      1) Thrombotic stroke usually occurs at night and is often discovered after awakening; it is likely caused by a decrease in cardiac output and blood pressure with less flow through an area of critical stenosis
      2) Embolic stroke is more likely to occur when the patient is active
   c. Visual changes: diplopia, blurring, or amaurosis fugax (i.e., the loss of a portion of the visual field)
2. Objective
   a. Hypertension is common
   b. May have an altered level of consciousness
   c. Hemiparesis or hemiplegia; more common with anterior circulation stroke
   d. Changes in speech: dysarthria, dysphasia, or aphasia
   e. Facial drooping
   f. Nystagmus
   g. Ataxia
3. Diagnostic
   a. Lipids: may be elevated
   b. Glucose
      1) Hypoglycemia may mimic stroke
      2) Hyperglycemia frequently seen with stroke
   c. Clotting profile: baseline before fibrinolytics
   d. CBC with differential and platelet count: to assess for anemia, thrombocytopenia, thrombocytosis, and polycythemia
   e. CT: rapid noncontrast within 25 minutes of coming through the emergency department door and read within 20 minutes of procedure
      1) Normal soon after ischemic stroke
      2) Identifies the location and character of subacute and old infarctions, the presence or absence of gross hemorrhage, and any mass lesions
      3) May show distortion or a shift of the ventricles
   f. ECG: dysrhythmias (e.g., atrial fibrillation as cause of cerebral emboli)
   g. Echocardiography: may show an intracardiac source of cerebral emboli (e.g., ventricular aneurysm)
   h. LP: may be performed to differentiate hemorrhagic from thrombotic stroke if there are no signs of intracranial hypertension
   i. Doppler carotid studies: if carotid stenosis is present
   j. Magnetic resonance imaging: shows the presence of early ischemic changes when a computed tomography scan still looks normal; can identify changes in cranial or spinal structures
   k. Cerebral angiography: identifies occlusion, stenosis, aneurysms, or hemorrhage in the arterial system

Collaborative management

1. Continue assessment
   a. ABCDs
   b. Vital signs: blood pressure, pulse, respiratory rate, and temperature
   c. Oxygen saturation
   d. Respiratory effort and excursion
   e. Cardiac rate and rhythm
   f. Level of consciousness, pupils, and motor function
   g. Clinical indications of intracranial hypertension; invasive ICP monitoring may be used
   h. Pain and discomfort level
   i. Accurate intake and output
   j. Close monitoring for the progression of symptoms
2. Maintain airway, oxygenation, and ventilation
   a. Positioning: head of bed elevated 30 degrees; place the patient in a side-lying position if nausea and vomiting are present
   b. Artificial airways as indicated
      1) Oral or nasopharyngeal airway to hold the tongue away from the hypopharynx for patients with altered consciousness
         a) Do not use oral airways in conscious patients because these airways stimulate the gag reflex
      2) Endotracheal intubation if required; use rapid-sequence intubation premedications
   c. Prevention of aspiration
      1) Positioning of the patient on his or her side
      2) Suctioning only as necessary, and limit duration of suctioning to 10 seconds
      3) Hyperoxygenation with 100% oxygen before and after suctioning

d. Oxygen by nasal cannula at 2 to 6 L/minute if required to maintain an SpO_2 level of 95% unless contraindicated; for patients with chronic obstructive pulmonary disease, use pulse oximetry to guide oxygen administration to an SpO_2 level of 90%
e. Mechanical ventilation may be necessary
  1) Recognize that positive pressure mechanical ventilation will increase ICP; the use of lower tidal volumes and PEEP may minimize this effect
3. Maintain MAP, CPP, and cerebral blood flow
  a. Identification and control of bleeding from the chest, abdomen, pelvis, extremities, and scalp
  b. IV access with two large-bore catheters for fluid and medication administration
  c. IV fluids as prescribed: avoid hypotonic fluids (e.g., D_5W), which may contribute to brain edema
  d. Measures to restore or maintain cerebral blood flow (Figure 6-26)
    1) Use the National Institutes of Health Stroke Scale (see Table 6-8) to assess changes in neurologic status
    2) Correct possible causes and contributing factors
      a) Assist with the electrical or pharmacologic conversion of atrial fibrillation or administer anticoagulants to prevent mural thrombi
      b) Administer antihypertensives to control blood pressure
        i) Maintain a systolic blood pressure of <185 mm Hg and a diastolic blood pressure of <110 mm Hg; however, hypotension must be avoided, because cerebral autoregulation is lost in the area of ischemia or infarction
        ii) Labetalol (Normodyne) is generally used, but nitroprusside (Nipride), hydralazine (Apresoline), or nicardipine (Cardene) may also be used
      c) Control hyperglycemia with IV insulin infusion
    3) Administer fibrinolytics as prescribed
      a) Goal: lysis of an occluding clot to restore blood flow to the compromised but potentially viable penumbra
      b) Indications: presentation within 3 hours of acute ischemic stroke symptoms: remember the seven Ds of stroke care (American Heart Association, 2005)
        i) Detection of early indications and determination of time of onset
        ii) Dispatch of emergency medical care
        iii) Delivery of the patient to the nearest facility that is capable of implementing the most current stroke guidelines
        iv) Door and rapid triage in the emergency department
        v) Data collected to help with decision making
          (a) Baseline imaging to exclude intracranial hemorrhage and other risk factors for intracranial hemorrhage
          (b) History, physical examination, and laboratory values
        vi) Decision made regarding whether the patient meets the criteria for fibrinolytics and does not have contraindications; see Table 4-25, but consider the following additions:
          (a) Awakening with symptoms of stroke so the time of onset cannot be determined
          (b) Seizure at the onset of stroke
          (c) Age of >75 years
          (d) National Institutes of Health Stroke Scale score of >22
          (e) Hypodensities on computed tomography scan
          (f) Subacute bacterial endocarditis
        vii) Drugs given within 3 hours of the onset of symptoms
      c) Drug and dosage: alteplase (Activase)
        i) Total dose: 0.9 mg/kg IV with a maximum dose of ≤90 mg
        ii) Bolus: 10% of this total dose given over the course of 1 minute
        iii) Infusion: remaining 90% of this total dose administered over the course of 60 minutes
    4) Administer anticoagulants and platelet aggregation inhibitors as prescribed if fibrinolytics are contraindicated or 24 hours after IV fibrinolytics
      a) Anticoagulants (e.g., heparin) are especially important if emboli are of cardiac origin (e.g., atrial fibrillation)
        i) Low-molecular-weight heparin given subcutaneously may be used for deep venous thrombosis prophylaxis
      b) Platelet aggregation inhibitors
        i) Oral agents (e.g., aspirin, clopidogrel [Plavix]) or IV agents (e.g., abciximab [ReoPro], eptifibatide [Integrilin]) as prescribed
        ii) Especially important for patients with carotid, intracranial, or vertebrobasilar artery stenosis
        iii) Contraindicated for 24 hours after IV fibrinolytics
4. Prevent, monitor, and treat clinical indications of intracranial hypertension (see Intracranial Hypertension section)
5. Control pain and discomfort
  a. Nonsteroidal antiinflammatory agents

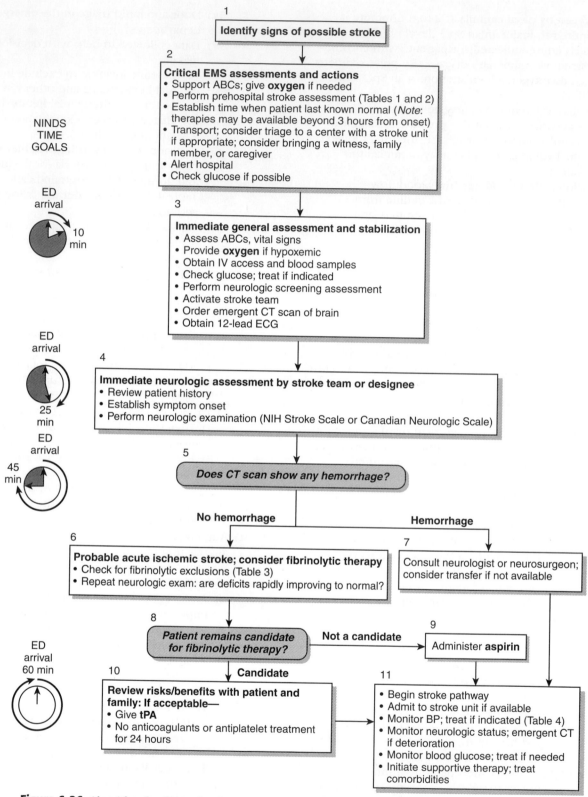

NINDS TIME GOALS

ED arrival
10 min

ED arrival
25 min

ED arrival
45 min

ED arrival
60 min

1
Identify signs of possible stroke

2
Critical EMS assessments and actions
• Support ABCs; give **oxygen** if needed
• Perform prehospital stroke assessment (Tables 1 and 2)
• Establish time when patient last known normal (*Note*: therapies may be available beyond 3 hours from onset)
• Transport; consider triage to a center with a stroke unit if appropriate; consider bringing a witness, family member, or caregiver
• Alert hospital
• Check glucose if possible

3
Immediate general assessment and stabilization
• Assess ABCs, vital signs
• Provide **oxygen** if hypoxemic
• Obtain IV access and blood samples
• Check glucose; treat if indicated
• Perform neurologic screening assessment
• Activate stroke team
• Order emergent CT scan of brain
• Obtain 12-lead ECG

4
Immediate neurologic assessment by stroke team or designee
• Review patient history
• Establish symptom onset
• Perform neurologic examination (NIH Stroke Scale or Canadian Neurologic Scale)

5
Does CT scan show any hemorrhage?

No hemorrhage   **Hemorrhage**

6
Probable acute ischemic stroke; consider fibrinolytic therapy
• Check for fibrinolytic exclusions (Table 3)
• Repeat neurologic exam: are deficits rapidly improving to normal?

7
Consult neurologist or neurosurgeon; consider transfer if not available

8
Patient remains candidate for fibrinolytic therapy?   **Not a candidate**

9
Administer **aspirin**

Candidate

10
Review risks/benefits with patient and family: If acceptable—
• Give **tPA**
• No anticoagulants or antiplatelet treatment for 24 hours

11
• Begin stroke pathway
• Admit to stroke unit if available
• Monitor BP; treat if indicated (Table 4)
• Monitor neurologic status; emergent CT if deterioration
• Monitor blood glucose; treat if needed
• Initiate supportive therapy; treat comorbidities

Figure 6-26 Algorithm for the goals of management of patients with suspected stroke. (From American Heart Association. [2005]. Part 9: Adult stroke. *Circulation, 112[24 suppl],* IV111–IV120.)

b. Narcotic analgesics

c. Anxiolytics

6. Prepare patient for procedures as indicated

   a. Nothing by mouth initially

   b. Nasogastric tube to low suction

   c. Foley catheter

7. Protect patient from injury

   a. Assistance during ambulation because patient may have postural imbalance related to hemiparesis or hemiplegia

   b. Frequent orientation and the provision of explanations of care because confusion, disorientation, and memory deficits may occur concomitantly with aphasia

   c. Anticonvulsants as prescribed

   d. Therapeutic hypothermia may be used for neuronal salvaging

8. Monitor for complications

   a. Related to fibrinolytic therapy: bleeding is the most catastrophic complication; any change in the level of consciousness after fibrinolytic therapy has started requires that the medication be stopped and the patient have a repeat head CT

   b. Persistent neurologic trauma

   c. Brain edema

   d. Seizures

   e. Fluid and electrolyte imbalance: DI or SIADH

Evaluation

1. Patent airway, adequate oxygenation (i.e., normal PaO_2, SpO_2, SaO_2) and ventilation (i.e., normal $PaCO_2$)

2. Absence of clinical indications of respiratory distress

3. Absence of clinical indications of hypoperfusion

4. Absence of clinical indications of infection or sepsis

5. Alert and oriented with no neurologic deficit

6. Absence of clinical indications of bleeding

7. Control of pain or discomfort

Typical disposition

1. If evaluation criteria met (i.e., transient ischemic attack with resolution): discharge with instructions

2. If evaluation criteria not met: admission to progressive care unit or critical care unit

Spinal Cord Injuries

Definition: damage to the spinal cord and nerve roots that may be temporary or permanent

1. Extrinsic damage: injury to bone and tissue

2. Intrinsic damage: hemorrhage, edema, or hypoxia (Emergency Nurses Association, 2007)

Predisposing factors

1. Trauma is the most common cause

   a. Risk factors for traumatic spinal cord injury include the following:

      1) Male gender

      2) Age of between 16 and 30 years

      3) Alcohol or other drug use

   b. Types of trauma include the following:

      1) Motor vehicle collisions

      2) Falls

      3) Diving into shallow water or hitting a submersed object

      4) Violence: assaults, gunshot wounds, and knife wounds

      5) Sports-related accidents (e.g., boxing, football)

      6) Industrial accidents

      7) Thrill-seeking behaviors

      8) Increased risk with alcohol or drug use

   c. Mechanisms of injury

      1) Hyperflexion

         a) The chin is forced to the chest

         b) Occurs most often at the C5 and C6 level

         c) Results from sudden deceleration

         d) Results in ligament tears, stretching of the spinal cord, and the dislocation or subluxation of intervertebral disks or bone fragments that compress the spinal cord or spinal nerve roots

      2) Hyperextension: also called *whiplash*

         a) The head is thrown backward

         b) Occurs most often in the cervical region

         c) Results from the forces of acceleration and deceleration

         d) Results in backward and downward movement, which stretches the spinal cord, disrupts the intervertebral disks, and tears the ligaments

            i) This ruptures the anterior ligaments

            ii) The posterior part of the vertebral body can fracture

      3) Rotation injury

         a) The spinal cord is rotated

         b) Can involve all parts of the vertebral column

         c) Results from rotational forces tearing the spinal ligaments

         d) Results in the displacement of the intervertebral disks and the compression of the spinal nerve roots

      4) Vertical compression

         a) Usually caused by falling or jumping and landing directly on the feet or the head

            i) Landing on the feet sends the impact traveling up to the spine, which causes fractures of the lower thoracic and lumbar vertebrae

            ii) Landing on the head can cause fractures of the cervical vertebrae

         b) The vertebral column is compressed

         c) Occurs primarily in area of T12 to L2

         d) Results in burst vertebra and intervertebral disks; bony fragments may impinge on the spinal cord

5) Penetrating trauma
   a) Can occur at any level
   b) Results from the spinal cord being injured by a penetrating object (e.g., bullet, knife)
   c) Results in the complete or incomplete transection of the spinal cord
2. Other disorders can lead to spinal cord injury as a result of the compression of the spinal cord or impaired tissue perfusion of the cord, including the following:
   a. Cervical spondylosis
   b. Myelitis
   c. Osteoporosis
   d. Tumors
   e. Vascular diseases
3. Specific cervical spine fractures
   a. Fracture of the odontoid process
   b. Bilateral fracture of the pedicles of C2 (hangman fracture)
   c. Burst fracture of the ring of C1 (Jefferson fracture)
   d. High cervical injury affects breathing
   e. Low cervical injury can affect the ability to take a deep breath, to cough, and to sigh (Emergency Nurses Association, 2007)

Pathophysiology

1. Acceleration, deceleration, or impact forces compress, shear, pull, or tear tissue around the spinal cord
2. Immediate microscopic bleeding around the cord—particularly in the gray matter—occurs, thus initiating the inflammatory response
3. Edema develops within an hour after the injury and spreads along sections of the cord
4. Edema and the resultant pressure cause a loss of cord function that can be temporary or permanent
5. Axons are demyelinated, which causes a loss of nerve conduction
6. Phagocytes that migrate to the injured area can scavenge some surviving axons, thereby creating more damage; macrophages can actually cause a cavity to form around scavenged neural tissue
7. Continuing inflammatory processes release mediators and cause further damage
8. This results in a complete or incomplete cord injury
9. Spinal shock occurs as a result of the loss of neurologic function below the level of the injury
   a. Flaccid paralysis
   b. Areflexia
   c. Loss of sensation
   d. Loss of autonomic function (e.g., sweating)

Clinical presentation

1. Subjective
   a. May relate a history of trauma or chronic illness that may predispose the patient to spinal cord injury
   b. Neck pain
   c. Paresthesia

2. Objective
   a. Hypotension and bradycardia may occur; spinal shock may be seen with cervical and high thoracic injuries
   b. Surface trauma may be present over the site of injury
   c. Step-off fractures may be palpated
   d. Varying degrees of motor and sensory dysfunction, depending on the location and extent of the injury
      1) Level of lesion: cervical and lumbar are more common than thoracic
         a) C1 to C2: ventilatory cessation and immediate death
         b) C3 to C5: quadriplegia with a total loss of ventilatory function; dependent on a mechanical ventilator dependent; remember: "C3, 4, 5 keeps the diaphragm alive"
         c) C5 to C6: quadriplegia with gross arm movements; the sparing of the diaphragm leads to diaphragmatic breathing; no intercostal or abdominal muscles to assist with coughing
         d) C6 to C7: quadriplegia with biceps muscles intact but no function of the intrinsic hand muscles; diaphragmatic breathing; no intercostal or abdominal muscles to assist with coughing
         e) C7 to C8: quadriplegia with triceps and biceps muscles intact but no function of the intrinsic hand muscles; diaphragmatic breathing; no intercostal or abdominal muscles to assist with coughing
         f) T1 to L2: paraplegia with a loss of varying amounts of intercostal and abdominal muscle; the lower the injury, the more intercostal function remains available
         g) Below L2: cauda equina injury; a mixed picture of motor and sensory loss with bowel and bladder dysfunction
      2) Complete versus incomplete
         a) Complete lesion: loss of sensory and motor function below the level of the lesion; irreversible
            i) Flaccid paralysis below the level of injury
            ii) Areflexia below the level of injury
            iii) Urinary retention or priapism
         b) Incomplete syndromes: varying degrees of paralysis and sensory loss below the level of injury with varying degrees of bowel and bladder paralysis (Figure 6-27 and Table 6-15)
   e. Spinal shock (occurs within minutes of the injury and may last from several days to months): results from the loss of inhibition of the descending tracts
      1) Clinical presentation
         a) Loss of all motor, sensory, and reflex responses
         b) Bradycardia and hypotension
         c) Loss of autonomic control
         d) Transient reflex depression below the level of the injury

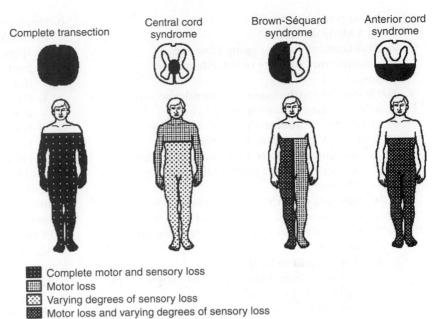

Figure 6-27 Complete and incomplete spinal cord injuries. (From Dennison, R. (2000). *Pass CCRN!* [2nd ed.]. St. Louis: Mosby. Figure 7-7, p. 364.)

- Complete transection
- Central cord syndrome
- Brown-Séquard syndrome
- Anterior cord syndrome

- ▨ Complete motor and sensory loss
- ▦ Motor loss
- ▨ Varying degrees of sensory loss
- ▨ Motor loss and varying degrees of sensory loss

e) Flaccid paralysis of all skeletal muscles below the level of the injury
f) Paralytic ileus
g) Urinary and fecal retention
h) Impairment of temperature regulation (i.e., vasodilation and inability to shiver): poikilothermia
i) Priapism may occur
2) May last from several days to months; when spinal shock is over, any or all of the following may occur:
   a) Flexor spasms caused by cutaneous stimulation

b) Reflex bowel and bladder emptying
c) Hyperactive deep tendon reflexes
3. Diagnostic
   a. CBC with differential
   b. Clotting panel
   c. Alcohol level
   d. Serum chemistries with glucose, BUN, and creatinine
   e. Radiography
      1) Cervical films: three views from the cervical vertebrae through the body of T1 are needed
         a) Cross-table lateral film

TABLE 6-15   Incomplete Spinal Cord Lesions

Type of Lesion	Motor Loss	Sensory Loss	Type of Injury
Central cord syndrome	• Weakness of all extremities but greater motor loss in upper extremities	• Varies depending on the number of undamaged spinal cord tracts	• Hyperextension
Brown-Séquard syndrome	• Ipsilateral motor loss below the lesion	• Ipsilateral loss of position and vibratory sense • Contralateral loss of pain and temperature sensation	• Rotational with dislocation of fracture fragments • Penetrating (e.g., knife or gunshot wound) • Tumor
Anterior cord syndrome	• Complete motor loss below the lesion	• Loss of pain and temperature sensation below the lesion; there is a sparing of proprioception, vibratory sense, and touch	• Hyperflexion
Posterior cord syndrome	• Motor function remains intact	• Loss of touch, vibratory sense, and proprioception below the lesion	• Hyperextension or disease processes
Cauda equina syndrome	• Varying amount of motor loss in the lower extremities • Bowel and bladder problems common	• Varying amount of sensory loss in the lower extremities	• Indirect trauma to the peripheral nerves associated with fracture

b) Anteroposterior film
c) Odontoid film
2) Thoracic and lumbar spine films for unconscious patients or if further injury suspected
3) Flexion–extension views: to identify soft-tissue injuries that can compress the cord
4) SCIWORA syndrome (Spinal *C*ord *I*njury With*Out* *R*adiographic *A*bnormality)
   a) Accounts for up to two thirds of severe cervical injuries among children <8 years old
   b) Inherent elasticity of pediatric cervical spine can allow severe spinal cord injury to occur without presence on radiography findings
   c) Diagnosis of exclusion
   d) MRI: may show hemorrhage or edema of the spinal cord
   e) Pseudosubluxation: anterior displacement may be up to 4 mm
   f) If suspected, management is to immobilize the pediatric patient for 1 to 3 weeks
f. CT: spine and head

Collaborative management

1. Continue assessment
   a. ABCDs
   b. Vital signs: blood pressure, pulse, respiratory rate, and temperature
   c. Oxygen saturation
   d. Respiratory effort and excursion
   e. Cardiac rate and rhythm
   f. Level of consciousness, pupils, and motor function
   g. Pain and discomfort level
   h. Accurate intake and output
   i. Close monitoring for the progression of symptoms
2. Maintain airway, oxygenation, and ventilation
   a. Positioning: do not tilt or hyperextend the head to maintain an open airway until the spine has been radiologically cleared; use the jaw-thrust technique
   b. Artificial airways as indicated
      1) Oral or nasopharyngeal airway to hold the tongue away from the hypopharynx in patients with altered consciousness
         a) Do not use a nasopharyngeal airway or nasal suctioning if a facial or skull fracture is present
         b) Do not use oral airways in conscious patients because these airways stimulate the gag reflex
      2) Endotracheal intubation if required
         a) Rapid-sequence intubation premedications
         b) The blind method for intubation may be required if the spine has not been radiologically cleared

c. Prevention of aspiration
   1) Position the patient on his or her side if the spine has been radiologically cleared
   2) Suctioning only as necessary, and limit the duration of suctioning to 10 seconds
   3) Hyperoxygenate with 100% oxygen before and after suctioning
   4) Do not suction by nose if there is evidence of head or facial trauma
d. Oxygen by nasal cannula at 2 to 6 L/minute if required to maintain an SpO_2 level of 95% unless contraindicated; for patients with chronic obstructive pulmonary disease, use pulse oximetry to guide oxygen administration to an SpO_2 level of 90%
e. Mechanical ventilation may be necessary
3. Maintain MAP, CPP, and blood flow to the spinal cord
   a. Identification and control of bleeding from the chest, abdomen, pelvis, extremities, and scalp
   b. IV access with two large-bore catheters for fluid and medication administration
   c. Intravenous fluids as prescribed
      1) Provide fluid resuscitation judiciously; often patients with spinal cord injury are hypotensive in the presence of normal volume, but xcessive fluid may increase cord edema and injury
      2) Avoid hypotonic fluids (e.g., D_5W), which may contribute to brain edema
   d. Low-dose pressor agents may be required to maintain an adequate blood pressure
   e. Elevation of the legs and the application of elastic stockings (i.e, TED) may help to improve venous return
4. Prevent further damage to the spinal cord
   a. Immediate immobilization by taping the patient to a back board and applying a Philadelphia cervical collar; do not flex, extend, or rotate the neck
      1) Log roll the patient from side to side
      2) Special beds may be used
   b. Prevent further spinal cord edema
      1) Corticosteroids as prescribed to prevent or limit damage to the spinal cord (this is controversial because supportive research evidence is limited)
         a) Drug: methylprednisolone (Solu-Medrol): 30 mg/kg over 15 minutes; pause for 45 minutes; maintenance dose of 5.4 mg/kg/hour for 23 hours
            i) Infuse for 24 hours if the patient is treated within 3 hours of injury
            ii) Infuse for 48 hours if the patient is treated 3 to 8 hours after the injury
         b) Contraindications
            i) Injury >8 hours old
            ii) Injury below L2
            iii) Injury to the cauda equina

2) Osmotic diuretics (e.g., mannitol [Osmitrol]) as prescribed

3) Therapeutic hypothermia may also be used to decrease oxygen consumption

5. Prepare the patient for procedures as indicated
   a. Nothing by mouth
   b. Nasogastric tube to low suction
   c. Foley catheter
   d. Tetanus immunization as indicated
   e. Close monitoring of body temperature for poikilothermism; warming or cooling may be necessary

6. Control pain and discomfort
   a. Nonsteroidal antiinflammatory drugs
   b. Narcotic analgesics
   c. Anxiolytics
   d. Gentle handling of paralyzed limbs

7. Monitor for complications
   a. Neurogenic shock: vasodilation, hypotension, or bradycardia
   b. Autonomic dysreflexia: a condition in which the blood pressure in a person with a spinal cord injury above T6 becomes excessively high as a result of the overactivity of the autonomic nervous system; eliminate noxious stimuli (e.g., full bladder or bowel) and administer antihypertensive agents
   c. Neurogenic bladder: the nerves that are supposed to carry messages from the brain to the bladder do not work properly; intermittent bladder catheterization is preferred to the use of a Foley catheter

Evaluation

1. Patent airway, adequate oxygenation (i.e., normal PaO_2, SpO_2, SaO_2) and ventilation (i.e., normal $PaCO_2$)
2. Absence of clinical indications of respiratory distress
3. Absence of clinical indications of hypoperfusion
4. Absence of clinical indications of infection or sepsis
5. Alert and oriented with no neurologic deficit
6. Control of pain or discomfort
7. Absence of clinical indications of bleeding

Typical disposition: admission to the critical care unit

Seizures

Definition: a sudden change in behavior that is characterized by changes in sensory perception or motor activity caused by an abnormal firing of nerve cells in the brain

1. Types of seizures (Table 6-16)
2. Epilepsy: a condition that is characterized by recurrent seizures that may include repetitive muscle jerking (i.e., convulsions)
3. Status epilepticus: seizure activity of ≥30 minutes caused by a single seizure or a series of seizures during which there is no return of consciousness between seizures
   a. Note that a more current definition is seizure activity of ≥10 minutes because treatment is generally

initiated within 10 minutes, thus preventing the continuation of seizure activity for 30 minutes

4. Febrile seizures: occur during the initial rapid rise in body temperature; usually within the first 24 hours of fever development
   a. Seizure is induced not by the actual temperature but by how rapidly the temperature rises
   b. Usually occur in children 6 months to 3 years old
   c. Rapid increase in temperature of >102°F

Predisposing factors

1. Most seizures are idiopathic
2. Preexisting history of seizure disorder
   a. Withdrawal from anticonvulsant medications
   b. Acute alcohol withdrawal
   c. Acute withdrawal from chronically used drugs that have sedative or depressant effects (e.g., barbiturates)
   d. Acute condition that lowers the seizure threshold
3. No preexisting history of seizure disorder
   a. Brain trauma: 50% risk of developing seizures after major head trauma
   b. Febrile illness with a fever of usually >102°F
   c. Processes that destabilize the cell membranes of the neurons
      1) Stroke: ischemic or hemorrhagic
      2) CNS infection: meningitis, encephalitis, or abscess
      3) Brain tumors
      4) Encephalopathy: anoxic (e.g., after cardiac arrest), hypertensive, or metabolic
         a) Hypoglycemia
         b) Hepatic failure
         c) Uremia
         d) Hyperosmolality
      5) Electrolyte imbalance
         a) Hyponatremia
         b) Hypocalcemia
         c) Hypomagnesemia
      6) Drug or alcohol withdrawal
      7) Drug toxicity: lidocaine, meperidine (Demerol), theophylline (TheoDur), salicylates, tricyclic antidepressants, or cocaine
      8) Sepsis
      9) Perinatal problems (i.e., anoxia or hypoglycemia at birth)

Pathophysiology

1. Disruption in the neuron cell membrane stability causes the neurons to fire more rapidly and with more amplitude
   a. With some types of seizures, patients have an "aura" (i.e., experiencing odd sensations before actual seizure activity)
2. When the discharges surpass the threshold for an action potential, the firing passes along to adjacent neurons (also known as *kindling*)

3. As a critical mass of neurons fire, this leads to the classic manifestations of seizures
4. Inhibitory processes in the cortex, the anterior thalamus, and the basal ganglia slow and eventually stop the firing
5. The inhibitory process also leads to CNS depression and impaired consciousness (i.e., the postictal phase)
6. Prolonged generalized seizures may deplete the brain of oxygen and glucose, which may produce hypoxia and neuronal death
   a. Early: hypersympathetic phase
      1) Cerebral blood flow increases
      2) Tachycardia and hypertension
      3) Blood pH and PaO_2 falls, $PaCO_2$ rises
      4) Glucose and potassium rise
   b. Late: after 25 to 30 minute of seizure activity
      1) Cerebral blood flow is unable to keep up with cerebral metabolic demands

2) Bradycardia, hypotension, dysrhythmias, and hypoglycemia
3) Marked elevations of creatine kinase and potassium
4) Ventricular fibrillation may occur
5) Rhabdomyolysis-induced renal failure

Clinical presentation
1. Subjective
   a. History may include a precipitating event or condition
   b. Patient may report aura before seizure
   c. Postictal period characterized by fatigue and muscle soreness
2. Objective
   a. Altered level of consciousness
   b. Tonic or clonic body movements
   c. Incontinence of urine or stool

TABLE 6-16   Types of Seizures

Type	Features	Duration
Generalized: loss of consciousness		
Absence (petit mal)	• Momentary loss of consciousness • Blank stare and cessation of activity • Eye blinking and lip smacking may occur • May lose muscle tone	Seconds
Tonic-clonic (grand mal)	• May be preceded by an aura or a cry as a result of forced expiration • Loss of consciousness • Symmetric tonic-clonic extremity movements • Possible apnea with cyanosis until tonic phase ends • May bite tongue or have an episode of incontinence • Postictal fatigue, muscle soreness, confusion, lethargy, and headache may occur	3-5 minutes
Myoclonic	• Short, abrupt muscle contractions of the arms, legs, and torso • Contractions may be symmetric or asymmetric	Seconds
Clonic	• Muscle contraction and relaxation but slower than with myoclonic seizure	Several minutes
Tonic	• Abrupt increase in muscle tone of torso and face • Flexion of arms and extension of legs	Seconds
Atonic	• Abrupt loss of muscle tone • May cause falling and injuries related to the fall	Seconds
Partial: focal at onset but may evolve into a generalized seizure		
Simple partial	• Consciousness not impaired • Abnormal unilateral movement of arm, leg, or both • Patient may sense abnormal smells or sounds or experience sensations such as numbness, tingling, and burning • Tachycardia or bradycardia, tachypnea, skin flushing, and epigastric discomfort may occur	Seconds to minutes
Complex partial	• Loss of consciousness, but eyes may be open • Lip smacking, chewing, and picking at clothing may occur • Mumbling or speaking in repetitive phrases • Posturing or jerking movements • Postictal confusion and amnesia common	Minutes

From Dennison, R. D. (2007). *Pass CCRN!* (3rd ed.). St. Louis: Mosby.

d. Involuntary motor activities: lip smacking, swallowing, or chewing

3. Diagnostic
    a. Evaluation of cause
       1) BUN: increased with uremia and hyperosmolality
       2) Liver function studies: increased with hepatic failure
       3) Drug and alcohol levels
       4) Anticonvulsant drug levels: subtherapeutic in noncompliant patients
    b. Electrolytes: hyperkalemia with prolonged generalized seizure activity
    c. Glucose: increased early and decreased late
    d. Creatine kinase: increased, especially if prolonged generalized seizure activity
    e. Lactic acid: increased, especially if prolonged generalized seizure activity
    f. ABGs: may show hypercapnia or hypoxemia
    g. Urine: may show myoglobinuria, especially if prolonged generalized seizure activity
    h. ECG: will show seizure activity
    i. CT and MRI or MRA: may indicate pathologic conditions (e.g., mass lesions)
    j. LP: may show meningitis as cause

Collaborative management

1. Continue assessment
    a. ABCDs
    b. Vital signs: blood pressure, pulse, respiratory rate, and temperature
    c. Oxygen saturation
    d. Respiratory effort and excursion
    e. Cardiac rate and rhythm
    f. Level of consciousness, pupils, and motor function
    g. Accurate intake and output
    h. Close monitoring for the progression of symptoms
2. Maintain airway, oxygenation, and ventilation
    a. Artificial airways as indicated
       1) Oral or nasopharyngeal airway to hold the tongue away from the hypopharynx in patients with altered consciousness
          a) Use a nasopharyngeal airway or nasotracheal intubation if the mouth cannot be opened; do not try to force the mouth open
       2) Endotracheal intubation if required
    b. Prevention of aspiration
       1) Position the patient on his or her side if the spine has been radiologically cleared
       2) Suction only as necessary, and limit the duration of suctioning to 10 seconds
       3) Hyperoxygenate with 100% oxygen before and after suctioning
    c. Oxygen by nasal cannula at 2 to 6 L/minute if required to maintain an SpO_2 level of 95% unless contraindicated; for patients with chronic obstructive pulmonary disease, use pulse oximetry to guide oxygen administration to an SpO_2 level of 90%

d. Mechanical ventilation may be necessary if drugs to suppress seizures depress ventilation

3. Maintain MAP, CPP, and cerebral blood flow
    a. IV access with two large-bore catheters for fluid and medication administration
    b. Intravenous fluids as prescribed: avoid hypotonic fluids (e.g., D_5W), which may contribute to brain edema
4. Assess for and eliminate causes or contributing factors
    a. Analyze serum for glucose, sodium, potassium, calcium, phosphorus, magnesium, and blood urea nitrogen
    b. Screen for drugs
       1) Barbiturates
       2) Tricyclic antidepressants
       3) Alcohol
    c. Obtain anticonvulsant drug levels
    d. Obtain blood cultures if the patient is hyperthermic
    e. Correct contributing factors that lower seizure threshold (e.g., hypoxemia, acid-base imbalance, electrolyte imbalance, hyperthermia, hypermetabolism)
5. Stop seizure activity
    a. Thiamine and D_5W if alcohol ingestion or hypoglycemia is suspected (thiamine is given with the dextrose to prevent Wernicke encephalopathy, especially with chronic malnutrition)
    b. Benzodiazepine or other drugs if seizures persist after dextrose and thiamine administration (Table 6-17)
       1) Benzodiazepine to stop the seizure (see Table 6-16)
          a) First choice: lorazepam (Ativan)
          b) Second choice: diazepam (Valium)
       2) Agents to prevent recurrence to be given after benzodiazepine
          a) Phenytoin (Dilantin)
          b) Fosphenytoin (Cerebyx)
          c) Phenobarbital (Luminal)
       3) Monitoring for respiratory depression; ventilation with manual resuscitation bag and mask or endotracheal intubation may be required
6. Protect the patient from injury and prevent complications during seizure
    a. Do not leave the patient
    b. Loosen the patient's constrictive clothing
    c. Remove pillow from under the patient's head
    d. Turn the patient to the side and maintain an open airway
    e. Do not restrain the patient; however, gentle guiding of the extremities is acceptable
    f. Pad side rails with blankets or pillows
    g. Maintain the patient's privacy
    h. Assess for injury
7. Monitor and document the duration of seizure activity, the patient's level of consciousness, and any drugs administered

TABLE **6-17**   Anticonvulsant Drugs

Drug	Intravenous Dosage	Time Until Stoppage of Seizure/Duration of Anticonvulsant Effect	Adverse Effects
Lorazepam (Ativan)	0.1 mg/kg (not to exceed 8 mg/kg) at a rate of ≤2 mg/min	6–10 minutes/12–24 hours	• Respiratory depression • Tachycardia • Hypotension • Dysrhythmias
Diazepam (Valium)	0.15–0.25 mg/kg at a rate of ≤5 mg/min	1–3 minutes/30 minutes	• Respiratory depression • Tachycardia • Hypotension • Dysrhythmias
Phenytoin sodium (Dilantin)	10–20 mg/kg at a rate of ≤50 mg/min; must be mixed with saline	30 minutes/24 hours	• Hypotension • Dysrhythmias or blocks • Hepatitis • Nephritis • Blood dyscrasias
Fosphenytoin (Cerebyx)	15–20 mg/kg of phenytoin equivalent at a rate of ≤150 mg/min may be administered intramuscularly	15 minutes/24 hours	• Hypotension (less risk than phenytoin) • Dysrhythmias (less risk than phenytoin) • Nephritis • Blood dyscrasias
Phenobarbital (Luminal)	20 mg/kg at a rate of ≤50 mg/min (not actively seizing) or ≤100 mg/min (actively seizing)	20–30 minutes/48 hours	• Respiratory depression • Hypotension • Angioedema • Thrombophlebitis

a. Aura: presence or absence and its nature if present
b. Cry: presence or absence
c. Onset: site of initial body movements, deviation of head and eyes, chewing, salivation, posturing, and sensory changes
d. Tonic phase: prolonged muscle contraction
e. Clonic phase: a rapid succession of alternating contractions and partial relaxations of a muscle
f. Relaxation phase: duration and behavior
g. Postictal phase: duration, patient's ability to remember the seizure, orientation, pupillary changes, headache, and injuries
h. Duration: from aura to relaxation
i. Drugs administered
8. Provide reassurance and comfort during the postictal period
a. Elevate the head of the bed 30 degrees
b. Reassure and reorient patient as he or she awakens
c. Provide privacy and a calm environment
d. Discretely clean the patient if he or she was incontinent
e. Allow the patient to sleep
f. Administer fluids cautiously
9. Monitor for complications
a. Acute respiratory failure
b. Aspiration
c. Injury
d. Renal failure related to rhabdomyolysis
e. Residual neurologic deficits

Evaluation

1. Patent airway, adequate oxygenation (i.e., normal PaO_2, SpO_2, SaO_2) and ventilation (i.e., normal $PaCO_2$)
2. Absence of clinical indications of respiratory distress
3. Absence of clinical indications of hypoperfusion
4. Absence of clinical indications of infection or sepsis
5. Alert and oriented with no neurologic deficit
6. Absence of seizure activity
7. Control of pain and discomfort

Typical disposition

1. If evaluation criteria met: discharge with instructions
   a. Pediatric patients with febrile seizure who are stable and whose fever is controlled may be discharged home with instructions
      1) Care of the child having a seizure
      2) Proper dosing of antipyretics
      3) Comfort and prescribed measures during a febrile illness
      4) Reassurance that febrile seizures have not been shown to cause neurologic damage and that children do not need to be treated prophylactically with antiseizure medications
      5) Return to emergency department if febrile seizure recurs
2. If evaluation criteria not met: admission to progressive care unit or critical care unit

Headaches

Definition: pain or discomfort in the head; headache is a manifestation of an underlying disorder and not a disease in itself

1. Primary headache: a headache for which no organic cause can be identified
   a. Tension
   b. Migraine
   c. Cluster
2. Secondary headache: a headache associated with an organic cause
   a. Tumor
   b. Aneurysm
   c. CNS infections (e.g., meningitis, encephalitis)
   d. Temporal arteritis

Precipitating factors

1. Tension headache: muscle tension as a result of physical strain (e.g., abnormal positioning, unusual physical activity) or emotional stress
2. Migraine headache
   a. Hormonal fluctuations (e.g., menstrual cycle)
   b. Foods: alcohol, chocolate, aged cheese, citrus fruits, or caffeine
   c. Low blood sugar
   d. Seasonal and environmental changes
   e. Stress or lack of sleep
3. Cluster headache: cyclic; may be seen more often during spring and fall

Pathophysiology

1. Tension: muscle tension
2. Migraine: vascular, with vasospasm, vasodilation, and tissue ischemia causing pain
3. Cluster: may be caused by trigeminal nerve dysfunction, but the cause is generally unknown
4. Temporal arteritis: a common form of systemic vasculopathy that affects patients who are >50 years old
   a. Chronic, systemic vasculitis of unknown origin that primarily affects the elastic lamina of medium- and large-sized arteries
   b. Marked by transmural inflammation of the intima, media, and adventitia
   c. Mural hyperplasia can result in arterial luminal narrowing and subsequent distal ischemia that causes temporal lobe headaches

Clinical presentation

1. Characteristics of secondary headaches that are likely to have a serious cause include sudden onset with rapid worsening, no previous history of similar headaches, fever, altered level of consciousness, indications of meningeal irritation (e.g., nuchal rigidity, Kernig sign, Brudzinski sign), age >50 years, and immunosuppression (Emergency Nurses Association, 2007)
2. Tension headache
   a. Subjective
      1) History of frequent headaches
         a) Episodic: the patient is affected <180 days per year but has at least 10 headaches per year that last between 30 minutes and 7 days
         b) Chronic: the patient is affected >15 days per month for >6 months or has >180 headaches per year that last between 30 minutes and 7 days
      2) Pain
         a) Described as tight pressure around the head; no throbbing
         b) Usually starts in occipital area and moves toward the frontal area
      3) May describe neck tension
   b. Objective
      1) Appears to be in mild to moderate distress
3. Migraine
   a. Subjective
      1) History of previous headaches
      2) Pain
         a) Often unilateral and described as throbbing
         b) May have had an aura that preceded the onset of the headache
      3) Complaints of nausea, vomiting, photophobia, or other neurologic symptoms (e.g., facial paresthesias)
   b. Objective
      1) Appears to be in moderate to severe distress
      2) Vomiting
      3) Speech difficulties may occur
4. Cluster
   a. Subjective
      1) History of previous headache
      2) Pain
         a) Cyclic headache
         b) Unilateral
         c) Periorbital or temporal
         d) Described as severe, sharp, burning, or boring
         e) Patting or rubbing affected area may relieve some of the discomfort
      3) Nasal congestion on affected side
      4) Photophobia
   b. Objective
      1) Appears to be in severe discomfort
      2) Eye changes: eyelid edema, red eye, or tearing on the affected side
      3) Sweating
      4) Pallor
5. Diagnostic
   a. CBC count with differential if patient has fever
   b. Erythrocyte sedimentation rate: increased in patients with temporal arteritis
   c. CT or MRI: head if sudden onset, nuchal rigidity, changes in level of consciousness, immunocompromise, or unusual presentation and pattern

d. LP: to rule out suspected meningitis; rule out possible subarachnoid hemorrhage first with computed tomography scanning

Collaborative management

1. Continue assessment
   a. ABCDs
   b. Vital signs: blood pressure, pulse, respiratory rate, and temperature
   c. Oxygen saturation
   d. Respiratory effort and excursion
   e. Cardiac rate and rhythm
   f. Level of consciousness, pupils, and motor function
   g. Pain and discomfort level
   h. Close monitoring for the progression of symptoms
2. Maintain airway, oxygenation, and ventilation
   a. Prevention of aspiration: position the patient on his or her side is the presence of nausea or vomiting
   b. Oxygen by nasal cannula at 2 to 6 L/minute if required to maintain an SpO_2 level of 95% unless contraindicated; for patients with chronic obstructive pulmonary disease, use pulse oximetry to guide oxygen administration to an SpO_2 level of 90%
3. Maintain adequate circulation and perfusion: IV access for fluid and medication administration
4. Control pain and discomfort
   a. Tension headache
      1) Quiet environment
      2) Mild analgesics: oral aspirin, acetaminophen (Tylenol), or nonsteroidal anti-inflammatory medication (e.g., ibuprofen [Motrin])
   b. Migraine
      1) Cool, calm, and dark environment
      2) Cold washcloth for forehead
      3) Pharmacologic agents as prescribed
         a) Dihydroergotamine (Dihydroergotamine-Sandoz, Migranal)
            i) Actions: α-adrenergic blocker constricts cerebral blood vessels
            ii) Cautions: may cause reflex tachycardia and high blood pressure; contraindicated during pregnancy
         b) Sumatriptan (Imitrex)
            i) Actions: selective binding to vascular receptors leads to cranial vasoconstriction
            ii) Cautions: tingling and hot sensations are common; use cautiously in patients with coronary artery disease
      4) Antiemetics: metoclopramide (Reglan), ondansetron (Zofran), or proclorperazine (Compazine)
   c. Cluster
      1) 100% oxygen for up to 15 minutes
      2) Intranasal lidocaine (4% topical or 2% viscous) to the most caudal aspect of the inferior nasal turbinate
      3) Calcium-channel blockers

d. Monitoring for complications
   1) Stroke
   2) Myocardial infarction or heart disease
   3) Pulmonary embolus or venous thromboembolism
   4) Hypertension
   5) Pre-eclampsia or gestational hypertension during pregnancy

Evaluation

1. Patent airway, adequate oxygenation (i.e., normal PaO_2, SpO_2, SaO_2) and ventilation (i.e., normal $PaCO_2$)
2. Absence of clinical indications of respiratory distress
3. Absence of clinical indications of hypoperfusion
4. Alert and oriented with no neurologic deficit
5. Control of pain and discomfort

Typical disposition

1. If evaluation criteria met: discharge with instructions for follow up
   a. Medications
   b. Follow up with primary care or neurologist as directed
   c. Return for worsening or new neurologic symptoms
2. If evaluation criteria not met: admission because a more serious condition should be suspected

Guillain-Barré Syndrome

Definition: an acute, rapidly progressing, symmetric demyelinating polyneuropathy in which the body's immune system attacks part of the peripheral nervous system; there are two types:
1. Acute motor axonal neuropathy: mainly a motor disease
2. Acute inflammatory demyelinating polyneuropathy: a demyelinating disease that affects motor and sensory neurons (this type is most common seen in the United States)

Predisposing factors

1. Viruses: cytomegalovirus, varicella-zoster virus, and Epstein-Barr virus
2. Bacteria: *Campylobacter jejuni* and *Mycoplasma pneumoniae*
3. Vaccines: rabies and H_1N_1 influenza
4. Trauma or surgery

Pathophysiology

1. Cell-mediated immune reaction
2. The antibody that forms damages the peripheral nerve myelin; lymphocytes help with the destruction of the myelin
3. Demyelination causes the slowing or cessation of nerve impulses; muscle innervation can no longer occur, and muscle wasting occurs
4. Involves the peripheral nerves, the ventral spinal nerve roots, and interstitial multifocal neuropathy (mostly motor); the only peripheral neuropathy affects the face

Clinical presentation
1. Subjective
   a. History of recent illness or immunization
   b. Complaints of sudden weakness and mild sensory disturbances of the legs
      1) Weakness that progresses in a symmetric ascending manner (i.e., the legs first, then the arms) and that evolves over days to weeks (peak effects occur between 1 and 4 weeks)
      2) Paresthesia
      3) Muscle cramping or ache in the hips, thighs, or back
   c. Dyspnea
   d. Dysphagia
2. Objective
   a. Wide blood pressure changes (i.e., hypertension or hypotension); may have orthostatic changes
   b. Clinical indications of respiratory distress
   c. Tachycardia that progresses to bradycardia
   d. Facial flushing
   e. Loss of sweating or episodic profuse diaphoresis
   f. Bell palsy or facial paresis
   g. Tenderness with deep tendon palpation
   h. Symmetric proximal and distal weakness
   i. Areflexia or decreased deep tendon reflexes
   j. No muscle atrophy (i.e., weakness develops too quickly)
3. Diagnostic
   a. CBC with differential to rule out other causes
   b. Hypercalcemia: seen with immobilization
   c. LP: increased protein

Collaborative management
1. Continue assessment
   a. ABCDs
   b. Vital signs: blood pressure, pulse, respiratory rate, and temperature
   c. Oxygen saturation
   d. Respiratory effort and excursion
   e. Cardiac rate and rhythm
   f. Level of consciousness, pupils, and motor function
   g. Pain and discomfort level
   h. Close monitoring for the progression of symptoms
2. Maintain airway, oxygenation, and ventilation
   a. Positioning with the head of the bed elevated
   b. Artificial airways as indicated: endotracheal intubation if required
   c. Oxygen by nasal cannula at 2 to 6 L/minute if required to maintain an SpO_2 level of 95% unless contraindicated; for patients with chronic obstructive pulmonary disease, use pulse oximetry to guide oxygen administration to an SpO_2 level of 90%
   d. Mechanical ventilation may be necessary
3. Maintain adequate circulation and perfusion: IV access for fluid and medication administration

4. Treat infection if present and prevent sepsis
   a. Antimicrobials as indicated
   b. Antipyretics and cooling methods to reduce fever
5. Control pain and discomfort
   a. Positioning for comfort
   b. Analgesics
   c. Anxiolytics or sedatives
6. Prepare patient for procedures as indicated
   a. Nothing by mouth
   b. Nasogastric tube to low suction
   c. Foley catheter
7. Monitor for complications
   a. Deep venous thrombosis
   b. Pulmonary embolism from prolonged immobilization
   c. Urinary retention
   d. Acute respiratory failure

Evaluation
1. Patent airway, adequate oxygenation (i.e., normal PaO_2, SpO_2, SaO_2) and ventilation (i.e., normal $PaCO_2$)
2. Absence of clinical indications of respiratory distress
3. Alert and oriented with no neurologic deficit

Typical disposition: admission to progressive care unit or critical care unit

Chronic Neurologic Disorders
Definitions
1. Amyotrophic lateral sclerosis (also known as *Lou Gehrig disease*): a progressive neurodegenerative disease of the upper and lower motor neurons of the cerebral cortex, the brainstem, and the spinal cord that results in total paralysis
2. Multiple sclerosis: the progressive demyelination of the central nervous system
3. Parkinson disease: the progressive degeneration of the neurons in the motor area of the brain
4. Myasthenia gravis: a progressive disorder of the peripheral nervous system that affects the transmission of nerve impulses to the voluntary muscles
   a. Two types
      1) Ocular myasthenia: confined to extrinsic ocular muscles
      2) Generalized myasthenia: generalized weakness
   b. Neonatal myasthenia can occur when the fetus acquires antibodies from a mother who is affected with myasthenia gravis

Predisposing factors
1. Amyotrophic lateral sclerosis
   a. Unknown cause, but viral infections, metabolic disorders, and trauma have been implicated
   b. More common among men than women
   c. Average age at diagnosis is 55 years

2. Multiple sclerosis
   a. Causes include possible genetic factors, autoimmunity, and childhood viral illness
   b. Affects women more than men; age of onset is 20 to 40 years
   c. More common in cold climates
3. Parkinson disease
   a. Primary: unknown
   b. Secondary
      1) Head trauma, especially repeated (e.g., as a result of boxing)
      2) Infection
      3) Neoplasm
      4) Encephalitis
      5) Carbon monoxide intoxication
      6) Heavy metals (e.g., mercury)
      7) Pesticides
      8) Hypoxia
      9) Cerebral ischemia
4. Myasthenia gravis
   a. Family history of autoimmune disorders; genetic markers may be associated with susceptibility
   b. Seen in adult women <40 years old and men >60 years old

Pathophysiology
1. Amyotrophic lateral sclerosis
   a. A progressive neurodegenerative disease that affects nerve cells in the brain and the spinal cord
   b. Progressive degeneration leads to the death of motor neurons; the brain's ability to initiate and control muscle movement is lost
   c. During the later stages of the disease, voluntary muscle action is affected, and total paralysis results
2. Multiple sclerosis
   a. A demyelinating chronic autoimmune disorder of the central nervous system
   b. The body's immune system attacks the protective myelin sheaths that surround the nerve cells of the brain and spinal cord, which results in damage that prevents the transmission of nerve impulses
3. Parkinson disease
   a. A neurodegenerative disease that involves the breakdown of the nerve cells in the motor area of the brain, which results in a shortage of dopamine
   b. The deficiency of dopamine in the basal ganglia affects the regulation of body movement
4. Myasthenia gravis
   a. Circulating acetylcholine receptor antibodies are present in 80% to 90% of patients with the generalized form of myasthenia gravis
   b. Immunoglobulin G autoantibodies prevent acetylcholine from binding with receptors at the neuromuscular junction

Clinical presentation
1. Amyotrophic lateral sclerosis
   a. Subjective
      1) Muscle weakness and stiffness (earliest sign)
         a) Muscle weakness in the arms, legs, or chest (i.e., trouble breathing) is the hallmark
      2) Twitching and cramping of muscles; impairment of the use of the arms and legs
   b. Objective
      1) Muscle twitches
      2) Thick speech
      3) Difficulty projecting the voice
      4) In advanced stages, problems with breathing and swallowing
   c. Diagnostic
      1) Serum: high-resolution serum protein electrophoresis; thyroid and parathyroid levels
      2) Urine: 24-hour collection for heavy metals
      3) Electrodiagnostic tests: electromyography and nerve conduction velocity
2. Multiple sclerosis
   a. Subjective
      1) Visual disturbances (e.g., diplopia, blurred vision)
      2) Muscle weakness, numbness, prickling sensations, and ataxia
      3) Facial hypesthesia and paresthesias
      4) Memory and concentration problems
   b. Objective
      1) Charcot triad: nystagmus, intention tremor, and scanning speech
      2) Abnormal reflexes: increased deep tendon reflexes, positive Hoffman sign, positive Babinski sign, and decreased cremasteric reflex
      3) Lhermitte sign: when the patient is laying down, the flexion of the neck causes an electrical shock-like sensation that radiates bilaterally down the arms, the back, and the lower trunk
      4) High steppage gait and scissors gait
      5) Decreased vibration and position sense
      6) Ataxia
      7) Decreased muscle strength and paralysis
   c. Diagnostic
      1) Serum: to rule out other causes
      2) Urine: urine gliotoxic activity
      3) CSF: increased total protein and immunoglobulin G levels
3. Parkinson disease
   a. Subjective
      1) Symptoms may start in one limb and spread to others, but asymmetry usually persists
      2) Stiffness
      3) Tremors, usually while resting
      4) Rigidity with repetitive motion (e.g., when brushing teeth)
      5) Gait slowing or difficulty with stepping; may fall
   b. Objective
      1) Expressionless face
      2) Decreased blink reflex
      3) Glabellar reflex: repeated gentle tapping on the glabella evokes the blinking of both eyes
      4) Akinesia, muscle rigidity, and tremors

5) Gait: difficulty taking the first step, then walks with a shuffling gait

6) Balance: when pulled backward, unable to maintain balance; postural instability occurs during later stages

c. Diagnostic

1) Serum: to rule out other causes

2) CT and MRI: to rule out other problems

3) Positron emission tomography scan: shows decreased dopaminergic activity

4. Myasthenia gravis

a. Subjective

1) Fatigue, especially after exercising

2) Insidious onset of weakness of the face, limbs, and trunk

3) Weakness of the eye muscles (may be the first symptom): ptosis or diplopia

b. Objective

1) Decreased muscle strength and paralysis

2) Ptosis

3) Dysarthria

4) Dysphagia

c. Diagnostic

1) Serum: to detect the presence of immune molecules or acetylcholine receptor antibodies (may not elevate with ocular-only myasthenia gravis)

2) Edrophonium (Tensilon) test: a drug that blocks the breakdown of acetylcholine and temporarily increases the levels of acetylcholine at the neuromuscular junction (myasthenia gravis temporarily improves)

3) Single fiber electromyography

Collaborative management

1. Continue assessment

a. ABCDs

b. Vital signs: blood pressure, pulse, respiratory rate, and temperature

c. Oxygen saturation

d. Respiratory effort and excursion

e. Cardiac rate and rhythm

f. Level of consciousness, pupils, and motor function

g. Close monitoring for the progression of symptoms

2. Maintain airway, oxygenation, and ventilation

a. Positioning: elevate the head of the bed

b. Artificial airways as indicated

1) Oral or nasopharyngeal airway to hold the tongue away from the hypopharynx in patients with altered consciousness

2) Endotracheal intubation if required

c. Prevention of aspiration: suction as indicated

1) Suction only as necessary, and limit the duration of suctioning to 10 seconds

2) Hyperoxygenate with 100% oxygen before and after suctioning

d. Oxygen by nasal cannula at 2 to 6 L/minute if required to maintain an SpO_2 level of 95% unless

contraindicated; for patients with chronic obstructive pulmonary disease, use pulse oximetry to guide oxygen administration to an SpO_2 level of 90%

e. Mechanical ventilation may be necessary

3. Maintain adequate circulation and perfusion: IV access for fluid and medication administration

4. Administer pharmacologic agents as prescribed to improve muscle strength or to slow progression

a. Amyotrophic lateral sclerosis

1) Anticholinesterase agents

2) Corticosteroids

3) Muscle relaxants

4) Antimicrobials as indicated

b. Multiple sclerosis

1) Immunosuppressive drugs, including corticosteroids

2) Antimicrobials as indicated

3) Corticotrophin (ACTH): may be beneficial for acute relapses

4) Interferon β-1a (Avonex, Rebif) or interferon β-1b (Betaseron): may slow the progression of multiple sclerosis

c. Parkinson disease

1) Dopaminergics (e.g., levodopa [L-dopa], carbidopa-levodopa [Sinemet], amantadine [Symmetrel])

2) Anticholinergics

3) Avoidance of neuroleptics agents (e.g., haloperidol [Haldol], prochlorperazine (Compazine), trimethobenzamide (Tigan), metoclopramide [Reglan])

4) Nonselective monoamine oxidase inhibitors are contraindicated because they may induce hypertensive crisis

d. Myasthenia gravis

1) Anticholinesterase agents (e.g., neostigmine [Prostigmin], pyridostigmine [Mestinon])

2) Immunosuppressive drugs, including corticosteroids

5. Prepare patient for procedures

a. Multiple sclerosis

1) LP

b. Myasthenia gravis

1) Plasmapheresis: a procedure during which abnormal antibodies are removed from the blood and high-dose IV immune globulins are given to provide the body with normal antibodies from donated blood; this temporarily modifies the immune system

2) Thymectomy: the removal of the thymus gland reduces symptoms in patients with an abnormal thymus

6. Monitor for complications

a. Acute respiratory failure

b. Aspiration pneumonitis

c. Orthostatic hypotension (Parkinson disease)

d. Failure to thrive in newborns from mothers with myasthenia gravis

Evaluation

1. Patent airway, adequate oxygenation (i.e., normal PaO_2, SpO_2, SaO_2) and ventilation (i.e., normal $PaCO_2$)
2. Absence of clinical indications of respiratory distress
3. Absence of clinical indications of hypoperfusion
4. Absence of clinical indications of infection or sepsis
5. Alert and oriented with no neurologic deficit
6. Control of pain and discomfort

Typical disposition: admission

1. Admission to a critical care unit may be required if the patient is in acute respiratory failure

LEARNING ACTIVITIES

1. **DIRECTIONS:** Complete the following crossword puzzle related to neurologic emergencies.

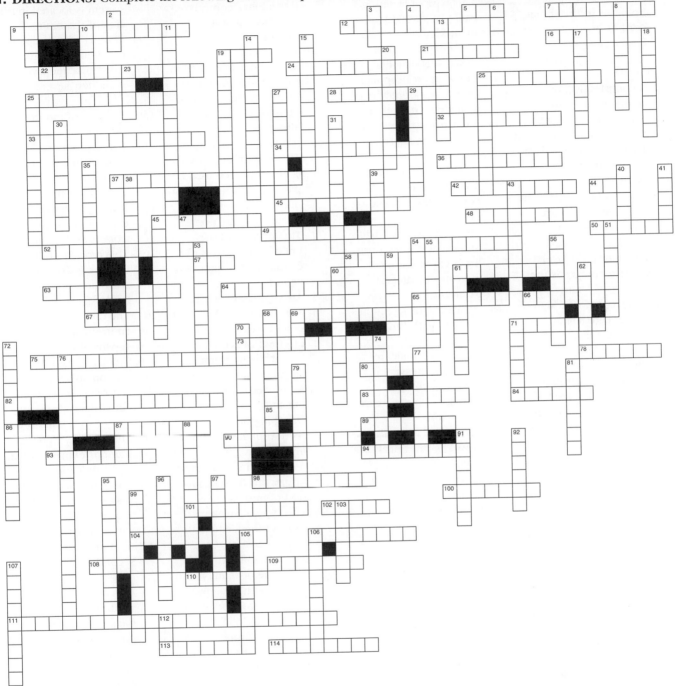

ACROSS

5. The innermost layer of the meninges is the _____ mater
7. Neurons that transmit impulses to the spinal cord or brain
9. Stroke causes _____-paresis/plegia
12. A complication of cerebral aneurysm that occurs most commonly after about 3 to 5 days; it is treated with calcium-channel blockers
16. Decreased amounts of this neurotransmitter in the basal ganglia are seen in patients with Parkinson disease
19. The outermost layer of the meninges is the _____ mater
21. This triad of vital sign changes are late signs of intracranial hypertension
22. The rupture of a cerebral aneurysm is sometimes referred to as a _____ *hemorrhage* because the blood vessels are located in this space
24. Diabetes _____ is a complication of head trauma or craniotomy that causes polyuria
25. A common oral anticonvulsant (generic)
26. This posturing is also referred to as *abnormal extension*
28. This type of herniation occurs with bilateral processes such as cerebral edema; also called *central herniation*
32. Involuntary movement of the eyes
33. This reflex is also referred to as *doll's eyes*

34. A primary neurotransmitter for the sympathetic nervous system
36. This type of irritation causes a shrill cry in infants
37. The enzyme that breaks down acetylcholine
42. The skin area supplied by the sensory fibers of a single spinal nerve
44. Mean arterial pressure − Intracranial pressure; normally 60 to 100 mm Hg (abbrev)
45. The cranial nerve that controls the sensations of the face
47. This sign involves pain in the neck when the leg is extended and indicates meningeal irritation
48. Muscle rigidity; seen in patients with Parkinson disease
49. The brain's ability to tolerate increases in volume without a corresponding increase in pressure
50. The cranial nerve that allows an individual to smile
52. A major risk factor for stroke
54. The most common type of cerebral aneurysm
57. A diagnostic study used to evaluate the brain's electrical activity (abbrev)
58. This area of the frontal lobe is responsible for motor speech
61. This lobe of the brain controls long-term memory
63. The cranial nerves, spinal nerves, and peripheral nerves constitute the _____ nervous system

64. Cerebrospinal fluid drainage from the nose
65. The posterior portion of these lobes controls voluntary motor function
66. This nerve originates at C3, C4, and C5 and innervates the diaphragm
67. The early signs of multiple sclerosis primarily affect the _____ (plural)
69. This respiratory pattern is characterized by a pause on inspiration and occurs with injury at the level of the pons
71. This portion of the brainstem controls the cardiac and respiratory centers
73. An unpleasant sensation
75. This disease is the result of a decreased amount or effect of acetylcholine at the neuromuscular junction (two words)
78. An unsteady or staggering gait
80. Drooping of the eyelid; seen in patients with myasthenia gravis
82. A chemical that acts as a bridge for the transmission of impulses
83. This type of stroke causes immediate neurologic deficits that are nonreversible
84. This type of rigidity occurs with meningeal irritation from infection or blood
85. This type of pressure is the pressure exerted from the intracranial contents
86. The testing of this reflex is also referred to as *caloric testing*
89. The unidirectional conduction of an impulse from one neuron to the next

90. The surgical opening of the cranium
93. The reticular activating system is located in this area of the brain
94. The primary symptom of hemorrhage from a cerebral aneurysm is sudden, severe _____
98. The loss of motor function
100. This type of headache is described as a band of pressure
101. The fold of the dura that separates the cerebral hemispheres from the cerebellum
102. This type of skull fracture is associated with raccoon eyes and Battle sign
104. The cranial nerve that controls pupillary constriction
106. Cranial nerve VIII
108. Cerebrospinal fluid is produced in capillary networks called _____ *plexuses*
109. The inability to understand or express verbal communication
110. This circle of blood vessels is formed by the internal carotid and vertebral arteries
111. A common cause of secondary brain injury (two words)
113. This type of cord syndrome causes more muscle weakness in the upper extremities than the lower extremities
114. The component of the neuron that conducts impulses toward the cell body

DOWN

1. The state of unconsciousness from which the patient cannot be awakened
2. A severe injury to the brain that causes prolonged unconsciousness, brainstem dysfunction, and profound residual deficits (abbrev)
3. This acts as a cushion for the brain and the spinal cord (abbrev)
4. This test should never be performed if the patient has clinical indications of intracranial hypertension (abbrev)
6. The component of the neuron that conducts impulses away from the cell body to other neurons or to end organs
8. This type of hematoma is caused by an arterial bleed and causes rapid deterioration
10. A subjective sensation that often precedes a seizure
11. The intrinsic ability of the cerebral blood vessels to dilate or constrict to stabilize cerebral blood flow
13. The description of the gait of patients with Parkinson disease
14. A gunshot or knife wound is likely to cause injury to half of the spinal cord and cause this type of injury (two words)
15. Inflammation of the meninges
17. These lobes control sensory function
18. These neurons transmit impulses away from the spinal cord or brain
19. The process that occurs in patients with multiple sclerosis

20. The sympathetic and parasympathetic nervous systems constitute the _____ nervous system
23. The spinal _____ extends from the brainstem to L2
25. This fontanelle closes at 2 months of age
26. This type of posturing is also referred to as *abnormal flexion*
27. The intrinsic ability of the cranium's contents to change to prevent increases in intracranial pressure
29. This type of stroke is caused by thrombus or embolism
30. This type of intracranial hematoma is caused by a venous bleed and causes symptoms that develop over several days
31. A loss of sensation
35. This type of encephalopathy is caused by a severe elevation of blood pressure
38. Whiplash causes spinal _____, which may cause spinal cord injury
39. This phase of a generalized seizure is characterized by prolonged muscle contraction
40. The cranial nerve that controls visual acuity
41. A side-to-side herniation
43. This type of cord syndrome causes complete motor loss and varied sensory loss
46. Difficulty with swallowing
51. This type of seizure is associated with a blank stare, smacking of the lips, and the cessation of activity
53. These nerve cells provide support, nourishment, and protection of the neurons

55. An abnormal weakness of an artery; most commonly occurs in the circle of Willis
56. May be mistaken for dementia or depression
59. Acute respiratory failure occurs with myasthenia _____
60. The part of the brain that coordinates muscle movement with sensory input
61. This test is used to look for myasthenia gravis; muscle weakness decreases when this drug is given
62. Four paired masses of gray matter in the deeper layers of each hemisphere are called the *basal* _____
68. The shifting of the brain within or out of the cranium
69. This degenerative neuromuscular disease selectively affects motor function (abbrev)
70. Uncal herniation causes dilation of the _____ pupil
71. The coating or sheath that speeds transmission along the axon; it is destroyed in patients with multiple sclerosis
72. This type of meningitis is highly contagious
74. This type of cell forms the blood-brain barrier
76. This complication of spinal cord injury at T6 or above causes hypertension and bradycardia and results from noxious stimuli below the level of the injury (two words)
77. Double vision
79. The speech impairment seen in patients with myasthenia gravis
81. The scoring system that is used to standardize the observation of responsiveness in neurologic patients

87. Focal cerebral ischemia that resolves within 24 hours (abbrev)
88. A common complication of chronic degenerative neuromuscular conditions
91. A complication of cerebral aneurysm that frequently occurs about 7 to 10 days after the bleed
92. This sign of Parkinson disease occurs at rest and goes away with movement and sleep
95. An abnormal sensitivity to light
96. A bruise on the brain
97. This hypothesis states that the cranium is an inexpansible vault and that, if one of the three intracranial volumes goes up, a reciprocal decrease in one or both of the other two volumes must occur to maintain normal intracranial pressure
99. This type of stroke is caused by aneurysm or arteriovenous malformation
103. This type of encephalopathy is most often caused by out-of-hospital cardiac arrest
105. This lobe of the brain controls vision
106. The middle layer of the meninges is the _____ mater; blood vessels and cerebrospinal fluid are located here
107. Herniation with a downward shift of the brain that causes the brainstem to be pushed through the foramen magnum
112. The most important assessment parameter for a patient with a neurologic condition (abbrev)

2. DIRECTIONS: Identify the following physiologic alterations as being associated with either the sympathetic or the parasympathetic nervous system.

	Sympathetic	Parasympathetic
Bronchodilation		
Coronary artery dilation		
Hypersalivation		
Increased blood glucose		
Increased perspiration		
Increased intestinal motility		
Pupil constriction		
Tachycardia		

3. DIRECTIONS: Identify the site of a lesion that would cause these respiratory patterns.

Pattern	Site of Lesion
Central nervous system hyperventilation	
Cheyne-Stokes	
Cluster	
Ataxic	
Apneustic	

4. DIRECTIONS: Name and identify the means of assessing the cranial nerves.

Number	Name	How to Assess
I		
II		
III		
IV		
V		
VI		
VII		
VIII		
IX		
X		
XI		
XII		

5. DIRECTIONS: List 10 factors that can increase intracranial pressure that can be eliminated.

1.	
2.	
3.	
4.	
5.	
6.	
7.	
8.	
9.	
10.	

6. DIRECTIONS: Match each of the following signs or symptoms with the neurologic conditions with which they are associations.

___ 1. Brainstem lesion	a. Kernig sign
___ 2. Chronic subdural hematoma	b. Babinski reflex
___ 3. Subarachnoid hemorrhage	c. Absence of doll's eyes reflex (oculocephalic reflex)
___ 4. Status epilepticus	d. Change in level of consciousness, pupillary changes, respiratory pattern changes, and the Cushing triad
___ 5. Dural tear	e. Periorbital edema
___ 6. Postcraniotomy	f. Battle sign
___ 7. Upper motor neuron lesion	g. Rhinorrhea
___ 8. Meningeal irritation	h. Personality change
___ 9. Intracranial hypertension	i. Pain described as the "worst headache of my life"
___ 10. Basal skull fracture	j. Myoglobinuria

7. DIRECTIONS: List five observations to make and interventions to perform when a patient is having a seizure.

Observations to Make	Interventions

8. DIRECTIONS: Label each statement as true or false.

	A child's occiput will cause hyperextension of the neck when the child is placed in a supine position.
	A child's brain absorbs more force of trauma than an adult's brain.
	Basal skull fractures are rare in children.
	Kids rarely have head trauma when struck by cars because the cars usually hit their legs.
	Same-level falls do not present a high risk for head injury in the older patient.
	Kyphosis can complicate cervical spine immobilization in older adults.

9. DIRECTIONS: Match the conditions on the right with the statements on the left. Conditions may be used more than once or not at all.

___ This condition is classified as acute, subacute, or chronic.	1. Contusion
___ A patient with this condition may or may not have a loss of consciousness.	2. Diffuse axonal injury
___ A classic sign of this problem is raccoon eyes.	3. Concussion
___ This consists of bruising of the brain.	4. Basal skull fracture
___ This is a fracture at the base of the skull.	5. Epidural hematoma
___ A disruption of the axons and their connections is caused by this problem.	6. Subdural hematoma
___ This is caused by bleeding between the skull and the dura mater.	
___ Seemingly minor trauma can cause this problem.	
___ A patient with this condition may lose consciousness, regain it briefly, and then rapidly deteriorate.	

10. DIRECTIONS: Match the incomplete spinal cord injury syndromes on the right with the descriptions on the left. Syndromes may be used more than once or not at all.

____ This is caused by the hemisection of the spinal cord.	1. Central cord syndrome
____ Severe bowel and bladder dysfunction accompany this syndrome.	2. Anterior cord syndrome
____ Older adults are prone to this spinal cord syndrome after falling.	3. Brown-Sequard syndrome
____ With this syndrome, the sense of position, proprioception, and vibration remain intact.	4. Cauda equina syndrome
____ This syndrome is uncommon.	5. Posterior cord syndrome
____ An injury to the lumbosacral nerve roots leads to this syndrome.	6. Conus medullaris syndrome
____ Patients with this syndrome have contralateral loss of pain and temperature sensation.	
____ Motor loss is worse in the upper extremities with this syndrome.	
____ This condition is caused by hyperflexion of the neck.	
____ With this syndrome, patients can only move the side of their body that they cannot feel.	

11. DIRECTIONS: Describe the teaching that you would provide to the parents of a child who is being dismissed from the emergency department after a febrile seizure.

1.
2.
3.
4.
5.

12. DIRECTIONS: Describe the classic signs of meningeal irritation, such as those that occur with meningitis or subarachnoid hemorrhage.

Sign	Description
Nuchal rigidity	
Brudzinski sign	
Kernig sign	

13. DIRECTIONS: When adapting the Glasgow Coma Scale for infants and small children, what score would the child obtain for the following responses?

1. Best verbal response: infant coos and babbles	
2. Best motor response: toddler yells "No!" when given a command	
3. Best verbal response: infant with irritable cry	

14. DIRECTIONS: Describe SCIWORA.

15. DIRECTIONS: Match the types of headache on the right with the statements on the left. The different types of headache may be used more than once or not at all.

___ One treatment for this type of headache is intranasal lidocaine.	1. Tension
___ Some patients experience an aura with this type of headache.	2. Migraine
___ This headache is often described as being "band-like" or like having the head in a vise.	3. Cluster
___ Menstrual cycles often bring on this type of headache.	
___ Patients with this headache often describe the pain as "deep" and "boring."	
___ Some patients with this type of headache exhibit Horner syndrome.	
___ Treatment with 100% oxygen often cures this headache.	
___ These headaches tend to occur frequently in people who have them.	
___ Vomiting often accompanies this type of headache.	
___ Mild analgesics should be enough to end this type of headache.	
___ Metaclopramine (Reglan) is often used to treat other symptoms that accompany this type of headache.	

LEARNING ACTIVITIES ANSWERS

1.

CONTRALATERAL · SUBARACHNOID · DECEREBRATE · OCULOCEPHALIC · CHOLINESTERASE · KERNIG · COMPLIANCE · HYPERTENSION · EEG · PERIPHERAL · RHINORRHEA · EYES · APNEUSTIC · PARESTHESIA · MYASTHENIAGRAVIS · NEUROTRANSMITTER · OCULOVESTIBULAR · MIDBRAIN · CRANIOTOMY · HEADACHE · PARALYSIS · TENSION · TENTORIUM · BASAL · OCULOMOTOR · ACOUSTIC · CHOROID · APHASIA · WILLIS · INTRACRANIAL · HYPERTENSION · CENTRAL · DENDRITE · TONSILLAR

PIA · AFFERENT · VASOSPASM · CUSHING · DOPAMINE · INSIPIDUS · PHENYTOIN · TENTORIAL · NYSTAGMUS · EPINEPHRINE · MENINGEAL · TRIGEMINAL · DERMATOME · DYSTONIA · FACIAL · SACCULAR · BROCA · TEMPORAL · FRONTAL · PHRENIC · MEDULLA · ATAXIC · PTOSIS · COMPLETE · ICP · SYNAPSE · NUCHAL

2.

	Sympathetic	Parasympathetic
Bronchodilation	X	
Coronary artery dilation	X	
Hypersalivation		X
Increased blood glucose	X	
Increased perspiration	X	
Increased intestinal motility		X
Pupil constriction		X
Tachycardia	X	

3.

Pattern	Site of Lesion
Central nervous system hyperventilation	Lower midbrain or upper pons
Cheyne-Stokes	Cerebral hemispheres, basal ganglia, cerebellum, or upper brainstem
Cluster	Lower pons or upper medulla
Ataxic	Medulla
Apneustic	Mid to lower pons

4.

I	Olfactory	• Evaluate the patient's ability to identify familiar odors
II	Optic	• Evaluate the patient's visual acuity with the use of the Snellen chart or newsprint • Evaluate the optic disc during the funduscopic examination
III	Oculomotor	• Evaluate the patient's ability to open the eyes widely • Check the size, shape, position, and reactivity of the pupils • Have the patient follow your finger with his or her eyes through the six cardinal positions of gaze • Look for abnormal eye movement
IV	Trochlear	• Have the patient follow your finger with his or her eyes through the six cardinal positions of gaze
V	Trigeminal	• Evaluate the ability of the patient to detect light touch, superficial pain, and temperature on the forehead, cheeks, and jaw • Touch the cornea with a wisp of cotton and check for bilateral blink • Palpate the strength of the masseter muscles with the patient clenching his or her teeth and the strength of the temporal muscles with the patient squeezing his or her eyes shut
VI	Abducens	• Have the patient follow your finger with his or her eyes through the six cardinal positions of gaze
VII	Facial	• Ask the patient to smile and assess facial symmetry • Test the patient's ability to taste salt and sugar on the anterior tongue
VIII	Acoustic	• Evaluate ability of the patient to hear when you are speaking at normal voice tones • Note any vertigo, nystagmus, nausea, vomiting, pallor, sweating, or hypotension
IX	Glossopharyngeal	• Evaluate patient's ability to speak, and note any hoarseness • Look for bilateral elevation of the palate with phonation • Test the patient's ability to taste sour and bitter on the posterior tongue • Evaluate the patient's ability to swallow • Test the gag reflex by stroking the patient's palate with a tongue blade • Evaluate the cough reflex by touching the patient's hypopharynx with a suction catheter
X	Vagus	• This is tested in the same way as the glossopharyngeal nerve

Continued

| XI | Spinal accessory | • Ask the patient to shrug his or her shoulders as you push down on them with your hands
• Palpate the sternocleidomastoid and trapezius muscles for size and symmetry |
| XII | Hypoglossal | • Look for midline alignment when the patient protrudes his or her tongue
• Look for fasciculations of the tongue |

5.

1. Neck twisting or flexion
2. Valsalva maneuver
3. Airway obstruction
4. Pain or noxious stimuli
5. Disturbing conversation
6. Noise
7. Bright lights
8. Tight tracheostomy ties or cervical collars
9. Seizure activity
10. Hyperthermia

6.

c Absence of doll's eyes reflex (oculocephalic reflex)	1. Brainstem lesion
h Personality change	2. Chronic subdural hematoma
i Pain described as the "worst headache of my life	3. Subarachnoid hemorrhage
j Myoglobinuria	4. Status epilepticus
g Rhinorrhea	5. Dural tear
e Periorbital edema	6. Postcraniotomy
b Babinski reflex	7. Upper motor neuron lesion
a Kernig sign	8. Meningeal irritation
d Change in level of consciousness, pupillary changes, respiratory pattern changes, and the Cushing triad	9. Intracranial hypertension
f Battle sign	10. Basal skull fracture

7.

Observations to Make
Preceding events: was there an aura?
Onset: • Body movements • Deviation of head and eyes • Chewing and salivation • Posture of body • Sensory changes
Tonic and clonic phases: • Progression of movements of the body • Skin color and airway • Pupillary changes • Incontinence • Duration of each phase
Level of consciousness during seizure
Postictal phase: • Duration • General behavior • Memory of events • Orientation • Pupillary changes • Headache • Aphasia • Injuries
Duration of entire seizure
Medications given and patient response

8.

False	The child's large occiput will cause extreme flexion.
True	Because the skull of a child is thinner and more pliable, the brain (not the skull) absorbs a great deal of the force of trauma.
False	Children actually seem to be prone to basal skull fractures.
False	Waddell's triad of injuries when children are hit by cars include extremity injury, thoracic and abdominal injury, and head injury.
False	The majority of falls in older adults are on the same level, and these patients have a high risk of acquiring a brain injury as a result of these injuries.
True	Kyphosis and lordosis will both make immobilization more difficult in older adult patients.

9.

6 These are classified as acute, subacute, or chronic.

3 A patient with this condition may or may not have a loss of consciousness.

4 A classic sign of this problem is raccoon eyes.

1 This consists of bruising of the brain.

4 This is a fracture at the base of the skull.

2 A disruption of the axons and their connections is caused by this problem.

5 This is caused by bleeding between the skull and the dura mater.

6 Seemingly minor trauma can cause this problem.

5 A patient with this condition may lose consciousness, regain it briefly, and then rapidly deteriorate.

10.

3 This is caused by hemisection of the spinal cord.
6 Severe bowel and bladder dysfunction accompany this syndrome.
1 Older adults are prone to this spinal cord syndrome after falling.
2 With this syndrome, the sense of position, proprioception, and vibration remain intact.
5 This syndrome is uncommon.
4 An injury to the lumbosacral nerve roots leads to this syndrome.
3 Patients with this syndrome have a contralateral loss of pain and temperature sensation.
1 Motor loss is worse in the upper extremities with this syndrome.
2 This condition is caused by hyperflexion of the neck.
3 With this syndrome, patients can only move the side of their body that they cannot feel.

11.

1. Care of the child who is having a seizure
2. Proper use and dosing of antipyretics
3. Comfort measures for the child with a febrile illness
4. Reassurance that febrile seizures have not been shown to cause neurologic damage
5. Return to the emergency department if the child has a seizure that lasts >5 minutes

12.

Nuchal rigidity	This is characterized by a stiff neck, and it is assessed by asking patient to touch the chin to the chest.
Brudzinski sign	Have the patient lie supine, and ask him or her to rapidly lift his or her head up from the bed. The sign is positive if the patient shows flexion of both thighs at the hips and flexion of the ankles and knees during this process.
Kernig sign	Have the patient lie supine and flex one hip at a 90-degree angle to the thigh. Extend the leg. A positive sign is when the patient will resist further movement and have pain and spasm in the hamstring.

13.

1. Best verbal response: infant coos and babbles	5
2. Best motor response: toddler yells "No!" when given a command	6
3. Best verbal response: infant with irritable cry	4

14.

Spinal nerve injury without vertebral damage
Usually seen in children <8 years old but can be seen in children up to the age of 17 years
Caused by the increased mobility of the child's spine as a result of the child having a large head, weak neck muscles, and incomplete vertebral (bony) development

15.

3 One treatment for this type of headache is intranasal lidocaine.
2 Some patients experience an aura with this type of headache.
1 This headache is often described as being "band-like" or like having the head in a vise.
2 Menstrual cycles often bring on this type of headache.
3 Patients with this headache often describe the pain as "deep" and "boring."
3 Some patients with this type of headache exhibit Horner syndrome.
3 Treatment with 100% oxygen often cures this headache.
1 These headaches tend to occur frequently in people who have them.
2 Vomiting often accompanies this type of headache.
1 Mild analgesics should be enough to end this type of headache.
2 Metaclopramine (Reglan) is often used to treat other symptoms that accompany this type of headache.

References and Selected Readings

Adams, R. J., Albers, G., Alberts, M. J., Benavente, O., Furie, K., Goldstein, L. B., et al. (2008). Update to the AHA/ASA recommendations for the prevention of stroke in patients with stroke and transient ischemic attack. *Stroke, 39(5)*, 1647-1652.

Altschul, D., Smith, M., & Sinson, G. P. (2009). Intracranial arteriovenous malformation. Retrieved April 9, 2009, from http://medscape.com/article/252426-overview.

American Heart Association. (2005). Part 9: Adult stroke. *Circulation, 112(24 suppl)*, IV111-IV120.

American Heart Association Stroke Council. (2009). Mission statement. Retrieved on April 9, 2009, from http://www.americanheart.org/presenter.jhtml?identifier=1197.

Anderson, H., & Kuljis, R. O. (2008). Alzheimer disease. Retrieved on April 9, 2009, from http://emedicine.medscape.com/article/1134817-overview.

Bader, M. K., Arbour, R., & Palmer, S. (2005). Refractory increased intracranial pressure in severe traumatic brain injury: Barbiturate coma and bispectral index monitoring. *AACN Clinical Issues, 16(4)*, 526-541.

Buttaro, T. M., Trybulski, J., Bailey, P. P., & Sandberg-Cook, J. (2003). *Primary care: A collaborative practice*. St. Louis: Mosby.

Clark, D. Y., Stocking, J., & Johnson, J. (Eds.). (2006). *Flight and ground transport nursing core curriculum* (2nd ed.). Denver: Air & Surface Transport Nurses Association.

Clem, K., & Morgenlander, J. C. (2008). Amyotrophic lateral sclerosis. Retrieved on April 3, 2009, from http://emedicine.medscape.com/article/791154-overview.

Crippen, D. W., & Shepard, S. (2008). Head trauma. Retrieved on April 9, 2009, from http://emedicine.medscape.com/article/433855-overview.

Dennison, R. D. (2007). *Pass CCRN!* (3rd ed.). St. Louis: Mosby.

Domino, F. J. (2008). *The 5-minute clinical consultant* (16th ed.). Philadelphia: Lippincott, Williams, & Wilkins.

Emergency Nurses Association. (2007). *Emergency nursing core curriculum* (6th ed). Philadelphia: Saunders.

Emergency Nurses Association. (2005). *Sheehy's manual of emergency care* (6th ed.). St Louis: Mosby.

Fryman, L., & Murray, L. (2007). Managing acute head trauma in a crowded emergency department. *Journal of Emergency Nursing, 33(3)*, 208-213.

Fultz, J. & Sturt, P. A. (2005). *Mosby's emergency nursing reference* (3rd ed.). St. Louis: Mosby.

Goldenberg, W. D., & Sinert, R. H. (2009). Myasthenia gravis. Retrieved on April 3, 2009, from http://emedicine.medscape.com/article/793136-overview.

Harper, J. P. (2007). Emergency nurses' knowledge of evidence-based ischemic stroke care: A pilot study. *Journal of Emergency Nursing, 33(3)*, 202-207.

Hauser, R. A., Pahwa, R., Lyons, K. E., & McClain, T. (2009). Parkinson's disease. Retrieved on April 9, 2009, from http://emedicine.medscape.com/article/1151267-overview.

Huang, J. (2008). Delirium and dementia. Retrieved on April 9, 2009, from http://www.merck.com/mmhe/sec06/ch083/ch083b.html.

Jarvis, C. (2008). *Physical examination and health assessment* (5th ed.). St. Louis: Saunders.

Josephson, L. (2004). Management of increased intracranial pressure: A primer for the non-neuro critical care nurse. *Dimensions of Critical Care Nursing, 23(5)*, 194-207.

Lazoff, M. (2008). Multiple sclerosis. Retrieved on April 9, 2009, from http://emedicine.medscape.com/article/793013-overview.

Kamienski, M. C. (2007). A 9-year-old boy with paresthesias in his hands and weak handgrips following a dirt bike crash. *Journal of Emergency Nursing, 33(3)*, 242-244.

Krock, A. B., & Massaro, L. (2008). Facilitating ED evaluation of patients with acute ischemic stroke. Journal of Emergency Nursing, *34(6)*, 519-522.

Merriam Webster Online. (2008). *Merriam-Webster medical dictionary*. http://medical.merriam-webster.com.

Miller, A., Rashid, R. M., & Sinert, R. H. (2007). Guillain-Barre syndrome. Retrieved on April 7, 2009, from http://emedicine.medscape.com/article/792008-overview.

National Institutes of Health (2009). NIH stroke scale. Retrieved May 16, 2010, from http://stroke.nih.gov/documents/NIH_Stroke_Scale_Booklet.pdf.

National Institute of Neurological Disorders and Stroke. (2009). Myasthenia gravis fact sheet. Retrieved on March 31, 2009 from http://www.ninds.nih.gov/disorders/myasthenia_gravis/detail_myasthenia_gravis.htm#124023153.

Newswanger, D. L., & Warren, C. R. (2004). Guillain-Barre syndrome. Retrieved on April 8, 2009, from http://www.aafp.org/afp/20040515/2405.html.

Oral, R. Yagmur, F., Nashelsky, M., Turkmen, M., & Kirby, P. (2008). Fatal abusive head trauma cases: Consequence of medical staff missing milder forms of physical abuse. *Pediatric Emergency Care, 24(12)*, 816-821.

Price, D. D., & Wilson, S. R. (2008). Epidural hematoma. Retrieved on April 7, 2009, from http://emedicine.medscape.com/article/824029-overview.

Price, S. A., & Wilson, L. M. (2003). *Pathophysiology: Clinical concepts of disease process* (6th ed.). St. Louis: Mosby.

Proehl, J. A. (2004). *Emergency nursing procedures* (3rd ed.). St. Louis: Saunders

Roppolo, L. P., Davis, D., Kelly, S. P., & Rosen, P. (2007). *Emergency medicine handbook: Critical concepts for clinical practice*. St. Louis: Mosby.

Scaletta, T. (2008). Subdural hematoma. Retrieved on April 8, 2009, from http://emedicine.medscape.com/article/828005-overview.

Somes, J., & Bergman, D. L. (2007). ABCDs of acute stroke intervention. *Journal of Emergency Nursing, 33(3)*, 228-234.

Taylor, K., & Paparella, K. (2008). Fatal errors with Cerebyx. *Journal of Emergency Nursing, 34(5)*, 460-461.

Wasserman, J. R., & Koenigsberg, R. A. (2007). Diffuse axonal injury. Retrieved on April 5, 2009, from http://emedicine.medscape.com/article/339912-overview.

Zebian, R. C., & Kazzi, A. A. (2009). Subarachnoid hemorrhage. Retrieved on April 9, 2009, from http://emedicine.medscape.com/article/794076-overview

Introduction

Constitutes 6% (nine items) of the CEN examination
The focus is on gastrointestinal conditions, including medical and traumatic conditions, commonly encountered in an emergency department setting
The continuum of age needs to be considered from infancy to older adulthood

Age-related Considerations

Neonates, infants, and children
1. These patients have a higher percentage of body water compared with adults and a higher metabolic rate; this makes them more susceptible to dehydration when they have vomiting or diarrhea
2. Nausea, vomiting, and diarrhea are major causes of fluid, electrolyte, and acid-base imbalances in these patients
3. Infants have immature kidney function which limits their ability to concentrate and dilute urine (Emergency Nurses Association [ENA], 2007)
4. Pain in children may be diffuse and seemingly not related to the injury or disease process
5. The kidneys are more mobile in these patients than in an adult and they are not well protected by fat (ENA, 2007)
6. Abdominal muscles are thinner and weaker than in adults
7. The liver is more anterior and not as well protected by the ribs as in adults
8. These patients often present with vague symptoms when they have significant abdominal injury
9. These patients can lose 25% to 40% of their circulating volume before they exhibit hypotension

Older adult
1. Metabolic rate slows with aging, which may contribute to obesity
2. Malnutrition, particularly protein malnutrition, is common in older adults; contributing factors include the following:
   a. Poverty
   b. Depression
   c. Fatigue
   d. Not wanting to cook for one person if living alone
3. Older patients frequently do not present with usual signs and symptoms

   a. May have less specific and/or less intense pain
   b. May have less temperature elevation
   c. May have less leukocytosis
4. Constipation is a common problem in older adults
   a. Gastrointestinal (GI) motility decreases with age
   b. Dehydration is a contributing factor
   c. Chronic laxative use may be a contributing factor
5. Older patients fear loss of independence so they frequently avoid coming to the ED or may be very anxious when coming to the ED

Selected Concepts in Gastrointestinal Anatomy and Physiology

General information about the gastrointestinal system
1. Functions of the GI system
   a. Digestion and absorption of nutrients
   b. Elimination of waste material
   c. Detoxification and elimination of bacteria, viruses, chemical toxins, and drugs
2. Processes of the GI system
   a. Ingestion
   b. Digestion
   c. Absorption
   d. Elimination
3. Structures of the GI system (Figure 7-1)
   a. Alimentary canal: from the mouth to the anus
      1) Oropharynx
      2) Esophagus
      3) Stomach
      4) Small intestine: divided into duodenum, jejunum, and ileum
      5) Large intestine: divided into cecum, ascending colon, transverse colon, descending colon, sigmoid colon, and rectum
   b. Accessory organs of digestion
      1) Liver
      2) Gallbladder
      3) Pancreas
4. Cell layers (Figure 7-2)
   a. All areas of the GI tract have the same cell layers (external to internal)
      1) Serosa: outermost layer that is frequently continuous with the peritoneum
      2) Muscularis: thin layer of smooth muscle between serosa and submucosa

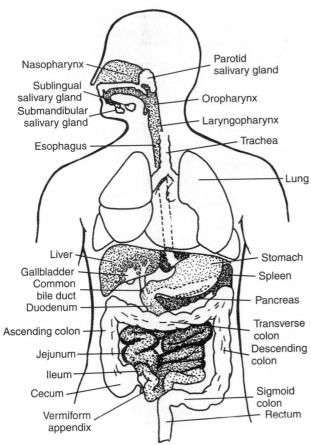

Figure 7-1 Structures of the gastrointestinal system. (From Kinney, M. R., Packa, D. R., & Dunbar, S. B. [1998]. *AACN's clinical reference for critical-care nursing* [4th ed.]. St. Louis: Mosby.)

Nasopharynx
Sublingual salivary gland
Submandibular salivary gland
Esophagus
Parotid salivary gland
Oropharynx
Laryngopharynx
Trachea
Lung
Liver
Gallbladder
Common bile duct
Duodenum
Ascending colon
Jejunum
Ileum
Cecum
Vermiform appendix
Stomach
Spleen
Pancreas
Transverse colon
Descending colon
Sigmoid colon
Rectum

e) Tongue: mucous glands and serous glands
f) Salivary glands
  i) Parotid glands (two)
  ii) Submandibular glands (two)
  iii) Sublingual glands (two)
2) Muscles of mastication
3) Pharynx
  a) Nasopharynx
  b) Oropharynx
  c) Laryngopharynx
c. Secretions: saliva
  1) Stimulated by thought, sight, smell, or taste
  2) Consists of the following:
    a) Ptyalin (amylase): begins the breakdown of polysaccharides (starches) to disaccharides
    b) Mucus: provides lubricant
  3) Volume: 1500 ml/day
d. Process
  1) The teeth break up the food into smaller pieces to increase surface area for digestive enzymes to act
  2) The masseter muscles are innervated by cranial nerve V (i.e., trigeminal)
  3) The tongue moves the food around in the mouth for better chewing and moves the food to the back of the throat to begin the process of swallowing
  4) Swallowing (deglutination)
e. Functions: summarized in Table 7-1
2. Esophagus
  a. Location
    1) Lies behind the trachea
    2) Passes through the thoracic cavity and the diaphragm; passes through the diaphragm at the diaphragmatic hiatus
  b. Description: hollow tube from the pharynx to the stomach; ≈25 cm in length and ≈2 cm in diameter
  c. Structure (Figure 7-3)
    1) Cell layers (external to internal)
      a) No serosa layer
      b) Muscularis
      c) Submucosa
      d) Mucosa: lined with mucous membrane that secretes a protective mucoid substance
    2) Sphincters
      a) Hypopharyngeal
        i) Also referred to as the upper esophageal sphincter (UES)
        ii) Made of cricopharyngeal muscle
      b) Gastroesophageal
        i) Also referred to as the lower esophageal sphincter (LES)
        ii) A physiologic rather than anatomic sphincter: last 2 to 4 cm of the esophagus
  d. Secretions: mucus
  e. Process: final phase of swallowing (involuntary)
    1) When a bolus of food enters the esophagus, the hypopharyngeal sphincter opens

3) Submucosa: dense irregular connective tissue that supports the mucosa
4) Mucosa: innermost layer that is exposed to dietary material
5. Peritoneum
  a. Covers the abdominal viscera
    1) Parietal layer lines the abdominal cavity wall
    2) Visceral layer covers the abdominal organs
    3) Peritoneal cavity is a potential space between the parietal and visceral layers
  b. There are two folds of the peritoneum
    1) Mesentery contains blood and lymph vessels and attaches the small intestine and part of the large intestine to the posterior abdominal wall
    2) The omentum contains fat and lymph nodes

Alimentary canal

1. Oropharynx
  a. Location: mouth to esophagus
  b. Description
    1) Oral cavity
      a) Lips
      b) Cheeks
      c) Palate
      d) Teeth

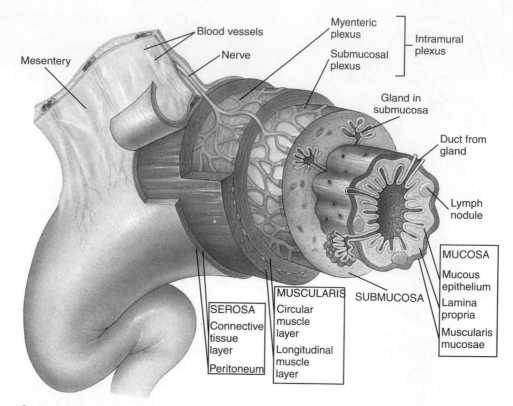

Figure 7-2 Cell layers of the gastrointestinal tract. (From Doughty, D. B., & Jackson, D. B. [1993]. *Gastrointestinal disorders: Mosby's clinical nursing series.* St. Louis: Mosby.)

2) Food is moved through the esophagus by gravity and peristaltic action; peristalsis is the alternating contraction and relaxation of muscle fibers which propels the substance in a wave-like motion through the esophagus, stomach, and intestines

3) The gastroesophageal sphincter opens and food enters the stomach

4) The process takes 5 to 10 seconds

  f. Functions: see Table 7-1

3. Stomach

  a. Location: inferior to the diaphragm with approximately 80% to 85% of the organ to the left of midline

  b. Description

    1) Largest dilation of the GI tract

    2) Approximately 25 to 30 cm in length and 10 to 15 cm at maximal diameter

    3) Relatively little muscle tone, which permits increased distention

  c. Structure (Figure 7-4)

    1) Anatomical divisions

      a) Cardia: portion of stomach that immediately adjoins the esophagus

      b) Fundus: dome-shaped portion of stomach that extends left of the cardia

      c) Greater curvature: lateral, convex side

      d) Body: major area (belly) of stomach

      e) Lesser curvature: medial, concave side

      f) Antrum: lower portion close to pylorus

2) Sphincters

  a) Cardiac: between esophagus and stomach

  b) Pyloric: between stomach and duodenum

3) Layers of stomach wall (external to internal)

  a) Serosa: continuous with the peritoneum

  b) Muscularis

  c) Submucosa

  d) Mucosa: contains rugae, which are thick folds on the interior of the stomach that do all of the following:

    i) Increase surface area for exposure

    ii) Allow for distention

    iii) Contain the openings of the gastric glands

4) Gastric glands

d. Secretions

  1) Description: gastric secretions are clear and contain water, salts, enzymes, hydrochloric acid (HCl)

  2) Gastric secretions are stimulated when a bolus of food enters the upper portion of the stomach

  3) Gastric secretions contain the following:

    a) HCl

      i) Stimulated by histamine, acetylcholine, gastrin

      ii) Functions

        (a) Denatures protein and break intermolecular bonds

TABLE 7-1 Functions of the Components of the Gastrointestinal System

Component	Function
Oropharynx	• Salivation • Ingestion • Mastication • Lubrication and moistening of food • First and second stages of swallowing
Esophagus	• Third stage of swallowing • Lubrication of food • Provision of vent for increased gastric pressures
Stomach	• Secretion of gastric enzymes • Mixing of food with gastric enzymes • Reduction of osmolality of food • Absorption of water • Movement of food through the pylorus
Small intestine	• Receipt of chyme from the stomach and movement of the chyme forward to facilitate proper absorption of proteins, carbohydrates, fats, electrolytes, vitamins, minerals, drugs, and water • Receipt of bile and pancreatic fluid to aid in digestion • Movement of chyme via peristalsis and segmentation • Bacteria in the small intestine to help break down and digest protein and, to some degree, fat
Large intestine	• Secretion of mucous to lubricate and protect intestinal lining • Movement of chyme through colon to rectum and initiate urge to defecate • Storage of feces • Elimination of digestive wastes: defecation • Absorption of water and electrolytes • Synthesis of vitamins (folic acid, riboflavin, vitamin K, nicotinic acid) • Metabolism of blood urea to ammonia
Liver	• Secretion of bilirubin, bile salts, cholesterol, fatty acids, calcium, and other electrolytes into bile • Storage of amino acids, glucose, vitamins, minerals (copper, iron), and blood • Vitamins: riboflavin, nicotinic acid, pyridoxine, vitamins A, D, E, K, B_{12} • Conversion of complex sugars to simple sugars • Conversion of carbohydrates to fats • Conversion stored glucose (glycogen) to glucose (process is called glycogenolysis) • Conversion of amino acids and fats to glucose (process is called gluconeogenesis) • Conversion of amino acids to fatty acids and triglycerides • Formation of phospholipids and cholesterol • Formation of lipoproteins from triglycerides and peptides. • Conversion of amino acids to plasma proteins (e.g., albumin, fibrinogen, globulins) • Phagocytosis of old RBCs • Formation of clotting factors and heparin • Conversion of ammonia to urea • Conversion of creatine to creatinine • Conversion of vitamin D_3 to 25-hydroxycholecalciferol • Detoxification of bacteria • Biotransformation of drugs to active and/or inactive metabolites • Deactivation of certain hormones
Gallbladder	• Collection, concentration, and storage of bile • Passageway for bile from liver to intestine • Regulation of bile flow • Release of bile

Pancreas	• Exocrine function
	  • Secretion of pancreatic juice for digestion of carbohydrates, proteins, and fats
	  • Secretion of bicarbonate to neutralize chyme
	• Endocrine function
	  • Secretion of insulin and glucagon

From Dennison, R. D. (2007). *Pass CCRN!* (3rd ed.). St. Louis: Mosby.

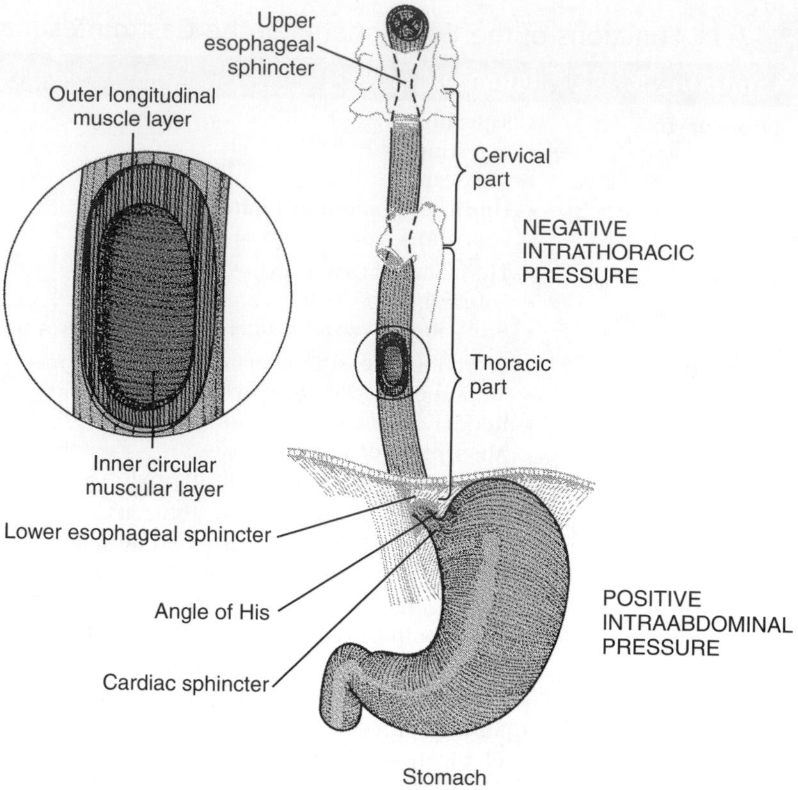

Figure 7-3 Anatomy of the stomach. (From Thompson, J. M., et al.: *Mosby's clinical nursing* [3rd ed.]. St. Louis: Mosby.)

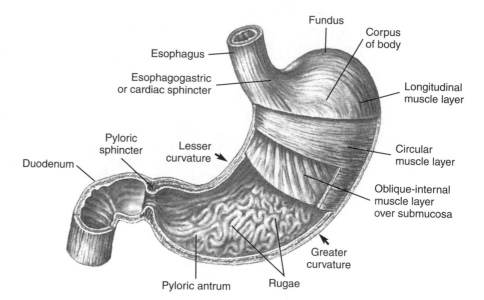

Figure 7-4 Anatomy of the esophagus. (From Beare, P. G., & Myers, J. L. [1994]. *Principles and practice of adult health nursing* [2nd ed.]. St. Louis: Mosby.)

(b) Activates a number of enzymes secreted by stomach

(c) Kills bacteria

b) Pepsinogen

i) Activated by HCl acid to form pepsin

ii) Function: catalyzes splitting of bonds between particular types of amino acids in protein chains

c) Intrinsic factor: mucoprotein necessary for intestinal absorption of vitamin B_{12} in the ileum; deficiency of vitamin B_{12} causes pernicious anemia

d) Mucus: contributes to the maintenance of the gastric mucosal barrier

e. Process

1) As food moves toward the pyloric sphincter at the distal end of the stomach, peristaltic waves increase in force and intensity

2) The food bolus becomes a substance known as chyme

3) Gastric motility is affected and controlled by various factors such as the quantity and pH of contents, autonomic nervous system activity, and gastric hormones

4) Chyme is pumped through the pyloric sphincter into the duodenum
5) The stomach empties as chyme moves through the pyloric channel
    a) Rate of gastric emptying proportional to the volume of the stomach's contents
    b) Regulation of gastric emptying affected by the following
       i) Consistency of the fluid chyme; liquids selectively move through the pylorus before solids
       ii) Receptiveness of the duodenum
    c) Factors inhibiting gastric emptying
       i) Chyme with high lipid content
       ii) High acidity in antrum
       iii) Emotions: pain, anxiety, sadness, hostility
       iv) Hormones: secretin and cholecystokinin
    d) Food usually stays in the stomach 2 to 6 hours after ingestion
f. Functions: see Table 7-1

4. Small intestine
  a. Description
    1) Length: 7 m; diameter: 2.5 cm
    2) Extends from pylorus to ileocecal valve
  b. Structure
    1) Divisions
      a) Duodenum: short segment only 30 cm long
      b) Jejunum: the next two fifths after the duodenum
      c) Ileum: the last three fifths after the duodenum
    2) Sphincters
      a) Pylorus: extends from stomach to duodenum
      b) Ileocecal: controls flow of contents into large intestine and prevents reflux from the large intestine back into the ileum
    3) Villi: fingerlike projections of mucosa and submucosa prominent in duodenum and jejunum increase surface area
  c. Secretions
    1) Stimulated by the presence of chyme in the duodenum and release of gastric hormones
  d. Process
    1) Movement of chyme
      a) During fasting and sleeping states: muscle contraction moves from antrum to ileum to sweep the gut of contents
      b) During eating state: slow, propulsive contractions (peristalsis) slowly push the chyme in the direction of the large intestine
      c) The movement of chyme from the small intestine to the large intestine regulated by gastroileal reflex; increased contractions in the ileum as the chyme nears the large intestine
      d) Movement of chyme through small intestine approximately 3 to 10 hours
  e. Function: see Table 7-1

5. Large intestine
  a. Description: length: 90 to 150 cm; diameter: 4 to 6 cm extending from ileum to anus
  b. Structure
    1) Divisions (Figure 7-5)
      a) Cecum
      b) Colon
        i) Ascending colon
        ii) Transverse colon
        iii) Descending colon
        iv) Sigmoid colon
      c) Rectum
    2) Flexures
      a) Hepatic: bend at the liver; in the right upper quadrant (RUQ)
      b) Splenic: bend at the spleen; in the left upper quadrant (LUQ)
    3) Sphincters
      a) Ileocecal: from small intestine to cecum
      b) Anal: internal and external anal sphincters
  c. Process
    1) Movement of intestinal contents
      a) Haustral shuttling: weak peristaltic contractions that move the chyme through the large intestine
      b) Phasic, random, nonpropulsive contractions: mixes the stool material and helps in the absorption of liquid contents without advancement toward the anus
      c) Spontaneous mass movements
        i) Stimulated by gastrocolic reflexes initiated when food enters the duodenum from the stomach, especially after the first meal of the day to move feces into the rectum

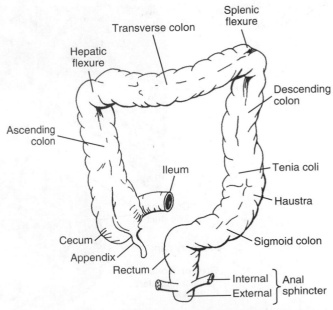

Figure 7-5 Anatomy of the colon. (From Kinney, M. R., Packa, D. R., & Dunbar, S. B. [1998]. *A-ACN's clinical reference for critical-care nursing* [4th ed.]. St. Louis: Mosby.)

ii) The defecation reflex occurs when feces enters the rectum; peristaltic waves in the rectum and relaxation of the internal and external anal sphincter occur

iii) Evacuation of the colon may be facilitated by Valsalva maneuver

2) Factors that enhance colonic motility
   a) High-residue diets
   b) Fluids
   c) Irritation of colon (e.g., spicy foods)
   d) Irritant laxatives

3) Factors that inhibit colonic motility
   a) Low-residue diet
   b) Anticholinergic drugs
   c) Opiates

4) Movement of fecal contents through small intestine in approximately 12 hours

5) Function: see Table 7-1

Accessory organs of digestion (Figure 7-6)

1. Liver
   a. Location: in RUQ, fitting snugly against right inferior diaphragm
   b. Description
      1) Largest organ in the body: 1.5 kg
      2) Attached to the abdominal wall by the falciform ligament, which also divides the left and right lobes
      3) Four main lobes
         a) Right: larger than left
         b) Left
         c) Caudate
         d) Quadrate
      4) Covered by a thick capsule of connective tissue (i.e., Glisson capsule); contains blood vessels, lymphatics
      5) Capsule covered by a layer of serosa continuous with the peritoneum
   c. Structure
      1) Lobes are divided into lobules; there are over 1 million lobules
         a) Hepatic cells (i.e., hepatocytes) are arranged in chains around a central vein: the hepatic cells remove oxygen, nutrients, and toxins from the blood
         b) Kupffer cells, which are responsible for phagocytosis, line the sinusoids; Kupffer cells are a part of the reticuloendothelium system; they destroy old or defective red blood cells and remove bacteria and foreign particles from the blood
         c) Ducts
            i) Bile canaliculi are located between the hepatic cells and empty bile into the small bile ducts
            ii) Small bile ducts join to form the right and left hepatic ducts

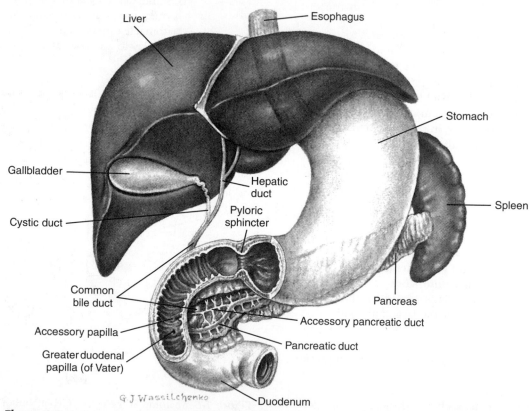

Figure 7-6 Accessory organs of the gastrointestinal system. (From Doughty, D. B., & Jackson, D. B. [1993]. *Gastrointestinal disorders: Mosby's clinical nursing series.* St. Louis: Mosby.)

iii) Left and right hepatic ducts merge to form the common hepatic duct

iv) Cystic duct from the gallbladder joins the common hepatic duct to form the common bile duct

v) The pancreatic duct joins the common bile duct and together empty into the duodenum through the ampulla of Vater

vi) The sphincter of Oddi is a valve in the common bile duct that regulates the passage of bile from the common bile duct into the duodenum

d. Secretions: bile is described under Gallbladder

e. Function: see Table 7-1

2. Gallbladder

a. Location

1) Attached to undersurface of liver

2) Connected to the upper portion of the duodenum by the common bile duct

b. Description

1) Saclike organ about 7 to 10 cm in length and 3 cm in diameter

2) Storage capacity of 50 to 70 ml

3) Layers (exterior to interior)

a) Serous layer: continuous with the peritoneum

b) Smooth muscle layer

c) Mucous membrane layer (has rugae, which allows an increase in gallbladder size)

4) The sphincter of Oddi

a) At terminal end of common bile duct, located at entrance into duodenum

b) Regulates the flow of bile and pancreatic juices into the intestine

c) Prevents reflux of intestinal contents into the duct

c. Structure

1) There are four anatomical divisions of the gallbladder

a) Fundus: distal portion of the body that forms a blind sac

b) Body: connects the fundus to the infundibulum

c) Infundibulum: connects the body to the neck

d) Neck: narrows into the cystic duct

2) The cystic duct merges with the common hepatic duct to form the common bile duct, which joins with the pancreatic duct to form ampulla of Vater

3) The sphincter of Oddi is at the terminal end of common bile duct, located at entrance into duodenum

a) Regulates the flow of bile and pancreatic juices into the intestine

b) Inhibits the entry of bile into the pancreatic duct

c) Prevents reflux of intestinal contents into the duct

d. Secretions

1) Bile: produced by the liver and stored in the gallbladder

a) The gallbladder contracts in response to the hormone cholecystokinin when food is present in the small intestine; release is stimulated when fatty food is present in the small intestine

b) The action of bile is to assist in the absorption of fats by emulsifying the fat and breaking down large fat droplets into small droplets

c) Bile is composed of the following:

i) Water

ii) Bile pigments

(a) The major bile pigment is bilirubin, a breakdown product of hemoglobin (Hgb)

iii) Bile salts

iv) High concentration of cholesterol

v) Some neutral fat, phospholipid, and inorganic salts

e. Process

1) Contraction of the gallbladder is stimulated by the hormone cholecystokinin

f. Function: see Table 7-1

3. Pancreas

a. Location: lies in the posterior curvature of the stomach behind duodenum and spleen

b. Description

1) Length: 15 to 20 cm; diameter: 5 cm

2) Anatomic divisions

a) Head: over the vena cava in the C-shaped curve of the curve of the duodenum

b) Body: behind duodenum and extends across the abdomen behind stomach

c) Tail: under the spleen

3) Not surrounded by a capsule

c. Structure

1) The acini are arranged around a small central lumen; they secrete their enzymes into the central lumen

2) These central lumina are drained into ductules

3) Ductules drain into intralobular ducts, which drain into interlobular ducts, which empty into the pancreatic duct (also called the duct of Wirsung)

4) The pancreatic duct runs from the tail to the head of the pancreas and unites with the common bile duct to form the ampulla of Vater, which empties into the duodenum

5) Cells have exocrine and endocrine functions

a) Acinar cells have exocrine (through a duct) functions

b) Alpha and beta cells of the islets of Langerhans have endocrine (ductless) functions

i) Alpha cells secrete glucagon

ii) Beta cells secrete insulin

iii) Delta cells secrete somatostatin

d. Secretions

1) Pancreatic secretions are triggered by the presence of undigested food in the small intestine

2) Acinar cells secrete a high concentration of sodium bicarbonate, water, sodium, potassium, and digestive enzymes (lipase, amylase, trypsin, ribonuclease, deoxyribonuclease)

   a) Trypsinogen: secreted in inactive form; activated in contact with bile salts

   b) Chymotrypsinogen: secreted in inactive form; activated in contact with bile salts

3) Secretions are controlled by the following

   a) Vagus nerve and parasympathetic nervous system

   b) Hormonal: secretin and cholecystokinin

e. Functions: see Table 7-1

Blood supply (Figure 7-7)

1. Arterial: aorta → aortic arch → thoracic arch → abdominal aorta

  a. Celiac artery: the following branches of the celiac artery supply these specified organs:

    1) Left gastric: supplies stomach, esophagus

    2) Hepatic to right gastric: supplies stomach

    3) Gastroduodenal: supplies stomach, duodenum

    4) Cystic: supplies gallbladder

    5) Splenic: supplies stomach, pancreas, spleen

  b. Superior mesenteric arteries supply the following:

    1) Jejunum, ileum, cecum

    2) Ascending colon, part of transverse colon

  c. Inferior mesenteric arteries supply the following:

    1) Transverse, descending, and sigmoid colon

    2) Rectum

  d. Hepatic artery and vein supply the liver

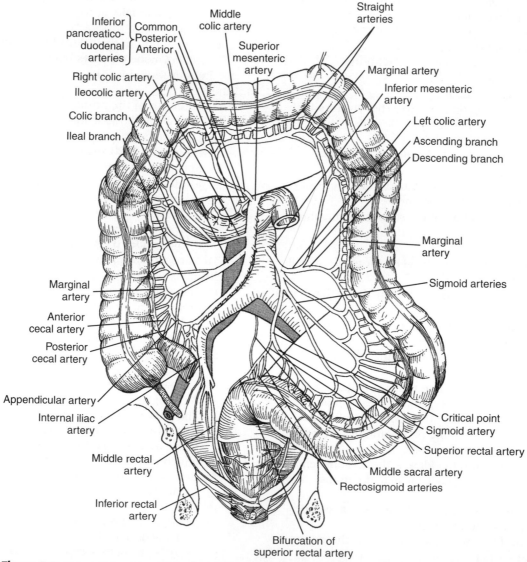

Figure 7-7 Arterial blood supply of the gastrointestinal system. (From Society of Gastroenterology Nurses and Associates. [1993]. *Gastroenterology nursing: A core curriculum.* St. Louis: Mosby.)

2. Venous
   a. Portal vein collects and delivers blood from entire venous drainage of GI tract to liver; branches: gastric; splenic; superior mesenteric; inferior mesenteric
   b. Portal vein subdivides into liver sinusoids, which then unite with branches from hepatic artery to form hepatic vein, which empties into inferior vena cava
   c. Partially metabolized digestive products are brought to liver sinusoids where hepatocytes complete the next stage of metabolism

Nervous innervation

1. Extrinsic
   a. Parasympathetic nervous system (PNS): increases the activity of the GI tract; innervated via the vagus nerve
   b. Sympathetic nervous system (SNS): decreases the activity of the GI tract; innervated via SNS fibers, which parallel the major blood vessels of the GI tract
2. Intrinsic
   a. Located inside the wall of GI tract
   b. Consists of extensions from extrinsic nerves of the autonomic nervous system (ANS)
   c. Form two major and three minor networks of plexuses

Functions of the gastrointestinal system

1. Ingestion
   a. Ingestion begins with the sensation of hunger, controlled by the feeding center of the hypothalamus
   b. Ingestion ends with the sensation of satisfaction provided by the satiety center also in the hypothalamus
   c. Food and liquids enter the alimentary tract at the mouth
2. Secretion of digestive enzymes
3. Digestion
   a. Carbohydrates: 4 kcal/g
      1) Digestion begins in the mouth, where polysaccharides (starch) are broken down to disaccharides (e.g., sucrose, lactose, maltose) by the action of ptyalin (amylase)
      2) The process continues when the disaccharides are broken down to monosaccharides (e.g., glucose, galactose, fructose) by the action of pancreatic amylase and intestinal enzymes (e.g., sucrase, lactase, maltase)
   b. Proteins: 4 kcal/g
      1) Digestion begins in the stomach where pepsin breaks down proteins into polypeptides
      2) The process continues when the polypeptides are broken down into peptides and amino acids in the small intestine by the action of trypsin, chymotrypsin, carboxypeptides from the pancreas, and aminopeptidases and dipeptidase from the intestinal villi

   c. Fats: 9 kcal/g
      1) Digestion of fats that are already emulsified (e.g., cream, butter) begins in the stomach by lipase
      2) Digestion of nonemulsified fat occurs in the small intestine with emulsification of the fat by bile and pancreatic lipase
      3) Fat is broken down into glycerol and fatty acids
4. Absorption
   a. Basic absorption mechanisms
      1) Active transport requires an energy source (e.g., ATP) to move substances into and out of the cell; substances absorbed by active transport include proteins, glucose, sodium, and potassium
      2) Passive diffusion is passive movement from an area of high solute concentration to an area of low solute concentration; substances absorbed by passive diffusion include free fatty acids and water
      3) Facilitated diffusion is movement that requires a carrier that moves into the cell without the requirement of energy; a substance absorbed by facilitated diffusion is fructose
      4) Nonionic transport is movement of solutes freely into and out of the cell; substances absorbed by nonionic transport include unconjugated bile salts, drugs
      5) Solvent drag is flow of water to higher osmotic concentration; it contributes to absorption and reduction in osmolality that occurs in jejunum
   b. Specific absorption in small intestine
      1) Electrolyte absorption: active transport from all areas of intestine
      2) Water absorption: small and large intestine
         a) Approximately 2 L of fluid is ingested daily
         b) Approximately 7 L of fluid is secreted by the GI tract daily
         c) Of these 9 L, 7500 ml are reabsorbed with only 1500 ml reaching the cecum
         d) Additional fluid is reabsorbed in the large intestinal but only 200 ml lost in the stool
      3) Carbohydrate absorption
      4) Protein absorption: amino acids absorbed by active transport in ileum and jejunum
      5) Fat absorption
         a) Micellar solubilization of fatty acid with bile salt to form micelle
         b) Diffusion of micelle into jejunal cell
         c) Delivery of fatty acids to circulation via lymphatic system
      6) Water-soluble vitamin absorption: all areas of small intestine by passive diffusion (absorption of B_{12} requires intrinsic factor)
      7) Fat-soluble vitamins absorption: absorbed in jejunum (bile salts required)
      8) Calcium absorption: mainly in duodenum (vitamin D required)
      9) Iron absorption: all areas of the intestine (especially in duodenum) by active transport; stored as protein-bound iron

5. Synthesis
   a. Bacteria in the large intestine produce vitamin K
   b. Peyer patches in the small intestine play a role in antibody synthesis
6. Effect on fluid and electrolyte balance
   a. Gastric losses are acidic; increased gastric losses (e.g., nasogastric suction, vomiting) cause metabolic alkalosis, hypokalemia, hyponatremia, hypovolemia
   b. Intestinal losses are alkaline: increased intestinal losses (e.g., biliary losses, pancreatic fistula, intestinal suction, diarrhea) cause metabolic acidosis, hypokalemia, hyponatremia, hypovolemia

Assessment of the Gastrointestinal System

Primary and secondary assessment (see Chapter 2)

Focused assessment

1. Chief complaint: identifies why the patient is seeking help
2. Symptoms
   a. Nonspecific problems/complaints
      1) Change in appetite
      2) Fatigue or weakness
      3) Unintentional weight loss or weight gain
      4) Fever, chills
   b. Abdominal pain: describe PQRST (Table 7-2)
      1) Provocation: relationship to food, drugs, activity, position, bowel movements, breathing, stress
      2) Palliation
         a) Ineffective or effective treatments
         b) Alleviating factors (e.g., position)

TABLE 7-2   Differentiation of Abdominal Pain

Condition	Location of Pain	Quality of Pain	Associated Symptoms
Gastritis	• Epigastric or slightly left of midline	• May be described as indigestion	• Nausea and vomiting • May have hematemesis • Abdominal tenderness
Peptic ulcer	• Epigastric or right upper quadrant (RUQ)	• Gnawing, burning	• Abdominal tenderness • Hematemesis (gastric) or melena (duodenal)
Pancreatitis	• Epigastric or LUQ • May radiate to back, flanks, or left shoulder	• Boring • Worsened by lying down	• Nausea and vomiting • Mild fever • Abdominal tenderness • May have Cullen sign (i.e., bluish discoloration at umbilicus), indicating intraperitoneal bleeding, or Grey Turner sign (i.e., bluish discoloration at flanks), indicating retroperitoneal bleeding
Cholecystitis	• Epigastric or RUQ • May be referred to below right scapula • Murphy sign: pain with deep breath while the nurse palpates under the right costal margin	• Cramping	• Nausea and vomiting • Abdominal tenderness in RUQ
Appendicitis	• Epigastric or periumbilical pain; later localizes to right lower quadrant (RLQ) • McBurney sign: pain with palpation at McBurney point (i.e., point at one third the distance between the right anterior iliac crest and the umbilicus) • Rovsing sign: pain in RLQ with palpation of left lower quadrant indicates peritoneal irritation	• Dull to sharp	• Anorexia, nausea, vomiting • Fever • Diarrhea • Leukocytosis. • Rebound tenderness indicates peritoneal irritation
Intestinal obstruction	• Epigastric or umbilical	• Spastic to dull	• Change in bowel habits • Melena or hematochezia. • Hyperactive to hypoactive bowel sounds

3) Quality: sharp, dull, tearing, cramping, burning, gnawing, stabbing, aching, colicky
  a) Visceral pain
    i) Dull, poorly localized
    ii) May be caused by organic lesions or functional disturbance within the GI tract
  b) Somatic pain
    i) Sharp, well localized
    ii) May be caused by inflammation of abdominal organs which cause peritoneal irritation
  c) Referred pain
    i) Pain experienced at a distance from the disease process
    ii) May be explained by the embryologic origins of the structures involved
4) Region: location
  a) May be poorly localized
  b) May be referred pain (Figure 7-8)
    i) Pain may be felt in a remote area that is supplied by the same nerve as the diseased or damaged organ.
    ii) Pain is usually sharp and localized but not over area of injury.
5) Radiation
6) Severity: 0 to 10 scale
7) Timing: constant, intermittent, duration
c. Abdominal distention
d. Change in bowel elimination
  1) Change in color of stools
    a) Clay-colored stools indicate biliary obstruction
    b) Tarry stools (i.e., melena) indicate upper GI bleeding
    c) Bright red bloody stools from rectum (i.e., hematochezia) indicate lower GI bleeding
  2) Change in consistency or frequency of stools
  3) Excessive flatus
  4) Use of laxative, enemas
  5) Relationship to food, drugs, alcohol
e. Nausea/vomiting
  1) Onset, duration
  2) Frequency
  3) Character and color; presence of blood in vomitus (i.e., hematemesis), bile, fecal matter

4) Palliation
  a) Ineffective or effective treatment
  b) Alleviating factors
5) Timing
  a) Time of day
  b) Relationship to food, odors, drugs, alcohol, activity, bowel movements
f. Abdominal trauma (e.g., gunshot, stab wounds)
g. Dentition problems (e.g., caries, gingivitis, poorly fitting dentures)
h. Painful swallowing
i. Dysphagia (i.e., difficulty swallowing)
j. Dyspepsia (i.e., indigestion)
k. Eructations (i.e., belching)
l. Flatulence (i.e., passing gas)
m. Edema
n. Abnormal bruising or bleeding
o. Jaundice
p. Change in color of urine: dark brown or orange urine may indicate biliary obstruction
q. Pruritus
r. Fecal incontinence
s. Rectal bleeding
t. Anal discomfort
3. History of present illness: use PQRST format
4. Past medical history
  a. GI, hematologic, or other medical conditions
  b. Eating disorders (e.g., obesity, bulimia, anorexia nervosa)
  c. Hepatic disease
    1) Cirrhosis
    2) Hepatitis
    3) History of blood transfusion
  d. Inflammatory bowel disease (e.g., ulcerative colitis, Crohn disease)
  e. Past injury: abdominal trauma
  f. Past surgical procedures
  g. Past diagnostic studies (e.g., endoscopy, radiographs, stool examination for occult blood)
5. Family history of medical illness or GI problems
6. Social history
  a. Occupation
  b. Educational level
  c. Stress level and usual coping mechanisms

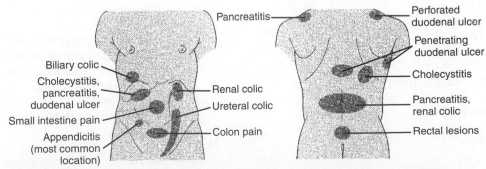

Figure 7-8 Common areas of referred abdominal pain. (From Beare, P. G., & Myers, J. L. [1994]. *Principles and practice of adult health nursing* [2nd ed.]. St. Louis: Mosby.)

d. Recreational and exercise habits
e. Dietary habits
1) Appetite
2) Usual foods
3) Number and time of meals, snacks
4) Fluid intake
5) Food restrictions
   a) Intolerances
   b) Prescribed restrictions
   c) Religious restrictions
6) Change in eating habits
f. Usual bowel habits
g. Caffeine intake
h. Tobacco use: record as pack-years (number of packs per day times the number of years patient has been smoking)
i. Alcohol use: record as alcoholic beverages consumed per month, week, or day
j. Exposure to toxins or infectious disease
k. Recent travel

7. Medication history
a. Prescribed drug, dose, frequency, time of last dose
b. Nonprescribed drugs
1) Over-the-counter drugs
2) Substance abuse
c. Patient understanding of drug actions, side effects
d. Drugs causing potential problems for patients with GI problems
1) Antibiotics
2) Aspirin
3) Nonsteroidal antiinflammatory drugs (NSAIDs) (e.g., ketorolac [Toradol], ibuprofen [Motrin])
4) Acetaminophen (Tylenol)
5) Many drugs have anorexia, nausea, vomiting as side effects
6) Many drugs are hepatotoxic
e. Drugs frequently used for GI problems
1) Antacids, H_2 receptor antagonists, proton-pump inhibitors
2) Stool softeners
3) Laxatives
4) Cathartics
5) Anticholinergics
6) Corticosteroids
7) Antidiarrheals
8) Antiemetics
9) Tranquilizers
10) Sedatives
11) Barbiturates

Vital signs include height and weight
Inspection
1. Landmarks (Figure 7-9)
a. Xiphoid
b. Costal margin
c. Midline
d. Umbilicus
e. Anterior superior iliac crest

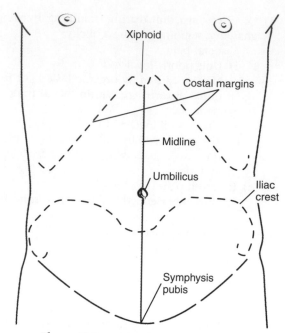

Figure 7-9 Landmarks of the abdomen.

f. Symphysis pubis
g. The abdomen may be divided into four quadrants (Figure 7-10): horizontal and vertical lines that intersect at the umbilicus

2. General survey
a. Apparent health status
b. Apparent age relative to chronologic age
c. Nutritional status
d. Level of consciousness
e. Stature/posture
1) Flexing of knees to relieve abdominal tension, frequently seen with peritonitis
2) Leaning forward to relieve abdominal pain, frequently seen in pancreatitis
f. Gait

3. Mouth
a. Lips: color, texture, lesions, swelling, symmetry
b. Gums: inflammation, retraction, hypertrophy, bleeding, lesions
c. Teeth: caries, state of repair, occlusion
1) Dentures: fit, gum ulceration
d. Tongue: swelling, laceration, lesions, coating
e. Mucosa: moisture, lesions, color
f. Odor
1) Fetor hepaticus: sweet fecal odor caused by hepatic failure (also known as the "breath of death")
2) Feculent breath: foul fecal odor caused by severe bowel obstruction
3) Severe halitosis: foul odor may be caused by poor dental hygiene, neoplasm of esophagus or stomach

4. Skin
a. Color: should be homogenous over the entire abdomen
1) Pallor: anemia

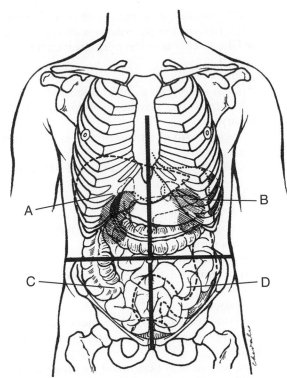

Figure 7-10 The abdomen divided into four quadrants. **A,** Right upper quadrant (RUQ). **B,** Left upper quadrant (LUQ). **C,** Right lower quadrant (RLQ). **D,** Left lower quadrant (LLQ). (From Abels, L. F. [1986]. *Critical care nursing*. St. Louis: Mosby.)

    2) Jaundice: seen with bilirubin greater than 3.0 mg/dl; associated with any of the following:
        a) Liver disease
        b) Biliary obstruction
        c) Excessive hemolysis
    3) Bluish: due to infiltration of the abdominal wall with blood
        a) Grey Turner sign: ecchymosis to flanks indicative of retroperitoneal bleeding (e.g., from pancreas, duodenum, kidneys, vena cava, aorta)
        b) Cullen sign: ecchymosis around umbilicus indicative of intraperitoneal bleeding (e.g., liver, spleen)
  b. Lesions or discoloration
    1) Scars: trauma, surgical procedures
    2) Striae:
        a) Initially pinkish or bluish, become silvery with time
        b) May be caused by pregnancy, obesity, ascites
        c) Purplish may be caused by Cushing disease
    3) Rash, ecchymosis, abrasions
    4) Spider angiomas: found just under the skin
        a) Central red spot and reddish extensions which radiate outward like a spider web
        b) Causes: B_{12} deficiency, liver disease, pregnancy
  c. Shiny, edematous abdomen

    1) Ascites: intraperitoneal fluid frequently associated with cirrhosis, intra-abdominal malignancy (e.g., liver, ovarian), or right ventricular failure
    2) Anasarca: entire body edematous; usually seen in end-stage heart failure or renal failure
  d. Stoma: location, color, drainage, condition of surrounding skin
  e. Draining wounds: location, drainage, condition of surrounding skin
  f. Fistula: location, drainage, condition of surrounding skin
5. Contour of abdomen
  a. Normal: flat from xiphoid process to pubic symphysis
  b. Scaffold: concave abdomen seen in malnutrition
  c. Distention or protuberance
    1) Diffuse and symmetrical
        a) Fat
        b) Flatus
        c) Fetus (i.e., pregnancy)
        d) Feces (i.e., obstruction)
        e) Fluid (i.e., ascites)
        f) Fatal growths (i.e., malignancy)
        g) Fibroids
    2) Distention in upper quadrants: gastric dilation, pancreatic cyst, malignancy
    3) Distention in lower quadrants: pregnancy, uterine fibroid, distended bladder, ovarian tumor
    4) Distention in one quadrant: hernia, tumor, cyst, obstruction, organomegaly
6. Abdominal girth: measurement of the distance around the abdomen at the umbilicus level
7. Hernia: abdominal, umbilical, or inguinal
8. Movement of abdomen
  a. Breathing: normal
  b. Peristalsis: abnormal to see waves of peristalsis across the abdomen: generally associated with intestinal obstruction
  c. Aortic pulsation: normally visible at the end of expiration in a supine patient especially if the patient is thin; pulsatile swelling in the epigastrium suggests an abdominal aortic aneurysm or an epigastric solid tumor overlying the aorta

Auscultation
1. Auscultation: done prior to percussion or palpation to prevent "stirring up" the abdomen
  a. Order for physical assessment of the abdomen: inspection, auscultation, percussion, palpation
2. Preparation: may be helpful to put pillow under knees to relax abdominal muscles
3. Bowel sounds: use diaphragm with light pressure for 1 minute in each of the four abdominal quadrants.
  a. Normal bowel sounds: bubbling or soft gurgling noises heard every 5 to 20 seconds in an irregular pattern; heard in all quadrants (also called borborygmi)
  b. Abnormal bowel sounds
    1) Very infrequent or absent bowel sounds

a) Functional obstruction: paralytic ileus
b) Advanced mechanical intestinal obstruction
2) Loud, hyperactive (but normally pitched) bowel sounds: hyperperistalsis (e.g., diarrhea, catharsis caused by GI bleeding)
3) High-pitched "rushing" bowel sounds: early mechanical small intestinal obstruction
4) Low-pitched "rushing" bowel sounds: early mechanical large intestinal obstruction
4. Vascular sounds: use of bell over specified areas
   a. Bruits
      1) Listen over midline and renal and femoral arteries.
      2) If bruit is noted, check circulation to extremities; if decreased blood flow is noted, aneurysm should be suspected.
   b. Venous hum: hum of medium tone created by blood flow in a large, engorged vascular organ such as liver or spleen
5. Peritoneal friction rub: scratchy sound heard over inflamed spleen or neoplastic liver

Percussion

1. Percussion tones normally heard over abdomen
   a. Dull: liver, full sigmoid colon, full bladder
   b. Flat: bone
   c. Tympany: gastric bubble, bowel
2. Organ borders
   a. Liver (dullness between right lung resonance and bowel tympany)
      1) Normal span 6 to 12 cm in the right midclavicular line
      2) Enlarged and tender in right ventricular failure (RVF), hepatitis, mononucleosis
      3) May be large or small in cirrhosis
      4) Absence of liver dullness: may indicate free air in peritoneum from bowel perforation
   b. Spleen (dullness under left diaphragm): if percussible, should be <7 cm at the left midaxillary line
   c. Stomach (tympany under left costal margin)
   d. Bladder (dullness above symphysis pubis): percussible only if enlarged
   e. Intestine (tympany over abdomen): may percuss dullness over lower left quadrant (LLQ) if sigmoid colon is full
3. Test for fluid wave as an indication of ascites

Palpation

1. Light palpation: use fingertips to depress 1 to 2 cm; note the following:
   a. Temperature, moisture
   b. Superficial skin reflexes: movement of the umbilicus toward the quadrant that is stroked
   c. Voluntary guarding: voluntarily splinting of abdominal muscles, especially when sensitive spot is touched; watch for nonverbal indicators of pain during palpation
   d. Involuntary guarding or rigidity
      1) Diffuse rigidity suggests an infectious, neoplastic, or inflammatory process in the peritoneal cavity

2) Rigid, boardlike abdomen is associated with acute perforation of a viscus with spillage of air or GI contents into the peritoneal cavity
   e. Tender areas
   f. Large masses
      1) If pulsating, refrain from additional abdominal palpation as this may be an abdominal aortic aneurysm
2. Deep palpation: with one hand on top of the other depress 4 to 5 cm
   a. Do not use deep palpation in the following situations:
      1) Polycystic kidneys
      2) After renal transplant
      3) Malignant tumor: may cause seeding
      4) Recent surgery
   b. Note the following:
      1) Direct tenderness: associated with local inflammation of the abdominal wall, the peritoneum, or a viscus
      2) Rebound (or indirect) tenderness (also referred to as Blumberg sign): associated with peritoneal irritation
         a) Assessment is performed by pressing into the tender area and then letting go
         b) If the pain is exacerbated when pressure is released, rebound tenderness is present
      3) Splenic tenderness
         a) Palpate left side of abdomen with patient in lateral decubitus position and note any tenderness
         b) The spleen is palpable only if significantly enlarged (e.g., injury, leukemia, mononucleosis, portal hypertension)
      4) Aortic pulsation: lateral expansion may indicate an aneurysm

Diagnostic studies

1. Serum chemistries
   a. Sodium: normal 136 to 145 mEq/L; elevated in dehydration from severe diarrhea or intestinal obstruction
   b. Potassium: normal 3.5 to 5.0 mEq/L; decreased in GI losses from upper or lower GI tract
   c. Chloride: normal 96 to 106 mEq/L
      1) Elevated in dehydration
      2) Decreased in vomiting, diarrhea, or intestinal obstruction
   d. Calcium: normal 9.0 to 10.5 mg/dl in adults and 8.8 to 10.8 mg/dl in children; decreased in acute pancreatitis
   e. Phosphorus: normal 3.0 to 4.5 mg/dl
      1) Elevated in intestinal obstruction
      2) Decreased in malnutrition or malabsorption syndromes
   f. Magnesium: normal adults 1.3 to 2.1 mEq/L; children 1.4 to 1.7 mEq/L; and infants 1.4 to 2 mEq/L; decreased in chronic diarrhea
   g. Glucose: normal 65 to 110 mEq/L; elevated in diabetes mellitus, pancreatitis

h. Blood urea nitrogen (BUN): normal 8 to 23 mg/dl
i. Creatinine: normal 0.6. to 1.1 mg/dl in females and 0.8 to 1.3 mg/dl in males
j. Bilirubin: normal 0.3 to 1.3 mg/dl; elevated in hepatic disease, biliary obstruction, or excessive hemolysis
k. Serum proteins
   1) Total protein: normal 6 to 8 g/dl
   2) Albumin: normal 3.5 to 5 g/dl; half-life is 19 to 20 days so poor indicator of acute changes in nutritional status
l. Serum lipids
   1) Cholesterol: normal 150 to 200 mg/dl
   2) Triglycerides: normal 40 to 150 mg/dl
m. Enzymes
   1) Alkaline phosphatase: normal 30 to 85 IU/L; elevated in cirrhosis, rheumatoid arthritis, biliary obstruction, liver tumor, hyperparathyroidism
   2) Amylase: normal 56 to 190 IU/L; elevated in acute pancreatitis, pancreatic cancer, pancreatic pseudocysts, perforated peptic ulcer, mesenteric thrombosis, ectopic pregnancy, renal failure, mumps
   3) Lipase: normal up to 1.5 u/ml; elevated in acute or chronic pancreatitis, duodenal ulcer, biliary obstruction, cirrhosis, hepatitis; stays elevated longer than amylase in pancreatitis
   4) Alanine aminotransferase (ALT): normal 5 to 36 units/ml
      a) Formerly called SGPT
      b) Elevated in hepatitis, cirrhosis, liver tumor, hepatotoxic drugs, cholestasis, infectious mononucleosis
   5) Aspartate aminotransferase (AST): normal 15 to 45 units/ml
      a) Formerly called SGOT
      b) Elevated in hepatitis, cirrhosis, acute pancreatitis, skeletal muscle disease or trauma, liver tumor
   6) Lactate dehydrogenase (LDH): normal 90 to 200 IU/L; elevated in hepatitis, hemolytic anemia, pancreatitis, muscular dystrophy, pulmonary infarction, myocardial infarction, pernicious anemia, renal disease
n. Serology for viral hepatitis
2. Hematology
   a. Hct: normal 40% to 52% for males; 35% to 47% for females
   b. Hgb: normal 13 to 18 g/dl for males; 12 to 16 g/dl for females
   c. WBCs: normal 5800 to 10,800 mm³
   d. Erythrocyte sedimentation rate: normal up to 15 mm/hr for males; up to 20 mm/hr for females
3. Clotting profile: may be abnormal in liver disease
   a. Activated partial thromboplastin time (aPTT): normal 25 to 38 seconds; therapeutic 1.5 to 2.5 times normal
   b. Prothrombin time (PT): normal 12 to 15 seconds; therapeutic 1.5 to 2.5 times normal
   c. International normalized ratio (INR): normal <2.0
   d. Platelets: normal 150,000 to 400,000/mm³
4. Urine
   a. Glucose: normal negative
   b. Ketones: normal negative
   c. Amylase: normal negative
   d. Bilirubin: normal negative
   e. Urobilinogen: normal 0.3 to 1.1 mg/dl for females and up to 2.1 mg/dl in males
      1) Elevated in hepatocellular disease
      2) Decreased in complete biliary obstruction
   f. Specific gravity: 1.005 to 1.030
   g. Osmolality: 50 to 1200 mOsm/L
5. Gastric contents analysis
6. Stool
   a. Fecal occult blood test: normal negative
   b. Ova, parasites, blood (OPB): normal negative; specimen must be warm
   c. Culture: normal intestinal flora
   d. Assay for *Clostridium difficile* toxin A or B: positive is diarrhea is caused *C. difficile,* an opportunistic infection caused primarily by suppression of normal flora by antibiotic therapy
7. Other diagnostic studies (Table 7-3, Figure 7-11)

Acute Abdomen

Definition: abnormal condition characterized by the acute onset of abdominal pain
Predisposing factors
1. Inflammation (e.g., appendicitis, cholecystitis)
2. Perforation of the GI tract (e.g., perforated ulcer, ruptured diverticulum)
3. Vascular problems (e.g., ruptured abdominal aortic aneurysm)
4. Gynecologic problems (e.g., ectopic pregnancy, pelvic inflammatory disease [PID])
5. Infectious disease (e.g., *Salmonella*)
6. Trauma

Pathophysiology: varies depending on illness or injury
Clinical presentation: varies depending on illness or injury
1. Subjective
   a. Pain
      1) Visceral
         a) Described often as cramping or "like gas"
         b) Comes and goes and may be difficult to localize, may be around the umbilicus or lower half of the abdomen
      2) Somatic
         a) Often described as sharp and intense
         b) Easily localized (usually)
      3) Referred

TABLE **7-3**   **Gastrointestinal Diagnostic Studies**

Study	Evaluates	Comments

Computed tomography (CT) of abdomen	• Diagnoses tumors, pancreatic cancer or cysts, pancreatitis, biliary tract disorders, obstruction versus nonobstructive jaundice, cirrhosis, liver metastases, ascites, lymph node metastases, aneurysm
	• Evaluates vasculature and focal points found on nuclear scans
	• Used to direct biopsy of tumors or aspiration of abscess
		• No special preparation required
		• Contrast medium may be used; if used:
		  • Check for allergy to iodine prior to the study
		  • Monitor for allergic reaction post-procedure
		  • Ensure hydration post-procedure

Endoscopic retrograde cholangiopancreatography (ERCP)	• Diagnoses biliary stones, ductal stricture, ductal compression, neoplasms of the pancreas and biliary system • Evaluates patency of biliary and pancreatic ducts, jaundice, pancreatitis, cholecystitis, hepatitis	• Same as for esophagogastroduodenoscopy • Contraindicated if patient is uncooperative or if bilirubin is >3.5 mg/dl • Monitor for clinical indications of pancreatitis (most common complication) after study • Monitor for clinical indications of sepsis
Endoscopy Colonoscopy	• Directly visualizes mucosa of areas of the GI tract • Colonoscopy diagnoses diverticular disease, obstruction, strictures, radiation injury, polyps, neoplasms, bleeding, ischemia • Colonoscopy or sigmoidoscopy may be used therapeutically for removal of polyps • Biopsies may be taken during any endoscopy	• Sedation may be prescribed, especially for colonoscopy • Bowel preparation with gastric irrigation (e.g., GoLYTELY) and cathartics required before lower GI endoscopy • Nothing by mouth (NPO) 4 to 8 hours prior to study • Keep NPO until gag reflex returns if sedation used • Monitor closely after procedure for clinical indications of perforation, hemorrhage
Flat plate of abdomen (may also be referred to as *KUB*)	• Diagnoses perforated viscous, paralytic ileus, mechanical obstruction, intra-abdominal mass • Evaluates the distribution of visceral gas (and identifies free air in the peritoneum indicative of bowel perforation) • Evaluates organ size	• No preparation required
Liver scan	• Diagnoses cirrhosis, hepatitis, tumors, abscesses, cysts, tuberculosis	• No preparation required
Magnetic resonance imaging (MRI)	• Evaluates liver, biliary tree, pancreas, spleen • Differentiation between cyst and solid mass • Diagnoses hepatic metastasis • Evaluates abscesses, fistulas, source of GI bleeding • Used for staging of colorectal cancer	• Cannot be used in patients with any implanted metallic device, including pacemakers • No special preparation required • Cannot be done on a patient being mechanically ventilated
Paracentesis	• Analysis of fluid removed during peritoneal tap • Diagnoses intraperitoneal bleeding with diagnostic peritoneal lavage	• Monitor for peritoneal leakage after tap • Monitor for clinical indications of infection or peritonitis after tap
Ultrasound of abdomen	• Evaluates the pancreas, biliary ducts, gallbladder, liver • Identifies tumor, abdominal abscesses, hepatocellular disease, splenomegaly, pancreatic or splenic cysts • Differentiates obstructive from nonobstructive jaundice	• All barium must have been cleared from the GI tract prior to ultrasonography • NPO for 8 hours prior to study • If for evaluation of gallbladder: fat-free meal the evening prior to study

TABLE 7-3   Gastrointestinal Diagnostic Studies—cont'd

Study	Evaluates	Comments
Focused assessment sonography for trauma (FAST)	• Evaluates abdomen for blood in the peritoneal space • Assesses the hepatorenal fossa, the spleno-renal fossa, the pericardial sac, and the pelvis (see Figure 7-11)	• Does not detect retroperitoneal bleeding; if this is suspected, the patient must have a CT • Positive test: >200 ml of blood • Does not diagnose hollow visceral organ injury, retroperitoneal injuries, or intraperitoneal injuries that are not associated with bleeding
Diagnostic peritoneal lavage (DPL)	• Used to detect intra-abdominal bleeding • Insert indwelling Foley catheter to drain bladder and a gastric tube to deflate the stomach prior to proceeding • Peritoneal catheter is inserted in the abdomen, usually below the umbilicus	• Especially good for hemodynamically unstable patient when rapid CT is not available • Gross bloody returns are positive for bleeding • If returns are not bloody, instill 1 L of warmed saline solution and let it drain out of the abdomen by gravity • Fluid may be sent to the lab for analysis of RBCs, WBCs, bile, amylase, food, or feces • Considered 98% accurate for intraperitoneal bleeding; does not assess retroperitoneal bleeding

From Dennison, R. D. (2007). *Pass CCRN!* (3rd ed.). St. Louis: Mosby.

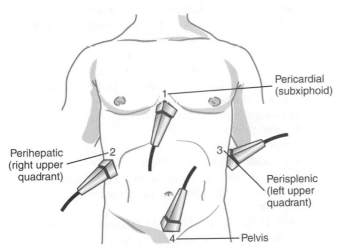

Figure 7-11 The FAST Examination includes ultrasound views of the following four sites: perihepatic (right upper quadrant), pericardial (subxiphoid), perisplenic (left upper quadrant), and pelvis. (From American Association of Critical-Care Nurses [2009]: *Advanced critical care nursing* [p. 1166, Figure 42-14A]. St. Louis: Mosby.)

TABLE 7-4   Potential Sources of Referred Abdominal Pain by Location

Condition	Location of Referred Pain
Fluid collection under the diaphragm	Top of the shoulder
Ruptured peptic ulcer	Back
Pancreas	Midline back or through to the back
Biliary tract	Right flank to the scapula
Dissecting or ruptured aneurysm	Lower back and thighs
Renal colic	Groin and external genitalia
Appendix	Right lower quadrant or epigastrium
Uterine disorders	Lower back
Rectal disease	Lower back

a) Difficult to describe; may be localized or diffuse (Table 7-4)
2. Objective
   a. Abdominal distention
   b. Guarding: contraction of abdominal muscles and discomfort with palpation of the abdomen
   c. Rigidity: palpation reveals hardness of abdominal muscles
   d. Rebound tenderness

3. Diagnostic
   a. CBC with differential: increased WBCs
   b. Radiographic: chest and abdomen
   c. Ultrasound: to evaluation of abdominal organs and spaces with sound waves
   d. Computed tomography (CT): chest and/or abdomen
   e. Endoscopy: use of an endoscope to view the upper or lower GI tract
   f. Angiography: view major blood vessels
   g. Radionuclide scans: to identify sources of intestinal bleeding

h. Stool for blood, mucous, parasites, bacteria
i. Urine for bacteria, blood, toxicology
j. See individual disease conditions

Collaborative management

1. Continue assessment
   a. ABCDs
   b. Vital signs: blood pressure, pulse, respiratory rate, and temperature
   c. Oxygen saturation
   d. Respiratory effort and excursion
   e. Cardiac rate and rhythm
   f. Pain, discomfort, or dyspnea level
   g. Accurate intake and output
   h. Serum electrolytes
   i. Level of consciousness
   j. Close monitoring for progression of symptoms
2. Prepare patient for diagnostic or surgical procedures as required
3. Treat infection if present
   a. Antimicrobials as indicated
   b. Surgical drainage, debridement, repair as required
4. Monitor for/prevent complications
   a. Infection
   b. Sepsis
   c. Hemorrhage
   d. Infertility if due to PID

Evaluation

1. Patent airway, adequate oxygenation (i.e., normal Pao_2, Spo_2, Sao_2) and ventilation (i.e., normal $Paco_2$)
2. Absence of clinical indications of infection/sepsis
3. Control of pain and discomfort

Typical disposition: admission

1. May require direct admission to surgery from the ED

Appendicitis

Definition: inflammation of the appendix

a. Acute: sudden onset of inflammation
b. Gangrenous: preperforation state
c. Chronic: lymphoid hyperplastic phenomena
d. Neonatal: very rare and seen mostly in preemies, symptoms similar to necrotizing enterocolitis, associated with Hirschsprung disease

Precipitating factors

1. Most common in males, age 10 to 30 years
2. Foreign bodies
3. Tumor of the cecum or appendix
4. Excessive lymphoid tissue growth
5. Recent barium enema

Pathophysiology

1. Obstruction of the lumen of the appendix occurs, most commonly from a fecalith (i.e., hardened accumulated feces)

2. The obstruction leads to distention of the appendix, venous engorgement, and eventual accumulation of mucus and bacteria
3. The appendix can become infected and gangrenous as bacteria invade the wall of the appendix

Clinical presentation

1. Subjective
   a. May present with vague complaints
   b. Anorexia
   c. Abdominal pain
      1) Increases over 6 to 12 hours
      2) Usually starts in periumbilical region and migrates to the RLQ
   d. Nausea, vomiting, and anorexia
   e. Infants: parents report infant being "fussy" and feeding poorly
   f. Young children: parents may report the child has had diarrhea and difficulty ambulating
2. Objective
   a. Low-grade fever common
   b. Responses to palpation
   c. Localized abdominal tenderness with palpation in RLQ
   d. Rebound tenderness with rupture/peritonitis
   e. Rovsing sign: palpating the left lower quadrant causes pain in the right lower quadrant
   f. Pain on palpation of McBurney point (two thirds of the way from umbilicus to anterior superior iliac spine)
   g. Psoas sign: pain on extension of right thigh with patient on left side (indicates retroperitoneal retrocecal appendix)
   h. Peritoneal signs: guarding, rigidity
   i. Hypoactive bowel sounds
3. Diagnostic studies
   a. CBC with differential: elevated WBCs
   b. Urinalysis: may show proteinuria and hematuria
   c. CT: abdominal helical CT highly sensitive and specific
   d. MANTRELS score (Box 7-1) (Mayo Clinic, 2007)
      1) Score of ≤3, there is <3.6% chance
      2) Scores of 4 to 6, there is a 32% chance
      3) Scores of 7 to 10, there is a 78% chance
   e. Ultrasound: to rule out PID

Collaborative management

1. Continue assessment
   a. ABCDs
   b. Vital signs: blood pressure, pulse, respiratory rate, and temperature
   c. Oxygen saturation
   d. Respiratory effort and excursion
   e. Cardiac rate and rhythm
   f. Pain and discomfort level
   g. Accurate intake and output
   h. Serum electrolytes
   i. Level of consciousness
   j. Close monitoring for progression of symptoms

BOX 7-1 MANTRELS Score

Characteristics	Score
M = Migration of pain to the RLQ	1
A = Anorexia	1
N = Nausea and vomiting	1
T = Tenderness in RLQ	2
R = Rebound pain	1
E = Elevated temperature	1
L = Leukocytosis	2
S = Shift of WBCs to the left	1
Total	10

2. Maintain airway, oxygenation, and ventilation
   a. Elevation of head of bed 30 to 45 degrees
   b. Oxygen by nasal cannula at 2 to 6 L/min to maintain SpO_2 of 95% unless contraindicated; for patients with chronic obstructive pulmonary disease (COPD), use pulse oximetry to guide oxygen administration to SpO_2 of 90%
3. Maintain adequate circulation
   a. IV access with two large-bore catheters for fluid and medication administration
   b. Hydration: intravenous fluids, usually 0.9% saline
4. Control pain and discomfort
   a. Position for comfort; flexing of knees with pillows for support help to relax abdominal muscles
   b. NSAIDs
   c. Analgesics
   d. Antiemetics
   e. Anxiolytics
5. Treat inflammation/infection (if present) and prevent sepsis
   a. Antimicrobials as indicated
   b. Antipyretics and cooling methods to reduce fever
6. Prepare patient for procedures (e.g., exploratory laparotomy and appendectomy) as indicated
   a. Nothing by mouth (NPO) and nasogastric (NG) tube attached to suction
   b. Explanation of procedures to patient and significant others
   c. Surgical consent
7. Monitor for complications
   a. Perforation
   b. Sepsis
   c. Preterm labor in pregnancy

Evaluation

1. Patent airway, adequate oxygenation (i.e., normal PaO_2, SpO_2, SaO_2) and ventilation (i.e., normal $PaCO_2$)
2. Absence of clinical indications of infection/sepsis
3. Control of pain and discomfort

Typical disposition: admission: may require direct admission to surgery from the ED

Upper Gastrointestinal Hemorrhage

Definitions

1. Gastritis: inflammation of the gastric mucosa of the stomach; may be acute or chronic and is a predisposing factor to peptic ulcer
2. Peptic ulcer: sharply defined erosion in mucosa, which may involve the submucosal and muscular layers of the esophagus ($\approx$5%), stomach ($\approx$15%), or duodenum ($\approx$80%)
   a. *Helicobacter pylori*: a bacterial infection that has now been identified as a common cause of recurrent ulcer disease
3. Esophageal varices: dilation of the submucosal esophageal veins
4. Mallory-Weiss tear: acute longitudinal tear of the esophagus caused by forceful retching
5. Boerhaave syndrome: spontaneous tear or rupturing of the esophagus associated with vomiting
6. Esophageal rupture: perforation or rupture of the esophagus

Predisposing factors

1. Gastritis or peptic ulcer
   a. Genetic predisposition
   b. Substance abuse: tobacco, alcohol
   c. Diet (e.g., caffeine, alcohol, dietary intolerance)
   d. Drugs and therapies:
      1) Drugs that alter the mucosal barrier: NSAIDs
      2) Drugs that decrease gastric mucosal renewal: corticosteroids, phenylbutazone (Butazolidine)
      3) Drugs that increase acid stimulation (e.g., coffee [because of peptides, not caffeine], nicotine)
      4) Hormones (e.g., estrogen)
   e. High physiologic stress situation (e.g., COPD, recent major surgery, myocardial infarction)
   f. Ingestion of strong acids or alkalis (referred to as corrosive gastritis)
2. Esophageal varices: portal hypertension as may occur with any of the following:
3. Cirrhosis
4. Hepatitis
5. Chronic right ventricular failure
6. Mallory-Weiss tear or Boerhaave syndrome: forceful retching or vomiting

Pathophysiology

1. Gastritis: inflammation of the stomach lining that causes mucosal bleeding, edema, and erosion
2. Peptic ulcer
   a. Injury is caused by exposure to hydrochloric acid, pepsin, and/or *H. pylori* bacteria; other factors include
      1) Increased acid production or inability to buffer acid
      2) Impaired mucosal barrier to acid
      3) Decreased gastric motility
   b. Ulceration occurs when there is injury to mucosa, allowing acid to diffuse back through the broken barrier

1) Gastric ulcers are more likely to present with hematemesis or perforation
2) Duodenal ulcers are more likely to present with melena, perforation, or scarring with obstruction

3. Esophageal varices
   a. Fibrotic liver changes and resistance to normal venous drainage of the liver to the portal vein (hepatic venous obstruction) causes increased pressure → portal hypertension → pressure transmitted to collateral circulation → dilation of the submucosal veins of the distal esophagus and stomach → predisposition to bleed (these vessels were not intended to tolerate this pressure) → bleeding frequently triggered by:
      1) Increased intra-abdominal pressure (e.g., Valsalva maneuver)
      2) Mechanical trauma (e.g., poorly chewed hard foods, insertion of nasogastric tube)
      3) Chemical trauma (e.g., gastroesophageal reflux)
      4) Coagulopathies

4. Mallory-Weiss tear or Boerhaave syndrome
   a. Result of a sudden rise in intraluminal esophageal pressure produced during retching and/or vomiting
   b. In Boerhaave syndrome, this increase in esophageal pressure is the result of neuromuscular incoordination causing failure of the cricopharyngeus muscle to relax

Clinical presentation

1. Subjective
   a. May have history of any of the following: epigastric pain, previous ulcer, previous GI bleeding, alcoholism, liver disease, forceful retching/vomiting
   b. Peptic ulcer: epigastric pain
      1) Gastric: pain usually occurs 30 minutes to 1 hour after meals
      2) Duodenal: pain usually occurs at night and 2 to 3 hours after meals
   c. Esophageal varices: report of painful bleeding by mouth
   d. May have symptoms of hypovolemia and/or anemia: dyspnea, chest pain, fatigue, weakness, thirst, anxiety

2. Objective
   a. Bleeding
      1) Peptic ulcer
         a) Hematemesis
            i) Gastritis: coffee-grounds appearance
            ii) Gastric peptic ulcer: bright red blood
         b) Melena: if duodenal peptic ulcer
         c) Severe anemia manifested by faintness, fatigue, and pallor may be the only indications when bleeding is slow and gradual
      2) Esophageal varices: bright, red blood gushing from mouth
   b. May have indications of liver disease (e.g., jaundice, spider angiomas, fetor hepaticus, ascites, hepatosplenomegaly)

c. Bowel sounds: may be hypoactive since blood in the GI tract has a cathartic effect
d. Clinical indications of hypoperfusion depending on degree of blood loss: tachycardia, tachypnea, hypotension, cool, clammy skin, decreased urine output, restlessness, confusion
e. Clinical indications of acute abdomen if ulcer perforates

3. Diagnostic studies
   a. BUN: elevated
   b. Bilirubin: may be elevated
   c. Albumin: may be decreased with liver disease
   d. AST, ALT, LDH: usually elevated due to liver disease
   e. Gastrin level: may be elevated in gastric ulcer
   f. Amylase: elevated if perforation occurs (causes penetration into the pancreas and causes acute pancreatitis)
   g. Total proteins, albumin, transferrin: may be decreased related to malnutrition
   h. Clotting studies: PT, aPTT prolonged if liver is affected
   i. Hgb, Hct: decreased but may take 4 to 6 hours after acute bleed
   j. Type and crossmatch: in preparation for possible need for blood
   k. Arterial blood gases (ABGs): metabolic acidosis with shock states
   l. Stool: positive for occult blood
   m. Chest radiograph: shows widened mediastinum, free air if lower esophagus, pneumothorax if pleura involved, left pleural effusion
   n. ECG: may show ischemia (e.g., ST-T wave changes)
   o. Flat plate of abdomen: free air under diaphragm indicates perforation of ulcer
   p. Gastroscopy: important in differentiating cause of upper GI bleeding
   q. Barium swallow: shows extravasation if perforation
   r. Angiography
      1) May reveal bleeding site or sites
      2) May include the placement of a catheter for intra-arterial administration of vasopressors (e.g., vasopressin [Pitressin])

Collaborative management

1. Continue assessment
   a. ABCDs
   b. Oxygen saturation
   c. Vital signs: blood pressure, pulse, respiratory rate, and temperature
   d. Cardiac rate and rhythm
   e. Discomfort and pain level
   f. Abdominal assessment: distention, rebound tenderness, rigidity
   g. Overt bleeding and laboratory indicator (hematocrit and hemoglobin) of bleeding
   h. Level of consciousness
   i. Accurate intake and output
   j. Close monitoring for progression of symptoms

2. Maintain airway, oxygenation, and ventilation
   a. Positioning on left side with head elevated to 30 to 45 degrees
   b. Oxygen by nasal cannula at 2 to 6 L/min to maintain SpO_2 of 95% unless contraindicated; for patients with COPD, use pulse oximetry to guide oxygen administration to SpO_2 of 90%
   c. Endotracheal intubation may be required to:
      1) Prevent pulmonary aspiration of blood
      2) Prevent potential obstruction of airway by displaced balloon if Sengstaken-Blakemore tube used
         a) Keep scissors at the bedside in case of tube migration or airway emergency; cut across all lumens and remove immediately
3. Maintain adequate circulation and perfusion
   a. IV access with two large-bore catheters for fluid and medication administration
   b. Fluid replacement
      1) Crystalloids: usually 0.9% saline; lactated Ringer solution is contraindicated in patients with liver disease
      2) Packed red blood cells (RBCs)
      3) Should be given early if significant blood loss is suspected to prevent tissue hypoxia
         a) Replacement of platelets, clotting factors, and calcium should be considered if multiple transfusions are given
   c. Control of bleeding
      1) Vasopressin (Pitressin) intravenous as prescribed
         a) Action: slows blood loss by constricting the splanchnic arteriolar bed and decreasing portal venous pressure
         b) Administration: IV, preferably through a central venous catheter
         c) Adverse effects of vasopressin: bradycardia; hypertension; water retention causing hyponatremia (syndrome of inappropriate secretion of antidiuretic hormone); chest pain; dysrhythmias; abdominal cramping and pain; oliguria
            i) Close monitoring of the blood pressure is essential as hypertension may increase bleeding
      2) Octreotide acetate (Sandostatin) as prescribed
         a) Action: reduces splanchnic blood flow, gastric acid secretion, GI mobility, and pancreatic exocrine function
         b) Administration: IV or subcutaneously
         c) Adverse effects of octreotide: pain or burning at injection site, abdominal pain, diarrhea
      3) Diagnostic/therapeutic endoscopy
         a) Diagnostic to identify the specific cause of the bleeding
         b) Therapeutic for peptic ulcer or Mallory-Weiss tear
            i) Endoscopic thermal therapy uses heat to cauterize the bleeding vessel
            ii) Endoscopic injection therapy uses hypertonic saline, epinephrine, or dehydrated alcohol to cause localized vasoconstriction of the bleeding vessel
         c) Therapeutic for esophageal varices
            i) Sclerosing agent is injected into the varix and surrounding tissue; the sclerosing agent causes variceal inflammation, venous thrombosis, and eventually scar tissue
            ii) Esophageal variceal ligation: rubber bands or O-rings are placed on the target vessels at gastroesophageal junction
      4) Stop bleeding in esophageal varices through measures that lower venous pressure
         a) β-Blockers (e.g., propranolol [Inderal]) as prescribed
         b) Placement of a multiple-lumen tube (e.g., Sengstaken-Blakemore) for balloon tamponade (Figure 7-12, Box 7-2) if bleeding cannot be controlled pharmacologically, endoscopically, or through use of transjugular intrahepatic portosystemic shunt (TIPS)
4. Prepare patient for procedures as indicated
   a. NPO
   b. NG tube with room-temperature saline lavage may be indicated
      1) Allows visualization during endoscopy
      2) Removes blood from GI tract to prevent digestion of the protein (i.e., Hgb) causing elevation of ammonia
   c. Foley catheter
   d. Endoscopy
5. Prevent further damage to the gastric mucosa caused by gastric irritants, hyperacidity, and/or impaired mucosal barrier
   a. Discontinuance of any gastric irritants
   b. Pharmacologic agents that decrease gastric acidity and/or protect gastric mucosa
      1) Antacids (e.g., magnesium hydroxide and aluminum hydroxide [Maalox, Mylanta])
      2) Histamine (H_2) receptor antagonist (e.g., ranitidine [Zantac], famotidine [Pepcid])
      3) Proton-pump inhibitors (e.g., omeprazole [Prilosec])
   c. Pharmacologic therapy for *H. pylori*: 2-week course with three drugs
      1) Bismuth subsalicylate (Pepto-Bismol) or a proton-pump inhibitor AND
      2) Metronidazole (Flagyl) and tetracycline (Achromycin) OR
      3) Clarithromycin (Biaxin) and amoxicillin (Amoxil)
6. Correct coagulopathies (may be caused by liver disease)
   a. Vitamin K as prescribed
   b. Close monitoring for bleeding
   c. Avoidance of invasive procedures and injections

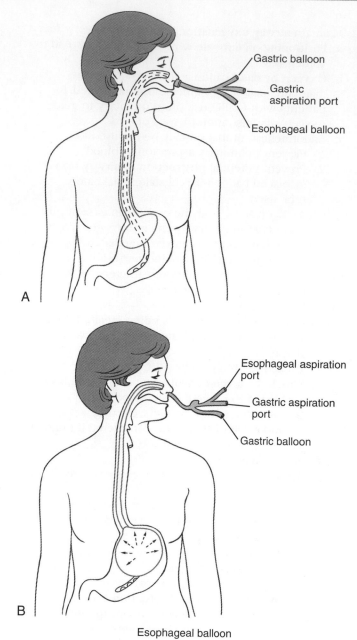

A

B

Figure 7-12 Esophageal tamponade tubes. **A,** Sengstaken-Blakemore tube. **B,** Linton tube. **C,** Minnesota tube. (From Thelan, L. A., Urden, L. D., Lough, M. E., & Stacy, K. M. [1998]. *Critical care nursing: Diagnosis and management* [3rd ed.]. St. Louis: Mosby.)

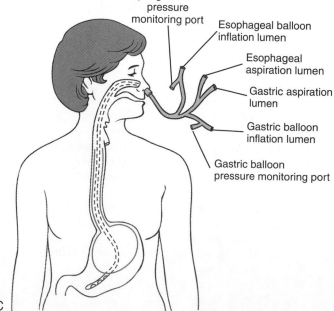

C

BOX 7-2   Balloon Tamponade for Esophageal Varices

Action	• Applies pressure to esophageal and intragastric varices
Tube	• Sengstaken-Blakemore (SB) tube (see Figure 7–12): esophageal balloon; gastric balloon; gastric suction
Lumens	• Gastric balloon: 200–500 ml for SB tube • Esophageal balloon: usually 20 mm Hg (25 cm H_2O) but may be as high as 30–40 mm Hg to control bleeding • Gastric suction: nonvented • Esophageal suction: nonvented

Insertion	• Generally done by physician but may be done by specifically trained nurse
	• Check balloon for leaks prior to insertion by inflating with air and putting in a basin of saline
	• Use viscous lidocaine or benzocaine/butamben/tetracaine (Cetacaine) to anesthetize the nose and posterior pharynx
	• Advance the catheter to ≈50-cm mark
	• Inflate the gastric balloon to ≈200–300 ml; double-clamp the lumen to prevent leakage
	• Pull back the catheter until resistance is felt, and then place nasal sponge at the nose to keep catheter pulled tight against the gastroesophageal junction
	  • A football helmet with face mask may also be used
	    • If a helmet is used, check fit closely; skin breakdown is frequently caused by an ill-fitting helmet
	    • 0.5–1.0 kg weight may be used, hung over the end of the bed
	• Inflate the esophageal balloon to a pressure of 20–40 mm Hg until bleeding is controlled; double-clamp the lumen to prevent leakage
	• Connect the suction lumens to intermittent low suction (these are nonvented)
	• Label all lumens
	• Obtain chest radiograph to check placement

Management	• Monitor and maintain airway
	  • Elevate head of bed to 45 degrees unless patient is unconscious; if patient is unconscious, elevated HOB 15 degrees on the left side
	  • Have suction equipment available
	  • Intubation is desirable but not absolutely required
	  • Suction the oropharynx and nasopharynx often as the patient cannot swallow with the tube in
	    • A small nasogastric tube may be inserted into the nostril opposite the SB tube to drain secretions that collect above the esophageal balloon
	• Maintain pressures at prescribed levels
	  • Periodic deflation at specific intervals (e.g., every 4 hours) may be prescribed since the pressures required to control bleeding exceed the pressure of capillary filling and ischemia or necrosis may occur
	    • Monitor closely for bleeding during any time of deflation
	• Have scissors at bedside to release pressure from esophageal balloon if it accidentally moves into the pharynx and acute respiratory distress occurs
	• Maintain traction on tube to keep gastric balloon pulled up against the gastroesophageal junction
	• Note amount of pressure/volume in each part of tube; maintain inflation of balloons
	• Ensure patency of the gastric suction lumen and keep connected to low intermittent suction to prevent aspiration or retention of blood in the gut, which is likely to increase ammonia levels

Complications	• Airway obstruction • Aspiration • Perforation of esophagus: sudden epigastric or substernal pain, respiratory distress, increased bleeding, shock • Dysrhythmias • Chest pain • Bronchopneumonia • Laceration, ulceration of stomach • Pressure necrosis of hypopharynx, esophagus, or upper stomach • Hiccoughs

From Dennison, R. D. (2007). *Pass CCRN!* (3rd ed.). St. Louis: Mosby.

7. Control pain and discomfort
    a. GI cocktail (viscous lidocaine, aluminum hydroxide, magnesium hydroxide, simethicone, and sorbitol [Mylanta], belladonna alkaloids and phenobarbital [Donnatal]) may be used initially for epigastric pain
    b. Analgesics
    c. Antiemetics
    d. Anxiolytics
8. Maintain fluid and electrolyte balance: evaluate sodium, potassium, calcium, magnesium and replace as prescribed
9. Monitor for complications
    a. Ulcer perforation
    b. Hypovolemic shock
    c. Hepatic encephalopathy (blood in gut causes elevated ammonia levels which are toxic to the brain)

Evaluation
1. Patent airway, adequate oxygenation (i.e., normal PaO_2, SpO_2, SaO_2) and ventilation (i.e., normal $PaCO_2$)
2. Absence of clinical indications of respiratory distress
3. Absence of clinical indications of infection/sepsis
4. Absence of clinical indications of bleeding
5. Stable hemodynamic status
6. Alert and oriented with no neurologic deficit
7. Control of pain and discomfort

Typical disposition: admission; may require admission to critical care unit or surgery

Gastroesophageal Reflux Disease and Esophagitis

Definition
1. Gastroesophageal reflux disease (GERD): persistent reflux of stomach content that occurs more than twice a week
    a. More serious form of gastroesophageal reflux (GER), also called acid reflux because digestive juices rise up with the food
    b. Can occur in all ages
2. Esophagitis: inflammation of the lining of the esophagus

Predisposing factors
1. GERD
    a. Obesity
    b. Pregnancy
    c. Smoking, alcohol
    d. Dietary factors
        1) Caffeine
        2) Fried or fatty foods
        3) Onions, garlic, spices
        4) Tomato-based sauces
        5) Citrus fruits
        6) Chocolate
        7) Mint flavoring
2. Esophagitis
    a. GERD
    b. Achalasia (i.e., neurogenic impairment of esophageal motility that affects the lower two thirds of the esophagus)

    c. Infection
    d. Medications (e.g., NSAIDs, potassium supplements)

Pathophysiology
1. Malfunction of the LES leads to reflux of acidic contents back up into the esophagus
2. When reflux occurs, food or fluid can be tasted in the back of the mouth and a burning sensation occurs when stomach acid refluxes back into the esophagus
3. Exposure to pepsin and trypsin enzymes along with bile salts causes a chemical irritation and initiation of the inflammatory process (i.e., esophagitis)

Clinical presentation
1. Subjective
    a. Burning or discomfort up and down epigastric area
        1) Increases when bending over
        2) May radiate to back, chest, and neck
        3) Worse about 30 minutes after eating
        4) May feel like something is stuck in upper chest area
    b. May complain of dyspnea
    c. May complain of excessive salivation (water brash)
2. Objective
    a. Cough
    b. Belching
    c. Sores in mouth; frequently herpes
    d. Halitosis
    e. Tenderness in epigastric area with palpation
    f. Wheezing
    g. Hoarseness
3. Diagnostic studies
    a. Upper GI/barium swallow: to evaluate motility and identify reflux
    b. Endoscopy: to evaluate the condition of the esophageal and gastric mucosa
    c. Esophageal manometry: to measure the function of the LES

Collaborative management
1. Continue assessment
    a. ABCDs
    b. Oxygen saturation
    c. Vital signs: blood pressure, pulse, respiratory rate, and temperature
    d. Discomfort and pain level
    e. Accurate intake and output
    f. Close monitoring for progression of symptoms
2. Maintain airway, oxygenation, and ventilation
    a. Elevation of the head of the bed to 30 to 45 degrees
    b. Oxygen by nasal cannula at 2 to 6 L/min to maintain SpO_2 of 95% unless contraindicated; for patients with COPD, use pulse oximetry to guide oxygen administration to SpO_2 of 90%
    c. Endotracheal intubation may be required to prevent pulmonary aspiration of blood

3. Maintain adequate circulation and perfusion
   a. IV access for fluid and medication administration
   b. Fluid replacement: usually 0.9% saline
4. Prevent further damage to the gastric mucosa caused by gastric irritants, hyperacidity, and/or impaired mucosal barrier
   a. Discontinuance of any gastric irritants
   b. Pharmacologic agents that decrease gastric acidity and/or protect gastric mucosa
      1) Antacids (e.g., magnesium hydroxide and aluminum hydroxide [Maalox, Mylanta])
      2) Histamine (H_2) receptor antagonist (e.g., ranitidine [Zantac], famotidine [Pepcid])
      3) Proton-pump inhibitors (e.g., omeprazole [Prilosec])
   c. Pharmacologic therapy for *H. pylori* (e.g., omeprazole + clarithromycin [Biaxin])
5. Control pain and discomfort
   a. GI cocktail (viscous lidocaine, aluminum hydroxide, magnesium hydroxide, simethicone, and sorbitol [Mylanta], belladonna alkaloids and phenobarbital [Donnatal])
   b. Analgesics
   c. Antiemetics
   d. Anxiolytics
6. Monitoring for complications
   a. Ulceration
   b. Perforation
   c. GI hemorrhage
   d. Shock
   e. Barrett esophagus: condition in which the color and composition of the cells lining the lower esophagus change because of repeated exposure to stomach acid; may lead to esophageal cancer

Evaluation
1. Patent airway, adequate oxygenation (i.e., normal PaO_2, SpO_2, SaO_2) and ventilation (i.e., normal $PaCO_2$)
2. Absence of clinical indications of respiratory distress
3. Absence of clinical indications of hypoperfusion
4. Control of pain and discomfort

Typical disposition: discharge home with instructions
1. Stop smoking
2. Avoid foods and beverages that worsen symptoms
3. If overweight, lose weight
4. Eat small, frequent meals
5. Wear loose-fitting clothes
6. Avoid lying down for 3 hours after a meal
7. Raise head of bed 6 to 8 inches by securing wood blocks under the bedposts
8. Follow-up with primary care or gastroenterologist as directed

Cholecystitis
Definition
1. Cholecystitis: inflammation of the gallbladder; gallstones usually present
   a. Cholelithiasis: presence of stones in the gallbladder

Predisposing factors
1. Cholecystitis
   a. Female gender, especially multiparous
   b. Usually over the age of 40 years
   c. Oral contraceptives/estrogen hormone replacement
   d. Sedentary lifestyle
   e. Obesity
   f. Familial tendency
   g. Tumor
2. Cholelithiasis
   a. Infection (most common is *Escherichia coli*)
   b. Cholesterol synthesis abnormalities
   c. Pregnancy
   d. Immobility

Pathophysiology
1. Usually associated with obstruction of the gallbladder by stones or sludge
2. Stasis of bile flow that leads to bacterial invasion and inflammatory process
3. Inflammation confined to the mucous lining of the gallbladder or extended through the entire wall
4. Gallbladder wall edema, ischemic injury from pressure buildup
5. About 20% develop secondary bacterial infection with enteric organisms; common enteric organisms include *E. coli, Klebsiella*
6. Any mechanism that alters the body's ability to keep cholesterol, bile salts, and calcium in solution can cause cholelithiasis; one or more components precipitate out of solution into stones as the bile becomes supersaturated with either cholesterol or calcium

Clinical presentation
1. Subjective
   a. Sharp constant pain that started in the mid abdomen
      1) May radiate to the back and right shoulder or go straight through to the back from the substernal area
   b. Usually occurs after eating a large meal or greasy/fried foods
   c. Anorexia, nausea, vomiting
2. Objective
   a. Low grade temperature (usually <38°C or <100.4°F)
   b. Jaundice may be present
   c. Murphy sign (i.e., inability to take a deep breath while the abdomen is palpated beneath the right costal arch below hepatic margin)
   d. Tenderness and guarding in RUQ with palpation
   e. Clay-colored stools, steatorrhea, dark amber urine if bile flow is obstructed
3. Diagnostic studies
   a. CBC with differential: WBCs elevated
   b. ALT, bilirubin: elevated
   c. Urinalysis: to rule out infection
   d. Urine bilirubin: elevated

e. Flat and upright abdominal radiographs

f. Ultrasound: to view stones

g. Hepatobiliary iminodiacetic acid (HIDA) scan: study of choice for diagnosis

h. Abdominal CT: to rule out other causes

Collaborative management

1. Continue assessment
   a. ABCDs
   b. Oxygen saturation
   c. Vital signs: blood pressure, pulse, respiratory rate, and temperature
   d. Discomfort and pain level
   e. Abdominal assessment: distention, rebound tenderness, rigidity
   f. Level of consciousness
   g. Accurate intake and output
   h. Close monitoring for progression of symptoms
2. Maintain airway, oxygenation, and ventilation
   a. Positioning with head elevated to 30 to 45 degrees
   b. Oxygen by nasal cannula at 2 to 6 L/min if needed to maintain SpO_2 of 95% unless contraindicated; for patients with COPD, use pulse oximetry to guide oxygen administration to SpO_2 of 90%
3. Maintain adequate circulation and perfusion
   a. IV access for fluid and medication administration
   b. Fluid replacement: usually 0.9% saline; lactated Ringer solution is contraindicated in patients with liver disease
4. Control pain and discomfort
   a. Analgesics
   b. Antiemetics
   c. Anxiolytics
   d. Antispasmodics (e.g., dicyclomine hydrochloride [Bentyl])
5. Prepare patient and assist with procedures
   a. NPO
   b. NG tube and connect to low suction as prescribed
   c. Foley catheter
6. Treat inflammation/infection and prevent sepsis: antibiotics may be prescribed
7. Monitoring for complications
   a. Empyema of gallbladder
   b. Gangrenous cholecystitis
   c. Perforation
   d. Peritonitis
   e. Ascending cholangitis: bacterial infection of the biliary tract
   f. Liver or subhepatic abscess
   g. Sepsis
   h. Biliary-enteric fistula
   i. Ileus

Evaluation

1. Patent airway, adequate oxygenation (i.e., normal PaO_2, SpO_2, SaO_2) and ventilation (i.e., normal $PaCO_2$)

2. Absence of clinical indications of respiratory distress
3. Absence of clinical indications of infection/sepsis
4. Control of pain and discomfort

Typical disposition

1. If evaluation criteria met: discharge with instructions
   a. Medications
   b. Low-fat diet
   c. Avoidance of fried foods
   d. Need to return to the ED if symptoms worsen
   e. Follow-up appointment with surgeon or primary care provider
2. If evaluation criteria not met: admission

Hepatic Failure/Encephalopathy

Definitions

1. Hepatic failure: inability of the liver to perform organ functions
2. Hepatic encephalopathy: neurologic failure as a result of hepatic failure

Precipitating factors

1. Acute liver failure
2. Viruses
   a. Herpes simplex
   b. Herpes zoster
   c. Epstein-Barr
   d. Adenovirus
   e. Cytomegalovirus
3. Hepatitis (Table 7-5)
4. Hepatotoxic drugs or toxins
5. Ischemia (e.g., shock, multiple organ dysfunction syndrome [MODS])
6. Trauma
7. Reye syndrome
8. Acute fatty liver of pregnancy
9. Acute hepatic vein occlusion

Pathophysiology

1. Cirrhosis: liver parenchymal cells are progressively destroyed and replaced with fibrotic tissue resulting in impaired hepatic function
   a. Distortion, twisting, and constriction of central section cause impedance of portal blood flow and portal hypertension
2. Fulminant hepatitis: liver cells fail to regenerate causing necrosis
3. Portal hypertension and impaired hepatic function
   a. Liver is unable to produce adequate amounts of bile; protein, carbohydrate, and fat metabolism is impaired
   b. Liver is unable to manufacture plasma proteins and inactivate hormones (e.g., aldosterone, estrogen)
   c. Increased circulating levels of aldosterone cause continuing retention of sodium and water by the kidney along with increased excretion of potassium; fluid and electrolyte imbalances occur (e.g., hypokalemia, hypocalcemia)

TABLE **7-5** Types of Viral Hepatitis

Type	Route	Incubation Period	Onset/Chronicity	Comments
A (HAV; infectious hepatitis)	Fecal-oral	2–6 weeks	Acute onset Chronicity does not develop	• 99% resolves but 1% becomes fulminant • Treatment is supportive
B (HBV; serum hepatitis)	Parenteral Sexual Perinatal	4–24 weeks	Insidious onset Chronicity develops in <5%	• 1% becomes fulminant • 15–25% develop liver cancer • Treatment includes interferon alfa-2b (Intron A); antivirals such as lamivudine (Epivir) or famciclovir (Famvir) may also be prescribed
C (HCV; non-A, non-B hepatitis; post transfusion hepatitis)	Parenteral Sexual Perinatal	2–20 weeks	Insidious onset Chronicity develops in 50–60%	• 20–50% develop cirrhosis • 20% develop liver cancer • 20% develop liver failure • Treatment includes interferon alfa-2b (Intron A) or peginterferon alpha-2b (Peg-Intron) and ribavirin (Virazole); may also include corticosteroids
D (HDV; Delta virus)	Superinfection or coinfection in patient with chronic hepatitis B	4–24 weeks	Acute onset Chronicity common with superinfection	• Up to 30% become fulminant • Most have worsening active hepatitis • Treatment is as for hepatitis B
E (HEV; enteric non-A, non-B hepatitis)	Fecal-oral Perinatal	2–8 weeks	Acute onset Chronicity does not develop	• Generally benign and self-limiting; however, 10–20% mortality when occurs during pregnancy
F (HFV)	Parenteral Sexual Perinatal			• Now considered a variant of hepatitis B
G (HGV)				• Very little known

From Dennison, R. D. (2007). *Pass CCRN!* (3rd ed.). St. Louis: Mosby.

    d. Liver is unable to detoxify toxins and drugs and to remove bacteria

    e. Cumulative drug effects frequently occur because the liver is unable to biotransform drugs into inactive and, with some drugs, active metabolites; reduced intravascular volume impairs the ability of the kidney to excrete the active and inactive metabolites

    f. Increased susceptibility to infection and sepsis occurs due to the following:

      1) Inability to store vitamins and manufacture clotting factors

      2) Fat-soluble vitamin (A, D, E, K) deficiencies may occur

      3) Clotting abnormalities occur since the liver manufactures all except two of the clotting factors

4. Hepatic encephalopathy may eventually occur as neurotoxics, such as ammonia, accumulate

Clinical presentation

1. Subjective
    a. History of precipitating event
    b. Family may report irritability, personality change, disorientation
    c. Weakness, fatigue
    d. Anorexia, nausea, vomiting
    e. Right upper quadrant dull abdominal pain
    f. Abdominal fullness
    g. Change in bowel habits
    h. Pruritus

2. Objective
    a. Emaciation
    b. Cardiovascular
      1) Tachycardia, dysrhythmias
      2) Bounding pulses
      3) Hypertension or hypotension
      4) Flushed skin
      5) Spider angioma: upper trunk, face, neck, arms

6) Jugular venous distention

7) Distended superficial vessels on abdomen (caput medusae)

c. Pulmonary

1) Tachypnea or hyperpnea

2) Decreased respiratory excursion if ascites present

d. Neurologic

1) Peripheral neuropathy

2) Slow, slurred speech

3) Asterixis: tremor of wrist when dorsiflexed (flapping tremor)

4) Hyperactive reflexes

5) Seizures

6) Positive Babinski reflex in encephalopathy

7) Extreme lethargy or coma in encephalopathy

e. Gastrointestinal

1) Fetor hepaticus: known as "breath of the dead"

2) Ascites

3) Hepatomegaly early; liver atrophy occurs later

4) Splenomegaly

5) Bowel sounds: diminished

6) Clay-colored (pale) stools if biliary obstruction

7) Steatorrhea (i.e., excessive fat in stool)

8) Esophageal varices and/or hemorrhoids

f. Renal

1) Oliguria

2) Dark amber urine

g. Hematologic/immunologic

1) Bruising or bleeding noted

2) Poor wound healing noted

h. Integumentary

1) Jaundice: usually noted in the sclera first

2) Petechiae

3) Bruises

4) Edema

i. Endocrine changes

1) Hypogonadism: testicular atrophy and reduced testosterone levels in men

2) Gynecomastia in men

3) Altered hair distribution

3. Diagnostic studies

a. Potassium: may be decreased

b. Sodium: may be decreased or normal

c. Calcium: may be decreased

d. Magnesium: may be decreased

e. BUN: may be elevated due to dehydration, hepatorenal syndrome, or GI bleeding

f. Glucose: may be elevated or decreased

g. Creatinine: may be elevated due to hepatorenal syndrome

h. Cholesterol: elevated

i. ALT, AST, LDH: elevated

j. Alkaline phosphatase: elevated

k. Bilirubin: elevated

l. Ammonia: elevated in encephalopathy

m. Total protein, serum albumin, fibrinogen: decreased

n. Hgb, Hct: decreased if hemorrhage or hypersplenism

o. WBC: decreased; if normal or elevated, infection may be present

p. Platelets: decreased in splenomegaly

q. Clotting studies: PT, PTT: prolonged

r. ABG: respiratory alkalosis; possible hypoxemia

s. Urine

1) Sodium: decreased

2) Bilirubin: elevated in biliary obstruction

3) Urobilinogen: elevated in hepatocellular disease; decreased in complete biliary obstruction

t. Chest radiograph: may show pleural effusion or atelectasis

u. Flat plate of abdomen: hepatosplenomegaly; abdominal haziness if ascites is present

v. Abdominal ultrasound: intra-abdominal fluid (ascites)

w. Liver scan: may show diffuse changes of cirrhosis

x. LP: may be done to rule out neurologic cause of altered consciousness; CSF shows increase in glutamine

4. Stages of encephalopathy (Box 7-3)

Collaborative management

1. Continue assessment

a. ABCDs

b. Oxygen saturation

c. Vital signs: blood pressure, pulse, respiratory rate, and temperature

d. Continuous cardiac monitor

e. Discomfort and pain level

f. Abdominal assessment: distention, rebound tenderness, rigidity

g. Level of consciousness

h. Accurate intake and output

i. Close monitoring for progression of symptoms

2. Maintain airway, oxygenation, and ventilation

a. Elevation of head of bed to 30 to 45 degrees, especially if ascites is present

b. Artificial airways as necessary in patients with altered consciousness and airway protective mechanisms (e.g., gag reflex); endotracheal intubation may be required

c. Oxygen by nasal cannula at 2 to 6 L/min to maintain SpO$_2$ of 95% unless contraindicated; for patients with COPD, use pulse oximetry to guide oxygen administration to SpO$_2$ of 90%

3. Maintain adequate circulation and perfusion

a. IV access with two large-bore catheters for fluid and medication administration

b. Fluid/electrolyte replacement

1) Crystalloids: usually 0.9% saline; lactated Ringer solution is contraindicated in patients with liver disease

2) Electrolyte replacement, especially potassium and magnesium as prescribed

c. Dextrose

1) Frequent monitoring of serum glucose and administration of dextrose as required

BOX 7-3 Stages of Encephalopathy

Stage I	• Mild confusion
	• Decreased attention span
	• Difficulty performing simple arithmetic computations (e.g., count backward from 100 by 7)
	• Decreased response time
	• Forgetfulness
	• Mood changes
	• Slurred speech
	• Personality changes
	• Irritability
	• Disruption in sleep-wake patterns
	• EEG normal
Stage II	• Lethargy
	• Confusion
	• Apathy
	• Aberrant behavior
	• Tremor and asterixis (also referred to as *liver flap*)
	• Inability to reproduce simple designs (constructional apraxia)
	• Slowing of normal EEG
Stage III	• Somnolent with diminished responsiveness to verbal stimuli
	• Severe confusion and incoherence following arousal
	• Speech incomprehensible
	• Tremor and asterixis
	• Hyperactive deep tendon reflexes
	• Hyperventilation
	• EEG abnormal
Stage IV	• No response to stimuli or abnormal (e.g., decorticate or decerebrate) posturing to stimuli
	• Areflexia except for pathologic reflexes
	• Positive Babinski reflex
	• Fetor hepaticus
	• EEG abnormal

From Dennison, R. D. (2007). *Pass CCRN!* (3rd ed.). St. Louis: Mosby.

2) Thiamine replacement should be considered especially when chronic alcohol ingestion is known or suspected to prevent Wernicke encephalopathy
   d. Multivitamins, folic acid, thiamine
4. Identify and treat cause of hepatic failure
   a. *N*-Acetylcysteine (Mucomyst) for acetaminophen (Tylenol) toxicity; must be administered within 24 hours of acetaminophen ingestion
   b. Antivirals (e.g., acyclovir [Zovirax]) as prescribed for hepatitis
   c. Avoidance of hepatotoxic drugs
5. Decrease portal hypertension
   a. β-Blockers as prescribed
6. Prevent and monitor for bleeding
   a. Avoidance of aspirin and NSAIDs
   b. Avoidance of invasive procedures and injections, if possible

   c. Vitamin K, fresh frozen plasma, and platelets as prescribed
7. Treat infection (if present) and prevent sepsis
   a. Antimicrobials (i.e., antibiotics, antivirals, antifungals) as prescribed
   b. Antipyretics and cooling methods to reduce fever
8. Observe for/treat alcohol withdrawal syndrome
   a. Close monitoring for clinical indications of alcohol withdrawal syndrome (Box 7-4)
   b. Sedatives as prescribed: most of these agents are hepatotoxic so doses are adjusted and liver enzymes are monitored
9. Monitor for complications
   a. Hemorrhage
   b. Infection; sepsis
   c. Acute renal failure
   d. Seizures

Evaluation
1. Patent airway, adequate oxygenation (i.e., normal PaO_2, SpO_2, SaO_2) and ventilation (i.e., normal $PaCO_2$)
2. Absence of clinical indications of respiratory distress
3. Absence of clinical indications of bleeding
4. Absence of clinical indications of hypoperfusion
5. Absence of clinical indications of infection/sepsis
6. Alert and oriented with no neurologic deficit
7. Control of pain and discomfort

Typical disposition: admission to the hospital; critical care unit admission may be required

Diverticulitis
Definitions
1. Diverticulum: a saccular dilation or outpouching of the mucosa through the circular smooth muscle of the intestinal wall
2. Diverticula: multiple diverticulum
3. Diverticulosis: the condition of having multiple diverticula that are not inflamed
4. Diverticulitis: infection of the diverticula
5. Meckel diverticulum: true congenital diverticulum where a small bulge in the small intestine is present at birth

BOX 7-4 Alcohol Withdrawal Syndrome

Early	Late
• Mild tachycardia	• Marked tachycardia
• Mild hypertension	• Marked hypertension
• Nausea, vomiting	• Hyperthermia
• Diaphoresis	• Dehydration
• Pruritus	• Delirium
• Visual disturbances	• Delusions
• Time disorientation	• Hallucinations
• Tremors	• Tonic-clonic seizures
• Anxiety, agitation	
• Sleep disturbances	

From Dennison, R. D. (2007). *Pass CCRN!* (3rd ed.). St. Louis: Mosby.

Predisposing factors

1. Low-fiber/high-fat diet
2. Risk increases with age (thought to be related to loss of muscle mass)
3. Chronic constipation
4. Previous episodes of diverticulitis
5. Hereditary factors

Pathophysiology

1. Smooth muscle of the intestinal wall thickens
   a. Affected area of the intestine is usually sigmoid colon
2. Outpouching appears with increased intraluminal pressure
3. Stool retention leads to bacterial accumulation in the diverticula, which then initiates the inflammatory process
4. Hardened stool masses (fecaliths) are formed
5. The inflammation leads to small perforations in the colon and spreads the inflammatory process into the surrounding intestinal tissue

Clinical presentation

1. Subjective
   a. Acute pain
   b. Constant
   c. Usually described as aching or crampy
   d. May be LLQ or generalized
   e. Change in bowel habits
   f. May report anorexia
2. Objective
   a. Low-grade temperature
   b. Abdominal tenderness with palpation of LLQ
   c. Palpable mass may be present
   d. Bowel sounds: usually decreased or normal; may be increased if obstruction present
   e. Clinical indications of peritoneal irritation (e.g., muscle guarding, tenderness, rebound tenderness) indicate perforation
   f. Older patients: may be afebrile, with normal WBCs, and no abdominal tenderness
3. Diagnostic studies
   a. CBC: elevated WBCs
   b. Urinalysis: to rule out urinary tract infection or other problems
   c. Flat and upright abdominal radiographs: rule out free air; may show edema and mass if present
   d. Ultrasound of abdomen: may be useful in diagnosis right side colonic diverticulitis
   e. CT: thickened fascia; muscular hypertrophy; localized colonic wall thickening with arrowhead-shaped lumen pointing to inflamed diverticula (i.e., arrowhead sign)
   f. Barium enema and colonoscopy: the preferred tests, although rarely done emergently (may cause perforation if done during acute episode)
   g. Stool for occult blood: may be positive

Collaborative management

1. Continue assessments
   a. ABCDs
   b. Oxygen saturation
   c. Vital signs: blood pressure, pulse, respiratory rate, and temperature
   d. Discomfort and pain level
   e. Abdominal assessment: distention, rebound tenderness, rigidity, bowel sounds
   f. Stools: color, consistency, frequency
   g. Level of consciousness
   h. Accurate intake and output
   i. Serum electrolytes
   j. Close monitoring for progression of symptoms
2. Maintain airway, oxygenation, and ventilation
   a. Position of comfort to facilitate breathing
   b. Deep breathing to aid in prevention of atelectasis
   c. Oxygen by nasal cannula at 2 to 6 L/min to maintain SpO_2 of 95% unless contraindicated; for patients with COPD, use pulse oximetry to guide oxygen administration to SpO_2 of 90%
3. Maintain adequate circulation and perfusion
   a. IV access with two large-bore catheters for fluid and medication administration
   b. Fluid/electrolyte replacement
      1) Crystalloids: usually 0.9% saline; lactated Ringer solution is contraindicated in patients with liver disease
      2) Electrolyte replacement, especially potassium and magnesium as prescribed
4. Treat infection (if present) and prevent sepsis
   a. Antimicrobials as prescribed
   b. Antipyretics and cooling methods to reduce fever
5. Control pain and discomfort
   a. Analgesics
   b. Antiemetics
   c. Anxiolytics
   d. Antispasmodics (e.g., dicyclomine hydrochloride [Bentyl])
6. Prepare patient for procedures as indicated
   a. NPO
   b. NG tube to low suction
   c. Foley catheter
7. Monitoring for complications
   a. Perforation
   b. Peritonitis
   c. Abscess/fistula formation
   d. Large bowel obstruction

Evaluation

1. Patent airway, adequate oxygenation (i.e., normal PaO_2, SpO_2, SaO_2) and ventilation (i.e., normal $PaCO_2$)
2. Absence of clinical indications of respiratory distress
3. Absence of clinical indications of infection/sepsis
4. Absence of clinical indications of hypoperfusion
5. Control of pain and discomfort

Typical disposition

1. If evaluation criteria met: discharge with instructions
   a. Clear liquids initially; then fiber is added to the diet progressing to high-fiber diet
   b. Increased fluid intake
   c. Weight reduction and exercise
   d. Follow-up with primary care as directed
   e. Instructions return to the ED for increasing pain, continued vomiting, unable to tolerate fluids, or blood in stool
2. If evaluation criteria not met: admission

Gastroenteritis

Definition: inflammation of the mucosal lining of the stomach and intestine

Predisposing factors

1. Infectious agents (85% of cases)
   a. Bacterial (e.g., *Salmonella, E. coli, C. difficile*)
   b. Viral (e.g., rotavirus, adenovirus)
   c. Parasitic (e.g., *Giardia, Microsporida*)
2. Introduction of new food in infants and small children
3. Antibiotics (change in normal flora within the GI tract allows proliferation of abnormal flora)
4. Laxatives
5. Ingestion of contaminated food or water
6. Crowded environments such as day care centers

Pathophysiology (Prescilla, 2009)

1. Viral diarrhea involves lysis of enterocytes, interference with absorption of electrolytes and carbohydrates
2. Bacterial gastroenteritis involves toxins produced by the pathogens and invasion and inflammation of mucosa lining
3. Parasitic organisms invade epithelial cells causing villus atrophy and malabsorption

Clinical presentation

1. Subjective
   a. History of recent travel or exposure to other ill people
   b. History of nausea/vomiting, watery diarrhea
   c. Crampy pain in abdomen
   d. Abdominal bloating
2. Objective
   a. Tachycardia
   b. Orthostatic hypotension
   c. Vomiting
   d. Frequent watery bowel movements; stool may contain blood or mucus
   e. Abdominal tenderness with palpation
   f. Bowel sounds: hyperactive
   g. Elevated temperature
3. Diagnostic studies
   a. CBC with differential: elevated WBCs
   b. BUN: increased if dehydrated
   c. Serum osmolality: increased if dehydrated
   d. Stool: for WBCs, ova and parasites, occult blood

Collaborative management

1. Continue assessments
   a. ABCDs
   b. Oxygen saturation
   c. Vital signs: blood pressure, pulse, respiratory rate, and temperature
   d. Discomfort and pain level
   e. Abdominal assessment: distention, rebound tenderness, rigidity, bowel sounds
   f. Level of consciousness
   g. Accurate intake and output
   h. Serum electrolytes
   i. Stools: color, consistency, frequency
   j. Close monitoring for progression of symptoms
2. Maintain airway, oxygenation, and ventilation
   a. Side-lying position if vomiting
   b. Suctioning as required
   c. Oxygen by nasal cannula at 2 to 6 L/min if required to maintain SpO_2 of 95% unless contraindicated; for patients with COPD, use pulse oximetry to guide oxygen administration to SpO_2 of 90%
3. Maintain adequate circulation and perfusion
   a. IV access with two large-bore catheters for fluid and medication administration
   b. Fluid replacement
      1) IV crystalloids: usually 0.9% saline
      2) Although initially NPO, oral fluids when vomiting stops
         a) Avoidance of carbonated, caffeinated, and high-sugar drinks
   c. Electrolyte replacement: especially potassium
4. Treat infection (if present) and prevent sepsis
   a. Antimicrobials as prescribed
   b. Antipyretics and cooling methods to reduce fever
5. Control pain and discomfort
   a. Antiemetics
   b. Antidiarrheals are not recommended because they prevent excretion of a microbe that may be the cause of the gastroenteritis
   c. Antispasmodics (e.g., dicyclomine hydrochloride [Bentyl])
   d. Anxiolytics
6. Monitor for complications
   a. Dehydration
   b. Electrolyte imbalance
   c. Hypovolemic shock

Evaluation

1. Patent airway, adequate oxygenation (i.e., normal PaO_2, SpO_2, SaO_2) and ventilation (i.e., normal $PaCO_2$)
2. Absence of clinical indications of infection/sepsis
3. Absence of clinical indications of dehydration
4. Absence of clinical indicators of hypoperfusion
5. Control of pain and discomfort
6. Reduction in frequency of stools
7. Reduction in episodes of vomiting

Typical disposition
1. If evaluation criteria met: discharge with instructions
   a. Clear liquids for 24 hours
   b. Bland foods after 24 hours using the BRAT diet: bananas, rice, applesauce without sugar, toast, tea
   c. Increased fluid intake
   d. Instructions to return to ED for bloody vomitus or diarrhea, weakness/fainting, intractable vomiting/diarrhea, or severe abdominal pain
2. If evaluation criteria not met: admission

Hernias
Definition: part of an internal organ bulges through a weakened area of a muscle
1. Reducible: hernia that can be pushed back into place
2. Irreducible/incarcerated: hernia that can no longer be pushed back into place
3. Strangulated: a surgical emergency because it is a hernia that is cutting off blood supply and will result in necrosis if not relieved
4. Indirect inguinal hernia: herniation through the umbilical ring following the spermatic cord through the inguinal canal
5. Direct inguinal hernia: when the bowel passes through an area of muscular weakness in the abdominal wall
6. Femoral hernia: herniation that occurs through the femoral ring
7. Umbilical: occurs through the umbilicus
8. Incisional: hernia through a previous surgical site
9. Hiatal: small opening in the diaphragm that allows the upper part of the stomach to move up into the chest
10. Congenital diaphragmatic: birth defect that needs repair

Predisposing factors
1. Straining
2. Heavy lifting
3. Coughing forcefully
4. Obesity
5. Pregnancy
6. Previous surgery
7. Congenital anomalies

Pathophysiology
1. Hernias can occur when the pressure in the compartment of the residing organ is increased and the boundary is weak or weakened

Clinical presentation
1. Subjective
   a. History of precipitating cause
   b. Complaint of bulging in the area of the hernia
   c. Discomfort ranging from mild to severe pain
   d. Nausea, vomiting (may be due to bowel obstruction)
2. Objective
   a. Obvious bulging hernia
   b. Abdominal distention may be present
   c. Asymptomatic hernia: no true tenderness; will enlarge with standing or increase in intra-abdominal pressure
   d. Bowel sounds: hypoactive bowel sounds suggest strangulation
   e. Toxic appearance: suggests strangulation
3. Diagnostic studies
   a. CBC with differential: elevated WBCs with left shift suggests strangulation
   b. Urinalysis: to rule out urinary tract causes
   c. Ultrasound: to distinguish between masses, intestinal wall, testicular swelling

Collaborative management
1. Continue assessments
   a. ABCDs
   b. Oxygen saturation
   c. Vital signs: blood pressure, pulse, respiratory rate, and temperature
   d. Discomfort and pain level
   e. Abdominal assessment: distention, rebound tenderness, rigidity, bowel sounds
   f. Level of consciousness
   g. Accurate intake and output
   h. Serum electrolytes
   i. Close monitoring for progression of symptoms
2. Maintain airway, oxygenation, and ventilation
   a. Side-lying position if vomiting; otherwise with head elevated to 30 to 45 degrees
   b. Suctioning as required
   c. Oxygen by nasal cannula at 2 to 6 L/min to maintain SpO_2 of 95% unless contraindicated; for patients with COPD, use pulse oximetry to guide oxygen administration to SpO_2 of 90%
3. Maintain adequate circulation and perfusion
   a. IV access for fluid and medication administration
   b. Fluid replacement: usually 0.9% saline
   c. Electrolyte replacement as indicated
4. Control pain and discomfort
   a. Analgesics
   b. Antiemetics
   c. Anxiolytics
5. Prepare patient for procedures as indicated
   a. NPO in preparation for possible surgery
   b. Conscious sedation if reduction to be attempted in the ED
   c. Surgery if irreducible in ED
6. Monitor for complications
   a. Intestinal ischemia
   b. Bowel obstruction
   c. Ovarian torsion in females with inguinal hernia

Evaluation
1. Patent airway, adequate oxygenation (i.e., normal PaO_2, SpO_2, SaO_2) and ventilation (i.e., normal $PaCO_2$)

2. Absence of clinical indications of respiratory distress
3. Absence of clinical indications of infection/sepsis
4. Absence of clinical indications of hypoperfusion
5. Control of pain and discomfort

Typical disposition

1. If evaluation criteria met (e.g., reducible hernia): discharge with instructions
   a. May be given a truss to wear to keep the hernia in place
   b. Follow-up with surgical consult as directed
2. If evaluation criteria not met (e.g., irreducible or strangulated hernias): admission; if strangulated hernia, may be taken directly to surgery

Intussusception/Volvulus

Definition

1. Intussusception: mechanical bowel obstruction caused when a loop of bowel telescopes within itself
2. Volvulus: complete twisting of a loop of intestine around its mesenteric attachment site

Predisposing factors

1. Intussusception
   a. Polyps
   b. Lymphoma
   c. Meckel diverticulum
   d. Hypertrophy of abdominal tissue
2. Volvulus
   a. Midgut volvulus (i.e., twisting of the midgut completely around the superior mesenteric artery) usually due to congenital intestinal malrotation
   b. Segmental volvulus can occur in patients of any age, usually with a predisposition because of abnormal intestinal conditions (e.g., adhesions)
   c. Malrotation diagnosed more often in infants <1 year
      1) Those asymptomatic and undiagnosed before age 2 years may never become symptomatic
      2) Malrotation will result in volvulus in one of three asymptomatic patients throughout lifetime

Pathophysiology

1. Intussusception
   a. A proximal segment of the bowel telescopes into a distal segment
   b. The mesentery of the intussusceptum is compressed, causing swelling of the bowel wall, and obstruction quickly occurs
   c. Venous engorgement and ischemia of the intestinal mucosa cause bleeding, which is an outpouring of mixed mucus and blood
      1) Results in the classic red "currant jelly" stool

2. Volvulus
   a. Malrotation of intestines in infants occurs during gestational development
   b. Normal embryos physiologic herniation of the gut through the umbilicus occurs at 6 weeks' gestation is accompanied by a 270-degree counterclockwise rotation of the developing intestine around the superior mesenteric artery (SMA)
   c. The intestine returns to the abdomen and assumes its normal adult anatomic position during weeks 10 to 12
   d. Malrotation usually caused by incomplete rotation of the intestine (<270 degrees of counterclockwise rotation, in weeks 5 to 12 of development)
   e. Malrotation predisposes infant to midgut volvulus and/or small bowel obstruction

Clinical presentation

1. Subjective
   a. Intussusception
      1) Parent reports that child cries inconsolably
      2) Sudden onset of crampy abdominal pain
      3) Intermittent episodes of pain may be the only symptoms in older children
      4) Lethargy
   b. Volvulus in infants
      1) Parent reports that child cries inconsolably, absence of stools, and failure to thrive
   c. Volvulus in adults: severe pain and bloating
2. Objective
   a. Intussusception
      1) Facial grimacing, legs drawn up to chest
      2) Vomiting
      3) Sausage-shaped abdominal mass
      4) Currant jelly stools
   b. Volvulus
      1) Abdominal distention in the epigastric area usually seen in infants <1 year
      2) Peristaltic waves may be visible
      3) Emesis: may be bile in color
      4) Clinical indications of shock: delayed capillary refill, weak pulses, tachycardia, hypotension, decreased urine output
      5) Bloody diarrhea and abdominal distention usually signify volvulus and possible gangrene
3. Diagnostic studies
   a. BUN: elevated if dehydrated
   b. Urinalysis: to rule out urinary tract cause of symptoms
   c. Flat plate of the abdomen: to rule out perforation
   d. Upper GI series: may show volvulus

Collaborative management

1. Continue assessments
   a. ABCDs

b. Oxygen saturation

c. Vital signs: blood pressure, pulse, respiratory rate, and temperature

d. Discomfort and pain level

e. Abdominal assessment: distention, rebound tenderness, rigidity, bowel sounds

f. Stools: color, consistency, frequency

g. Accurate intake and output

h. Serum electrolytes

i. Close monitoring for progression of symptoms

2. Maintain airway, oxygenation, and ventilation

a. Side-lying position if vomiting; otherwise with head elevated to 30 to 45 degrees

b. Suctioning as required

c. Oxygen by nasal cannula at 2 to 6 L/min to maintain SpO_2 of 95% unless contraindicated; for patients with COPD, use pulse oximetry to guide oxygen administration to SpO_2 of 90%

3. Maintain adequate circulation and perfusion

a. IV access for fluid and medication administration

b. Fluid replacement: usually 0.9% saline

c. Electrolyte replacement as indicated

4. Control pain and discomfort

a. Analgesics

b. Antiemetics

c. Anxiolytics

5. Prepare patient for procedures as indicated

a. NPO in preparation for possible surgery

b. If patient has intussusception

1) Hydrostatic reduction: enema using barium or water-soluble contrast and air pressure to force the invaginated portion of the bowel out into its normal position

2) Surgical correction with resection of ischemic/gangrenous bowel

c. If patient has a volvulus prepare for procedures

1) Infants with a volvulus: surgical intervention (emergent surgery if symptomatic)

2) Adults and children with a sigmoid volvulus: endoscopic derotation of the sigmoid colon may be done instead of surgery

6. Monitoring for complications

a. Dehydration, hypovolemic shock

b. Bowel necrosis

c. Perforation

d. Peritonitis

e. Sepsis

Evaluation

1. Patent airway, adequate oxygenation (i.e., normal PaO_2, SpO_2, SaO_2) and ventilation (i.e., normal $PaCO_2$)

2. Absence of clinical indications of respiratory distress

3. Absence of clinical indications of infection/sepsis

4. Absence of clinical indications of hypoperfusion

5. Alert and oriented with no neurologic deficit

6. Control of pain and discomfort

Typical disposition

1. Infant: admission

2. Adults and children: may be discharged home or admitted for 23-hour observation if nonsurgical reduction is successful; admission if nonsurgical reduction unsuccessful

Pyloric Stenosis

Definition: gastric outflow obstruction

Predisposing factors

1. Neonates (also called infantile pyloric stenosis): usually diagnosed within the first 12 weeks of life; occurs four times as often in males

a. Erythromycin (Emycin) use in first 2 weeks of life

b. Turner syndrome: occurs in females where one of the X chromosomes is defective or absent in some or all cells

c. Phenylketonuria: genetic disorder characterized by an inability of the body to utilize the essential amino acid, phenylalanine

d. Trisomy 18: extra chromosome with the 18th pair of chromosomes

2. Adults

a. Transient: edema from peptic ulcer disease (PUD)

b. Chronic: scarring from PUD or carcinoma

Pathophysiology

1. Hypertrophy and hyperplasia of the muscular layers of the pylorus occur, causing the gastric antrum to narrow

2. This leads to a lengthening of the pyloric canal and the whole pylorus becomes thickened

3. The mucosa will then become edematous and thickened

4. If unrecognized, the stomach will become markedly dilated in response to near-complete obstruction

Clinical presentation

1. Subjective

a. Parents of infant or child report:

1) Although there was no vomiting at birth, there was a gradual onset of vomiting

2) Infant is fussy and seems to be hungry after feeding

3) Infrequent, hard stools

4) Weight loss

5) Decreased urination

b. Adults report:

1) Abdominal bloating

2) Vomiting

2. Objective

a. Tachycardia, hypotension may be present

b. Projectile vomiting

c. Jaundice

d. May have visible peristalsis (noticeable prior to emesis)

e. Palpable epigastric (RUQ) mass that is hard and mobile; may be olive shaped

f. Bowel sounds: hypoactive; may increase prior to emesis

g. Succussion splash: splashing sound audible when the patient is rocked from side to side

h. Clinical indications of dehydration: poor skin turgor, dry, sticky mucous membrane, decreased urine output

i. Restlessness or lethargy

3. Diagnostic studies
   a. Electrolytes: hypokalemia, hypochloremia
   b. Bilirubin: elevated
   c. ABG: metabolic alkalosis
   d. Flat plate of abdomen: air in stomach
   e. Ultrasound: dilated stomach and pyloric thickening
   f. Upper GI: shows gastric retention at 3 to 4 hours, one or two thin barium tracts and nonprogression of peristaltic wave from stomach to duodenum

Collaborative management

1. Continue assessment
   a. ABCDs
   b. Oxygen saturation
   c. Vital signs: blood pressure, pulse, respiratory rate, and temperature
   d. Discomfort and pain level
   e. Abdominal assessment: distention, rebound tenderness, rigidity, bowel sounds
   f. Accurate intake and output
   g. Serum electrolytes
   h. Stools: color, consistency, frequency
   i. Level of consciousness
   j. Close monitoring for progression of symptoms

2. Maintain airway, oxygenation, and ventilation
   a. Side-lying position if vomiting; otherwise with head elevated to 30 to 45 degrees
   b. Suctioning as required
   c. Oxygen by nasal cannula at 2 to 6 L/min to maintain SpO_2 of 95% unless contraindicated; for patients with COPD, use pulse oximetry to guide oxygen administration to SpO_2 of 90%

3. Maintain adequate circulation and perfusion
   a. IV access for fluid and medication administration
   b. Fluid replacement: usually 0.9% saline initially
   c. Electrolyte replacement as indicated: potassium chloride most likely to be required

4. Control pain and discomfort
   a. Analgesics
   b. Antiemetics
   c. Anxiolytics
   d. Antispasmodics: atropine may be used to shorten the of pyloric canal and decrease thickening over several weeks (Hernanz-Schulman, 2003)

5. Prepare patient for procedures as indicated
   a. NPO in preparation for possible surgery
   b. Oral gastric tube to drain or low wall suction as prescribed to decompress dilated stomach
   c. Foley catheter to monitor output accurately
   d. Surgery

6. Monitoring for complications
   a. Malnutrition
   b. Dehydration
   c. Failure to thrive

Evaluation

1. Patent airway, adequate oxygenation (i.e., normal PaO_2, SpO_2, SaO_2) and ventilation (i.e., normal $PaCO_2$)
2. Absence of clinical indications of respiratory distress
3. Absence of clinical indications of infection/sepsis
4. Absence of clinical indications of dehydration
5. Absence of clinical indications of hypoperfusion
6. Alert and oriented with no neurologic deficit
7. Control of pain and discomfort

Typical disposition: admission for surgery

Irritable Bowel Syndrome (IBS)

Definition: functional disorder characterized by cramping, abdominal pain, bloating, constipation and/or diarrhea; as opposed to inflammatory bowel disease, there is no inflammation or structural changes

Predisposing factors

1. Affects women more than men
2. Symptoms may be triggered by any of the following:
   a. Specific foods
      1) Wheat, rye, barley, chocolate, milk products, or alcohol
      2) Drinks with caffeine, such as coffee, tea, or colas
   b. Large meals
   c. Medicines
   d. Stress, conflict, or emotional upsets

Clinical presentation

1. Subjective
   a. Abdominal cramping
   b. Bloating and gas
   c. Change in frequency and/or appearance of bowel movements (may have mucus in stool)
   d. Feeling of uncontrollable urgency to have a bowel movement
   e. Report of diarrhea, constipation, or both

2. Objective
   a. Healthy appearance
   b. Palpation of the abdomen may reveal tenderness
   c. Digital rectal examination: negative

3. Diagnostic studies
   a. No specific diagnostic test
   b. Laboratory and radiographic studies are done to rule out other diagnosis
   c. Pelvic in women to rule out ovarian tumors and cysts or endometriosis, which may mimic IBS
   d. Colonoscopy: to rule out as inflammatory bowel disease and structural conditions such as bowel obstruction

Collaborative management

1. Continue assessment
   a. ABCDs
   b. Vital signs: blood pressure, pulse, respiratory rate, and temperature
   c. Discomfort and pain level
   d. Abdominal assessment: distention, bowel sounds
   e. Stools: color, consistency, frequency
   f. Serum electrolytes
   g. Close monitoring for progression of symptoms
2. Maintain airway, oxygenation, and ventilation
   a. Position of comfort
   b. Oxygen by nasal cannula at 2 to 6 L/min as indicated to maintain SpO_2 of 95% unless contraindicated; for patients with COPD, use pulse oximetry to guide oxygen administration to SpO_2 of 90%
3. Maintain adequate circulation and perfusion
   a. IV access for fluid and medication administration
   b. Fluid replacement as indicated: usually 0.9% saline
   c. Electrolyte replacement as indicated: potassium chloride most likely to be required
4. Control pain and discomfort
   a. Analgesics
   b. Antiemetics
   c. Anxiolytics
   d. Antispasmodics
5. Treat depression
   a. Tricyclic antidepressants as prescribed
   b. Cognitive-behavioral therapy
6. Monitoring for complications
   a. Masking of more serious problem: bleeding, fever, weight loss, and persistent severe pain are not symptoms of IBS and indicate another problem
   b. Constipation
   c. Dehydration
   d. Depression

Evaluation

1. Patent airway, adequate oxygenation (i.e., normal PaO_2, SpO_2, SaO_2) and ventilation (i.e., normal $PaCO_2$)
2. Absence of clinical indications of infection/sepsis
3. Absence of clinical indications of dehydration
4. Control of pain and discomfort

Typical disposition

1. Discharged home with instructions
   a. Avoidance of gas-producing and diarrhea-producing foods
   b. Increased fiber intake to prevent constipation
   c. Increased fluid intake
   d. Medications as directed
   e. Probiotics
   f. Followup with primary care provider and/or counselor

Inflammatory Bowel Disease

Definition: chronic inflammation of the GI tract; two types include the following:

1. Crohn disease (i.e., regional enteritis)
   a. Affects segmental areas along the entire wall of the GI tract
   b. Can affect the GI tract from the mouth to the anus, but most commonly affects the ileum
   c. Characterized by repeated bouts of exacerbation and remission
2. Ulcerative colitis
   a. Affects the mucosa and submucosa of the colon and rectum
   b. Characterized by repeated bouts of exacerbation and remission
3. See Table 7-6 for comparison

Precipitating factors

1. Exaggerated inflammatory response to an unidentified microorganism (e.g., bacteria, fungi, or virus)

TABLE 7-6 Differentiation of Crohn Disease and Ulcerative Colitis

Crohn Disease	Ulcerative Colitis
• Can occur anywhere in the GI tract but commonly found in the ileum	• Found only in the colon and rectum
• Usually affects right side of colon	• Usually affects left side of colon
• Inflammation and fissures extend transmurally	• Inflammation confined to mucosa except in rare cases
• Bleeding rare	• Gross rectal bleeding
• Abscess and fistulas	• No fistulas
• Significant perianal lesion may be present	• Significant perianal lesions do not occur
• Endoscopic view: patchy discrete ulcerations separated by normal bowel areas; cobblestone appearance from projections of inflamed tissue surrounded by ulceration	• Endoscopic view: mucosa hyperemic, dark red with the inflammation uniform and diffuse
• Sarcoidlike granulomas can be found in bowel wall and lymph nodes	• Sarcoidlike granulomas do not occur

Adapted from Merck Manuals Online. (2007). Inflammatory bowel disease. Retrieved on March 27, 2009, from http://www.merck.com/mmpe/sec02/ch018/ch018a.html#CBBDCBAD.

2. Autoimmune
3. Genetic predisposition
4. Psychological stressors
5. Onset of symptoms usually age 15 to 30 years
6. More prevalent in Jewish population

Pathophysiology

1. Crohn disease
   a. Begins with inflammation and abscesses, which progress to tiny focal lesions
   b. The mucosal lesions may develop into deep longitudinal and transverse ulcers with intervening mucosal edema, creating a characteristic cobblestone appearance to the bowel
   c. Inflammation spreads transmurally leading to lymph edema and thickening of the bowel wall and mesentery
   d. Mesenteric fat will extends onto the serosal surface of the bowel and the mesenteric lymph nodes enlarge
   e. Abscesses are common, fistulas develop and often penetrate into adjoining structures (e.g., loops of bowel, bladder)
   f. Skip lesions develop: disease will be scattered throughout the GI tract and in between there is normal bowel tissue
2. Ulcerative colitis
   a. Starts in the rectum and can remain localized to the rectum but often will extend proximally and may involve the entire colon
   b. Inflammation affects the mucosa and submucosa with a well defined border between normal and affected tissue; the muscularis will be involved in severe conditions
   c. Mucous membrane is erythemic, finely granular, and friable, with scattered areas of hemorrhage
   d. Large mucosal ulcers develop with copious purulent exudate
   e. Areas of normal or hyperplastic inflammatory mucosa (pseudo polyps) project above areas of ulcerated mucosa

Clinical Presentation

1. Subjective
   a. Abdominal pain
   b. In ulcerative colitis: reports of bloody diarrhea (15 to 20 times/day) with or without pus
   c. In Crohn disease: report of diarrhea (3 to 5 times/day) usually without blood but stools may contain fat (i.e., steatorrhea)
   d. Diarrhea
   e. Weight loss
   f. Fever
2. Objective
   a. Elevated temperature: may indicate infection, perforation, abscess, or fistula
   b. In Crohn disease: right-sided tenderness with palpation
   c. In ulcerative colitis: left-sided tenderness with palpation
   d. May have clinical indications of dehydration
   e. May have clinical indications of infection or sepsis
   f. May have clinical indications of acute abdomen if perforation occurs
3. Diagnostic studies
   a. CBC: decreased Hgb and Hct may indicate bleeding
   b. BUN: may be elevated due to dehydration
   c. Electrolytes: may show electrolyte imbalance, especially hypokalemia
   d. Flat plate of abdominal (KUB): to look for free air
   e. Abdominal CT or MRI to look for complications such as abscess
   f. Endoscopy: for diagnosis of inflammatory bowel disease
   g. Stool sample for occult blood, WBCs, culture and sensitivity (C&S) if indicated

Collaborative management

1. Continue assessment
   a. ABCDs
   b. Oxygen saturation
   c. Vital signs: blood pressure, pulse, respiratory rate, and temperature
   d. Discomfort and pain level
   e. Abdominal assessment: distention, rebound tenderness, rigidity, bowel sounds
   f. Stools: color, consistency, frequency
   g. Accurate intake and output
   h. Serum electrolytes
   i. Level of consciousness
   j. Close monitoring for progression of symptoms
2. Maintain airway, oxygenation, and ventilation
   a. Position of comfort
   b. Oxygen by nasal cannula at 2 to 6 L/min if indicated to maintain SpO_2 of 95% unless contraindicated; for patients with COPD, use pulse oximetry to guide oxygen administration to SpO_2 of 90%
3. Maintain adequate circulation and perfusion
   a. IV access for fluid and medication administration
   b. Fluid replacement as indicated: usually 0.9% saline
   c. Electrolyte replacement as indicated: potassium chloride most likely to be required
   d. Vitamin replacement: B_{12}, folic acid, vitamin D more likely to be needed
4. Control pain and discomfort
   a. Analgesics
   b. Antiemetics
   c. Anxiolytics
   d. Antidiarrheals, anticholinergics, antispasmodics
   e. NPO status
5. Treat inflammation and infection (if present) and prevent sepsis
   a. Corticosteroids as prescribed
   b. Antimicrobials (i.e., antibiotics and antifungals) as prescribed
   c. Antipyretics and cooling methods to reduce fever
6. Prepare patient for procedures as indicated
   a. NPO

b. NG tube to low suction
c. Foley catheter
d. Endoscopy
e. Colectomy may be required for serious complications
7. Monitoring for complications
   a. Anemia
   b. Perforation
   c. Toxic megacolon (i.e., dilation of the colon >5 cm)
   d. Abscess
   e. Sepsis

Evaluation

1. Patent airway, adequate oxygenation (i.e., normal Pao_2, Spo_2, Sao_2) and ventilation (i.e., normal $Paco_2$)
2. Absence of clinical indications of respiratory distress
3. Absence of clinical indications of infection/sepsis
4. Absence of clinical indications of dehydration
5. Absence of clinical indications of hypoperfusion
6. Alert and oriented with no neurologic deficit
7. Control of pain and discomfort

Typical disposition

1. If evaluation criteria met: discharge with instructions
2. If evaluation criteria not met: admission

Pancreatitis

Definition: inflammatory process of the pancreas that can involve peripancreatic tissues and/or remote organ systems

1. Acute: usually reversible inflammatory episode of the pancreas with little to no necrotic damage to tissue. Hypovolemia may occur from fluid leak into peritoneal cavity
2. Chronic: progressive and irreversible destruction of the pancreas. Extensive necrosis of pancreas and peripancreatic tissue and fat; erosion into blood vessels; hemorrhage occurs

Predisposing factors

1. Obstruction of common bile duct
2. Alcoholism
3. Hypertriglyceridemia
4. Medications (e.g., thiazides, estrogen, steroids, antibiotics, opiates)
5. Peptic ulcer with perforation
6. Cancer, especially tumors of pancreas or lung
7. Injury to pancreas
8. Pregnancy: third trimester; ectopic pregnancy
9. Ovarian cyst
10. Infections (e.g., mumps, mononucleosis, hepatitis)

Pathophysiology

1. Etiologic factor triggers activation of pancreatic enzymes and pancreatic cell injury → autodigestion of pancreas is caused by the escape of prematurely activated proteolytic enzymes from the acinar space or cells into the periacinal tissue → trypsin causes edema, necrosis, and hemorrhage
   a. Elastase causes hemorrhage
   b. Phospholipase A causes fat necrosis and damages the pulmonary capillary endothelium; may lead to acute respiratory distress syndrome (ARDS)
   c. Kallikreins are peptidases (enzymes that cleave peptide bonds in proteins) that cause edema, vascular permeability, smooth muscle contraction, shock
2. Damage to the acinar cells occurs
3. Erosion into vessels may cause hemorrhage
4. Inflammatory process causes necrosis of fat in pancreas and exudates with high albumin content, leading to hypoalbuminemia and ascites; fat necrosis results in precipitation of calcium, leading to hypocalcemia
5. Release of necrotic toxins may cause sepsis and/or systemic inflammatory response syndrome (SIRS)

Clinical presentation

1. Subjective
   a. May have history of recent heavy meal or a drinking binge
   b. Epigastric pain
      1) Aggravated by eating, alcohol, walking, supine position
      2) Lessened by sitting up and leaning forward
      3) Sharp, boring through to the back; may radiate to the back
   c. Anorexia
   d. Dyspepsia, flatulence
   e. Nausea, vomiting, retching
   f. Dyspnea
   g. May report weight loss
   h. Weakness
2. Objective
   a. Tachycardia, hypotension
   b. Elevated temperature: usually low grade (e.g., 37.8°–39°C)
   c. Abdominal distention, tenderness, guarding
   d. Jaundice: if biliary obstruction
   e. Grey Turner sign: ecchymosis over flank area
   f. Cullen sign: ecchymosis at umbilicus
   g. Chvostek sign: unilateral spasm of facial muscles when cheek tapped, indicating tetany (hypocalcemia)
   h. Trousseau sign: carpal spasm occurs when upper arm compressed with tourniquet or blood pressure cuff indicating tetany (hypocalcemia)
   i. Ascites may be present
   j. Rebound tenderness with palpation: suggests peritoneal irritation
   k. Epigastric mass may be palpable
   l. Decreased bowel sounds
   m. Breath sounds may be diminished: possibly related to atelectasis, pleural effusion, or ARDS; crackles may also be heard
   n. Stools: steatorrhea (i.e., bulky, pale, foul-smelling, floating)

3. Diagnostic studies
   a. Electrolytes: decreased potassium, calcium, magnesium
   b. Glucose: elevated if endocrine function of the pancreas is compromised
   c. Triglycerides: may be elevated
   d. Amylase and lipase: elevated
   e. Albumin: decreased
   f. BUN: may be elevated due to hypovolemia
   g. Liver panel: elevated if liver or biliary disease
   h. Hct: decreased with hemorrhage; elevated with hemoconcentration due to third-spacing
   i. WBCs: usually elevated with shift to the left
   j. ABGs: metabolic acidosis; respiratory complications may cause respiratory acidosis and hypoxemia
   k. Urine: amylase usually elevated
   l. Stool: increase in fecal fat
   m. ECG: may suggest myocardial infarction (e.g., ST-T wave elevations)
   n. Chest radiograph: bilateral or only left pleural effusion, elevated left hemidiaphragm, left atelectasis
   o. Flat plate of abdomen: may show gall stones, ileus, bowel dilation, calcified pancreatic stones
   p. Abdominal ultrasound: swelling, edema, gallstones, pseudocysts, or peripancreatic fluid collections
   q. CT with contrast: enlargement, edema, or necrosis of the pancreas
   r. MRI: inflammatory changes within the pancreas
   s. HIDA scan: may identify hepatocellular disease from biliary obstruction as cause of pancreatitis

Collaborative management
1. Continue assessment
   a. ABCDs
   b. Oxygen saturation
   c. Vital signs: blood pressure, pulse, respiratory rate, and temperature
   d. Discomfort and pain level
   e. Abdominal assessment: distention, rebound tenderness, rigidity, bowel sounds
   f. Accurate intake and output
   g. Serum electrolytes
   h. Level of consciousness
   i. Close monitoring for progression of symptoms
2. Maintain airway, oxygenation, and ventilation
   a. Elevation of head of bed 30 to 45 degrees, on side if vomiting
   b. Suctioning as required
   c. Oxygen by nasal cannula at 2 to 6 L/min to maintain SpO_2 of 95% unless contraindicated; for patients with COPD, use pulse oximetry to guide oxygen administration to SpO_2 of 90%
3. Maintain adequate circulation and perfusion
   a. IV access for fluid and medication administration
   b. Fluid replacement as indicated: usually 0.9% saline; colloids (e.g., albumin) as prescribed
   c. Electrolyte replacement as indicated: calcium and potassium most likely to be required

4. Control pain and discomfort
   a. Analgesics
   b. Antiemetics
   c. Anxiolytics
   d. Close monitoring for alcohol withdrawal syndrome (see Box 7-4) if indicated; sedatives, thiamine, and multivitamins as prescribed
5. Prepare patient for procedures as indicated
   a. NPO
   b. NG tube to low suction
   c. Foley catheter as indicated for close monitoring of urine output
6. Treat inflammation and infection (if present) and prevent sepsis
   a. Antimicrobials as prescribed; not used routinely but may be prescribed if infection or abscess suspected
   b. Antipyretics and cooling methods to reduce fever
   c. Pharmacologic agents that decrease gastric acidity and/or protect gastric mucosa
      1) Antacids (e.g., magnesium hydroxide and aluminum hydroxide [Maalox, Mylanta])
      2) Histamine (H_2) receptor antagonist (e.g., ranitidine [Zantac], famotidine [Pepcid])
      3) Proton-pump inhibitors (e.g., omeprazole [Prilosec])
7. Monitoring for complications
   a. Hypovolemic shock
   b. Electrolyte imbalances
   c. Acute respiratory distress syndrome
   d. Disseminated intravascular coagulation
   e. Sepsis
   f. Peritonitis

Evaluation
1. Patent airway, adequate oxygenation (i.e., normal PaO_2, SpO_2, SaO_2) and ventilation (i.e., normal $PaCO_2$)
2. Absence of clinical indications of respiratory distress
3. Absence of clinical indications of infection/sepsis
4. Absence of clinical indications of dehydration
5. Absence of clinical indications of hypoperfusion
6. Control of pain and discomfort

Typical disposition: admission
1. Critical care unit admission may be required in acute pancreatitis
2. Preparation for surgery may be required for hemorrhagic or necrotizing pancreatitis

Intestinal Infarction/Obstruction/Perforation
Definitions
1. Intestinal infarction: necrosis of the intestinal wall resulting from ischemia
2. Intestinal obstruction: failure of the intestinal contents to progress forward through the lumen of the bowel
   a. Functional obstruction: caused by loss of peristalsis; usually referred to as paralytic ileus

b. Structural (i.e., mechanical) obstruction: caused by factors that occlude the bowel lumen
3. Intestinal perforation: penetration of the lumen of the intestine with resultant spillage of intestinal contents into the peritoneal cavity

Predisposing factors
1. Infarction
2. Emboli (e.g., atrial fibrillation)
3. Strangulated intestinal obstruction
4. Intra-abdominal infection
5. Cirrhosis
6. Paralytic ileus
7. Adhesions
8. Incarcerated hernia
9. Volvulus
10. Inflammatory bowel disease
11. Intussusception
12. Perforation

Pathophysiology
1. Infarction
   a. Decrease in blood flow to major mesenteric vessels causes vasoconstriction, vasospasm
   b. Prolonged ischemia increases the permeability of the bowel and edema of the intestinal wall
      1) Normal bowel flora (e.g., *E. coli, Klebsiella*) may penetrate the bowel wall causing peritonitis
   c. Edema of intestinal wall may cause full thickness necrosis and bowel perforation with leakage of normal bowel flora into the peritoneal cavity and peritonitis
2. Obstruction
   a. Obstruction of bowel preventing adequate forward movement of bowel contents
   b. Impairment in digestion
   c. Sequestration of gas and fluids proximal to the obstruction
   d. Shifting of fluids from bowel into the peritoneal cavity
   e. Dehydration, hypovolemia, shock
3. Perforation
   a. Leakage of GI content into peritoneal cavity causing infection and inflammation
   b. Peritonitis and potentially sepsis

Clinical presentation
1. Infarction
   a. Subjective
      1) Anorexia
      2) Abdominal pain
         a) Severe cramping periumbilical or nonspecific diffuse
         b) Abdominal pain related to mesenteric ischemia; may be referred to as abdominal angina
      3) Patient report of weight loss
      4) Urgency to have a bowel movement

   b. Objective
      1) Tachycardia, tachypnea
      2) Hypotension
      3) Pallor
      4) Abdominal distention, rigidity, guarding, rebound tenderness with perforation and peritoneal irritation
      5) Hypoactive or absent bowel sounds
      6) Vomiting: persistent, may be bloody
      7) Urgent diarrhea: may be bloody
      8) Clinical indications of dehydration
      9) Elevated temperature
   c. Diagnostic studies
      1) BUN: elevated due to dehydration
      2) Alkaline phosphatase: elevated
      3) Amylase: elevated
      4) Hct: elevated
      5) WBC: elevated
      6) ABGs: metabolic acidosis
      7) Stool: guaiac positive
      8) Angiography: occlusion of the arterial supply
2. Obstruction
   a. Small bowel
      1) Subjective
         a) Severe sharp episodic pain; steady, severe, localized pain may signal strangulation
         b) Patient report of changes in bowel habits
            i) Partial bowel obstruction: normal stools or diarrhea
            ii) Complete obstruction: absence of stools
      2) Objective
         a) Vomiting early: may be projectile and/or fecal
            i) Clear gastric fluid: obstruction at the pylorus
            ii) Gastric contents and bile:
               (a) Obstruction in the proximal small intestine
               (b) Paralytic ileus
            iii) Brown fecal: obstruction in the distal small intestine
         b) Abdominal distention
         c) Clinical indications of dehydration
         d) Bowel sounds: high-pitched that increase early and decreased in later stages
      3) Diagnostic studies
         a) Sodium: decreased, increased, normal depending on hydration status
         b) Potassium: decreased
         c) Chloride: decreased
         d) BUN: elevated
         e) Hct: elevated
         f) WBCs: elevated
         g) ABGs: metabolic acidosis
         h) Flat plate of abdomen: shows dilated loops of gas-filled bowel
         i) CT and MRI are done to differentiate cause and location

b. Large bowel
   1) Subjective
      a) Dull pain
      b) Patient report of change in bowel habits: thin, ribbonlike stools progressing to constipation to absence of stools with watery discharge
      c) Report of decrease in flatus
   2) Objective
      a) Vomiting late
      b) Abdominal distention
      c) Bowel sounds: low-pitched that are increased early and decreased in later stages
      d) Melena: may occur if large bowel obstruction is caused by ulcerative colitis, cancer, or diverticulitis
   3) Diagnostic studies
      a) Sodium: may be decreased, increased, or normal depending on hydration level and serum osmolality
      b) Potassium: decreased
      c) Chloride: decreased
      d) BUN: elevated with dehydration
      e) Hct: may be elevated due to dehydration or decreased due to hemorrhage; large intestinal tumor frequently causes slow bleeding
      f) WBCs: elevated
      g) ABG: metabolic acidosis
      h) Stools: may be positive for occult blood in large bowel obstruction due to ulcerative colitis, cancer, or diverticulitis
      i) Flat plate of abdomen: shows dilated loops of gas-filled bowel
3. Perforation
   a. Subjective
      1) Abdominal pain
      2) Anorexia, nausea
   b. Objective
      1) Tachycardia, tachypnea
      2) Fever
      3) Vomiting
      4) Abdominal tenderness
      5) Rigid, "boardlike" abdomen, guarding, rebound tenderness
      6) Absence of liver dullness due to free air in peritoneum
      7) Bowel sounds: diminished or absent
   c. Diagnostic studies
      1) WBCs: increased
      2) Hct: may increase with dehydration or decrease with hemorrhage
      3) Potassium: decreased
      4) Sodium: may be normal, increased, or decreased depending on hydration
      5) Chloride: decreased
      6) BUN: increases with dehydration
      7) Flat plate of abdomen: free air in peritoneum may be seen
      8) Barium enema: may show point of obstruction
      9) Endoscopy: visualization obstruction

Collaborative management

1. Continue assessment
   a. ABCDs
   b. Oxygen saturation
   c. Vital signs: blood pressure, pulse, respiratory rate, and temperature
   d. Discomfort and pain level
   e. Abdominal assessment: distention, rebound tenderness, rigidity, rebound tenderness
   f. Accurate intake and output
   g. Serum electrolytes
   h. Level of consciousness
   i. Close monitoring for progression of symptoms
2. Maintain airway, oxygenation, and ventilation
   a. Elevation of head of bed 30 to 45 degrees, on side if vomiting
   b. Suctioning as required
   c. Oxygen by nasal cannula at 2 to 6 L/min to maintain SpO_2 of 95% unless contraindicated; for patients with COPD, use pulse oximetry to guide oxygen administration to SpO_2 of 90%
3. Maintain adequate circulation and perfusion
   a. IV access for fluid and medication administration
   b. Fluid replacement as indicated: usually 0.9% saline; colloids (e.g., albumin) and/or blood products as prescribed
   c. Electrolyte replacement as indicated: calcium and potassium most likely to be required
4. Control pain and discomfort
   a. Analgesics
   b. Antiemetics
   c. Anxiolytics
   d. Position of comfort: encourage knee flexing while in supine position to relax abdominal muscles
5. Prevent perforation of bowel if obstruction present
   a. NPO
   b. NG tube or orogastric tube to decompress the stomach, prevent vomiting, and reduce the risk of aspiration
   c. Pharmacologic agents as prescribed to enhance GI motility in partial intestinal obstruction (e.g., metoclopramide HCl [Reglan])
   d. Surgery is indicated for vascular obstruction, complete bowel obstruction, and bowel perforation
6. Treat infection (if present) and prevent sepsis
   a. Antimicrobials as prescribed
   b. Antipyretics and cooling methods to reduce fever
   c. Prevention of leakage of intestinal bacteria and risk of peritonitis and sepsis if perforation has occurred
      1) Keep the patient immobilized to reduce the chemical irritation to the peritoneum
      2) Give antibiotics preoperatively
7. Monitor for complications
   a. Respiratory distress secondary to abdominal distention
   b. Hemorrhage and hemorrhagic shock
   c. Peritonitis, sepsis, septic shock

Evaluation

1. Patent airway, adequate oxygenation (i.e., normal Pao_2, Spo_2, Sao_2) and ventilation (i.e., normal $Paco_2$)
2. Absence of clinical indications of respiratory distress
3. Absence of clinical indications of infection/sepsis
4. Absence of clinical indications of dehydration
5. Absence of clinical indications of hypoperfusion
6. Alert and oriented with no neurologic deficit
7. Control of pain and discomfort

Typical disposition: admission

1. Critical care unit admission may be required
2. Preparation for surgery may be required for intestinal perforation, ischemia/infarction, and complete bowel obstruction

Abdominal Trauma

Definition: trauma that occurs between the nipple line to mid-thigh

Predisposing factors

1. Penetrating trauma (e.g., motor vehicle collision; assault; sharp instruments [e.g., knife; gunshot wound; impalement])
2. Blunt trauma (e.g., motor vehicle collision, assault, fall, sports injury)
3. Iatrogenic trauma
   a. Peritoneal tap
   b. Endoscopy
   c. Biopsy
   d. Cardiopulmonary resuscitation

Pathophysiology

1. Seldom a single-organ injury
2. High-velocity penetrating trauma
   a. Extensive destruction of contact tissue
   b. Severe associated blast effect on the surrounding tissues
   c. Liver most often affected by penetrating trauma
3. Blunt trauma
   a. Due to direct injury, crushing force between two objects, acceleration/deceleration, shearing, twisting
   b. Pressure injury
   c. Spleen most often affected by blunt trauma; pancreas frequently injured with spleen

Clinical presentation

1. Subjective
   a. Abdominal pain: may be poorly localized or referred
      1) Kehr sign: left shoulder pain indicative of splenic rupture caused by blood below diaphragm that irritates the phrenic nerve
      2) Rovsing sign: pain in RLQ with palpation of LLQ indicates peritoneal irritation
2. Objective
   a. Seatbelt sign: ecchymosis across the lower abdomen caused by seatbelt

   b. Hematoma: note location; hematoma in flank area may be seen in renal injury
   c. Entrance and exit wounds if gunshot involved
   d. Grey Turner or Cullen sign: may be seen
   e. Coopernail sign (ecchymosis of scrotum or labia): indicative of fractured pelvis
   f. Abdominal tenderness to palpation
   g. Rigid abdomen: may indicate intra-abdominal bleeding
   h. Diminished femoral pulses: may be seen in vascular injury
   i. Ballance sign (i.e., resonance over right flank with patient on left side): indicative of ruptured spleen
   j. Loss of liver dullness: indicates perforation with free air in peritoneum
   k. Bowel sounds: diminished or absent
   l. Clinical indications of hypoperfusion or shock
   m. Clinical indications of perforation
   n. Specifics related to organ injured (Table 7-7)
3. Diagnostic studies
   a. Glucose: elevated due to stress
   b. Amylase: elevated if injury to pancreas or bowel
   c. ALT, AST, LDH: may be elevated if liver injury
   d. Hgb, Hct: decreased with hemorrhage
   e. WBCs: elevated with infection or spleen injury
   f. Platelets: elevated if spleen is injured
   g. PT, aPTT: may be prolonged
   h. Drug and alcohol screens: may be positive
   i. Hematuria indicates renal trauma
   j. Myoglobinuria: crush injury or muscle breakdown occurring
   k. Stool: to check for occult blood
   l. Chest radiograph: to rule out concurrent thoracic injury; identify free air under diaphragm
   m. Flat plate of abdomen: may show free air in peritoneum if stomach or bowel is perforated
   n. IVP: if hematuria is present to look for renal trauma
   o. Angiography: may show vascular injury
   p. CT or MRI: to identify areas of injury
   q. Focused abdominal sonography for trauma (FAST)
      1) Detects fluid or blood in the pericardium, abdomen, or pelvis
      2) Allows visualization of the spleen and liver
   r. Diagnostic peritoneal lavage (DPL): may be done to assess for intra-abdominal bleeding though FAST is usually the preferred screening study
      1) Assist with placement of peritoneal catheter; if gross blood if obtained with catheter insertion, immediate exploratory laparotomy is indicated
      2) Instill 1 L of normal saline over 15 to 20 minutes
      3) Move the patient side to side after fluid instillation to distribute the lavage fluid
      4) Drain
      5) Send for analysis

TABLE 7-7   Clinical Indications of Organ Injury

Organ	Suspect Injury to this Organ if:	Clinical Indications of Injury	Complications
Liver	• Seatbelt sign • Hematoma or ecchymosis in right upper quadrant (RUQ) • Lower right rib fracture • Blunt or penetrating trauma • Acceleration/deceleration motor vehicle collision (MVC) • Presence of other abdominal injuries	• RUQ pain • Guarding right side • Referred pain to right shoulder • Increase in abdominal girth and rigidity • Increased pain in RUQ with inspiration • Tachycardia, hypotension • Increased WBCs • Liver enzymes: elevated (e.g., alanine aminotransferase, aspartate aminotransferase, lactate dehydrogenase) • Decreased Hgb and Hct • Abnormal clotting studies • Chest radiograph: may show elevated diaphragm on right side • Injury evident on FAST • DPL: positive	• Shock • Infection, sepsis • Subdiaphragmatic abscess • Atelectasis • Pneumonia • ARDS • Hepatic failure
Spleen	• Seatbelt sign • Local sign of injury (left upper quadrant [LUQ]) • Lower left rib fractures • Left pneumothorax • Blunt or penetrating trauma to abdomen • Acceleration/deceleration MVC • Presence of other abdominal injuries	• LUQ pain, tenderness, and guarding • Increased abdominal girth and rigidity • Kehr sign • Ballance sign • Increased pain LUQ with inspiration • Tachycardia, hypotension • Decreased Hgb and Hct • Injury evident on FAST • Positive DPL	• Shock • Atelectasis • Pneumonia • ARDS • Sepsis • Subdiaphragmatic abscess
Pancreas	• Seatbelt sign • Other abdominal injuries • MVC • Blunt or penetrating trauma to abdomen	• Epigastric, back, or shoulder pain • Abdominal tenderness and guarding • Increased abdominal girth • Decreased bowel sounds • Electrolyte imbalances: hyperglycemia or hypoglycemia • Elevated serum lipase • Elevated WBCs • DPL: may be positive for amylase	• Shock • Diabetes • Pancreatitis • Pancreatic abscess, pseudocyst, or fistula • Atelectasis • Pneumonia • ARDS
Stomach	• Penetrating trauma to abdomen • Presence of other abdominal injuries	• Epigastric or LUQ pain and tenderness • Hematemesis or bloody aspirate from nastogastric tube • Rebound tenderness • Tachycardia, hypotension • Elevated WBCs • DPL: positive • Abdominal flat plate: free air	• Atelectasis • Pneumonia • ARDS • Gastric fistula

Continued

TABLE 7–7 Clinical Indications of Organ Injury—cont'd

Organ	Suspect Injury to this Organ if:	Clinical Indications of Injury	Complications
Intestine	• Seatbelt sign • Presence of other abdominal injuries • Blunt trauma with deceleration. • Penetrating injury	• Local sign of injury (e.g., ecchymosis, abrasion) • Nausea, vomiting • Abdominal pain: may be referred or rebound • Absent bowel sounds • Elevated WBCs • DPL: positive for blood and fecal matter • Abdominal flat plate: free air • Positive fecal occult blood test	• Ileus • Peritonitis • Sepsis • Abscess • Intestinal ischemia, infarction, obstruction, perforation • Fistula
Abdominal vessels	• Other abdominal injuries • Blunt or penetrating abdominal injury • Sudden deceleration in MVC or fall	• Abdominal distention and guarding • Increased abdominal girth and rigidity • Abdominal bruit • Diminished femoral pulses if aorta or iliac injury • Mottled lower extremities • Cullen sign • Decreased Hgb and Hct • Tachycardia, hypotension (i.e., shock)	• Shock • Mesenteric ischemia or infarction • Sepsis

From Dennison, R. D. (2007). *Pass CCRN!* (3rd ed.). St. Louis: Mosby.

a) Considered positive if lavage fluid is grossly bloody or contains the following:
  i) RBCs >100,000 mm³
  ii) WBCs >500 mm³
  iii) Amylase >175 units/dl
  iv) Bile, bacteria, intestinal content
b) Major limitation of peritoneal lavage: does not detect diaphragmatic or retroperitoneal injuries
s. Specifics related to organ injured (see Table 7-7)

Collaborative management

1. Continue assessment
  a. ABCDs
  b. Oxygen saturation
  c. Vital signs: blood pressure, pulse, respiratory rate, and temperature
  d. Clinical indications of bleeding
  e. Discomfort and pain level
  f. Abdominal assessment: distention, rebound tenderness, rigidity, rebound tenderness
  g. Level of consciousness
  h. Accurate intake and output
  i. Close monitoring for progression of symptoms
2. Maintain airway, oxygenation, and ventilation
  a. Cervical spine stabilization as indicated
  b. BLS, ACLS as required
  c. Artificial airway, including endotracheal intubation, may be required
  d. Oxygen at 100% by nonrebreathing mask may be required to maintain SpO₂ of 95%
  e. Mechanical ventilation may be required
3. Maintain adequate circulation and perfusion
  a. IV access with two large-bore catheters for fluid and medication administration
  b. Fluid replacement
    1) Crystalloids
      a) Isotonic crystalloids: 0.9% saline or lactated Ringer solution
      b) Rate determined by acuity; rapid infusion may be required
    2) Packed RBCs
    3) Should be given early if significant blood loss is suspected to prevent tissue hypoxia
      a) Replacement of platelets, clotting factors, and calcium should be considered if multiple transfusions are given
    4) Colloids (e.g., albumin) may also be required
  c. Control hemorrhage
    1) Impaled objects should be stabilized and only removed in surgery
    2) Pressure to bleeding sites; apply pressure around the wound if there is an object in place and there is bleeding around the wound
  d. Cover any eviscerated organs with saline-soaked pads
4. Prepare patient for procedures as indicated
  a. NPO
  b. NG or orogastric tube to low suction

c. Foley catheter to evaluate hourly urine output unless contraindicated; contraindications include the following:
   1) Blood around the urinary meatus
   2) Perineal or scrotal hematoma
   3) Displacement of the prostate gland noted during rectal examination by physician
d. Arterial catheter and/or pulmonary artery catheter in patient with hemodynamic instability
e. Exploratory laparotomy for any of the following
   1) Penetrating injury invading the peritoneum
   2) Clinical indications of perforation (e.g., acute abdomen)
   3) Hemorrhage and/or shock
   4) Massive hematuria
   5) Evisceration
   6) Positive peritoneal lavage
   7) Surgical indications on CT or angiography
5. Control pain and discomfort
   a. Analgesics; caution must be exercised until diagnosis is made because the patient need to identify areas of pain, discomfort
   b. Antiemetics
   c. Anxiolytics
   d. Positioning: encourage knee flexing while in supine position to relax abdominal muscles in patients with peritoneal irritation
   e. Nonpharmacologic pain relief methods (e.g., distraction, repositioning)
6. Treat infection (if present) and prevent sepsis
   a. Antimicrobials as prescribed

b. Antipyretics and cooling methods to reduce fever
c. Tetanus toxoid if surface trauma and if >5 years since last immunization
d. Aseptic wound care as indicated
7. Prepare patient for exploratory laparotomy as indicated.
8. Monitor for complications.
   a. Respiratory complications (e.g., atelectasis, ARDS)
   b. Perforation, peritonitis
   c. Infection, sepsis, septic shock
   d. Hemorrhage, hypovolemic shock
   e. Multiple organ dysfunction syndrome (i.e., ARDS, disseminated intravascular coagulation, acute tubular necrosis, hepatic failure, myocardial failure, cerebral failure)

Evaluation
1. Patent airway, adequate oxygenation (i.e., normal Pao_2, Spo_2, Sao_2) and ventilation (i.e., normal $Paco_2$)
2. Absence of clinical indications of respiratory distress
3. Absence of clinical indications of infection/sepsis
4. Absence of clinical indications of bleeding, hypovolemia
5. Absence of clinical indications of hypoperfusion
6. Alert and oriented with no neurologic deficit
7. Control of pain and discomfort

Typical disposition: admission
1. Critical care unit admission may be required
2. Preparation for emergent surgery may be required

LEARNING ACTIVITIES

1. DIRECTIONS: Complete the following crossword puzzle related to gastrointestinal emergencies.

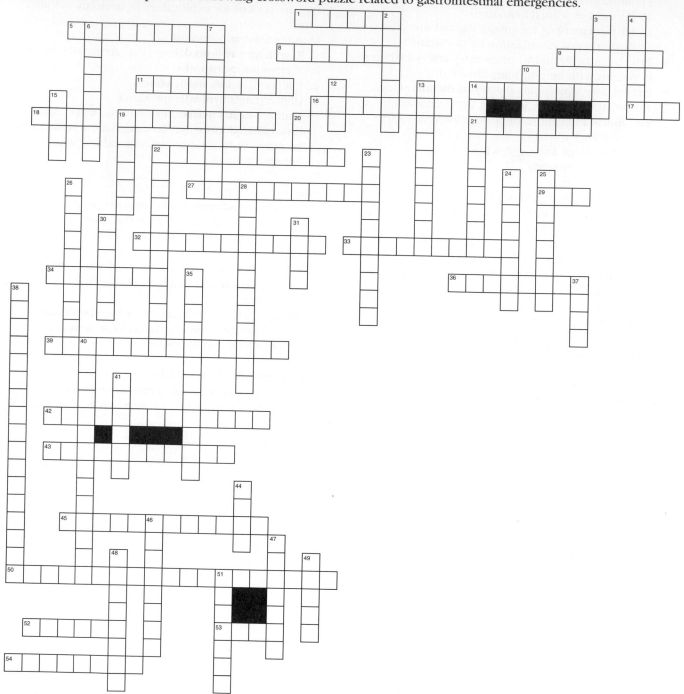

ACROSS

1. Tarry stools
5. Inflammation of the stomach lining that causes mucosal bleeding, edema, and erosion
8. An obstruction here is manifested by persistent vomiting
9. *Helicobacter* _____ is a bacteria associated with peptic ulcer
11. A flapping tremor seen in hepatic encephalopathy
14. _____ sign is indicative of splenic rupture
16. This location of peptic ulcer is frequently manifested by pain at night and melena
17. Pain of diverticulitis is usually more pronounced here
18. _____ sign is caused by phrenic nerve irritation by subphrenic blood
19. An osmotic laxative frequently used in hepatic encephalopathy (generic)
21. _____ tenderness indicates that pain is more severe on release than with pressure
22. Vomiting blood

27. This group of drugs may be used to decrease portal hypertension
29. Liver tenderness is associated with tenderness in this quadrant (abbreviation)
32. This drug is used in GI hemorrhage to cause vasoconstriction (generic)
33. A drug used in GI hemorrhage to suppress gastrin (generic)

34. This location of peptic ulcer is frequently manifested by pain with meals and hematemesis
36. A deficiency of this vitamin commonly seen in alcoholism
39. Abnormal function of the brain
42. A drug commonly used for suicide gesture that is a major cause of hepatic failure in adolescents (generic)

43. The location of pain in acute pancreatitis
45. Acute longitudinal tear of the esophagus associated with forceful retching (two words)
50. This type of tube has three lumens and is used to create a tamponade effect in bleeding esophageal varices (two words)
52. When part of an internal organ bulges through a weakened area of a muscle

53. This sphincter is located at the terminal end of the common bile duct at the duodenum
54. Chronic constipation frequently causes older patients to use this type of drug habitually

DOWN
2. An abnormal accumulation of fluid in the peritoneal cavity
3. _____ sign is a bluish discoloration around the umbilicus; indicative of intra-abdominal bleeding
4. Hypertension of this circulation system is seen in cirrhosis
6. Generalized, massive edema
7. A drug that acts as mucosal barrier used to protect the gastric mucosa (generic)
10. The form of fluid replacement that is indicated for acute hemorrhage
12. A flat plate of the abdomen is also referred to as a ___

13. H_2 receptor antagonist (generic)
14. Loud, hyperactive bowel sounds
15. This disorder is caused by the reflux of gastric secretions back up into the esophagus (abbreviation)
19. Most specific laboratory test for pancreatitis
20. This syndrome is characterized by cramping, abdominal pain, and constipation or diarrhea (abbreviation)
22. Electrolyte imbalance seen in acute pancreatitis
23. This type of anemia is caused by a deficiency of intrinsic factor
24. Cramping type pain that is difficult to localize

25. IV proton-pump inhibitor (brand name)
26. Belching
28. Burney sign is seen in this condition
30. This type of ulcer causes erosion in the mucosa of the esophagus, stomach, or duodenum
31. A stent is placed between the hepatic and portal veins in this procedure performed in patients with esophageal varices (abbreviation)
35. Release of this acid is stimulated by the hormone gastrin
37. This test may cause pancreatitis (abbreviation)
38. This inflammatory bowel disease affects the large intestine (two words)
40. A common cause of acute pancreatitis

41. This type of hernia allows the upper stomach to slide into the thoracic cavity
44. A type of ultrasound important in trauma care
46. This type of pain is when the location of pain is a distance from the disease process
47. Sharp, intense pain that is usually easily located
48. A "maneuver" that facilitates evacuation of the colon
49. This inflammatory bowel disease affects any area of the alimentary tract
51. Elevated _____ levels cause neurologic changes in patients with hepatic encephalopathy

2. DIRECTIONS: Explain why children are prone to serious abdominal injuries after a traumatic event.

3. DIRECTIONS: List the types of abdominal pain and give a description of each.

Type of Pain	Description

4. DIRECTIONS: Describe the following "signs" and identify what they indicate.

Sign	Description	Indicates
Ballance		
Grey Turner		
Cullen		
Coopernail		
Kehr		
Chvostek		
Trousseau		

5. DIRECTIONS: List three general causes of jaundice.

a.

b.

c.

6. DIRECTIONS: List five classic indications of an "acute abdomen."

a.

b.

c.

d.

e.

7. DIRECTIONS: List five causes of acute abdomen.

a.

b.

c.

d.

e.

8. DIRECTIONS: List five most likely causes for upper GI hemorrhage.

a.

b.

c.

d.

e.

9. DIRECTIONS: List four interventions for any patient with acute hemorrhage (regardless of location).

a.

b.

c.

d.

10. DIRECTIONS: List three classifications of drugs that are used to prevent ulcers and an example of each one.

Type	Example

11. DIRECTIONS: Match the following clinical manifestations of hepatic failure with the pathophysiologic change (answers may be used more than once).

___ 1. Splenic engorgement	a. Petechiae, purpura, bleeding
___ 2. Stretching of the liver capsule	b. Jaundice
___ 3. Decrease in the metabolism of testosterone	c. Third-spacing
___ 4. Decrease in metabolism of aldosterone	d. Testicular atrophy
___ 5. Decrease in production of plasma proteins	e. Gynecomastia
___ 6. Decrease in metabolism of estrogen	f. Anemia, leukopenia, thrombocytopenia
___ 7. Decreased production of clotting factors	g. Dull RUQ pain
___ 8. Decrease in conjugation and excretion of bilirubin	

12. DIRECTIONS: Complete the following table. You may include more than one condition for each but include only conditions discussed in this chapter.

Clinical Finding	Condition
Elevated lipase, amylase	
Sudden, painless hematemesis	
Decreased protein	
Rebound tenderness	
Jaundice	
Hypocalcemia	
Bleeding tendencies	
Elevated ammonia	
Bloody diarrhea	
Hyperbilirubinemia	
Fetor hepaticus	
High-pitched rushing bowel sounds	
Management	**Condition**
Irrigate NG tube until clear	
Sclerosis during endoscopy	
Aldosterone-antagonist diuretics	
NPO status	
Sengstaken-Blakemore tube	
Volume and blood replacement	

13. DIRECTIONS: Explain why a patient with cholecystitis would complain of clay-colored stools, steatorrhea, or dark amber urine.

14. DIRECTIONS: Differentiate among the terms *diverticula, diverticulosis,* and *diverticulitis.*

Term	Description
Diverticula	
Diverticulosis	
Diverticulitis	

15. DIRECTIONS: Describe the 10 types of hernias.

Type of Hernia	Description

16. DIRECTIONS: Identify whether the listed signs or symptoms occur in either of the following inflammatory bowel diseases.

Manifestation	Crohn Disease	Ulcerative Colitis
Diarrhea		
Crampy abdominal pain		
Fever		
Weight loss		
Rectal bleeding		
Tenesmus		
Malabsorption/nutritional problems		

17. DIRECTIONS: Describe the classic signs of intussusception and possible complications. What is a problem with assessing for the classic signs?

Classic Signs	Complications

18. DIRECTIONS: List contraindications for inserting a Foley catheter in a patient with abdominal trauma.

LEARNING ACTIVITIES ANSWERS

1.

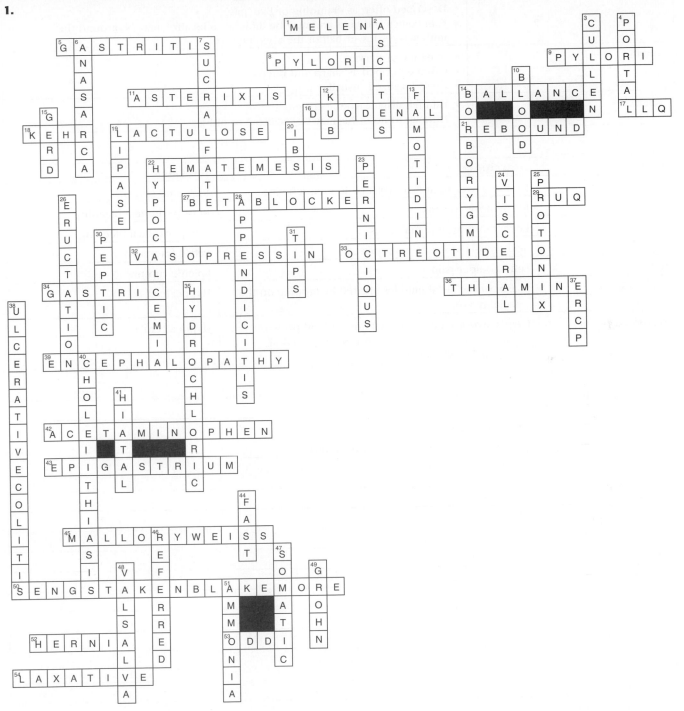

2.

Almost 50% of children will have multisystem injuries following trauma because their body organs are all in close proximity to each other and because there is less protection from bones, fat, and connective tissue.

3.

Type of Pain	Description
Visceral	• Stretching of a hollow organ or body cavity • Described often as cramping or like "gas" • Pain comes and goes and may be difficult to localize, may be around the umbilicus or lower half of the abdomen
Somatic	• Irritation of nerves • Often described as sharp and intense • Easily localized (usually)
Referred	• Pain felt distant from its origin • Difficult to describe; may be localized or diffuse

4.

Sign	Description	Indicates
Ballance	Dullness over right flank with patient on left side	Ruptured spleen
Grey Turner	Ecchymosis to flank	Retroperitoneal bleeding
Cullen	Ecchymosis around umbilicus	Intraperitoneal bleeding
Coopernail	Ecchymosis of scrotum or labia	Pelvic fracture
Kehr	Left shoulder pain	Splenic rupture
Chvostek	Spasm of the facial muscles elicited by tapping on the facial nerve	Hypocalcemia
Trousseau	Carpal spasm induced by inflating a blood pressure cuff on the upper arm to a pressure exceeding systolic blood pressure	Hypocalcemia

5.

a. Liver disease (e.g., cirrhosis, hepatitis)
b. Biliary obstruction (e.g., cholelithiasis)
c. Excessive hemolysis (e.g., hemolytic blood transfusion reaction)

6.

Abdominal pain
Rebound tenderness
Abdominal distention
Rigid, "boardlike" abdomen
Diminished bowel sounds
Fever
Leukocytosis
Nausea, vomiting

7.

Appendicitis
Bowel obstruction
Cholecystitis
Diverticulitis
Gastroenteritis
Pelvic inflammatory disease
Perforated ulcer
Peritonitis
Ruptured abdominal aneurysm
Ruptured ectopic pregnancy

8.

a. Peptic ulcer
b. Esophageal varices
c. Mallory-Weiss tear
d. Gastritis
e. Vascular tumor

9.

a. Administer oxygen (maintain Sao$_2$ of at least 95%)
b. Insert at least 2 large gauge (16 or 18) intravenous catheters
c. Obtain blood samples for H&H and type and crossmatch
d. Initiate normal saline infusion initially and then blood when prescribed and available

10.

Type	Example
Antacids	Calcium carbonate (Tums, Rolaids) Aluminum hydroxide, magnesium hydroxide, simethicone (Maalox Advanced) Aluminum hydroxide, magnesium hydroxide, simethicone, and sorbitol (Mylanta)
Histamine (H$_2$) receptor antagonists	Cimetidine (Tagamet) Ranitidine (Zantac) Famotidine (Pepcid)
Proton-pump inhibitors	Omeprazole (Prilosec) Lansoprazole (Prevacid) Esomeprazole (Nexium)

11.

f, a. 1. Splenic engorgement Remember that splenic engorgement causes thrombocytopenia and, therefore, clotting abnormalities.	a. Petechiae, purpura, bleeding
g. 2. Stretching of the liver capsule	b. Jaundice
d. 3. Decrease in the metabolism of testosterone	c. Third-spacing
c. 4. Decrease in metabolism of aldosterone	d. Testicular atrophy
c, a.5. Decrease in production of plasma proteins Remember that many plasma proteins are actually clotting factors	e. Gynecomastia
e. 6. Decrease in metabolism of estrogen	f. Anemia, leukopenia, thrombocytopenia
a. 7. Decreased production of clotting factors	g. Dull RUQ pain
b. 8. Decrease in conjugation and excretion of bilirubin	

12.

Sign/Symptom	Condition
Elevated lipase, amylase	Acute pancreatitis
Sudden, painless hematemesis	Esophageal varices
Decreased protein	Acute pancreatitis, liver disease, malnutrition
Rebound tenderness	Peritonitis
Jaundice	Liver disease, biliary obstruction, hemolysis
Hypocalcemia	Acute pancreatitis
Bleeding tendencies	Liver disease
Elevated ammonia	Hepatic failure, hepatic encephalopathy
Bloody diarrhea	Intestinal infarction
Hyperbilirubinemia	Liver disease, biliary obstruction, hemolysis
Fetor hepaticus	Hepatic failure
High-pitched rushing bowel sounds	Small bowel obstruction
Management	**Condition**
Irrigate NG tube until clear	Upper GI bleed
Neomycin and lactulose	Hepatic failure; hepatic encephalopathy
Sclerosis during endoscopy	Esophageal varices
Aldosterone-antagonist diuretics	Hepatic failure; hepatic encephalopathy
NPO status	Pancreatitis
Sengstaken-Blakemore tube	Esophageal varices
Volume and blood replacement	GI bleed

13. The patient has obstruction of bile flow.

14.

Term	Description
Diverticula	Saccular dilation or outpouching of intestinal mucosa through the circular smooth muscle of the abdominal wall
Diverticulosis	The condition of having multiple noninflamed diverticula
Diverticulitis	Infection or inflammation of the diverticula

15.

Type of Hernia	Description
Reducible	A hernia that can be pushed back into place
Irreducible/incarcerated	A hernia that can no longer be pushed back into place
Strangulated	A surgical emergency: an incarcerated hernia that has had its blood supply cut off
Indirect inguinal hernia	Herniation through the umbilical ring following the spermatic cord through the inguinal canal
Direct inguinal hernia	Where the bowel passes through an area of muscular weakness in the abdominal wall
Femoral hernia	Herniation that occurs through the femoral ring
Umbilical hernia	Occurs through the umbilicus
Incisional hernia	Hernia through a previous surgical site
Hiatal hernia	Small opening in the diaphragm that allows the upper part of the stomach to move up into the chest
Congenital diaphragmatic	Birth defect that needs repair

16.

Manifestation	Crohn Disease	Ulcerative Colitis
Diarrhea	Common	Common
Crampy abdominal pain	Common	Common
Fever	Common	During acute attacks
Weight loss	Common, may be severe	Rare
Rectal bleeding	Infrequent	Common
Tenesmus	Rare	Common
Malabsorption/nutritional problems	Common	Minimal incidence

17.

Classic Signs	Complications
Abdominal pain Sausage-shaped abdominal mass Currant jelly stools	Dehydration Hypovolemic shock Bowel necrosis Sepsis Perforation Peritonitis
The problem with assessing for the classic manifestations of intussusception is that that they only occur in about 20% of children with this disorder	

18.

Blood around the urinary meatus
Perineal or scrotal hematoma
Displacement of the prostate gland noted during rectal examination by physician

References and Suggested Readings

Buttaro, T. M., Trybulski, J., Bailey, P. P., & Sandberg-Cook, J. (2003). *Primary care: A collaborative practice*. St. Louis: Mosby.

Clark, D. Y., Stocking, J., & Johnson, J. (Eds.). (2006). *Flight and ground transport nursing core curriculum* (2nd ed.). Denver, CO: Air and Surface Transport Nurses Association.

Craig, S. (2008, September). Appendicitis, acute. Retrieved on March 24, 2009, from http://emedicine.medscape.com/article/773895-overview.

Dennison, R. D. (2007). *Pass CCRN!* (3rd ed.). St. Louis: Mosby.

Domino, F. J. (2008). *The 5-minute clinical consultant* (16th ed.). Philadelphia: Lippincott Williams and Wilkins.

Emergency Nurses Association. (2007). *Emergency nursing core curriculum* (6th ed.). Philadelphia: Saunders.

Emergency Nurses Association. (2005). *Sheehy's manual of emergency care* (6th ed.). St. Louis: Mosby.

Fass, R. (2007, May/June). Symptom assessment tools for gastroesophageal reflux disease (GERD) treatment. *Journal of Clinical Gastroenterology, 41(5)*, 437-444.

Fultz, J., & Sturt, P. A. (2005). *Mosby's emergency nursing reference* (3rd ed.). St. Louis: Mosby.

Hernanz-Schulman, M. (2003, May). Infantile hypertrophic pyloric stenosis. *Radiology, 227(2)*, 319-331. Epub 2003 Mar 13.

Jarvis, C. (2008). *Physical examination and health assessment* (5th ed.). St. Louis: Saunders.

King, L. (2007, October). Pediatrics, intussusception. Retrieved on March 26, 2009, from http://emedicine.medscape.com/article/802424-overview.

Markowitz, J. E., Dancel, L. D., & Shukla, P. C. (2008, May). Volvulus: overview. Retrieved on March 26, 2009, from http://emedicine.medscape.com/article/932430-overview.

Mayo Clinic Website. (2007). Appendicitis. Retrieved on March 24, 2009, from http://www.mayoclinic.com/health/appendicitis/DS00274.

McCarthy, D. (2007, July). Do drugs or bugs cause GERD? [Presentations: Current Status] *Journal of Clinical Gastroenterology, 41*(suppl. 2), S59-S63.

Merck Manuals Online. (2007). Inflammatory bowel disease. Retrieved on March 27, 2009, from http://www.merck.com/mmpe/sec02/ch018/ch018a.html#CBBDCBAD.

Merriam Webster Online. (2007-2008). Merriam-Webster's medical dictionary. http://medical.merriam-webster.com.

Nick, B. A., & Askew, K. (2008, November). Hernias. Retrieved on March 26, 2009, from http://emedicine.medscape.com/article/775630-overview.

Prescilla, R. P. (2009, January). Gastroenteritis. Retrieved on March 26, 2009, from http://emedicine.medscape.com/article/964131-overview.

Price, S. A., & Wilson, L. M. (2003). *Pathophysiology: Clinical concepts of disease process* (6th ed.). St. Louis: Mosby.

Proehl, J. A. (2004). *Emergency nursing procedures* (3rd ed.). St. Louis: Saunders.

Roppolo, L. P., Davis, D., Kelly, S. P., & Rosen, P. (2007). *Emergency medicine handbook: Critical concepts for clinical practice*. St. Louis: Mosby.

Singh, J., Kass, D. A., & Sinert, R. (2008, January). Pediatrics, pyloric stenosis. Retrieved on March 27, 2009, from http://emedicine.medscape.com/article/803489-overview.

CHAPTER 8

Orthopedic and Wound Emergencies

Introduction

This content constitutes 9% (13 items) of the CEN examination

The focus is on orthopedic conditions and wounds that are commonly encountered in an ED setting

The continuum of age needs to be considered from infancy through older adulthood

Age-Related Considerations (Emergency Nurses Association [ENA], 2003, 2007)

Neonates, infants, and children

1. Infants: appear bowlegged (i.e., genu varum) from 2 to 3 years of age
2. Children have open epiphyses until after adolescence; injury may affect healing and growth formation
3. Bones in infants and young children are more narrow and flexible; significant force may cause incomplete fractures
4. Possible child abuse should always be considered; surface trauma is the most evident sign of nonaccidental trauma
5. Children may have a pigeon-toed walk that is normal at this stage, and they may appear flat-footed
6. Children between 18 and 36 months of age may appear knock-kneed (i.e., genu valgum)
7. Ligaments in children are more resistant to trauma; dislocations are rare at this age, and, if they occur, there is usually a fracture involved as well
8. Limping in children is rare; if it occurs, look for a possible hip disorder

Older adult

1. Joint stiffness as a result of aging contributes to decreased mobility
2. Aging changes affect posture, balance, and strength
3. Falls are the most common cause of fractures among older adults
4. Older adults have a diminished ability to respond to traumatic stressors
5. Medications for the older adult may affect bleeding and healing
6. Slower metabolism and body functions also slow healing in older adults

Selected Concepts in Anatomy and Physiology

General information about the musculoskeletal system

1. Provides the supporting framework of the human body
2. Responsible for movement
3. Consists of bones, joints, skeletal muscles, tendons, ligaments, bursae, and connective tissue

Bones

1. Provide protection to vital organs and enable the body to move
2. Serve as a primary storage site for calcium and phosphate and help with the regulation of these substances
3. Continually going through a turnover process that consists of deposition and absorption at a constant rate, except during childhood development, when more deposition occurs
4. Bone tissue consists of three types of cells:
   a. Osteoblasts: cells that build new bones
      1) Form type I collagen to produce osteoid
      2) Responsible for the mineralization of the osteoid matrix, which then develops into new bone tissue
   b. Osteocytes: cells that maintain bone tissue
      1) Derived from osteoblasts; they represent the final stage of bone maturation
      2) Mature bone cells that provide a pathway for chemical exchange in bone tissue
      3) Most abundant cells found compact bone tissue
   c. Osteoclasts: cells that maintain bone reabsorption
      1) Formed by the fusion of the monocyte–macrophage cell line
      2) Remove bone tissue by removing the mineralized matrix
5. There are two types of bone in the body:
   a. Cortical (i.e., dense)
      1) Hard outer layer of bone tissue that gives the smooth, white, solid appearance
      2) Accounts for 80% of the total bone mass in adults
   b. Trabecular or cancellous (i.e., spongy)
      1) Porous tissue found on the inside of the bone
      2) Composed of rod- and plate-like elements that make the bone lighter and that allow room for blood vessels and marrow

3) Accounts for 20% of the total bone mass in adults

6. Hormones regulate bone metabolism
   a. Increased levels of parathyroid hormone cause calcium and phosphate to be absorbed and moved into the bloodstream
   b. Vitamin D affects bone deposition and absorption

Connective tissue

1. Cartilage is dense connective tissue that is found in various areas
2. Ligaments are fibrous bands or sheets that connect bone to bone, that provide stability for the joint, and that aid in movement
3. Tendons are composed of collagen fibers that are packed tightly together to form a tough band of fibrous tissue
   a. Tendons connect muscle to bone, thereby enabling flexion and extension movements

Joints

1. The areas where two bones connect
2. They provide either stability or movement
3. Joints are held together by various types of soft tissue, including joint capsules, fibrous bands, ligaments, tendons, fasciae, and muscles
4. There are three types of joints:
   a. Fibrous joints: joints that connect bones without allowing movement
      1) Skull
      2) Pelvis
      3) Spinous processes
      4) Vertebrae
   b. Cartilaginous joints: joints that make use of cartilage to connect bones and that allow for minimal movement
      1) Spine
      2) Ribs
   c. Synovial joints: fluid-filled joints that are lubricated and that allow bones to move freely

Spinal cord

1. Center for spinal reflexes that provides a pathway for impulses to travel back and forth to the brain
2. Composed of white and gray matter
   a. White matter provides a conducting pathway for afferent and efferent impulses
   b. Gray matter is responsible for sensory perception and cord reflexes
   c. Spinal cord vertebra and 31 pairs of spinal nerves
      1) Seven cervical vertebrae (C1–C7) and 8 nerve pairs
      2) Twelve thoracic vertebrae (T1–T12) and 12 thoracic nerve pairs
      3) Five lumbar vertebrae (L1–L5) and 5 lumbar nerve pairs
      4) Five sacrum vertebrae (S1–S5) and 5 sacral nerve pairs

5) Five coccyx vertebrae bones fused together at the base of the spine and 1 coccyx nerve pair

Injuries to the musculoskeletal system

1. May be limb or life threatening
2. Are frequently a secondary injury with a low priority during the initial stabilization of an unstable patient with multiple traumatic injuries
3. May cause the following complications:
   a. Early
      1) Thrombophlebitis caused by immobility and venous stasis
      2) Pain
      3) Compartment syndrome, which occurs when perfusion pressure falls below tissue pressure in a closed anatomic space
      4) Neurovascular deficits as a result of the soft-tissue swelling of surrounding vessels and nerves
   b. Long-term complications associated with delayed stabilization and surgical interventions
      1) Acute respiratory distress syndrome
      2) Sepsis
      3) Infections
      4) Delayed bone healing
      5) Permanent disability

Orthopedic Assessment

Primary and secondary assessment (see Chapter 2)

Focused assessment

1. Chief complaint: identifies why the patient is seeking help and the duration of the problem
2. Symptoms related to orthopedic disorders
   a. Changes in neurovascular status
   b. Deformities
   c. Gait and ability to bear weight
   d. Range of motion
3. History of present illness
   a. Mechanism of injury or illness
   b. Motor and sensory deficits distal to the injury
   c. Provocation and palliation
   d. Quality and quantity
   e. Region and radiation
   f. Severity
   g. Timing
   h. Associated symptoms
      1) Swelling
      2) Tenderness
      3) Numbness
      4) Weakness
4. Past medical history
   a. Previous illnesses and injuries
      1) Arthritis: involves the breakdown of cartilage, which can cause pain, swelling, and stiffness (Price & Wilson, 2003)
      2) Systemic lupus erythematous: inflammatory autoimmune disorder that can affect joints and cause symptoms similar to those of arthritis

3) Paget disease: alteration of the normal bone growth process of breakdown and rebuilding so that bone breaks down more quickly and grows back softer; can cause the bone to bend and break more easily (Price & Wilson, 2003)

4) Sjögren syndrome: autoimmune disorder that causes chronic inflammation that can affect joints

5) Osteopenia: low bone density

6) Osteoporosis: brittle and weak bones

7) Pre-existing disabilities

b. Previous surgical procedures

c. Allergies and types of reactions

d. Previous diagnostic studies (e.g., radiologic and computed tomography [CT] scans)

5. Social history
   a. Usual activity level and ability to perform activities of daily living
   b. Recreational habits
   c. Exercise habits
   d. Dietary habits
   e. Tobacco use; smoking can weaken bones (Torpy, 2006)

6. Medication history
   a. Prescribed drug, dose, frequency, and time of last dose
      1) Check for medications that can cause bone loss (e.g., corticosteroids)
   b. Nonprescribed drugs
      1) Over-the-counter drugs, including herbal supplements
      2) Substance abuse (e.g., cocaine, amphetamines)
   c. Patient understanding of drug actions and side effects

General survey

1. Apparent health status
2. Level of consciousness
3. Nutritional status
4. Stature and posture
5. Gait
6. Deformity

Inspection

1. Uncontrolled bleeding or open wounds
2. Foreign bodies
3. Angulations and deformities
4. Discolorations (ENA, 2005)
   a. 24 to 48 hours after injury: the area can appear reddish blue to purple, depending on how deep the injury is and the amount of bleeding
   b. 5 to 7 days after injury: the outer area takes on a greenish hue
   c. 7 to 10 days after injury: the outer area is yellowish
   d. 10 to 14 days after injury: the outer area is brownish
   e. 2 to 4 weeks after injury: no injury is evident
5. Comparison of extremities for symmetry, size, and alignment
   a. Valgus: a deformity in which the angle of the part is away from the midline of the body to an abnormal degree (*Dorland's Illustrated Medical Dictionary*, 2003)

b. Varus: a deformity in which the angle of the part is toward the midline of the body to an abnormal degree (*Dorland's Illustrated Medical Dictionary*, 2003.)

Palpation

1. Neurovascular status: PMS
   a. P: palpable pulses
   b. M: movement
   c. S: sensation and tenderness
2. Skin
   a. Temperature
   b. Presence of edema and any pitting
3. Muscles
   a. Symmetry
   b. Tone
      1) Note the normal degree of tension or contraction
      2) Assess by pulling selected muscle groups through passive range-of-motion testing
      3) Recognize that tone may decrease with fatigue, infections, or neurologic, metabolic, or musculo-skeletal problems (ENA, 2005)
      4) Recognize that tone may increase with injury, spasms, or tremors associated with electrolyte disorders or neurologic conditions (ENA, 2005)
   c. Muscle strength: assess from proximal to distal
4. Capillary refill
   a. Assess distal to any injury
   b. Normal is <2 seconds

Auscultation: Doppler pulses present
Diagnostic studies

1. Laboratory studies
   a. CBC
      1) Decreased hemoglobin and hematocrit levels may indicate chronic anemia or acute bleeding
      2) Leukocytosis can occur with wound infection
   b. Electrolyte imbalances (ENA, 2005)
      1) Alkaline phosphates can increase with increased metabolic bone activity
      2) Calcium can increase with prolonged immobility or immobilization, Paget disease, and metastatic bone cancer
      3) Vitamin deficiencies can occur with decreased calcium absorption
   c. Troponin increases with skeletal muscle damage
   d. Creatine kinase increases with muscle damage
   e. Lactate dehydrogenase increases with skeletal muscle damage
   f. Uric acid level increases with gout and acute tissue destruction
   g. C-reactive protein increases with acute inflammatory processes
   h. C-reactive protein, antinuclear antibodies, and serum rheumatoid factor will be positive with rheumatoid arthritis
   i. Bone reabsorption test

1) C-telopeptide: a fragment of the protein matrix
2) N-telopeptide: a fragment of the protein matrix
3) Deoxypyridinoline: a collagen breakdown product with a ring structure
4) Pyridinium crosslink: collagen breakdown products, including deoxypyridinoline

j. Bone formation tests (Lab Tests Online, n.d.)
   1) Bone-specific alkaline phosphatase: isoenzyme type of alkaline phosphatase; associated with osteoblasts and thought to be involved in bone mineralization
   2) Osteocalcin (bone gamma-carboxyglutamic acid-containing protein [BGLAP]): protein created by osteoblasts; the noncollagen part of new bone structure; some of this substance will enter the bloodstream

2. Imaging studies
   a. Radiographic studies: complete views to rule out fracture
      1) Need two views of the injured extremity
      2) Joints above and below the injury must be visible
      3) WEAK: *W*rist, *E*lbow, *A*nkle, *K*nee joints; mnemonic to help one to remember to obtain comparative films for these joints for patients who are <16 years old (ENA, 2007)
      4) Spinal cord injury without radiographic abnormality (SCIWRA): common with cervical injuries in pediatric patients <8 years old; recommend magnetic resonance imaging (MRI) to rule out (Roppolo, Davis, Kelly, & Rosen, 2007)
   b. CT
   c. Arteriogram: used to locate vascular injury
   d. MRI: used to visualize soft tissue
   e. Bone scan: nuclear scan test that looks at bone mineral density
   f. Doppler sonography

General Principles of Wound Care

1. Determine priorities: Airway, Breathing, Circulation, and Disability (ABCDs)
2. Position for comfort
3. Clean around the injured area, and consider shaving it
4. Give anesthetic if necessary (Table 8-1)
5. Clean the wound itself with large volume of normal saline; flush the area for ≥5 minutes if highly contaminated
6. Soak puncture wounds for 10 to 15 minutes; other wounds should not be soaked
7. Remove debris and debride if needed before closing wound
8. Dress with antibiotic ointment as indicated or directed
9. Splint as indicated
10. Administer analgesics as required
11. Administer antibiotics as prescribed
12. Provide the patient and significant others with discharge instructions
13. Assist with suture removal (Table 8-2)
14. When removing sutures, be sure to pull the suture across the wound rather than away from the wound

General Orthopedic Management

Six Ps of neurovascular assessment
1. Pain
2. Pallor
3. Polar (i.e., cold)

TABLE 8-1   Common Anesthetics

Agent	Onset	Duration	Contraindications	Maximum Dose for Adults
Lidocaine (1%-2%)	1-5 min	30-60 min	Allergies	4.5 mg/kg (300 mg maximum)
Lidocaine (1%-2%) with epinephrine 1:100,000 or 1:200,000	1-5 min	2-6 hr	Allergies; do not use in areas of poor circulation or for digits, nasal tip, ears, or penis	7 mg/kg (500 mg maximum)
Bupivacaine 0.25% (Marcaine)	5 min	2-4 hr (Windle, 2008); 8-16 hr (ENA, 2007)	Allergies	2.5 mg/kg (175 mg maximum)
Bupivacaine 0.25% with epinephrine 1:200,000	5 min	3-7 hr (Windle, 2008); 8-16 hr (ENA, 2007)	Allergies; do not use in areas of poor circulation or for digits, nasal tip, ears, or penis	225 mg
Eutectic mixture of local anesthetics (EMLA) cream (lidocaine 2.5% and prilocaine 2.5%)	30-60 min; reaches maximum peak within 3 hr	Lasts 1-2 hours after the removal of the actual cream	Allergies; do not apply near eyes or to open wounds	Do not use for >4 hr

Adapted from Emergency Nurses Association. (2007). *Emergency nursing core curriculum* (6th ed.). Philadelphia: Saunders.

TABLE 8-2 Suture Removal Guidelines

Laceration Area	Adults	Children
Eyelids	Cutaneous, 5 days (Ing, 2007); other, 10–14 days	Varies
Face	3–5 days	3–4 days
Scalp	5–8 days	5–6 days
Neck	3–5 days	3–4 days
Chest	7–10 days	6–8 days
Abdomen	7–10 days	6–8 days
Back	10–12 days	7–10 days
Joint surfaces (i.e., knee, elbow, wrist)	10–12 days	7–10 days
Nonjoint surfaces of the upper arms and legs (i.e., thigh, lower leg, foot)	7–10 days	6–8 days
Palm of hand or sole of foot	7–12 days	7–10 days

Adapted from Emergency Nurses Association. (2007). *Emergency nursing core curriculum* (6th ed.). Philadelphia: Saunders.

4. Pulses
5. Paresthesia
6. Paralysis

Four Rs of fractures (ENA, 2007)
1. Recognition
2. Reduction
3. Retention
4. Rehabilitation

RICE (ENA, 2007)
1. Rest
   a. No weight bearing
   b. Avoidance of use of extremity
2. Ice to area four times a day or as directed
3. Compression
   a. Application of elastic bandage to area
   b. Rewrapping twice a day
   c. Removal at night
4. Elevation of injured extremity above the level of the heart for at least the first 24 hours after injury

Cold therapy (Proehl, 2004)
1. Injuries of <24 to 48 hours should have cold packs applied before splint application
2. Cold therapy stiffens collagen and reduces the tendency for ligament and tendons to deform
3. Cold therapy decreases muscle spasms, inflammation, and blood flow, thus limiting hemorrhage and swelling; it also increases the pain threshold
4. Cold packs should be applied for 20 to 30 minutes at a time (longer use could cause frostbite or tissue injury) for up to 48 hours after the initial injury.

5. For chronic injuries or pain, ice is used after exercise
6. Cold therapy should be discontinued if the skin blanches and then turns red after use

Heat therapy (Proehl, 2004)
1. Heat is generally used for chronic injuries or injuries that have no inflammation or swelling; it should not be used for an acute injury until 48 hours after the injury occurs
2. Before exercising, patients with chronic pain or injuries should use heat therapy to increase the elasticity of joint connective tissues and to stimulate blood flow
3. Heat therapy increases circulation aids in relaxing tight muscles or spasms
4. Heat should be applied to an injury for 15 to 30 minutes at a time; to prevent burns, do not place the heat source directly on the skin
5. Heat therapy should be avoided if neurologic or vascular compromise or disease, infection, or bleeding disorders are present unless directed by the primary care provider

Immobilization
1. The goal of immobilization is to protect the damaged bone while maintaining anatomic position
2. Immobilization will facilitate the healing process, protect the extremity from further insult, and help decrease pain

Splints and casts (Proehl, 2004)
1. The goals of splints and casts are to reduce mobility and to help with reducing edema
2. There are numerous types of splints that can be modified to immobilize almost any type of fracture (Table 8-3):
   a. Soft splints: nonrigid
   b. Hard splints: firm and rigid
   c. Air splints: inflatable
   d. Traction splints: support fractures while providing traction
   e. Pneumatic antishock garments: controversial but used to stabilize fractures and to control bleeding
3. Immobilization of joints proximal and distal to the injured area when preparing to splint
4. Padding for splints
5. Support of limb during splinting process to maintain alignment, decrease movement, and decrease pain and discomfort during the application of the splint
6. Assessment of neurovascular status before and after splinting extremity
7. Monitoring for complications that can result from casting and splinting (Table 8-4)
   a. Ischemia
   b. Plaster burns
   c. Pressure sores
   d. Infection
   e. Dermatitis
   f. Joint stiffness

TABLE 8-3 Types of Splints

Splint	Indications	Application	Illustration
Long arm posterior sling	Distal humerus or proximal radius/ulna fractures, elbow sprains/ dislocations	From palmar crease along ulnar aspect of forearm to posterior humerus below axilla Thumb should point upward (neutral supination/ pronation) Use arm sling with shoulder range-of-motion exercises	A
Coaptation (sugar tong)	Distal radius/ulna fractures (most often Colles type), severe wrist injuries	From palmar crease along volar forearm, around elbow to dorsal forearm ending at MCP joints Thumb should point upward (neutral supination/pronation); wrist should be neutral for splint	B
Thumb spica	First phalangeal and metacarpal fractures/ dislocations, scaphoid injuries, gamekeeper's thumb, de Quervain's tendinitis	From tip of thumb (remains exposed for neurovascular checks) ending distal to antecubital fossa with the wrist in neutral position Thumb should be neutral (as if holding a soda can); thumb should be slightly adducted with gamekeeper's thumb	C
Radial gutter	Second or third (index and long finger) phalangeal (severe) and metacarpal fractures; carpal fractures/ dislocations	From distal index and long fingers along radial aspect of hand ending distal to antecubital fossa Cut large holes for Thumb and thenar eminence; 90 degrees flexion at MCP with slight extension at wrist	D

Continued

TABLE **8-3** Types of Splints—cont'd

Splint	Indications	Application	Illustration
Ulnar gutter	Fourth or fifth phalangeal (severe) and metacarpal fractures; carpal fractures/dislocations	• From distal ring and little fingers along ulnar aspect of hand ending distal to olecranon • Reduce boxer's fractures with splint in place; 90 degrees flexion at MCP with slight extension at wrist	E
Volar wrist	Wrist sprains; carpal tunnel syndrome; minor carpal fractures; NOT distal radius/ulna	• From palmar crease along volar aspect of hand and wrist ending at widest part of forearm flexors • Avoid excessive pressure over carpal tunnel, especially with carpal tunnel syndrome; do not immobilize thumb	F Ace wrap / Plaster / Webril / Stockinette/Webril
Dorsal finger	Mallet finger (avulsion fracture of dorsal aspect of distal phalanx or rupture of extensor tendon)	• Rigid object (splint, paper clip, popsicle stick) taped over DIP joint in full extension • Tape should be applied to both distal phalanx and middle phalanx to maintain joint in extension	G
Posterior knee splint (long leg splint)	Distal femur fractures; patellar fractures; knee injuries; proximal tibia fractures	• From distal tibia/fibula to mid thigh (medial/lateral or posterior); may extend past ankle (tibia fractures) • Use medial/lateral for MCL/LCL or meniscal injuries, posterior for ACL/PCL injuries, both for severe injuries	H

TABLE 8-3	Types of Splints—cont'd		
Splint	**Indications**	**Application**	**Illustration**
Posterior ankle	Achilles injuries; often used with stirrup splint for ankle fractures (see Bulky Jones)	From toes along plantar surface of foot behind ankle, ending just distal to popliteal fossa Should place ankle in plantar flexion with Achilles injury; may crack at apex if used alone for ankle injuries	I
Bulky Jones	Any lower leg, ankle, or foot injury with significant swelling	From metatarsal heads along medial and lateral aspect of lower leg; should cross ankle at malleoli Ankle should be neutral at 90 degrees of flexion; use posterior splint for additional strength, but avoid circumferential splint The cotton roll should be completely unrolled and split in half (with regard to thickness). It is then rerolled loosely to make application easier. After applying the stockinette, wrap the extremity loosely from toes to knee with the split cotton roll. A layer of Webril is applied to compress the cotton roll. Each Webril layer is overlaid by half of its width. The splint (posterior splint in combination with a sugar tong splint) is applied over the bulky Jones dressing and covered with an Ace wrap in the usual fashion	J K

MCP, metacarpophalangeal; *DIP,* distal interphalangeal; *MCL,* medial collateral ligament; *LCL,* lateral collateral ligament; *ACL,* anterior cruciate ligament; *PCL,* posterior cruciate ligament.
From Roppolo, L. P., Davis, D., Kelly, S. P., & Rosen, P. (2007). *Emergency medicine handbook: Critical concepts for clinical practice* (pp. 197-200). St. Louis: Mosby.

TABLE 8-4	Orthopedic Initial Immobilizing Devices and Techniques
Site	**Initial Immobilization**
Clavicle	Sling and swathe or figure-eight splint
Shoulder dislocation	
• Anterior	Splint to the body in the position found with an elastic bandage
• Posterior	Sling and swathe
Scapula	Sling and swathe
Humerus	Rigid splint with sling and swathe
Elbow	Rigid splint with sling and swathe in the position found
Forearm	Rigid splint with sling or air splint
Wrist	Rigid splint with sling
Hand and fingers	Rigid splint in the position of function
Spine	Full immobilization: long spine board, stiff cervical collar, and lateral head support
Pelvis	Long spine board, circumferential binding, or pneumatic antishock garment (PASG)
Hip	Long spine board, traction splint, or secure the affected leg to the unaffected leg
Femur	Traction splint, rigid splint, or PASG
Patella	Soft or padded rigid splint applied posteriorly in the position found
Tibia and fibula	Rigid splint or air splint
Ankle	Air splint or pillow
Foot	Air splint or pillow

Adapted from Proehl, J. A. (2004). *Emergency nursing procedures* (3rd ed.). St. Louis: Saunders.

Reduction of orthopedic injury

1. Obtain consent for procedure
2. Administer analgesics and anesthetics as directed
3. Apply postreduction immobilization devices

Tetanus immunization (Ing, 2007)

1. If the patient has never been immunized, administer 250 units of human tetanus immune globulin intramuscularly
2. If no tetanus shot has been given during the previous 10 years, administer tetanus toxoid 0.5 ml intramuscularly
3. For puncture wounds or contaminated wounds, administer tetanus toxoid 0.5 ml intramuscularly if the last immunization occurred ≥5 years prior

General Discharge Instruction

Aftercare of splints and casts (Roppolo et al., 2007)

1. Keep splint or cast dry
2. Maintain rest, ice, compression, and elevation (i.e., RICE)
3. Do not insert sharp objects into the cast or splint; if the skin under the casted or splinted area is itching, blow cool air down the cast or splint to sooth the area
4. Wiggle the digits every hour while awake
5. Return to the ED if any of the following occurs:
   a. Numbness or tingling
   b. Decreased sensation
   c. Temperature changes in digits
   d. Foul odor from cast or splint
   e. Foreign body lodged in cast or splint.

Crutch-walking techniques (Proehl, 2004)

1. Balance is the key to using crutches properly
2. There should be 1 to 1½ inches between the axilla and the top of the crutches
3. Hand rests should be positioned so that elbows are slightly bent (30 degrees of flexion) and so that the weight can be supported on the hands and wrists; the patient should never rest their weight on the axillary area, because this can cause damage to the axillary nerves
4. Crutches should be 12 inches forward and 6 inches to the side of the body when walking
5. When going up stairs, the uninjured leg goes up on the first step and is then followed with the injured leg and the crutches
6. When going down stairs, the crutches are placed down one step and then followed with the injured leg and then the uninjured leg

Use of a cane (Proehl, 2004)

1. With the patient standing upright, the appropriately sized cane will reach the patient's wrist when the cane is placed on the floor; the handgrips should be level with the ulnar side of the wrist
2. The cane is held with the elbow slightly bent in the hand opposite from the injured side
3. The cane and the injured leg should move together and touch the ground at the same time when walking; the cane is kept 4 to 5 inches forward
4. When going up stairs, the uninjured leg is moved first and followed by the cane and the injured leg
5. When going down stairs, the cane is placed on the step first and followed by the injured leg and then the uninjured leg

Walker (Proehl, 2004)

1. Walkers are used for patients who are unable to use crutches or a cane
2. When the patient is standing, the handgrips of the walker should be level with the wrist crease; the

patient should have a 15- to 25-degree bend of the elbow when grasping the handles to walk

3. If the patient can bear weight on only one leg, have him or her move the affected leg and the walker forward together using the arms to support his or her body weight, and then have him or her step up to the walker with the unaffected leg

Specific Orthopedic Emergencies

Low back pain
Definition: pain in the lower back region that is most commonly related to muscle strain, spasms, and ligament inflammation
1. Usually benign; affects up to 80% of the population at least once

Predisposing factors
1. Repetitive motions
2. Heavy lifting
3. Prolonged standing or sitting; poor posture
4. Increases with age

Clinical presentation
1. Subjective
   a. Recent injury or activity
      1) Acute: <7 days (ENA, 2007)
      2) Subacute: 7 days to 7 weeks (ENA, 2007)
      3) Chronic: >7 weeks (ENA, 2007)
   b. May report previous injuries
   c. Pain in lower back
   d. Stress at home or work
2. Objective
   a. Change in posture, gait, and stance
   b. May have spine abnormality
   c. Swelling, tenderness, and spasms
      1) Tenderness over the sciatic notch with radiation to the leg may indicate irritation of the sciatic nerve or nerve roots
   d. Limited spinal range of motion or painful arc
   e. Diminished knee and ankle reflexes in patients with radicular symptoms; determine if there is spinal cord compromise and, if so, at what level
   f. Weakness with dorsiflexion of the great toe and ankle may indicate L5 and some L4 root dysfunction
3. Diagnostic studies (Buttaro, Trybulski, Bailey, & Sandberg-Cook, 2003)
   a. Straight-leg raise test if the patient complains of pain that radiates down the legs; place the patient supine and raise affected leg with knee fully extended
      1) Considered positive if lifting the leg produces or worsens pain in that leg
      2) Pain that occurs when the angle is between 30 and 60 degrees is an indication of nerve root irritation
      3) If the patient has a popliteal compression, bending the knee while maintaining hip flexion should relieve the pain and pressure in the popliteal region
      4) If the patient has nerve root or sciatic nerve irritation, moving the knee back in full extension

during the straight-leg raise and dorsiflexing the ankle will increase the pain; this is known as *Lasegue sign*
   b. Radiography: provides details of the bone structures; used to check for instability, tumors, and fractures
   c. CT: provides more detail (e.g., herniated disc)
   d. MRI: provides detail of the disc and the nerve root; useful for finding tumors or spinal infections

Collaborative management
1. Continue assessment
   a. ABCDs
   b. Vital signs: blood pressure, pulse, respiratory rate, and temperature
   c. Pain or discomfort level
   d. Activity and range of motion
   e. Gait
2. Prevent and/or treat pain and discomfort
   a. Positioning for optimal comfort; pelvic tilt may alleviate or reduce pain (ENA, 2007)
   b. Medications as prescribed and indicated
      1) Analgesics
      2) Nonsteroidal anti-inflammatory drugs (NSAIDs)
      3) Muscle relaxants (e.g., cyclobenzaprine [Flexeril])
   c. Ice for acute injury for first 48 hours
3. Monitor for complications
   a. Bowel or bladder problems
   b. Motor weakness, numbness, tingling, and increasing pain in the legs

Evaluation
1. Alert and oriented with no neurovascular deficit
2. Control of pain, discomfort, or dyspnea

Typical disposition
1. If evaluation criteria met: discharge with instructions
   a. Mobilization and activity; bed rest is not recommended beyond 24 hours
   b. Use of proper body mechanics
   c. No lifting of objects >25 pounds until pain has resolved
   d. Home safety (e.g., rails in the tub and shower)
   e. Back strengthening exercises as directed
   f. Generally able to return to normal activities within 7 to 10 days
   g. Referral: arrange for assistive devices as needed (e.g., cane, elastic back brace)
   h. Follow up with primary care provider or specialist as instructed
2. Admission to the hospital for pain management if pain is intractable

Bursitis (Roppolo et al., 2007)
Definition: an inflammation of the bursa
1. There are >150 bursae in the human body
2. A bursa is a tiny, fluid-filled sac that contains a small amount of synovial fluid and that acts as a lubricant

to cushion movement between bones, tendons, and muscles

3. Common sites of bursitis are the shoulder, elbow, hip, knee, and heel

Predisposing factors

1. Repetitive use or trauma
2. Autoimmune disorders
3. Infection

Clinical presentation

1. Subjective
   a. Joint pain that improves with initial movement; continued activity or use increases pain
      1) Shoulder bursitis: anterior or lateral shoulder pain that worsens with overhead activities
      2) Hip bursitis: pain and tenderness over the trochanter
      3) Knee bursitis: pain and tenderness over the anterior knee with localized edema; severe pain is uncommon unless the condition is caused by infection
      4) Heel bursitis: heel pain that worsens with weight bearing; often a history of poorly fitting shoes
   b. Deep aching that interrupts sleep
   c. New recent activity or increased frequency of use of the involved joint
   d. Decreased range of motion
   e. Preexisting illnesses (e.g., arthritis, previous bursitis)
2. Objective
   a. Swelling and redness at site
   b. Area warm to touch
   c. May have limited strength as a result of pain with movement
   d. If the knee is affected, may be able to palpate a moving mass (i.e., housemaid's knee)
3. Diagnostic studies
   a. Ultrasound of area shows thickening and surrounding inflammation
   b. Needle aspiration of fluid from bursa
      1) CT or ultrasound may be needed to guide the aspiration of deep bursa
   c. Increased erythrocyte sedimentation rate if bursitis is related to autoimmune or inflammatory process (e.g., rheumatoid arthritis)

Collaborative management

1. Continue assessment
   a. ABCDs
   b. Pain and discomfort level
   c. Activity and range of motion
   d. Neurovascular assessment: 6 Ps
2. Reduce pain, discomfort, and/or inflammation
   a. Initial compression dressings and elevation with rest
   b. Rest for several days followed by range-of-motion exercises
   c. Cold therapy for the first 48 hours
   d. Analgesics and NSAIDs as prescribed

e. Antibiotics as prescribed if infection is suspected
3. Monitor for complications
   a. Infection of bursa
   b. Chronic bursitis

Evaluation

1. Control of pain and discomfort
2. Return to activities of daily living (ADL)
3. Normal neurovascular status
4. No indications of infection

Typical disposition

1. If evaluation criteria met: discharge with instructions
   a. Medications and rest as directed
   b. Joint rest or exercise as directed; exercise is recommended after pain subsides to restore and maintain function
   c. Avoidance of excessive exercise and repetitive movements that exacerbate the condition
      1) Take frequent breaks when doing repetitive tasks
      2) Use cushioned chairs when sitting and cushioned or foam pads under the knees when kneeling
      3) Avoid leaning, kneeling, or sitting on hard surfaces for any extended period
      4) Wear low-heeled shoes and replace running shoes as soon as the soles wear out
   d. Referral: may require evaluation by an orthopedist
2. If evaluation criteria not met: admission so that the bursa can be surgically drained if infected

Tendinitis
Definition: the inflammation to a tendon related to repetitive stress

1. Elbow (ENA, 2007)
   a. Lateral epicondylitis (i.e., tennis elbow)
   b. Medial epicondylitis (i.e., golfer's elbow)
2. Shoulder: rotator cuff tendinitis
3. Knee: patellar tendinitis (i.e., jumper's knee)
4. Heel: Achilles tendinitis (i.e., Achilles heel)

Predisposing factors

1. Previous history of tendinitis
2. Pain that increases with motion
3. Repetitive use of area

Clinical presentation

1. Subjective
   a. History that is likely to reveal the following:
      1) Repetitive motion that involves the affected area
      2) Previous episodes of tendinitis
   b. Pain
      1) Deep ache that increases in severity with motion
         a) May occur at night
      2) Pressure with rolling motion over tendon
2. Objective
   a. Swelling at site

b. Tenderness with palpation
c. Tenderness with rolling motion over tendon
3. Diagnostic studies
   a. Radiographs may be requested to look for calcific deposits, which can be caused by tendinitis

Collaborative management

1. Continue assessment
   a. ABCDs
   b. Pain and discomfort level
   c. Range of motion and function
2. Prevent and/or treat pain and discomfort
   a. Sling or brace to help rest the tendon
   b. Ice for the first 48 hours for acute tendonitis
   c. Compression dressings to support the tendon; remove twice a day
   d. Elevation of the affected joint if appropriate
   e. NSAIDs
3. Monitor for complications
   a. Recurrence of tendinitis
   b. Chronic inflammation of the tendon

Evaluation

1. Control of pain and discomfort
2. Return to ADLs
3. Absence of indications of inflammation or infection

Typical disposition: discharge with instructions

1. Use of splint or brace as directed
2. Cold and heat applications as directed
3. Prevention
   a. Warm up by exercising at a relaxed pace before more intense exercise
   b. Keep all muscles strong and flexible with regular exercise and stretching
   c. Avoid repetitive motion and the overuse of the extremities
4. Referrals
   a. Physical therapy: to stretch and strengthen the tendon
   b. Surgery: in rare insistences, the patient may require follow up for the surgical removal of inflamed tissue

Gout
Definition: urate or calcium crystals are deposited into a joint, which causes a crystal-induced arthritis

1. Three stages of gout: asymptomatic hyperuricemia, acute, and tophaceous (ENA, 2007)

Predisposing factors (Roppolo et al., 2007)

1. Male-to-female occurrence ratio is 9:1
2. Obesity
3. Alcohol use
4. Diabetes
5. Hypertension
6. Thiazides
7. High consumption of foods rich in purines

Clinical presentation

1. Subjective
   a. Joint pain: affects insteps, ankles, heels, knees, wrists, fingers, and elbows (ENA, 2007)
      1) Pain that began in one joint and that moves into more joints
         a) Monoarticular: first occurrence is usually in the first metatarsophalangeal joint
      2) Pain occurrence that increases in frequency and severity
         a) Polyarticular: lower extremities most common
      3) Clothing, movement, or weight bearing causes intolerable pain
2. Objective
   a. Affected joints are swollen, red, and tender when palpated or touched
   b. May have a fever (may be >101° F)
   c. Reluctance to use or move affect joint
3. Diagnostic studies (Roppolo et al., 2007)
   a. CBC: WBC and erythrocyte sedimentation rate (ESR) increased during acute episodes
   b. Uric acid levels: may be increased or normal
   c. Radiographs: may show soft-tissue swelling and bone erosion
      1) Chronic gout may have rat-bitten appearance (ENA, 2007)
      2) Pseudogout may show degenerative changes and calcification (ENA, 2007)
   d. Synovial fluid analysis: definitive test
      1) Gout
         a) Monosodium urate crystals are found; these are needle shaped and look yellow when aligned parallel to the axis of a red compensator; they will turn blue when aligned across the polarization direction (ENA, 2007)
      2) Pseudogout: calcium pyrophosphate crystals are found; these are rhomboid shaped, weakly positively birefringed, and difficult to see; they will not change color with alignment like monosodium urate crystals do

Collaborative management

1. Continue assessment
   a. ABCDs
   b. Pain and discomfort level
   c. Range of motion and activity level
   d. Neurovascular assessment: 6 Ps
2. Prevent and/or treat pain and discomfort
   a. NSAIDs (e.g., ibuprofen [Motrin])
   b. Steroids
      1) Oral (e.g., prednisone [Deltasone]) may be prescribed
      2) Injection into affected joint
   c. Colchicine (Colcrys) may be given to young, healthy patients with acute gout
3. Monitor for complications
   a. Recurring attacks of gout
   b. Damage to joints and cartilage

c. Kidney stones
d. Uncontrollable pain
e. Medication side effects

Evaluation
1. Control of pain and discomfort
2. Improvement in range of motion

Typical disposition: discharge with instructions
1. Weight reduction for obese patients
2. Avoidance of precipitating factors (e.g., alcohol, thiazides, high-purine diet)
3. Increase in fluid intake to prevent stone formation
4. Medications as prescribed (including information about side effects)
5. Avoidance of aspirin because it interferes with uric acid excretion
6. Referral: follow up with primary care provider

Carpal tunnel syndrome
Definition: compression neuropathy of the median nerve at the wrist; this is the most common nerve entrapment syndrome
Predisposing factor is thought to be repetitive motion, but the exact mechanism is not known
Clinical presentation
1. Subjective
   a. Pain
   b. Paresthesia, numbness, and weakness
   c. History of repetitive action motion
   d. Tinel sign: tapping lightly over the medial nerve causes a sensation of tingling that indicates nerve irritation
   e. Phalen test: push the back of the hands together for 1 minute to compress the carpal tunnel; this test is positive if a tingling sensation is felt in the distribution of the medial nerve over the hand
2. Objective
   a. Soft-tissue swelling may occur
   b. Muscle tingling
   c. Atrophy in the surrounding muscles
   d. Red shiny skin above the affected area
3. Diagnostic studies
   a. Wrist radiography: to rule out bony abnormalities
   b. Nerve conduction studies

Collaborative management
1. Continue assessment
   a. ABCDs
   b. Pain and discomfort level
   c. Muscle strength
   d. Neurovascular assessment: 6 Ps
2. Prevent and/or treat pain and discomfort
   a. Rest or reduced activity
   b. Ice to affected area
   c. Elevation
   d. Compression dressings applied to the area
   e. NSAIDs

3. Maintain joint function
   a. Splint at night
   b. Physical therapy
4. Monitor for complications
   a. Permanent nerve damage

Evaluation
1. Control of pain and discomfort
2. Improvement of range of motion
3. Return to ADLs

Typical disposition: discharge with instructions
1. Immobilization and elevation of affected area (i.e., RICE)
2. Removal of compression dressings twice a day
3. Referrals
   a. Orthopedist follow-up
   b. Physical therapy may be scheduled

Joint effusion
Definition: the collection of fluid in the joints as a result of an inflammatory process; usually occurs in the knee
Predisposing factors
1. Recent or past trauma
2. New activity or the repetitive use of the joint
3. Medication use (e.g., loop diuretics)
4. Recent surgery
5. Hemophilic patient with minimal blunt trauma to the knee who is at risk for bleeding into the joint (i.e., hemarthrosis)
6. If septic arthritis is present, the patient may have a history of substance abuse

Clinical presentation
1. Subjective
   a. Patient reports a history of repetitive joint use or trauma
   b. Pain at joint site
   c. Chills and malaise
   d. Inability to bear weight
2. Objective
   a. Tenderness at site with palpation
   b. Fever
   c. Swelling and redness at joint site
   d. Decreased range of motion
3. Diagnostic studies
   a. ESR increased
   b. WBC may be increased
   c. Arthrocentesis
      1) WBC of 20,000 to 60,000/mm^3 with normal glucose level indicates inflammatory process; ≥100,000/mm^3 with decreased glucose level indicates infection
   d. Rapid plasma reagin, hepatitis B, and C-reactive proteins: to rule out other causes
   e. Joint radiography: to compare extremities

Collaborative management
1. Continue assessment
   a. ABCDs

b. Pain and discomfort level
c. Range of motion and activity
d. Neurovascular status
e. Skin changes in color, integrity, or size
2. Prevent and/or treat pain and discomfort
   a. Rest or reduced activity
   b. Ice applied to affected area
   c. Compression dressings applied to area
   d. Elevation of the affected limb
   e. Analgesics, NSAIDs, or both
3. Maintain joint function
   a. Immobilization of affected joint
   b. Preparation for possible arthrocentesis
      (i.e., joint aspiration)
   c. Antibiotics as indicated
4. Monitor for complications
   a. Uncontrollable pain
   b. Meniscus tear
   c. Sepsis

Evaluation

1. Control of pain and discomfort
2. Improvement in range of motion
3. Return to ADLs
4. Neurovascular assessment: 6 Ps
5. Absence of indications of inflammation or infection

Typical disposition: discharge with instructions

1. RICE
2. Any prescribed medications
3. Indications for the need for reevaluation by the primary care provider

Costochondritis

Definition: the inflammation of a rib and sternal junction that causes pain and tenderness; usually more than one of the seven costochondral junctions are affected when this condition occurs (Flowers & Wippermann, 2007)

1. Differential from Tietze syndrome: Tietze syndrome has the same symptoms, but the patient will have swelling at the rib–cartilage junction

Predisposing factors

1. Repetitive minor trauma
2. Chest surgery or trauma
3. History of IV substance abuse
4. Recent upper respiratory infection that caused force-ful coughing

Clinical presentation

1. Subjective
   a. Onset usually insidious, with a history of repeated minor trauma or new activity
   b. Chest pain
      1) Sharp, aching, or pressure type of pain; tenderness with palpation
      2) May be severe

3) May radiate to either arm
4) Worsens on deep inspiration, coughing, or trunk movement
5) Lessens with shallow breathing, decreased movement, and the application of heat
2. Objective
   a. Redness and warmth at the site of tenderness
   b. Absence of chest swelling or crepitus
   c. Chest tenderness with palpation
3. Diagnostic studies
   a. Chest radiography: to rule out other possible causes
   b. Other diagnostic studies (e.g., CBC, ESR, C-reactive protein): to rule out other possible causes

Collaborative management

1. Continue assessment
   a. ABCDs
   b. Breath sounds
   c. Oxygen saturation
   d. Pain and discomfort level
2. Prevent and/or treat pain and discomfort
   a. Rest
   b. Analgesics and NSAIDs as prescribed
   c. Muscle relaxants as prescribed
3. Maintain normal ventilatory function
   a. Deep breathing exercises, incentive spirometry, or both
4. Monitoring for complications
   a. Uncontrollable pain
   b. Atelectasis and/or pneumonia
   c. Chronic costochondritis (rare)

Evaluation

1. Absence of clinical indications of respiratory distress
2. Control of pain, discomfort, or dyspnea

Typical disposition: discharge with instructions

1. Rest and perform deep-breathing exercises every 1 to 2 hours
2. Avoid activities that aggravate or increase symptoms
3. Referral: follow up with primary care provider in 1 week

Osteoarthritis

Definition: degeneration and loss of articular cartilage that results in joint pain

1. Most common form of arthritis; commonly affects the knee, hand, spine, and hip
2. Also referred to as *degenerative joint disease* and *osteoarthrosis* (Mayo Clinic, 2007))
3. Symptoms gradually worsen over time; usually occur in one joint, but can occur in more than one

Predisposing factors

1. Age: >40 years (men, usually <45; women, >55 years)
2. Gender: females have a greater tendency to develop this condition, but the reason why is unclear
3. History of bone deformities, illnesses (e.g., Paget disease), or injuries (e.g., sports injuries)
4. Obesity

Clinical presentation

1. Subjective
   a. Gradual onset of symptoms
   b. History of stiffness in the morning and asymmetric joint pain that is better with rest and that increases with activity; pain typically worse later in the day
   c. Pain and grating sensations with movement
2. Objective
   a. Joint enlargement and/or deformity
   b. Limited range of motion of the affected joints
   c. Crepitus may be palpated
   d. Swelling or hard lumps (i.e., bone spurs)
   e. Heberden nodes: nodular swelling of the distal interphalangeal joint if affected
   f. Bouchard nodes: nodular swelling of the proximal interphalangeal joint if affected
3. Diagnostic studies
   a. Radiography
      1) Narrowing of the space within the joint as a result of cartilage breakdown
      2) Cyst formation
      3) Bone hypertrophy
   b. Joint fluid analysis: to differentiate between inflammation and arthritis
      1) Inflammation: cell count usually >2000 cells/mm³
      2) Osteoarthritis: cell count <500 cells/mm³
   c. Arthroscopy: to view the joint space

Collaborative management

1. Continue assessment
   a. ABCDs
   b. Pain and discomfort level
   c. Range of motion
2. Reduce pain, discomfort, and/or inflammation
   a. Rest of joint and avoidance of activity that requires repetitive joint movement
   b. Hot and cold therapy
      1) Heat relieves stiffness
      2) Cold relieves muscle spasms
   c. Analgesics and NSAIDs as prescribed
   d. Pain-relieving creams (e.g., methyl salicylate topical [ArthriCare], capsaicin topical [Zostrix]) may be used
   e. Initial compression dressings and elevation with rest
   f. Rest of joint for several days followed by range-of-motion exercises
   g. Cold therapy for the first 48 hours
   h. Antibiotics as prescribed if infection is suspected
3. Restore normal joint function
   a. Counseling regarding weight loss
   b. Exercise recommended to increase endurance and strengthen muscle
4. Monitor for complications
   a. Uncontrollable pain
   b. Stress fractures
   c. Bleeding or infection into the joint
   d. Depression

Evaluation

1. Control of pain or discomfort to a level that allows the patient to continue with normal activities of daily living
2. Stabilization of stress fractures

Typical disposition: discharge with instructions

1. Regular exercise
2. Calcium to preserve bone mass
3. Referral: primary care provider or orthopedist for further definitive testing as indicated

Osteoporosis

Definition: a weakening of the bone that is characterized by low bone mass and the structural deterioration of bone tissue that leads to the bones being brittle and susceptible to injury (National Osteoporosis Foundation, 2008)

1. Low bone density without a fracture does not cause pain, so osteoporosis may not be recognized

Predisposing factors

1. Aging
2. Gender: female
3. Low body mass: small and thin frame
4. Family history of osteoporosis and/or fractures
5. Diet low in calcium and vitamin D; increased intake of protein, caffeine, or carbonated beverages
6. Low estrogen or testosterone levels
7. Inactive lifestyle
8. Medications (e.g., steroids, anticonvulsants)

Clinical presentation

1. Subjective
   a. Bone pain: if a patient with osteoporosis presents with pain, fracture and other causes of pain will need to be ruled out
      1) Pain started after feeling a "pop"
2. Objective
   a. Height loss of more than 1½ to 2 inches during the prior 10 years
   b. Fracture that occurred with minimal or no trauma (i.e., pathologic fracture)
      1) Common sites for fracture: vertebra, proximal femur, and wrist
      2) Hip pain and limp: may indicate hip or pelvic fracture
      3) Vertebral compression fracture
         a) Dowager's hump: thoracic spine kyphotic deformity that results from multiple vertebral compression fractures
      4) Colles fracture of wrist if there is a history of fall; this is frequently the first sign of osteoporosis in women <65 years old (ENA, 2007)
   c. May have indications of secondary osteoporosis
      1) Band keratopathy: result of the precipitation of calcium salts on the corneal surface; may indicate possible hyperparathyroidism (Taravella, 2006)

2) Exophthalmos (i.e., lid lag), goiter, tremors, weight loss, and moist, warm skin indicate hyperthyroidism (Buttaro et al., 2003)

3) Decreased facial or axillary hair may indicate hypogonadism

4) Blue sclera may indicate osteogenesis imperfecta (Buttaro et al., 2003)

3. Diagnostic studies
   a. Radiography: to rule out fracture
   b. CT and MRI: to rule out fractures
   c. Bone mineral density (BMD)

Collaborative management

1. Continue assessment
   a. ABCDs
   b. Fall risk: balance, gait, reflexes, and poor visual acuity
   c. Pain and discomfort level
2. Prevent and/or treat pain and discomfort
   a. Rest or reduced activity
3. Promote safe mobility and prevent or treat stress fractures
   a. Calcium and vitamin D
   b. Antiresorptive medications: bisphosphonates (e.g., alendronate [Fosamax], ibandronate [Boniva])
   c. Appropriate treatment of fractures and analgesics as prescribed
4. Monitor for complications
   a. Chronic pain
   b. Stress fractures

Evaluation

1. Control of pain or discomfort
2. Stabilization of fractures

Typical disposition

1. If evaluation criteria met: discharge with instructions
   a. Prevention of falls
      1) Careful when lifting, bending, going up and down stairs, and ambulating
      2) Remove loose carpet, throw rugs, and so on that may increase the potential for falls
      3) Remove obstacles that may cause tripping
      4) Brighter lighting
   b. Deceleration of progression
      1) Calcium and vitamin D supplements as directed
      2) Healthy, balanced diet
      3) Regular weight-bearing exercise
   c. Referrals
      1) Physical therapist
      2) Nutritionist
      3) Endocrinologist if the cause is hyperparathyroidism or hyperthyroidism
      4) Pain specialist if there is persistent chronic pain
2. If evaluation criteria not met (e.g., unstable fracture): admission

Specific Orthopedic Trauma

Contusions and hematomas

Definitions: a contusion is a closed wound in which a ruptured blood vessel has hemorrhaged into the surrounding tissue; this may form a hematoma

1. Presence of necrotic tissue and hematoma initiates an inflammatory reaction that can cause edema and possible further cell death

Predisposing factors

1. Blunt trauma
2. Coagulopathy

Clinical presentation

1. Subjective
   a. Soreness or pain at site
      1) Tender with palpation
      2) Pain may or may not increase with activity
2. Objective
   a. Swelling
   b. Skin discoloration (ENA, 2007)
      1) 24 to 48 hours after injury: reddish blue or purple
      2) 5 to 7 days after injury: greenish outside that is moving inward toward center
      3) 7 to 10 days after injury: yellowish
      4) 10 to 14 days after injury: brown
      5) 2 to 4 weeks after injury: healed and area back to normal
   c. Increased tenderness with palpation of the area
3. Diagnostic studies
   a. Radiography: to rule out fracture
   b. CBC: to rule out blood loss
   c. Coagulation profile: to rule out coagulopathy

Collaborative management

1. Continue assessment
   a. ABCDs
   b. Pain and discomfort level
   c. Indications of bleeding
   d. Neurovascular assessment: 6 Ps
2. Reduce pain, discomfort, and/or inflammation
   a. Rest for several days followed by range-of-motion exercises
   b. Ice: cold therapy for the first 48 hours
   c. Compression dressings
   d. Elevation with rest
   e. Analgesics and NSAIDs as prescribed
3. Restore normal regional function and prevent further injury
   a. Splint extremity
4. Monitor for complications
   a. Ischemia caused by vascular compression
   b. Compartment syndrome

Evaluation

1. Control of pain and discomfort
2. Alert and oriented with no neurologic deficit

Typical disposition: discharge with instructions
1. RICE
2. Splint care and application
3. Proper use of physical assistive devices (e.g., crutches) if indicated
4. Proper use of analgesics and NSAIDs

Sprain
Definition: an injury that occurs as a result of the tearing or stretching of ligaments that support moveable joints
1. First degree: involves a few ligaments (ENA, 2007)
2. Second degree: partial ligament tear (ENA, 2007)
3. Third degree: complete disruption of the ligament (ENA, 2007)

Predisposing factors
1. History of bone disease
2. Injury
3. Obesity

Clinical presentation
1. Subjective
   a. History of injury
   b. Pain or tenderness at site
   c. Activity intolerance
2. Objective
   a. Swelling or deformity at site
   b. Decreased range of motion (ROM)
   c. Increased tenderness at site with palpation
3. Diagnostic studies
   a. Radiography: to rule out fractures or dislocations
   b. Ottawa rules for knee, ankles, and feet help to determine if radiography films are needed (Table 8-5)
      1) These rules were developed by a emergency medical team in Ottawa, Canada (Stiell, et al., 1992)

Collaborative management
1. Continue assessment
   a. ABCDs
   b. Pain and discomfort level
   c. Neurovascular checks: 6 Ps
2. Reduce pain, discomfort, and/or inflammation
   a. Rest for several days followed by range-of-motion exercises
   b. Ice: cold therapy for the first 48 hours
   c. Compression dressings
   d. Elevation with rest
   e. Analgesics and NSAIDs as prescribed
   f. Antibiotics as prescribed if infection is suspected
3. Restore normal regional function
   a. Application of immobilization device (e.g., splint, cast)
4. Monitor for complications
   a. Uncontrolled pain
   b. Neurovascular compromise

Evaluation
1. Control of pain and discomfort
2. Alert and oriented with no neurovascular deficit

Typical disposition: discharge with instructions
1. RICE
   a. Cold therapy four times a day
2. Care and use of splint if applicable
3. No weight bearing; use of crutches if required
4. Referral: follow up with primary care provider or orthopedist as indicated

Fractures
Definition: a break in the continuity of bone
1. Two categories: closed (also called *simple*) or open (also called *compound*)
2. Types of fractures
   a. Pathologic: occurs because of a bone pathology (e.g., osteoporosis, malignancy)

TABLE 8-5   Ottawa Rules

Area	Indications for Radiography	Associated Signs
Ankle	• Acute ankle pain plus one of the associated signs	• Bony tenderness at the posterior tip of the medial malleolus • Bony tenderness at the posterior edge of the lateral malleolus • Inability to bear weight both immediately after the injury and in the ED
Knee	• Age of ≥50 yr • Tenderness at the head of the fibula • Isolated tenderness of the patella • Inability to flex knee to 90 degrees • Inability to bear weight immediately after injury or in the ED	
Foot	• Pain in the midfoot region plus one of the associated signs	• Bony tenderness at the base of the fifth metatarsal • Bony tenderness at the navicular or cuboid • Inability to bear weight immediately after injury or in the ED

From Stiell, I. G., Greenberg, G. H., McKnight, R. D., Nair, R. C., McDowell, I., & Worthington, J. R. (1994). Implementation of the Ottawa ankle rules. *Journal of the American Medical Association, 271,* 827-832.

b. Displaced: ends of bone are not aligned

c. Transverse: fracture is directly across the bone

d. Oblique: fracture is angled across the bone

e. Spiral: fracture resulted from a twisting motion

f. Comminuted: bone broken into fragments

g. Avulsion: a separation of a bone fragment from the bone

h. Impact: the compression of the bone with shortening

i. Torus or buckle fracture: an incomplete fracture in which one side of the bone may buckle upon itself without disrupting the other side

j. Compression: one bone forced against another

k. Greenstick: periosteum divided on only one side

l. Epiphyseal: fracture through the epiphyseal plate

m. Nursemaid's elbow: subluxation of the radial head (usually seen in children who are 2-3 years old; caused by the pulling of the arm)

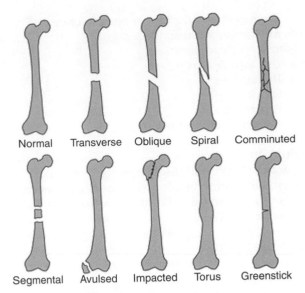

Figure 8-1 Types of fractures.

Predisposing factors

1. Aging: the chance of fracture increases with age.
2. Falls
3. Osteoporosis or bone malignancy
4. Smoking weakens the bones and can delay healing
5. Low body weight may lead to a higher risk of hip fracture
6. Previous fractures
   a. Spine fracture usually indicates osteoporosis and a particularly high risk of additional spine fractures

Clinical presentation

1. Subjective
   a. May have a medical history that predisposes to fracture (e. g., immune disorders, osteoporosis)
   b. May have a history of the injury: location, time, and circumstances
   c. Pain or spasm in the area
   d. Activity intolerance or limited movement
2. Objective
   a. Deformity or swelling
   b. Changes in gait and limited ROM
   c. Spasms may be palpated or seen during inspection
   d. Tenderness, instability, or crepitus with palpation
   e. May have a break in the skin integrity or an obvious open fracture as part of a compound fracture
   f. May have associated injuries (e.g., chest, abdomen)
   g. May have neurovascular compromise: 6 Ps
3. Diagnostic studies
   a. Radiography of extremity
      1) See types of fractures (Figure 8-1)
         a) Must have complete views and be able to see joints above and below injury
         b) For children, opposite extremity view also required to evaluate the epiphyseal configuration
      2) May require stress views
   b. CT and possibly MRI for more complex complications

Collaborative management

1. Continue assessment
   a. ABCDs
   b. Pain and discomfort level
   c. Neurovascular assessment: 6 Ps
   d. Clinical indications of bleeding
2. Reduce pain, discomfort, and/or inflammation
   a. Rest with immobilization
   b. Ice: cold therapy for the first 48 hours
   c. Compression dressings
   d. Elevation with rest
   e. Analgesics and NSAIDs as prescribed; regional blocks may also be used
3. Restore normal regional function and prevent further injury
   a. Immobilization of the joints above and below the fracture
      1) Splint in position found unless pulseless distal to injury; in that case, reposition extremity and recheck pulse
   b. Medical antishock trousers (MAST)
      1) Although controversial, these are still sometimes used to stabilize pelvic and lower-extremity fractures
      2) If used, close monitoring for vascular compromise is required
   c. Wound management for open fractures
      1) Cover wound with sterile dressing
      2) Avoid bacteriostatic cleansers (e.g., Betadine), which may inhibit wound healing
   d. Closed reduction may be performed
      1) Obtain informed consent
      2) Monitor vital signs and ventilation during procedural sedation and analgesia
      3) Apply a postreduction immobilization device

e. Tetanus immunization for open fractures

f. Antibiotics as prescribed

4. Monitor for complications
   a. Uncontrolled pain
   b. Hemorrhage
   c. Shock
   d. Fat emboli
   e. Compartment syndrome

Evaluation

1. Control of pain and discomfort
2. Alert and oriented with no neurovascular deficit
3. Absence of clinical indicators of hypoperfusion
4. Fracture stabilized

Typical disposition

1. If evaluation criteria met: discharge with instructions
   a. RICE
   b. Assistive devices (e.g., crutches)
   c. Cast or splint care
   d. Medications (e.g., analgesics, antibiotics)
2. If evaluation criteria not met: admission for surgical reduction, fracture stabilization, or the management of concurrent injuries or illnesses

Dislocations

Definition: the surfaces of the bones that form a joint are t longer in contact and lose their anatomic position

1. Sternoclavicular joint: this is a rare injury; if it occurs, consider underlying thoracic trauma
2. Anterior shoulder: seen among younger patients and can recur
3. Posterior shoulder: uncommon injury; associated with seizures and ethanol abuse
4. Elbow or knee: neurovascular compromise can occur; the permanent loss of some function is common
5. Posterior hip: common; extremity flexed and adducted with loss of ROM
6. Anterior hip:
   a. Deformity with wide abduction and the external rotation of the extremity
   b. The affected leg will appear to be shorter than the unaffected leg
   c. Femoral head necrosis can occur, thus making this a true emergency

Predisposing factors

1. Trauma
2. Previous dislocation
3. More common among younger adults

Clinical presentation

1. Subjective
   a. History of mechanism of injury
   b. Intense pain
2. Objective
   a. Obvious deformity
   b. Decreased range of motion

c. Changes in length of affected extremity as compared with the unaffected one

d. May have neurovascular compromise with diminished or absent pulses, delayed capillary refill, muscle weakness, tingling, or coolness distal to site

e. Tenderness with palpation

3. Diagnostic studies
   a. Radiography
      1) To verify dislocation and rule out fracture
      2) To check successful reduction after a reduction procedure

Collaborative management

1. Continue assessment
   a. ABCDs
   b. Pain and discomfort level
   c. Neurovascular status: 6 Ps
2. Reduce pain, discomfort, and/or inflammation
   a. Immobilization
   b. Ice: cold therapy for the first 48 hours
   c. Elevation
   d. Analgesics and NSAIDs as prescribed
3. Restore normal regional function and prevent further injury
   a. Reduction
      1) Obtain informed consent
      2) Monitor vital signs and ventilation during conscious sedation
      3) Apply a postreduction immobilization device (e.g., sling)
      4) Perform neurovascular checks before and after reduction
      5) May require consultation with orthopedist
4. Monitor for complications
   a. Hemorrhage
   b. Compartment syndrome

Evaluation

1. Control of pain and discomfort
2. Alert and oriented with no neurovascular deficit
3. Absence of clinical indicators of hypoperfusion
4. Dislocation resolved

Typical disposition

1. If evaluation criteria met: discharge with instructions
   a. Rest and apply ice as directed
   b. Use of immobilization device as directed
   c. Medications (e.g., NSAIDs)
   d. Follow up with orthopedics provider
2. If evaluation criteria not met: admission for surgical reduction

Traumatic amputations

Definition: the loss of body part that occurs as a result of an accident

1. Amputations with straight, clean cuts have a better chance for reattachment
2. Crush injuries usually have extensive soft-tissue damage and possible muscle damage, which creates a

more difficult reattachment challenge with decreased success

Predisposing factors
1. Greater incidence in farm and factory work settings
2. Motor vehicle collisions
3. Use of lawnmowers, saws, and power tools

Clinical presentation
1. Subjective
   a. Pain
   b. Mechanism of injury
2. Objective
   a. Obvious injury and wound
   b. Deformities and angulation of stump and amputated part
   c. Uncontrolled bleeding and blood loss
   d. Neurovascular compromise of stump
   e. Possible contamination of stump and amputated part
3. Diagnostic studies
   a. Two radiography views: injury site and amputated part
   b. Blood type and crossmatch blood

Collaborative management
1. Continue assessment
   a. ABCDs
   b. Pain and discomfort level
   c. Neurovascular assessment: 6 Ps
   d. Clinical indications of bleeding
2. Ensure adequate airway, breathing, and ventilation
   a. Positioning and/or artificial airway to maintain the patency of the airway
   b. Oxygen by nasal cannula at 2 to 6 L/minute if to maintain an SpO_2 level of 95% unless contraindicated; for patients with chronic obstructive pulmonary disease (COPD), use pulse oximetry to guide oxygen administration to an SpO_2 level of 90%
3. Maintain adequate circulation and perfusion
   a. Intravenous access with two large-bore catheters for fluid and medication administration
   b. Fluid replacement
      1) Crystalloids: usually 0.9% saline
      2) Red packed cells or other blood products as prescribed
         a) Should be given early if significant blood loss is suspected to prevent tissue hypoxia
         b) Replacement of platelets, clotting factors, and calcium should be considered if multiple transfusions are given
      3) Colloids as prescribed
   c. Control of bleeding
      1) Direct pressure to control hemorrhage; tourniquets are not recommended
      2) Minimization of movement of stump to decrease risk of renewed hemorrhage
4. Restore normal regional function and prevent further injury
   a. Stump care
      1) Handle stump and amputated part gently
      2) Clean stump and amputated part gently with a large amount of normal saline
      3) Do not rub the stump; apply a moist sterile dressing and wrap in a light compression dressing (e.g., ACE bandage)
      4) Splint and elevate the stump
   b. Surgery for reimplantation if possible
      1) Ensure that the patient receives nothing by mouth
      2) Preserve the amputated extremity or digit for reimplantation
         a) Wrap the part in a moist, sterile, saline gauze dressing
         b) Place the part in a plastic bag and seal the bag
         c) Place the plastic bag in ice water
         d) Label the plastic bag with the patient's name and ID number as well as the date, and send it to the operating department with the patient
         e) Monitor the bag closely, and do not let the amputated part freeze
5. Reduce pain, discomfort, and/or inflammation
   a. Analgesics and NSAIDs as prescribed
6. Treat infection if present, and prevent sepsis
   a. Antibiotics as prescribed if infection is suspected
   b. Antipyretics and cooling methods to reduce fever
   c. Tetanus immunization as indicated
7. Monitor for complications
   a. Inability to reimplant amputated part
      1) Factors that affect the success of reattachment include the following:
         a) Contamination of the area
         b) Prolonged time period between the injury and the cooling of the area and the amputated part
         c) Degloving or avulsion of tissue
      2) With cooling, amputated body parts may be viable for up to 12 hours, and digits may be viable for up to 24 hours (ENA, 2007)
   b. Infection and sepsis

Evaluation
1. Control of pain and discomfort
2. Absence of clinical indications of hypoperfusion
3. Absence of clinical indications of infection or sepsis
4. Alert and oriented with no neurovascular deficit

Typical disposition: admission; may go directly from ED to surgery for control of bleeding and/or for the reattachment of the amputated part

Specific Orthopedic Life-Threatening Complications
Hemorrhage from fractures
Definition: blood loss that occurs as a result of a fracture
1. May or may not be visible; can continue for up to 48 hours

2. Estimated blood loss that occurs with fractures (Table 8-6)

Predisposing factors
1. Traumatic injury
2. History of coagulopathy
3. Medications that affect clotting (e.g., aspirin, NSAIDs)

Clinical presentation
1. Subjective
   a. May have history of coagulopathy and/or use of medications that affect clotting
   b. Pain
   c. Mechanism of injury
2. Objective
   a. Tachycardia
   b. Hypotension
   c. Swelling and possible discoloration in the affected area
   d. Clinical indications of hypoperfusion (e.g., pale and cool skin, decrease in urine output, changes in mentation or level of consciousness)
3. Diagnostic studies
   a. CBC: low hemoglobin and hematocrit levels
   b. Coagulation profile
   c. Blood type and crossmatch blood
   d. Radiography of the injured area

Collaborative management
1. Continue assessment
   a. ABCDs
   b. Hemodynamic status
   c. Neurovascular assessment: 6 Ps
   d. Pain and discomfort level
2. Maintain airway, oxygenation, and ventilation
   a. Positioning and/or artificial airway to ensure patency of the airway
   b. Oxygen by nasal cannula at 2-6 liters/minute to maintain SpO_2 of 95% unless contraindicated; for patients with COPD, use pulse oximetry to guide oxygen administration to SpO_2 of 90%
3. Maintain adequate circulation and perfusion
   a. Measures to control bleeding
      1) Direct pressure to control the hemorrhage; tourniquets are not recommended
      2) Immobilization of the area to decrease blood loss
      3) Elevation and ice applied to the area
   b. IV access with two large-bore catheters for fluid and medication administration
      1) Fluid replacement
         a) Crystalloids: usually 0.9% saline
         b) Red packed cells or other blood products as prescribed
            i) Should be given early if significant blood loss is suspected to prevent tissue hypoxia
            ii) Replacement of platelets, clotting factors, and calcium should be considered if multiple transfusions are given
         c) Colloids as prescribed
4. Reduce pain, discomfort, and/or inflammation
   a. Analgesics and NSAIDs as prescribed
   b. Antibiotics as prescribed if infection is suspected
   c. Tetanus immunization as indicated
5. Monitor for complications
   a. Hypovolemia
   b. Hypovolemic shock
   c. Hypoperfusion of organs

Evaluation
1. Absence of clinical indications of bleeding
2. Absence of clinical indications of hypoperfusion
3. Absence of clinical indications of infection or sepsis
4. Alert and oriented with no neurovascular deficit
5. Control of pain and discomfort

Typical disposition: admission; may go from ED to surgery
Compartment syndrome
Definition: the condition that occurs when interstitial pressure exceeds capillary pressure, thus causing localized muscle and nerve ischemia
1. Results in vascular and neurologic compromise
2. Occurs more often in the lower arm or lower leg or the hand or foot area
   a. Occurrence in the upper arm or upper leg is associated with prolonged compression
3. If untreated, compartment syndrome can lead to tissue necrosis, permanent functional impairment, and, in severe cases, renal failure and death (Paula & Chiang, 2006)

Predisposing factors
1. Long-bone injury
2. Crush injuries
3. Venous or vascular injuries
4. Circumferential or electrical burns
5. Prolonged overuse of the extremity (e.g., marathon runner)
6. Recent surgery
7. Cast, splint, or PASG
8. Environmental injuries (e.g., frostbite, snakebite)

TABLE 8-6 Estimated Blood Loss From Factures

Site	Estimated Blood Loss
Forearm	0.5–1 L
Tibia	0.5–1.5 L
Elbow	0.5–1.5 L
Knee	1–1.5 L
Femur	1–2 L
Humerus	1–2 L
Hip	1.5–2.5 L
Pelvis	1.5–4.5 L

Adapted from Clark, D. Y., Stocking, J., & Johnson, J. (Eds.). (2006). *Flight and ground transport nursing core curriculum* (2nd ed.). Denver, CO: Air & Surface Transport Nurses Association.

Clinical presentation

1. Subjective
   a. Pain
      1) Occurrence with passive stretching (flexion) is earliest sign
      2) At rest or with any motion
      3) Out of proportion to injury
      4) Progressive in nature
   b. Numbness
2. Objective
   a. Pallor
   b. Distal muscle weakness
   c. Paralysis: results from ischemia
   d. Delayed capillary refill and loss of pulses are late findings
3. Diagnostic studies
   a. Measurement of compartment pressures
   b. Radiography: to rule out fractures
   c. CT if the condition is suspected to be in the pelvic area or the thigh
   d. Creatine phosphokinase (CPK) and urine myoglobin: increased levels indicates muscle damage (i.e., rhabdomyolysis)
   e. Ultrasound: to evaluate arterial flow and to rule out deep vein thrombosis (DVT) and arterial occlusion

Collaborative management

1. Continue assessment
   a. ABCDs
   b. Pain and discomfort level
   c. Neurovascular assessment: 6 Ps
2. Relieve pressure and prevent neurovascular compromise
   a. Removal of all external compression (e.g., bandages, clothing) that may compromise circulation
   b. Do not elevate: can compromise circulation
   c. Avoidance of ice: causes vasoconstriction
   d. Compartment pressure monitoring: a catheter is inserted into the compartment and then attached to a transducer for the continuous monitoring of pressure
      1) Pressures of ≤10 mm Hg are normal
      2) Pressures of >30 to 35 mm Hg suggest the need for fasciotomy
   e. Fasciotomy as indicated
3. Reduce pain, discomfort, and/or inflammation
   a. Analgesics and NSAIDs as prescribed
   b. Antibiotics as prescribed if infection is suspected
   c. Tetanus immunization as indicated
4. Monitor for complications
   a. Loss of limb
      1) Changes in the quality of the pulses indicate worsening of the problem
   b. Sepsis
   c. Myonecrosis: necrotic damage to the muscle tissue

Evaluation

1. Absence of clinical indications of hypoperfusion
2. Absence of clinical indications of infection or sepsis
3. Alert and oriented with no neurovascular deficit
4. Control of pain and discomfort

Typical disposition: admission
Fat embolism syndrome
Definition: fat droplets enter the bloodstream and circulate, thus causing occlusions; there are two theories regarding how this occurs:

1. The mechanical theory
   a. Large fat droplets are released into the venous system and deposited in the pulmonary capillary beds
   b. They then travel through arteriovenous shunts to the brain, thereby causing the microvascular lodging of the droplets
   c. Local ischemia and inflammation occurs with the concomitant release of inflammatory mediators, platelet aggregation, and vasoactive amines
2. The biochemical theory
   a. Hormonal changes are caused by trauma, which triggers a release of free fatty acids as chylomicrons
   b. During the acute phase, reactants cause chylomicrons to coalesce and to create the physiologic reactions described in the mechanical theory

Predisposing factors

1. Long-bone and pelvic fractures
2. Parenteral lipid infusion
3. Recent steroids

Clinical presentation

1. Subjective
   a. Symptoms may take 12 to 72 hours after injury to occur
   b. Dyspnea
   c. Palpitations
   d. Possible syncope
2. Objective
   a. Tachypnea
   b. Tachycardia
   c. Hypotension
   d. Fever of 101.4°F to 104°F
   e. Crackles
   f. Cough
   g. Restlessness
   h. Petechial hemorrhages in buccal membranes, chest, neck, shoulders, anterior axillary folds, and possibly face
3. Diagnostic studies
   a. Pulse oximetry: SpO_2 decreased
   b. ABGs
      1) SaO_2 and PaO_2 decreased
      2) $PaCO_2$ decreases initially as a result of hyperventilation and then increases as respiratory failure occurs

   c. CBC
     1) May show anemia
     2) May show low platelet count
   d. ESR: increased
   e. Urinalysis: fat globules maybe found
   f. Chest radiography: initially normal followed by increasing haziness and interstitial edema
   g. V/Q studies: show V/Q mismatch

Collaborative management

1. Continue assessment
   a. ABCDs
   b. Hemodynamic status
   c. Neurologic status
   d. Pain and discomfort level
2. Maintain airway, oxygenation, and ventilation
   a. Positioning and/or artificial airway to ensure patency of the airway
   b. Oxygen by nasal cannula at 2-6 liters/minute to maintain SpO_2 of 95% unless contraindicated; for patients with COPD, use pulse oximetry to guide oxygen administration to SpO_2 of 90%
   c. Intubation and mechanical ventilation if unable to maintain oxygenation (SpO_2 of $\geq$90%) or ventilation ($PaCO_2$ of 35–45 mm Hg)
   d. IV steroids may be prescribed (controversial)
3. Maintain adequate circulation and perfusion
   a. IV access with two large-bore catheters for fluid and medication administration
   b. Fluid replacement: usually 0.9% saline
4. Control pain and discomfort
   a. NSAIDs
   b. Narcotic analgesics
   c. Anxiolytics
5. Monitor for complications
   a. Pulmonary infarction
   b. Cerebral infarction
   c. Myocardial infarction
   d. Dysrhythmias
   e. Acute respiratory distress syndrome

Evaluation

1. Patent airway: adequate oxygenation (i.e., normal PaO_2, SpO_2, and SaO_2) and ventilation (i.e., normal $PaCO_2$)
2. Absence of clinical indications of respiratory distress
3. Absence of clinical indications of hypoperfusion
4. Control of pain and discomfort
5. Alert and oriented with no neurovascular or neurologic deficit

Typical disposition: admission to the critical care unit
Septic arthritis
Definition: infectious arthritis caused by bacterial, fungal, or viral infection

1. Pathogenic causes
   a. Bacteria are most common cause and are usually associated with acute course
   b. Fungi or viruses are associated with chronic course

2. Most frequently affected joints are knee, hip, shoulder, wrist, elbow, and finger

Predisposing factors

1. Recent injury to a joint
2. Recent infection or sepsis
3. Joint surgery or replacement
4. Diabetes
5. Immunocompromise
6. Aging

Clinical presentation

1. Subjective
   a. Severe joint pain, especially with palpation or passive range-of-motion exercises
   b. Malaise
   c. Chills
   d. Irritability
2. Objective
   a. Tachycardia and tachypnea; may have mild hypertension
   b. Redness and swelling of the affected area
   c. Tenderness and warmth at the site with palpation
   d. Significantly elevated temperature
3. Diagnostic studies
   a. CBC: increased WBC
   b. Blood cultures: to determine cause and organism
   c. Synovial fluid analysis: to detect organism and rule out other causes (e.g., gout)
   d. Radiography of affected joints

Collaborative management

1. Continue assessment
   a. ABCDs
   b. Pain and discomfort level
   c. Clinical indications of sepsis: fever, tachycardia, tachypnea, confusion, and coagulopathy
2. Reduce pain, discomfort, and/or inflammation
   a. Analgesics and NSAIDs as prescribed
   b. Splinting of affected joint initially; limitation of activity
   c. Fluid aspiration from affected joint to relieve pressure and for culture
     1) Aspiration may need to be done several times to relieve pressure
     2) Surgery may be required
3. Treat infection and prevent sepsis
   a. Antimicrobial therapy initially that is specific for the most likely organism and then specific to culture results
4. Monitor for complications
   a. Permanent joint damage
   b. Sepsis and septic shock

Evaluation

1. Control of pain and discomfort
2. Absence of clinical indications of infection or sepsis

Typical disposition: admission to the hospital for IV antimicrobials and possibly for surgery

Osteomyelitis

Definition: the acute or chronic inflammation of the bone

1. Direct contiguous inoculation: caused by direct contact of the tissue with bacteria as a result of trauma or surgery (King & Johnson, 2006)
2. Hematogenous: caused by bacterial seeding from the blood (King & Johnson, 2006)

Predisposing factors

1. Surgery
2. Trauma
3. Immunocompromise
4. IV substance abuse

Clinical presentation

1. Subjective
   a. Pain and tenderness, especially with movement and the palpation of the site
2. Objective
   a. Swelling, redness, and warmth at the site
   b. Fever
   c. May palpate a deformity
   d. Tenderness with palpation
   e. Impaired range of motion
3. Diagnostic studies
   a. Needle aspiration or bone biopsy: definitive diagnosis (Domino, 2008)
   b. CBC: increased WBC in acute cases but may not be increased in chronic cases
   c. ESR and C-reactive protein: increased but nonspecific
   d. Radiography: shows overlying soft-tissue edema at 3 to 5 days after infection starts (King & Johnson, 2006)
      1) Bony changes 14 to 21 days after start and initially manifested as periosteal elevation (King & Johnson, 2006)
   e. Bone scan

Collaborative management

1. Continue assessment
   a. ABCDs
   b. Pain and discomfort level
   c. Clinical indications of sepsis: fever, tachycardia, tachypnea, confusion, and coagulopathy
2. Reduce pain, discomfort, and inflammation
   a. NSAIDs
   b. Narcotic analgesics
   c. Anxiolytics
   d. Splinting of affected joint initially and limitation of activity
3. Treat infection and prevent sepsis
   a. IV antibiotics for up to 6 weeks
   b. Antipyretics and cooling methods to reduce fever
4. Monitor for complications
   a. Bone abscess
   b. Cellulitis

   c. Fracture
   d. Sepsis and septic shock

Evaluation

1. Absence of clinical indications of infection and sepsis
2. Control of pain, discomfort, or dyspnea

Typical disposition: admission

1. May go directly to surgery for drainage and removal of necrotic tissue
2. Referrals: orthopedist and infectious disease specialist

Specific Wound Emergencies

Lacerations

Definition: an open wound of the skin caused by blunt or penetrating trauma

1. There are three phases of wound healing:
   a. Inflammation phase: occurs within 6 hours of tissue damage
      1) Clotting factors are activated
      2) Release of prostaglandins and histamine, which cause vasodilation and an increase in vascular permeability
   b. Proliferation phase: the wound is infiltrated with new blood vessels that are supported by connective tissue
   c. Maturation phase: involves re-epithelialization, wound contraction, and connective-tissue re-organization

Predisposing factors

1. Blunt or penetrating trauma
2. Immunocompromise

Clinical presentation

1. Subjective
   a. Mechanism of injury, location, and time of occurrence
   b. Pain and tenderness
2. Objective
   a. Bleeding
   b. Wound: note appearance, depth, and condition of surrounding tissue
   c. Range of motion
   d. Neurovascular compromise distal to injury
3. Diagnostic studies
   a. CBC: may see increase in WBC if wound infection is present
   b. Culture and sensitivity of wound drainage
   c. Radiography: to evaluate the bone in the area and to check for foreign bodies

Collaborative management

1. Continue assessment
   a. ABCDs
   b. Clinical indications of bleeding
   c. Neurovascular assessment: 6 Ps
   d. Clinical indications of infection: fever, redness, swelling, and purulent drainage
   e. Pain and discomfort level

2. Maintain airway, oxygenation, and ventilation
   a. Positioning and/or artificial airway to ensure patency of the airway
   b. Oxygen by nasal cannula at 2-6 liters/minute to maintain SpO$_2$ of 95% unless contraindicated; for patients with COPD, use pulse oximetry to guide oxygen administration to SpO$_2$ of 90%
3. Maintain adequate circulation and perfusion
   a. Measures to control bleeding
      1) Direct pressure to control hemorrhage; tourniquets are not recommended
      2) Immobilization of area to decrease blood loss
      3) Elevation and ice applied to the area
   b. IV access with two large-bore catheters for fluid and medication administration
      1) Fluid replacement as indicated
         a) Crystalloids: usually 0.9% saline
         b) Red packed cells or other blood products as prescribed
            i) Should be given early if significant blood loss is suspected to prevent tissue hypoxia
            ii) Replacement of platelets, clotting factors, and calcium should be considered if multiple transfusions are given
         c) Colloids as prescribed
4. Reduce pain, discomfort, and inflammation
   a. NSAIDs
   b. Narcotic analgesics
   c. Anxiolytics
   d. Splinting of affected joint initially and limitation of activity
5. Treat impaired skin integrity and prevent infection
   a. General wound cleaning and irrigation with normal saline
   b. Suturing
      1) Assist with topical analgesia
      2) Assist with suturing
   c. Antibiotics as prescribed
   d. Dressings and splints as indicated
   e. Tetanus immunization
6. Monitor for complications
   a. Bleeding and possible hypovolemia
   b. Uncontrolled pain
   c. Infection and sepsis

Evaluation
1. Absence of clinical indications of bleeding
2. Absence of clinical indications of hypoperfusion
3. Absence of clinical indications of infection or sepsis
4. Control of pain and discomfort

Typical disposition: discharge with instructions
1. Elevation for 48 hours
2. Wound management: keep wound and dressing clean and dry for 48 hours
3. Application of ice and heat as directed
4. Instructions to return to the ED if indications of infection occur (e.g., increased redness, swelling, purulent discharge, fever)

5. Instructions to return for suture removal as directed (see Table 8-2)
6. Sunblock on the area for at least 5 months after the area is healed to prevent permanent pigment discoloration

Abrasions
Definition: the partial-thickness denudation of an area of skin
Predisposing factor: trauma; note the following:
1. Mechanism of injury
2. Location
3. Time
4. Treatment before arrival

Clinical presentation
1. Subjective
   a. Pain
2. Objective
   a. Wound; note the following:
      1) Depth
      2) Extent of tissue involved
      3) Presence of embedded debris
   b. May be associated injuries present
3. Diagnostic studies
   a. CBC: WBC increased if infection present
   b. Radiography of affected area

Collaborative management
1. Continue assessment
   a. ABCDs
   b. Clinical indications of bleeding
   c. Clinical indications of infection: fever, redness, swelling, and purulent drainage
   d. Neurovascular assessment: 6 Ps
   e. Pain and discomfort level
2. Ensure adequate circulation
   a. Application of direct pressure to control bleeding
3. Reduce pain, discomfort, and inflammation
   a. NSAIDs
   b. Narcotic analgesics
   c. Anxiolytics
   d. Position for comfort
4. Treat impaired skin integrity and prevent infection
   a. Cleansing of the area and application of a nonadherent dressing; dirt and debris can cause a permanent tattooing effect if they are not removed within 24 hours of injury
      1) General wound cleaning and irrigation with normal saline
         a) Clean extremity wounds within 4 to 6 hours of injury (ENA, 2007)
         b) Clean facial wounds within 8 hours of injury (ENA, 2007)
   b. Antibiotics as prescribed
   c. Tetanus immunization as indicated
5. Monitor for complications
   a. Bleeding and hypovolemia
   b. Infection
   c. Uncontrolled pain

Evaluation
1. Absence of clinical indications of infection or sepsis
2. Control of pain and discomfort

Typical disposition: discharge with instructions
1. Dressing changes with the application of ointment as directed
2. Instructions to return to the ED if indications of infection occur (e.g., increased redness, swelling, purulent discharge, fever)
3. Avoidance of direct sunlight to the area for 6 months, because it may cause pigment changes
4. Medications as prescribed
5. Referrals: follow up with primary care provider

Avulsions
Definition: full-thickness tissue loss that prevents wound-edge approximation (e.g., degloving)
Predisposing factors: trauma; note the following:
1. Mechanism of injury
2. Time
3. Location
4. Treatment before arrival

Clinical presentation
1. Subjective
   a. Pain and tenderness
2. Objective
   a. Obvious wound injury
   b. Bleeding
   c. May have neurovascular compromise distal to the injury
   d. Tenderness with palpation
3. Diagnostic studies
   a. CBC: WBC increased if infection is present
   b. Radiography: indicated for severe avulsions or degloving to rule out fractures

Collaborative management
1. Continue assessment
   a. ABCDs
   b. Clinical indications of bleeding
   c. Clinical indications of infection: fever, redness, swelling, and purulent drainage
   d. Neurovascular assessment: 6 Ps
   e. Pain and discomfort level
2. Ensure adequate circulation
   a. Application of direct pressure to control bleeding
3. Restore normal regional function and prevent further injury
   a. Sterile dressing applied to area (ENA, 2007)
      1) Small avulsion: petroleum jelly gauze and light compression dressing
      2) Large avulsion: petroleum jelly gauze, layered dressing, and a metal protector
         a) Gelfoam as needed for bleeding
   b. For degloving injuries, realign the tissue and cover it with sterile dressing to prevent further injury to the area

   c. Elevation of the area
   d. Ice applied to the area as directed
4. Reduce pain, discomfort, and inflammation
   a. NSAIDs
   b. Narcotic analgesics
   c. Anxiolytics
   d. Positioning for comfort
5. Treat impaired skin integrity and prevent infection
   a. Antibiotics as prescribed
   b. Tetanus immunization as indicated
6. Monitor for complications
   a. Bleeding and hypovolemia
   b. Shock
   c. Infection and sepsis
   d. Neurovascular compromise

Evaluation
1. Absence of clinical indications of hypoperfusion
2. Absence of clinical indications of infection or sepsis
3. Control of pain and discomfort

Typical disposition
1. If evaluation criteria met: discharge with instructions
   a. Ice therapy and elevation to control swelling and bleeding
   b. General wound care instructions
   c. Return to the ED if indications of infection occur (e.g., increased redness, swelling, purulent discharge, fever)
   d. Medications as directed
   e. Follow up with primary care provider
2. If evaluation criteria not met (e.g., degloving): admission from ED to surgery

Puncture wounds
Definition: a wound caused by a small object penetrating the skin
1. Bleed minimally
2. Tend to seal off, thus setting up the potential for infection
   a. If near a joint, can place that joint at risk

Predisposing factors
1. Stepping on a sharp object
2. Working with power injectors or sprays
3. Penetrating trauma with a sharp object (accidental or intentional)

Clinical presentation
1. Subjective
   a. Pain related to puncture wound; determine the following:
      1) Type of object that caused the injury
      2) Time of injury
      3) Treatment before arrival
2. Objective
   a. Puncture wound; note the following:
      1) Location
      2) Estimate of wound depth
   b. May have associated injuries
   c. May involve the presence of foreign bodies

d. May involve neurovascular compromise distal to the injury

e. May involve a decrease in the range of motion

3. Diagnostic studies
   a. CBC: WBC increased if infection present
   b. Radiography: to assess for fractures and foreign bodies

Collaborative management

1. Continue assessment
   a. ABCDs
   b. Clinical indications of infection: fever, redness, swelling, and purulent drainage
   c. Pain and discomfort level
2. Reduce pain, discomfort, and inflammation
   a. NSAIDs
   b. Narcotic analgesics
   c. Anxiolytics
   d. Positioning for comfort
3. Treat impaired skin integrity and prevent infection
   a. Wound management
      1) Gently cleanse the area
      2) Soak puncture wounds
      3) Assist with local anesthetics for exploration
      4) Assist with wound debridement if indicated
   b. Antibiotics as prescribed
   c. Tetanus immunization as indicated
4. Monitor for complications
   a. Infection

Evaluation

1. Absence of clinical indications of infection or sepsis
2. Control of pain and discomfort

Typical disposition: discharge with instructions

1. Wound management: soak the wound two or three times a day (ENA, 2007)
   a. Wounds with packing should not be soaked
2. Instructions to return to the ED if indications of infection occur (e.g., increased redness, swelling, purulent discharge, fever)
3. Referrals: follow up with primary care provider

Foreign body object (FBO)
Definition: objects such as wood, metal, glass, pins, and needles that become embedded in various body parts
Predisposing factors
1. Trauma
2. Occupational hazards

Clinical presentation

1. Subjective
   a. Description of injury
      1) Object and estimate of depth
      2) Time of injury
      3) Treatment before arrival
   b. Pain and tenderness
2. Objective
   a. Open wound with embedded object
   b. May have neurovascular impairment

3. Diagnostic studies
   a. CBC: WBC increased if infection present
   b. Radiography
      1) To view FBO and surrounding tissue
         a) Natural wood splinters or clothing type material not visualized
      2) To check for other injuries, such as fractures or an object being embedded in bone (depending on the length of the object)

Collaborative management

1. Continue assessment
   a. ABCDs
   b. Pain and discomfort level
   c. Neurovascular assessment: 6 Ps
2. Ensure adequate circulation: apply direct pressure to control bleeding if applicable
3. Reduce pain, discomfort, and inflammation
   a. NSAIDs
   b. Narcotic analgesics
   c. Anxiolytics
   d. Positioning for comfort
4. Treat infection and prevent sepsis
   a. Wound management
      1) Gently clean area do not soak area if the FBO is wood, because soaking will cause object to swell
      2) Assist with local anesthetic for exploration
      3) Apply dressing to area as prescribed
   b. Antibiotics as prescribed
   c. Tetanus immunization as indicated
5. Monitor for complications
   a. Residual of FBO still embedded
   b. Uncontrolled pain
   c. Fracture possible depending on object
   d. Infection

Evaluation

1. No evidence of FBO in tissue
2. Control of pain and discomfort

Typical disposition: discharge with instructions

1. Wound management
2. Medications as prescribed
3. Return to the ED if indications of infection occur (e.g., increased redness, swelling, purulent discharge, fever)
4. Referral: follow up with primary care provider

Missile injuries
Definition
1. Injuries that result from projectile penetrating objects, including gunshot wounds, stab wounds, and other high-pressure penetrating wounds
2. Entry and exit wounds have no bearing on the amount of damage that may occur
3. Forensic considerations include documentation, reporting to law enforcement, and carefully preserving and handling evidence

Predisposing factors

1. Stab wounds: note mechanism of injury, the depth, the angle of entry, and the amount of force
2. Gunshot wounds: note the movement of the bullet, the type of weapon, the distance from the weapon, the characteristics of the bullet, and possible bone and tissue injuries
   a. Low-velocity bullets travel at speeds of <1000 feet/second
   b. Medium-velocity bullets travel at speeds of 1000 to 2000 feet/second
   c. High-velocity bullets travel at speeds of >2000 feet/second
   d. Look for entry and exit wounds (do not differentiate)
3. High-pressure wounds (e.g., paint guns)
   a. Note the substance type, the injury depth, and the amount of pressure
4. Projectile missiles (e.g., nail gun, bolt from machinery)

Clinical presentation

1. Subjective
   a. Pain
   b. History of events
      1) Mechanism of injury
      2) Time of injury
      3) Treatment before arrival
2. Objective
   a. Wound
      1) Location
      2) Extent of tissue damage
      3) Contamination of wound (e.g., paint or grease gun)
      4) Look for entrance and exit wounds
         a) Document the description of the sites
         b) Do not distinguish in charting which is the entrance and which is the exit
   b. Amount of bleeding if present
   c. May have associated injuries
   d. May have neurovascular impairment
3. Diagnostic studies
   a. CBC
      1) Increased WBC indicates infection
      2) Decreased hemoglobin and hematocrit levels suggest bleeding
   b. Radiography: to assess any impaled objects (e.g., bullets) and underlying injuries
   c. Toxicology screen as indicated (e.g., lead)

Collaborative management

1. Continue assessment
   a. ABCDs
   b. Clinical indications of bleeding
   c. Clinical indications of infection: fever, redness, swelling, and purulent drainage
   d. Clinical indications of sepsis: fever, tachycardia, tachypnea, confusion, and coagulopathy
   e. Neurovascular assessment: 6 Ps
   f. Pain and discomfort level

2. Ensure adequate circulation
   a. Application of direct pressure to control bleeding
   b. IV access with two large-bore catheters for fluid and medication administration
      1) Fluid replacement
         a) Crystalloids: usually 0.9% saline
         b) Blood and blood products may be needed
   c. Surgery: prepare the patient and family
3. Reduce pain, discomfort, and inflammation
   a. NSAIDs
   b. Narcotic analgesics
   c. Anxiolytics
4. Treat impaired skin integrity and prevent infection
   a. Wound management
      1) Clean and irrigate with normal saline (do not soak)
      2) Assist with local anesthetic and debridement as needed
         a) High-pressure injection wounds often require debridement
      3) Apply dressing
   b. Antibiotics as prescribed
   c. Tetanus immunization as indicated
5. Monitor for complications
   a. Allergic reaction to toxin (e.g., high-powered paint gun injection)
   b. Neurovascular impairment
   c. Hypovolemia and shock

Evaluation

1. Absence of clinical indications of hypoperfusion
2. Absence of clinical indications of infection or sepsis
3. Control of pain and discomfort

Typical disposition

1. If evaluation criteria met: discharge with instructions
   a. Elevation of affected part
   b. Wound management
   c. Instructions to return to the ED if indications of infection occur (e.g., increased redness, swelling, purulent discharge, fever)
   d. Medications as prescribed
   e. Referrals: follow up with primary care provider
2. If evaluation criteria not met: admission to progressive care unit or critical care unit

Snake bite (Medline Plus, 2008)
Definition: a bite from one of the two types of venomous snakes in the United States

1. Pit vipers are in the family Crotalidae; this family includes rattlesnakes, copperheads, and cottonmouths (water moccasins)
   a. Get their common name from a small "pit" between the eye and nostril that detects heat and that allows the snake to sense prey at night; they have cat-like pupils and a triangular head
   b. Deliver venom through two fangs that they can retract at rest and spring into biting position rapidly

1) Fang marks may or may not leave accessory teeth marks

c. Account for the vast majority of all venomous bites in the United States

d. Copperheads have milder and less dangerous venom that sometimes may not require antivenin treatment.

2. Coral snakes are members of the poisonous family Elapidae
   a. Two of the species are found mainly in the Southern states
   b. Have black, red, and yellow bands on their body, black heads, slender bodies, and round, black eyes
   c. Have small mouths, fixed fangs, and short teeth; they lack the characteristic fang marks of pit vipers, which sometimes make the bite hard to detect
      1) Bites will leave scratch marks or tiny puncture marks
   d. May cause respiratory paralysis as one of the effects of the neurotoxic venom

Predisposing factors: outdoor activities
Clinical presentation

1. Subjective
   a. Report of being bitten by a snake
      1) Time of injury
      2) Location of bite
      3) Description of snake
      4) Treatment before arrival
   b. May or may not have pain initially
      1) Rattlesnake bites tend to be painful
      2) Coral snake bite may not involve any pain initially
   c. Nausea and vomiting may occur
   d. Blurred vision may occur
2. Objective
   a. Swelling and redness at site
   b. Petechiae and ecchymosis
   c. Neurologic changes
   d. Renal failure may occur
3. Symptoms of envenomation
   a. Local: fang marks, edema, pain, petechiae, ecchymosis, loss of function of limb, and necrosis
   b. Systemic: nausea, vomiting, diaphoresis, syncope, metallic or rubbery taste in the mouth, paralysis, visual disturbances, muscle twitching, hemorrhage, renal failure, and death
4. Envenomation severity grade (Clark et al., 2007)
   a. Minimal: moderate pain, edema of 2.5 to 15 cm, redness, and no systemic symptoms; no antivenin needed
   b. Moderate: severe pain, tenderness, edema of 25 to 40 cm, redness, petechiae, vomiting, fever, and weakness; may give 20 ml of antivenin
   c. Severe: widespread pain, tenderness, edema of 40 to 50 cm, rapid swelling, bruising, vertigo, central nervous system and visual disturbances, and shock; may give 50 to 90 ml of antivenin

5. Diagnostic studies
   a. CBC: decreased hemoglobin and hematocrit levels in <50% of cases (Domino, 2008)
   b. Clotting studies: decrease in platelet count
   c. Electrolytes
   d. ABGs: may show hypoxemia in the presence of systemic indications of envenomation
   e. Urinalysis: may show increased myoglobin level

Collaborative management

1. Continue assessment
   a. ABCDs
   b. Vital signs: blood pressure, pulse, respiratory rate, and temperature
   c. Oxygen saturation
   d. Respiratory effort and excursion
   e. Cardiac rate and rhythm
   f. Pain and discomfort level
   g. Level of consciousness
   h. Neurovascular assessment: 6 Ps, measurement of extremity girth every 15 minutes
2. Maintain airway, oxygenation, and ventilation
   a. Positioning and/or artificial airway to ensure patency of the airway
   b. Oxygen by nasal cannula at 2-6 liters/minute to maintain SpO_2 of 95% unless contraindicated; for patients with COPD, use pulse oximetry to guide oxygen administration to SpO_2 of 90%
3. Ensure adequate circulation and perfusion
   a. IV access with two large-bore catheters for fluid and medication administration
      1) Fluid replacement: usually 0.9% saline
   b. Immobilization of bitten part in neutral position at level of injury
      1) Below the level of the heart can increase swelling at site
      2) Above the level of the heart may allow venom to travel throughout the body
   c. Antivenin: works best if given within 4 hours of bite
      1) Skin test before administration 0.02 ml of 1:10 dilution or 1:100 dilution if patient has suspected sensitivity to equine serum (Clark, Stocking, & Johnson, 2006)
      2) Antivenin pretreatment drugs as prescribed
4. Reduce pain, discomfort, and inflammation
   a. NSAIDs
   b. Narcotic analgesics
   c. Anxiolytics
   d. Positioning for comfort
5. Restore normal regional function and prevent further injury
   a. Avoidance of ice or any other type of cooling on the bite; this may increase tissue necrosis and the toxicity of the venom
   b. Avoidance of tourniquets; these cut blood flow completely and may result in the loss of the affected limb

c. Avoidance of incisions into the wound; these have not been proven to be useful and may cause further injury

6. Treat impaired skin integrity and prevent infection
   a. Antibiotics as prescribed
   b. Tetanus immunization as indicated
7. Monitoring for complications
   a. Compartment syndrome
   b. Skin infections
   c. Coagulopathy
   d. Anaphylaxis or anaphylactic shock
   e. Serum sickness (usually 1–2 weeks after treatment with antivenin)

Evaluation

1. Absence of clinical indications of hypoperfusion
2. Absence of clinical indications of infection or vsepsis
3. Control of pain or discomfort
4. Alert and oriented with no neurovascular deficit

Typical disposition

1. If evaluation criteria met: discharge with instructions
   a. Wound care
   b. Instruction to return to the ED if indications of infection occur (e.g., increased redness, swelling, purulent discharge, fever)
   c. Prevention of recurrence
      1) Wear high-top shoes and long pants when hiking or in wooded areas
      2) Do not approach or bother snakes when encountering them in the outdoor environment
      3) Be familiar with venomous species when participating in outdoor activities in which snakes may be encountered
   d. Referrals: follow up with primary care provider

2. If evaluation criteria not met: admission to progressive care unit or critical care unit

Tick bite

Definition: a bite from a small, blood-sucking, parasitic arachnid that can carry and transmit blood-borne diseases such as Rocky Mountain spotted fever and Lyme disease (*Merriam-Webster*, 2008)

Predisposing factors

1. Spending time outdoors
2. Having pets that spend time outside
3. Walking through wooded areas, shrubs, and areas with tall grass

Clinical presentation (Medline Plus, 2008)

1. Subjective
   a. Report of a tick bite or the finding of a tick on the body
   b. Weakness
   c. Muscle and joint pain
   d. Headache
   e. Chills
   f. Flu-like symptoms: shortness of breath, nausea, vomiting, chills, and numbness
2. Objective
   a. Presence of a tick
   b. Fever
   c. Skin rash
   d. Specific to Lyme disease (Table 8-7)
3. Diagnostic studies
   a. Electrocardiogram
   b. Clotting studies
   c. Lyme antibody titers

TABLE 8-7	Lyme Disease	
Stages	**Symptoms**
Stage 1 • Primary • 1 to 4 weeks	• Lack of energy (most common symptom) • Nonspecific flu-like symptoms: headache, stiff neck, fever, chills, and muscle and joint pain • Swollen lymph nodes • Symptoms usually disappear within 2 weeks if untreated
Stage 2 • Secondary • 1 to 4 months	• Tired and fatigued • Additional skin rashes; may develop systemic dissemination • Pain, weakness, or numbness in the arms or legs • Paralysis of the facial nerves (Bell palsy) • Poor memory and reduced ability to concentrate • Conjunctivitis • Palpitations or, in rare cases, serious heart problems
Stage 3 • Tertiary • Weeks to years after the initial bite	• Swelling and pain (inflammation) in the joints, especially in the knees • Numbness and tingling in the hands, feet, or back • Severe fatigue • Neurologic complications: memory loss, mood changes, sleep problems, and poor coordination • Chronic Lyme arthritis, which causes recurring episodes of swelling, redness, and fluid buildup in one or more joints that lasts ≤6 mo at a time

Data from http://www.nlm.nih.gov/medlineplus/ency/article/001319.htm.

Collaborative management

1. Continue assessment
   a. ABCDs
   b. Vital signs: blood pressure, pulse, respiratory rate, and temperature
   c. Oxygen saturation
   d. Respiratory effort and excursion
   e. Cardiac rate and rhythm
   f. Pain and discomfort level
2. Prevent and treat infection
   a. Removal of tick if present
      1) May use viscous Lidocaine at site before removal
      2) Do not squeeze tick
      3) Gently remove with a blunt angled, medium sized forceps; use a steady upward pulling motion
      4) Once tick removed, inspect the bite area for retained parts; if found, remove
   b. Washing of area with antiseptic soap
   c. Antibiotics are rarely indicated unless patient has obvious disease process
   d. Tetanus immunization as indicated
3. Monitor for complications
   a. Lyme disease
   b. Neurologic complications
   c. Myocarditis
   d. Arthritis

Evaluation

1. Complete removal of tick
2. Absence of clinical indications of hypoperfusion
3. Absence of clinical indications of infection or sepsis
4. Control of pain and discomfort

Typical disposition: discharge with instructions

1. How to prevent tick bites
   a. Wear long sleeves and long pants in wooded areas or areas with tall grass
   b. Tuck pant legs into socks or boots when walking in these areas
   c. Use tick repellant when outdoors in areas where ticks may be
   d. Inspect all areas of the body for ticks after possible exposure

Spider bite
Definition: a bite from a poisonous spider

1. Although all spiders are poisonous, most are harmless to humans because they are small and their venom is weak; the black widow and the brown recluse are the exceptions, and they are found in warm climates

Predisposing factors: exposure to woodpiles, sheds, and basements, where spiders are common
Clinical presentation

1. Black widows have neurotoxic venom that produces pain and paresthesia
   a. The black widow has a shiny black body with a red hourglass shape on the ventral side of the abdomen
   b. Subjective
      1) Pain: a sharp pinprick followed by dull, numbing pain that progresses to severe pain in 15 to 60 minutes and that increases in 12 to 48 hours
      2) Cramping, nausea, vomiting, and intense abdominal pain are common, with similar pain in the back, thorax, and groin
      3) Dyspnea may occur
   c. Objective
      1) Presence of tiny fang marks
      2) Swelling
      3) Fever
      4) Tremors
      5) Systemic anaphylactic reaction may occur within 30 minutes
2. Brown recluse bite causes extensive localized skin necrosis and cellulitis
   a. The brown recluse is brown with a violin-shaped marking on the dorsal aspect of the cephalothoraxes; it has three eyes instead of four (most spiders have four eyes)
   b. Subjective
      1) Vague history of pain that began 3 to 4 hours after the bite
      2) Nausea and vomiting
      3) Chills
      4) Joint pain (i.e., arthralgias)
      5) Malaise
   c. Objective
      1) May have no changes at the site or may have a large necrotic area (i.e., ≤ 30 cm)
      2) Fever
3. Diagnostic studies
   a. Black widow: increase in WBCs (i.e., leukocytosis)
   b. Brown recluse: decrease in RBCs (i.e., hemolytic anemia) and platelets (i.e., thrombocytopenia)
   c. Urinalysis: blood (i.e., hematuria), myoglobin (i.e., myoglobinuria), and protein (i.e., proteinuria) may appear in the urine after either type of bite

Collaborative management

1. Continue assessment
   a. ABCDs
   b. Skin condition at bite site: note rash, vesicles, or necrosis
   c. Pain and discomfort level
2. Maintain airway, oxygenation, and ventilation
   a. Positioning and/or artificial airway to ensure patency of the airway
   b. Oxygen by nasal cannula at 2 to 6 liters/minute to maintain SpO_2 of 95% unless contraindicated; for patients with COPD, use pulse oximetry to guide oxygen administration to SpO_2 of 90%
3. Maintain adequate circulation and perfusion
   a. IV access with two large-bore catheters for fluid and medication administration
   b. Fluid replacement: usually 0.9% saline
   c. Ice to a black widow bite to slow absorption

d. Antivenin
   1) Sensitivity test for black widow bites before administration
   2) Antivenin pretreatment drugs as prescribed
e. Dapsone and steroids maybe given for brown recluse bite (ENA, 2007)
4. Reduce pain, discomfort, and inflammation
   a. NSAIDs
   b. Narcotic analgesics
   c. Anxiolytics
   d. Benzodiazepines, opiates, and muscle relaxants to relieve cramping from black widow bites
5. Restore normal regional function and prevent further injury
   a. Immobilization of bitten part in neutral position at level of injury
   b. Cleansing of brown recluse bite area with mild soap
6. Prevent and treat impaired skin integrity and infection
   a. Antibiotics as prescribed
   b. Tetanus immunization as indicated
7. Monitor for complications
   a. Anaphylaxis and anaphylactic shock
   b. Tissue necrosis and infection (could result in the loss of digits or a limb)
   c. Coagulopathies (e.g., disseminated intravascular coagulation)
   d. Rhabdomyolysis
   e. Renal failure

Evaluation

1. Absence of clinical indications of hypoperfusion
2. Absence of clinical indications of infection or sepsis
3. Control of pain and discomfort
4. Alert and oriented with no neurovascular deficit

Typical disposition

1. If evaluation criteria met: discharge with instructions
   a. Wound care for spider bite
   b. Medication instructions
   c. Instructions regarding indications of inflammation or infection
   d. Follow up with primary care provider
   e. Instruction regarding prevention
      1) Wear protective clothing and remain attentive when venturing into areas in which there may be spiders
      2) Carefully remove cobwebs and spiders from under and behind beds or other areas
      3) Use caution when putting on clothing or shoes that have been kept in storage
2. If evaluation criteria not met (e.g., patients exhibiting systemic toxicity): admission to progressive care unit or critical care unit

Hymenopteran stings (Janson & Iseke, 2007)

Definition: a sting by a member of the hymenoptera family, which represents 14,000 species, including bees, hornets, wasps, and ants
1. Reactions from hymenoptera venom can cause local to severe reactions; these bites are toxic to certain individuals

Predisposing factors: outdoor activities

Clinical presentation

1. Subjective
   a. Report of sting or bite
   b. May report a history of allergic reactions or problems with stings
   c. Local reaction: pain at site
   d. Toxic reaction: nausea, vomiting, diarrhea, and syncope (consider with $\geq$10 stings); symptoms usually resolve within 48 hours
   e. Systemic (anaphylactic) reaction: dyspnea, itching, and chills
2. Objective
   a. Local reaction: swelling at site
   b. Systemic (anaphylactic) reaction
      1) Stridor or wheezing
      2) Fever
      3) Tachycardia
      4) Hypotension
      5) Change in level of consciousness
      6) Medications (e.g., β-blockers) may mask the indications of anaphylaxis
   c. Delayed hypersensitivity reaction: $\leq$1 week (Janson & Iseke, 2007)
      1) Joint effusions
      2) Serum sickness
      3) Purpura
      4) Heart failure
      5) Renal failure or nephrotic syndrome
      6) Jaundice or bruising (related to hemolytic anemia or thrombocytopenia)
3. Diagnostic studies
   a. CBC: increased WBC with severe reactions
   b. Clotting studies: may show clotting abnormalities
   c. Chemistry
      1) May show electrolyte imbalance
      2) May show increased blood urea nitrogen and creatinine levels

Collaborative management

1. Continue assessment
   a. ABCDs
   b. Vital signs: blood pressure, pulse, respiratory rate, and temperature
   c. Oxygen saturation
   d. Respiratory effort and excursion
   e. Cardiac rate and rhythm
   f. Neurovascular assessment
   g. Pain and comfort level

2. Maintain airway, oxygenation, and ventilation
   a. Positioning and/or artificial airway to ensure patency of the airway
   b. Oxygen by nasal cannula at 2-6 liters/minute to maintain SpO_2 of 95% unless contraindicated; for patients with COPD, use pulse oximetry to guide oxygen administration to SpO_2 of 90%
3. Maintain adequate circulation and perfusion
   a. IV with two large-bore catheters for fluid and medication administration
      1) Fluid replacement: usually 0.9% saline
   b. Measures to reduce toxin absorption
      1) Removal of stinger, if present, by scraping the skin; do not squeeze the skin
      2) Cleansing of the area
      3) Ice to delay the local reaction and to slow absorption
   c. Steroids may be used for hypersensitivity reactions
   d. Epinephrine and diphenhydramine (Benadryl) for patients with a history of allergy or for anaphylactic reactions
4. Reduce pain, discomfort, and inflammation
   a. Analgesics as prescribed for pain
   b. Antihistamines as prescribed for itching
5. Restore normal regional function and prevent further injury
   a. Immobilization of affected area in neutral position at level of injury
6. Monitor for complications
   a. Anaphylaxis or anaphylactic shock
   b. Myocardial infarction
   c. Stroke
   d. Renal failure
   e. Coagulopathies (e.g., disseminated intravascular coagulation)

Evaluation
1. Absence of clinical indications of hypoperfusion
2. Absence of clinical indications of infection or sepsis
3. Control of pain and discomfort

Typical disposition
1. If evaluation criteria met: discharge with instructions
   a. Wound care
   b. Instruction regarding indications of anaphylaxis that indicate the need to return to the ED
   c. Medications as prescribed
   d. Referrals: follow up with primary care provider
2. If evaluation criteria not met (e.g., anaphylaxis): admission

Human bite
Definition: a laceration or puncture wound caused by human teeth
1. May be self-inflicted or caused by another person
2. High risk for infection

Predisposing factors
1. Violence

Clinical presentation
1. Subjective
   a. Report of bite
      1) Description of incident
      2) Time of bite
      3) Location of bite
      4) Circumstances surrounding the bite (e.g., is it part of a crime?)
   b. Pain
2. Objective
   a. Wound; note the following:
      1) Size and depth of the wound
      2) Range of motion and function of the affected part
      3) Swelling, redness, debris, or discharge
   b. May involve neurovascular compromise

Diagnostic studies
1. CBC: increased WBC with infection
2. Saliva residue swab
3. Culture and sensitivity for any drainage
4. Radiography: for FBO

Collaborative management
1. Continue assessment
   a. ABCDs
   b. Clinical indications of bleeding
   c. Clinical indications of infection
   d. Pain and discomfort level
   e. Wound: take pictures if it is associated with a crime
2. Reduce pain, discomfort, and inflammation
   a. NSAIDs
   b. Narcotic analgesics
   c. Anxiolytics
   d. Positioning for comfort
3. Prevent and treat infection
   a. Irrigation of wound with a large amount of normal saline
   b. Debridement and wound closure; this will usually delay closure to decrease infection
   c. Tetanus immunization if indicated
4. Restore normal regional function and prevent further injury
   a. Immobilization of affected area in neutral position at level of injury
5. Monitor for complications
   a. Hemorrhage
   b. Infection
   c. Neurovascular compromise

Evaluation
1. Absence of clinical indications of infection or sepsis
2. Control of pain and discomfort
3. Alert and oriented with no neurovascular deficit

Typical disposition: discharge with instructions
1. Wound care instructions
2. Instructions to return to the ED if indications of infection occur (e.g., increased redness, swelling, purulent discharge, fever)

3. Antibiotics as prescribed
4. Follow up with primary care provider

Skin infections (e.g., those related to wounds)
Definition: a breakdown in skin integrity caused by bacteria, fungi, or viruses
Predisposing factors
1. Infections related to wounds may be an initial problem or occur later

Specific infections
1. Staphylococcal infections *(Staphylococcus aureus)*: gram positive, usually localized, and associated with most skin infections in superficial subcutaneous tissue
   a. Cause: common bacteria found on the skin that can cause an infection when there is a break in the skin or if the bacteria are trapped in a pore or follicle
   b. Symptoms: vary but can include redness, rash, nausea, vomiting, diarrhea, headache, and aches
   c. Onset: can be from 2 days to 33 days
   d. Management: antibiotics and good hand-washing techniques
2. *Pasteurella multocida*: a necrotizing infection that is also seen with animal bites
   a. Cause: cellulitis, osteomyelitis, sinusitis, and pleuritis
   b. Symptoms: swelling and redness at the site, tenderness, discharge, fever, and chills
   c. Onset: 3 hours to 3 days
   d. Management: antibiotics (e.g., penicillin)
3. Cat scratch fever *(Afipia felis* or *Bartonella henselae)*: an infection that usually occurs as a result of a bite, scratch, or lick from a cat and that occurs because an estimated 40% of cats carry bacteria in their saliva
   a. Cause: cat or dog scratches; occurs more commonly after dealing with kittens
   b. Symptoms: regional or local lymphadenitis, fever, nausea, vomiting, and fatigue
   c. Onset: 2 to 3 weeks after exposure, lymph nodes start to swell
   d. Management: antibiotics are not usually indicated unless the patient is immunocompromised
      1) Antipyretics
      2) Analgesics
      3) Heat applied to area
4. Wound botulism *(Clostridium botulinum)*: a neurologic disorder that can cause life-threatening neuroparalysis as a result of a neurotoxin produced by the bacteria *Clostridium botulinum*
   a. Cause: seen with crush injuries or major trauma
   b. Symptoms: include weakness, blurred vision, difficulty swallowing or speaking, dry mucous membranes, dilated pupils, and progressive muscular paralysis
   c. Onset: incubation period of 4 to 14 days
   d. Management:
      1) Debridement of wound
      2) Antitoxin therapy
      3) Antibiotics (e.g., high-dose penicillin)
5. Gas gangrene *(Clostridium perfringens)*: an infection of the muscle tissue by toxin-producing clostridia
   a. Cause: a history of intestinal or gallbladder surgery or minor trauma to old scars that contain spores
   b. Symptoms: soft-tissue crepitus, pain, thin and watery brown drainage, increased pulse, nausea, vomiting, diarrhea, and coma
   c. Onset: incubation period of 1 day to 6 weeks
   d. Management:
      1) Tetanus toxoid if indicated
      2) Antibiotics
      3) Surgical wound debridement
6. Tetanus *(Clostridium tetani)*: an infectious disease caused by the contamination of wounds with bacteria that live in the soil.
   a. Cause: the organism is found in soil and in human and animal intestines; it enters through a break in the skin
   b. Symptoms
      1) Early symptoms include restlessness, headache, muscle spasms, and pain
      2) Later symptoms include extreme stiffness, tonic spasms, exaggerated reflex activity, general convulsions, and respiratory depression
   c. Onset: incubation period of 2 days to several months (average onset, 6–10 days)
   d. Management: antitoxins, antibiotics, and vaccine
7. Rabies: neurotoxin virus; found in the saliva of rabid animals
   a. Cause: bites from infected animals
   b. Symptoms: malaise, fever, headache, lymphadenitis, photophobia, muscle spasms, coma, osteomyelitis, abscess, and necrotizing fasciitis
   c. Onset: incubation period of 10 days to several months
   d. Management:
      1) Cleansing of the wound with virus-killing soap
      2) Rabies immune globulin given
      3) Rabies vaccine given in a series during the first 28 days after the bite occurs; give the first vaccine on day 1 and then follow with vaccinations on days 3, 7, 14, and 28
8. Group A streptococcus: found in the throat and on the skin; can be life threatening; causes necrotizing fasciitis and toxic shock syndrome
   a. Cause: spread by direct person-to-person contact
   b. Symptoms:
      1) Necrotizing fasciitis, fever, severe pain, swelling, heat, and redness at wound site
         a) Known for rapidly attacking tissue and destroying muscle and flesh
      2) Streptococcal toxic shock syndrome includes fever, dizziness, and confusion
   c. Onset: 1 to 3 days after exposure
   d. Management:
      1) Necrotizing fasciitis: antibiotics (e.g., beta-lactam) and supportive therapy for shock

2) Streptococcal toxic shock syndrome: antibiotics, immunoglobulin G, and supportive therapy for shock
9. Diagnostic studies
   a. CBC: WBC increased with bacterial infection
   b. Wound culture and sensitivity

Collaborative management

1. Continue assessment
   a. ABCDs
   b. Vital signs: blood pressure, pulse, respiratory rate, and temperature
   c. Clinical indications of infection
   d. Pain and discomfort level
2. Prevent and treat infection
   a. Irrigation of wound with large amount of normal saline
   b. Incision and drainage as necessary
   c. Antibiotics as prescribed
   d. Tetanus immunization if indicated
   e. Adherence to Centers for Disease Control and Prevention guidelines for bites

3. Reduce pain, discomfort, and inflammation
   a. Topical anesthetic as directed
   b. NSAIDs
   c. Narcotic analgesics
4. Monitor for complications
   a. Infection
   b. Coagulopathies

Evaluation

1. Control of pain and discomfort
2. Stable hemodynamic status

Typical disposition: discharge with instructions

1. Wound care
2. Instruction to return to the ED if indications of infection occur (e.g., increased redness, swelling, purulent discharge, fever)
3. Counseling regarding maintenance of immunizations as recommended by the Centers for Disease Control and Prevention
4. Referral: follow up with primary care provider or specialist as instructed

LEARNING ACTIVITIES

1. DIRECTIONS: Complete the following crossword puzzle related to orthopedic and wound emergencies.

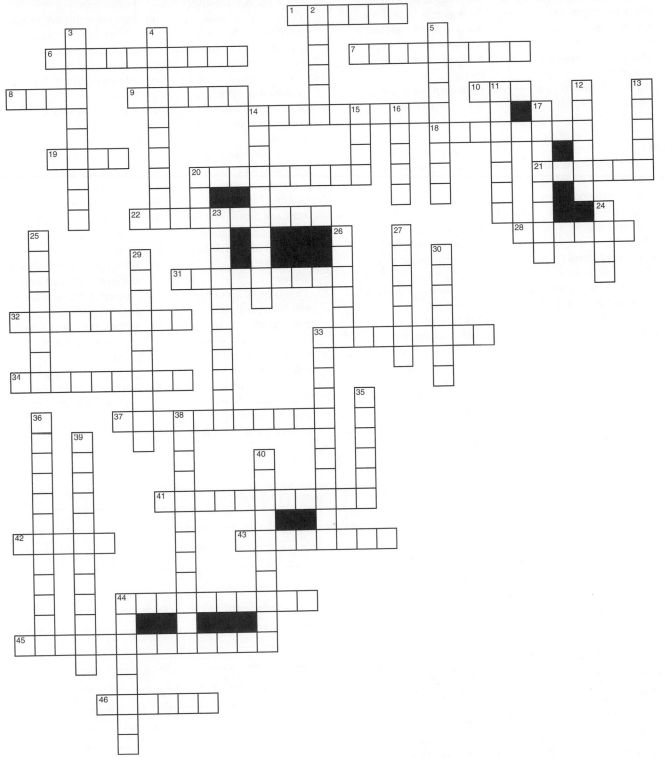

ACROSS

1. Fracture resulting from a twisting motion
6. When the periosteum is divided on only one side
7. The term for full-thickness tissue loss that prevents wound-edge approximation
8. A bone _____ is a test that looks at bone mineral density
9. This structure joins muscle to bone
10. Bullets that travel at speeds of <1000 feet/ second are referred to as _____ *velocity bullets*

14. This fever is associated with *Afipia felis* or *Bartonella henselae* (two words)
18. This occurs when there is a bone fragment separated from the bone
19. This is a mnemonic to remember for comparing joint films in patients less than <16 years old

DOWN

2. With this disease, the bone breaks down more quickly, which causes it to grow back softer
3. Fracture directly across the bone
4. Low bone density
5. These nodes cause swelling of the proximal interphalangeal joints seen in osteoarthritis
11. Fracture at an angle across the bone
12. This sign involves tingling in the wrist as a result of the tapping of the median nerve; it is indicative of carpal tunnel syndrome

20. Dense connective tissue that is found in various locations in the body, including the external ear
21. A deformity in which the body part is turned outward from the midline to an abnormal degree
22. A type of bone that is spongy
28. Lateral epicondylitis is referred to as _____ *elbow*

13. A deformity in which the body part is turned inward from the midline to an abnormal degree
14. Pit vipers are in this family of snakes
15. The mnemonic for common interventions for orthopedic injuries
16. Fracture with buckling of the bone
17. This type of snake is poisonous and has cat-like eyes (two words)
20. Follow these guidelines for bites (acronym)
23. This is the first drug that is given when a patient is having an anaphylaxic reaction

31. Knock-kneed (two words)
32. Fracture that occurs when the ends of the bone are not aligned
33. These nodes cause swelling of the distal interphalangeal joints seen in osteoarthritis
34. The procedure used to realign a fracture
37. When one bone is forced against another

24. Small, blood-sucking, parasitic arachnid
25. Coral snakes are in this family of snakes
26. Fracture that is straight and in good alignment
27. Medial epicondylitis is referred to as _____ *elbow*
29. This type of spider has a red hourglass shape on the ventral side of the abdomen (two words)
30. Patellar tendonitis is referred to as _____ *knee*
33. Bees, wasps, hornets, and fire ants are also known by this name

41. A syndrome that results in neurovascular compromise
42. The area at which two bones connect
43. Bowlegged (two words)
44. The medicine used in gout (generic)
45. Acute or chronic inflammation of the bone
46. Another name for a torus fracture

35. Fracture with compression of the bone with shortening
36. Brittle and weak bones
38. Fracture that results from weakness of the bone
39. When giving orthopedic discharge instructions, proper crutch walking must be clearly _____
40. Subluxation of the radial head is sometimes referred to as _____ *elbow*
44. Fracture that involves the bone piercing the skin

2. DIRECTIONS: Name the type of fracture described.

Description	Type of Fracture
Fracture that is angled across the bone	
Periosteum that is divided on only one side	
Bone that is broken and piercing the skin	
Fracture that is directly across the bone	
Fracturing off of a bone fragment	
Bone that is broken into fragments	
Compression of the bone with shortening	
Fracture that results from a twisting motion	
Fracture that is straight and in good alignment	
Fracture that occurs as a result of a bone deficit	
Fracture through the epiphyseal plate	
Fracture in which the bone buckles	
Fracture in which one bone is forced against another	
Fracture in which the ends of the bone are not aligned	

3. DIRECTIONS: Fill in the following table regarding common anesthetics used for the management of wounds.

Agent	Onset	Duration	Contraindications	Maximum Dose for Adults
Lidocaine (1%–2%)				
Lidocaine (1%–2%) with epinephrine 1:100,000 or 1:200,000				
Bupivacaine 0.25% (Marcaine)				
Bupivacaine 0.25% with epinephrine 1:200,000				
Eutectic mixture of local anesthetics (EMLA) cream (lidocaine 2.5% and prilocaine 2.5%)				

4. DIRECTIONS: Fill in the wound complication table.

Infection	Causative Organism	Incubation Period	Symptoms
Wound botulism			
Gas gangrene			
Tetanus			

5. DIRECTIONS: Complete the following table regarding estimated blood loss from fractures.

Site	Estimated Blood Loss
Forearm	
Tibia	
Elbow	
Knee	
Femur	
Humerus	
Hip	
Pelvis	

6. DIRECTIONS: Name the "six Ps" of neurovascular assessment.

1.
2.
3.
4.
5.
6.

7. DIRECTIONS: Name the "four Rs" of fractures.

1.
2.
3.
4.

8. DIRECTIONS:: Complete the following chart about specific wound infections.

Specific Wound Infection	Causative Organism	Cause	Symptoms	Onset or Incubation Period	Management
Cat-scratch fever					
Gas gangrene					
Group A strep-tococcus					
Pasteurella multocida					
Rabies					
Staphylococcal infections					
Tetanus					
Wound botulism					

LEARNING ACTIVITIES ANSWERS

1.

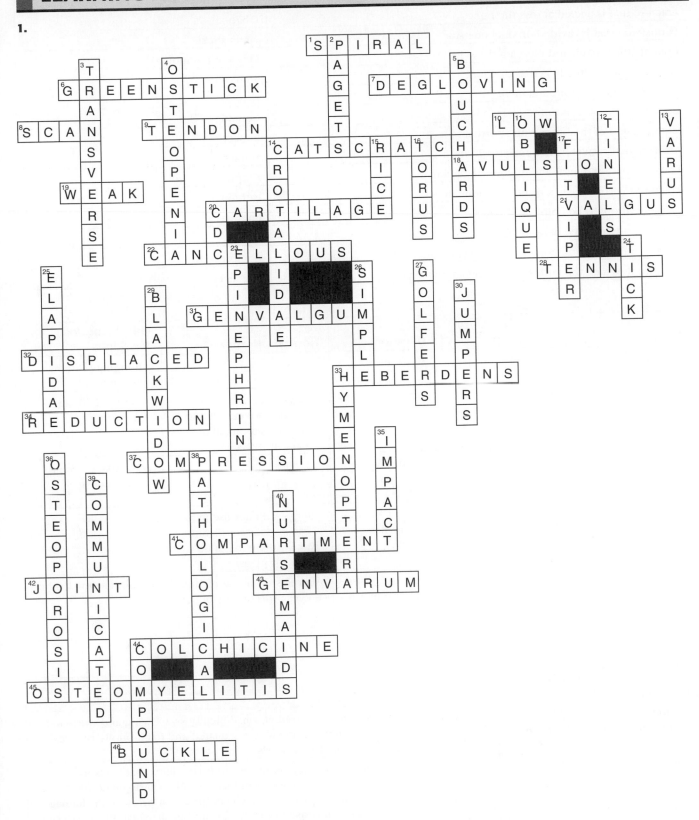

2.

Description	Type of Fracture
Fracture that is angled across the bone	Oblique
Periosteum that is divided on only one side	Greenstick
Bone that is broken and piercing the skin	Open or compound
Fracture that is directly across the bone	Transverse
Fracturing off of a bone fragment	Avulsion
Bone that is broken into fragments	Comminuted
Compression of the bone with shortening	Impact
Fracture that results from a twisting motion	Spiral
Fracture that is straight and in good alignment	Simple or closed
Fracture that occurs as a result of a bone deficit	Pathologic
Fracture through the epiphyseal plate	Epiphyseal
Fracture in which the bone buckles	Torus
Fracture in which one bone is forced against another	Compression
Fracture in which the ends of the bone are not aligned	Displaced

3.

Agent	Onset	Duration	Contraindications	Maximum Dose for Adults
Lidocaine (1%–2%)	1–5 min	30–60 min	Allergies	4.5 mg/kg (300 mg maximum)
Lidocaine (1%–2%) with epinephrine 1:100,000 or 1:200,000	1–5 min	2–6 hr	Allergies; do not use in areas of poor circulation or for digits, nasal tip, ears, or penis	7 mg/kg (500 mg maximum)
Bupivacaine 0.25% (Marcaine)	5 min	2–4 hr (Windle); 8–16 hr (ENA)	Allergies	2.5 mg/kg (175 mg maximum)
Bupivacaine 0.25% with epinephrine 1:200,000	5 min	3–7 hr (Windle); 8–16 hr (ENA)	Allergies; do not use in areas of poor circulation or for digits, nasal tip, ears, or penis	225 mg
EMLA cream (lidocaine 2.5% and prilocaine 2.5%)	30–60 min; reaches maximum peak within 3 hr	Lasts 1–2 hours after removal of the actual cream	Allergies; do not apply near eyes or to open wounds	Do not use for >4 hr

4.

Infection	Causative Organism	Incubation Period	Symptoms
Wound botulism	*Clostridium botulinum*	4–14 days	Weakness, blurred vision, difficulty swallowing and speaking, dry mucous membranes, dilated and fixed pupils, progressive motor paralysis
Gas gangrene	*Clostridium perfringens*	1 day–6 weeks	Rapidly developing tense and hard edema that leads to hypoxia, thrombosis of local vessels, soft-tissue crepitus, severe pain, thin and watery brown or brown-gray drainage, fever, increased heart rate, vomiting, diarrhea, anorexia, coma
Tetanus	*Clostridium tetani*	2 days–several mo (average, 6–14 days)	Restlessness, headache, muscle spasms, pain (neck, back, face); progresses to extreme stiffness, tonic spasms of the voluntary muscles, convulsions, respiratory depression

5.

Site	Estimated Blood Loss
Forearm	0.5–1 L
Tibia	0.5–1.5 L
Elbow	0.5–1.5 L
Knee	1–1.5 L
Femur	1–2 L
Humerus	1–2 L
Hip	1.5–2.5 L
Pelvis	1.5–4.5 L

6.

1. Pain
2. Pallor
3. Pulselessness
4. Polar
5. Paresthesia
6. Paresis/paralysis

7.

1. Recognition
2. Reduction
3. Retention
4. Rehabilitation

8.

Specific Wound Infection	Causative Organism	Cause	Symptoms	Onset or Incubation Period	Management
Cat-scratch fever	*Afipia felis* or *Bartonella henselae*	• Organism that is found in the saliva of cats and dogs • More commonly results from kittens licking, biting, or scratching	• Lymphadenitis • Fever • Nausea and vomiting • Fatigue	• Onset 2–3 wk after exposure	• Analgesics • Antipyretics • Heat therapy • Antibiotics for immunocompromised individuals
Gas gangrene	*Clostridium perfringens*	• Infection of the muscle tissue caused by toxin-producing clostridia • History of intestinal or gallbladder surgery	• Soft-tissue crepitus • Pain • Thin, watery drainage • Increased pulse • Nausea, vomiting, and diarrhea • Coma	• Incubation period of 1–6 days	• Tetanus toxoid • Antibiotics • Surgical wound debridement
Group A streptococcus	Group A streptococcal bacteria	• Found in the throat and on the skin • Spread by direct person-to-person contact	• Necrotizing fasciitis • Toxic shock syndrome	• Onset 1–3 days after exposure	• Antibiotics • Supportive therapy for shock • Immunoglobulin G for toxic shock syndrome

Continued

Specific Wound Infection	Causative Organism	Cause	Symptoms	Onset or Incubation Period	Management
Pasteurella multocida	*Pasteurella multocida*	• Animal bites	• Swelling and redness at the site • Tenderness and possible discharge at the site • Fever and chills	• Onset 3 hr–3 days after exposure	• Antibiotics
Rabies	Neurotoxic virus	• Found in the saliva of rabid animals	• Malaise • Fever • Headache • Photophobia • Lymphadenitis • Muscle spasms • Osteomyelitis • Abscess • Necrotizing fasciitis • Coma	• Incubation period of 10 days–several mo	• Clean wound with virus-killing soap • Rabies immunoglobulin • Rabies vaccine series on days 1, 3, 7, 14, and 28
Staphylococcal infections	*Staphylococcus aureus*	• Common bacteria found on the skin that can cause infection via a break in the skin	• Various • Redness and swelling • Nausea and vomiting • Diarrhea • Headache • General aches	• Onset varies from 2 days to 3–4 wk	• Antibiotics • Good hand washing
Tetanus	*Clostridium tetani*	• Bacteria in the soil	• Restlessness • Headache • Muscle spasms • Stiffness and tetany • Pain • Exaggerated reflex activity • Convulsions • Respiratory depression	• Incubation period of 2 days–several mo (average, 6–10 days)	• Antitoxins • Antibiotics • Vaccine
Wound botulism	*Clostridium botulinum*	• Crush injuries and major trauma	• Weakness • Blurred vision • Difficulty speaking and swallowing • Dry mucous membranes • Dilated pupils • Progressive paralysis	• Incubation period of 4–14 days	• Debridement • Antitoxins • Antibiotics

References and Suggested Readings

Arnold, T. (2007, June 7). Spider envenomations, brown recluse. Retrieved October 23, 2008, from http://www.emedicine.com/EMERG/topic547.htm.

Bower, M. (2001). Managing dog, cat, and human bite wounds. *Nurse Practitioner, 26(4),* 36-38, 41-42, 45.

Brinker, D., Hancox, J. D., & Bernardon, S. (2003). Assessment and initial treatment of lacerations, mammalian bites, and insect stings. *AACN Clinical Wound Care: Heart Failure, 14(4),* 401-410.

Brusch, J. L. (2008). Septic arthritis. Retrieved September 4, 2008, from http://www.emedicine.com/med/topic3394.htm.

Buttaro, T. M., Trybulski, J., Bailey, P. P., & Sandberg-Cook, J. (2003). *Primary care: A collaborative practice.* St. Louis: Mosby.

Cassinelli, E., Young, B., Vogt, M., Pierce, M., & Deeney, V. (2005). Spica cast application in the emergency room for select pediatric femur fractures. *Journal of Orthopaedic Trauma, 19(10),* 709-716.

Clark, D. Y., Stocking, J., & Johnson, J. (Eds.). (2006). *Flight and ground transport nursing core curriculum* (2nd ed.). Denver, CO: Air & Surface Transport Nurses Association.

Daley, B. J., & Barbee, J. (2008). Snakebite. Retrieved September 5, 2008, from http://www.emedicine.com/med/topic2143.htm.

Dennison, R. D. (2007). *Pass CCRN!* (3rd ed.). St. Louis: Mosby.

Domino, F. J. (2008). *The 5-minute clinical consultant* (16th ed.). Philadelphia: Lippincott, Williams, & Wilkins.

Dorland's Illustrated Medical Dictionary (30th ed.). (2003). St. Louis: W.B. Saunders.

Elzik, M., Dirschl, D., & Dahners, L. E. (2008). Hemorrhage in pelvic fractures does not correlate with fracture length. *Journal of Trauma: Injury, Infection, and Critical Care, 65(2),* 436-441.

Emergency Nurses Association. (2007). *Emergency nursing core curriculum* (6th ed.). Philadelphia: Saunders.

Emergency Nurses Association. (2003). *Emergency nursing pediatric course provider manual* (3rd ed.). Park Ridge, IL: Author.

Emergency Nurses Association. (2005). *Sheehy's manual of emergency care* (6th ed.). St. Louis: Mosby.

Flowers, L. K., & Wippermann, B. D. (2007). Costochondritis. Retrieved September 5, 2008, from http://www.emedicine.com/emerg/topic116.htm.

Foresman-Capuzzi, J., Tadduni, G. T., & Callahan T. (2006). A 56-year-old man sustains high pressure injection trauma to his hand. *Journal of Emergency Nursing, 32(4),* 310-312.

Fultz, J., & Sturt, P. A. (2005). *Mosby's emergency nursing reference* (3rd ed.). St. Louis: Mosby.

Harrahill, M. (2006). Posterior hip dislocation with femoral head fracture: An unusual injury. *Journal of Emergency Nursing, 32(5),* 451-453.

Ing, E. (2007). Lacerations, eyelid. Retrieved August 31, 2008, from http://www.emedicine.com/oph/topic219.htm.

Janson, P. A., & Iseke, R. (2007). Hymenoptera stings. Retrieved September 5, 2008, from http://www.emedicine.com/med/topic1058.htm#section~followup.

Jarvis, C. (2008). *Physical examination and health assessment* (5th ed.). St. Louis: Saunders.

King, R. W., & Johnson, D. (2006). Osteomyelitis. Retrieved September 5, 2008, from http://www.emedicine.com/emerg/topic349.htm.

Kirkland, L. (2007). Fat embolism. Retrieved September 10, 2008, from http://www.emedicine.com/med/topic652.htm.

Lab Tests Online. (2008). Inside the lab. Retrieved August 31, 2008, from http://www.labtestsonline.org/index.html.

Marx, J. (2002). *Rosen's emergency medicine: Concepts and clinical practice* (5th ed.). St. Louis: Mosby.

Mayo Clinic. (2007). Osteoarthritis. Retrieved September 5, 2008, from http://www.mayoclinic.com/health/osteoarthritis/DS00019.

Medline Plus. (2008). Snake bites. Retrieved September 5, 2008, from http://www.nlm.nih.gov/medlineplus/ency/article/000031.htm.

Merriam-Webster Online. (2008). *Merriam-Webster's medical dictionary.* Retrieved September 5 from http://medical.merriam-webster.com.

Mullins, J., & Harrahill, M. (2008). Dog bites: A brief case review. *Journal of Emergency Nursing, 34(5),* 490-491.

National Osteoporosis Foundation. (2008). Retrieved September 5, 2008, from http://www.nof.org/osteoporosis/index.htm.

Norvelle, J. G., & Steele, M. (2008). Carpal tunnel syndrome. Retrieved August 31, 2008, from http://www.emedicine.com/emerg/topic83.htm

O'Dell, M. L. (1998). Skin infections: An overview. *American Family Physician.* Retrieved September 3, 2008, from http://www.aafp.org/afp/980515ap/odell.html.

Paula, R., & Chiang, W. K. (2006). Compartment syndrome, extremity. Retrieved September 4, 2008, from http://www.emedicine.com/emerg/topic739.htm.

Price, S. A., & Wilson, L. M. (2003). *Pathophysiology: Clinical concepts of disease process* (6th ed.). St. Louis: Mosby.

Proehl, J. A. (2004). *Emergency nursing procedures* (3rd ed.). St. Louis: Saunders.

Roppolo, L. P., Davis, D., Kelly, S. P., & Rosen, P. (2007). *Emergency medicine handbook: Critical concepts for clinical practice.* St. Louis: Mosby.

Schmidt, J. M. (2005). Antivenom therapy for snakebites in children: Is there evidence? *Current Opinion in Pediatrics, 17(2),* 234-238.

Schwartz, R. A. (2008, August 8). Black widow spider bite. Retrieved October 25, 2008, from http://www.emedicine.com/derm/topic599.htm.

Selfe, T., & Taylor, A. G. (2008). Acupuncture and osteoarthritis of the knee: A review of randomized, controlled trials. *Family & Community Health. Complementary Practice and Products, 31(3),* 247-254.

Stephenson, J. (2007) Rabies and snake bites. *Journal of the American Medical Association, 297(7),* 686.

Stiell, I. G., Greenberg, G. H., McKnight, R. D., Nair, R. C., McDowell, I., & Worthington, J. R. (1992). A study to develop clinical decision rules for the use of radiography in acute ankle injuries. *Annals of Emergency Medicine, 21(4),* 384-390.

Stiell, I. G., Greenberg, G. H., McKnight, R. D., Nair, R. C., McDowell, I., & Worthington, J. R. (1994). Implementation of the Ottawa ankle rules. *Journal of the American Medical Association, 271(11),* 827-832.

Taravella, M. (2006). Keratopathy, band. Retrieved September 5, 2008, from http://www.emedicine.com/oph/topic105.htm.

Torpy, J. M. (2006). Osteopenia and preventing fractures. *Journal of the American Medical Association, 296(21).* Retrieved August 31, 2008, from http://jama.ama-assn.org/cgi/content/full/296/21/2644.

Windle, M. L. (2008). Local anesthetic agents, infiltrative administration. Retrieved August 31, 2008, from http://www.emedicine.com/proc/topic149178.htm

Zeglin, D. (2005). Brown recluse spider bites: Managing the effects, which can include necrotic arachnidism and loxoscelism. *American Journal of Nursing, 105(2),* 64-68.

Zimmerman, P. G., & Herr, R. (2006). *Triage nursing secrets.* St. Louis: Mosby.

CHAPTER 9

Genitourinary, Gynecologic, and Obstetric Emergencies

Introduction

This content constitutes 6.5% (10 items) of the CEN examination

The focus is on genitourinary (GU), gynecologic (GYN), and obstetric (OB) conditions commonly encountered in an ED setting

The continuum of age needs to be considered from infancy to older for GU and GYN conditions

Consider the possibility of pregnancy in all women of childbearing age when they present to the ED

Age-Related Considerations

Neonates, infants, and children

1. Children with urinary tract infection (UTI) may present with enuresis
2. Children are at higher risk for testicular torsion
3. Presence of sexually transmitted infections (STIs) (previously referred to as sexually transmitted diseases [STDs]) in children may indicate abuse and should be further investigated
4. Incidence of STIs is increasing in teens

Older adult

1. Immobility increases risk for UTIs and renal stones
2. Epididymitis is usually associated with *Escherichia coli* rather than STI

Pregnancy-Related Changes

Cardiovascular

1. Heart rate increases by 15 to 20 beats per minutes (bpm) due to increased blood volume that occurs during pregnancy
   a. Increase in total blood volume may mask hemorrhage
2. Blood pressure decreases; systolic BP will decrease 0 to 15 mm Hg while diastolic BP will decrease 10 to 20 mm Hg
   a. Elevated progesterone levels cause a relaxation of smooth muscles which decreases systemic vascular resistance and blood pressure.
3. Cardiac output (CO) increases 30% to 50%
4. Normal hematocrit in the pregnant patient is approximately 32% to 34% since circulating plasma increases, which causes a dilutional anemia
5. White blood cells can be up to 20,000 mm³, primarily due to an increase in neutrophils, which occurs with a slight increase in lymphocytes

6. Increased clotting factors and hypercoagulability occur with an increased risk of disseminated intravascular coagulation (DIC)
7. Selective uterine vasoconstriction in response to hemorrhage can cause fetal hypoxia
8. Heart is displaced more horizontally so that the apex is displaced laterally

Airway/breathing

1. Upper airway engorgement occurs with pregnancy
2. Enlarging uterus will elevate the diaphragm which decreases lung capacity
3. Respiratory rate and tidal volume both increase to result in an increase in minute ventilation
4. Oxygen consumption increases

Gastrointestinal

1. Abdominal organs become displaced as the uterus enlarges
2. Pelvic veins become engorged
3. Progesterone relaxation of gastrointestinal smooth muscle level causes a decrease in gastric motility and emptying; may cause paralytic ileus
4. Abdominal injuries may be masked

Selected Concepts in Anatomy and Physiology

General information about the GU and GYN systems

1. The GU system consists of a group of organs that are involved in reproduction and production and elimination of urine
2. The term *genitourinary* refers to two different systems (Figure 9-1)
   a. "Genito" refers to the genital organs and the reproductive system
   b. "Urinary" refers to the system responsible for removal of nitrogenous waste products from the blood in the form of urine
      1) The primary function is to help maintain homeostasis by controlling the composition and volume of blood by removing and restoring selected amounts of water and solutes
      2) Urinary system is made up of two kidneys, two ureters, one urinary bladder, and one urethra; each kidney excretes urine through a ureter and urine is stored in the urinary bladder and expelled from the body through the urethra

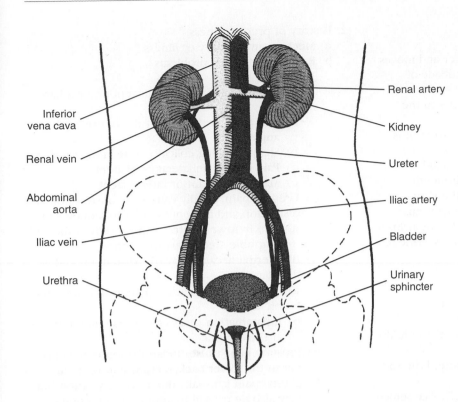

Figure 9-1 The kidneys and other structures of the urinary tract. (From Long, B. C., Phipps, W. J., & Cassmeyer, V. [1993]. *Medical-surgical nursing: A nursing process approach* [3rd ed.] St. Louis: Mosby).

Kidneys

1. There are two kidneys, which are reddish, bean-shaped organs averaging approximately 12 cm long and 6 cm wide
2. The kidney is held in place by connective tissue surrounded by a thick layer of adipose tissue
3. The kidneys are located on the posterior wall of the abdominal cavity just above the waist line between the level of the twelfth thoracic vertebra (T12) and the third lumbar vertebra (L3)
4. The kidneys are composed of three types of tissue called the capsule, cortex, and medulla
   a. The capsule is the outermost cover of the kidneys.
   b. The cortex forms an outer layer on the kidneys and contains the glomerulus and the proximal and distal tubules
   c. The medulla forms the inner kidney renal columns and is made up of the collecting tubes; the renal pyramids and papillae are part of the medulla tissue
5. Functions of the kidney
   a. Filter metabolic wastes products in the form of urine
      1) The entire volume of blood in the body is filtered through the kidney approximately 60 times each day
   b. Urine is formed by the activities of the kidneys
   c. Regulate the composition and volume of blood (e.g., fluid and electrolytes) by removing select amounts of water and solutes
   d. Balance acid base by controlling blood pH
   e. Regulation of blood pressure is influenced by aldosterone and antidiuretic hormone (ADH) and by secreting the enzyme renin
   f. Participates in activation of vitamin D

Ureters

1. A musculomembranous tubular structure that is continuous with the renal pelvis
2. The ureters are approximately 12 inches long and form the upper part of the renal pelvis of each kidney
3. The ureters move the urine from the kidneys to the bladder by the process of peristalsis
4. Urine enters the ureters from the kidney a drop at a time and is pushed by waves of muscular contraction toward the urinary bladder and enters through the base

Urinary bladder

1. A musculomembranous sac, which acts as a reservoir for the urine
2. Size of the bladder depends on the amount of fluid it contains
3. Located in the lower portion of the abdominal cavity just behind the symphysis pubis
4. The base of the bladder is known as the trigone, which is solid, nonstretchable, and triangular in shape
5. The rest of the wall of the bladder is stretchable and forms a spherical sac when filled
6. The mucosal lining of the bladder is composed of epithelial cells that are cuboidal and when the bladder fills these cells stretch and flatten, which is why they are called transitional epithelium
7. The voiding reflex occurs when the transitional epithelium reaches a certain degree of stretch; when the limit of stretch is reached a message is sent via the spinal cord to the brain, which initiates the voiding reflex
   a. When it is inconvenient to void the transitional cells can reorganize and undergo more stretching until the limit of the urinary bladder is reached; at that time the bladder must be emptied

Urethra

1. Begins at the anterior base of the bladder and moves urine from the urinary bladder to the outside of the body
2. Female urethra is short and opens directly to the outside of the body.
3. Male urethra is longer and has two curvatures; it is divided into three sections
   a. Prostatic portion enters the prostate gland
   b. Membranous portion enters the peritoneum
   c. Penile portion forms in the shaft of the penis
4. The urethral sphincters are two circular muscular structures that prevent urine from leaving the urinary bladder; when relaxed, the sphincters allow urine to be forced through them

Male genital organs

1. Scrotum is the sac which contains the testes
2. Testes produce sperm and testosterone
3. Vas deferens allows communication from the epididymis to ejaculatory duct
4. Spermatic cord is a protective sheath around the vas deferens
5. Seminal vesicles and the prostate gland produce semen
6. Bulbourethral gland secretes an alkaline component of semen to neutralize vaginal secretions
7. Epididymis stores sperm until it is mature
8. Penis is the male sex organ, which contains the urethra, the route for urine excretion during voiding and semen during ejaculation during sexual organism
   a. Glans penis is important for sexual arousal

Female genital organs

1. Mons pubis is a subcutaneous pad over the symphysis pubis for protection
2. Labia majora and minora consist of folds of adipose and connective tissue that protect and lubricate external genitalia
3. Clitoris is an erectile tissue for sexual stimulation
4. Skene glands provide lubrication and protection
5. Vagina is a muscular tube to allow menstrual blood flow, sexual intercourse, and fetal delivery
6. Vaginal introitus is the opening of the vagina
7. Bartholin glands secretes alkaline mucus that improves viability and motility of sperm
8. Cervix is the neck of the uterus leading from the vagina
9. Uterus is a hollow, muscular organ; site for fertilized egg implantation; protects fetus
10. Fallopian tubes serve as a passage for an ovum to uterus for fertilization and implantation
11. Ovaries produce ova, estrogen, and progesterone

Physical Assessment

Primary and secondary assessment (see Chapter 2)

Focused assessment

1. Chief complaint: identifies why the patient is seeking help and the duration of the problem

2. History of present illness
   a. Mechanism of injury or illness
   b. Pain related to GU problems
      1) PQRST
      2) Renal pain can be due to distention or inflammation
         a) Dull ache in the area of the costovertebral angle
         b) Sharp, stabbing, colicky nature in the flank area
         d) Pain can be unilateral or bilateral
         c) May be constant or intermittent
      3) Ureteral pain: usually caused by obstruction and distention and presents similar to kidney pain
         a) Pain in lower ureters can present in the suprapubic area, penis, or urethra
      4) Bladder pain: caused by overdistention and inflammation
         a) Overdistention causes pain in the suprapubic area
         b) Inflammation causes sharp pain and burning at the urethra
      5) Prostate pain: causes inflammation that can occur in the lower back, rectum, and perineum
      6) Scrotal pain is usually due to inflammation but may also be caused by trauma and torsion
   c. Pain related to GYN problems
      1) PQRST
         a) Provocation related to activity or position
      2) Fallopian tube or ovary: caused by distention or inflammation
         a) Visceral pain: pain from internal organs
         b) Dull, steady, and poorly localized
      3) Uterus caused by contractions and spasms
         a) Visceral pain that is localized in midline
         b) Waxing and waning severity
      4) Peritoneal (localized) caused by inflammation
         a) Pain is sharp and well-defined
      5) Peritoneal (generalized) is related to blood accumulation from a ruptured ectopic or ovarian cyst
         a) Pus from a pelvic infection spreading through the abdomen with guarding and rigidity causes rebound tenderness
   d. Vaginal bleeding between periods or after menopause or during pregnancy
      1) Onset: date and time
      2) Course since onset
      3) Relationship to activity or time of day
      4) Color: pink, red, dark red, brown, other
      5) Characteristics: thin, thick, mixed with mucus; if clots, how many and how large
      6) Amount: stain on underwear or saturation of how any pads and/or tampons in a specific time period
      7) Associated symptoms: pain, cramping, abdominal distention, pelvic fullness, changes in bowel habits, weight loss or gain
   e. Vaginal discharge
      1) Onset: date and time
      2) Course since onset

3) Color: white, yellowish-green, gray, other
4) Consistency: thin, curdlike, purulent
5) Odor: "fishy" foul
6) Amount
7) Associated symptoms: vulvar itching, vaginal itching, rash, pain with sexual intercourse, dysuria, abdominal pain, pelvic fullness, fever

f. Nausea and vomiting
g. Fever, chills
h. Headache
i. Weight gain or loss
j. Edema
k. Changes in micturition (i.e., urination)
  1) Changes in urine volume
    a) Anuria: absence of urine output (<100 ml/24 hr)
    b) Polyuria: increased urine output (>2500 ml/24 hr)
    c) Oliguria: decreased urine output (100 to 400 ml/24 hr)
  2) Urgency: feeling need to void immediately
  3) Hesitancy: difficulty starting urine flow
  4) Dysuria: painful, burning or difficult urination
  5) Nocturia: excessive urination at night (more than twice)
  6) Retention: incomplete emptying of bladder
  7) Incontinence: inability to control urination
  8) Enuresis: incontinence of urine in bed at night
l. Changes in urine appearance (Merck Source, 2005; Terris, 2008)
  1) Clear to light yellow: dilute or normal
  2) Dark yellow or amber: can indicate dehydration
  3) Dark yellow to orange can be caused by vitamin B and some laxatives
  4) Orange: can be caused by medications (e.g., phenazopyridine [Pyridium], rifampin [Rifadin])
  5) Orange pink: may indicate uric acid crystals
  6) Cloudy: possible infection (i.e., pyuria)
  7) Pink to red: blood in urine (i.e., hematuria)
  8) Blue/green: may indicate a blue dye such as methylene blue
  9) Brown or black: may be caused by excessive L-dopa or melanin excretion as well as copper or phenol poisoning.
    a) Ingestion of large amounts of rhubarb, blackberries, or beets can cause dark brownish black urine
    b) Dark brown may indicate presence of bilirubin
  10) Tea, rust, or wine colored may indicate rhabdomyolysis and myoglobinuria or hemoglobinuria (i.e., heavy pigments)

3. Past medical history
a. Past illnesses and injuries
b. Past surgical procedures (include GU, GYN, and OB)
c. Past diagnostic studies (e.g., radiologic and CT)
d. Preexisting illness
e. Menstrual history
  1) Age menses initiated (i.e., menarche)
  2) Date of first day of last menstrual period (LMP)
  3) Usual menstrual pattern
  4) Discomfort before or during menses (i.e., dysmenorrhea)
  5) Unusually heavy menstrual flow (i.e., metrorrhagia)
  6) Dysfunctional bleeding between periods or after menopause (i.e., menorrhagia)
f. OB history
  1) Number of pregnancies
    a) Gravida: total number of pregnancies (if pregnant currently include in number)
    b) Parity or para: number of pregnancies that have lasted at least 20 weeks
    c) Primigravida: first pregnancy
    d) Nullipara: no live births
    e) Primipara: given birth to one live child
    f) Multipara: more than one live birth
  2) Spontaneous or therapeutic abortions
  3) Full term and preterm deliveries
  4) Number of living children
g. Currently pregnant (women of childbearing age)
  1) Date of first day of LMP
  2) Results of pregnancy test
  3) Date of test and was it a urine or serum test
  4) Expected date of confinement (EDC)
  5) Prenatal care
h. Exposure to sexually transmitted infections (STIs)
i. Allergies and type of reaction
j. Immunization

4. Social history
a. Usual activity level
b. Ability to perform activities of daily living (ADLs)
c. Sexual history
  1) Multiple partners
  2) Unprotected sexual intercourse

5. Medication history
a. Prescribed drugs, doses, frequency, time of last dose
b. Nonprescribed drugs
  1) Over-the-counter drugs including herbal supplements
  2) Substance abuse (e.g., cocaine, amphetamines)
c. Patient's understanding of drug actions, side effects

General survey

1. Level of consciousness
2. Vital signs
3. Nutritional status
4. Stature/posture
5. Gait
6. Odor

Inspection

1. Skin color
   a. Yellowish-gray color seen in renal failure
   b. Pallor seen in anemia
   c. Petechiae and bruising may be seen in renal failure as a result of platelet dysfunction
2. Skin turgor
   a. Recoil should be immediate
   b. Decrease indicates interstitial dehydration (late sign)
3. Scars, lesions, hernias
4. Abdominal distention
5. Signs of infection
6. Uncontrolled bleeding or open wounds
7. Edema: generalized, facial, peripheral, sacral
8. Vaginal bleeding: amount, passage of clots or tissue, color, odor
9. Foreign bodies

Auscultation

1. Heart sounds
2. Lung sounds
3. Bowel sounds
4. Fetal heart tones if pregnant

Palpation

1. Abdominal tenderness, guarding
2. Costovertebral angle (CVA) (i.e., formed on either side of the vertebral column between the last rib and the lumbar vertebrae) tenderness
3. Rebound tenderness
4. If pregnant
   a. Uterine size
   b. Fundal height
   c. Contractility
   d. Any irritability

Pelvic assessment

1. Visual inspection of external genitalia looking for any abnormalities such as excoriation, erythema, and lesions or vesicles
2. Inspect vaginal mucosa for color, lesions, discharge, and presence of edema
3. Inspect and palpate
   a. Bartholin gland: located inside each labium near the opening of the vagina, which produces fluid that is secreted through small ducts and lubricates the vagina; if it becomes clogged a cyst may form and the area becomes tender.
   b. Skene gland: located on the anterior wall of the vagina, around the lower end of the urethra; It drains into the urethra and near the urethral opening
4. Inspect vagina and cervix for bleeding, discharge, erosion, lesions, and ulcerations
5. Bimanual examination is performed to palpate for uterus size, shape, cervical motion tenderness, adnexal, and masses

System-Specific Tasks

General GYN emergency interventions

1. Prepare vaginal or cervical specimens
2. Assess characteristics of vaginal discharge/bleeding
3. Interview victim of sexual assault
4. Collect forensic evidence from sexual assault victims

Laboratory studies

1. Serum
   a. CBC with differential
      1) Decreased hemoglobin and hematocrit: indicates possible blood loss
      2) Increased WBC count with left shift if bacterial infection present
   b. ESR: increase indicates infection
   c. Type and cross-match
   d. Rh factor: Rh-negative pregnant women are given Rho (immune globulin; i.e., RhoGAM)
   e. Coagulation profile (e.g., PT, aPTT, fibrin split products)
   f. Serum and urine toxicology screen
   g. Thyroid function test
   h. Liver enzymes
2. STI screening
   a. Gonorrhea culture
   b. Chlamydia culture
   c. Wet mount
   d. Cytologic smear
   e. Test for syphilis
   f. HIV screen
3. hCG pregnancy test
4. Radiographic studies
   a. Chest radiograph
   b. Abdominal radiograph (i.e., flat plate of abdomen [also referred to as KUB])
   c. Ultrasound
      1) Bladder scan: measures bladder volume
      2) Sonogram: uses ultrasonic waves to image an internal body structure, monitor a developing fetus, or generate localized deep heat to the tissues

General OB emergency interventions

1. Perform neonatal resuscitation following emergency delivery
2. Place a patient in labor with a prolapsed cord in a knee-chest position
3. Assist with emergency delivery of fetus
4. Assess for presence of fetal heart tones (normal 110 to 160 bpm)
5. Obtain laboratory studies
   a. CBC: to assess for anemia
   b. Glucose challenge or tolerance testing: to assess for gestational diabetes
   c. Antibody screen: to assess potential incompatibility in blood type between mother and fetus (e.g., Rh factor antibodies)

d. Coagulation studies: to assess for thrombocytopenia

e. Kleihauer-Betke test: to defect fetal red cells in the maternal circulation

f. Urine analysis: to determine presence of protein, glucose, or bacteria

SPECIFIC GEN/GYN/OB EMERGENCIES

Urinary Tract Infections

Definition: inflammation of the urinary mucosa that can occur anywhere in the urinary tract; the most common nosocomial infection

1. Cystitis: infection of the urinary bladder; may be called lower UTI
2. Urethritis: infection of the urethra

Predisposing factors

1. Previous history of UTI
2. Diabetes mellitus
3. Female gender: females have 10 times the risk of men because women have a shorter urethra
   a. Sexually active women have greater risk than non-sexually active women
4. In men under 50 years old, UTIs are most frequently associated with STIs (Howe & Pillow, 2009)
5. Pregnant women with diabetes have a higher risk of UTIs
6. Circumcision in males reduces risk of UTIs

Pathophysiology

1. Pathogens (usually bacteria) enter the urinary tract
   a. Most likely gram negative
   b. Route
      1) Most likely route is ascending from perineal area to lower urinary tract
      2) From the blood
         a) Rare
         b) Usually associated with previous damage to the urinary tract
2. Colonization of the epithelium of the urinary tract
3. Inflammation of the urinary tract

Clinical presentation

1. Subjective
   a. Usually abrupt onset
   b. Dysuria and burning with urination (pain usually referred to distal urethra)
   c. Frequency and urgency with urination, but voiding in small amounts
   d. Nocturia
   e. Change in color of urine (e.g., hematuria)
   f. Lower abdominal pain and back pain; back pain may indicate pyelonephritis
   g. Dizziness, nausea, vomiting, chills
   h. Urinary incontinence
2. Objective
   a. Malodorous or cloudy urine
   b. Elevated temperature
   c. May have orthostatic blood pressure changes due to hypovolemia since patient may attempt to decrease symptoms by decreasing need to urinate
   d. Suprapubic tenderness
   e. Flank pain with percussion or palpitation may indicate pyelonephritis
   f. CVA tenderness with palpation or percussion
3. Diagnostic studies
   a. Urine dip: positive leukocytes and nitrates
   b. Urine analysis and culture
      1) WBCs: increased
      2) Leukocyte esterase activity: increased
      3) Nitrites: increased
      4) Bacteria: positive
   c. Urine pregnancy test for women of childbearing age
   d. BUN and creatinine: to evaluate renal function

Collaborative management

1. Continue assessment
   a. ABCDs
   b. Vital signs: blood pressure, pulse, respiratory rate, and temperature
   c. Pain and discomfort level
   d. Accurate intake and output
   e. Level of consciousness
   f. Close monitoring for progression of symptoms
2. Maintain airway, oxygenation, and ventilation
   a. Position of comfort
   b. Oxygen by nasal cannula at 2 to 6 L/min to maintain SpO_2 of 95% unless contraindicated; for patients with COPD, use pulse oximetry to guide oxygen administration to SpO_2 of 90%
3. Maintain adequate circulation and perfusion
   a. Increased oral fluids
   b. IV access for fluid and medication administration as indicated
      1) IV fluids if dehydrated and/or unable to take oral fluids
   c. Close monitoring for indications of sepsis (i.e., fever, confusion, widened pulse pressure)
4. Administer drugs and therapies to treat cause
   a. Antimicrobials (e.g., ciprofloxacin [Cipro], trimethoprim-sulfamethoxazole [Bactrim])
   b. Pelvic examination as indicated to evaluate possible cause
   c. Foley catheter may be indicated to monitor closely for impairment in urinary elimination
5. Control pain and discomfort
   a. Analgesics (e.g., phenazopyridine [Pyridium]); note that phenazopyridine is available over the counter
   b. Antipyretics for fever as indicated
6. Monitor for complications
   a. Pyelonephritis
   b. Sepsis, septic shock
   c. Deep vein thrombosis (DVT) and pulmonary embolism (PE)

Evaluation

1. Patent airway, adequate oxygenation (i.e., normal Pao_2, Spo_2, Sao_2) and ventilation (i.e., normal $Paco_2$)
2. Absence of clinical indicators of hypoperfusion
3. Absence of clinical indications of sepsis
4. Control of pain, discomfort

Typical disposition

1. If evaluation criteria met: discharge with instructions
   a. Instructions related to when to call primary care provider
      1) Symptoms continue after 3 days of antibiotics
      2) Symptoms return within 14 days
      3) Fever >100.5°F while on antibiotics
      4) Pink or red color in urine after 3 days
   b. Instructions related to drug therapy
      1) Complete entire course of antimicrobials
         a) Take at night if possible so that drug will remain in bladder longer
      2) Inform the patient that phenazopyridine:
         a) Changes color of urine to orange or pink for up to 24 hours after last dose
         b) May stain contact lenses and clothing
         c) Should be taken after meals
   c. Measures to prevent recurrence
      1) Copious oral fluids to promote bacterial excretion
      2) Avoidance of long periods without urinating
      3) Urination after intercourse
      4) For women
         a) Cleanse perineal area from front to back
         b) Avoid bubble baths, feminine hygiene sprays, douching
         c) Wear cotton panties
2. If evaluation criteria not met (i.e., urosepsis): admission

Pyelonephritis

Definition: ascending urinary infection of the upper urinary tract involving the kidneys, tubules, glomeruli, and renal pelvis
Predisposing factors

1. Seen more often in infants, young sexually active women, and older men with obstructive uropathy
2. Underlying urinary tract abnormalities
3. Recurrent UTIs
4. Sexual intercourse
   a. New sexual partner
   b. Recent spermicidal use
5. Diabetes
6. Congenital urinary tract anomalies
7. Urinary catheterization
8. Pregnancy
9. Stress incontinence
10. Neurogenic bladder
11. Immunosuppression
12. Urinary or ureteral obstruction
13. Prostatic enlargement

Pathophysiology (Shoff, Green-McKenzie, Behrman, & Moore-Shepherd, 2007)

1. Results from bacterial invasion of the renal parenchyma
   a. Most common cause is reflux of urine into one or both kidneys
   b. Infection is influenced by bacterial factors and host factors
      1) *Escherichia coli* accounts for 70% to 90% of uncomplicated UTIs and 21% to 54% of complicated UTIs
2. Infection spreads to cortex with WBC infiltration and inflammation
3. The kidney becomes grossly edematous and abscesses may form
   a. Renal carbuncle: a cortical abscess in the periphery of the kidneys usually caused by *Staphylococcus aureus*
4. Scar tissue replaces the infected/inflamed areas if untreated
5. Chronic pyelonephritis is a major cause of renal failure and end-stage renal failure

Clinical presentation (Domino, 2008; ENA, 2007)

1. Subjective
   a. Sudden onset
   b. Recent history of a UTI or STI
   c. Frequency, urgency, dysuria, nocturia
   d. Flank, back, or abdominal pain or tenderness
   e. Report of cloudy, foul-smelling urine
   f. Fever, chills, malaise
   g. Nausea and vomiting
   h. Fatigue
   i. Children may present with history of decreased urination, bed wetting (i.e., enuresis), irritability, loss of energy
   j. Infants may present with irritability, cool skin, jaundice to gray skin color, decrease in number of wet diapers, poor feeding
2. Objective
   a. Elevated temperature
      1) Older adults frequently will not have a temperature elevation
   b. Orthostatic hypotension
   c. Tenderness over affected flank area with palpation
   d. CVA tenderness with palpation
   e. Behavior changes in children or infants (e.g., restless, not active)
3. Diagnostic studies
   a. CBC: note leukocytosis
   b. Electrolytes: note sodium and potassium levels
   c. BUN and creatinine: to evaluate renal function
   d. Blood cultures: used to rule out septicemia, but not to diagnosis or manage pyelonephritis
   e. Urinalysis: pyuria with or without leukocyte casts and mild proteinuria
   f. Urine culture: to identify causative organism
   g. CT of abdomen and pelvis with and without contrast media
   h. Renal ultrasound
   i. IVP to rule out obstruction

Collaborative management

1. Continue assessment
   a. ABCDs
   b. Vital signs: blood pressure, pulse, respiratory rate, and temperature
   c. Oxygen saturations as indicated
   d. Pain and discomfort level
   e. Accurate intake and output
   f. Serum electrolytes
   g. Level of consciousness
   h. Close monitoring for progression of symptoms
2. Maintain airway, oxygenation, and ventilation
   a. Position of comfort
   b. Oxygen by nasal cannula at 2 to 6 L/min to maintain SpO_2 of 95% unless contraindicated; for patients with COPD, use pulse oximetry to guide oxygen administration to SpO_2 of 90%
3. Maintain adequate circulation and perfusion
   a. Increased oral fluids
   b. IV access for fluid and medication administration as indicated
      1) IV fluids if dehydrated and/or unable to take oral fluids
   c. Close monitoring for indications of sepsis (i.e., fever, confusion, widened pulse pressure)
4. Control pain and discomfort
   a. Analgesics
   b. Antiemetics; nasogastric tube may be needed for uncontrolled vomiting
5. Administer drugs and therapies to treat cause
   a. In and out catheterization for urine culture; Foley catheter may be indicated to monitor closely for impairment in urinary elimination
   b. Antimicrobials (e.g., ciprofloxacin [Cipro], trimethoprim-sulfamethoxazole [Bactrim])
   c. Antipyretics and cooling methods to reduce fever
6. Monitor for complications
   a. Renal calculi
   b. Lower UTIs
   c. Papillary necrosis (necrotizing papillitis)
   d. Perinephric abscess
   e. Preterm labor in pregnant women

Evaluation

1. Patent airway, adequate oxygenation (i.e., normal PaO_2, SpO_2, SaO_2) and ventilation (i.e., normal $PaCO_2$)
2. Absence of clinical indicators of hypoperfusion
3. Absence of clinical indications of sepsis
4. Alert and oriented with no neurologic deficit
5. Control of pain, discomfort

Typical disposition

1. If evaluation criteria met: discharge with instructions
   a. If no improvement in 48 to 72 hours, need for re-evaluation for urinary tract obstruction or urinary calculus
   b. Increased oral fluid intake
   c. Foods and fluids to acidify the urine (e.g., meat, fish, eggs, cereals)
   d. Rest
   e. Antimicrobials and antipyretics
2. If evaluation criteria not met (e.g., high fever, severe pain, immunosuppression, pregnancy, sepsis): admission

Urinary Calculi

Definition: masses of crystals composed of minerals that are normally excreted in the urine, which can be found anywhere; may also be referred to as kidney stones

Predisposing factors

1. Previous urinary calculi
2. Gout or high-purine diet
3. History of hypercalcemia
4. Recent UTIs
5. Ingestion of increased amount of involved mineral
6. Dehydration
7. Immobility
8. Medications such as antacids, vitamin D, laxatives, high doses of aspirin
9. Hyperparathyroidism
10. Multiple myeloma

Pathophysiology

1. Precipitation of a poorly soluble salt occurs around a mucoprotein, which forms a crystalline structure; types of calculi include the following
   a. Calcium: caused by too much calcium in the urine such as with hypercalcemia and demineralization of bone (e.g., immobility, bone malignancy)
      1) The majority of calculi are calcium oxalate or calcium phosphate
   b. Uric acid: caused by too much uric acid in the urine such dehydration, gout, and antineoplastic agents
   c. Struvite: mechanism not well understood but thought to occur as a result of an interaction between protein breakdown products and infection causing bacteria in the urine
   d. Cystine: caused by a genetic disease called cystinuria
2. Size varies
   a. Most (80% to 90%) are small and exit spontaneously in the urine
   b. Larger calculi are not able to be expelled and are trapped most frequently in the renal pelvis or at the ureterovesicular junction
3. Consequences
   a. Trauma to the urinary tract
   b. Obstruction, which may lead to postrenal failure if bilateral or at bladder neck or urethra
   c. Infection

Clinical presentation

1. Subjective
   a. Pain
      1) Usually described as dull and constant
      2) Worsens with voiding

3) May radiate to abdomen, groin, scrotal, and labial areas
  b. Dysuria
  c. Fever and chills
  d. Nausea and vomiting
  e. May have noticed blood in urine
2. Objective
  a. Tachycardia
  b. Blood pressure may be decreased, normal, or increased
  c. Elevated temperature
  d. CVA pain with palpation
  e. May have cool, clammy skin
  f. Restlessness
  g. Abdominal distention if obstruction present
  h. Hematuria
3. Diagnostic studies
  a. BUN and creatinine: to assess renal function
  b. Electrolytes: to assess for hypercalcemia
  c. Uric acid levels: to assess for hyperuricemia
  d. Urine dip: positive for blood
  e. Urinalysis
    1) pH >7 suggests struvite stone (ENA, 2007)
    2) pH <5 suggests uric acid stone (ENA, 2007)
  f. Urine culture: to check for UTI
  g. Stone analysis
  h. KUB, renal CT, IVP: to identify calculus location
  i. Helical CT: 97% accurate in detection of calculi and preferred over IVP (ENA, 2005)

Collaborative management

1. Continue assessment
  a. ABCDs
  b. Vital signs: blood pressure, pulse, respiratory rate, and temperature
  c. Oxygen saturation
  d. Pain and discomfort level
  e. Accurate intake and output
  f. Serum electrolytes
  g. Close monitoring for progression of symptoms
2. Maintain airway, oxygenation, and ventilation
  a. Position of comfort
  b. Oxygen by nasal cannula at 2 to 6 L/min if indicated to maintain SpO_2 of 95% unless contraindicated; for patients with COPD, use pulse oximetry to guide oxygen administration to SpO_2 of 90%
3. Identify type of stone and prevent urinary tract obstruction
  a. IV access for fluid and medication administration
    1) IV fluids (usually 0.9% saline): typically 1 L over 30 to 60 minutes, then decrease fluids to 200 to 500 ml/hr
  b. Frequent assessment of urine quantity and quality
  c. Straining of urine for calculi
4. Control pain and discomfort
  a. Analgesics
    1) Ketorolac [Toradol]) is analgesic of choice (ENA, 2005)

2) Narcotics analgesics (e.g., morphine) may be given
  b. Antiemetics (e.g., ondansetron [Zofran], promethazine [Phenergan]) as indicated
  c. Anxiolytics as indicated
5. Treat infection (if present) and prevent sepsis: antimicrobials as indicated
6. Monitor for complications
  a. UTI, urosepsis
  b. Urinary tract obstruction
  c. Acute renal failure
  d. Recurrence of calculi

Evaluation

1. Patent airway, adequate oxygenation (i.e., normal PaO_2, SpO_2, SaO_2) and ventilation (i.e., normal $PaCO_2$)
2. Absence of clinical indicators of hypoperfusion
3. Absence of clinical indications of infection/sepsis
4. Alert and oriented with no neurologic deficit
5. Control of pain, discomfort
6. Absence of clinical indications of bleeding

Typical disposition

1. If evaluation criteria met discharge with instructions
  a. Increased oral fluid intake
  b. Foods and fluids to acidify the urine (e.g., meat, fish, eggs, cereals)
  c. Rest
  d. Importance of straining urine if calculus has not yet been passed
  e. Dietary changes to prevent recurrent calculi (depends on analysis of calculus)
2. If evaluation criteria not met (i.e., urosepsis, severe pain): admission

Urinary Retention

Definition: mechanical or physiologic obstruction of urine passage

Predisposing factors

1. Urethral obstruction (i.e., benign prostatic hypertrophy [BPH], urethral stricture)
2. Bladder neoplasm
3. Neurogenic bladder (i.e., multiple sclerosis, spinal cord injuries)
4. Medications with anticholinergic or sympathomimetic properties can induce urinary retention
5. Cauda equina syndrome (i.e., compression of the nerve root)

Clinical presentation

1. Subjective
  a. Past medical history of urinary retention
  b. Lower abdominal discomfort
  c. Inability to pass urine
  d. Dribbling
  e. Decreased (<30 ml/hr) or absent urinary output for 2 consecutive hours
  f. Frequency, hesitancy, urgency

2. Objective
   a. Distended bladder and tenderness with palpation
   b. Enlarged prostate
   c. Bimanual examination reveals distended and potentially prolapsed bladder
3. Diagnostic study: bladder scan

Collaborative management

1. Continue assessment
   a. ABCDs
   b. Vital signs: blood pressure, pulse, respiratory rate, and temperature
   c. Oxygen saturation
   d. Pain and discomfort level
   e. Accurate intake and output
   f. Close monitoring for progression of symptoms
2. Maintain airway, oxygenation, and ventilation
   a. Position of comfort
   b. Oxygen by nasal cannula at 2 to 6 L/min if indicated to maintain SpO_2 of 95% unless contraindicated; for patients with COPD, use pulse oximetry to guide oxygen administration to SpO_2 of 90%
3. Maintain adequate circulation and perfusion
   a. Increased oral fluids
   b. IV access for fluid and medication administration if indicated
      1) Isotonic fluids for replacement of postobstructive diuresis
4. Control pain and discomfort
   a. Analgesics if indicated
   b. Anxiolytics
5. Treat infection (if present) and prevent sepsis
   a. Antimicrobials as indicated
   b. Antipyretics and cooling methods to reduce fever
6. Maintain urinary elimination
   a. Bethanechol (Urecholine) may be prescribed
   b. Relief of bladder distention
      1) Foley catheter insertion; if unable to pass Foley catheter, insertion of suprapubic catheter may be necessary to bypass bladder outlet obstruction
      2) Slow drainage (500 ml every 3 hours) to avoid micturition syncope
7. Prepare patient for procedures and possible surgery
8. Monitor for complications
   a. Venous obstruction due to distended urinary bladder
   b. Postrenal failure

Evaluation

1. Patent airway, adequate oxygenation (i.e., normal PaO_2, SpO_2, and SaO_2) and ventilation (i.e., normal $PaCO_2$)
2. Absence of clinical indicators of hypoperfusion
3. Absence of clinical indications of infection/sepsis
4. Control of pain and discomfort

Typical disposition

1. If evaluation criteria met: discharge with instructions
   a. May be discharged with Foley or suprapubic catheter in place
   b. Follow-up with urologist
2. If evaluation criteria not met: admission

Testicular Torsion

Definition: abnormal twisting of the spermatic cord due to rotation of a testis, which causes strangulation, ischemia, and possible infarction of the testis

Predisposing factors (Mbibu, Maitama, Ameh, Khalid, & Adams, 2004)
1. Age
   a. May occur in neonates
   b. Two thirds of all cases occur between 12 and 18 years of age
   c. Rare in men over 25 to 30 years of age
2. Congenital abnormality
3. Trauma
4. Sexual activity
5. Undescended testicle
6. Rapid movement
7. Physical trauma
8. Paraplegia
9. Previous contralateral testicular torsion
10. More common in winter; cold air may be associated with increased risk

Pathophysiology (Price & Wilson, 2003)

1. Sudden, forceful contraction of the cremaster muscle
2. Sudden twisting of the spermatic cord
   a. The tunica vaginalis normally envelops the testis and attaches to the epididymis and spermatic cord
      1) Intravaginal twisting (most common type of testicular torsion in adolescents): results from an abnormality of the tunica
      2) Extravaginal torsion (most common in neonates): loose attachment of the tunica vaginalis to the scrotal lining causes spermatic cord rotation above the testis
3. Testis rotates on its vascular pedicle, twisting the arteries and veins in the spermatic cord
4. Interruption of circulation to the testis
5. Venous engorgement and ischemia develop, which may progress to testicular infarction

Clinical presentation

1. Subjective
   a. Severe sudden onset of unilateral scrotal pain and tenderness
      1) Usually occurs with physical activity but can occur during sleep
      2) May radiate into lower abdominal and inguinal canal
      3) Not relieved by elevation of the testis

(a) Phren sign: reduction in pain by manual elevation of the testis helps to distinguish epididymitis from testicular torsion
  b. Nausea and vomiting
  c. May have prior history of testicular pain that resolved spontaneously
2. Objective
  a. Possible tachycardia
  b. Elevated temperature possible
  c. Scrotum is erythematous and edematous
  d. Affected testis is tender and elevated
  e. Absent cremasteric reflex (i.e., stroking or pinching of medial thigh causes the cremasteric muscle to contract causing the testis to rise)
3. Diagnostic studies
  a. CBC: WBC may be increased
  b. Urinalysis: normal
  c. Doppler studies: color Doppler will show lack of intratesticular blood flow
  d. Doppler ultrasound will show rotation or distortion
    1) Can rule out hydrocele, which is a collection of serous fluid that results from a defect or irritation in the tunica vaginalis of the scrotum

Collaborative management

1. Continue assessment
  a. ABCDs
  b. Vital signs: blood pressure, pulse, respiratory rate, and temperature
  c. Pain and discomfort level
  d. Scrotal swelling and erythema
  e. Close monitoring for progression of symptoms
2. Maintain airway, oxygenation, and ventilation
  a. Position of comfort
  b. Oxygen by nasal cannula at 2 to 6 L/min if required to maintain SpO_2 of 95% unless contraindicated; for patients with COPD, use pulse oximetry to guide oxygen administration to SpO_2 of 90%
3. Maintain adequate circulation and perfusion
  a. IV access with two large-bore catheters for fluid and medication administration
    1) Intravenous fluids: usually 0.9% saline
  b. Control of bleeding
4. Control pain and discomfort
  a. Analgesics
  b. Anxiolytics
5. Prepare patient and assist with manual detorsion
  a. Immediate urology consult
  b. Sedation or cord block
  c. Affected testis is rotated laterally (usually has internally twisted medially)
  d. Confirmation of restoration of flow with ultrasound
6. Prepare patient for surgical intervention and admission to operating room
  a. Preoperative antibiotics
  b. Consent for surgical detorsion and surgical fixation
    1) If surgical fixation is done within 4 hours of onset, salvage rate of testicle is 80%

    2) After 12 hours, salvage is 20% and ischemic testicle must be removed
7. Monitor for complications
  a. Atrophic testis
  b. Infarction and necrosis of affected testis

Evaluation

1. Patent airway, adequate oxygenation (i.e., normal PaO_2, SpO_2, and SaO_2) and ventilation (i.e., normal $PaCO_2$)
2. Absence of clinical indicators of hypoperfusion
3. Absence of clinical indications of infection/sepsis
4. Control of pain, discomfort
5. Resolution of torsion

Typical disposition: admission; may transport to OR for emergent surgery

Epididymitis

Definition: inflammation of the epididymis, generally in adult males
Predisposing factors

1. Age: generally in adults
  a. In men younger than 40 years, usually due to STIs
  b. Over 40 years, urinary pathogens most likely cause; voiding dysfunction is likely
2. STI
3. UTI
4. Prostatitis and urethritis
5. Trauma
  a. Surgical
  b. Insertion of urinary catheter
  c. Kick to groin

Pathophysiology

1. Infection travels up the urethra to the epididymis
  a. Causative organism usually *Neisseria gonorrheae* or *Chlamydia trachomatis* in sexually active heterosexual men younger than 35 to 40 years
  b. Enterobacteriaceae usually the cause in older men with voiding dysfunction
2. Trauma causes inflammation of traumatized tissue

Clinical presentation

1. Subjective
  a. Onset can be slow or sudden
  b. Dysuria
  c. Scrotal pain
    1) Phren sign: pain lessened when testis is elevated
  d. Fever and chills
2. Objective
  a. Tachycardia
  b. Elevated temperature
  c. Gait: duck waddle
  d. Urethral discharge
  e. Involved area swollen and tender, especially over posterolateral scrotum; discomfort in epididymitis distinct from testicular parenchyma
  f. Scrotal induration

3. Diagnostic studies
   a. Urine cultures
   b. Urethral smear for gram stain and culture for *N. gonorrheae* or *C. trachomatis*
   c. Ultrasound in pediatric cases to exclude other causes
   d. Scrotal ultrasound or Doppler studies will show good flow state in epididymis

Collaborative management

1. Continue assessment
   a. ABCDs
   b. Vital signs: blood pressure, pulse, respiratory rate, and temperature
   c. Pain and discomfort level
   d. Accurate intake and output
   e. Close monitoring for progression of symptoms
2. Maintain airway, oxygenation, and ventilation
   a. Position of comfort
   b. Oxygen by nasal cannula at 2 to 6 L/min if indicated to maintain SpO_2 of 95% unless contraindicated; for patients with COPD, use pulse oximetry to guide oxygen administration to SpO_2 of 90%
3. Maintain adequate circulation and perfusion
   a. Increased oral fluid intake
   b. IV access for fluid and medication administration
      1) IV fluids: usually 0.9% saline
   c. Control of bleeding
4. Control pain and discomfort
   a. Elevation of scrotum
   b. Application of ice packs to scrotum
   c. Bed rest for 1 to 2 days
   d. Analgesics
      1) Nonsteroidal antiinflammatory agents (NSAIDs) (e.g., ibuprofen [Motrin], naproxen [Naprosyn])
      2) Narcotic analgesics
   e. Anxiolytics
5. Treat infection and prevent sepsis
   a. Antimicrobials (e.g., ceftriaxone [Rocephin], levofloxacin [Levaquin]) as indicated
   b. Antipyretics and cooling methods to reduce fever
6. Monitor for complications
   a. Infection
   b. Pain control

Evaluation

1. Patent airway, adequate oxygenation (i.e., normal PaO_2, SpO_2, and SaO_2) and ventilation (i.e., normal $PaCO_2$)
2. Absence of clinical indicators of hypoperfusion
3. Absence of clinical indications of infection/sepsis
4. Control of pain and discomfort

Typical disposition: discharge home with instructions

1. Medications and management
2. Prevention
3. Abstinence of sexual intercourse until both partners are treated if caused by STI

Epididymo-orchitis

Definition: inflammation of both the epididymis and testis, usually from infection

1. Orchitis, which is usually caused by the mumps virus, is rarely seen today because of the mumps vaccine

Predisposing factors

1. Recent GU instrumentation
2. STI
3. UTI
4. Reflux of urine
5. Mumps if bilateral orchitis

Pathophysiology

1. Spread of infection from the epididymis to the testis
   a. Common causative agents
      1) *Staphylococcus*
      2) *Streptococcus*
      3) *E. coli*
      4) *Streptococcus pneumoniae*
      5) *Pseudomonas*
2. Inflammation, swelling, and tissue trauma

Clinical presentation

1. Subjective
   a. Scrotal pain: slow or sudden onset
   b. Dysuria
   c. Fever, chills
   d. Fatigue
   e. Malaise
   f. Myalgias
   g. Nausea
   h. Headache
2. Objective
   a. Elevated temperature
   b. Urethral discharge
   c. Scrotum erythematous, swollen
   d. Tenderness with palpation
   e. Scrotal induration
   f. Testicular enlargement
3. Diagnostic studies
   a. Diagnosing mumps orchitis can be comfortably made based on history and physical examination alone
      1) If epididymo-orchitis is suspected, then obtain urine dip, urinalysis, and urethral cultures
      2) Diagnosing mumps orchitis can be confirmed with serum immunofluorescence antibody testing
   b. Urine culture: usually negative for pyuria
   c. Urethral smear for gram stain (culture for *N. gonorrhea* or *C. trachomatis*)
   d. Color Doppler ultrasonography

Collaborative management

1. Continue assessment
   a. ABCDs
   b. Vital signs: blood pressure, pulse, respiratory rate, and temperature

c. Pain and discomfort level
d. Accurate intake and output
e. Serum electrolytes
f. Level of consciousness
g. Close monitoring for progression of symptoms
2. Maintain airway, oxygenation, and ventilation
   a. Position of comfort
   b. Oxygen by nasal cannula at 2 to 6 L/min if indicated to maintain SpO$_2$ of 95% unless contraindicated; for patients with COPD, use pulse oximetry to guide oxygen administration to SpO$_2$ of 90%
3. Maintain adequate circulation and perfusion
   a. Increased oral fluids
   b. IV access for fluid and medication administration as indicated
4. Control pain and discomfort
   a. Warm soaks to scrotum
   b. Elevate scrotum
   c. NSAIDs
   d. Ice packs
5. Treat infection and prevent sepsis
   a. Antibiotics (e.g., ceftriaxone [Rocephin])
   b. Steroids may be prescribed
   c. STI testing should be considered
6. Monitor for complications
   a. Urethritis
   b. Hydrocele
   c. Abscess
   d. Hemospermia (i.e., blood in sperm)
   e. Oligospermia (i.e., low sperm count)
   f. Testicular atrophy and sterility

Evaluation

1. Patent airway, adequate oxygenation (i.e., normal PaO$_2$, SpO$_2$, and SaO$_2$) and ventilation (i.e., normal PaCO$_2$)
2. Absence of clinical indicators of hypoperfusion
3. Absence of clinical indications of infection/sepsis
4. Control of pain and discomfort

Typical disposition: discharge with instructions

1. Bed rest
2. Medicines as prescribed
3. Elevation of the scrotum
4. Ice on the affected testis for 10 to 15 minutes, 4 times a day, until pain resolves
5. Jock strap to support testes
6. Follow up with urologist

Prostatitis

Definition: inflammation of the prostate gland
Predisposing factors

1. Recent UTI
2. Trauma (e.g., horseback riding, bicycle)
3. Catheterization
4. Cystoscopy
5. Urethral dilatation
6. Transurethral resection of the prostate (TURP)

7. Transrectal biopsy
8. STI

Pathophysiology

1. Usually an extension of urinary tract infection
2. May occur following manipulation of prostate or urethra
3. Acute bacterial
   a. Sudden onset
   b. Usually gram-negative enteric bacteria: *E. coli* (most common), *Klebsiella, Enterobacter, Serratia, Proteus, Pseudomonas, Enterococcus*
   c. Radiation (e.g., therapy for malignant pelvic disease)
4. Chronic bacterial
   a. Symptoms are often absent
   b. Chronic more commonly caused by *C. trachomatis*, usually *E. coli* if chronic cause is bacterial (least common)

Clinical presentation

1. Subjective
   a. Low back pain, perineal, suprapubic or rectal pain, ejaculatory pain
   b. Discomfort may be constant or intermittent
   c. Fever, chills, malaise
   d. Dysuria, frequency and urgency
   e. Urinary retention
   f. Hematuria
2. Objective: prostate by rectal examination
   a. Tender
   b. Warm
   c. Swollen
3. Diagnostic studies
   a. Urinalysis
      1) Greater than 10 to 12 WBC per high-power field of prostatic secretions (prostatic massage is contraindicated).
      2) Gram-negative rods usually show up in urine culture
   b. Prostate specific antigen (PSA) elevated in acute prostatitis
   c. CT or ultrasound if malignancy suspected
   d. Transrectal ultrasound if abscess or calculi suspected
   e. Needle biopsy or aspiration for culture

Collaborative management

1. Continue assessment
   a. ABCDs
   b. Vital signs: blood pressure, pulse, respiratory rate, and temperature
   c. Pain and discomfort level
   d. Close monitoring for progression of symptoms
2. Maintain airway, oxygenation, and ventilation
   a. Position of comfort
   b. Oxygen by nasal cannula at 2 to 6 L/min if indicated to maintain SpO$_2$ of 95% unless contraindicated; for patients with COPD, use pulse oximetry to guide oxygen administration to SpO$_2$ of 90%
3. Maintain adequate circulation and perfusion
   a. Increased oral fluids

b. IV access for fluid and medication administration
   1) IV fluids: usually 0.9% saline
4. Control pain and discomfort
   a. Analgesics
   b. Antipyretics
   c. Stool softeners
   d. Heat therapy
   e. Suprapubic catheter for severe urinary retention
5. Treat infection and prevent sepsis
   a. Antibiotics (e.g., doxycycline [Vibramycin], trimethoprim-sulfamethoxazole [Bactrim], ciprofloxacin [Cipro])
   b. Prostatic massage contraindicated (due to discomfort and potential for bacteremia)
6. Monitor for complications
   a. Prostatic abscess
   b. Urinary retention
   c. Epididymitis
   d. Chronic bacterial prostatitis
   e. Metastatic infections

Evaluation

1. Patent airway, adequate oxygenation (i.e., normal PaO_2, SpO_2, and SaO_2) and ventilation (i.e., normal $PaCO_2$)
2. Absence of clinical indicators of hypoperfusion
3. Absence of clinical indications of infection/sepsis
4. Control of pain and discomfort

Typical disposition

1. If evaluation criteria met: discharge with instructions
   a. Antibiotics for 3 to 4 weeks
   b. Analgesics
   c. Stool softeners
   d. Heat therapy
   e. Sitz bath
   f. Follow up with primary care provider
2. If evaluation criteria not met: admission

Benign Prostatic Hypertrophy (BPH)

Definition: benign enlargement of the prostate gland

1. Can lead to obstructive urinary symptoms

Predisposing factors

1. Age: most common cause of urinary tract obstruction in older men; BPH is present in 50% of men at age 60 years and 90% of men by age 85 years
2. Diet high in fat and red meat
3. Recent urinary stone or urinary surgery
4. Medications (e.g., antihistamines, opioids, anticholinergic drugs, tricyclic antidepressants, muscle relaxants) may exacerbate symptoms and cause urinary retention

Pathophysiology

1. Increased estrogens and decreased testosterone with age
2. BPH has both static and dynamic components
   a. Static component: increased prostate size
   b. Dynamic component: increased smooth muscle tone in prostate, prostate capsule, and bladder neck

3. Urinary bladder response to resistance to urinary flow
   a. Compensatory phase: bladder muscle hypertrophies
   b. Decompensation: residual urine, urinary obstructive symptoms

Clinical presentation

1. Subjective
   a. Urinary frequency and urgency
   b. Nocturia
   c. Dysuria
   d. Decreased force of urinary stream
   e. Hesitancy in initiating stream
   f. Overflow incontinence
   g. Intermittent stream, dribbling after voiding
2. Objective
   a. Lower abdominal or suprapubic area tenderness
   b. May have enlarged or normal-sized prostate
   c. May have rubbery nodules on palpation
   d. Distended bladder noted with percussion
3. Diagnostic studies
   a. BUN and creatinine: to evaluate renal function
   b. Urinalysis and urine dip
      1) Sediment
      2) Changes in urine pH related to chronic residual urine
   c. Urinary cytology, upper urinary tract imaging, and cystoscopy if hematuria present
   d. Post-void residual urine measurement or bladder scan
   e. PSA: likely to be elevated in prostate cancer but a normal level does not rule out cancer

Collaborative management

1. Continue assessment
   a. ABCDs
   b. Vital signs: blood pressure, pulse, respiratory rate, and temperature
   c. Pain and discomfort level
   d. Accurate intake and output
   e. Close monitoring for progression of symptoms
2. Maintain airway, oxygenation, and ventilation
   a. Position of comfort
   b. Oxygen by nasal cannula at 2 to 6 L/min if indicated to maintain SpO_2 of 95% unless contraindicated; for patients with COPD, use pulse oximetry to guide oxygen administration to SpO_2 of 90%
3. Maintain adequate circulation and perfusion
   a. Increased oral fluids
   b. IV access for fluid and medication administration if indicated
      1) IV fluids: usually 0.9% saline
4. Maintain urinary elimination
   a. If patient is unable to void, insertion of urinary catheter; may need Coude catheter or flexible cystoscopy
   b. α1-Blockers (e.g., terazosin [Hytrin], tamsulosin [Flomax], doxazosin [Cardura])

    c. Avoidance of anticholinergic drugs, narcotics, and skeletal muscle relaxants in older patients with BPH

    d. Procedures as indicated

       1) Transurethral microwave therapy (TUMT)

       2) Transurethral resection of prostate (TURP)

5. Treat infection (if present) and prevent sepsis: antimicrobials as indicated

6. Monitor for complications

    a. Urinary tract infection and retention

    b. Pyelonephritis

    c. Postrenal failure

    d. Nephrolithiasis

    e. Prostatitis

Evaluation

1. Patent airway, adequate oxygenation (i.e., normal Pao_2, Spo_2, and Sao_2) and ventilation (i.e., normal $Paco_2$)

2. Absence of clinical indicators of hypoperfusion

3. Absence of clinical indications of infection/sepsis

4. Control of pain and discomfort

5. Absence of impairment in urinary elimination

Typical disposition

1. If evaluation criteria met: discharge with instructions

    a. Limitation of fluid intake in evening

    b. Avoidance of bladder irritants (e.g., caffeine, alcohol)

    c. Pelvic floor exercises (to help stop dribbling)

    d. NSAIDs daily may aid in prevention (St. Sauver et al., 2006)

    e. Follow-up with urologist as scheduled

2. If evaluation criteria not met: admission for surgery

Priapism

Definition: prolonged penile erection lasting more than 4 to 6 hours in absence of sexual stimulation; considered a medical-urologic emergency

Predisposing factors

1. Trauma (e.g., bicycling)

2. Prolonged sexual activity

3. Hematologic and oncologic conditions

    a. Common in males with sickle cell anemia

    b. Leukemia

4. Dehydration

5. Medications

    a. Intracavernosal injection therapy (e.g., prostaglandin E_1)

    b. Oral phosphodiesterase (PDE)-5 inhibitors (e.g., sildenafil [Viagra], tadalafil [Cialis], vardenafil [Levitra])

    c. Psychotropic drugs (e.g., phenothiazines, trazodone [Desyrel])

    d. Antihypertensives (e.g., prazosin [Minipres])

    e. Heparin

6. Neurologic causes (e.g., spinal cord injuries)

7. Tumors

Pathophysiology

1. Ischemic (low-flow) priapism: most common type of priapism

    a. Caused by decreased venous outflow and vascular stasis

    b. 30% to 50% of cases are idiopathic

2. Nonischemic (high-flow) priapism: rare occurrence and often painless

    a. Caused by fistula between cavernosal artery and corporal tissue

    b. Not associated with long-term erectile dysfunction

3. Stuttering (intermittent, recurrent) priapism

    a. May be central (when related to sleep disorders) or local (hematologic disorder)

    b. Caused by clumping of erythrocytes leading to veno-occlusion in sinusoids of corpus cavernosum

       1) Often seen in sickle cell disease

    c. Short-lived, self-limiting episodes of prolonged and painful erections usually occurring at night

    d. Commonly less than 3 hours, but some episodes are prolonged and require acute medical attention

4. Malignant priapism: rare clinical entity in which prolonged erection is due to an invasion of the corpora cavernosa by a malignant neoplasm

Clinical presentation

1. Subjective

    a. History of trauma, drug use, or hematologic problems

    b. Persistent erection that is painful and prolonged

    c. Urination difficulty during erection

    d. Stuttering priapism may present as nocturnal painful erections

2. Objective

    a. May be hypotensive if due to PDE inhibitors used for erectile dysfunction

    b. Erect penis

    c. Bladder distention

    d. Findings in low-flow priapism

       1) Soft glans

       2) Painful penile shaft

       3) Aspirate of the corpus cavernosum is thick and dark

    e. Findings in high-flow priapism

       1) Firm glans

       2) Some discomfort of penile shaft

       3) Aspirates of corpus cavernosum will be bright red

3. Diagnostic studies

    a. CBC: may show hematologic disorder

    b. Peripheral blood smear: to rule out chronic myeloid leukemia

    c. Urine toxicology screen

    d. Blood analysis of corpus cavernosum aspirate

       1) Low glucose concentration in low-flow priapism

       2) Normal glucose concentration in high-flow priapism

3) Abnormal blood gas analysis of aspirated blood from corpus cavernosum (hypoxia, hypercarbia, acidosis)
  e. Penile Doppler ultrasound
    1) Low arterial flow in ischemic (low-flow) priapism
    2) Elevated flow in nonischemic (high-flow) priapism

Collaborative management
1. Continue assessment
   a. ABCDs
   b. Vital signs: blood pressure, pulse, respiratory rate, and temperature
   c. Oxygen saturation
   d. Pain and discomfort level
   e. Accurate intake and output
   f. Close monitoring for progression of symptoms
2. Maintain airway, oxygenation, and ventilation
   a. Position of comfort
   b. Oxygen by nasal cannula at 2 to 6 L/min if indicated to maintain SpO_2 of 95% unless contraindicated; for patients with COPD, use pulse oximetry to guide oxygen administration to SpO_2 of 90%
3. Maintain adequate circulation and perfusion
   a. Increased oral fluids
   b. IV access for fluid and medication administration
     1) IV fluids: usually 0.9% saline
4. Control pain and discomfort
   a. Bed rest
   b. Narcotic analgesics
   c. Ice to penis
   d. Anxiolytics
5. Establish and maintain urinary flow
   a. Foley catheter insertion; suprapubic catheterization may be required
6. Administer drugs and therapies for treatment of cause
   a. Intracavernous injections may be done for priapism caused by drug injections into the penis to treat impotence
     1) Sympathomimetic agents are injected to constrict or narrow the blood vessels in the penis, allowing less blood to flow into the penis and more to flow out; thus the priapism subsides.
   b. Aspiration can be done for priapism caused by ischemia
     1) Local anesthetic is applied and then excess blood is drained from the penis using a small needle and syringe
     2) May be done as an adjunct to intracavernous injections
   c. Surgery when other options are unsuccessful
7. Procedures and surgery as indicated (Merck, 2008)
8. Monitor for complications
   a. Compartment syndrome
   b. Erectile dysfunction

Evaluation
1. Patent airway, adequate oxygenation (i.e., normal PaO_2, SpO_2, and SaO_2) and ventilation (i.e., normal $PaCO_2$)
2. Absence of clinical indicators of hypoperfusion
3. Absence of clinical indications of infection/sepsis
4. Control of pain and discomfort
5. Absence of impairment in urinary elimination
6. Absence or penile erection

Typical disposition
1. If evaluation criteria met: discharge with instructions for follow-up
2. If evaluation criteria not met: admission for procedure or surgery

Phimosis
Definition: tightened foreskin of the penis is unable to retract over the glans
Predisposing factors
1. Congenital
2. Inflammation
3. Trauma
4. Poor hygiene

Pathophysiology
1. Foreskin is tightened and cannot be retracted
2. Excess oil gland secretion and smegma accumulates with resultant inflammation and infection

Clinical presentation
1. Subjective
   a. Painful erections
   b. Ballooning of foreskin with voiding
2. Objective
   a. Foreskin cannot retract
     1) Gentle retraction applied to normal but nonretractable infant foreskin leads to puckering of distal part of the foreskin with narrow portion proximal to preputial tip
     2) Gentle retraction applied to foreskin with true phimosis leads to cone-shaped foreskin with fibrotic, circular band forming most distal and narrowest part of prepuce
   b. Decrease in urine flow
3. Diagnostic studies: none required

Collaborative management
1. Continue assessment
   a. ABCDs
   b. Vital signs: blood pressure, pulse, respiratory rate, and temperature
   c. Pain and discomfort level
   d. Accurate intake and output
   e. Color, warmth of distal end of penis
   f. Close monitoring for progression of symptoms
2. Maintain airway, oxygenation, and ventilation
   a. Position of comfort

b. Oxygen by nasal cannula at 2 to 6 L/min if indicated to maintain SpO_2 of 95% unless contraindicated; for patients with COPD, use pulse oximetry to guide oxygen administration to SpO_2 of 90%
3. Maintain adequate circulation and perfusion
   a. Assessment and reporting of any change in color or warmth of distal end of penis
4. Control pain and discomfort
   a. Analgesics
   b. Steroids
   c. Anxiolytics
5. Prepare for admission if surgery indicated (i.e., circumcision)
6. Monitor for complications
   a. Balanitis (i.e., inflammation of the glans)
   b. Posthitis (i.e., inflammation of the prepuce)

Evaluation

1. Patent airway, adequate oxygenation (i.e., normal PaO_2, SpO_2, SaO_2) and ventilation (i.e., normal $PaCO_2$)
2. Absence of clinical indicators of hypoperfusion
3. Absence of clinical indications of infection/sepsis
4. Control of pain and discomfort
5. Absence of impairment in urinary elimination
6. Successful retraction of foreskin

Typical disposition

1. If evaluation criteria met: discharge with instructions
   a. No sexual activity until healing complete
2. If evaluation criteria not met: admission for circumcision

Urethral Injury

Definition: injury to urethra
Predisposing factors

1. Gender: occurs most often in males due to longer urethra
2. Surgical trauma, particularly vaginal
3. Childbirth
4. Blunt or penetrating trauma
5. Straddle injuries
6. Pelvic fractures
7. Instrumentation (e.g., urethral catheterization, dilation with sounds)

Pathophysiology

1. Posterior segment injuries are usually seen in pelvic trauma as a result of shearing forces applied at the prostatomembranous junction during blunt trauma
   a. Pelvic displacement can lead to tearing or stretching of the membranous urethra.
   b. Urethral rupture should be considered early with pelvic trauma
2. Anterior segment injuries occur usually from a blunt force blow to the perineum, which produces a crushing effect on the tissue; common with straddle injuries

3. Complete rupture of the urethra seen more often in children due to the decreased elasticity of their urethra

Clinical presentation

1. Subjective
   a. History of injury
   b. Pain especially with voiding
   c. Inability to void
   d. Hematuria
2. Objective
   a. Tachycardia
   b. Pallor
   c. Blood at urinary meatus
   d. Bladder distention
   e. Butterfly-shaped hematoma of lower abdominal or perineum
3. Diagnostic studies
   a. CBC: decreased hemoglobin and hematocrit with bleeding; serial hematocrit indicated if suspect pelvic injury (ENA, 2007)
   b. Coagulation profile
   c. Urinalysis: will show hematuria
   d. Abdominal and pelvis radiology
   e. Cystography for patency and minor injury
   f. Pelvic ultrasound
   g. CT
   h. IVP

Collaborative management

1. Continue assessment
   a. ABCDs
   b. Vital signs: blood pressure, pulse, respiratory rate, and temperature
   c. Oxygen saturation
   d. Pain and discomfort level
   e. Accurate intake and output
   f. Close monitoring for progression of symptoms
2. Maintain airway, oxygenation, ventilation, and perfusion, since other injuries may be present
   a. Airway, oxygenation, circulation support using BLS, ACLS if needed
      1) Airway with cervical spine immobilization if suspected cervical injury
   b. Oxygen by nasal cannula at 2 to 6 L/min if indicated to maintain SpO_2 of 95% unless contraindicated; for patients with COPD, use pulse oximetry to guide oxygen administration to SpO_2 of 90%
      1) 100% nonrebreather may be required to maintain SpO_2 depending on coexisting trauma
   c. Intubation and mechanical ventilation as indicated
   d. IV access with two large-bore catheters for fluid and medication administration
      1) Normal saline or lactated Ringer solution by rapid infusion until blood is available; colloids (e.g., albumin, hetastarch, or dextran) may also be used
      2) Blood and blood products if indicated
   e. Control of bleeding; surgery may be required

3. Control pain and discomfort
    a. NSAIDs
    b. Narcotic analgesics
    c. Anxiolytics
4. Establish and maintain urinary flow
    a. Suprapubic catheterization is preferred
    b. If Foley catheter insertion requested, stop if any resistance and ask physician to insert
5. Treat infection (if present) and prevent sepsis
    a. Antimicrobials as indicated
    b. Antipyretics and cooling methods to reduce fever
    c. Tetanus immunization
6. Assist in preparation of diagnostic studies
7. Monitor for complications
    a. Fistula
    b. Stricture
    c. Persistent urinary leakage
    d. Infection, sepsis

Evaluation
1. Patent airway, adequate oxygenation (i.e., normal PaO_2, SpO_2, and SaO_2) and ventilation (i.e., normal $PaCO_2$)
2. Absence of clinical indicators of hypoperfusion
3. Absence of clinical indications of infection/sepsis
4. Control of pain and discomfort
5. Absence of clinical indications of bleeding
6. Absence of urinary impairment

Typical disposition: admission to the hospital and surgery as indicated: may need to be transferred to another hospital if services not available

Ruptured Bladder
Definition: rupture of the urinary bladder
Predisposing factors
1. Blunt or penetrating trauma
    a. Blunt trauma 70% to 80%, with 40% to 68% needing surgical repair
    b. High incidence with vertebral and flank injury
    c. Seldom occurs as lone trauma
2. OB trauma
3. Iatrogenic injury secondary to surgical GYN, urologic, and orthopedic procedures near the urinary bladder
4. Spontaneous or idiopathic bladder injuries of unknown origin

Pathophysiology (Platter & Vaccaro, 2008)
1. Five types of bladder rupture
    a. Type I: Bladder contusion
        1) Most common bladder injury that occurs from incomplete tear of bladder mucosa
        2) Cystography is normal
    b. Type II: Intraperitoneal rupture
        1) Results from trauma to lower abdomen when bladder is distended
        2) Bladder dome is weakest portion making it easy to rupture
    c. Type III: Interstitial injury (rare)
        1) Caused by a tear of the intact serosa surface

    d. Type IV: Extraperitoneal
        1) Almost always associated with pelvic fractures
        2) Usually close to base of bladder anterolaterally
    e. Type V: Combined extra peritoneal and intraperitoneal rupture
2. Extravasation of blood and urine into peritoneal cavity or pelvis, which may cause peritonitis and sepsis

Clinical presentation
1. Subjective
    a. History of trauma
    b. Abdominal pain or tenderness
    c. Inability to void
2. Objective
    a. Tachycardia
    b. Pallor
    c. Suprapubic bruising or hematoma
    d. Abdominal distention with rigidity
    e. Rebound tenderness with palpation
    f. Clinical indications of hypoperfusion or shock
3. Diagnostic studies
    a. CBC: serial hematocrit for suspected or confirmed bleeding
    b. Coagulation profile
    c. Type and cross-match
    d. Urinalysis
    e. Abdominal series
    f. Pelvic CT

Collaborative management
1. Continue assessment
    a. ABCDs
    b. Vital signs: blood pressure, pulse, respiratory rate, and temperature
    c. Oxygen saturation
    d. Pain and discomfort level
    e. Accurate intake and output
    f. Close monitoring for progression of symptoms
2. Maintain airway, oxygenation, ventilation, and perfusion, since other injuries may be present
    a. Airway, oxygenation, circulation support using BLS, ACLS if needed
        1) Airway with cervical spine immobilization if suspected cervical injury
    b. Oxygen by nasal cannula at 2 to 6 L/min if indicated to maintain SpO_2 of 95% unless contraindicated; for patients with COPD, use pulse oximetry to guide oxygen administration to SpO_2 of 90%
        1) 100% nonrebreather may be required to maintain SpO_2 depending on coexisting trauma
    c. Intubation and mechanical ventilation as indicated
    d. IV access with two large-bore catheters for fluid and medication administration
        1) Normal saline or lactated Ringer solution by rapid infusion until blood is available; colloids (e.g., albumin, hetastarch, or dextran) may also be used
        2) Blood and blood products if indicated
    e. Control of bleeding; surgery may be required

3. Control pain and discomfort
   a. Position of comfort unless contraindicated
   b. Analgesics
   c. Anxiolytics
4. Establish and maintain urinary flow
   a. Suprapubic catheterization is preferred
   b. If no blood at urinary meatus, Foley catheter insertion may be requested; stop if any resistance and ask physician to insert
5. Treat infection (if present) and prevent sepsis
   a. Antimicrobials as indicated
   b. Antipyretics and cooling methods to reduce fever
   c. Tetanus immunization
6. Assist in preparation for diagnostic studies and surgery
7. Monitor for complications
   a. Hypovolemic shock
   b. Peritonitis, sepsis

Evaluation

1. Patent airway, adequate oxygenation (i.e., normal Pao_2, Spo_2, and Sao_2) and ventilation (i.e., normal $Paco_2$)
2. Absence of clinical indicators of hypoperfusion
3. Absence of clinical indications of infection/sepsis
4. Control of pain and discomfort
5. Absence of clinical indications of bleeding

Typical disposition

1. If evaluation criteria met: discharge with instructions for follow-up and further testing and/or treatment
2. If evaluation criteria not met: admission to progressive care unit or critical care unit

Renal Trauma
Definition

1. Injury to the kidney caused by blunt or penetrating trauma
2. Considered in any patient with back, chest, or abdominal trauma
3. Extrarenal and intrarenal bleeding can occur

Predisposing factors

1. Motor vehicle collision: the kidney is the organ most likely to be injured in a lateral impact collision
2. Falls
3. Pedestrian injuries
4. Assault
5. Industrial injury
6. Sports-related injury
7. Gunshot wounds
8. Stab wounds

Pathophysiology

1. Anatomic issues
   a. The right kidney is more vulnerable to injury than the left as it is lower
   b. Fracture of ribs 11 and 12 may cause penetration of the kidney

c. Renal trauma is almost always accompanied by other system problems
   1) Injury to the left kidney is frequently accompanied by injury to spleen
   2) Injury to the right kidney is frequently accompanied by injury to liver
2. Classifications (Figure 9-2)
   a. Class I: caused by compression of the kidneys between the lower ribs and the vertebral column
      1) Contusion: hematuria, but normal urologic studies
      2) Hematoma: subcapsular, nonexpanding
      3) May have minor cortical laceration, but not into parenchyma
   b. Class II: caused by fractures of ribs 10 to 12 or the transverse process of the vertebrae
      1) Hematoma: perirenal, nonexpanding, confined to the retroperitoneum
      2) Laceration: less than 1 cm parenchymal depth and without urinary extravasation
   c. Class III
      1) Laceration of more than 1 cm parenchymal depth without urinary extravasation
   d. Class IV
      1) Laceration extending through the renal cortex, medulla, and collecting system
      2) Vascular injury to the renal artery or vein with contained hemorrhage
   e. Class V
      1) Lacerations that are extensive at various sites in the renal parenchyma resulting in a completely shattered kidney
      2) Vascular injury with avulsion of the renal hilum resulting in devascularization of the kidney
3. Severity
   a. Minor: contusions, shallow cortical lacerations
   b. Major: deep cortical lacerations, caliceal laceration
   c. Critical: renal fracture, renal vascular injury

Clinical presentation

1. Subjective
   a. Mechanism of injury
   b. Pain or tenderness
      1) Flank or upper abdominal quadrant pain; persistent flank pain may indicate renal artery thrombosis
      2) CVA pain
      3) Renal colic: pain radiating from flank area into groin, external genitalia or thigh
2. Objective
   a. May have altered LOC
   b. May have vomiting
   c. Oliguria
   d. Hematuria: gross or microscopic
   e. Abrasion or hematoma over posterior aspect of rib 11 or 12
   f. Entrance/exit wound if penetrating trauma
   g. Abdominal and flank tenderness

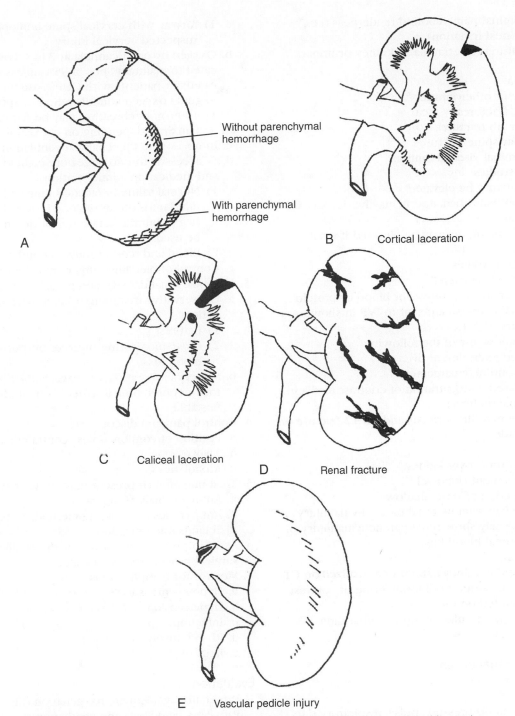

Without parenchymal hemorrhage

With parenchymal hemorrhage

A

B   Cortical laceration

C   Caliceal laceration

D   Renal fracture

E   Vascular pedicle injury

Figure 9-2 Renal trauma. **A,** Renal contusion. **B,** Cortical laceration. **C,** Caliceal laceration. **D,** Renal fracture. **E,** Vascular pedicle injury. (From Dennison, R. [2007]. *Pass CCRN!* [3rd ed.]. Drawing by Ann M. Walthall.).

h. Palpated flank swelling or mass
i. Abdominal distention or asymmetry
j. Decreased or absent bowel sounds
k. External genitalia ecchymosis
l. Blood at urinary meatus
m. Clinical indications of retroperitoneal bleeding
    1) Back pain
    2) Clinical indications of hemorrhage (i.e., tachycardia, hypotension, oliguria)

    3) Grey-Turner sign: ecchymosis over the flank indicative of retroperitoneal bleeding
n. Clinical indications of extravasated urine
    1) Midline bulging (i.e., over distended bladder)
    2) Lower quadrant, flank, or thigh distortion (i.e., fluid collection)
    3) Lower abdominal pain or mass (i.e., bladder rupture)

4) Abdominal pain, rebound tenderness (i.e., peritoneal irritation)
5) Hematuria (i.e., trauma to kidney or urinary tract)
6) Anuria

o. Presence of other injuries
   1) Pelvic fractures
   2) Lower rib fractures
   3) Lumbar spine fractures
   4) Abdominal visceral injuries

3. Diagnostic studies
   a. Potassium: may be elevated
   b. Hemoglobin and hematocrit: may be decreased if hemorrhage
   c. BUN and creatinine: may be elevated if renal damage
   d. Coagulation studies
   e. Type and cross-match
   f. Urinalysis: may be positive for blood or protein
   g. CT with IV contrast superior to IVP in showing renal injury
   h. IVP may show any of the following
      1) Delayed excretion of dye
      2) Renal outline enlargement
      3) Decreased concentration of contrast media in renal parenchyma
   i. Chest film may show rib 11 and rib 12 fracture on affected side
   j. KUB
      1) Rib fractures over kidney
      2) Displacement of bowel
      3) Obliteration of renal shadow
   k. Ultrasound: may show renal parenchyma injury
   l. Renal scan may show renal parenchyma injury or defect in renal blood flow
   m. Arteriogram
      1) Indicated if kidney cannot be visualized on CT or if extravasation of bloody urine or contrast media noted on CT
      2) May show vascular disruption, infarction, hematoma

Collaborative management

1. Continue assessment
   a. ABCDs
   b. Vital signs: blood pressure, pulse, respiratory rate, and temperature
   c. Oxygen saturation
   d. Respiratory effort and excursion
   e. Cardiac rate and rhythm
   f. Pain and discomfort level
   g. Accurate intake and output
   h. Serum electrolytes
   i. Level of consciousness
   j. Close monitoring for progression of symptoms
2. Maintain airway, oxygenation, ventilation, and perfusion
   a. Airway, oxygenation, circulation support using BCLS, ACLS if needed

1) Airway with cervical spine immobilization if suspected cervical injury
   b. Oxygen by nasal cannula at 2 to 6 L/min if indicated to maintain SpO_2 of 95% unless contraindicated; for patients with COPD, use pulse oximetry to guide oxygen administration to SpO_2 of 90%
      1) 100% non-rebreather may be required to maintain SpO_2 depending on coexisting trauma
   c. Intubation and mechanical ventilation as indicated
   d. IV access with two large-bore catheters for fluid and medication administration
      1) Normal saline or lactated Ringer solution by rapid infusion until blood is available; colloids (e.g., albumin, hetastarch, or dextran) may also be used
      2) Blood and blood products if indicated
   e. Control of bleeding; surgery may be required
3. Minimize renal damage and preserve renal function
   a. Conservative treatment if hemodynamically stable patient
      1) Bed rest
      2) Close monitoring of urine output and blood loss
   b. Surgery exploration, drainage, and/or partial or total nephrectomy if patient is hemodynamically unstable
4. Control pain and discomfort
   a. Position of comfort unless contraindicated
   b. Analgesics
   c. Anxiolytics
5. Treat infection (if present) and prevent sepsis
   a. Antimicrobials as indicated
   b. Antipyretics and cooling methods to reduce fever
   c. Tetanus immunization
6. Assist in preparation for diagnostic studies and/or surgical procedures as indicated
7. Monitor for complications
   a. Hypovolemic shock
   b. Hypertension
   c. Infection, sepsis
   d. Rhabdomyolysis
   e. Ileus

Evaluation

1. Patent airway, adequate oxygenation (i.e., normal PaO_2, SpO_2, and SaO_2) and ventilation (i.e., normal $PaCO_2$)
2. Absence of clinical indicators of hypoperfusion
3. Absence of clinical indications of infection/sepsis
4. Control of pain and discomfort
5. Absence of clinical indications of bleeding
6. Absence of impairment in urinary elimination

Typical disposition

1. If evaluation criteria met: discharge with instructions for follow-up
2. If evaluation criteria not met: admission to the hospital and surgery as indicated: may need to be transferred to another hospital if services not available

Foreign Bodies in Urethra, Vagina, or Rectum

Definition: Foreign body object placed in or around urethra, vagina, or rectum

1. Note that embarrassment and fear of punishment may prevent patient's request for help until there is pain or discomfort

Predisposing factors

1. More common in young children
2. Sexual exploration and/or abuse

Clinical presentation

1. Subjective
   a. History of inserting foreign body into cavity
   b. Pain
   c. Dysuria or inability to void
   d. Constipation
2. Objective
   a. May be tachycardic and hypotensive
   b. Abdominal distention
   c. Presence of bloody urine or stool
   d. Blood at urinary meatus or urethral discharge
   e. Visualization of object
3. Diagnostic studies
   a. Urinalysis: hematuria
   b. Cultures: to assess for infection
   c. KUB
   d. Cystoscopy or sigmoidoscopy
   e. Pelvic examination: to assess for foreign body

Collaborative management

1. Continue assessment
   a. ABCDs
   b. Vital signs: blood pressure, pulse, respiratory rate, and temperature
   c. Oxygen saturation
   d. Pain and discomfort level
   e. Changes in urinary or bowel elimination
   f. Close monitoring for progression of symptoms
2. Maintain airway, oxygenation, and ventilation
   a. Position of comfort
   b. Oxygen by nasal cannula at 2 to 6 L/min if indicated to maintain SpO_2 of 95% unless contraindicated; for patients with COPD, use pulse oximetry to guide oxygen administration to SpO_2 of 90%
3. Maintain adequate circulation and perfusion
   a. Increased oral fluids
   b. IV access for fluid and medication administration
      1) IV fluids: usually 0.9% saline
   c. Control of bleeding
4. Control pain and discomfort
   a. NSAIDs
   b. Narcotic analgesics
   c. Anxiolytics
5. Treat infection (if present) and prevent sepsis
   a. Antimicrobials as indicated
   b. Antipyretics and cooling methods to reduce fever
   c. Tetanus immunization
6. Prepare patient and assist with removal of object
   a. If unable to remove, surgery is indicated
7. Monitor for complications
   a. Infection
   b. Trauma to GU tract or lower GI tract

Evaluation

1. Patent airway, adequate oxygenation (i.e., normal PaO_2, SpO_2, and SaO_2) and ventilation (i.e., normal $PaCO_2$)
2. Absence of clinical indications of infection/sepsis
3. Control of pain and discomfort
4. Absence of clinical indications of bleeding
5. Absence of impairment in urinary or bowel elimination
6. Successful removal of object

Typical disposition

1. If evaluation criteria met: discharge with instructions
   a. Medications as prescribed
   b. Increased fluid intake
   c. To return if:
      1) Urine does not clear up, urine output decreases, or other symptoms start
      2) Significant hematuria or rectal bleeding
2. If evaluation criteria not met: admission for endoscopic or surgical procedure

Pelvic Pain

Definition: pain in pelvis; common complaint that can have many origins; may or may not be related to GYN causes

Predisposing factors

1. Sexually active female, particularly with multiple sexual partners
2. Trauma

Pathophysiology

1. Varies depending on cause
2. Can originate from several areas
   a. Lower intestinal tract
   b. Reproductive system
   c. Urinary system
   d. Nervous system
   e. Musculoskeletal system

Clinical presentation

1. Subjective and objective (Tables 9-1 and 9-2)
2. Diagnostic studies
   a. Pelvic examination
   b. Urine pregnancy test to rule out ectopic pregnancy
   c. Pelvic ultrasound

Collaborative management

1. Continue assessment
   a. ABCDs
   b. Vital signs: blood pressure, pulse, respiratory rate, and temperature

TABLE 9-1 Gynecologic Causes of Pelvic Pain

Cause	Timing and Type	Onset	Location	Nausea, Vomiting	Fever	Contributing Factors	Aggravating Factors	Vaginal discharge
Degenerating tumor	Constant and full or sudden sharp	Slow	Generalized and/or midline	No	No	Fibroids, pelvic congestion	Stress, menses	No
Ectopic pregnancy	Constant and sharp	Rapid	Pelvis	Maybe	No	PID; infertility; IUD, previous pelvic problems; advanced maternal age	Activity and movement	No, but may have slight bleeding
Incomplete, threatened, or septic abortion	Constant and cramping or sharp	Rapid	General pelvic area	No	Maybe	Previous abortion	Activity and movement	Possibly
Endometriosis	Constant during menses and sharp	Week before menses	Bilateral posterior pelvis	No	Yes	Delay in child-bearing or no child-bearing; congenital	Adhesions; coitus, bowel movements	Bleeding
Mittelschmerz	Mid-menses cycle and sharp	Rapid	Generalized and/or midline	No	No	Ruptured graafian follicle		No
Ruptured ovarian cyst	Constant and sharp	Rapid	Pelvis	No	No	Common occurrence during coitus	Activity and movement	No
Pelvic Inflammatory Disease (PID)	Constant and sharp	Rapid	Bilateral pelvis	Nausea	Yes	STIs; multiple partners; previous PID	Coitus; menses; activity and movement	Yes
Premenstrual Syndrome (PMS)	Premenstrual and cramping	Rapid	Generalized and/or midline	Nausea	No	History of PMS		No
Primary Dysmenorrhea	Onset of menses and cramping	Rapid	Generalized	No	No	History of primary dysmenorrhea	Activity and movement	No
Septic pelvis thrombosis	Constant throbbing and sharp	Rapid	Pelvis	No	Yes	Pregnancy or postpartum	Position	No
Torsion of ovary, cyst, or tumor	Constant and sharp	Rapid	Unilateral or bilateral pelvis	Nausea and vomiting	Maybe	Cyst; fibroids	Activity, movement, and position	No
Tubal-ovarian abscess	Constant and sharp	Rapid	Unilateral or bilateral pelvis	Nausea	Yes	History of PID or gonorrhea	Activity and movement	Purulent

Adapted from: Emergency Nurses Association. (2007). *Emergency nursing core curriculum* (6th ed.). Philadelphia: Saunders.

TABLE 9-2   Nongynecologic Causes of Pelvic Pain

Causes	Timing and Type	Onset	Location	Nausea, Vomiting	Fever	Contributing Factors	Aggravating Factors	Vaginal Discharge
Appendicitis	Constant that starts dull and becomes sharp	Slow, then rapid	Periumbilical, RLQ	Nausea	Low grade	None	Activity and movement	No
Diverticulitis	Intermittent cramping	Slow	LLQ	No	Maybe	Food that obstruct a diverticulum	Diet	No
DKA	Constant pain that is severe and sharp	Rapid	Diffuse	N/V	Maybe	DM	Hyperglycemia, Acidosis	No
Gastroenteritis	Constant and cramping	Rapid	Diffuse	N/V	Maybe	Viral infection, Diet	Peristalsis, Eating	No
Strangulated hernia	Intermittent pain that can be dull or sharp	Slow	Generalized	N/V	Yes	Defect in fascia, muscle or peritoneum that traps bowel	Peristalsis	No
Intussusception	Intermittent and cramping	Slow	Lower abdomen	Vomiting	Maybe	Family history	Eating	No
Leaking AAA	Constant and severe	Rapid	Maybe, referred	None	No	NTM, family history	HTN, bleeding hypoxia	No
Peritonitis	Constant that starts vague then becomes sharp	Slow or rapid	Variable	Nausea	Yes	None	Activity and movement	No
Sickle cell crisis	Constant and severe	Rapid	Diffuse	N/V	Yes	Dehydration, hypoxia, stress, infection	Position	No
Small bowel obstruction	Intermittent at first then constant. Pain ranges from bloating, cramping, or severe	Slow	Diffuse	N/V later stage	No	Any bowel abnormality, cancer, impaction	Eating, movement and activity if perforation	No
Urethral stone	Intermittent and sharp	Rapid	Unilateral flank to groin	Maybe	No	Patient or family history of stones	Peristaltic movement of ureter	No
UTI	Intermittent and burning	Rapid	Pelvis	None	Maybe	Frequent coitus, poor hygiene, multiple partners	Voiding	No
Volvulus	Intermittent then constant and severe	Rapid	Diffuse or localized	N/V	No	Previous surgery	Peristalsis	No

Adapted from: Emergency Nurses Association. (2007). *Emergency nursing core curriculum* (6th ed.). Philadelphia: Saunders.

c. Oxygen saturation
d. Respiratory effort and excursion
e. Cardiac rate and rhythm
f. Pain and discomfort level
g. Accurate intake and output
h. Evidence of bleeding
i. Close monitoring for progression of symptoms
2. Maintain airway, oxygenation, and ventilation
   a. Position of comfort
   b. Oxygen by nasal cannula at 2 to 6 L/min if indicated to maintain SpO_2 of 95% unless contraindicated; for patients with COPD, use pulse oximetry to guide oxygen administration to SpO_2 of 90%
3. Maintain adequate circulation and perfusion
   a. IV access with two large-bore IV catheters for fluid and medication administration
      1) IV fluids: usually 0.9% saline
   b. Control of any bleeding
4. Control pain and discomfort
   a. NSAIDs
   b. Narcotic analgesics
   c. Anxiolytics
   d. Rest
   e. Application of heat
5. Treat infection (if present) and prevent sepsis
   a. Antimicrobials as indicated
   b. Antipyretics and cooling methods to reduce fever
6. Prepare for and assist with procedures
   a. Preparation for pelvic examination
      1) Bimanual examination for uterine or adnexal mass, uterine enlargement, or tenderness
   b. Preparation for possible surgical intervention
7. Monitor for complications
   a. Uncontrolled pain
   b. Hemorrhage
   c. Sepsis

Evaluation
1. Patent airway, adequate oxygenation (i.e., normal PaO_2, SpO_2, and SaO_2) and ventilation (i.e., normal $PaCO_2$)
2. Absence of clinical indicators of hypoperfusion
3. Absence of clinical indications of infection/sepsis
4. Control of pain and discomfort
5. Absence of clinical indications of bleeding

Typical disposition
1. If evaluation criteria met: discharge with instructions
   a. Activity as tolerated
   b. Instructions to return to the ED for fever higher than 100.6°F (38.1°C), if bleeding occurs or increases, for increased pain (ENA, 2007)
   c. Follow up with primary care provider or GYN provider
2. If evaluation criteria not met: admission for diagnostic or surgical procedures

Endometriosis
Definition: development of endometrial tissue outside the uterus

Predisposing factors
1. Most likely in European American women of child-bearing age
2. May have genetic predisposition

Pathophysiology
1. Exact cause and mechanism unknown; may be caused by the following factors:
   a. Embryonic epithelial cells
   b. Backflow of menstrual fluid through the fallopian tubes
   c. Spread of endometrial tissue by lymphatic or vascular system
2. Endometrial tissue develops outside the uterus; most likely sites of growth include the bladder, ovaries, fallopian tubes, bowel, and broad ligament
3. Endometrial tissue reacts to hormonal changes and sloughs off with menses causing pelvic pain
4. Bleeding causes inflammation and pain in tissues
5. Infertility is common and may result from mechanical blockage of the fallopian tubes with the endometrial implants

Clinical presentation
1. Subjective
   a. Lower back, intestinal, or pelvic pain
   b. Dysmenorrhea
   c. Dyspareunia
   d. Dysuria
   e. Heavy menstrual periods and/or spotting and bleeding between periods
   f. Painful bowel movements or painful urination during menstrual periods
2. Objective
   a. Tenderness with pelvic examination
   b. May have other masses
3. Diagnostic studies
   a. Laparoscopic visualization
   b. Biopsy

Collaborative Management
1. Continue assessment
   a. ABCDs
   b. Vital signs: blood pressure, pulse, respiratory rate, and temperature
   c. Oxygen saturation
   d. Pain and discomfort level
   e. Evidence of bleeding
   f. Accurate intake and output
   g. Close monitoring for progression of symptoms
2. Maintain airway, oxygenation, and ventilation
   a. Position of comfort
   b. Oxygen by nasal cannula at 2 to 6 L/min if indicated to maintain SpO_2 of 95% unless contraindicated; for patients with COPD, use pulse oximetry to guide oxygen administration to SpO_2 of 90%
3. Maintain adequate circulation and perfusion

a. IV access with two large-bore IV catheters for fluid and medication administration
   1) IV fluids: usually 0.9% saline
b. Control of bleeding
4. Control pain and discomfort
   a. NSAIDs
   b. Narcotic analgesics
   c. Anxiolytics
5. Treat infection (if present) and prevent sepsis
   a. Antimicrobials as indicated
   b. Antipyretics and cooling methods to reduce fever
6. Monitor for complications
   a. Uncontrolled pain
   b. Infertility

Evaluation

1. Patent airway, adequate oxygenation (i.e., normal PaO_2, SpO_2, and SaO_2) and ventilation (i.e., normal $PaCO_2$)
2. Absence of clinical indicators of hypoperfusion
3. Absence of clinical indications of infection/sepsis
4. Control of pain and discomfort
5. Absence of clinical indications of bleeding

Typical disposition

1. If evaluation criteria met: discharge with instructions
   a. Increases fluid intake
   b. Reporting of any signs of infection
   c. Referral to gynecologist
      1) Hormone therapy to control the growth of endometriosis
      2) Surgery to remove growths or control the size of very large endometriosis and to relieve pain
2. If evaluation criteria not met: admission for further diagnostic or surgical procedures

Dysfunctional Uterine Bleeding (DUB)

Definition: irregular menstruation without anatomic lesions of uterus; also referred to as menorrhagia or abnormal uterine bleeding
Predisposing factors
1. Most cases in adolescents secondary to immature hypothalamic-pituitary-ovarian axis
   a. The pituitary and ovarian hormones equally control the other's circulating level to sustain a self-perpetuating monthly endocrine cycle
2. Oral contraceptives and intrauterine devices
3. Thyroid, adrenal, or pituitary disease can cause absence of ovulation
4. Adenosis (maternal diethylstilbestrol [DES] exposure)
5. Trauma or contact irritation (e.g., repeated intercourse)
6. Endometriosis
7. Polycystic ovary syndrome
8. Intrauterine masses or functional cysts
9. Bleeding disorders
10. Liver disease
11. Obesity
12. Diabetes mellitus

Pathophysiology

1. Normal menstrual flow is 2 to 8 days with 20 to 80 ml of blood loss
2. Postmenopausal may indicate carcinoma
3. Types by symptomatology
   a. Regular menstrual cycles with heavy bleeding >10 days
   b. Menstrual periods more frequent than every 21 days
   c. Intermenstrual bleeding with spotting or breakthrough bleeding between menstrual periods
   d. Irregular menstrual periods (except from those that commonly occur in first 2 years after menarche)
   e. Postmenopausal bleeding
4. Types by cause
   a. Hormonal: infrequent or lack of ovulation, chronic estrus, and endometrial stimulation are usually hormonal
      1) Anovulatory cycle: ovulation fails to occur (most common)
      2) Luteal phase defect: when ovulation occurs the corpus luteum is inadequate
   b. Mechanical problems (e.g., polyps, fibroids)
   c. Malignancies
      1) Gestational trophoblastic disease
         a) Hydatidiform moles
         b) Tumor forms at conception instead of fetus, usually benign
         c) Choriocarcinomas: can originate from a hydatidiform mole or tissue from previous miscarriage or normal delivery that remained
      2) Uterine, cervical, or vaginal malignancy

Clinical presentation

1. Subjective
   a. Prolonged and excessive bleeding
      1) Mild dysfunctional bleeding: patient has history of increased duration of menses, decreased length of menstrual cycle, and moderate increase in bleeding during menses
      2) Moderate dysfunctional bleeding: patient has a history of repeated episodes of prolonged menses, decreased length of menstrual cycle to occur every 2 to 3 weeks, and moderate to severe bleeding
      3) Severe dysfunctional bleeding: patient has a history of menses so prolonged that timing of cycle not clear and very heavy bleeding
   b. No premenstrual symptoms (e.g., breast fullness, abdominal bloating, mood changes, edema, weight gain, menstrual cramps)
2. Objective
   a. Painless vaginal bleeding
   b. May have vulvar, vaginal, or cervical lesions
3. Diagnostic studies
   a. Coagulation profile: to detect bleeding disorder
   b. Thyroid hormones (T_3, T_4, TSH): endocrine disorder

c. Beta hCG
  1) Serum is quantitative and gives more accurate fetal development information
  2) Urinalysis is qualitative
d. Ultrasound: ectopic pregnancy, miscarriage
  1) Snowstorm pattern on ultrasound (gestational trophoblastic disease)
e. Vaginal cultures for infection (e.g., cervicitis, endometritis, vaginitis)
f. LH-FSH ratio: polycystic ovary syndrome
g. Pap smear and colposcopy: malignancy

Collaborative management

1. Continue assessment
   a. ABCDs
   b. Vital signs: blood pressure, pulse, respiratory rate, and temperature
   c. Oxygen saturation
   d. Respiratory effort and excursion
   e. Cardiac rate and rhythm
   f. Pain and discomfort level
   g. Accurate intake and output
   h. Color, consistency, and quantity of vaginal bleeding
   i. Level of consciousness
   j. Close monitoring for progression of symptoms
2. Maintain airway, oxygenation, and ventilation
   a. Position of comfort
   b. Oxygen by nasal cannula at 2 to 6 L/min if indicated to maintain SpO_2 of 95% unless contraindicated; for patients with COPD, use pulse oximetry to guide oxygen administration to SpO_2 of 90%
3. Maintain adequate circulation and perfusion
   a. IV access with two large-bore IV catheters for fluid and medication administration
     1) IV fluids: usually 0.9% saline
   b. Control of bleeding
     1) Preparation for pelvic examination
       a) Bimanual examination for uterine or adnexal mass, uterine enlargement or tenderness
     2) Preparation for possible surgical intervention
       a) Dilation and curettage (D&C)
     3) Hormone replacement therapy
   c. Iron supplements as prescribed
4. Control pain and discomfort
   a. NSAIDs
   b. Narcotic analgesics
   c. Anxiolytics
5. Treat infection (if present) and prevent sepsis: antimicrobials as indicated
6. Monitor for complications
   a. Anemia
   b. Endometrial hyperplasia
   c. Endometrial carcinoma

Evaluation

1. Patent airway, adequate oxygenation (i.e., normal PaO_2, SpO_2, and SaO_2) and ventilation (i.e., normal $PaCO_2$)
2. Absence of clinical indications of respiratory distress
3. Absence of clinical indicators of hypoperfusion
4. Absence of clinical indications of infection/sepsis
5. Control of pain and discomfort
6. Absence of clinical indications of bleeding

Typical disposition

1. If evaluation criteria met: discharge with instructions
   a. Activity as tolerated
   b. Instructions to return to the ED for fever higher than 100.6°F (38.1°), if bleeding occurs or increases, for increased pain. (ENA, 2007)
   c. Follow up with primary care provider or GYN provider
2. If evaluation criteria not met: admission for diagnostic or surgical procedures

Vaginal Discharge

Definition: discharge from vagina

1. Infections are identified as the cause in 80% to 90% patients presenting with vaginal discharge
   a. Candidiasis 25%
   b. Trichomonas 25%
   c. Bacterial vaginosis 50%

Predisposing factors

1. Infection
   a. Can be result of changes in pH
     1) Normal vaginal pH is 3.8 (ENA, 2007)
     2) When the pH is less acidic, there is a predisposition to infection
   b. Multiple sex partners
   c. Unprotected sex
   d. Poor hygiene
   e. Diabetes
2. Atrophic vaginitis caused by decreased estrogen levels
3. Foreign body

Clinical presentation

1. Subjective
   a. Report of vaginal discharge: large amount with trichomonas
   b. Dyspareunia
   c. Dysuria
   d. Vaginal odor particularly with vaginosis and trichomonas
   e. Vulvar burning
   f. Pruritus is common with *Candida*
2. Objective
   a. Vaginal discharge
     1) White with *Candida*
     2) Yellow-gray and frothy with trichomonas
     3) Gray with vaginosis
   b. Erythema and possible swelling of vaginal area
   c. Abdominal tenderness with palpation
   d. On pelvic examination
     1) Severe mucosal erythema and excoriation seen with *Candida*
     2) No or minimal erythema with vaginosis
     3) Petechiae with trichomonas

3. Diagnostic studies
   a. Discharge: amount, color, pH, odor
      1) Sight amount, yellowish-white, pH 3.5 to 4.5 usually no odor is normal
      2) Vaginal discharge clear with a pH 6 to 8 prepubertal or postmenopausal
      3) Moderate amount, gray-white and thin, pH 5 to 5.5 with a "cheesy" odor (vaginosis)
      4) White, thick, and curd discharge with a pH 4 to 5 usually no odor (*Candida*)
      5) Moderate amount of yellow-green, frothy discharge with a pH 6 to 7; has a fishy smell (*Trichomonas*)
   b. Vaginal acidity measured with Nitrazine paper
      1) Normal 3.8 to 4.2
      2) <4.5 with bacterial vaginosis (5 to 6) or trichomonas (6 to 7)
      3) <4.5 with fungal infection (4 to 5) or physiologic discharge
      4) Blue = bacteria, yellow = yeast
   c. Microscopic examination of discharge
      1) Budding filaments with *Candida*, mycelia on KOH, "yeasty" odor
      2) Mobile protozoa with *Trichomonas*
      3) Clue cells and whiff test with vaginosis
      4) Few WBCs is normal

Collaborative management

1. Continue assessment
   a. ABCDs
   b. Vital signs: blood pressure, pulse, respiratory rate, and temperature
   c. Oxygen saturation
   d. Pain and discomfort level
   e. Close monitoring for progression of symptoms
2. Maintain airway, oxygenation, and ventilation
   a. Position of comfort
   b. Oxygen by nasal cannula at 2 to 6 L/min if indicated to maintain SpO_2 of 95% unless contraindicated; for patients with COPD, use pulse oximetry to guide oxygen administration to SpO_2 of 90%
3. Maintain adequate circulation and perfusion
   a. Increased oral fluids
   b. IV access for fluid and medication administration if indicated
4. Control pain and discomfort
   a. Position of comfort
   b. Analgesics if required
   c. Anxiolytics if required
5. Treat infection (if present) and prevent sepsis
   a. Antimicrobials as indicated
   b. Antipyretics and cooling methods to reduce fever
6. Prepare and assist with pelvic examination
7. Monitor for complications
   a. Pelvic inflammatory disease (PID)
   b. Sepsis

Evaluation

1. Absence of clinical indicators of hypoperfusion
2. Absence of clinical indications of infection/sepsis
3. Control of pain and discomfort

Typical disposition: discharge with instructions

1. Prescribed medications
2. Good personal hygiene
3. Safe sexual practices
4. Follow up with primary care or GYN as directed

Sexually Transmitted Infections (STIs)

Definition: infection that has a high probability of being transmitted through sexual contact (i.e., vaginal, oral, or anal); previously known as:
1. Venereal disease
2. Sexually transmitted disease (STD)

Predisposing factors

1. Unprotected sex
2. Multiple sexual partners
3. STI can be also be transmitted from an infected person to a noninfected individual through sharing needles in IV drug use, childbearing, and breastfeeding

Specifics to type of STI (Table 9-3)

1. Chancroid (Mehta and Silverberg, 2007)
   a. Caused by *Haemophilus ducreyi*
   b. Clinical presentation
      1) Produces an area of ulceration on the penis, anus, cervix, vagina, vulva, or perineum
         a) Soft dirty-looking irregularly shaped ulcers with undefined margins, excavated depth, yellow to gray base
         b) Purulent hemorrhagic secretions
         c) Similar ulcers on opposing labia (kissing ulcers)
      2) Progresses to painful inguinal adenopathy within 3 to 14 days
   c. Diagnostic studies: gram stain and culture
   d. Management
      1) Antibiotic therapy: ceftriaxone (Rocephin), azithromycin (Zithromax), ciprofloxacin (Cipro) (contraindicated in pregnancy or lactation)
      2) Treatment of sexual partners
2. Gonorrhea (GC) (Behrman & Shoff, 2008)
   a. Caused by *N. gonorrheae*
   b. Clinical presentation
      1) Genital pain and discharge; maybe found in numerous organs and tissue and misdiagnosed
         a) Gonococcal cervicitis
         b) PID
         c) Salpingitis
         d) Prostatitis, epididymitis
         e) Pharyngitis
         f) Conjunctivitis

TABLE 9-3   Sexually Transmitted Infections

STI	Cause	Lesions	Discharge	Odor	Rash	Pain	Medication	Complications
Chancroid	*Haemophilus ducreyi*	Ulcers without defined edges	None	Foul odor from lesion	No	Yes, increasing with voiding	Ceftriaxone (Rocephin) Erythromycin (Erythrocin) Ciprofloxacin (Cipro)	Increased infection rate of HIV, Secondary infection, Fistula
Chlamydia	*Chlamydia trachomatis*	None	Off white – Mucopurulent	Sometimes from cervix being infected	Erythema of cervix	Men burning with urination. Women-none	Azithromycin (Zithromax) Doxycycline (Vibramycin) Erythromycin (Erythrocin)	PID, Infertility, Ectopic pregnancy, Epididymitis, Cervicitis, Salpingitis, Conjunctivitis, Urethral stricture, Reiter syndrome
Gonorrhea	*Neisseria gonorrhea*	None	Yellow, mucopurulent	Usually	Possibly itching and redness	Male – dysuria Women – if PID	Ceftriaxone (Rocephin) Cefixime (Suprax).	PID, Abscesses, Chronic pelvic pain, Damage to fallopian tubes, Epididymitis
Genital herpes	Herpes Simplex virus type 2	Multiple shallow vesicles	Purulent	No unless another infection present	May have redness	Yes	Acyclovir (Zovirax) Famcyclovir (Famvir)	May past to others Newborn infections as they pass through the birth canal
Genital warts	*Human papillomavirus*	No lesions, but will have small, flesh-colored or gray swellings	Pink-gray. Soft.	No	No	No pain, but itching and discomfort	Imiquimod 5% cream (Aldara), Trichloro-acetic acid (Tri-chlor), or liquid nitrogen	Cervical cancers If large enough can interfere with urination

| Syphilis | *Treponema pallidum* | Chancre | None | No | Rash, often appearing as rough, red or reddish-brown, penny-sized sores | None | Benzathine PCN (Bicillin CR) Doxycycline (Vibramycin) | Increases risk of HIV Without treatment can cause pregnancy complications, cardiac problems Late stage can cause: Stroke Infection and inflammation of the membranes and fluid surrounding the brain and spinal cord (meningitis) Poor muscle coordination Numbness Paralysis Deafness or visual problems Personality changes Dementia |
| Trichomonas | *Trichomonas vaginalis* | None | Greenish-gray; thin frothy | Malodorous | Yes | Severe pruritus | Metronidazole (Flagyl) | Increased risk of HIV, and low birth weight or premature births |

2) Men and women both may present asymptomatic

3) Burning sensation may occur with urination

4) Vaginal or penile discharge: white, yellow, or green

5) Men may have painful or swollen testicles

6) Women usual have mild or vague symptoms; possible irregular bleeding between menses

c. Diagnostic studies

1) Gram stain shows gram-negative diplococci

2) Positive cultures

3) Consider testing for syphilis and chlamydia

d. Management

1) Antibiotic therapy: ceftriaxone (Rocephin), cefixime (Suprax)

a) As of 2007, the CDC no longer recommends fluoroquinolone antibiotics (ciprofloxacin [Cipro], ofloxacin [Floxin], and levofloxacin [Levaquin]) because the prevalence of fluoroquinolone resistance in *N. gonorrhoeae* has been increasing

2) Treatment of sexual partners

3. *Chlamydia* (CDC, 2008; Mayo Clinic, 2008): most common STI

a. Caused by *C. trachomatis*

1) Can occur in the rectum, urethra, cervix, and throat

2) Commonly coexists with gonorrhea

3) Consider Fitz-Hugh-Curtis syndrome in women who present with RUQ tenderness (Frumovitz, 2006)

b. Clinical presentation

1) Men and women may be asymptomatic

2) Women

a) In women, bacteria will start in the cervix and urethra, then spread to the fallopian tubes (may still be asymptomatic)

b) Women may report having abnormal vaginal discharge and/or dysuria

c) Women may also present with complaints of lower abdominal pain, low back pain, nausea, fever, pain during intercourse, bleeding between menstrual periods

3) Men

a) Men may present with complaints of penile discharge, itching, or burning at the opening of the penis

b) Testicular pain and swelling uncommon

c. Diagnostic studies

1) Culture for *Chlamydia* and gonorrhea

2) Chlamydia gram stain shows gram-negative diplococci

3) Positive cultures

d. Management

1) Antibiotic therapy: one-time dose of azithromycin (Zithromax) or one week of doxycycline (Vibramycin)

4. Genital herpes (Mayo Clinic, 2008)

a. Caused by infection caused by herpes simplex virus (HSV)

1) Genital herpes usually caused by HSV-2

2) Virus lives on nerve root; recurrent and incurable

b. Clinical presentation

1) Painful lesions appear on an erythematous base as vesicles that ulcerate, crust over, then heal; vesicles form on cervix, vagina, vulva, perineum, buttock, and penis

2) May also have fever, headache, photophobia, malaise, myalgia, lymphadenopathy, and waddling gait

c. Diagnostic studies

1) Blood test

2) Culture of viral lesions

d. Management

1) Acyclovir (Zovirax)

2) Warm baths

3) Topical anesthetic ointments

4) Treatment of sexual partners

5. Genital warts (Mayo Clinic, 2008)

a. Caused by the human papillomavirus (HPV)

1) >100 types of HPV have been identified

2) >40 types are passed through sexual contact (CDC, 2009)

3) HPV can affect men and women

b. Clinical presentation

1) Classified as low- and high-risk HPV

a) Low-risk HPV may never have symptoms

b) Having high-risk HPV does not mean a patient will have symptoms or cancer; it is an indication for screening and monitoring for risk

c) HPV types 16 and 18 together cause about 70% of cervical cancers (CDC, 2008)

2) Patient presents complaining of genital or anal itching, burning, and discomfort; warts may be visible

c. Diagnostic studies (CDC, 2008)

1) Often based on findings from the history and physical examination

2) PAP smear: if abnormal, patient will usually be scheduled to follow up with GYN specialist

3) Colposcopy may be done to examine cervix closer

4) Schiller test: cervix is swabbed with an iodine solution; healthy cells will turn brown and abnormal cells will turn white or yellow

5) Biopsy will not be done in the ED, but may be scheduled to further examine cervical tissue for cancer

d. Management

1) Warts may resolve on own; patients present to the ED when they become painful

2) Imiquimod 5% cream (Aldara) applied to area as prescribed (it destroys wart tissue)

3) Other procedures usually not done in the ED

a) Cryosurgery (freezing with liquid nitrogen)

b) Trichloroacetic acid (Tri-Chlor)

6. Syphilis (Mayo Clinic, 2008)

a. Caused by the spirochete *Treponema pallidum*

1) Slow evolving infection that can be latent for years

b. Clinical presentation by stages
   1) First stage (primary stage)
      a) Painless ulcerations or pustules on genitals several weeks after exposure
   2) Second stage
      a) Lasts 1 to 2 months
      b) Malaise, lethargic, fever, rash on palms and soles of feet, headache, bone and joint pain, white sores in mouth, anorexia
   3) Third stage (latent stage)
      a) May not appear for 20 years
      b) Soft rubbery tumors attack all areas of the body (e.g., brain, nerves, eyes, heart, blood vessels, liver, bones, and joints)
      c) Coordination problems, paralysis, numbness, gradual blindness, and dementia can occur (CDC, 2008)
      d) Can be transmitted to fetus in pregnancy
c. Diagnostic studies
   1) Lesion cultures positive
   2) Lumbar puncture and cerebral spinal fluid testing in third stage
   3) Serum blood test for syphilis can be drawn to test for an antigen-antibody reaction occurrence (rarely done in the ED)
      a) Rapid plasma reagin test (RPR)
      b) Venereal Disease Research Laboratory test (VDRL)
d. Management
   1) Antibiotic therapy: penicillin G benzathine (Bicillin CR) intramuscular
      a) If patient has had syphilis >1 year, will probably require additional doses and be referred to primary care
      b) If allergic to penicillin, there are other antibiotics available (see CDC guidelines)
   2) Treatment of sexual partners

Collaborative management
1. Continue assessment
   a. ABCDs
   b. Vital signs: blood pressure, pulse, respiratory rate, and temperature
   c. Pain and discomfort level
   d. Accurate intake and output
   e. Close monitoring for progression of symptoms
2. Maintain airway, oxygenation, and ventilation
   a. Position of comfort
   b. Oxygen by nasal cannula at 2 to 6 L/min if indicated to maintain SpO_2 of 95% unless contraindicated; for patients with COPD, use pulse oximetry to guide oxygen administration to SpO_2 of 90%
3. Maintain adequate circulation and perfusion
   a. IV access for fluid and medication administration
4. Control pain and discomfort
   a. Analgesics if required
   b. Anxiolytics if required
5. Treat infection and prevent sepsis

a. Assessment for other STIs
b. Antimicrobials as indicated
c. Antipyretics and cooling methods to reduce fever
6. Monitor for complications
   a. Other STIs
   b. Pyelonephritis
   c. PID
   d. Infertility

Evaluation
1. Patent airway, adequate oxygenation (i.e., normal PaO_2, SpO_2, and SaO_2) and ventilation (i.e., normal $PaCO_2$)
2. Absence of clinical indications of infection/sepsis
3. Control of pain and discomfort

Typical disposition: discharge with instructions
1. Education on STIs and safe sex
2. Emphasis on need to continue with prescribed medications including treatment of sexual partners if indicated
3. Follow up with primary care or GYN as directed

Pelvic Inflammatory Disease (PID)
Definition: acute or chronic inflammation of the fallopian tubes and supporting structures
1. Condition may include any combination of inflammatory disorders within female upper genital tract
   a. Mucopurulent cervicitis
   b. Endometritis
   c. Salpingitis
   d. Tubal-ovarian abscess
   e. Pelvic peritonitis
2. Fitz-Hugh-Curtis syndrome: RUQ pain occurring in PID related to perihepatitis (Frumovitz & Ascher-Walsh, 2006)

Predisposing factors (Crossman, 2006)
1. Infection, usually STI
   a. Increased number of sexual partners
   b. No use of barrier contraceptives
2. Intrauterine device (IUD)
   a. IUD long considered a risk factor for PID and infertility
   b. IUD causes in the United States thought likely due to insertion of device
3. Risk increases during or shortly after menses
4. Douching
5. Smokers have twice the risk of nonsmokers
6. Adolescents are at higher risk because they tend to seek health care later

Pathophysiology
1. Usually caused by *C. trachomatis* or *N. gonorrheae* infection of the cervix or vagina that then spreads into the endometrium, fallopian tubes, ovaries, and adjacent structures
2. Less commonly, direct spread from a nearby infection such as appendicitis or diverticulitis may occur

Clinical presentation

1. Subjective
   a. Fever and chills
   b. Abdominal pain
   c. Vaginal discharge
   d. Irregular bleeding
   e. Nausea and vomiting
   f. Dysuria
2. Objective
   a. Elevated temperature may or may not be present
      1) If fever present, it is usually >101.3°F
   b. Stooped over or shuffled gait
   c. Muscle guarding
   d. Rebound tenderness
   e. Cervical discharge
   f. Pelvic mass
   g. Tenderness on palpation of cervix, uterus
3. Diagnostic studies
   a. No historical, physical, or laboratory findings can conclusively diagnose PID
   b. Abnormal laboratory studies may provide supportive but not confirmatory evidence; all laboratory studies may be normal in patient with PID
   c. Minimum diagnostic criteria: uterine tenderness or adnexal tenderness or cervical motion tenderness with one or more of the following:
      1) Oral temperature >101°F (>38.3°C)
      2) Abnormal cervical or vaginal mucopurulent discharge
      3) Presence of WBCs on saline microscopy of vaginal secretions
      4) Elevated ESR
      5) Elevated C-reactive protein (CRP)
      6) Laboratory documentation of cervical infection
   d. Diagnosis of PID unlikely if normal cervical discharge and no WBCs on wet prep
      1) Most specific criteria
         a) Histopathology evidence of endometritis on endometrial biopsy
         b) Transvaginal sonography or MRI techniques showing thickened fluid-filled tubes with or without free pelvic fluid or tubo-ovarian complex, or Doppler studies suggesting pelvic inflammation (e.g., tubal hyperemia)
         c) Laparoscopic abnormalities consistent with PID

Collaborative management

1. Continue assessment
   a. ABCDs
   b. Vital signs: blood pressure, pulse, respiratory rate, and temperature
   c. Pain and discomfort level
   d. Accurate intake and output
   e. Close monitoring for progression of symptoms
2. Maintain airway, oxygenation, and ventilation
   a. Position of comfort
   b. Oxygen by nasal cannula at 2 to 6 L/min if indicated to maintain SpO_2 of 95% unless contraindicated; for patients with COPD, use pulse oximetry to guide oxygen administration to SpO_2 of 90%
3. Maintain adequate circulation and perfusion
   a. Increased oral fluids
   b. IV access for fluid and medication administration
      1) IV fluids: usually 0.9% saline
4. Control pain and discomfort
   a. NSAIDs
   b. Narcotic analgesics
   c. Anxiolytics
5. Treat infection and prevent sepsis
   a. Antimicrobials as indicated
   b. Antipyretics and cooling methods to reduce fever
6. Prepare patient for diagnostic testing and possible surgical intervention
7. Monitor for complications
   a. Infertility
   b. Chronic pelvic pain
   c. Ectopic pregnancy
   d. Pelvic abscess

Evaluation

1. Patent airway, adequate oxygenation (i.e., normal PaO_2, SpO_2, and SaO_2) and ventilation (i.e., normal $PaCO_2$)
2. Absence of clinical indicators of hypoperfusion
3. Absence of clinical indications of infection/sepsis
4. Control of pain and discomfort

Typical disposition: discharge with instructions

1. Avoidance of sex until treatment completed
2. Evaluation of sex partners for STI
3. Prevention of PID: precautions used to prevent STIs
4. Antibiotic prophylaxis with doxycycline may decrease infection related to IUD insertion
5. Follow up with primary care or GYN as directed

Bartholin Cyst/Abscess

Definition: accumulation of material in mucus-producing Bartholin gland in vulva; may involve the vulva, labia majora, and vagina

Predisposing factors

1. Unknown

Pathophysiology

1. Bacteria from the vagina enters the gland
   a. Anaerobic isolates from Bartholin gland abscesses are most common and may include
      1) *Bacteroides fragilis*
      2) *Clostridium perfringens*
      3) *Peptostreptococcus* sp.
      4) *Fusobacterium* sp.
   b. Aerobic isolates from Bartholin gland abscesses often polymicrobial and may include:
      1) *N. gonorrheae* (most common)
      2) *C. trachomatis*

3) *E. coli*
4) *Pseudomonas aeruginosa*
5) *Staphylococcus aureus*
6) *Streptococcus faecalis*

2. Blockage of distal duct of Bartholin gland causes:
   a. Retention of secretions
   b. Dilation of duct
   c. Formation of cyst (enlargement without inflammation)
3. May progress to a local infection with abscess formation and may spread to nearby tissue, such as the labia and vagina

Clinical presentation (Merck Source, 2008)
1. Subjective
   a. May be asymptomatic
   b. Pain particularly with activity and intercourse
2. Objective
   a. Swelling in labia area on one side
      1) If abscess, severe vulvar pain
   b. Vulvar asymmetry
   c. Vulvar erythema
   d. Tenderness or pain with palpation
   e. Possible fever
   f. May have altered gait
3. Diagnostic study
   a. Biopsy in women >40 years to rule out cancer (rare)

Collaborative management
1. Continue assessment
   a. ABCDs
   b. Vital signs: blood pressure, pulse, respiratory rate, and temperature
   c. Pain and discomfort level
   d. Accurate intake and output
   e. Close monitoring for progression of symptoms
2. Maintain airway, oxygenation, and ventilation
   a. Position of comfort
   b. Oxygen by nasal cannula at 2 to 6 L/min if indicated to maintain SpO_2 of 95% unless contraindicated; for patients with COPD, use pulse oximetry to guide oxygen administration to SpO_2 of 90%
3. Maintain adequate circulation and perfusion
   a. Fluids by mouth
   b. IV access for fluid and medication administration as indicated
4. Control pain and discomfort
   a. Position of comfort
   b. NSAIDs
   c. Narcotic analgesics
5. Treat infection (if present) and prevent sepsis
   a. Antimicrobials as indicated
   b. Antipyretics and cooling methods to reduce fever
   c. Incision and drain as indicated
6. Monitor for complications
   a. Recurring cyst
   b. Nonhealing lesion
   c. Scarring

Evaluation
1. Absence of clinical indicators of hypoperfusion
2. Absence of clinical indications of infection/sepsis
3. Control of pain and discomfort

Typical disposition: discharge with instructions
1. Sitz bath for comfort
2. Antibiotics and analgesic as directed
3. Instructions related to safe sex practices
4. Follow up with gynecologist

Sexual Assault and Rape
Definitions
1. Sexual assault: a wide range of unwanted behaviors up to but not including penetration, which are attempted or carried out against a victim's will or when a victim cannot consent due to age, disability, or the influence of alcohol or drugs. It may include actual or threatened physical force, weapons, coercion.
2. Rape: definitions vary by state, but most define it as nonconsensual oral, anal, or vaginal penetration of the victim by body parts or objects using force, threats of bodily harm, or by taking advantage of a victim who incapacitated or incapable of giving consent.
3. Generally defined as felonies.
   a. Only 36% of rapes, 34% of attempted rapes, and 26% of sexual assaults were reported to the police. Reasons include:
      1) Self-blame or guilt
      2) Shame, embarrassment, privacy issues
      3) Humiliation or fear of the perpetrator or other individual's perceptions
      4) Fear of not being believed or of being accused of playing a role in the crime
      5) Lack of trust in the criminal justice system

Predisposing factors (National Institute of Justice, 2008)
1. Majority of victims are women
2. Most perpetrators are known to their victims
3. History of multiple sexual partners
4. Substance abuse (alcohol, drugs)
5. Age: among female rape victims surveyed, 54% were younger than age 18; 32.4% were ages 12 to 17; 21.6% were younger than age 12
6. College students
7. Disabled persons

Clinical presentation
1. Subjective
   a. History of assault
      1) Location, time, date
      2) Any weapons or penetrating foreign bodies
      3) Consensual sex within the past week
      4) Post-assault hygiene (e.g., showering, cleaning self up in any way)
   b. Voluntary or involuntary use of drugs or alcohol
      1) Date rape drugs include:

      a) Ketamine hydrochloride (Ketaset or Ketalar)
      b) Gamma-hydroxybutyric acid (GHB)
      c) Flunitrazepam (Rohypnol)
   c. Past medical history
   d. Immunization status
2. Objective
   a. Level of consciousness, behavior
   b. All areas for
     1) Abrasions, scrapes, scratches
     2) Ecchymosis
     3) Bite marks
     4) Laceration
   c. All areas for tenderness
   d. Forensic examination if assault occurred <72 hours earlier
3. Chain of evidence collection (ENA, 2005) (http://samfe.dna.gov/operational_issues/evidence_collection_kit/)
   a. Use gloves for all evidence collection including touching of clothing
   b. Obtain a good history of the events
   c. Properly label all evidence with hospital name, patient name, and identification number in a sealed approved container for evidence collection
     1) Date and time of collection and signature of individual collecting evidence
     2) Description of specimen and site it was collected from
   d. Place any objects removed during evidence collection in an evidence bag by itself and label
   e. Do not cut through clothing and if impossible, remove by cutting around stains, holes, tears, etc. Fold clothing without shaking and place in evidence bag
   f. Air-dry evidence taken from victim
   g. Collect evidence before any procedures (e.g., voiding, catheter insertion)
   h. Have patient remove while standing on a paper sheet (ENA, 2007)
   i. Collect fingernail scrapings, oral evidence, pubic hair, and pelvic and anal examination
   j. If moisture needed to collect evidence, lightly moisten a cotton tip swab to decrease the chance of diluting DNA evidence
   k. After cotton tips specimen, dry place bulb end first into envelope and sealed properly (do NOT lick envelopes to seal because it will leave your DNA)
   l. Do not place moist evidence in glass or plastic because mold may grow
     1) When collecting specimens, they are stored in glass or paper bags
  m. Slide specimen collection as indicated
   n. Use Woods light to examine for stains on body and clothes if indicated
   o. Photograph sites before collection of evidence using 35 mm camera
   p. Document physical evidence and findings
   q. Allow patient time to shower and clean up after examination

4. Diagnostic studies
   a. Blood, urine, and cultures per protocols
   b. Pregnancy testing
   c. STI testing
     1) RPR: screen for syphilis
   d. HIV testing
   e. Serum and urine toxicology testing

Collaborative management
1. Continue assessment
   a. ABCDs
   b. Vital signs: blood pressure, pulse, respiratory rate, and temperature
   c. Pain and discomfort level
   d. Level of consciousness
   e. Emotional status
   f. Close monitoring for progression of symptoms
2. Assist with forensic examination and management
   a. Physical examination and evidence collection as above
   b. Prophylaxis for pregnancy in females within 72 hours
     1) Ethinil estradiol (Ovral) 2 tablets now, repeat in 12 hours
       a) Antiemetic to prevent nausea and vomiting
   c. Prophylaxis for STIs in all victims includes all of the following:
     1) Ceftriaxone (Rocephin) 125 mg–250 mg IM
     2) Azithromycin (Zithormax) 1 g by mouth
     3) Metronidazole (Flagyl) 2 g by mouth
     4) Doxycycline (Vibramycin) 100 mg twice daily for 7 days
   d. IV fluids and hydration as indicated
   e. Tetanus immunization as indicated
   f. Hepatitis B immunization series if not already immunized
3. Monitor for complications
   a. STIs
   b. Pregnancy
   c. Anxiety/fear
   d. Posttraumatic stress syndrome

Evaluation
1. Patent airway, adequate oxygenation (i.e., normal Pao_2, Spo_2, and Sao_2) and ventilation (i.e., normal $Paco_2$)
2. Absence of clinical indicators of hypoperfusion
3. Absence of clinical indications of infection/sepsis
4. Control of pain and discomfort
5. Absence of extreme emotional crisis

Typical disposition: discharge home with instructions
1. Medical follow-up in 2 to 4 weeks to repeat STI and pregnancy testing
2. Counseling
3. Education patient on STI signs and symptoms
4. Safe sex practices
5. How to care for injuries at home

Spontaneous Abortion

Definition: involuntary loss of pregnancy prior to viability; types of abortions include the following

1. Threatened: slight vaginal bleeding with mild uterine cramping, cervical os is closed, uterus enlarged and soft
2. Inevitable: moderate vaginal bleeding with moderate cramping, cervical os is open 3 cm or greater, gross rupture of membranes
3. Imminent: appearance of symptoms that signal the impending loss of the products of conception
4. Missed: slight vaginal bleeding, no cramping or contraction and cervical os is closed -retention of dead products of conception
5. Incomplete: heavy vaginal bleeding with severe cramping, cervical os open some but not all of uterine contents have been passed
6. Complete: slight vaginal bleeding with mild uterine cramping, cervical os is closed, products of conception have been completely expelled
7. Septic: malodorous vaginal bleeding, no cramping or contractions, cervical os closed, fever, ascending infection present
8. Habitual: recurrent, patient has had two or more consecutive spontaneous abortions

Predisposing factors

1. Genetic factors (e.g., trisomy, monosomy)
2. Endocrine abnormalities (e.g., thyroid disorders, diabetes)
3. Reproductive tract abnormalities (e.g., incompetent cervix, fibroids)
4. Infection (e.g., toxoplasmosis, syphilis)
5. Systemic (e.g., lupus, chronic renal failure)
6. Environmental (e.g., toxins, smoking, alcohol)
7. Increasing maternal age
8. Previous history of abortion

Clinical presentation

1. Subjective
   a. Bleeding
   b. Low abdominal pain and cramping
   c. May have foul smelling vaginal discharge
   d. Fever, chills
2. Objective
   a. Elevated temperature
   b. Distended "doughy-feeling" abdomen or peritoneal signs may suggest ruptured ectopic pregnancy with hemoperitoneum
   c. Detection of fetal heart tones in viable pregnancy
      1) Detected at 10 to 12 weeks' gestation
   d. Pelvic examination
      1) Dilated cervix on speculum examination
      2) Tender adnexal mass may suggest ectopic pregnancy; bulging cul-de-sac may suggest ruptured ectopic pregnancy with hemoperitoneum
      3) Passed tissue (spontaneous abortion versus decidual reaction)

3. Diagnostic studies
   a. Beta-hCG quantitative (serum)
   b. Ultrasound (sonogram)
   c. Blood type and Rh factor
      1) RhoGAM may be recommended if Rh-negative mother

Collaborative management

1. Continue assessment
   a. ABCDs
   b. Vital signs: blood pressure, pulse, respiratory rate, and temperature
   c. Oxygen saturation
   d. Respiratory effort and excursion
   e. Cardiac rate and rhythm
   f. Clinical indications of bleeding
   g. Pain and discomfort level
   h. Accurate intake and output
   i. Close monitoring for progression of symptoms
2. Maintain airway, oxygenation, and ventilation
   a. Position of comfort
   b. Oxygen by nasal cannula at 2 to 6 L/min to maintain SpO_2 of 95% unless contraindicated; for patients with COPD, use pulse oximetry to guide oxygen administration to SpO_2 of 90%
   c. Oropharyngeal or nasopharyngeal airway or endotracheal intubation may be required especially if altered LOC or pulmonary edema
3. Maintain adequate circulation and perfusion
   a. IV access for fluid and medication administration
      1) IV fluids: usually 0.9% saline
   b. Control of bleeding
   c. Rh immune globulin
4. Control pain and discomfort
   a. Bed rest
   b. Analgesics
   c. Anxiolytics
   d. Vaginal or pelvic rest
   e. Reassurance
5. Prepare for procedures and surgical intervention
   a. Oxytocin (Pitocin) to expel uterine contents (incomplete) as prescribed
   b. D&C for inevitable, missed, septic, incomplete abortion as indicated
6. Monitor for complications
   a. Bleeding
   b. Infection
   c. Depression

Evaluation

1. Patent airway, adequate oxygenation (i.e., normal PaO_2, SpO_2, SaO_2) and ventilation (i.e., normal $PaCO_2$)
2. Absence of clinical indications of respiratory distress
3. Absence of clinical indicators of hypoperfusion
4. Absence of clinical indications of infection/sepsis
5. Control of pain and discomfort
6. Absence of clinical indications of bleeding

Typical disposition

1. If evaluation criteria met: discharge with instructions (Valley, Jackson-Williams, & Fly, 2006)
   a. Rest
   b. Instructions to return to the ED if the following symptoms occur:
      1) Profuse vaginal bleeding
      2) Severe pelvic pain
      3) Temperature above 100.4°F (38°C)
   c. Patient may experience intermittent menstrual-like flow and cramps during the following week.
   d. After spontaneous abortion it may take 4 to 5 weeks before the next menstrual period occurs
   e. Patient can resume regular activities when able but should refrain from sexual intercourse, tampons, and douching for 2 weeks
   f. Follow-up with obstetrician/gynecologist
2. If evaluation criteria not met (e.g., uncontrolled bleeding or pain): admission

Pregnancy-Induced Hypertension (PIH)

Definition: hypertension that is unique to pregnancy

1. Defined as systolic blood pressure (SBP) >140 mm Hg or diastolic blood pressure (DBP) >90 mm Hg present at least twice 6 hours or more apart with the patient lying in the left lateral position
2. PIH can range from mild to severe; in severe forms the patient can develop preeclampsia, eclampsia, or HELLP syndrome

Predisposing factors

1. First-time pregnancy
2. Women whose sisters and mothers had PIH
3. Women carrying multiple babies
4. Teenage pregnancy
5. Pregnancy in women over age 40 years
6. Women who have high blood pressure or kidney disease prior to pregnancy
7. Obesity

Pathophysiology (Gibson & Carson, 2007)

1. The exact mechanism not understood
2. Preeclampsia is primarily an endothelial dysfunction
3. Hypertension occurs because of vasospasms
4. Classic triad in preeclampsia is hypertension, proteinuria, and edema occurring after the 20th week of pregnancy
5. Eclampsia is a worsening of preeclampsia characterized by convulsion
6. HELLP syndrome is a more severe form of preeclampsia characterized by hemolysis, elevated liver enzymes, and low platelets

Clinical presentation

1. Subjective
   a. Headache
   b. RUQ abdominal pain
   c. Excessive or too rapid weight gain
   d. Swelling and edema of upper extremity, face, ankles
      1) Persistent edema unresponsive to resting supine
   e. Visual disturbances
      1) Double vision
      2) Blurred vision
      3) Sudden blindness
   f. Dyspnea
   g. Ringing or buzzing sound in ears
   h. Vomiting
   i. Drowsiness
   j. Fever
2. Objective
   a. Hypertension that decreases when patient placed in left lateral position
   b. Facial, hand, and ankle edema
   c. Papilledema
   d. RUQ tenderness with palpation
   e. Hyperreflexia of lower extremities
3. Diagnostic studies
   a. CBC: check for increase in hematocrit, anemia, and thrombocytopenia
   b. Serum creatinine: increase indicates decreasing renal function
   c. Coagulation profile: PT/aPTT, fibrin degradation products to evaluate for disseminated intravascular coagulation
   d. Urine dip and urine analysis
      1) Urine protein dipstick: proteinuria 1+
      2) 24-hour urine collection for total protein
      3) Creatinine clearance
   e. Additional tests when HELLP syndrome suspected
      1) Platelet count
      2) Alanine aminotransferase (ALT)
      3) Aspartate aminotransferase (AST)
      4) Serum lactic dehydrogenase (LDH): >600 U/L
      5) Serum glutamic oxaloacetic transaminase (SGOT): >72 U/L
   f. Ultrasound to assess for small gestational age, oligohydramnios, and accelerated placental calcification

Collaborative management

1. Continue assessment
   a. ABCDs
   b. Vital signs: blood pressure, pulse, respiratory rate, and temperature
   c. Oxygen saturation
   d. Respiratory effort and excursion
   e. Cardiac rate and rhythm
   f. Fetal heart tones
   g. Pain and discomfort level
   h. Accurate intake and output
   i. Serum electrolytes
      1) Clinical indications of magnesium toxicity (i.e., loss of deep tendon reflexes, respiratory depression)
   j. Level of consciousness
   k. Close monitoring for progression of symptoms

2. Maintain airway, oxygenation, and ventilation
   a. Oxygen by nasal cannula at 2 to 6 L/min to maintain SpO_2 of 95% unless contraindicated; for patients with COPD, use pulse oximetry to guide oxygen administration to SpO_2 of 90%
3. Maintain adequate circulation and perfusion
   a. Best rest: left lateral decubitus (to prevent vena cava compression)
   b. IV access for fluid and medication administration
   c. Antihypertensive therapy to maintain diastolic pressure 90 to 100 mm Hg
      1) Hydralazine (Apresoline)
      2) Labetalol (Trandate)
      3) Nitroprusside (Nipride)
4. Control pain and discomfort: analgesics
5. Prevent/treat seizures
   a. Seizure precautions: minimize stimulation
   b. Magnesium sulfate prophylaxis for seizures
   c. Diazepam (Valium) if seizure occurs
6. Monitor for complications
   a. Maternal
      1) Acute renal failure (anuria)
      2) Disseminated intravascular coagulation (DIC)
      3) Stroke
      4) Encephalopathy
      5) Heart failure
      6) Hepatocellular damage
      7) Ruptured liver
      8) Pulmonary edema
   b. Fetal complications
      1) Placental insufficiency can lead to ischemia, which can cause progressive fetal hypoxia and malnutrition
      2) Dysmaturity: intrauterine growth retardation (IUGR)
      3) Oligohydramnios: deficiency of amniotic fluid level
      4) Intrapartum fetal distress
      5) Fetal intolerance to labor
      6) Increased risk of placental abruption

Evaluation

1. Patent airway, adequate oxygenation (i.e., normal PaO_2, SpO_2, and SaO_2) and ventilation (i.e., normal $PaCO_2$)
2. Absence of clinical indicators of hypoperfusion
3. Alert and oriented with no neurologic deficit
4. Control of pain and discomfort
5. Alert and oriented with no neurologic deficit
6. Absence of seizures
7. Absence of clinical indications of fetal distress

Typical disposition

1. If evaluation criteria met: discharge with instructions
   a. Bed rest
   b. Modified activity recommended, though no supportive evidence
   c. Salt restriction not recommended because it may contribute to hypovolemia

   d. Return to the ED for headaches, visual disturbances, RUQ pain, increase in edema, vaginal bleeding, contractions
   e. Follow-up with obstetrician/gynecologist
2. If evaluation criteria not met: admission

Bleeding in Late Pregnancy
Definition: bleeding that occurs after the 20th week of pregnancy
1. Placenta previa: an abnormally implanted placenta in the lower uterine segment; cause unknown
   a. Classification is based on the degree to which the cervical os is covered by the placenta
      1) Total: internal os is completely covered by placental tissue
      2) Partial: internal os is partially covered by placental tissue
      3) Marginal: the edge of the placenta is at the margin of the internal os
      4) Low lying: the placenta lies abnormally low on the uterine wall but is not yet over the cervix
2. Abruptio placenta: a premature separation of the placenta from the uterine wall; cause unknown

Predisposing factors
1. Placenta previa
   a. Multiparity
   b. Multiple gestations
   c. Advanced maternal age
   d. Previous placenta previa
   e. Previous uterine or placenta abnormalities
2. Abruptio placentae
   a. Maternal hypertension
   b. Vascular disease
   c. Poor nutrition
   d. Maternal smoking or substance abuse (e.g., cocaine use)
   e. Recent intercourse
   f. Acute external trauma

Clinical presentation
1. Subjective
   a. Decreased fetal movement
   b. Sudden onset of painless bright red bleeding in placenta previa
   c. Dark red vaginal bleeding and cramping or painful contractions in abruptio placenta
2. Objective
   a. May have orthostatic hypotension
   b. Abdominal contractions
   c. Placenta previa: bright red bleeding from vaginal area
   d. Abruptio placentae
      1) Dark red bleeding from vaginal area
      2) Increasing fundal height
      3) Port-wine–colored amniotic fluid
      4) Decreased or deceleration of fetal heart rate
3. Diagnostic studies
   a. CBC: decreased hematocrit in abruptio placenta

b. Coagulation studies: platelet count, fibrinogen level

c. Blood type and antibody screen: women who are Rh negative should receive RhoGAM

d. Kleihauer-Betke test: to identify fetal cells in the maternal circulation as evidence of fetomaternal hemorrhage

e. Sonogram: to rule out placenta previa

f. Continuous fetal heart monitoring

Collaborative management

1. Continue assessment
   a. ABCDs
   b. Vital signs: blood pressure, pulse, respiratory rate, and temperature
   c. Oxygen saturation
   d. Respiratory effort and excursion
   e. Cardiac rate and rhythm
   f. Pain and discomfort level
   g. Accurate intake and output
   h. Serum electrolytes
   i. Level of consciousness
   j. Abdominal height of fundus and abdominal girth
   k. Fetal heart tones
   l. Close monitoring for progression of symptoms
2. Maintain airway, oxygenation, and ventilation
   a. Oxygen by nasal cannula at 2 to 6 L/min if indicated to maintain SpO_2 of 95% unless contraindicated; for patients with COPD, use pulse oximetry to guide oxygen administration to SpO_2 of 90%
3. Maintain adequate circulation and perfusion
   a. IV access for fluid and medication administration
      1) IV fluids: usually 0.9% saline
   b. Control of bleeding
4. Control pain and discomfort
   a. Analgesics
   b. Antiemetic
   c. Position on left side
5. Administer drugs and therapies to prevent maternal and/or fetal death
   a. Avoidance of cervical examinations
   b. Tocolytics (e.g., terbutaline [Brethine]) for placenta previa
   c. RhoGAM if indicated
   d. Preparation for possible delivery and resuscitation
6. Monitor for complications
   a. DIC
   b. Hemorrhagic shock
   c. Maternal or fetal death

Evaluation

1. Patent airway, adequate oxygenation (i.e., normal PaO_2, SpO_2, and SaO_2) and ventilation (i.e., normal $PaCO_2$)
2. Absence of clinical indicators of hypoperfusion
3. Absence of clinical indications of infection/sepsis
4. Control of pain and discomfort
5. Absence of clinical indications of bleeding
6. Absence of clinical indications of fetal distress

Typical disposition: admission to labor and delivery and possibly for surgery (i.e., cesarean section) or emergency vaginal delivery if delivery imminent and possible newborn resuscitation

Hyperemesis Gravidarum

Definition: intractable vomiting in pregnancy with weight loss and ketosis

Predisposing factors

1. Can occur at any time throughout pregnancy, but more common at the end of the first trimester (weeks 8 to 12)
2. History of hyperemesis in previous pregnancy
3. Primigravidas
4. Multiple gestations
5. Previous abortions or unsuccessful pregnancies
6. Preexisting diabetes
7. Weight >170 pounds (77.3 kg)
8. Prepregnancy eating disorders
9. Chronic liver, kidney, thyroid, or gastrointestinal disease
10. Chronic hypertension
11. Triggered by various odors, taste or sight of food

Pathophysiology

1. Associated with high estrogen levels
2. Can lead to fluid and electrolyte imbalances, weight loss, and ketosis
3. In severe cases can lead to neurologic disturbances, liver damage, retinal hemorrhage and renal damage

Clinical presentation

1. Subjective
   a. Nausea and vomiting
   b. Alteration in taste
   c. Fatigue
   d. Weight loss
2. Objective
   a. Orthostatic hypotension
   b. Vomiting
   c. Pale
   d. Diaphoretic
3. Diagnostic studies
   a. CBC with differential: may have elevated hematocrit due to dehydration
   b. Electrolytes: may have hyponatremia, hypokalemia, hypochloremic alkalosis
   c. Liver panel: 50% AST and ALT 1 to 2 times normal
   d. Thyroid panel: elevated free thyroxine levels, suppressed TSH levels
   e. Urinalysis: ketonuria, elevated specific gravity if dehydrated

Collaborative Management

1. Continue assessment
   a. ABCDs
   b. Vital signs: blood pressure, pulse, respiratory rate, and temperature
   c. Pain and discomfort level

d. Frequency and character of vomitus
e. Accurate intake and output
f. Serum electrolytes
g. Fetal heart tones
h. Close monitoring for progression of symptoms
2. Maintain airway, oxygenation, and ventilation
   a. Head of bed at 30 degrees
   b. Oxygen by nasal cannula at 2 to 6 L/min to maintain SpO_2 of 95% unless contraindicated; for patients with COPD, use pulse oximetry to guide oxygen administration to SpO_2 of 90%
3. Maintain adequate circulation and perfusion
   a. IV access for fluid and medication administration
      1) IV fluids: usually 0.9% saline
4. Control nausea and vomiting
   a. Pharmacologic agents as prescribed
      1) Antiemetics (e.g., [phenothiazines [Phenergan, Compazine], ondansetron [Zofran], dimenhydrinate [Dramamine])
      2) Antihistamines (e.g., diphenhydramine [Benadryl], doxylamine [Aldex], meclizine [Antivert])
      3) Metoclopramide (Reglan)
      4) Pyridoxine (vitamin B_6)
      5) Thiamine (vitamin B_1) to prevent Wernicke encephalopathy
   b. Frequent small meals
   c. Reassurance that symptoms are self-limited and may represent higher estrogen levels, which are associated with improved pregnancy outcome
5. Monitor for complications
   a. Dehydration
   b. Ketosis
   c. Electrolyte imbalance
   d. Wernicke encephalopathy
   e. Retinal hemorrhage
   f. Mallory-Weiss tear (i.e., esophageal tear, which tends to resolve with cessation of vomiting)
   g. Esophageal rupture

Evaluation
1. Patent airway, adequate oxygenation (i.e., normal PaO_2, SpO_2, and SaO_2) and ventilation (i.e., normal $PaCO_2$)
2. Absence of clinical indications of respiratory distress
3. Absence of clinical indicators of hypoperfusion
4. Absence of electrolyte imbalance
5. Control of pain and discomfort
6. Absence of clinical indications of fetal distress
7. Control of vomiting

Typical disposition
1. If evaluation criteria met: discharge with instructions
   a. Dietary guidelines
      1) Avoid greasy and spicy foods, and possibly odors
      2) Eat dry carbohydrates (i.e., crackers) on awakening, soft, low-fat foods and protein snack at bedtime
      3) Drink carbonated beverages
      4) Avoid fluids with meals may help

b. Medicines as prescribed
c. Prophylactic thiamine supplementation recommended
d. Alternative therapies may be recommended
   1) Acupressure including sea bands
   2) Ginger
   3) Hypnosis
e. Instructions to return to the ED for persistent vomiting
f. Follow-up with obstetrician
2. If evaluation criteria not met: admission

Preterm Labor (PTL)
Definition: regular uterine contractions prior to the 37th week of gestation; contractions occur every 10 minutes or less and each contraction lasts at least 30 seconds

Predisposing factors
1. Prior preterm labor
2. Multiple gestations
3. Infection
4. Dehydration
5. Premature rupture of membranes (PROM)
6. Incompetent cervix: painless dilation of cervix (usually seen in second trimester)
7. Excessive uterine enlargement
8. Uterine distention
9. Substance abuse
10. Malposition

Clinical presentation
1. Subjective
   a. Menstrual-like cramps
   b. Low dull backache
   c. Abdominal and/or pelvic pressure
   d. Abdominal cramping with or without diarrhea
   e. Increase or change in vaginal discharge
   f. Uterine contractions that are often painless
   g. Change in vaginal discharge
2. Objective
   a. Elevated temperature
   b. Cervix may be dilated
   c. Fetal heart tones and rate (may increase or decrease)
3. Diagnostic studies
   a. CBC, urine drug screen, blood type and screen if cesarean section considered
   b. Urinalysis and culture
   c. External electronic fetal monitoring
   d. Cervical culture for group B streptococci, gonorrhea, *Chlamydia* if rupture of membranes
   e. Vaginal fluid samples for wet mount (bacterial vaginosis, *Trichomonas*)
   f. pH and fern testing for ruptured membranes

Collaborative management
1. Continue assessment
   a. ABCDs
   b. Vital signs: blood pressure, pulse, respiratory rate, and temperature

c. Pain and discomfort level

d. Accurate intake and output

e. Serum electrolytes

f. Level of consciousness

g. Fetal heart tones

h. Close monitoring for progression of symptoms

2. Maintain airway, oxygenation, and ventilation
   a. Oxygen by nasal cannula at 2 to 6 L/min to maintain SpO_2 of 95% unless contraindicated; for patients with COPD, use pulse oximetry to guide oxygen administration to SpO_2 of 90%

3. Maintain adequate circulation and perfusion
   a. Nothing by mouth if delivery imminent
   b. IV access for fluid and medication administration
      1) Intravenous fluids: usually 0.9% saline

4. Control pain and discomfort
   a. Analgesics
   b. Steroids
   c. Tocolytics for contractions (e.g., terbutaline [Brethine], magnesium)

5. Monitor for complications
   a. Prematurity (reflects gestational age)
   b. Low birth weight (<2500 g)
   c. Respiratory distress syndrome (e.g., hyaline membrane disease)
   d. Intraventricular hemorrhage
   e. Necrotizing enterocolitis
   f. Sepsis
   g. Seizures
   h. Bronchopulmonary dysplasia
   i. Developmental abnormalities

Evaluation

1. Patent airway, adequate oxygenation (i.e., normal PaO_2, SpO_2, and SaO_2) and ventilation (i.e., normal $PaCO_2$)

2. Absence of clinical indicators of hypoperfusion

3. Control of pain and discomfort

4. Absence of clinical indications of fetal distress

Typical disposition: admission to labor and delivery

Postpartum Hemorrhage

Definition: blood loss of 500 ml or more within the first 24 hours after delivery

1. Types
   a. Early postpartum hemorrhage: occurs within 24 hours
   b. Late postpartum hemorrhage: occurs between 24 hours and 6 weeks
   c. Severe postpartum hemorrhage = blood loss >1000 ml or resulting in hemodynamic instability

2. Causes
   a. Four Ts mnemonic (Smith, 2006)
      1) Tone: uterine atony (most common cause)
      2) Trauma: uterine inversion, uterine rupture, lacerations, hematomas, episiotomy
      3) Tissue: retained placenta,
      4) Thrombin: coagulopathies (rare cause)

   b. ATTIRE mnemonic: in order of frequency
      1) Atony
      2) Tissue: retained placenta
      3) Trauma: lacerations, hematomas, episiotomy
      4) Inversion
      5) Rupture
      6) Erythrocytes: coagulopathies

Predisposing factors

1. Uterine atony (most common cause)
2. Birth trauma
   a. Difficulty removing placenta
   b. Use of forceps
3. Coagulopathies
4. Uterine inversion
5. Preeclampsia
6. Placenta previa
7. Multiple gestation
8. Obesity
9. Hypertensive disorders
10. Antepartum hemorrhage

Clinical presentation

1. Subjective
   a. Excessive vaginal bleeding
   b. Lightheadedness
   c. Syncope
2. Objective
   a. Tachycardia
   b. Tachycardia and narrow pulse pressure may occur early with severe postpartum hemorrhage
   c. Hypotension
   d. Oliguria may appear late
   e. Bimanual examination
      1) Boggy uterus
      2) Uterus enlarged with accumulated blood
      3) Hematomas
   f. Earliest clinical sign of placental separation may be absence of backflow pressure when applying pressure to blood in umbilical cord for 10 to 15 cm toward placenta
3. Diagnostic studies
   a. CBC with differential: low hemoglobin and hematocrit indicates possible bleeding
   b. Coagulation profile: abnormalities may indicate DIC or other hematologic problems
   c. Pelvic and vaginal sonography

Collaborative management

1. Continue assessment
   a. ABCDs
   b. Vital signs: blood pressure, pulse, respiratory rate, and temperature
   c. Oxygen saturation
   d. Respiratory effort and excursion
   e. Cardiac rate and rhythm
   f. Pain and discomfort level
   g. Accurate intake and output
   h. Serum electrolytes

i. Level of consciousness
j. Vaginal bleeding and consistency (e.g., clots, tissue)
k. Fetal heart tones
l. Close monitoring for progression of symptoms
2. Maintain airway, oxygenation, and ventilation
   a. Oxygen by nasal cannula at 2 to 6 L/min if indicated to maintain SpO_2 of 95% unless contraindicated; for patients with COPD, use pulse oximetry to guide oxygen administration to SpO_2 of 90%
   b. Artificial airway may be required
3. Maintain adequate circulation and perfusion
   a. IV access with two large-bore IV catheters for fluid and medication administration
      1) Intravenous fluids: usually 0.9% saline or lactated Ringer solution
   b. Control of bleeding
      1) Methylergonovine (Methergine) for bleeding
         a) Acts directly on smooth muscles of the uterus to increases tone, and on the rate and amplitude of contractions to slow blood loss
      2) Massage of uterine fundus
   c. May need bimanual massage of uterus
   d. Dilation and curettage (D&C) as indicated
4. Control pain and discomfort
   a. Analgesics
5. Monitor for complications
   a. Hypovolemic shock
   b. Infection

Evaluation

1. Patent airway, adequate oxygenation (i.e., normal PaO_2, SpO_2, and SaO_2) and ventilation (i.e., normal $PaCO_2$)
2. Absence of clinical indicators of hypoperfusion
3. Absence of clinical indications of infection/sepsis
4. Control of pain and discomfort
5. Absence of clinical indications of bleeding
6. Absence of clinical indications of fetal distress

Typical disposition: admission and possible surgery

Emergency Delivery

Definition: unplanned event causes delivery of fetus
Predisposing factors

1. Prior preterm labor
2. Multiple gestations
3. Increased parity
4. Hydramnios: too much amniotic fluid
5. Oligohydramnios: not enough amniotic fluid
6. Placenta previa
7. Hydrocephalus (i.e., enlarged fetus head)
8. Previous delivery complications
9. Uterine anomalies

Clinical presentation

1. Subjective
   a. Regular contractions or abdominal pain
   b. A feeling of a gush of water or rupture of membranes

2. Objective
   a. Color and amount of vaginal bleeding
   b. Stage of labor
      1) Stage I: from onset of regular contractions to full cervical dilation (dilation)
      2) Stage II: from full cervical dilation until infant crowns (infant delivery)
      3) Stage III: from time infant is delivered until the placenta is delivered (placenta delivery)
      4) Stage IV: 4 hours post placenta delivery (recovery stage)
   c. Fetal heart tones (FHTs)
   d. Fundus height, tone, and contractions
      1) Timing and characteristics of contractions
   e. Pelvic examination if not delivering emergently
      1) Effacement (thinning of cervix, normal is 2 cm)
      2) Dilation of cervix (in centimeters 1 to 10)
      3) Consistency of cervix (soft or firm)
      4) Station of fetal head: describes how far the head of the fetus has descended into the birth canal (measured in plus and minus)
      5) Membranes intact or ruptured
3. Diagnostic studies
   a. CBC
   b. Type and cross-match
   c. Ferning test for amniotic fluid
   d. pH test for amniotic fluid
   e. Ultrasound: to confirm or rule out possibility of breech if time permits

Collaborative management

1. Continue assessment
   a. ABCDs
   b. Vital signs: blood pressure, pulse, respiratory rate, and temperature
   c. Oxygen saturation
   d. Respiratory effort and excursion
   e. Cardiac rate and rhythm
   f). Pain and discomfort level
   g. Accurate intake and output
   h. Serum electrolytes
   i. Level of consciousness
   j. Vaginal bleeding and consistency (e.g., clots, tissue)
   k. Fetal heart tones
   l. Close monitoring for progression of symptoms
2. Maintain airway, oxygenation, and ventilation
   a. Oxygen by nasal cannula at 2 to 6 L/min to maintain SpO_2 of 95% unless contraindicated; for patients with COPD, use pulse oximetry to guide oxygen administration to SpO_2 of 90%
      1) If unable to maintain SpO_2 of 95%, place on 100% oxygen by face mask
   b. Intubation and mechanical ventilation as indicated
3. Maintain adequate circulation and perfusion
   a. IV access with two large-bore IV catheters for fluid and medication administration
      1) Intravenous fluids: usually 0.9% saline or lactated Ringer solution

4. Control pain and discomfort
   a. Position of comfort
   b. Analgesics
5. Assist patient and physician with delivery
   a. Coaching of breathing
   b. Immediate delivery if head is visible
6. Stabilization of the newborn after delivery (Figure 9-3)
   a. Keep infant warm (prevent heart loss and monitor temperature)
   b. Clamp the umbilical cord in two places approximately 4 to 5 cm from the infant's umbilicus
   c. Do not cut umbilical cord until pulsation stops
   d. Perform overall evaluation: Apgar scores at 1, 5, and 10 minutes
   e. Assess for delivery of placenta (usually within 30 minutes of the newborn)
7. Monitor for complications
   a. Birth trauma
   b. Fetal hypoxia during labor
   c. Placenta abruption
   d. Postpartum hemorrhage
   e. Infant breathing problems after delivery

Evaluation

1. Patent airway, adequate oxygenation (i.e., normal PaO_2, SpO_2, and SaO_2) and ventilation (i.e., normal $PaCO_2$)
2. Absence of clinical indications of respiratory distress
3. Absence of clinical indicators of hypoperfusion
4. Absence of clinical indications of infection/sepsis
5. Control of pain and discomfort
6. Absence of clinical indications of bleeding
7. Absence of clinical indications of fetal distress

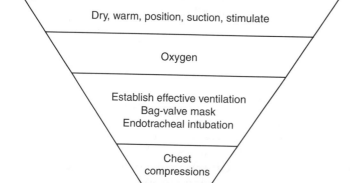

Neonatal resuscitation inverted pyramid

Dry, warm, position, suction, stimulate

Oxygen

Establish effective ventilation
Bag-valve mask
Endotracheal intubation

Chest
compressions

Meds

Figure 9-3 Neonatal resuscitation inverted pyramid. (From Hazinski, M. F., Field, J. M., & Gilmore, D. [Eds.] [2005]. *Handbook of emergency cardiovascular care for healthcare providers*, p. 70, Dallas, TX: Copyright © 2006 American Heart Association. Reprinted with permission.

Typical disposition

1. Mother: admission to the hospital
2. Neonate: admission to the nursery or neonatal intensive care as indicated

Complicated Deliveries

Breech presentation: fetal buttocks or the lower extremities present into the maternal pelvis

1. There are three types:
   a. Frank (most common): both fetal thighs are flexed and both lower extremities are extended at the knees
   b. Complete: both fetal thighs are flexed and one or both knees are flexed
   c. Incomplete (i.e., footling): when one or both fetal thighs are extended and one or both knees or feet are below the buttocks
2. Collaborative management (Mason, 2010)
   a. Cesarean section is preferred if there is time but delivery must be completed in the ED if the fetus has been delivered to the level of the umbilicus
   b. OB support should be immediately requested with any breech presentation
   c. Spontaneous delivery should be allowed to level of umbilicus
   d. After the umbilicus is visualized, a generous portion of the umbilical cord should be gently extracted
   e. The fetus is rotated to align shoulders in an anterior-posterior position to deliver the shoulders
   f. The buttocks are then rotated to the mother's front to deliver the head
   g. The fetus's head is flexed and suprapubic pressure is applied to the mother's uterus
   h. Gentle pressure is applied to the shoulders to deliver the head
   i. The neonate is suctioned and the cord is clamped

Shoulder dystocia

1. After delivery of the head, the shoulders cannot pass through the pelvis; can lead to cord compression and fetal distress
2. Collaborative management
   a. OB support is requested
   b. Mother's legs are hyperflexed over the abdomen (i.e., McRoberts maneuver) to disengage the anterior shoulder
   c. If this positioning is unsuccessful, suprapubic pressure is applied

Umbilical cord prolapse

1. Umbilical cord slips down into the vagina or externally after the membranes have ruptured; causes sudden fetal bradycardia and severe recurrent variable decelerations unresponsive to position
2. Collaborative management
   a. Insertion of a gloved hand into vagina to separate presenting part and release it off the cord
   b. Placement of the patient in Trendelenburg or knee chest position

c. High-flow oxygen

d. Tocolytics to decrease contractions

Amniotic fluid embolism

1. Rare occurrence when the barrier between amniotic fluid and maternal circulation is broken
2. Clinical indications include
   a. Sudden onset of dyspnea and/or chest pain
   b. Hypoxemia (i.e., decreased SpO_2)
   c. Pulmonary edema
   d. Clinical indications of shock
   e. Coagulopathy
3. Collaborative management
   a. High flow oxygen by nonrebreathing mask
   b. Intubation and mechanical ventilation with positive end-expiratory pressure (PEEP) may be required
   c. IV administration of crystalloids; blood and blood products may be required

Uterine inversion

1. Rare but potentially fatal complication of the third state of labor; may be caused by excessive traction on the umbilical cord in an attempt to expedite delivery of the placenta
2. Clinical indication is a pear-shaped, bleeding mass noted vaginally and that the uterine fundus is not in its usual position
3. Collaborative management
   a. Manual replacement of uterus with a closed fist
   b. Placenta should not be removed since pulling on it may cause hemorrhage; it should be put back in the vaginal vault with the uterus
   c. IV administration of crystalloids; blood and blood products may be required
   d. Oxytocic agents (e.g., oxytocin [Pitocin]) to promote uterine tone

Neonatal Resuscitation

Definition: perinatal asphyxia and extreme prematurity are the most common complications of pregnancy that require resuscitation of the neonate

Predisposing factors

1. Prematurity
2. Breech presentation
3. Multiple gestations
4. Placental insufficiency
5. Delivery complications
6. Substance abuse by mother

Clinical presentation

1. Objective: depressed infant
2. Diagnostic studies
   a. CBC
   b. Glucose
   c. ECG
   d. Venous or arterial pH
   e. STI screening
   f. Pelvic ultrasound

Collaborative management

1. Continue assessment
   a. ABCDs
   b. Vital signs: blood pressure, pulse, respiratory rate, and temperature
   c. Oxygen saturation
   d. Respiratory effort and excursion
   e. Cardiac rate and rhythm
   f. Level of consciousness
   g. Apgar scores at 1, 5, and 10 minutes
   h. Close monitoring for progression of symptoms
2. Maintain airway, breathing, and circulation
   a. Airway: position head in neutral position and bulb suction mouth first, then the nose
   b. Breathing
      1) Blow by oxygen with 100%
      2) If inadequate response after 30 to 60 seconds, bag-valve-mask (BVM) ventilation with 100%
      3) If no improvement, intubation
   c. Circulation: assess heart rate by listening to apical pulse with stethoscope, pulse in umbilicus, or brachial pulse
      1) If heart less than 60 bpm after 100% oxygen administration for 30-60 seconds, start CPR
   d. IV access or umbilical access: administer normal saline
   e. Neonatal resuscitation medications (Figure 9-4)
      1) Epinephrine
      2) Naloxone (Narcan)
      3) Glucose
3. Communicate with family and allow them to see infant as soon as possible
4. Monitor for complications
   a. Infant death
   b. Anoxic encephalopathy

Evaluation

1. Patent airway, adequate oxygenation (i.e., normal PaO_2, SpO_2, and SaO_2) and ventilation (i.e., normal $PaCO_2$)
2. Absence of clinical indications of respiratory distress
3. Absence of clinical indicators of hypoperfusion
4. Absence of clinical indications of fetal distress

Typical disposition

1. Admission to the neonatal ICU; consider transfer to Level III neonatal unit if not available at present hospital and newborn is a premature

Trauma in Pregnancy

Definition: blunt or penetrating trauma in a pregnant woman

1. Trauma is the leading cause of death in women of childbearing age and vehicular collisions represent the leading cause of maternal injury.
2. The frequency with, which women sustain injury increases with each trimester
3. Anatomic and physiologic changes in pregnancy can mask or mimic injury

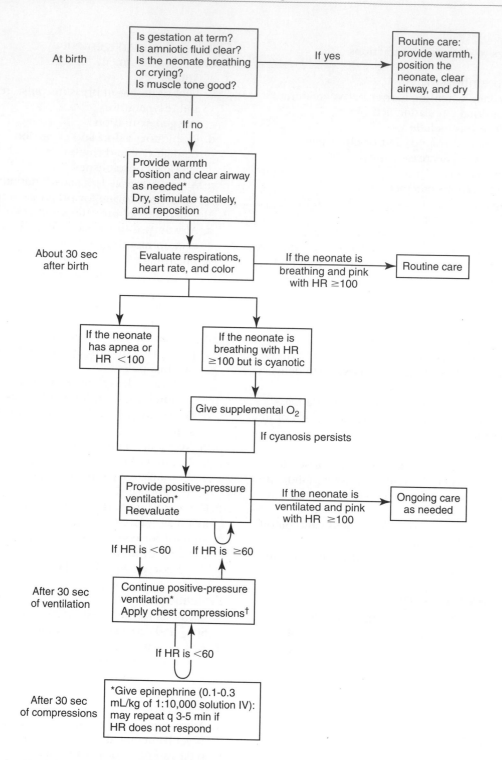

*Endotracheal intubation may be considered at any of several steps.
†Reassess heart rate about every 30 sec. Continue chest compressions until the spontaneous HR is ≥60 beats/min.
HR = heart rate.

Figure 9-4 Algorithm for resuscitation of neonates. (From The Merck Manual of Diagnosis and Therapy, Online Medical Library, edited by Robert Porter. Copyright © 2004-2010 by Merck Sharp & Dohme Corporation, a subsidiary of Merck & Co., Inc., Whitehouse Station, NJ. Available at http://www.merck.com/mmpe.)

Predisposing factors

1. Blunt or penetrating trauma
2. Domestic violence
3. Accidental injury

Clinical presentation

1. Subjective
   a. Mechanism of injury
   b. Contractions
   c. Vaginal bleeding
   d. Fetal movement
2. Objective: dependent on extent and location of injury
   a. May have ecchymosis of breasts, abdomen, and upper extremities
   b. May have injuries at more than one site in varying stages of healing may be observed
   c. May have ecchymosis on lower abdomen due to seatbelt injury
   d. May feel uterine contractions
   e. May have vaginal bleeding
3. Diagnostic studies
   a. CBC: remember pregnancy-induced leukocytosis and anemia occur normally
   b. Electrolyte and glucose levels
   c. Blood type and cross-match
   d. Rhesus (Rh) blood group determination: RhoGAM if Rh-negative
   e. Urinalysis
   f. Kleihauer-Betke testing: to detect fetal-to-maternal hemorrhage
   g. Vaginal fluid: pH and ferning
   h. Possible diagnostic peritoneal lavage (DPL)
   i. Radiographic imaging as necessary (need to limit fetal exposure)
      1) Abdominal, pelvis, and transvaginal ultrasound
      2) CT of head, chest, and spine as indicated

Collaborative management

1. Continue assessment
   a. ABCDs
   b. Vital signs: blood pressure, pulse, respiratory rate, and temperature
   c. Oxygen saturation
   d. Respiratory effort and excursion
   e. Cardiac rate and rhythm
   f. Pain and discomfort level
   g. Level of consciousness
   h. Clinical indications of bleeding
   i. Fundal height
   j. Doppler FHTs
   k. Close monitoring for progression of symptoms
2. Maintain airway, oxygenation, and ventilation: approach the pregnant trauma patient as you would any other patient
   a. ABCDs with cervical spine immobilization
   b. Oxygen by nasal cannula at 2 to 6 L/min to maintain SaO_2 of 95% unless contraindicated
   c. Intubation and mechanical ventilation may be necessary

3. Maintain adequate circulation and perfusion
   a. IV access: two large-bore, short IV catheters; blood for type and cross-match
   b. Normal saline or lactated Ringer solution by rapid infusion until blood is available; colloids (e.g., albumin, dextran) may also be used
   c. Blood and blood products as indicated
   d. Control of bleeding
   e. Positioning of patient on left lateral by elevating backboard under the right hip to deflect the uterus off of the vena cava
4. Control pain and discomfort: analgesics as indicated
5. Treat infection (if present) and prevent sepsis
   a. Antimicrobials as indicated
   b. Antipyretics and cooling methods to reduce fever
6. Provide comfort
   a. Placement of padding around patient with care not to alter spinal immobilization
   b. Analgesics
7. Monitor fetal status
   a. Contractions
   b. FHTs
   c. Fundal height
8. Prepare patients for procedures (e.g., sterile speculum examination if no vaginal bleeding) as indicated
9. Monitor for complications
   a. Rupture of amniotic membranes can lead to preterm labor, and cord prolapse
   b. Retroperitoneal hemorrhage
   c. Uterine rupture (palpation of fetal part with abdomen assessment)
   d. Amniotic fluid embolism
   e. Placenta abruption
   f. Maternal death
      1) Leading cause of fetal death
      2) Second leading cause of fetal death is unrecognized or poorly managed maternal shock

Evaluation

1. Maternal hemodynamic status stable
   a. Patent airway, adequate oxygenation (i.e., normal PaO_2, SpO_2, and SaO_2) and ventilation (i.e., normal $PaCO_2$)
   b. Absence of clinical indications of respiratory distress
   c. Absence of clinical indicators of hypoperfusion
   d. Absence of clinical indications of infection/sepsis
   e. Alert and oriented with no neurologic deficit
   f. Control of pain and discomfort
   g. Absence of clinical indications of bleeding
   h. Alert and oriented with no neurologic deficit
2. Fetal hemodynamic status stable

Typical disposition

1. If evaluation criteria met (e.g., injuries are minor), discharge with instructions
   a. Instructions to return to ED if any cramping, bleeding, or contractions
2. If evaluation criteria not met: admission

LEARNING ACTIVITIES

1. DIRECTIONS: Complete the following crossword puzzle related to genitourinary, gynecologic, and obstetric emergencies.

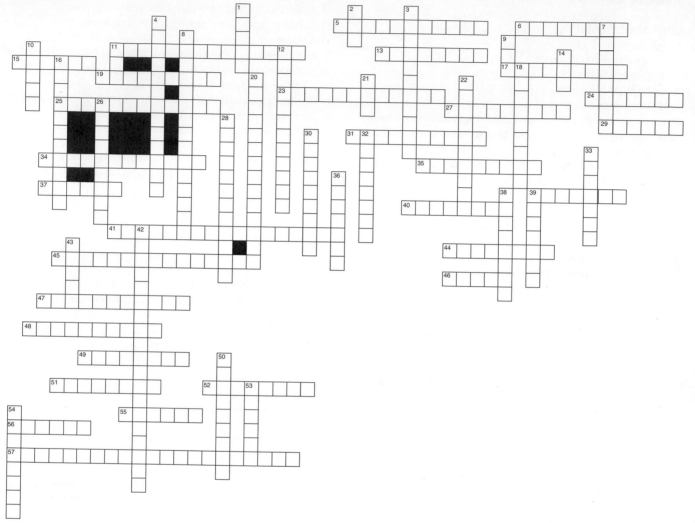

ACROSS

5. Another term for urination
6. Incontinence of urine in bed at night
11. UTI involving the kidney
13. Excessive urination at night
15. The neck of the uterus
17. Blood in the urine
19. These tubes serve as a passage for an ovum to the uterus for fertilization and implantation
23. Low sperm count
24. This area of the kidney contains the collecting ducts

25. Discomfort before and during menses
27. Difficulty starting the flow of urine
29. This organ produces sperm and testosterone
31. This structure stores sperm until it is mature
34. This hormone causes relaxation of GI smooth muscle in pregnancy
35. Inflammation of the glans of the penis
37. A complication of dysfunctional uterine bleeding
39. Another term for stone
40. This type of pain is from internal organs

41. This causes sudden twisting of the spermatic cord (two words)
44. When the foreskin of the penis adheres to the glans and will not retract
45. This is a urinary antisepsis that decreases urinary burning; causes urine to be orange (generic)
46. Epididymitis in the older adult is usually associated with this gram negative bacterium (abbrev)
47. Dysfunctional uterine bleeding
48. Type of abortion when cervical os is closed

49. Decrease in the volume of urine
51. This type of placenta previa is when the edge of the placenta is at the margin of the internal os
52. Prolonged erection in the absence of sexual stimulation
55. This area of the kidney contains the glomerulus
56. Given to Rh-negative mother to prevent the development of antibodies to Rh-negative fetus
57. Intractable vomiting in pregnancy with weight loss and ketosis

DOWN

1. This structure produces ova, estrogen, and progesterone
2. A serious coagulopathy, which may occur in the postpartum period (abbrev)
3. Pregnancy with proteinuria, edema, and hypertension
4. This gland secretes an alkaline component of semen
7. Type of abortion when symptoms signal impending loss of the products of conception
8. This type of medication can cause urinary retention

9. This hormones causes the reabsorption of water in the distal tubule
10. This syndrome is characterized by hemolysis, elevated liver enzymes, and thrombocytopenia
11. Test used to identify prostate cancer but non-specific (abbrev)
12. Inability to control urination
14. Sexually transmitted infection was previously referred to as ___ (abbrev)
16. This allows communication from the epididymis to the ejaculatory duct

18. Seizure in a patient with preeclampsia
20. Test to detect fetal RBCs in the maternal circulation (two words)
21. This benign enlargement of the prostate gland may cause postrenal failure
22. Type of abortion when the cervical os is open 3 cm or greater with rupture of membranes
26. Given in eclampsia to prevent recurrent seizures
28. Unusually heavy menstrual flow
30. Inflammation of the prepuce of the penis
32. Increase in the volume of urine

33. Painful urination
36. Feeling the need to void immediately
38. This structure is erectile and is the female equivalent of the man's penis
39. Given for hypermagnesemia
42. Involuntary loss of fetus prior to viability (two words)
43. This sign helps to differentiate testicular torsion from epididymitis
50. α_1–blocker used for BPH (generic)
53. Absence of urine output (<100 ml/24 hr)
54. Inflammation of the testes is usually caused by mumps

2. DIRECTIONS: List four types of urinary stones.

a.	
b.	
c.	
d.	

3. DIRECTIONS: List five possible causes of pyelonephritis.

a.	
b.	
c.	
d.	
e.	

4. DIRECTIONS: Describe the following signs or assessment findings and what they indicate.

Sign or Assessment Findings	Description	Indicates
Phren sign		
Absent cremasteric reflex		
Grey-Turner sign		
Chancre		
Asterixis		
Oligohydramnios		
Macrosomia		
Kleihauer-Betke		

5. DIRECTIONS: Describe the five types of bladder ruptures.

a.	
b.	
c.	
d.	
e.	

6. DIRECTIONS: Complete the following table for gynecologic causes of pelvic pain.

Cause	Timing and Type	Onset	Location	Nausea, Vomiting	Fever	Contributing and Aggravating Factors	Vaginal Discharge
Degenerating tumor							
Ectopic pregnancy							
Incomplete, threatened, or septic abortion							
Endometriosis							
Mittelschmerz							
Ruptured ovarian cyst							
PID							
PMS							
Primary dysmenorrhea							
Septic pelvis thrombosis							
Torsion of ovary, cyst, or tumor							
Tubal-ovarian abscess							

7. DIRECTIONS: Complete the following chart on types and characteristics of spontaneous abortions.

Type of Abortion	Vaginal Bleeding	Cervical Os Open	Passage of Products of Conception*
Threatened			
Inevitable			
Incomplete			
Complete			
Missed			
Septic			

*May be visible or need to send clots to lab for verification.

8. DIRECTIONS: Match the following.

___ 1. Ketamine (Ketalar)		a. Primarily an endothelial dysfunction
___ 2. Terazosin (Hytrin)		b. Carbohydrate intolerance
___ 3. Bethanechol (Urecholine)		c. Painless dilation of cervix
___ 4. Ruptured ectopic pregnancy		d. Complication of preeclampsia
___ 5. Placental insufficiency		e. Medication used to treat BPH
___ 6. Polyhydramnios		f. Painless, bright red vaginal bleeding occurs after 20th week
___ 7. Incomplete breech		g. Children may present with bed wetting
___ 8. HELLP syndrome		h. Compression of the nerve root
___ 9. PIH		i. Given for urinary retention
___ 10. Placenta previa		j. Foreskin balloons with voiding
___ 11. Amniotic fluid embolism		k. One or both fetal thighs are extended and one or both knees or feet are below the buttocks
___ 12. Kleihauer-Betke		l. "Date rape" drug
___ 13. Incompetent cervix		m. Premature separation of placenta from uterine wall
___ 14. Frank breech		n. Too much amniotic fluid
___ 15. Placenta abruption		o. Used to detect fetal-to-maternal hemorrhage
___ 16. Phimosis		p. Polycythemia
___ 17. Cauda equina syndrome		q. Rare occurrence when the barrier between amniotic fluid and maternal circulation is broken
___ 18. Gestational diabetes		r. Both fetal thighs are flexed and both lower extremities are extended at the knees
___ 19. Hyperviscosity		s. Causes fetal hypoxia and malnutrition
___ 20. Pyelonephritis		t. Distended, doughy-feeling abdomen

LEARNING ACTIVITIES ANSWERS

1.

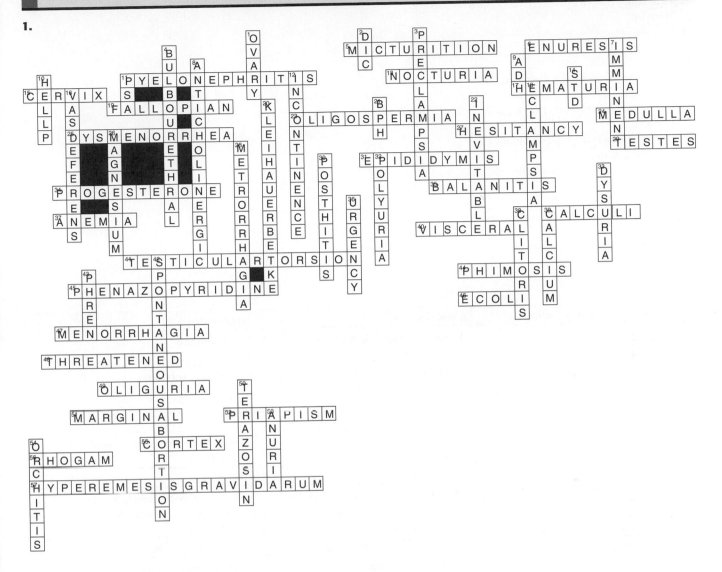

2.

a. Calcium
b. Uric acid
c. Struvite
d. Cystine

3.

a. Underlying urinary tract abnormalities
b. Recurrent UTIs
c. Sexual intercourse
d. Diabetic
e. Congenital urinary tract anomalies
f. Catheterization
g. Pregnancy, especially if bacteriuria
h. Spermicidal use
i. Stress incontinence
j. Multiple sclerosis (bladder not contracting)
k. Immunosuppression
l. Urinary or ureteral obstruction
m. Prostatic enlargement

4.

Sign or Assessment Findings	Description	Indicates
Phren sign	Elevation of testicle leading to intense pain	Epididymitis
Absent cremasteric reflex	Stroking or pinching of medial thigh causes the cremasteric muscle to contract causing the testicle to rise	Testicular torsion
Grey-Turner sign	Ecchymosis over the flank	Indicative of retroperitoneal bleeding
Chancre	Painless ulcer or lesion	Syphilis
Asterixis	Hand flapping tremors induced by extending the arm and dorsiflexing the wrist	Seen in hepatic failure with increased ammonia levels
Oligohydramnios	Deficiency of amniotic fluid level	PIH fetal complication
Macrosomia	Large for gestation age	Gestational diabetes fetal complication
Kleihauer-Betke	Testing done to detect fetal-to-maternal hemorrhage	Trauma in pregnancy

5.

Type I is a bladder contusion—most common bladder injury that occurs from incomplete tear of bladder mucosa
Type II is a intraperitoneal rupture—results from trauma to lower abdomen when bladder is distended
Type III is an interstitial injury—rare—caused by a tear of the intact serosa surface
Type IV is extraperitoneal—almost always associated with pelvic fractures
Type V is combined extraperitoneal and intraperitoneal rupture

6.

Cause	Timing and Type	Onset	Location	Nausea, Vomiting	Fever	Contributing and Aggravating Factors	Vaginal discharge
Degenerating tumor	Constant and full or sudden sharp	Slow	Generalized and/or midline	No	No	*Fibroids, pelvic congestion *Stress, menses	No
Ectopic pregnancy	Constant and sharp	Rapid	Pelvis	Maybe	No	*PID; infertility; IUD, previous pelvic problems; advanced maternal age *Activity and movement	No, but may have slight bleeding
Incomplete, threatened, or septic abortion	Constant and cramping or sharp	Rapid	General pelvic area	No	Maybe	*Previous abortion *Activity and movement	Possibly
Endometriosis	Constant during menses and sharp	Week before menses	Bilateral posterior pelvis	No	Yes	*Delay in child-bearing or no child-bearing; congenital *Adhesions; coitus, bowel movements	Bleeding
Mittelschmerz	Mid-menses cycle and sharp	Rapid	Generalized and/or midline	No	No	Ruptured graafian follicle	No
Ruptured ovarian cyst	Constant and sharp	Rapid	Pelvis	No	No	*Common occurrence during coitus *Activity and movement	No
PID	Constant and sharp	Rapid	Bilateral pelvis	Nausea	Yes	*STIs; multiple partners; previous PID *Coitus; menses; activity and movement	Yes
Premenstrual syndrome (PMS)	Premenstrual and cramping	Rapid	Generalized and/or midline	Nausea	No	*History of PMS	No
Primary dysmenorrhea	Onset of menses and cramping	Rapid	Generalized	No	No	*History of primary dysmenorrhea *Activity and movement	No
Septic pelvis thrombosis	Constant throbbing and sharp	Rapid	Pelvis	No	Yes	*Pregnancy or postpartum *Position	No
Torsion of ovary, cyst, or tumor	Constant and sharp	Rapid	Unilateral or bilateral pelvis	Nausea and vomiting	Maybe	*Cyst; fibroids *Activity, movement, and position	No
Tubal-ovarian abscess	Constant and sharp	Rapid	Unilateral or bilateral pelvis	Nausea	Yes	*History of PID or gonorrhea *Activity and movement	Purulent

7.

Type of Abortion	Vaginal Bleeding	Cervical Os Open	Passage of Products of Conception**
Threatened	Yes	No	No
Inevitable	Yes	Yes	No
Incomplete	Yes	Yes	Yes
Complete	Yes	Yes or no	Yes
Missed	No	No	No
Septic	Yes	No	Maybe

8.

l. 1. Ketamine (Ketalar)	a. Primarily an endothelial dysfunction
e. 2. Terazosin (Hytrin)	b. Carbohydrate intolerance
i. 3. Bethanechol (Urecholine)	c. Painless dilation of cervix
t. 4. Rupture ectopic pregnancy	d. Complication of preeclampsia
s. 5. Placenta insufficiency	e. Medication used to treat BPH
n. 6. Polyhydramnios	f. Painless bright red vaginal bleeding occurs after 20th week
k. 7. Incomplete breech	g. Children may present with bed wetting
d. 8. HELLP syndrome	h. Compression of the nerve root
a. 9. PIH	i. Given for urinary retention
f. 10. Placenta previa	j. Foreskin balloons with voiding
q. 11. Amniotic fluid embolism	k. One or both fetal thighs are extended and one or both knees or feet are below the buttocks
o. 12. Kleihauer-Betke	l. "Date rape" drug
c. 13. Incompetent cervix	m. Premature separation of placenta from uterine wall
r. 14. Frank breech	n. Too much amniotic fluid
m. 15. Placenta abruption	o. Used to detect fetal-to-maternal hemorrhage
j. 16. Phimosis	p. Polycythemia
h. 17. Cauda equina syndrome	q. Rare occurrence when the barrier between amniotic fluid and maternal circulation is broken
b. 18. Gestational diabetes	r. Both fetal thighs are flexed and both lower extremities are extended at the knees
p. 19. Hyperviscosity	s. Causes fetal hypoxia and malnutrition
g. 20. Pyelonephritis	t. Distended doughy-feeling abdomen

References and Suggested Readings

Behrman, J., & Shoff, W. (2008). Gonorrhea. Retrieved November 30, 2008, from http://www.emedicine.com/EMERG/topic220.htm.

Bissinger, R. L., & Ohning, L. (2006, August). Neonatal resuscitation. Retrieved November 21, 2008, from http://www.emedicine.com/ped/topic2598.htm.

Buttaro, T. M., Trybulski, J., Bailey, P. P., & Sandberg-Cook, J. (2003). *Primary care: A collaborative practice.* St. Louis: Mosby.

Cantu, S. (2006, April). Phimosis and Paraphimosis. Retrieved November 18, 2008, from http://www.emedicine.com/emerg/topic423.htm.

Centers for Disease Control and Prevention Website. (2007). Chlamydia: CDC fact sheet. Retrieved January 15, 2008, from http://www.cdc.gov/std/chlamydia/STDFact-Chlamydia.htm.

Centers for Disease Control and Prevention Website. (2008). Genital herpes: CDC fact sheet. Retrieved January 15, 2008, from http://www.cdc.gov/std/Herpes/STDFact-Herpes.htm.

Centers for Disease Control and Prevention Website. (2008). HPV: CDC fact sheet. Retrieved January 15, 2008, from http://www.cdc.gov/std/HPV/STDFact-HPV.htm.

Centers for Disease Control and Prevention Website. (2008). Syphilis: CDC fact sheet. Retrieved January 15, 2008, from http://www.cdc.gov/std/syphilis/STDFact-Syphilis.htm#symptoms.

Chang, K. (2006). Pregnancy, trauma. Retrieved December 6, 2008, from http://www.emedicine.com/emerg/TOPIC484.HTM.

Chmielewski, N., & Gregg, M. (2008). A 25-year-old woman with a headache 4 days postpartum. *Journal of Emergency Nursing, 34(1),* 41–43.

Clark, Y., Stocking, J., & Johnson, J. (Eds.). (2006). *Flight and ground transport nursing core curriculum* (2nd ed.). Denver, CO: Air and Surface Transport Nurses Association.

Covington, D., & Rickabaugh, B. (2006). Caring for the patient with a spontaneous abortion. *Journal of Emergency Nursing, 32(6),* 513-515.

Crossman, S. (2006). The challenges of pelvic inflammatory disease. *American Family Physicians, 73(5),* 859.

Cummings, J. M., & Bouiller, J. (2006, July). Urethral injury. Retrieved November 24, 2008, from http://www.emedicine.com/med/topic3082.htm.

Dennison, R. (2007). *Pass CCRN!* (3rd ed.). St. Louis: Mosby.

Domino, J. (2008). *The 5-minute clinical consultant* (16th ed.). Philadelphia: Lippincott Williams and Wilkins.

Douglass, M. (2007). Emergency contraception. *Journal of Emergency Nursing, 33(2),* 140-142.

DynaMed Editorial Team. Pelvic inflammatory disease. Last updated October 5, 2008. Retrieved November 17, 2008, from http://www.ebscohost.com/dynamed.http://www.ebscohost.com/dynamed.

Emergency Nurses Association. (2007). *Emergency nursing core curriculum* (6th ed). Philadelphia: Saunders.

Emergency Nurses Association. (2005). *Sheehy's manual of emergency care* (6th ed). St Louis: Mosby.

Ernoehazy, W., & Murphy-Lavoie, H. (2008). Sexual assault. Retrieved November 30, 2008, from http://www.emedicine.com/emerg/TOPIC527.HTM.

Frumovitz, M. M., & Ascher-Walsh, J. (2006, August). Fitz-Hugh-Curtis syndrome. Retrieved November 23, 2008, from http://www.emedicine.com/med/topic797.htm.

Fultz, J., & Sturt, P. (2005). *Mosby's emergency nursing reference* (3rd ed.). St. Louis: Mosby.

Gibson, P., & Carson, M. P. (2007). Hypertension and pregnancy. Retrieved December 4, 2008, from http://www.emedicine.com/MED/topic3250.htm.

Gowda, A., & Nzerue, M. (2008, September). Pyelonephritis, chronic. eMedicine. Retrieved November 21, 2008, from http://www.emedicine.com/med/topic2841.htm.

Howe, S., & Pillow, M. T. (2009, April). Urinary tract infection: Male. Retrieved August 24, 2009, from http://emedicine.medscape.com/article/778578-overview.

Jarvis, C. (2008). *Physical examination and health assessment* (5th ed.). St. Louis: Saunders.

Jenis, A. (2006). Pregnancy, breech delivery. Retrieved December 1, 2008, from http://www.emedicine.com/emerg/TOPIC868.HTM.

Lab Test Online. (2008). Inside the lab. Retrieved August 31, 2008, from http://www.labtestsonline.org/index.html.

Leman, P. (2002, June). Validity of urinalysis and microscopy for detecting urinary tract infection in the emergency department. *European Journal of Emergency Medicine, 9(2):* 141-147.

Lindsey, J. L., & Rivera, V. R. (2008). Missed abortion. Retrieved December 3, 2008, from http://www.emedicine.com/med/topic3309.htm.

Marx, J. (2002). *Rosen's emergency medicine: Concepts and clinical practice* (5th ed.). St. Louis: Mosby.

Mason, D. (2010). Obstetric emergencies. In P. K. Howard and R. Steinmann (Eds.), *Sheehy's emergency nursing. Principles and practice* (6th ed., pp. 619-629). St. Louis: Mosby Elsevier.

Mayo Clinic Website. (2008). Diseases and conditions. Retrieved November 30, 2008, from http://www.mayoclinic.com/health/DiseasesIndex/DiseasesIndex.

Mbibu, N., Maitama, Y., Ameh, , Khalid, L. M., & Adams, L. M. (2004). Acute scrotum in Nigeria: An 18-year review. *Tropical Doctor, 34(1),* 34-36.

Mehta, A., & Silverberg, M. A. (2007). Chancroid. Retrieved November 30, 2008, from http://www.emedicine.com/emerg/TOPIC95.HTM.

Merck Source. (2002-2008). Retrieved November 17, 2008, from http://www.mercksource.com/pp/us/cns/cns_home.jsp.

Merriam-Webster Online. (2007-2008). Merriam-Webster's medical dictionary. http://medical.merriam-webster.com.

Moore, L. (2008). Amniotic fluid embolism. Retrieved December 5, 2008, from http://www.emedicine.com/Med/topic122.htm.

Mudgil, S., & Cohen, L. (2007, August). Pelvic inflammatory disease/tubo-ovarian abscess. Retrieved November 27, 2008, from http://www.emedicine.com/radio/topic543.htm.

Mycyk, M. (2007). Orchitis. Retrieved December 1, 2008, from http://www.emedicine.com/emerg/topic344.htm.

National Institute of Justice. (2008). Retrieved November 27, 2008, from http://www.ojp.usdoj.gov/nij/topics/crime/rape-sexual-violence/campus/increased-risk.htm.

Newton, R. (2006). Trauma and pregnancy. Retrieved December 6, 2008, from http://www.emedicine.com/med/topic3268.htm.

Owens, M. K., & Clenney, T. L. (2004). Management of vaginitis. Retrieved November 30, 2008, from http://www.aafp.org/afp/20041201/2125.html.

Platter, L., & Vaccaro, J. P. (2008, August). Bladder, trauma. Retrieved November 30, 2008, from http://www.emedicine.com/Radio/topic81.htm.

Prahlow, J., & Barnard, J. J. (2004, September). Pregnancy-related maternal deaths. *American Journal of Forensic Medicine and Pathology. 25(3),* 220-236.

Price, S., & Wilson, L. M. (2003). *Pathophysiology: Clinical concepts of disease process* (6th ed.). St. Louis: Mosby.

Proehl, J. (2004). *Emergency nursing procedures* (3rd ed.). St. Louis: Saunders.

Rackley, R., Vasavada, S. P., Firoozi, F., & Ingber, M. S. (2009, May). Neurogenic bladder. Retrieved August 25, 2009, from http://emedicine.medscape.com/article/453539-overview.

Roppolo, L. P., Davis, D., Kelly, S. P., & Rosen, P. (2007). *Emergency medicine handbook: Critical concepts for clinical practice.* St. Louis: Mosby.

Rudkin, S., & Kazzi, A. A. (2008, September) Hydrocele. Retrieved November 23, 2008, from http://www.emedicine.com/emerg/topic256.htm.

Rupp, T. J., & Zwanger, M. (2008, November). Testicular torsion. Retrieved August 10, 2009, from http://cmedicine.medscape.com/article/778086-overview.

Savaris, R., Teixeira, L. M., Torres, T., Edelweiss, M., Moncada. J., & Schachter, J. (2007). Comparing ceftriaxone plus azithromycin or doxycycline for pelvic inflammatory disease: a randomized controlled trial. *Obstetrics and Gynecology, 110(1):* 53-60.

Schecter, J., & Hipp, A. (2008). Bartholin gland diseases. Retrieved December 4, 2008, from http://www.emedicine.com/emerg/topic54.htm.

Smith, J. R. (2006). Postpartum hemorrhage. Retrieved November 20, 2008, from http://www.emedicine.com/Med/topic3568.htm.

Shoff, W., Green-McKenzie, J., Behrman, J., & Moore-Shepherd, S. (2007). Pyelonephritis, acute. Retrieved November 25, 2008, from http://www.emedicine.com/Med/topic2843.htm.

Solheim, J. (2006). A 44-year-old pregnant patient who had and needed HELLP. *Journal of Emergency Nursing, 32(5),* 412-414.

St. Sauver, J. L., Jacobson, J., McGree, M., Lieber, M. M., & Jacobsen, S. J. (2006, October). Protective association between nonsteroidal anti-inflammatory drug use and measures of benign prostatic hyperplasia. *American Journal of Epidemiology, 164(8):* 760-768.

Terris, M. K. (2008). The significance of abnormal urine color. Retrieved November 17, 2008, from http://urology.stanford.edu/about/articles/abnormal_urine.html.

Turok, K., Ratcliffe, S., & Baxley, (2003). Management of gestational diabetes. *American Family Physicians.* Retrieved November 18, 2008, from http://www.aafp.org/afp/20031101/1767.html.

Valley, V.T., Jackson-Williams, L., & Fly, C.A. (2006). Abortion, inevitable. Retrieved November 30, 2008, from http://www.emedicine.com/emerg/topic6.htm.

Wharton, P., Chaudhry, A. H., & French, M. (2006, Feb 25). A case of mumps epididymitis. *Lancet, 367(9511)*, 702.

You, W., & Zahn, M. (2006, March). Postpartum hemorrhage: Abnormally adherent placenta, uterine inversion, and puerperal hematomas. *Clinical Obstetrics and Gynecology. 49(1)*, 184–197.

Valentini, R. P. (2006). Goodpasture's syndrome. Retrieved December 5, 2008, from http://www.emedicine.com/PED/topic888.htm.

Zimmerman, P., & Herr, R. (2006). *Triage nursing secrets.* St. Louis: Mosby.

CHAPTER 10

Maxillofacial and Ocular Emergencies

Introduction

This content constitutes 4% (6 items) of the CEN examination

The focus is on maxillary, facial, dental, and ocular injuries that are commonly encountered in an ED setting

The continuum of age needs to be considered from infancy through older adulthood

Age-Related Considerations

Neonates, infants, and children

1. Airway compromise may occur rapidly in infants and small children as a result of immature and less rigid airway structures
   a. Small amounts of edema and secretions can rapidly occlude the airway
   b. The tongue is the most common cause of airway obstruction in small children and infants
2. Infants are obligate nose breathers
   a. Any swelling or blocking of the nares can cause respiratory distress
3. Retractions may be common in some infants (especially those born prematurely), but they can also indicate respiratory distress
   a. Supraclavicular retractions indicate labored effort
4. Foreign body objects in the nose, ear, and mouth occur most often in children, especially if they are <3 years old
   a. These objects can cause airway compromise and respiratory distress and should be suspected if there is a sudden onset of any of following:
      1) Wheezing or stridor
      2) Drooling
      3) Vomiting
      4) Decreasing level of consciousness
5. Infants who present with difficulty feeding and irritability may have dental or ear, nose, and throat problems
6. Pediatric dental abnormalities have been linked to maternal tetracycline use during pregnancy (Fultz & Sturt, 2005)
7. Falls are a common cause of facial injuries in children
   a. Midface fractures are uncommon in children and infants; their occurrence represents significant force and probably intracranial trauma
8. Eye injuries in children and infants are related to shaking or direct trauma

9. Viral and bacterial conjunctivitis can occur at any age but is more common among children
10. It is hard to detect vision loss in infants and very young children; visual impairment may go unnoticed for a period of time
    a. May be more noted when the child is old enough that a head tilt is noticeable, which is how children compensate for double vision
11. Unexplained crying in an infant could be the result of a corneal abrasion (Emergency Nurses Association [ENA], 2007)
12. Neonates delivered vaginally can contract sexually transmitted infections as they come through the birth canal

Older adults

1. Falls are the most common cause of head and facial injuries among older adults
   a. Senses such as vision and hearing decrease with aging, which makes older adults more prone to falls and accidents
      1) The eyes do not accommodate or adjust to distance as well as aging occurs
      2) Eye problems (e.g., cataracts, glaucoma, detached retina) increase with aging
   b. Decreased mobility and flexibility
2. Facial bleeding is more profuse with aging
3. Posterior epistaxis is more common with aging
4. Ludwig angina is rare but more common among older immunocompromised patients
5. Ocular injuries and disorders are more common among geriatric patients
6. Eye dryness is common and related to a decrease in lacrimal secretions that occurs with aging
7. There is an increased pain threshold among older patients (McCleane, 2007)

Selected Concepts in Anatomy and Physiology

Functions of facial bones

1. Protect the brain
2. House and protect the sense organs of smell, sight, and taste
3. Provide a frame for soft tissues of the face, which facilitate eating, facial expression, breathing, and speech

Primary bones of the face

1. Mandible
   a. Structure
      1) U-shaped facial bone
      2) Only mobile bone of the facial skeleton
      3) Formed by intramembranous ossification
      4) Composed of two hemimandibles that are joined at the midline by a vertical symphysis
         a) The hemimandibles fuse to form a single bone by the age of 2 years
         b) Each hemimandible is composed of a horizontal body with a posterior vertical extension called the *ramus*
   b. Houses the lower teeth
   c. Essential for mastication
2. Maxilla: two maxillary bones joined at the midline to form the middle third of the face
   a. Houses the teeth
   b. Forms the roof of the oral cavity
   c. Forms the floor of and contributes to the lateral wall and roof of the nasal cavity
   d. Houses the maxillary sinus
   e. Contributes to the inferior rim and floor of the orbit
3. Frontal bone
   a. Forms the anterior portion of the cranium
   b. Houses the frontal sinuses
   c. Forms the roof of the ethmoid sinuses, the nose, and the orbit
4. Nasal bones
   a. The nasal bones are paired and approximately quadrangular to form the anterosuperior bony roof of the nasal cavity
   b. Articulate with the nasal process of the frontal bone superiorly, the frontal process of the maxillary bone laterally, and with one another medially
   c. The inferior border forms the superior margin of the piriform aperture
   d. The external surface is convex except for the most superior portion, where a concavity forms as the margin turns superiorly to articulate with the frontal bone
   e. The external nasal artery is located in a vertical groove on the internal surface
5. Zygoma
   a. Forms the lateral portion of the inferior and lateral orbital rim and the lateral wall of the orbit
   b. Forms the anterior zygomatic arch
   c. The masseter muscle, which functions to close the mandible for mastication and speech, is suspended from the anterior zygomatic arch
   d. The zygomatic bone has three lateral processes
      1) Inferior: a concave process that projects medially to articulate with the zygomatic process of the maxilla and that forms the lateral portion of the infraorbital rim
         a) The concave process projects superiorly to form the frontal process, which articulates with the frontal bone
      2) Posterior: a temporal process that articulates with the zygomatic process of the temporal bone to form the zygomatic arch
      3) Medial: a smooth orbital plate that forms the lateral floor and lateral wall of the orbit
         a) Articulates posteriorly with the greater wing of the sphenoid bone

Ear

1. Organ used for hearing
2. The ear has three parts: external, middle, and inner (Figure 10-1)
   a. The external or outer ear consists of the following:
      1) Pinna (i.e., auricle): outside part of the ear
      2) External auditory canal: connects the outer ear to the middle ear
   b. Tympanic membrane (i.e., eardrum): divides the external and middle ear
   c. The middle ear (i.e., tympanic cavity): consists of ossicles, which are small bones that are connected together to transmit sound waves to the inner ear:
      1) Malleus (i.e., hammer)

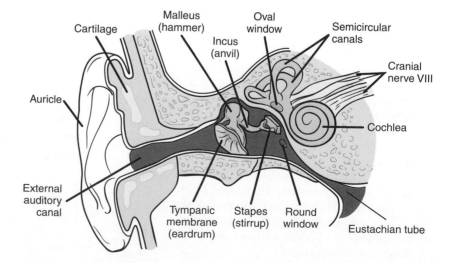
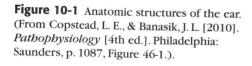

Figure 10-1 Anatomic structures of the ear. (From Copstead, L. E., & Banasik, J. L. [2010]. *Pathophysiology* [4th ed.]. Philadelphia: Saunders, p. 1087, Figure 46-1.).

2) Incus
3) Stapes
  d. Eustachian tube: a canal that links the middle ear with the throat area, which helps to equalize the pressure between the outer ear and the middle ear
  e. The inner ear consists of the following:
    1) Cochlea: contains the nerves for hearing
    2) Vestibule: contains receptors for balance
    3) Semicircular canals: contain receptors for balance

Nose
1. Organ responsible for smell
2. The internal part of the nose lies above the roof of the mouth
3. The nose has several parts:
  a. External meatus: a triangular-shaped projection in the center of the face
  b. External nostrils: two chambers divided by the septum
  c. Septum
    1) Made primarily of cartilage and bone and covered by mucous membranes
    2) Gives shape and support to the outer part of the nose
  d. Nasal passages: lined with mucous membranes and tiny hairs (i.e., cilia) that help to filter air
  e. Turbinates: shelf-like structures on the inside of each nostril that provide moisture, warmth, airflow for breathing, and natural defenses against infection
  f. Sinuses: four pairs of air-filled cavities that are lined with mucous membranes
    1) The ethmoid sinus is located inside the face around the area of the bridge of the nose; it is present at birth

2) The maxillary sinus is located inside the face around the area of the cheeks; it is present at birth
3) The frontal sinus is inside the face in the area of the forehead; it develops at the age of ≈7 years
4) The sphenoid sinus is located deep in the face behind the nose; it develops during adolescence

Pharynx (i.e., throat)
1. A ring-like muscular tube that helps with the formation of speech and that acts as the passageway for air, food, and liquid
2. The pharynx consists of the larynx, the epiglottis, the tonsils, and the adenoids
  a. Larynx (i.e., voice box)
    1) A cylindric grouping of cartilage, muscles, and soft tissue that contains the vocal cords
    2) The upper opening into the trachea
  b. Epiglottis
    1) A flap of soft tissue located just above the vocal cords
    2) Folds down over the vocal cords to prevent food and irritants from entering the lungs
  c. Tonsils and adenoids
    1) Lymph tissue located at the back and sides of the mouth
    2) Protect against infection

Ocular structures
1. The eye is a slightly asymmetric sphere (Figure 10-2)
  a. Size
    1) At birth, the eye is ≈18 mm horizontally and ≈17 mm vertically; the anteroposterior diameter is ≈16.5 mm

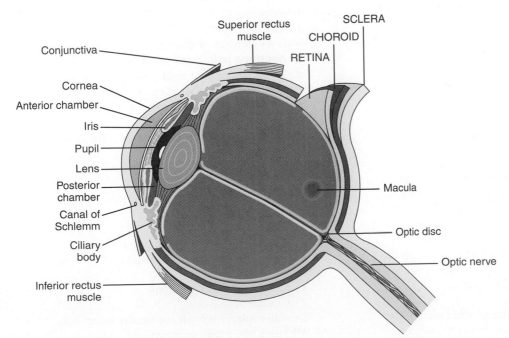

Figure 10-2 Anatomic structures of the eye. (From Copstead, L. E., & Banasik, J. L. [2010]. *Pathophysiology* [4th ed.]. Philadelphia: Saunders, p. 1094, Figure 46-4.).

2) It reaches adult dimensions by ≈13 years; the average adult eye is ≈25 mm horizontally and ≈23 mm vertically, with an anteroposterior diameter of ≈21 to 26 mm (Toris et al., 1999)

2. Pupil: the black opening in the center of the iris that allows light to enter the eye

3. Iris: the colored circular muscle that controls pupil size to allow more or less light into the eye, depending on environmental conditions

4. Cornea: the transparent covering of the iris and the pupil
   a. Provides protection of the iris and pupil
   b. Acts as the first and most powerful lens of the optic system
   c. Works in conjunction with the crystalline lens

5. Sclera: the white supporting structure of the eye

6. Lens: transparent biconvex structure
   a. Works with the cornea to refract light and focus it on the retina
   b. It can change shape to adjust for distance, thereby allowing it to focus on objects at various distances

7. Ciliary body
   a. Responsible for accommodation, aqueous humor production, and the production and maintenance of the lens zonules
   b. Receives parasympathetic innervation from the oculomotor nerve

8. Aqueous humor
   a. Responsible for providing most of the nutrients for the lens and the cornea
   b. Involved in waste management for these areas

9. Conjunctiva: clear membrane that covers the sclera and the inside of the eyelid
   a. Helps to lubricate the eye
   b. Prevents the entry of microbes

10. Uvea: vascular layer that provides nourishment for the eye

11. Vitreous humor
    a. Clear, gelatin-like substance located between the lens of the eye and the retina; thins with aging
    b. Light rays carrying images to the brain must pass through this clear gel on the way to the retina

12. Retina
    a. The layer of tissue that lines the inside of the back of the eye and that transmits information carried by light rays to the brain via the optic nerve
    b. A partial or complete loss of vision can occur with disease or injury that clouds the vitreous humor or that damages the retina

13. Optic nerve: the cranial nerve (II) responsible for vision

14. Choroid: the vascular layer of the eye between the retina and the sclera that provides oxygen and nourishment to the outer layer of the retina

15. Fovea centralis
    a. Located in the center of the macula area of the retina
    b. Responsible for sharp central vision when performing activities that require attention to detail

16. Zonules of Zinn
    a. Ring of fibrous strands that connect the ciliary body to the crystalline lens

Cranial nerves (Table 10-1; Figure 10-3)

Physical Assessment

Primary and secondary assessment (see Chapter 2)
Focused assessment

1. Chief complaint: identifies why the patient is seeking help and the duration of the problem
2. Possible subjective/objective findings
   a. Airway compromise
   b. Breathing difficulties
   c. Bleeding or hemorrhage
   d. Dyspnea
   e. Deformity, asymmetry, or dislocation
   f. Facial, dental, or ocular pain
   g. Eye discharge
   h. Diplopia or photophobia
   i. Change in visual acuity, clarity, or fields
   j. Nasal discharge
   k. Dysphonia
   l. Dysphagia
   m. Drooling
   n. Headache
   o. Foreign body in eye, nose, mouth, or pharynx
   p. Trismus (i.e., the inability to open the mouth completely)
   q. Misalignment of the teeth
3. History of present illness
   a. Mechanism of injury or illness
   b. Provocation and palliation
   c. Quality and quantity
   d. Region and radiation
   e. Severity
   f. Timing
   g. Sensory deficits or changes
      1) Auditory: pain, tinnitus, or hearing loss
      2) Visual: decreased light perception, visual deficits, or decreased extraocular movement
      3) Tactile: changes in sensation, numbness, tingling, or pain
      4) Gustatory: changes in taste of salty, sweet, bitter, or sour
4. Medical history
   a. Past illnesses and injuries
      1) Diabetes
      2) Hematologic conditions
      3) Neurologic conditions
      4) Immunosuppressive illnesses
      5) Maxillofacial or ocular trauma
   b. Past surgical procedures
      1) Dental or otolaryngologic
      2) Ocular
   c. Dental, otolaryngologic, or ocular infections
   d. Allergies and types of reactions

TABLE **10-1**   The Cranial Nerves

Number	Name	Memory Jogger: Name	Functions
I	Olfactory	On	Sensory • Smell
II	Optic	Old	Sensory • Vision
III	Oculomotor	Olympus'	Motor • Upward lateral eye movement (Figure 10-2) • Pupillary constriction • Eyelid elevation
IV	Trochlear	Towering	Motor • Downward medial eye movement (Figure 10-2)
V	Trigeminal	Tops	Sensory • Sensation of scalp and face • Sensation of cornea of eye Motor • Temporal and masseter muscles
VI	Abducens	A	Motor • Lateral eye movement (Figure 10-2)
VII	Facial	Fin	Sensory • Taste on anterior two thirds of tongue Motor • Muscles of facial expression • Eyelid closure • Lacrimal and salivary glands
VIII	Acoustic	And	Sensory • Hearing • Equilibrium and balance
IX	Glossopharyngeal	German	Sensory • Taste on posterior third of tongue • Pharynx Motor • Parotid gland
X	Vagus	Viewed	Sensory • Pharynx, larynx, and neck Motor • Palate, larynx, and pharynx • Swallowing • Cardiac muscle • Secretory glands of pancreas and gastrointestinal tract
XI	Spinal accessory	Some	Motor • Shoulder and neck movement • Sternocleidomastoid and trapezius muscles
XII	Hypoglossal	Hops	Motor • Tongue

From Dennison, R. D. (2007). *Pass CCRN!* (3rd ed.). St. Louis: Mosby.

e. Past diagnostic studies (e.g., radiologic and computed tomography [CT])

5. Social history
   a. Poor nutrition
   b. Poor dental care and health maintenance
   c. Risk-taking behaviors
   d. Trauma from abuse or altercation
   e. Occupational hazards
   f. Hobbies, sports, and recreational activities
   g. Corrective lenses: contact lenses or glasses
   h. Swimming: may increase risk for ocular and ear infections

6. Medication history
   a. Prescribed drug, dose, frequency, and time of last dose
   b. Nonprescribed drugs
      1) Over-the-counter drugs, including herbal supplements

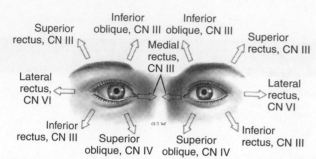

Figure 10-3 The six cardinal positions of gaze and the cranial nerves that control eye movement. CN, Cranial nerve. (From Dennison, R. [2007]. *Pass CCRN!* [3rd ed.]. St. Louis: Mosby, p. 472, Figure 7-25.).

2) Substance abuse (e.g., cocaine, amphetamines, ethanol)
c. Allergies
d. Immunization status
e. Patient's understanding of drug actions and side effects
f. Tobacco abuse

General survey
1. Airway problems
2. Apparent health status
3. Level of consciousness
4. Hygiene or odors
5. Discomfort or distress

Inspection
1. Bleeding or open wounds
2. Foreign bodies
3. Angulations and symmetry
4. Deformities and fractures
5. Ecchymosis
6. Herpetiform vesicular eruption (i.e., herpes)
7. Dental: teeth and gingiva
   a. Dental caries
   b. Missing teeth
   c. Gingivitis
8. Ear
   a. External and internal structures
   b. Otoscopic examination
      1) Tympanic membrane: pearly gray
      2) Cone of light at 5 o'clock position
      3) Mobility: assessed with pneumatic otoscope
9. Nose
   a. Patency of each nostril
   b. Nasal mucosa: color and presence of lesions
10. Mouth and pharynx
    a. Lips and buccal mucosa
    b. Dorsum, sides, and undersurface of tongue
    c. Floor of mouth, salivary glands, salivary duct openings, and hard palate
    d. Anterior and posterior pillars, tonsils, and uvula

11. Neck
    a. Range of motion
    b. Jugular veins
    c. Tracheal position
12. Ocular
    a. Vision: visual acuity and visual fields
    b. Tearing and discharge
    c. Eyelid swelling
    d. Conjunctiva, sclera, and lid: color or inflammation
    e. Cornea: color or inflammation
    f. Pupils: size, equality, shape, reactivity, and accommodation
    g. Extraocular movement: intact, limited, or discomfort with movement
13. Balance and gait: instability
14. Drainage from ears and nose for blood and cerebrospinal fluid
    a. Otorrhea: any drainage from the ears
    b. Rhinorrhea: any drainage from the nose
    c. Blood and cerebrospinal fluid (CSF) can mix together, thus making it difficult to assess for cerebrospinal fluid
       1) Halo sign: take a drop of drainage and place it on filter paper or a white sheet; blood will stay in the center of the drop, and cerebrospinal fluid will separate to the outside to demonstrate what is known as the "halo sign"
       2) Glucose: CSF will test positive for glucose

Palpation
1. Face and neck for swelling, deformities, tenderness, and crepitus
2. Paranasal sinuses: maxillary, frontal, and ethmoid for tenderness
3. Lymph nodes: enlargement or tenderness
4. Temporomandibular joint: crepitus or tenderness

Cranial nerves (Table 10-1; Figure 10-3)
Vital signs: include the assessment of blood pressure and heart rate with the patient in both lying and sitting positions if hemorrhage is noted or suspected
Diagnostic studies
1. Laboratory
   a. ABGs: if actual or suspected airway compromise
   b. CBC
      1) Decreased hemoglobin and hematocrit levels occur with bleeding
      2) Leukocytosis can occur with infection
   c. ESR elevates with infection
   d. C-reactive protein level elevates with infection and inflammation
   e. Blood typing and cross matching if hemorrhage noted or suspected
   f. Coagulation profile if hemorrhage noted or suspected
   g. Cultures if infection suspected

2. Imaging
   a. Upper face
      1) CT
      2) Skull series
      3) Water's view radiograph: frontal view of the maxillary sinus, orbits, nasal structures, and zygoma with direct comparison of the sides
   b. Middle face
      1) CT
      2) Water's view radiograph
   c. Lower face
      1) Panographic radiograph: panoramic view of the mouth
         a) Position of wisdom teeth, jaw, and joint problems
         b) Receding bone levels indicate periodontal disease
         c) Abscesses
         d) Sinus problems
      2) Right and left lateral oblique views of the mandible
      3) Elongated Towne projection radiograph
   d. CT of the condyle is indicated if fracture is suspected and accompanying radiographic findings are negative
   e. Chest radiograph: to rule out foreign bodies and concurrent injuries
   f. Cervical spine and odontoid views: for suspected neck injuries
3. Visual
   a. Visual acuity
      1) Snellen chart: tested at 20 feet
      2) Rosenbaum card: handheld card for measuring visual acuity that is held 14 inches away from the patient's face
      3) If vision is <20/400, test with a finger count at 4 feet away from patient
      4) Peripheral vision testing using confrontation
   b. Contact lenses should be removed before examination
      1) If patient is unable to remove the lenses, gently remove them manually or with a suction cup
      2) Do not instill topical anesthetics until contact lenses are removed
   c. Fluorescein examination: fluorescein dye is applied to the inside lower eyelid to visualize the cornea with a Wood lamp
      1) Removal of contact lenses required before examination
      2) Vitreous humor leakage present with a positive Seidel sign, which is a sickle-shaped scotoma appearing as an upward or downward extension of the blind spot when fluorescence is applied to the eye (ENA, 2007)
   d. Refraction test: measures the ability to see specific objects at a distance

e. Pupillary dilation: dilates pupil to allow for the examination of the retina
f. Slit-lamp examination: provides a stereoscopic magnified view of the eye structures in detail
g. Tonometry: measures intraocular pressure
h. Ocular sonography: provides imaging of the eye and the intraocular structures

System-Specific Tasks

Eye irrigation
1. Eyewash fountain
   a. Method
      1) Have the patient place his or her face in the middle of two streams of sterile saline to flush the eyes and eyelids
      2) Ask the patient to blink eyes continuously in the stream and to move the eyes in all directions to flush them thoroughly
      3) Irrigate for at least 15 minutes
   b. The fountains must be able to provide at least 1.5 L/minute to both eyes at the same time; this is a higher flow than manual or contact irrigation can provide
2. Manual irrigation method
   a. Position the patient and drape him or her to prepare for the procedure
   b. Instill topical anesthetic in the eye unless contraindicated
   c. Prepare irrigant with intravenous tubing
   d. Gently retract the patient's eyelid and begin the irrigation with direct flow in all directions over the globe of the eye
   e. Hold the eyelid open; a Desmarres lid retractor may be used
   f. Irrigate each eye with at least 1 L of saline; in the presence of stronger alkali or acids, more irrigant is needed to correct the eye pH to 7.0
3. Contact lens irrigation (Morgan lens): method
   a. Position and drape the patient
   b. Apply topical anesthetic unless contraindicated
   c. Check for foreign body object before irrigation if suspected
   d. Prepare intravenous irrigant with intravenous tubing hooked to the Morgan lens, and run some irrigant through to lubricate the lens
   e. Have the patient look downward and slip the lens under the upper lid, then gently pull the lower lid outward until the lens is in place; let the lower lid return to place and cover the lens
   f. Irrigate the affected eye with 1 to 2 L of fluid; adjust the rate for patient comfort
   g. When done, gently remove the lens by having the patient look up; pull the lower lid out, and the lens will pop up off the eye surface; have patient look down, and slide the lens out
4. Irrigation drainage must be kept away from the patient and others

Ear irrigation

1. Examine the ear with an otoscope before irrigation
2. Instill ceruminolytic drops and wait at least 10 minutes before starting irrigation
3. Do not insert the tip of the irrigation device beyond the cartilaginous portion of the canal
4. In adults, pull the pinna upward and back; in children, pull the pinna downward and back to straighten the ear canal
5. Point the irrigation stream toward the posterosuperior aspect of the canal and not directly at the tympanic membrane
   a. In the left ear, point the stream toward the 1 o'clock position
   b. In the right ear, point the stream toward the 11 o'clock position
6. Stop the irrigation if the patient complains of discomfort, vertigo, or nausea

SPECIFIC MAXILLOFACIAL AND OCULAR EMERGENCIES

Odontalgia (i.e., dental pain)

Definitions

1. Toothache: refers to pain around the tooth and jaw; usually related to inflammation of the pulp from a cavity deep within the dentin
2. Tooth eruption: in infants and children, when the primary teeth are erupting through gums and when the third molars (i.e., wisdom teeth) erupt
3. Periostitis: pain and bleeding ≤24 hours after tooth extraction
4. Alveolar osteitis or alveolitis (i.e., dry socket): pain for 2 to 3 days after tooth extraction caused by localized inflammation that results when the clot is dislodged

Predisposing factors

1. Poor oral hygiene
2. Dental caries
3. Gum disease

Pathophysiology

1. Dental caries
   a. Bacterial plaque causes acids that break down the dental enamel
   b. As decay progresses, there is invasion of the dentin and the pulp
   c. Inflammation leads to pulpitis and pulpal necrosis
   d. Abscess formation may occur
2. Tooth eruption: pericoronitis (i.e., gingival inflammation)
3. Alveolar osteitis: inflammation

Clinical presentation

1. Subjective
   a. Pain
      1) Sharp and progressively worse
      2) May radiate to gum, jaw, ear, temple, and neck
      3) Worsened by hot or cold applied to area
      4) Not relieved by over-the-counter analgesics
2. Objective
   a. Discoloration of teeth
   b. Decaying teeth
   c. May have halitosis
   d. Tenderness with tapping of affected tooth
3. Diagnostic: diagnosis made with the evaluation of the patient's clinical presentation and an assessment

Collaborative management

1. Continue assessment
   a. ABCDs
   b. Vital signs: blood pressure, pulse, respiratory rate, and temperature
   c. Pain and discomfort level
   d. Clinical indications of infection: fever, redness, swelling, and purulent drainage
   e. Close monitoring for the progression of symptoms
2. Ensure adequate airway, oxygenation, ventilation, and circulation
   a. Application of direct pressure to control bleeding if applicable
   b. IV access as indicated for fluid and medication administration; crystalloids as prescribed
3. Control pain, discomfort, and inflammation
   a. Topical analgesics (e.g., lidocaine gel, oil of wintergreen)
   b. Oral analgesics: non-narcotic or narcotic as prescribed
   c. Dental nerve block: assist as requested
   d. With alveolitis: irrigation of socket and application of gauze moistened with eugenol (oil of clove) daily (ENA, 2007)
4. Control bleeding after extraction
   a. Pressure dressing of cotton wrapped in gauze to site applied for 30 minutes (ENA, 2007)
   b. Hemostatic agent to socket: oxidized cellulose, topical thrombin, and microfibrillar collagen
   c. Lidocaine with epinephrine to anesthetize
   d. Suturing as indicated
5. Treat infection and prevent sepsis
   a. Antimicrobials
   b. Irrigation with Waterpik as indicated
6. Monitor for complications
   a. Airway compromise
   b. Infection or sepsis
   c. Uncontrolled pain

Evaluation

1. Patent airway, adequate oxygenation (i.e., normal PaO_2, SpO_2, SaO_2) and ventilation (i.e., normal $PaCO_2$)
2. Absence of clinical indications of respiratory distress
3. Absence of clinical indications of dehydration or shock
4. Absence of clinical indications of infection or sepsis
5. Control of pain and discomfort

Typical disposition: discharge with instructions
1. Good oral hygiene
2. Importance of regular dental checkups
3. For extractions
   a. If bleeding recurs from extraction site, recommendation to bite on gauze for 30 minutes
   b. Avoidance of hot foods and things that are hard or chewy
4. Dental referral and follow-up appointment

Gingival Emergencies

Definitions
1. Pericoronitis: an inflammation of the gingival tissue around a tooth that is usually caused by tooth eruption or impaction
2. Acute necrotizing ulcerative gingivitis (ANUG) (i.e., trench mouth or Vincent angina): a noncontagious infection of the gums that occurs with the overgrowth of normal mouth bacteria
3. Ludwig angina: a diffuse cellulitis of the sublingual, submental, and submandibular tissue of the mandible

Predisposing factors
1. Tooth eruption
2. Tooth decay
3. Poor dental hygiene
4. Immunosuppression
5. Poor nutrition

Pathophysiology
1. Pericoronitis: inflammation
2. ANUG: inflammation or infection caused by mixed anaerobic bacteria
3. Ludwig angina
   a. Existing dental infection or cellulitis that usually involves the lower second or third molars
      1) Usually caused by streptococci (e.g., *Streptococcus bacilli*) and *Bacteroides melaninogenicus*
   b. Descending infection can spread from the jaw to the mediastinum

Clinical presentation
1. Subjective
   a. General
      1) Pain that ranges from mild to severe
      2) Difficulty chewing
      3) Fever or chills
   b. Pericoronitis
      1) Nonspecific pain or pain when opening the mouth
      2) Earache on the affected side
   c. ANUG
      1) Fever, sore throat, bad taste in the mouth (i.e., metallic), or odor
      2) Painful gingivostomatitis or bleeding gums
      3) Headache
   d. Ludwig angina
      1) Difficulty talking (i.e., dysphasia) and swallowing (i.e., dysphagia)
2. Objective
   a. General: red, swollen, or bleeding gums
   b. Pericoronitis
      1) Temperature of >100°F
      2) Red, swollen gums around the affected tooth
      3) Trismus (i.e., difficulty opening the mouth)
   c. ANUG
      1) Temperature of >101°F
      2) Spontaneous bleeding from the gums and swollen gums
      3) Fetid breath and gray ulcers on the tonsil bases
      4) Lymphadenopathy
   d. Ludwig angina
      1) Temperature of >101°F
      2) Stridor
      3) Dyspnea
      4) Swelling of the neck, jaw, floor of the mouth toward the palate, and tongue; the swollen tissue is firm to palpation
      5) Swelling into the mediastinal area may be noted
      6) May have an altered level of consciousness
3. Diagnostic
   a. CBC with differential: increased WBC count
   b. ESR: increased with infection
   c. ABGs: indicated in the presence of dyspnea or possible airway compromise
   d. Mandibular Panorex
   e. CT: neck
   f. Lateral soft neck films may be needed

Collaborative management
1. Continue assessment
   a. ABCDs
   b. Vital signs: blood pressure, pulse, respiratory rate, and temperature
   c. Oxygen saturation
   d. Respiratory effort and excursion
   e. Cardiac rate and rhythm
   f. Pain and discomfort level
   g. Clinical indications of infection: fever, redness, swelling, or purulent drainage
   h. Level of consciousness
   i. Close monitoring for the progression of symptoms
2. Maintain airway, oxygenation, and ventilation
   a. Airway, oxygenation, and circulation support with the use of BLS or ACLS if needed
      1) Positioning with the head of stretcher up 60 to 90 degrees (i.e., Fowler position)
      2) Artificial airway may be required in patients with Ludwig angina
   b. 100% oxygen by face mask may be required; intubation and mechanical ventilation as indicated

3. Maintain adequate circulation and perfusion
   a. IV access for fluid and medication administration; crystalloids may be given if there is any compromise of the airway or circulation
4. Control pain, discomfort, and inflammation
   a. Irrigation of the mouth
      1) Pericoronitis: warmed normal saline
      2) ANUG: half-strength hydrogen peroxide or chlorhexidine (Peridex)
   b. Topical anesthetics
   c. Local anesthetics maybe needed for patients with Ludwig angina
   d. Analgesics and narcotics may be required
5. Treat infection and prevent sepsis
   a. Antimicrobials (e.g., penicillin) as indicated
   b. Antipyretics and cooling methods to reduce fever
6. Assist with procedures as indicated
   a. Pericoronitis: debridement, excision of the gingival flap, and extraction of the molar; the patient is usually referred to a dentist
   b. ANUG: possible debridement and gingival curettage
   c. Ludwig angina: intraoral incision and drainage under conscious sedation
7. Monitor for complications
   a. Pericoronitis: cellulitis, abscess, and Ludwig angina
   b. ANUG: abscesses and underlying alveolar bone destruction
   c. Ludwig angina: airway compromise and septicemia

Evaluation

1. Patent airway, adequate oxygenation (i.e., normal PaO_2, SpO_2, SaO_2) and ventilation (i.e., normal $PaCO_2$)
2. Absence of clinical indications of respiratory distress
3. Absence of clinical indications of infection or sepsis
4. Absence of clinical indications of hypoperfusion
5. Control of pain and discomfort
6. Alert and oriented with no neurologic deficit

Typical disposition: discharge with instructions

1. If evaluation criteria met: discharge with instructions
   a. Good oral hygiene and proper care of gums
   b. Good nutrition
   c. Antimicrobials and analgesics as prescribed
   d. Follow up with oral surgeon as directed
2. If evaluation criteria not met (e.g., Ludwig angina, airway compromise, sepsis): admission

Dental Abscess

Definition: a collection of pus in a dental cavity that is formed as a result of the disintegration of tissue

1. Periapical abscess: acute inflammation that originates in the dental pulp and that spreads beyond bone tissue; this is common in children
2. Periodontal abscess: bony destruction at the periodontal membrane

Predisposing factors

1. Dental caries and plaque
2. Baby bottle tooth decay
3. Poor dental hygiene
4. Trauma or surgical infection
5. Conditions that cause immunocompromise

Pathophysiology

1. Extension of pulpal necrosis from a decayed tooth or trauma
2. Development of a pocket of plaque and food debris that becomes pus between the tooth and the gingiva
3. May be confined or spread to the face and neck

Clinical presentation

1. Subjective
   a. Pain and swelling
   b. Thermal sensitivity with periapical abscess
   c. Fever, chills, and malaise
   d. Gingival bleeding
2. Objective
   a. Edema of the face and neck
   b. Temperature of >99°F
   c. Increased teeth mobility with periapical abscess
   d. Tenderness to percussion
   e. Swollen red gums
   f. Swelling noted in the pharynx
   g. Lymphadenopathy
3. Diagnostic
   a. CBC with differential: increased WBC count
   b. Blood cultures before antibiotic therapy
   c. Culture and sensitivity of any drainage
   d. Periapical radiography or Panorex to view the teeth and the surrounding structures
   e. Lateral and anteroposterior neck radiographs to view the airway if cellulitis is present

Collaborative management

1. Continue assessment
   a. ABCDs
   b. Vital signs: blood pressure, pulse, respiratory rate, and temperature
   c. Oxygen saturation
   d. Respiratory effort and excursion
   e. Cardiac rate and rhythm
   f. Pain and discomfort level
   g. Clinical indications of infection: fever, redness, swelling, or purulent drainage
   h. Level of consciousness
   i. Close monitoring for the progression of symptoms
2. Assist with procedures as indicated
   a. Incision and drainage; may leave a drain tube in place
   b. Culture of drainage
3 Control pain, discomfort, and inflammation
   a. Analgesics
   b. Oral rinses with warm normal saline
   c. Corticosteroids as prescribed for inflammation

4. Treat infection and prevent sepsis
   a. Antimicrobials
   b. Antipyretics and cooling methods to reduce fever
5. Monitor for complications
   a. Airway compromise
   b. Sepsis

Evaluation

1. Patent airway, adequate oxygenation (i.e., normal PaO_2, SpO_2, SaO_2) and ventilation (i.e., normal $PaCO_2$)
2. Absence of clinical indications of respiratory distress
3. Absence of clinical indications of sepsis
4. Absence of clinical indications of hypoperfusion
5. Control of pain or discomfort
6. Alert and oriented with no neurologic deficit

Typical disposition

1. If evaluation criteria met: discharge with instructions
   a. Avoidance of manipulation of drain or packing if in place
   b. Oral rinses with warm saline every 1 to 2 hours during the day
   c. Medications as prescribed
   d. Good oral hygiene
   e. Soft diet for a few days
   f. Follow-up referral with a dentist or an endodontist
2. If evaluation criteria not met (e.g., airway compromise): admission

Foreign Body in the Ear, Nose, or Throat

Definition: when an object is swallowed or stuck in the ear, nose, or throat

Predisposing factors

1. Most common among children between the ages of 1 and 3 years
   a. Most common foreign bodies in children: buttons, coins, and food (e.g., nuts)
      1) Small toy parts such as screws, stuffed animal or doll eyes and noses, and other pieces that can be removed or taken apart are dangerous
      2) Vegetable matter may swell and cause removal to be more difficult
      3) Small, interesting, shiny objects are likely to attract children's attention and could easily become foreign bodies
      4) Small batteries are easily swallowed and dangerous because they are toxic
2. Insects
3. Esophageal strictures

Pathophysiology

1. Ear foreign bodies can produce local irritation and tissue inflammation
2. Nose foreign bodies can cause airway compromise in infants and bleeding trauma in children and adults
3. Throat foreign bodies can lodge in the larynx and cause airway obstruction or in the esophagus and cause dysphagia or nausea

Clinical presentation

1. Subjective
   a. History of foreign body insertion
   b. Pain and discomfort
   c. Ear
      1) Decreased hearing
      2) Buzzing in ear
      3) Sensation of fullness
      4) Discharge from ear
   d. Nose
      1) Sudden onset of moderate to severe respiratory distress
      2) Chronic cough
      3) Wheezing with expiration
      4) Feeling of something being in the nose
   e. Throat (esophageal)
      1) Sensation of foreign body
      2) Usually the patient will have no difficulty talking unless the foreign body is causing airway obstruction (see Chapter 5 for information about foreign body objects in the airway)
      3) Retching without nausea
      4) Children may present with drooling, nausea, vomiting, and difficulty talking if the obstruction is high; a foreign body may also affect the airway
2. Objective
   a. Ear
      1) Foul odor from the affected ear
      2) Affected ear canal is edematous with erythema
      3) Visible object
      4) Purulent drainage or bleeding from the affected canal
   b. Nose
      1) Stridor
      2) Wheezing
      3) Impaired phonation
      4) Unequal breath sounds
   c. Throat
      1) Retching
3. Diagnostic
   a. Otoscopic examination
   b. Lateral neck and chest radiography
   c. Fiberoptic laryngoscope

Collaborative management

1. Continue assessment
   a. ABCDs
   b. Vital signs: blood pressure, pulse, respiratory rate, and temperature
   c. Oxygen saturation
   d. Respiratory effort and excursion
   e. Pain and discomfort level
   f. Level of consciousness
   g. Close monitoring for the progression of symptoms
2. Ensure adequate airway, oxygenation, ventilation, and circulation
   a. Airway maintenance
      1) Chin lift and head tilt
      2) Jaw thrust if suspect cervical spine injury

3) Abdominal or chest thrusts to dislodge foreign body as indicated
   4) Suctioning of airway as indicated
   b. Oxygen by nasal cannula at 2 to 6 L/minute if indicated to maintain SpO_2 rate of 95% unless contraindicated; for patients with chronic obstructive pulmonary disease (COPD), use pulse oximetry to guide oxygen administration to an SpO_2 rate of 90%
   c. Intubation and mechanical ventilation as indicated
   d. IV access with two large-bore catheters for fluid and medication administration; isotonic crystalloids as indicated
   e. Application of direct pressure if bleeding is present
3. Reduce and relieve pain, discomfort, and inflammation
   a. Ear
      1) Analgesics
      2) Neomycin and polymixin B sulfates and hydrocortisone (Cortisporin) drops
   b. Nose
      1) Upright position
      2) Cool-mist oxygen
      3) Reassurance and coaching of patient to breathe through the mouth and to not take deep sharp breaths because this may lodge object further inward
   c. Throat
      1) Position of comfort
      2) IV glucagon as prescribed to relax the smooth muscle of the distal esophagus
4. Assist with the removal of the object
   a. Ear
      1) Irrigation of ear canal with normal saline
         a) Mixture of alcohol and water if the material is organic to the reduce swelling of the foreign body
         b) Mineral oil or 2% lidocaine solution for live insects
      2) Suctioning if indicated
      3) Direct visual removal
      4) Ear curette
      5) Flashlight to attract live insects out of the ear canal
   b. Nose
      1) Gentle pressure to close the unaffected nostril and then instructions for the patient to try to blow the object out; if unsuccessful, proceed to removal
      2) Topical vasoconstrictor
      3) Alligator forceps removal
      4) Fiberoptic laryngoscope
   c. Throat
      1) May gradually pass on own
      2) IV glucagon as prescribed to relax the esophagus to allow the item to pass on down
      3) Esophagoscopy with conscious sedation
5. Treat infection (if present) and prevent sepsis
   a. Antimicrobials as indicated
   b. Antipyretics and cooling methods to reduce fever

6. Monitor for complications
   a. Airway obstruction
   b. Perforated tympanic membrane
   c. Infection of ear canal or nasal passages
   d. Epistaxis

Evaluation

1. Patent airway, adequate oxygenation (i.e., normal PaO_2, SpO_2, SaO_2) and ventilation (i.e., normal $PaCO_2$)
2. Absence of clinical indications of respiratory distress
3. Stable hemodynamic status
4. Control of pain and discomfort
5. Alert and oriented with no neurologic deficit
6. Removal of foreign body

Typical disposition: discharge with instructions

1. Discuss prevention with patient or parents (Cleveland Clinic Foundation, n.d.)
   a. Closely observe infants and toddlers
   b. Monitor the eating habits of infants and toddlers and the size and texture of their food
   c. Keep small shiny objects out of the reach of infants and toddlers
   d. Avoid food hazards: hot dogs, candies, nuts, grapes, raw peas, beans, popcorn, and marshmallows
   e. Keep household hazards (e.g., buttons, coins, beads, jewelry, marbles, toothpicks, razors, and broken or uninflated balloons) out of children's reach
   f. Read toy labels and follow guidelines for age recommendations
   g. Inspect toys often and look for loose or broken parts and pieces
2. Consultation with an otolaryngologist and follow up as needed

Labyrinthitis

Definition: an inflammatory process that affects the labyrinths of the inner ear
Predisposing factors
1. Acute febrile illness
2. Chronic otitis media
3. Recent ear surgery
4. Trauma to the head or cervical spine
5. Hypertension
6. Diabetes
7. Stroke
8. Migraine

Pathophysiology (Strasnick & Steinberg, 2008)

1. The labyrinth is made up of an outer osseous framework that surrounds a membranous network that contains the peripheral sensory organs for balance and hearing, which include the utricle, the saccule, the semicircular canals, and the cochlea
   a. Inflammation can result from viral or bacterial causes

2. When infectious microorganisms or inflammatory mediators invade the labyrinth, it can cause damage to the vestibular and auditory end organs, which results in labyrinthitis

Clinical presentation

1. Subjective
   a. Upper respiratory tract infection symptoms (preceding or concurrent)
   b. Ear pain (i.e., otalgia) or pressure
   c. Neck pain or stiffness
   d. Vertigo (more prominent with head movement)
   e. Decreased unilateral or bilateral hearing; hearing loss is rare but can also occur
   f. Nausea or vomiting
2. Objective
   a. Otorrhea (i.e., drainage from the ear)
   b. Facial weakness or asymmetry
   c. Altered gait
   d. Ear pain or tenderness with palpation and examination
   e. Orthostatic blood pressure changes
3. Diagnostic
   a. CBC and blood cultures if infection suspected
   b. Noncontrast CT scan: to visualize fibrosis and calcification of the membranous labyrinth in a patient with chronic labyrinthitis
      1) Useful to rule out causes such as mastoiditis
   c. MRI: to rule out stroke, brain abscess, and other potential causes of vertigo and hearing loss
   d. Forced hyperventilation: to see if symptoms can be reproduced
   e. Dix-Hallpike test
      1) Performed to test whether head movement causes vertigo
      2) Nystagmus (i.e., jerky movement of the eyes) indicates a positive result

Collaborative management

1. Continue assessment
   a. ABCDs
   b. Vital signs: blood pressure, pulse, respiratory rate, and temperature
   c. Pain and discomfort level
   d. Clinical indications of dehydration
   e. Close monitoring for the progression of symptoms
2. Control discomfort and anxiety
   a. Rest
   b. Anxiolytics
   c. Antiemetics
3. Ensure safety by assisting with ambulation
4. Maintain adequate hydration: IV for fluid administration
5. Treat infection and prevent sepsis
   a. Antimicrobials
   b. Antipyretics and cooling methods to reduce fever
6. Monitor for complications
   a. Falls
   b. Dehydration

Evaluation

1. Patent airway, adequate oxygenation (i.e., normal PaO_2, SpO_2, SaO_2) and ventilation (i.e., normal $PaCO_2$)
2. Absence of clinical indications of hypoperfusion
3. Vertigo or disequilibrium diminished or resolved
4. Alert and oriented with no neurologic deficit
5. Absence of injury related to fall

Typical disposition: discharge with instructions

1. Treatment of acute episode: lie quietly with the eyes closed
2. Fluids
3. Medications as prescribed
4. Follow up with primary care provider or specialist as directed

Ménière Disease

Definition: an increase in the volume and pressure of the fluid in the vestibular system located within the inner ear; also known as *endolymphatic hydrops*

Predisposing factors

1. Food allergy
2. Exposure to loud noise levels over the course of several years
3. Stress
4. Increased salt intake
5. Metabolic dysfunction
6. Viral infection
7. Hereditary factors

Pathophysiology

1. Rare idiopathic disease with unknown origins
2. Volume and pressure of the fluid in the inner ear increases, thereby causing symptoms
3. Characterized by attacks of vertigo, tinnitus, a feeling of fullness in the ear, and a fluctuation of hearing ability
   a. Duration of acute attacks can be from minutes to hours; usually 2 to 3 hours and settle within 1 to 2 days
   b. Acute episodes usually occur in clusters (approximately 6–11 times a year)
   c. Periods of remission may last for several months

Clinical presentation

1. Subjective
   a. Classic triad: vertigo, hearing loss, and tinnitus
   b. Fullness in the ears
   c. Feeling of spinning or that objects are spinning
   d. Nausea and vomiting
   e. Sensitivity to noise
   f. Anxiety and diaphoresis
   g. Blurred vision and headache
   h. Sudden unexplained falls without vertigo or loss of consciousness (drop attacks)
2. Objective
   a. Horizontal nystagmus (i.e., involuntary rapid movement of the eyes from side to side) during attack

b. Falling toward the affected side

c. Vomiting

d. Hearing loss in the affected ear

e. Diaphoretic and pale skin

3. Diagnostic

   a. Serum analysis to help rule out other causes

   b. Auditory testing (e.g., tuning fork)

   c. Vestibular testing (e.g., cold water caloric, nystagmogram)

   d. MRI to rule out acoustic tumor, which presents with the same symptoms

Collaborative management

1. Continue assessment

   a. ABCDs

   b. Vital signs: blood pressure, pulse, respiratory rate, and temperature

   c. Pain and discomfort level

   d. Clinical indications of dehydration

   e. Level of consciousness

   f. Close monitoring for the progression of symptoms

2. Relieve vertigo and nausea

   a. Antihistamines (e.g., meclizine [Antivert]): reduce vertigo by providing strong vestibular repression

   b. Anticholinergics: relieve nausea and vomiting by suppressing conduction in the vestibular cerebellar pathways

   c. Diuretics: decrease inner ear volume and thus decrease vertigo

   d. Corticosteroids: treat possible autoimmune disorders of the inner ear

   e. Vasodilators: when labyrinthitis ischemia is suspected to be cause

   f. Benzodiazepines: facilitate inhibitory γ-aminobutyric acid neurotransmission and other inhibitory transmitters, which may decrease vertigo

3. Ensure safety during attacks

   a. Bed rest with the eyes closed

   b. Limitation of activity during episodes

   c. Assistance with ambulation

   d. Side rails in place

4. Monitor for complications

   a. Progressive hearing loss

   b. Injury to self during attack

Evaluation

1. Patent airway, adequate oxygenation (i.e., normal PaO_2, SpO_2, SaO_2) and ventilation (i.e., normal $PaCO_2$)

2. Absence of clinical indications of hypoperfusion

3. Vertigo or disequilibrium diminished or resolved

4. Alert and oriented with no neurologic deficit

5. Absence of injury caused by fall

Typical disposition: discharge with instructions

1. Bed rest and limitation of noise

2. Maintenance of safety with movement

   a. Limit activity

   b. Change positions slowly

   c. Avoid quick or sudden movements

3. Avoidance of triggers (e.g., salt, caffeine, alcohol)

4. Medications as prescribed

5. Follow up with primary care provider

6. Instructions related to prevention

   a. Limit stress

   b. Reduce salt intake

   c. Avoid significant noise or use hearing protection

   d. Avoid use of ototoxic medicines (e.g., aspirin, quinine [Qualaquin])

Otitis Externa

Definition: an inflammation of the external ear canal; also known as *swimmer's ear*

Predisposing factors

1. Conditions that cause irritation or trauma or an infectious agent

   a. Prolonged swimming

   b. Hearing aids

   c. Impacted cerumen or insufficient production of cerumen

   d. Exposure to water with a high bacterial count

2. Excessive moisture and maceration of the skin: whitish-colored appearance of the skin tissue as a result of excess moisture

3. Sweating

4. Allergies

5. Stress

6. Previous ear infections

7. Aggressive cleaning of the ear canal

8. Anatomic abnormalities (e.g., narrow canal)

9. Previous ear surgery (e.g., tympanostomy)

Pathophysiology

1. Acute condition usually caused by bacteria, but a chronic condition that lasts >3 months is usually viral in origin

2. Disruption of the skin surface or of the cerumen protective barrier in the external ear canal

   a. Sometimes involves the pinna or the tympanic membrane

3. Cellulitis of the skin and subdermis of the ear canal develops with acute inflammation and varying degrees of edema

Clinical presentation

1. Subjective

   a. Pain: otalgia (i.e., earache)

     1) May radiate from the ear to the head, jaw, and neck

     2) No relief with nonsteroidal anti-inflammatory drugs or analgesics

   b. Pruritus and swelling of the ear

   c. Drainage from the ear

   d. Sensation of canal fullness with or without hearing loss

   e. Tinnitus (i.e., ringing in the ear) may be present

2. Objective
    a. Temperature (may be >99°F)
    b. Tenderness of tragus and pinna with palpation
    c. Erythema in canal
    d. Regional cellulitis of auricle, pinna, and adjacent skin may be present
        1) Cellulitis may be present as a result of dermatologic disorders (e.g., eczema)
    e. Visible otorrhea
        1) Green exudate from gram-negative bacteria (e.g., *Pseudomonas*)
        2) Yellow exudate possibly from *Staphylococcus aureus*
        3) Fluffy white or black exudate from fungal agents (e.g., *Aspergillus, Candida*)
    f. Conductive hearing loss
        1) Sensorineural: loss occurs when there is damage to the inner ear (cochlea) or to the nerve pathways from the inner ear (retrocochlear) to the brain
            a) Permanent loss
            b) Involves a reduction in sound level or in the ability to hear faint sounds
            c) Also affects the understanding of speech or the ability to hear clearly
        2) Conductive: occurs when sound is not conducted efficiently through the ear canal
            a) Involves a reduction in sound level or a decreased ability to hear faint sounds
            b) Usually can be treated
    g. Lymphadenopathy: periauricular or cervical
    h. Tympanic membrane usually appears normal
3. Diagnostic
    a. Otoscopic examination
    b. Culture the ear if persistent otitis externa is unresolved after antibiotic treatment
    c. Whisper test: a screening test that involves standing behind the patient and whispering and then having the patient repeat what was said
    d. Rinne test: test of air conduction versus bone conduction of sound with the use of a tuning fork (air conduction > bone conduction normal)
    e. Weber test: vibration is heard equally on both sides when the tuning fork is held in the middle of the forehead (i.e., no lateralization)

Collaborative management
1. Continue assessment
    a. ABCDs
    b. Vital signs: blood pressure, pulse, respiratory rate, and temperature
    c. Pain and discomfort level
    d. Clinical indications of dehydration
    e. Close monitoring for the progression of symptoms
2. Control pain, discomfort, and inflammation
    a. Analgesic
    b. Cortisporin (neomycin, polymixin B with hydrocortisone) otic drops
    c. Warm, moist compresses to the affected ear

3. Treat infection and prevent sepsis
    a. Topical antibiotics
    b. Oto-Wick saturated with antibiotic if significant swelling is present
        1) Wick will fall out on its own in a few days after the swelling decreases (Domino, 2008)
    c. Antipyretics
4. Monitor for complications
    a. Ear canal stenosis (related to fibrosis)
    b. Tympanic membrane perforation
    c. Conductive hearing loss
    d. Opportunistic bacterial or fungal infection
    e. Furuncle: infected hair follicles
    f. Regional lymphadenitis

Evaluation
1. Absence of clinical indications of infection or sepsis
2. Control of pain and discomfort

Typical disposition: discharge with instructions
1. Warm compresses to the affected ear as directed
2. Instillation of medications into the ear as directed
3. Efforts to keep the ear dry
4. Avoidance of insertion of objects into the affected ear
5. Prevention of recurrence
    a. Use of a bathing cap
    b. Avoidance of earplugs, earphones, headphones
6. Follow up with primary care provider or specialist as directed

Otitis Media
Definition: an inflammation of the middle ear
Predisposing factors
1. Serous otitis media
2. Bottle-fed infants
3. Barotrauma
4. Eustachian tube dysfunction
5. Recent upper respiratory infection
6. Recent air travel
7. Passive smoke

Pathophysiology
1. Pathogens can enter the Eustachian tube from the nasopharynx, which is also the primary route for the clearing of middle ear secretions
    a. Common pathogens: *Streptococcus pneumonia, Haemophilus influenzae, Streptococcus pyogenes,* and *Moraxella catarrhalis* (ENA, 2007)
2. Inflammatory edema of the nasopharynx causes obstruction of the Eustachian tube
3. Exudative and transudative fluids collect in the middle ear, thereby allowing for the overgrowth of nasopharyngeal bacteria in the middle ear

Clinical presentation

1. Subjective
   a. History of recent upper respiratory symptoms
   b. Rapid onset of ear pain, fever, and irritability
   c. Decreased hearing or fullness in ear
   d. Vertigo and dizziness
   e. In infants: difficulty feeding, fussiness, and pulling at ear
2. Objective
   a. Bulging or retracting of tympanic membrane
   b. Limited or absent mobility of tympanic membrane with pneumatic otoscopy
   c. Air-fluid level behind the tympanic membrane
   d. Otorrhea: white or yellowish from the tympanic membrane
      1) Large amount of purulent exudate indicates rupture of the membrane
   e. Erythema of tympanic membrane and pharynx
   f. Bullous myringitis: bleb on the eardrum
3. Diagnostic
   a. CT: may show clouding of the mastoid cells or isolated radiolucent areas in the mastoid if mastoiditis present
   b. MRI: to evaluate otogenic intracranial complications
   c. Blood cultures if sepsis is suspected

Collaborative management

1. Continue assessment
   a. ABCDs
   b. Vital signs: blood pressure, pulse, respiratory rate, and temperature
   c. Pain and discomfort level
   d. Close monitoring for the progression of symptoms
2. Reduce and relieve pain, discomfort, and inflammation
   a. Analgesics
   b. Nonsteroidal anti-inflammatory drugs
   c. Topical decongestants and otic analgesics (e.g., antipyrine, benzocaine, dehydrated glycerin [Auralgan])
3. Treat infection and prevent sepsis
   a. Antimicrobials as prescribed
   b. Antipyretics
4. Assist with procedures as indicated (usually performed by an otolaryngologist)
   a. Tympanocentesis: effusion aspiration from the middle ear for recurrent otitis
   b. Myringotomy: if tympanic membrane bulging in a patient with recurrent otitis
5. Monitor for complications
   a. Hearing loss
   b. Mastoiditis
   c. Meningitis

Evaluation

1. Control of pain and discomfort
2. Absence of clinical indications of infection or sepsis

Typical disposition: discharge with instructions

1. Medications as prescribed
2. Follow up with primary care provider in 2 weeks for a recheck of the ear
3. Follow up in 2 to 3 days if no improvement or worsening of symptoms
4. Prevention
   a. In infants
      1) For infants who are bottle feeding, keep the head elevated
      2) Limit pacifier use when the infant or child is falling asleep
   b. Avoidance of cigarette smoke

Ruptured Tympanic Membrane

Definition: a rupture or tear of the tympanic membrane

Predisposing factors

1. Otitis media
2. Acoustic or head injury
3. Foreign body in ear
4. Barotrauma (e.g., air travel, scuba diving)

Pathophysiology

1. Can be caused by invading organism or traumatic injury
   a. Injury may be a result of a sudden change in pressure
2. Healing usually occurs spontaneously
3. Hearing loss is usually temporary

Clinical presentation

1. Subjective
   a. History of recent air travel, upper respiratory infection, or trauma
   b. Sharp, sudden pain in the ear that is quickly resolved
   c. Hearing loss
   d. Tinnitus
   e. Vertigo that usually resolves quickly
   f. Nausea or vomiting with vertigo
   g. Drainage from the ear
2. Objective
   a. Temperature of >100°F if related to infection
   b. Altered gait
   c. Ataxia
   d. Decreased hearing in affected ear
   e. Otoscopic examination
      1) Perforation of tympanic membrane: slit appearance
      2) Discharge: clear, bloody, or purulent
   f. May have nystagmus
3. Diagnostic
   a. Culture ear drainage
   b. Tuning fork examination to evaluate hearing: Rinne or Weber
   c. Radiography: skull, temporal bone, and cervical spine as indicated

Collaborative management

1. Continue assessment
   a. ABCDs
   b. Vital signs: blood pressure, pulse, respiratory rate, and temperature
   c. Pain and discomfort level
   d. Hearing
   e. Close monitoring for the progression of symptoms
2. Control pain, discomfort, and inflammation
   a. Nonsteroidal anti-inflammatory drugs
   b. Analgesics
   c. Warm compresses to the affected ear
   d. Communication: speak clearly and toward the unaffected ear
3. Treat infection if present
   a. Antimicrobials as indicated
   b. Antipyretics and cooling methods to reduce fever
   c. Gentle removal of blood and debris from the ear canal
4. Monitor for complications
   a. Hearing loss
   b. Otitis media

Evaluation

1. Absence of clinical indications of infection or sepsis
2. Control of pain and discomfort

Typical disposition: discharge with instructions

1. Warm compresses as directed
2. Efforts to keep ear canal dry
3. Medications as prescribed
4. Follow up with otolaryngologist as directed

Sinusitis and Rhinosinusitis

Definition

1. Sinusitis: an inflammation of the mucous membranes that line the paranasal sinuses, which include the maxillary sinuses, the frontal sinus, and the ethmoid sinus
2. Rhinosinusitis: an inflammation of the mucosa of the nasal cavity and the paranasal sinuses

Predisposing factors

1. Deviated septum
2. Nasal polyps, tumors, and foreign bodies
3. Allergic rhinitis
4. Asthma

Pathophysiology

1. Usually caused by upper respiratory infections (e.g., parainfluenza, adenovirus, influenza, rhinovirus)
2. Mucosal edema occurs, thereby causing a decrease in mucus transport; this leads to a stagnation of secretions
3. Stagnant secretions, decreased pH, and lowered oxygen tension promote bacterial or viral overgrowth

Clinical presentation

1. Subjective
   a. Pain
   b. Headache that worsens when the patient bends forward
   c. Facial pain: dull, achy pressure
2. Objective
   a. Red, swollen nasal mucous
   b. Purulent nasal drainage
   c. Conjunctivitis
   d. Puffy eyes in children
   e. Tenderness with palpation over the sinus areas
   f. Malodorous breath
   g. Purulent secretions in the nasal cavity
3. Diagnostic
   a. Diagnosis is usually made by clinical assessment
   b. Sinus cultures: if recurrent sinus infections
   c. Radiography
      1) Water's view
      2) Caldwell view
      3) Lateral view

Collaborative management

1. Continue assessment
   a. ABCDs
   b. Vital signs: blood pressure, pulse, respiratory rate, and temperature
   c. Pain and discomfort level
   d. Close monitoring for the progression of symptoms
2. Control pain, discomfort, and inflammation
   a. Nonsteroidal anti-inflammatory drugs
   b. Analgesics
   c. Nasal steroids
   d. Decongestants
3. Relieve nasal obstruction
   a. Vaporizer
   b. Saline nasal sprays
   c. Preparation for surgery as indicated
4. Treat infection if present and prevent sepsis
   a. Antibiotics: controversial because of antibiotic resistance and because most sinusitis is viral in nature rather than bacterial; must distinguish between the two (Domino, 2008)
   b. Antipyretics and cooling methods to reduce fever
5. Monitor for complications
   a. Dehydration
   b. Orbital cellulitis
   c. Cavernous sinus thrombosis
   d. Meningitis
   e. Osteomyelitis

Evaluation

1. Patent airway, adequate oxygenation (i.e., normal PaO_2, SpO_2, and SaO_2) and ventilation (i.e., normal $PaCO_2$)
2. Absence of clinical indications of respiratory distress
3. Absence of clinical indications of infection or sepsis
4. Control of pain and discomfort

Typical disposition: discharge with instructions
1. Increased fluid intake to prevent and treat dehydration
2. Humidification at home: humidifier or vaporizer
3. Nasal decongestants for only 2 to 3 days, because longer use can lead to rebound congestion (ENA, 2007)
4. Follow up with primary care provider as directed
5. For recurrent frequent sinus problems, follow up with allergist

Cavernous Sinus Thrombosis

Definition: thrombosis of one or both of the cavernous sinuses (Sharma & Bessman, 2008)
1. Late complication of an infection of the central face or the paranasal sinuses

Predisposing factors
1. Midfacial cellulitis
2. Paranasal infection
3. Bacteremia
4. Trauma
5. Ear or maxillary tooth infection
6. Chronic sinusitis

Pathophysiology
1. The cavernous sinuses receive venous blood from the superior and inferior ophthalmic veins and the sphenoid and middle cerebral veins
2. Blood empties into the inferior petrosal sinuses and then into the internal jugular veins and the sigmoid sinuses through the superior petrosal sinuses
3. There are no valves to prevent blood from flowing forward or backward, depending on the prevailing pressure gradients
4. Infections of the face, including of the nose, tonsils, and orbits, cause thrombosis of the cavernous sinuses
   a. Most likely organisms are *Staphylococcus aureus* and *Streptococcus*
5. Overwhelming sepsis or neurologic infection may occur
   a. High rates of morbidity and mortality

Clinical presentation
1. Subjective
   a. History of sinus or midface infection for at least the preceding 5 days
   b. Symptoms may be very subtle
   c. Headache
2. Objective
   a. Periorbital edema (may be earliest finding)
      1) Ptosis (i.e., drooping of eyelid)
      2) Mydriasis (i.e., excessive dilation of the pupil)
      3) Eye muscle weakness as a result of palsy of cranial nerve III
      4) Exophthalmos (i.e., abnormal protrusion of the eyeball)
   b. Sluggish pupillary response if increased intracranial pressure
   c. Meningeal signs
      1) Nuchal rigidity (i.e., neck stiffness)
      2) Kernig sign: when the patient is lying supine, he or she cannot extend the leg at the knee when the thigh is flexed at a right angle to the trunk
      3) Brudzinski sign: when passive flexion of the neck causes flexion of the legs
3. Diagnostic
   a. CBC with differential: may show leukocytosis
   b. CT: with contrast to confirm or differentiate other problems (e.g., orbital cellulitis)
   c. Magnetic resonance venography: absence of venous flow in the affected cavernous sinus

Collaborative management
1. Continue assessment
   a. ABCDs
   b. Vital signs: blood pressure, pulse, respiratory rate, and temperature
   c. Oxygen saturation
   d. Cardiac rate and rhythm
   e. Pain and discomfort level
   f. Close monitoring for the progression of symptoms
2. Treat infection
   a. Aggressive antimicrobial therapy: patient usually receives intravenous antibiotics for 3 to 4 weeks
   b. Antipyretics and cooling methods to reduce fever
3. Control pain and discomfort
   a. Nonsteroidal anti-inflammatory drugs
   b. Narcotic analgesics
   c. Corticosteroids to reduce inflammation and edema
4. Monitor for complications
   a. Meningitis
   b. Septic emboli
   c. Blindness
   d. Cranial nerve palsies
   e. Sepsis and shock

Evaluation
1. Patent airway, adequate oxygenation (i.e., normal PaO_2, SpO_2, and SaO_2) and ventilation (i.e., normal $PaCO_2$)
2. Absence of clinical indications of hypoperfusion
3. Absence of clinical indications of infection or sepsis
4. Control of pain and discomfort

Typical disposition: admission, possibly to the critical care unit

Epistaxis

Definition: an acute hemorrhage of the nostril, nasal cavity, or nasopharynx; usually unilateral, even when bleeding from both nares occurs
Predisposing factors
1. Trauma
   a. Nose picking is the most common cause

b. Forceful blowing

c. Hitting of the nose

2. Foreign bodies
3. Sinus infections and rhinitis
4. Hypertension
5. Coagulopathy
6. Alcohol abuse and liver disease
7. Drugs that affect clotting (e.g., aspirin, NSAIDs, warfarin [Coumadin])
8. Substance abuse (e.g., cocaine, inhalants)

Pathophysiology

1. Classified as anterior or posterior (Evans & Rothenhaus, 2007)
   a. Anterior bleeds are more common (90%)
      1) Majority originate in the Kiesselbach plexus of the nasal septum through the internal and external carotids; can originate anterior to the inferior turbinate
      2) Area is very vascular
   b. Posterior is less common
      1) Originate from the sphenopalatine artery branches (i.e., "the arteries of the epistaxis") found in the posterior nasal cavity or the nasopharynx (i.e., the roof of the nasal chamber)
      2) Bleeding is more profuse and difficult to control
      3) Bleeding around any anterior nasal packing suggests a posterior bleed

Clinical presentation

1. Subjective
   a. Recent predisposing factors
   b. Reported nose bleeding
      1) Constant oozing seen with anterior bleed
      2) Profuse bleeding with blood draining into pharynx seen with posterior bleed
      3) Identification of which nare started bleeding first
2. Objective
   a. Bleeding
      1) Obvious bleeding from nares
      2) Bleeding visualized in the anterior nasal cavity or the pharynx
      3) Blood visualized behind the tympanic membrane: indicates tympanic membrane rupture
      4) Blood from the lacrimal ducts, which are connected to the nasal sinuses
   b. Tachycardia
   c. BP changes: may be hypertensive but may have orthostatic hypotension if significant blood loss
   d. Nasal mucosa and turbinates edematous with erythema
3. Diagnostic
   a. CBC
      1) Hemoglobin and hematocrit levels: may be decreased
      2) Platelet level: to rule out coagulopathy
   b. Coagulation profile: bleeding times
   c. Typing and cross matching if persistent heavy bleeding is present

d. CT scan or nasopharyngoscopy: if tumor is suspected

Collaborative management

1. Continue assessment
   a. ABCDs
   b. Vital signs: blood pressure, pulse, respiratory rate, and temperature
   c. Oxygen saturation
   d. Respiratory effort and excursion
   e. Cardiac rate and rhythm
   f. Clinical indications of bleeding
   g. Clinical indications of dehydration
   h. Close monitoring for the progression of symptoms
2. Maintain airway, oxygenation, ventilation, and perfusion
   a. 100% oxygen by face mask or blow by to maintain an SpO_2 of 95% unless contraindicated; for patients with COPD, use pulse oximetry to guide oxygen administration to an SpO_2 of 90%
   b. Intubation and mechanical ventilation if patient is unable to maintain airway
   c. Circulating volume replacement
      1) Two large-bore IV catheters
      2) Normal saline or lactated Ringer solution by rapid infusion until blood is available
      3) Colloids (e.g., albumin, hetastarch, dextran) may also be used
      4) Blood and blood products may be required
3. Control hemorrhage
   a. Pressure
      1) Grasp and pinch patient's entire nose
      2) Maintain continuous pressure over Little area (i.e., the area on the anterior portion of the nasal septum that is rich in capillaries) for ≥10 minutes with the use of a nosebleed clip, or have the patient hold the pressure
   b. Positioning: place the patient in high Fowler position and have him or her lean forward
   c. Topical vasoconstrictors: cocaine, epinephrine, or lidocaine
   d. Antihypertensives to control elevated blood pressure which may be contributing to bleeding
4. Assist with procedures to control bleeding
   a. Rapid control of massive bleeding may require the insertion of an epistaxis balloon or a Foley catheter and otolaryngology consultation
   b. If bleeding can be visualized, topical anesthetic is applied and chemical cautery performed with a silver nitrate stick
   c. If attempts to control bleeding with pressure and cautery fail, the anterior nasal cavity will be packed
      1) Cellulose (i.e., Merocel) tampon packing: removed in 1 to 2 days
      2) Oxidized cellulose (Oxycel) packing: dries up; patient can blow it out in a few days
      3) Long ribbon of petrolatum gauze: removed in 1 to 2 days
   d. Otolaryngology specialist should be consulted for posterior nasal bleeds

1) Double-balloon catheter (e.g., Nasostat, Epistat)
2) May also include anterior packing in combination with a balloon with the use of petrolatum gauze
3) Vasoconstrictors and anesthetic agents may be used, but monitor for side effects
5. Control pain and discomfort
   a. Topical anesthetics for procedures as indicated
   b. Analgesics
   c. Anxiolytics
6. Prevent infection
   a. Antibiotics as prescribed: nasal packing prevents the sinuses from draining, so an antibiotic may be prescribed
7. Monitor for complications
   a. Hemorrhage
   b. Hypovolemia and shock
   c. Septal hematoma
   d. Septal necrosis

Evaluation
1. Patent airway, adequate oxygenation (i.e., normal PaO_2, SpO_2, and SaO_2) and ventilation (i.e., normal $PaCO_2$)
2. Absence of clinical indications of respiratory distress
3. Absence of clinical indications of hypoperfusion
4. Absence of clinical indications of bleeding
5. Absence of clinical indications of infection or sepsis
6. Control of pain and discomfort

Typical disposition
1. If evaluation criteria met: discharge with instructions
   a. Antibiotics as prescribed
   b. Analgesics
   c. Return to the ED if any signs of bleeding or airway problems
   d. Follow up with otolaryngologist if discharged home with anterior packing
2. If evaluation criteria not met (e.g., posterior bleeds or difficult to control anterior bleeds): admission likely

Pharyngitis
Definitions
1. Pharyngitis: an inflammation of the pharynx
2. Laryngitis: an inflammation of the larynx
3. Tonsillitis (i.e., exudate pharyngitis): an inflammation of the tonsils

Predisposing factors
1. Upper respiratory infection
2. Recurrent streptococcal pharyngitis
3. Recurrent tonsillitis
4. Smoking or substance abuse
5. Nasal obstruction

Pathophysiology
1. Viral pharyngitis

a. Rhinovirus and adenovirus are the most common causes
b. Less common causes: Epstein-Barr virus, herpes simplex virus, influenza virus, parainfluenza virus, and corona virus (Aung & Ojha, 2009)
2. Bacterial pharyngitis
   a. Streptococcal pharyngitis
      1) Caused by group A β-hemolytic streptococci
         a) There are >80 M-protein types of group A β-hemolytic streptococci that have been isolated (Simon, 2008)
      2) Group A β-hemolytic streptococci pharyngitis is spread via respiratory secretions
      3) Incubation period is 2 to 5 days
   b. Other causes of bacterial pharyngitis: *Neisseria gonorrhoeae, Clostridium diphtheriae, Haemophilus influenzae, Moraxella catarrhalis,* and group C and G streptococci (Simon, 2008)
3. Laryngitis
   a. Inflammation caused by overuse, irritation, or infection
   b. Considered chronic if it lasts >3 weeks
      1) Chronic laryngitis is caused by irritants over time (e.g., chronic sinus drainage, excessive alcohol use)
4. Tonsillitis: usually viral in nature

Clinical presentation
1. Subjective
   a. Sore throat
   b. Pain
      1) With swallowing
      2) May radiate to jaw, ears, and neck
      3) May involve headache or body aches
   c. Fever and chills
   d. May have postnasal drip
2. Objective
   a. Elevated temperature
   b. Harsh cough
   c. Flushed face
   d. Pharynx is edematous with erythema
   e. Petechiae of the palatine tonsils
   f. Cervical lymphadenopathy
   g. May or may not have exudates in pharynx and on tonsils (i.e., pharyngitis, tonsillitis)
   h. Streptococcal pharyngitis
      1) Scarlatina rash: a fine red rash that feels similar to sandpaper; it blanches to the touch and lasts 2 to 5 days
      2) Strawberry appearance to the tongue caused by enlarged papillae
      3) Foul breath
   i. Laryngitis
      1) Dysphonia (i.e., hoarseness) or aphonia (i.e., no voice)
      2) Dyspnea and stridor maybe present
      3) Swelling of larynx and epiglottis
      4) Larynx erythemic

3. Diagnostic studies
   a. Rapid *Streptococcus* screen: 98% accurate if a good swab of the throat is obtained
   b. Throat culture

Collaborative management
1. Continue assessment
   a. ABCDs
   b. Vital signs: blood pressure, pulse, respiratory rate, and temperature
   c. Oxygen saturation
   d. Respiratory effort and excursion
   e. Pain and discomfort level
   f. Close monitoring for the progression of symptoms
2. Control pain and discomfort
   a. Analgesics
   b. Topical anesthetics: 2% viscous lidocaine, benzocaine spray (Cetacaine), or phenol spray (Chloraseptic)
   c. Corticosteroids: decrease swelling and inflammation
   d. Zinc throat lozenges
   e. Ice to the anterior neck
   f. Warm saline or salt-water gargles
3. Treat infection and prevent sepsis
   a. Increased oral fluids; intravenous fluids may be required
   b. Antimicrobials
   c. Antipyretics
4. Monitor for complications
   a. Sinusitis
   b. Otitis media
   c. Peritonsillar abscess
   d. Retropharyngeal abscess

Evaluation
1. Patent airway, adequate oxygenation (i.e., normal PaO_2, SpO_2, and SaO_2) and ventilation (i.e., normal $PaCO_2$)
2. Absence of clinical indications of respiratory distress
3. Absence of clinical indications of hypoperfusion
4. Absence of clinical indications of infection or sepsis
5. Control of pain and discomfort

Typical disposition: discharge with instructions
1. Warm saline or salt-water gargles for comfort
2. Increased fluid intake
3. Rest in a warm environment with humidification
4. Ice to the anterior neck
5. Avoidance of use of voice for patients with laryngitis
6. Antipyretics for fever
7. Antimicrobials as directed
8. Follow up with primary care provider as directed

Peritonsillar Abscess
Definition: the colonization of the peritonsillar area by aerobic and anaerobic bacteria that results in the formation of an abscess
Predisposing factors
1. Recurrent tonsillitis
2. Immunosuppression
3. Recent upper respiratory infection

Pathophysiology
1. Infection begins superficially and then progresses into the deep soft tissues
   a. Most common aerobic cause: *Streptococcus* species (usually *Streptococcus pyogenes*)
   b. Most common anaerobic cause: *Prevotella* species and *Peptostreptococcus* species
2. The abscess forms between the palatine tonsil and its capsule, most commonly at the superior pole

Clinical presentation
1. Subjective
   a. Pain and discomfort
      1) Sore throat and pain with swallowing
      2) Otalgia
   b. Difficulty swallowing own saliva or drooling
   c. Fever and chills
   d. Throat feels swollen
   e. Bad breath and bad taste in mouth
2. Objective
   a. Temperature of >100°F
   b. Tachycardia
   c. Drooling
   d. Trismus: (i.e., difficulty opening the mouth)
   e. "Hot potato"/muffled voice: sounds like the patient is talking with hot food in the mouth
   f. Anterior cervical lymphadenopathy; lymph nodes tender to palpation
   g. Erythema and swelling of tonsils and uvula (with possible deviation and asymmetry)
   h. Exudate on the tonsil or the posterior pharynx
   i. Torticollis (i.e., twisting of the neck related to cervical muscle contraction)
3. Diagnostic
   a. Monospot: to rule out mononucleosis if the diagnosis is unclear
   b. Needle aspiration of abscess
   c. Culture and sensitivity of drainage from abscess

Collaborative management
1. Continue assessment
   a. ABCDs
   b. Vital signs: blood pressure, pulse, respiratory rate, and temperature
   c. Oxygen saturation
   d. Respiratory effort and excursion
   e. Pain and discomfort level
   f. Clinical indications of dehydration
   g. Close monitoring for the progression of symptoms
2. Maintain airway, oxygenation, ventilation, and perfusion
   a. 100% oxygen by face mask or blow by to maintain an SpO_2 of 95% unless contraindicated; for patients with COPD, use pulse oximetry to guide oxygen administration to an SpO_2 of 90%
   b. Positioning: place the patient in high Fowler position to optimize breathing and decrease effort

c. Suctioning: provide patient with Yankauer tonsil tip
d. Intubation and mechanical ventilation if patient is unable to maintain airway
e. Replacement of vascular volume
1) Two large-bore IV catheters
2) Normal saline for hydration as needed
3. Control pain and discomfort
a. Analgesics
b. Ice collar to the anterior neck
c. Topical anesthetic spray: benzocaine (Hurricaine), phenol (Chloraseptic), aminobenzoate, and tetracaine (Cetacaine)
4. Prepare the patient and assist with procedures
a. Positioning: high Fowler position
b. Needle aspiration for symptom relief and culture
c. Incision and drainage
1) Lidocaine and epinephrine solution for anesthetic; usually will use a No. 11 blade
2) Yankauer suction available during procedure
5. Treat infection and prevent sepsis
a. Antimicrobials
b. Antipyretics
6. Monitor for complications
a. Airway obstruction
b. Rupture of abscess leading to aspiration pneumonitis
c. Sepsis
d. Extension of infection into mediastinum
e. Poststreptococcal sequelae (secondary infection)

Evaluation
1. Patent airway, adequate oxygenation (i.e., normal PaO_2, SpO_2, and SaO_2) and ventilation (i.e., normal $PaCO_2$)
2. Absence of clinical indications of respiratory distress
3. Absence of clinical indications of hypoperfusion
4. Absence of clinical indications of infection or sepsis
5. Control of pain and discomfort

Typical disposition
1. If evaluation criteria met: discharge with instructions
a. Ice collar applied to neck
b. Rest with the head elevated
c. Medications as prescribed
d. Instructions to return to the ED immediately for uncontrolled fever or any swallowing or airway difficulties develop
2. If evaluation criteria not met: admission

Retropharyngeal Abscess
Definition: the colonization of the retropharyngeal area by aerobic and anaerobic bacteria that results in the formation of an abscess
Predisposing factors
1. Seen primarily in children <6 years old but may be seen in adults
2. Upper respiratory infections

3. Sinusitis
4. Otitis
5. Instrumentation trauma or other trauma (e.g., oral intubation, fishbone)

Pathophysiology
1. Retropharyngeal space is posterior to the pharynx
a. Anteriorly it is bound by the buccopharyngeal fascia
b. Posteriorly it is bound by the prevertebral fascia
c. Laterally it is bound by the carotid sheaths
d. Extends superiorly to the base of the skull and inferiorly to the mediastinum
2. Infection usually spreads from the tonsils, throat, sinuses, adenoids, nose, or middle ear
a. Causative organisms
1) Aerobic: β-hemolytic streptococci and *Staphylococcus aureus*
2) Anaerobic: *Bacteroides* and *Veillonella*
3) Gram negative: *Haemophilus parainfluenzae* and *Bartonella henselae*
3. May cause airway obstruction

Clinical presentation
1. Subjective
a. Sudden onset of symptoms: <24 hours
b. Severe pain
1) Sore throat
a. Odynophagia (i.e., painful swallowing)
b. Dysphagia
c. Fever and chills
d. Neck stiffness and swelling
e. Agitation or fussiness in infant
2. Objective
a. In adults
1) Temperature of >101°F
2) Posterior pharyngeal swelling
3) Nuchal rigidity
4) Cervical adenopathy
5) Drooling
6) Stridor possible
b. In infants and children
1) Elevated temperature
2) Cervical adenopathy
3) Neck stiffness or torticollis
4) Drooling
5) Neck mass; be cautious because it may rupture if palpated
6) May have torticollis (i.e., twisting of the neck related to cervical muscle contraction)
7) Lethargy or altered level of consciousness
8) Associated signs, including tonsillitis, pharyngitis, and otitis media
3. Diagnostic
a. CBC: elevated WBC count (occasionally normal)
b. C-reactive protein: elevated
c. Culture of abscess

d. Chest radiography will show aspiration pneumonia and mediastinitis if present

e. Lateral neck radiography: widening of retropharyngeal space
   1) Swelling of >7 mm at C2 and of >14 cm at C6 (ENA, 2007)

f. CT if difficulty viewing retropharyngeal space on plain film

Collaborative management

1. Continue assessment
   a. ABCDs
   b. Vital signs: blood pressure, pulse, respiratory rate, and temperature
   c. Oxygen saturation
   d. Respiratory effort and excursion
   e. Cardiac rate and rhythm
   f. Pain and discomfort level
   g. Clinical indications of dehydration
   h. Close monitoring for the progression of symptoms

2. Maintain airway, oxygenation, ventilation, and perfusion
   a. 100% oxygen by face mask or blow by to maintain an SpO_2 of 95% unless contraindicated; for patients with COPD, use pulse oximetry to guide oxygen administration to an SpO_2 of 90%
   b. Positioning: high Fowler position to optimize breathing and decrease effort
   c. Suctioning: Yankauer tonsil tip suction
   d. Rapid-sequence intubation and mechanical ventilation if patient is unable to maintain airway
      1) If unable to intubate patient, needle or surgical cricothyrotomy is indicated
   e. Emergent otolaryngology consult
   f. Replacement of vascular volume
      1) Two large-bore IV catheters
      2) Normal saline for hydration as needed

3. Control pain and discomfort: analgesics

4. Treat infection and prevent sepsis
   a. Antibiotics: clindamycin (Cleocin) and metronidazole (Flagyl)
   b. Antipyretics

5. Monitor for complications
   a. Airway obstruction and laryngospasm
   b. Bleeding around or rupture of the abscess
   c. Pneumonia
   d. Jugular thrombosis
   e. Sepsis or septic shock

Evaluation

1. Patent airway, adequate oxygenation (i.e., normal PaO_2, SpO_2, and SaO_2) and ventilation (i.e., normal $PaCO_2$)
2. Absence of clinical indications of respiratory distress
3. Absence of clinical indications of hypoperfusion
4. Absence of clinical indications of infection or sepsis
5. Control of pain and discomfort

Typical disposition: admission

Diphtheria

Definition: an infection caused by *Corynebacterium diphtheriae* that can affect the respiratory tract, the skin, the throat, the heart, and the nerves

Predisposing factors

1. *C. diphtheriae* is an aerobe that is found in the human throat
2. Crowded environments
3. Poor hygiene
4. Lack of immunization or partial immunization

Pathophysiology

1. *C. diphtheriae* is usually a harmless disease that is caused by a lysogenized phage (i.e., a cell that carries an extra gene of the virus)
2. Transmission
   a. Transmitted by direct contact or airborne droplets
   b. *C. diphtheriae* can survive on dry inanimate surfaces for ≥7 days
   c. Patient is considered contagious until 4 days after receiving medication for treatment
   d. If untreated, the disease can spread for ≤2 weeks after exposure
   e. Incubation period is 2 to 5 days

Clinical presentation

1. Subjective
   a. Recent travel to endemic area
   b. Fever
   c. Sore throat or difficulty swallowing
   d. Headache
   e. Malaise, anorexia, or nausea
   f. Sweating and pallor
2. Objective
   a. Tachycardia
   b. Temperature of >101°F
   c. Respiratory distress: increased effort
   d. Bluish-white membrane on the tonsils and soft palate after 2 to 3 days that will change color to greenish or black with hemorrhage
   e. Cervical lymphadenopathy; lymph nodes tender to palpation
   f. Marked edema of submandibular area can present as a "bull neck" appearance in patients with severe disease
   g. Cranial neuropathies
3. Diagnostic
   a. CBC with differential: elevated WBC count (leukocytosis) and decreased platelet count (i.e., thrombocytopenia)
   b. ECG: first-degree AV block and ST and T wave abnormalities may occur
   c. Chest radiography: subglottic narrowing
   d. Throat culture: from beneath the membrane
      1) Black culture on tellurite plate

2) Granules stain metachromatically (i.e., methylene blue)

e. Schick skin test: injection procedure that is similar to tuberculosis tine test but rarely used

f. Gel diffusion precipitin test: to test for toxin

Collaborative management

1. Continue assessment
   a. ABCDs
   b. Vital signs: blood pressure, pulse, respiratory rate, and temperature
   c. Oxygen saturation
   d. Respiratory effort and excursion
   e. Clinical indications of dehydration
   f. Close monitoring for the progression of symptoms
2. Maintain airway, oxygenation, ventilation, and perfusion
   a. 100% oxygen by face mask or blow by to maintain an SpO_2 of 95% unless contraindicated; for patients with COPD, use pulse oximetry to guide oxygen administration to an SpO_2 of 90%
   b. Rapid-sequence intubation and mechanical ventilation if patient is unable to maintain airway
      1) If unable to intubate patient, needle or surgical cricothyrotomy is indicated
   c. Circulating volume replacement
      1) Two large-bore IV catheters
      2) Normal saline for hydration as needed
3. Treat infection and prevent sepsis
   a. Immediate equine antitoxin (possible before diagnosis is confirmed)
      1) Diphtheria antitoxin available through the Centers for Disease Control and Prevention
         a) Sensitivity testing before actual administration of antitoxin (either intradermal or via mucous membrane)
   b. Antibiotics: erythromycin (E-Mycin) or penicillin G used only to halt further toxin production or to prevent carrier state
   c. Antipyretics
4. Control pain and discomfort
   a. Topical anesthetic agents
   b. Analgesics
   c. Antitussives
5. Monitor for complications
   a. Airway obstruction
   b. Recurrent laryngeal nerve palsy
   c. Septicemia
   d. Endocarditis
   e. Myocarditis

Evaluation

1. Patent airway, adequate oxygenation (i.e., normal PaO_2, SpO_2, and SaO_2) and ventilation (i.e., normal $PaCO_2$)
2. Absence of clinical indications of respiratory distress
3. Absence of clinical indications of hypoperfusion
4. Absence of clinical indications of infection or sepsis
5. Control of pain and discomfort

Typical disposition: admission

1. Identification of close contacts: culture and provide prophylactic antibiotics
2. Tetanus-diphtheria (booster if >5 years since last booster)
   a. If no previous immunization, then start a three-shot series of immunizations per the Centers for Disease Control and Prevention guidelines

Conjunctivitis

Definition: an inflammation of the conjunctiva marked by hyperemia and mucopurulent drainage

Predisposing factors

1. Allergic
   a. Ocular exposure to allergen
      1) Usually inhaled (i.e., airborne) allergens
      2) Also contact allergens
2. Viral
   a. Exposure to viruses (e.g., the common cold)
   b. Adenovirus types 3, 4, and 7 and herpes simplex
3. Bacterial
   a. Exposure to bacteria
   b. Incompletely opened tear duct
   c. Herpetic conditions
   d. Neonates are at risk for conjunctival chlamydia and *N. gonorrhoeae* during vaginal delivery

Pathophysiology

1. Allergic
   a. Associated with a type 1 hypersensitivity
   b. Also known as *atopic* or *seasonal allergic conjunctivitis*
   c. Allergic response on ocular and tarsal conjunctival surfaces
      1) Causes a cross linkage of membrane-bound immunoglobulin E and triggers mast cell degranulation
      2) Then there is a cascade of allergic and inflammatory mediators that is released
   d. Histamine is the primary contributor to the development of distinct signs and symptoms
2. Viral (Scott & Luu, 2007)
   a. Adenoviral conjunctivitis is the most common cause
   b. Adenoviral conjunctivitis subtypes: epidemic keratoconjunctivitis (i.e., pink eye) and pharyngoconjunctival fever
   c. Transmission via contact with infected upper respiratory droplets, fomites, and contaminated swimming pools
3. Bacterial
   a. Invading bacteria produce exotoxins
   b. This induces an antigen–antibody immune reaction causing inflammation
   c. Common bacteria: *Staphylococcus aureus*, *Haemophilus influenzae*, *Streptococcus pneumoniae*, and *Pseudomonas aeruginosa*

Clinical presentation

1. Subjective
   a. May or may not have pain in the affected eye
   b. Gritty sensation in the affected eye

c. Redness, itching, and burning of the affected eye
d. Drainage from the affected eye
e. Photophobia
2. Objective
   a. Red or pink conjunctiva
   b. Purulent discharge (bacterial)
   c. Watery discharge (allergic)
   d. Eyelid edema
   e. Chemosis (i.e., swelling of the conjunctiva)
3. Diagnostic
   a. Cultures of discharge
   b. Fluorescein stain: herpes simplex shows corneal dendrites (branching pattern)

Collaborative management
1. Continue assessment
   a. ABCDs
   b. Pain and discomfort level
   c. Drainage from the affected eye
   d. Close monitoring for the progression of symptoms
2. Control pain and discomfort
   a. Nonsteroidal anti-inflammatory drugs for a viral cause
   b. Cool compresses for a viral cause
   c. Warm compresses for a bacterial cause
   d. Antihistamines and topical vasoconstrictors for an allergic cause
   e. Avoidance of the rubbing of the eye
3. Treat infection and prevent sepsis or further complications
   a. Broad-spectrum antibiotic ointment or drops for a bacterial cause
   b. Instructions regarding the cleansing of the eye by wiping gently from the inner eye to the outer eye
   c. Fluoroquinolone if the patient wears contact lens
   d. Ophthalmology referral for herpes simplex
4. Monitor for complications
   a. Corneal ulceration
   b. Decreased vision

Evaluation
1. Absence of clinical indications of infection or sepsis
2. Control of pain and discomfort
3. Absence of visual deficit

Typical disposition: discharge with instructions
1. Instillation of medication; do not touch the dropper of the medication bottle to the eye
2. Frequent hand washing with good technique
3. Avoidance of eye makeup for a week; throw away eye makeup and start with new products
4. Allergic and viral
   a. Identification and removal of irritants
   b. Cold compresses during waking hours for comfort
   c. Avoidance of eye rubbing, which worsens symptoms
   d. Avoidance of allergens
5. Bacterial
   a. Considered contagious until the patient has been taking antibiotics for 24 hours; the patient should stay home from school or work
   b. Avoidance of the touching of the eye
      1) If the eye is accidentally touched, thorough hand washing should be performed immediately
   c. Warm compresses as directed
6. Consult ophthalmologist as directed or if any of the following occur:
   a. Painful red eye
   b. Prominent light sensitivity
   c. Pupil irregularity or sluggish response to light
   d. Chronic condition with vision impairment
   e. Fluorescein stain that is positive for ulcers
   f. Papillary conjunctival changes

Iritis and Uveitis
Definitions
1. Iritis and uveitis: inflammatory processes that include the iris and the uveal layer of the anterior segment of the eye
   a. Posterior uveitis is also known as *choroiditis* (rare)
2. Iridocyclitis: the ciliary body and the iris are inflamed

Predisposing factors
1. Spondyloarthropathies
2. Systemic immune illnesses (e.g., lupus, rheumatic disease)

Pathophysiology
1. Immunologically mediated breakdown of the blood aqueous barrier that results in inflammation in the anterior chamber
2. Symptoms of acute anterior uveitis may develop over 1 to 2 days without affecting vision
3. Types
   a. Infectious
   b. Noninfectious
   c. Human leukocyte antigen association
   d. Idiopathic

Clinical presentation
1. Subjective
   a. Unilateral eye pain
      1) Gradual onset
      2) Photophobia
   b. Blurred vision
   c. Excessive tearing
   d. Edema of the upper eyelid
   e. Redness
2. Objective
   a. Redness
   b. Cornea that is clear to hazy
   c. Pupil of the affected eye is constricted (i.e., miosis), sluggish, and irregular in shape
   d. Ciliary flushing: a ring of red or violet around the cornea of the eye
   e. Hypopyon: an effusion of pus in the anterior chamber
3. Diagnostic
   a. Vision testing: decreased visual acuity
      1) Visual acuity testing with a pinhole at first presentation for acute anterior uveitis
   b. Slit-lamp examination: inflammatory cells in the anterior chamber; this is the hallmark assessment

1) Muddy to grayish appearance from endothelial deposits known as *keratic precipitates* can occur

c. Tonometry: intraocular pressure is low to slightly elevated

d. Fundus examination: interior surface of the eye

e. Fluorescein stain

Collaborative management

1. Continue assessment
   a. ABCDs
   b. Pain and discomfort level
   c. Visual acuity
   d. Close monitoring for the progression of symptoms
2. Control pain and discomfort
   a. Nonsteroidal anti-inflammatory drugs
   b. Analgesics
   c. Dark room
   d. Warm compresses
   e. Rest
   f. Eye shield or dark glasses for photosensitivity; eye should not be patched
   g. Cycloplegic agents for mydriasis, pain reduction, photophobia, and the treatment of pupillary synechiae (i.e., a condition in which the iris adheres to the cornea)
3. Reduce inflammation
   a. Nonsteroidal anti-inflammatory drugs
   b. Topical corticosteroids
   c. Fluorometholone (Flarex) ointment at bedtime (Fultz & Sturt, 2005)
4. Monitor for complications
   a. Macular edema
   b. Permanent vision loss

Evaluation

1. Absence of clinical indications of infection or sepsis
2. Control of pain and discomfort
3. Absence of visual deficit

Typical disposition: discharge with instructions

1. Use of eye shield for affected eye or to wear dark sunglasses
2. Importance of resting the eyes (i.e., no reading)
3. Instructions regarding how to instill eye drops
4. Immediate referral to an ophthalmologist

Periorbital Cellulitis

Definition: a spreading inflammation of the subcutaneous or connective tissue around the eyes

Predisposing factors

1. Trauma: usually lacerations or insect bites
2. Infections (e.g., conjunctivitis, hordeolum, impetigo)
3. Diabetes
4. Immunocompromise

Pathophysiology

1. Infections as a result of hematogenous spread during bacteremia caused by nasopharyngeal pathogens
2. Pathogens with traumatic causes
   a. *Staphylococcus aureus* and *Streptococcus pyogenes* (i.e., group A streptococci)
3. Nontraumatic pathogenic causes
   a. *Streptococcus pneumoniae* and *H. influenzae*

Clinical presentation

1. Subjective
   a. History of underlying illness that increases risk of infection
   b. Pain: increases with eye movement
   c. Fever and chills
   d. Redness and rapid swelling of the eyelid
2. Objective
   a. Elevated temperature
   b. Periorbital erythema and edema
   c. Decreased pupil reflexes
   d. Erythema and tenderness of the lids without evidence of orbital congestion
   e. Vesicles if associated with herpetic infection
   f. Break in the skin overlying the area of cellulitis may be present if the condition is caused by trauma
3. Diagnostic
   a. CBC with differential if sepsis is suspected
   b. Blood cultures
   c. Culture of discharge
   d. CT of orbits to rule out orbital and subperiosteal involvement
   e. MRI to rule out cavernous sinus thrombosis
   f. Lumbar puncture if *H. influenzae* type b or *Streptococcus pneumoniae* is suspected to rule out meningitis

Collaborative management

1. Continue assessment
   a. ABCDs
   b. Vital signs: blood pressure, pulse, respiratory rate, and temperature
   c. Oxygen saturation
   d. Cardiac rate and rhythm
   e. Pain and discomfort level
   f. Clinical indications of dehydration
   g. Close monitoring for the progression of symptoms
2. Control pain and discomfort
   a. Analgesics
   b. Bed rest
   c. Warm compresses
3. Treat infection and prevent sepsis
   a. Antibiotics: IV, oral, and optic ointments or drops
   b. Antipyretics and cooling methods to reduce fever
4. Monitor for complications
   a. Blindness
   b. Cavernous sinus thrombosis
   c. Intracranial abscess

Evaluation

1. Absence of clinical indications of infection or sepsis
2. Control of pain and discomfort

3. Absence of visual deficit
4. Absence of clinical indications of hypoperfusion

Typical disposition

1. If evaluation criteria met (i.e., mild): discharge with instructions
   a. Oral and optic antibiotics as directed
   b. Warm compresses
   c. Follow up with ophthalmologist within 24 hours
   d. Instructions to return to the ED immediately for increased pain or swelling or worsening of symptoms
2. If evaluation criteria not met: admission for IV antibiotics
   a. Orbital abscesses require surgery

Glaucoma

Definition: an abnormally high fluid pressure in the eye

Predisposing factors

1. Higher incidence among African Americans, Asians, Hispanics, and Alaskan natives
2. Aging
3. Family history of glaucoma
4. Myopia: nearsightedness
5. Eye trauma
6. Corticosteroids
7. Medical conditions: diabetes, hypertension, and hypothyroidism
8. Acute episodes may be precipitated by anticholinergic or sympathomimetic medications (Fultz & Sturt, 2005)

Pathophysiology

1. Usually a slow increase in intraocular pressure within the aqueous chamber
2. Ischemia occurs as the pressure increases
3. Damage to the retina and optic nerve results if the condition is not treated; peripheral vision loss may progress to total blindness
4. Types: open angle and acute closed angle (Figure 10-4)

   a. Open-angle glaucoma: occurs over time as drainage channels gradually become clogged
   b. Acute closed-angle glaucoma: occurs when pressure increases suddenly because the filtering angle becomes closed and blocks off the drainage channels

Clinical presentation

1. Subjective
   a. Primary open-angle glaucoma: usually asymptomatic during the early stages
   b. Acute closed-angle glaucoma: presents with severe ocular pain
   c. Eye redness
   d. Headache: may be mistaken for a migraine
      1) Migraine pain usually has a pulsating quality, whereas glaucoma pain is described as a continuous boring pain (Fultz & Sturt, 2005)
      2) New onset of migraines among individuals ≥50 years is unusual
   e. Decreased vision and halos
   f. Nausea and vomiting
   g. Excessive tearing
2. Objective
   a. Cornea hazy or cloudy
   b. Affected pupil midline and sluggish or nonreactive
   c. Intraocular pressure >20 mm Hg
   d. Globe feels like a rock when palpated
3. Diagnostic
   a. Visual testing: visual acuity decreased
   b. Slit-lamp examination: provides a stereoscopic magnified view of the eye structures in detail
   c. Intraocular pressure measurement
      1) Schiotz (indentation)
      2) Applanation tonometry
   d. Gonioscopy: examination performed by an ophthalmologist to determine whether the drainage angle of filtration is open or closed

Collaborative management

1. Continue assessment
   a. ABCDs

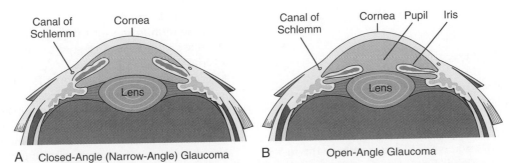

Figure 10-4 Closed-angle (narrow-angle) glaucoma compared with open-angle glaucoma. **A,** In closed-angle glaucoma, the outflow of aqueous humor is obstructed by the iris roof of the dilated pupil. **B,** In open-angle glaucoma, the obstruction to the outflow of aqueous humor is in the drainage canals. (From Copstead, L. E., & Banasik, J. L. [2010]. *Pathophysiology* [4th ed.]. Philadelphia: Saunders, p. 1164, Figure 46-11.).

b. Vital signs: blood pressure, pulse, respiratory rate, and temperature
c. Pain and discomfort level
d. Visual acuity
e. Intraocular pressure
f. Close monitoring for the progression of symptoms
2. Control pain and discomfort
   a. Analgesics
   b. Antiemetics
3. Decrease intraocular pressure pharmacologically
   a. β-Blockers (e.g., timolol [Timoptic]) decrease the production of aqueous humor
   b. Cholinergic agents (e.g., pilocarpine [Salagen]) constrict pupils, thereby resulting in an improved outflow of aqueous humor
      1) 2% solution for light-colored eyes
      2) 4% solution for dark-colored eyes
   c. Carbonic anhydrase inhibitors (e.g., acetazolamide [Diamox]) decrease the secretion of aqueous humor
4. Monitor for complications
   a. Visual impairment
      1) Blind spots in the peripheral vision
      2) Tunnel vision
      3) Total blindness

Evaluation

1. Control of pain and discomfort
2. Decrease in intraocular pressure
3. Absence of visual deficit

Typical disposition

1. If evaluation criteria met: discharge with instructions
   a. Medications and proper instillation of eye drops
   b. Follow up with ophthalmologic consultant
2. If evaluation criteria not met: admission for surgery

Central Retinal Artery Occlusion

Definition: the occlusion of the central artery of the retina that results in sudden unilateral blindness
1. Amaurosis fugax (also known as *transient monocular blindness*): the temporary loss of vision in one eye caused by a lack of blood flow to the retina

Predisposing factors

1. Systemic hypertension
2. Diabetes mellitus
3. Cardiac valvular disease or anomalies
4. Embolism
5. Increased intraocular pressure (e.g., glaucoma)
6. Coagulopathies

Pathophysiology (Graham & Ebrahim, 2009)

1. Visual loss occurs when the blood supply to the inner layer of the retina is lost
2. During the acute stage, the obstruction of the central retinal artery will cause edema in the inner layer of the retina and a degeneration of the cell nucleus that is marked by the clumping of the chromosomes

3. Ischemic necrosis will then occur, and the retina becomes opacified and takes on a yellowish-white appearance
4. Amaurosis fugax is thought to be the result of a clot of plaque in the carotid artery that has broken off and traveled to the retinal artery; unlike central retinal artery occlusion, spontaneous improvement usually occurs within minutes (Fultz & Sturt, 2005)

Clinical presentation

1. Subjective
   a. History of a preexisting condition that contributes to central retinal artery occlusion
   b. No pain
   c. Sudden unilateral loss of vision
2. Objective
   a. Visual acuity limited to light perception in the affected eye
   b. Dilated and nonreactive pupil
   c. Ophthalmoscopic examination
      1) Optic nerve examination to look for signs of temporal arteritis
         a) Afferent pupillary defect and a pale and swollen optic nerve with splinter hemorrhages
      2) Cherry-red spot
      3) Ground-glass appearance of the retina; this may take hours to develop
      4) Emboli can be seen in ≈20% of patients
3. Diagnostic
   a. CBC: anemia, polycythemia, and platelet disorders
   b. ESR: elevated
   c. Clotting profile: coagulopathy may be evident
   d. Blood cultures: to rule out bacterial endocarditis and septic emboli
   e. Fluorescein angiogram: shows a delay in arteriovenous transit time and retinal arterial filling

Collaborative management

1. Continue assessment
   a. ABCDs
   b. Vital signs: blood pressure, pulse, respiratory rate, and temperature
   c. Visual acuity
   d. Intraocular pressure
   e. Close monitoring for the progression of symptoms
2. Decrease intraocular pressure to promote retinal arterial flow
   a. IV access with two large-bore IV catheters; normal saline for hydration as needed
   b. β-Blockers (e.g., timolol [Timoptic]) decrease the production of aqueous humor
   c. Cholinergic agents (e.g., pilocarpine [Salagen]) constrict pupils, thereby resulting in an improved outflow of aqueous humor
      1) 2% solution for light-colored eyes
      2) 4% solution for dark-colored eyes
   d. Carbonic anhydrase inhibitors (e.g., acetazolamide [Diamox]) decrease the secretion of aqueous humor

e. Carbogen gas in 3- to 10-minute treatments every 2 hours; this substance dilates the retinal arterioles and increases oxygen delivery to ischemic tissues

f. Gentle digital globe massage (only to be performed by a physician)

g. Hyperbaric oxygen chamber may be beneficial if used within 2 to 12 hours of the onset of the condition

h. Fibrinolytics and anticoagulants: tissue plasminogen activator (Activase) and heparin

i. Surgery though salvage of vision is rare after 2 hours from the time of onset

3. Monitor for complications

a. Cerebrovascular accident as a result of emboli traveling to the brain

b. Vision loss as a result of emboli or the progression of temporal arteritis

Evaluation

1. Absence of clinical indications of hypoperfusion
2. Absence of clinical indications of infection or sepsis
3. Control of pain and discomfort
4. Absence of visual deficit

Typical disposition: admission and possible surgery

Corneal Ulcer or Abrasion

Definition

1. Corneal ulcer: a defect in the epithelial layer of the cornea with underlying inflammation
2. Corneal abrasion: the partial or complete removal of the epithelium of the cornea, most commonly as a result of eye injury
3. Keratitis: the acute infection or chronic nonulcerative infiltration of the deep layers of cornea with uveal inflammation

Predisposing factors

1. Contact lens wear
2. Dryness of the eyes
3. Foreign bodies
4. Inflammation

Pathophysiology

1. Corneal ulcer
   a. Necrosis of corneal tissue can occur as a result of the invasion of bacteria, fungi, or viruses
   b. Ulcers tend to heal and leave scar tissue in the injured area, which causes opacification of the cornea and decreased visual acuity
2. Corneal abrasion
   a. Superficial abrasions do not involve the Bowman membrane
   b. Deep abrasions penetrate the Bowman membrane without rupture of the Descemet membrane
   c. Usually heals in 24 to 48 hours as a result of the rapid migration and proliferation of the corneal epithelium

3. Keratitis
   a. Inflammation of the cornea that involves the transparent dome-like portion of the eyeball in front of the iris and pupil

Clinical presentation

1. Subjective
   a. Pain or discomfort in the eye
      1) Photophobia
   a. Ciliary muscle spasms
   b. Red eyes
   c. Excessive tearing or pus draining from the eye
   d. Visual disturbance: blurring
2. Objective
   a. White patch visible on the cornea
   b. Excessive tearing or blinking
   c. Red, swollen upper and lower eyelids
   d. Purulent discharge may be seen
3. Diagnostic
   a. Visual acuity: usually normal
   b. Fluorescein stain of cornea: damaged area will take up stain
   c. Scraping of ulcer for culture

Collaborative management

1. Continue assessment
   a. ABCDs
   b. Pain and discomfort level
   c. Visual acuity
   d. Close monitoring for the progression of symptoms
2. Control pain and discomfort
   a. Analgesics
   b. Cool compresses to the affected eye
   c. Cycloplegic drops to relieve ciliary spasms
3. Treat inflammation and prevent infection
   a. Topical antibiotic drops or ointment
   b. Eye patching usually not performed today
   c. Corticosteroid drops
   d. Tetanus immunization
   e. Dark room or sunglasses to decrease photophobia and to rest the eyes
4. Monitor for complications
   a. Corneal scarring
   b. Loss of vision
   c. Loss of eye

Evaluation

1. Absence of clinical indications of infection or sepsis
2. Control of pain and discomfort
3. Absence of visual deficit

Typical disposition: discharge with instructions

1. Cool compresses to the affected eye as directed
2. Avoidance of touching and rubbing of the affected eye
3. Frequent hand washing to limit the spread of infection

Blepharitis

Definition: an acute or chronic inflammation of the lid margin

Predisposing factors
1. Seborrheic dermatitis
2. Bacterial infection
3. Rosacea
4. Allergies
5. Infestation of lice in the lashes

Pathophysiology
1. Anterior blepharitis involves the eyelid skin, the eyelashes, and the associated glands; the two main types are as follows:
    a. The seborrheic type, which is associated with seborrhea of the scalp and brows
    b. The staphylococcal type, which is associated with *Staphylococcus epidermidis* or *Staphylococcus aureus*
2. Posterior blepharitis involves the eyelids and the meibomian glands
    a. May be caused by staphylococci or dysfunction of the meibomian glands (strong association with rosacea)
    b. Involves inflammation of the meibomian glands and their orifices along with the dilation of the glands, the plugging of the orifices, and abnormal secretions

Clinical presentation
1. Subjective
    a. Watery, itchy eyes
    b. Gritty, burning sensations
    c. Crusted eyelashes in the morning
    d. Photosensitivity
2. Objective
    a. Crusting of the eyelid
    b. Scaling and whitening of the eyelashes
    c. Swelling and redness of eyelid
    d. Loss of or misdirected eyelashes
    e. Ulcerations along the eyelid margins
3. Diagnostic
    a. Biopsy may be indicated to rule out malignancy

Collaborative management
1. Continue assessment
    a. ABCDs
    b. Vital signs: blood pressure, pulse, respiratory rate, and temperature
    c. Pain and discomfort level
    d. Visual acuity
    e. Close monitoring for the progression of symptoms
2. Control pain and discomfort
    a. Analgesics: topical ointment or drops
    b. Warm compresses
    c. Good hand-washing technique

3. Treat infection if present and prevent sepsis
    a. Antibiotic ophthalmic ointment (e.g., Bacitracin [Ocu-Tracin], erythromycin [E-Mycin])
    b. Oral antibiotics as prescribed
4. Monitor for complications
    a. Excess tearing or dry eyes
    b. Chronic pink eye

Evaluation
1. Absence of clinical indications of infection or sepsis
2. Control of pain and discomfort
3. Absence of visual deficit
4. Decrease in redness and tearing

Typical disposition: discharge with instructions
1. Medications as prescribed
2. Good hand-washing technique
3. Warm compresses
4. Follow up with ophthalmologist

Hordeolum and Chalazion

Definitions
1. Hordeolum: a bacterial infection that develops near the root of an eyelash; also referred to as a *sty*
2. Chalazion: a small circumscribed cyst of the eyelid that is formed by the retention of secretions of the meibomian gland; may be accompanied by inflammation

Predisposing factors
1. Diabetes
2. Debilitating illness
3. Chronic blepharitis
4. Seborrhea
5. High serum lipid levels

Pathophysiology
1. Hordeolum
    a. Infection of the sebaceous glands of the eye
    b. Staphylococcal organisms are the most common cause
2. Chalazion
    a. Inflammation of the meibomian gland
    b. May follow internal hordeolum

Clinical presentation
1. Subjective
    a. Painful swelling of one eye
    b. Redness
2. Objective
    a. Localized tender area of swelling
    b. Eruption either on the internal or external side of the eyelid
3. Diagnostic
    a. None; diagnosed by physical assessment

Collaborative management

1. Continue assessment
   a. ABCDs
   b. Pain and discomfort level
   c. Visual acuity
   d. Close monitoring for the progression of symptoms
2. Control pain and discomfort
   a. Analgesics
   b. Warm compresses to the eyelids
3. Treat inflammation and infection
   a. Antibiotics if prescribed; though hordeolum is a bacterial infection, antibiotics are not usually prescribed
   b. Preparation for incision and drainage if indicated
4. Monitor for complications: systemic infection

Evaluation

1. Absence of clinical indications of infection or sepsis
2. Control of pain and discomfort
3. Absence of visual deficit

Typical disposition: discharge with instructions

1. Warm compresses
2. Medications as prescribed
3. Follow up with ophthalmologist as directed

Extraocular Foreign Bodies

Definition: foreign bodies on the surface of the eye

1. Usually related to occupation or trauma
2. Metal is of great concern because rust may invade the cornea

Predisposing factors

1. Trauma
2. Industrial related

Clinical presentation

1. Subjective
   a. Pain
   b. Sensation of foreign body
   c. Blurring of vision
2. Objective
   a. Red, tearing eye
   b. Visualization of foreign bodies
   c. Visual acuity may be abnormal
3. Diagnostic
   a. Visual acuity can be normal to slightly abnormal
   b. Fluorescein stain: damaged area takes up stain
   c. Slit-lamp examination

Collaborative management

1. Continue assessment
   a. ABCDs
   b. Vital signs: blood pressure, pulse, respiratory rate, and temperature
   c. Pain and discomfort level
   d. Visual acuity
   e. Pupil size, shape, and reactivity
   f. Close monitoring for the progression of symptoms
2. Control pain and discomfort
   a. Analgesics
   b. Topical anesthetics, especially before foreign body removal
   c. Gentle irrigation of the eye with normal saline
3. Prepare the patient and assist with removal
   a. Foreign body removal: moist cotton-tipped swab, sterile needle, or foreign body removal instrument
   b. If rust ring is present, removal of foreign body with ophthalmic drill
4. Treat infection
   a. Topical antibiotics
   b. Tetanus immunizations
5. Monitor for complications
   a. Infection
   b. Scarring
   c. Corneal ulcer

Evaluation

1. Absence of clinical indications of infection
2. Control of pain and discomfort
3. Absence of visual deficit
4. Successful removal of foreign body

Typical disposition

1. If successful removal in the ED: discharge with instructions
2. If unable to remove in the ED: admission for surgery

Retinal Detachment

Definition: the separation of the sensory retina from the pigment epithelium (Figure 10-5)

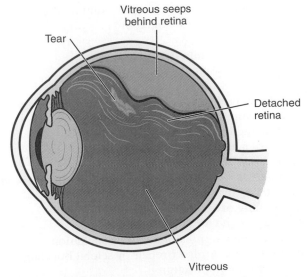

Figure 10-5 Retinal detachment. (From Copstead, L. E., & Banasik, J. L. [2010]. *Pathophysiology* [4th ed.]. Philadelphia: Saunders, p. 1098, Figure 46-9.).

Predisposing factors

1. Can occur at any age but more likely among patients >40 years old
2. Trauma
3. Extremely nearsighted
4. History of retinal detachment in the other eye
5. Family history of retinal detachment
6. Previous cataract surgery
7. History of eye diseases or disorders

Pathophysiology

1. Tear in the retina
2. Blood or serous fluid accumulates between the sensory retina and the pigment epithelium, thereby causing decreased blood and decreased oxygen to get to the eye
3. Retina is unable to perceive light

Clinical presentation

1. Subjective
   a. Painless gradual or sudden loss of vision unilaterally
   b. Sudden or gradual increase in the number of "floaters" in the visual field
   c. Light flashes in the eye
   d. Appearance of a curtain over the field of vision
2. Objective
   a. Decreased visual acuity
   b. Loss of a portion of the visual field
   c. Afferent pupillary defect: unequal dilation and constriction with examination
3. Diagnostic
   a. Visual acuity: decreased
   b. Slit-lamp examination: provides a stereoscopic magnified view of the eye structures in detail
   c. Tonometry: intraocular pressure decreased
   d. Funduscopic examination: to examine the retina
   e. Ophthalmic ultrasonography

Collaborative management

1. Continue assessment
   a. ABCDs
   b. Vital signs: blood pressure, pulse, respiratory rate, and temperature
   c. Pain and discomfort level
   d. Visual acuity
   e. Intraocular pressure
   f. Close monitoring for the progression of symptoms
2. Prevent permanent blindness
   a. Patching of both eyes
   b. Bed rest and a calm environment
   c. Emergency ophthalmologist consultation
   d. Preparation for laser repair or scleral buckling
3. Monitor for complications
   a. Loss of vision, including permanent blindness in the affected eye

Evaluation

1. Absence of visual deficit

Typical disposition: admission for surgery

Orbital Fracture

Definition: a fracture of the orbital floor, the orbital rim, or both

Predisposing factors

1. Greater risk among males than females
2. Blunt trauma: altercation, sports related, industrial, or explosion
3. Exophthalmos

Pathophysiology

1. Usually caused by blunt trauma and associated with the entrapment and ischemia of nerves or penetration into the sinuses
2. Fractures occur when a blow to the eye increases pressure in the orbit and results in a weakening of the orbital floor
3. If the orbital fracture pushes into the maxillary sinus or the ethmoid bone, it will cause a "blow out" fracture (Figure 10-6)
4. Periorbital fat and extraocular muscles may become trapped in the fracture, thereby causing problems with ocular movement
5. If the medial wall is fractured, the medial rectus becomes entrapped, causing a lateral gaze dysfunction

Clinical presentation

1. Subjective
   a. Pain
   b. Diplopia

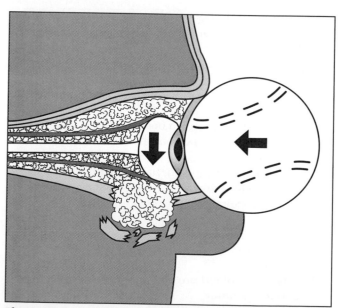

Figure 10-6 Mechanism of a blow-out fracture caused by the impact of a ball. The periorbital fat is forced through the floor of the orbit. (From Emergency Nurses Association. [2005]. *Sheehy's manual of emergency care* [6th ed.] St. Louis: Mosby, p. 746, Figure 40-3.).

c. Paresthesia or anesthesia of the cheek and upper gum on the affected side related to infraorbital nerve damage
2. Objective
    a. Subconjunctival hemorrhage
    b. Periorbital hematoma and edema
    c. Lateral and upward gaze dysfunction as a result of the entrapment of the medial and inferior rectus muscles
    d. Crepitus with palpation
3. Diagnostic
    a. CT provides better definition of orbital injuries as compared with plain films
    b. Water's view: best displays inferior orbital rims, nasoethmoidal bones, and maxillary sinuses
    c. Caldwell projection provides the best view of the lateral orbital rim and the ethmoid bone
    d. Lateral views: show air–fluid levels in the posterior of the maxillary sinus when performed with the patient upright
    e. Cervical spine radiographs: if there are severe facial injuries or mechanism consistent with orbital fracture or neck pain
    f. Slit-lamp examination: to rule out eye injury

Collaborative management

1. Continue assessment
    a. ABCDs
    b. Vital signs: blood pressure, pulse, respiratory rate, and temperature
    c. Oxygen saturation
    d. Respiratory effort and excursion
    e. Cardiac rate and rhythm
    f. Pain and discomfort level
    g. Visual acuity
    h. Tonometry
    i. Close monitoring for the progression of symptoms
2. Maintain airway, oxygenation, ventilation, and perfusion
    a. Airway with cervical spine immobilization as indicated
    b. 100% oxygen by face mask; intubation and mechanical ventilation as indicated
        1) Oxygen by nasal cannula at 2 to 6 L/minute if indicated to maintain an SpO_2 rate of 95% unless contraindicated; for patients with COPD, use pulse oximetry to guide oxygen administration to an SpO_2 rate of 90%
        2) Two large-bore IV catheters
        3) Normal saline for hydration as needed
    c. Consultation with ophthalmology, otolaryngology, and plastic surgery
3. Control pain and discomfort
    a. Elevation of head of stretcher
    b. Analgesics
        1) Nonsteroidal anti-inflammatory drugs
        2) Narcotic analgesics
    c. Ice to the affected area
    d. Instructions to the patient to not blow the nose
4. Treat infection if present and prevent sepsis
    a. Antimicrobials as prescribed
    b. Tetanus immunization

5. Major complications
    a. Bleeding
    b. Loss of vision
    c. Infraorbital nerve damage
    d. Infection

Evaluation

1. Patent airway, adequate oxygenation (i.e., normal PaO_2, SpO_2, SaO_2) and ventilation (i.e., normal $PaCO_2$)
2. Absence of clinical indications of respiratory distress
3. Absence of clinical indications of infection
4. Absence of clinical indications of hypoperfusion
5. Absence of visual deficit
6. Control of pain and discomfort

Typical disposition: admission for surgery

1. Limitation of physical activity for 3 to 6 weeks after surgery; no contact sports should occur during this period

Ocular Chemical Burn

Definition: an injury to the eye that is caused by a tissue-injuring chemical

1. True ocular emergency

Predisposing factors

1. Occupations (e.g., auto mechanic, industrial worker, brick cleaner)
2. Chemical exposure

Pathophysiology

1. Ocular burn severity correlates directly to exposure duration and the causative agent
    a. Chemical burn severity relates to the solution pH, the contact duration, the solution quantity, and the solution penetrability
    b. Burn severity results from the depth and degree of epithelial damage and limbal ischemia
2. Alkalines produce coagulation necrosis with total cellular disruption
    a. Penetrate more rapidly than acids
    b. Saponification (i.e., a chemical reaction that occurs in fat hydrolysis) of the cell membrane fatty acids causes cell disruption and death
    c. Damaged tissues stimulate an inflammatory response that causes further tissue damage by the release of proteolytic enzymes (i.e., liquefactive necrosis)
    d. Irreversible damage if the pH is >11.5
3. Acids cause the immediate denaturation of tissue proteins
    a. Acid burns are usually nonprogressive and superficial
    b. Hydrofluoric acid is an exception; it can rapidly cross the cell membrane and act much like an alkali

Clinical presentation

1. Subjective
    a. Severe, burning pain

b. Varying degrees of visual loss
c. Photophobia
2. Objective
    a. Visual acuity: decreased
    b. Corneal whitening or haziness
    c. Chemosis (i.e., swelling of the conjunctiva)
    d. Eyelid edema
3. Diagnostic should be performed after the rinsing of the eye
    a. Visual acuity: chart and hand motion perception
    b. Slit-lamp examination
    c. Funduscopic examination
    d. Fluorescein staining after irrigation to view injury

Collaborative management

1. Continue assessment
    a. ABCDs
    b. Vital signs: blood pressure, pulse, respiratory rate, and temperature
    c. Pain and discomfort level
    d. Visual acuity
    e. Ocular pH
    f. Close monitoring for the progression of symptoms
2. Prevent permanent damage to the eye and loss of vision
    a. Immediate eye irrigation with copious amounts of normal saline until the pH reaches 7.0 to 7.4
        1) Specifically for hydrofluoric acid burn: irrigate the eyes for 30 minutes with saline followed by a 1% aqueous solution of calcium gluconate (50 ml of 10% solution in 450 ml of saline) over 1 to 2 hours (ENA, 2007)
    b. Medications to decrease intraocular pressure
        1) Miotics (e.g., pilocarpine [Isopto Carpine])
        2) Topical β-blockers (e.g., timolol [Timoptic])
        3) Carbonic anhydrase inhibitors (e.g., acetazolamide [Diamox])
3. Control pain and discomfort
    a. Analgesics
    b. Cycloplegic agents: relax the ciliary muscle
    c. Topical corticosteroids as prescribed
    d. Patching of eyes is usually not indicated
4. Treat and prevent infection
    a. Antimicrobials as prescribed
    b. Tetanus prophylaxis
5. Monitor for complications
    a. Permanent visual impairment
    b. Corneal ulcerations
    c. Entropion (i.e., the eyelids fold inward)

Evaluation

1. Absence of clinical indications of hypoperfusion
2. Control of pain and discomfort
3. Absence of visual deficit

Typical disposition

1. For minor burns: discharge with instructions
    a. Rest

b. Medications as prescribed
c. Follow up with ophthalmology as directed
2. For serious burns: admission

Hyphema

Definition: blood in the anterior chamber of eye between the cornea and the iris

Predisposing factors

1. Blunt trauma
2. Blood-vessel abnormality
3. Cancer of the eye
4. Severe inflammation of the iris
5. Blood-clotting disturbances
6. Leukemia

Pathophysiology

1. Blood vessels of the iris rupture
2. Blood leaks into the clear aqueous fluid of the anterior chamber; most hyphemas fill less than one third of the anterior chamber
3. Uncomplicated hyphemas typically resolve in 5 to 6 days; if there is a large clot, the aqueous outflow can be obstructed, and secondary glaucoma will occur
4. Grading of hyphema
    a. Grade 1: layered blood in less than one third of the anterior chamber
    b. Grade 2: blood filling one third to one half of the anterior chamber
    c. Grade 3: layered blood filling one half to less than 100% of the anterior chamber
    d. Grade 4: anterior chamber completely filled with clotted blood; this is referred to as *blackball hyphema* or *8-ball hyphema*

Clinical presentation

1. Subjective
    a. Mechanism of injury
    b. Blurred vision
    c. Pain
    d. Photophobia
2. Objective
    a. Blood visualized at the bottom of the iris
    b. Afferent pupillary defect (i.e., affected pupil dilates [rather than normal constriction] to light)
    c. Decreased extraocular movements
3. Diagnostic
    a. Visual acuity: decreased
    b. Tonometry: intraocular pressure may be increased
    c. Ultrasound testing

Collaborative management

1. Continue assessment
    a. ABCDs
    b. Vital signs: blood pressure, pulse, respiratory rate, and temperature
    c. Pain and discomfort level
    d. Visual acuity
    e. Intraocular pressure
    f. Close monitoring for the progression of symptoms

2. Control pain and discomfort
   a. Positioning: patient should be upright unless contraindicated (e.g., suspected spine injury)
   b. Analgesics
   c. Rigid eye shield over the affected eye
   d. Cycloplegic: decreases inflammation and discomfort by dilating the pupil and relaxing the ciliary body; thought to improve the healing process by compressing the iris vessels, which decreases pupil movement, thereby decreasing stress to the vessels
3. Decrease intraocular pressure
   a. Bed rest with the head of the stretcher elevated 30 to 45 degrees
   b. Ocular diuretics may be prescribed
      1) Carbonic anhydrase inhibitors (e.g., acetazolamide [Diamox])
      2) Osmotic diuretics (e.g., mannitol)
   c. Avoidance of aspirin or nonsteroidal anti-inflammatory drugs
4. Monitor for complications
   a. Acute glaucoma
   b. Impaired vision
   c. Recurring bleeding

Evaluation
1. Control of pain and discomfort
2. Absence of visual deficit
3. Decrease in intraocular pressure

Typical disposition: admission to the hospital
1. Ophthalmology consult

Eyelid Laceration
Definition: a laceration of the eyelid that may involve the lid margin, be extramarginal, or cause tissue loss
Predisposing trauma
Clinical presentation
1. Subjective
   a. Mechanism of injury
   b. Visual disturbances
2. Objective
   a. Laceration of the eyelid
   b. Bleeding
   c. Protrusion of fat from the eyelid
   d. Levator muscle deficit
3. Diagnostic
   a. Visual acuity testing
   b. Extraocular movement testing
   c. Fluorescein staining
   d. Funduscopic examination
   e. Slit-lamp examination

Collaborative management
1. Continue assessment
   a. ABCDs with cervical immobilization if trauma related
   b. Vital signs: blood pressure, pulse, respiratory rate, and temperature
   c. Pain and discomfort level

d. Visual acuity
e. Clinical indications of bleeding
f. Close monitoring for the progression of symptoms
2. Control hemorrhage: direct pressure on the eye
3. Control pain and discomfort
   a. Analgesic
   b. Cold packs to the affected eye
4. Prevent and treat infection
   a. Cleansing of the wound with saline
   b. Wound closure: consultation with plastic surgery for repair if tissue is missing
5. Monitor for complications
   a. Infection
   b. Underlying eye injury

Evaluation
1. Absence of clinical indications of infection
2. Control of pain and discomfort
3. Absence or loss of eyelid motor function

Typical disposition: discharge with instructions if no other injury
1. Elevation of head of bed to decrease swelling
2. Antibiotic ointment as prescribed
3. Follow up with ophthalmology as directed

Globe Rupture or Impaled Objects
Definition: a rupture of the eye globe with or without an impaled object
1. A full-thickness injury to the cornea, sclera, or both is considered an open globe injury

Predisposing factors
1. Blunt injury during a motor vehicle collision, an assault, or another trauma
   a. Workplace accidents
   b. Sports activities: basketball, water sports, baseball, racquet sports, martial arts, wrestling, and archery
2. Penetrating trauma
   a. Gunshot and stab wounds
   b. Incidents that involve sharps or projectiles
3. Anterior chamber deepens and the iris diaphragm falls backwards

Pathophysiology
1. Occurs when a blunt object impacts the orbit, thereby causing anteroposterior compression of the globe and raising intraocular pressure to a point at which the sclera tears
2. Usually occur at the sites where the sclera is thinnest (i.e., insertions of the extraocular muscles, the limbus, and around the optic nerve)
3. Represents a major ophthalmologic emergency and always requires surgical intervention
4. Damage to the posterior eye segment is associated with an increased risk of permanent visual loss

Clinical presentation
1. Subjective
   a. Mechanism of injury

b. Pain
c. Sudden visual loss or change
d. Diplopia
2. Objective
   a. Asymmetry of the globe
   b. Extrusion of aqueous or vitreous humor
   c. Pupil herniation: indicates disruption of the iris
   d. Impaled object can be seen in place
3. Diagnostic
   a. Visual acuity: decreased
   b. CT: to detect occult rupture, associated optic nerve injury, and small foreign bodies, visualize the globe and orbit anatomy

Collaborative management

1. Continue assessment
   a. ABCDs
   b. Vital signs: blood pressure, pulse, respiratory rate, and temperature
   c. Pain and discomfort level
   d. Visual acuity
   e. Intraocular pressure
   f. Close monitoring for the progression of symptoms
2. Maintain airway, oxygenation, ventilation, and perfusion
   a. Airway with cervical spine immobilization as indicated
   b. Oxygen by nasal cannula at 2 to 6 L/minute or 100% via face mask if indicated to maintain an SpO_2 rate of 95% unless contraindicated; for patients with COPD, use pulse oximetry to guide oxygen administration to an SpO_2 rate of 90%
   c. Intubation and mechanical ventilation as indicated
   d. Replacement of vascular volume
      1) Two large-bore IV catheters
      2) Normal saline for hydration as needed
3. Control pain and discomfort
   a. Semi-Fowler position immediately unless contraindicated (e.g., spinal injury)
   b. Analgesics
      1) Do not apply topical anesthetics
   c. Antiemetics for nausea
4. Preserve vision
   a. Ophthalmology consult
   b. Eye shield to protect from further injury
   c. Prevention of further injury
      1) Do not pry the eyes open if rupture is expected
      2) Do not remove the impaled object; stabilize it in place
   d. Preparation for surgery as indicated
5. Treat and prevent infection
   a. Antimicrobials as prescribed
   b. Tetanus prophylactic
6. Monitor for complications
   a. Loss of vision, including permanent blindness
   b. Blindness

Evaluation

1. Absence of clinical indications of infection or sepsis
2. Control of pain and discomfort
3. Absence of clinical indications of hypoperfusion
4. Absence of visual deficit

Typical disposition: admission for surgery

Snow Blindness

Definition: a burn of the cornea that occurs as a result of ultraviolet type B light rays
Predisposing factors
1. Spending time outside on a highly reflective snow field or surface
   a. Usually occurs at high altitudes on highly reflective snow fields
2. Sun-tanning beds: from artificial light ultraviolet type B lights
3. Welder's arc (i.e., flash burn, welder's flash, or arc eye)
4. Carbon arcs
5. Photographic flood lamps
6. Electric sparks
7. Halogen desk lamps

Pathophysiology: radiation burn of the cornea
Clinical presentation
1. Subjective
   a. History of precipitating event: symptoms may take 6 to 12 hours to appear
   b. Pain and tearing
   c. Red, swollen eyelids
   d. Gritty feeling in the eyes
   e. Seeing halos around lights
   f. Hazy vision
2. Objective
   a. Eyelids edematous with erythema
   b. Eyelids tender to touch
   c. Patient demonstrates difficulty opening the eyelids
3. Diagnostic
   a. Visual acuity: decreased
   b. Fluorescein stain

Collaborative management

1. Continue assessment
   a. ABCDs
   b. Vital signs: blood pressure, pulse, respiratory rate, and temperature
   c. Pain and discomfort level
   d. Visual acuity
   e. Close monitoring for the progression of symptoms
2. Control pain and discomfort
   a. Analgesics
   b. Cool compresses to the eyelids
3. Treat and prevent infection
   a. Antibiotic drops
   b. Patching of both eyes
4. Monitor for complications
   a. Corneal burn
   b. Infection

Evaluation
1. Control of pain and discomfort
2. Absence of visual deficit
   a. Alert and oriented with no neurovascular deficit

Typical disposition: discharge with instructions
1. Sunglasses when exposed to ultraviolet type B light rays

Tooth Fracture, Subluxation, and Avulsion

Definitions: all may include injury to the lips, mouth, teeth, and jawbone
1. Fractured tooth: damage to the enamel, the dentin, or both
   a. Ellis classification of fractured teeth (Figure 10-7)
      1) Ellis I: involves enamel only
      2) Ellis II: involves enamel and dentin
      3) Ellis III: involves enamel, dentin, and pulp
   b. Subluxation
   c. Avulsed tooth: complete displacement of the tooth from the alveolar socket

Predisposing factors
1. Falls
2. Athletic injuries
3. Altercations
4. Motor vehicle collisions

Clinical presentation
1. Subjective
   a. Pain
   b. Headache
   c. Nausea and vomiting
2. Objective
   a. Obvious injury to the tooth
   b. Bleeding with an avulsed tooth
   c. Displacement of the tooth
   d. Changes in level of consciousness
3. Diagnostic
   a. Panoramic oral radiography
   b. Facial radiography

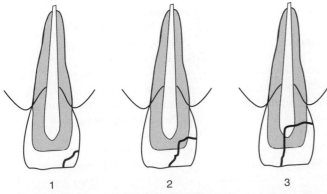

Figure 10-7 Ellis classification of tooth fractures. **1,** Enamel injury. **2,** Dentin injury. **3,** Pulp injury. (Modified from McQuillan, K.A., Makic, M. B. F., & Whalen, E. [2009]. *Trauma nursing* [4th ed.]. Philadelphia: Saunders, p. 529, Figure 21-16.).

Collaborative management
1. Continue assessment
   a. ABCDs
   b. Vital signs: blood pressure, pulse, respiratory rate, and temperature
   c. Oxygen saturation
   d. Pain and discomfort level
   e. Close monitoring for the progression of symptoms
2. Ensure the viability of the tooth
   a. Referral to dentist or oral surgeon
3. Control pain and discomfort
   a. Nonsteroidal anti-inflammatory drugs
   b. Fractured tooth
      1) Ellis II or III: zinc oxide or calcium hydroxide paste (Dycal)
      2) Analgesics
   c. Avulsed tooth
      1) Reimplantation of the avulsed tooth; the success rate of this treatment is high if the tooth is replaced within 30 minutes of injury
      2) Analgesics
      3) Avoidance of hot or cold substances, which increase discomfort
4. Monitor for complications
   a. Airway compromise
   b. Uncontrolled pain

Evaluation
1. Patent airway, adequate oxygenation (i.e., normal PaO_2, SpO_2, and SaO_2) and ventilation (i.e., normal $PaCO_2$)
2. Control of pain and discomfort

Typical disposition: discharge with instructions
1. No solid foods for 24 hours
2. Follow up with dental referral as directed

Larynx Fracture

Definition: a fracture of the larynx that is caused by direct trauma to the neck
Predisposing factors
1. Motor vehicle collisions
2. Clothesline injuries
3. Strangulation
4. Blunt trauma to the neck

Pathophysiology
1. Mechanism of injury reflects the causative agent
2. Direct transfer of severe forces to the larynx
3. Mechanism can produce many injuries, including mucosal tears, dislocations, and fractures
4. Can lead to life-threatening airway problems

Clinical presentation
1. Subjective
   a. Neck pain
   b. Dyspnea

c. Dysphonia, aphonia, and dysphasia

d. Odynophonia (i.e., pain and soreness in the throat with use of the voice)

e. Odynophagia (i.e., pain with swallowing)

2. Objective
a. Hematoma and ecchymosis
b. Subcutaneous emphysema
c. Stridor
d. Hemoptysis
e. Laryngeal tenderness with palpation and deformity

3. Diagnostic
a. CBC with differential
b. ABGs
c. Direct laryngoscopy: provides a detailed visual examination of the larynx; may allow for the visualization of vocal cord immobility
d. Fiber-optic laryngoscopy: edema and hematoma indicate that the patient requires immediate tracheotomy
e. Chest and cervical spine radiography to rule out cervical injury
f. CT of the neck: to rule out fractures, hematomas, and dislocations
g. Esophagoscopy: provides visualization of the esophageal mucosa for traumatic lacerations

Collaborative management

1. Continue assessment
a. ABCDs
b. Vital signs: blood pressure, pulse, respiratory rate, and temperature
c. Oxygen saturation
d. Respiratory effort and excursion
e. Cardiac rate and rhythm
f. Pain and discomfort level

g. Close monitoring for the progression of symptoms

2. Maintain airway, oxygenation, ventilation, and perfusion
a. Airway with cervical spine immobilization as indicated
b. Oxygen by nasal cannula at 2 to 6 L/minute or 100% via face mask if indicated to maintain an SpO_2 rate of 95% unless contraindicated; for patients with COPD, use pulse oximetry to guide oxygen administration to an SpO_2 rate of 90%
c. Rapid-sequence intubation and mechanical ventilation if patient is unable to maintain airway
   1) Tracheotomy indicated if edema and hematoma are present
d. Replacement of vascular volume
   1) Two large-bore intravenous catheters
   2) Normal saline for hydration as needed

3. Control pain and discomfort
a. Nonsteroidal anti-inflammatory drugs
b. Analgesics

4. Decrease edema and trauma of larynx (Table 10-2)

5. Monitor for complications
a. Infection
b. Bleeding
c. Granuloma formation

Evaluation

1. Patent airway as well as adequate oxygenation (i.e., normal PaO_2, SpO_2, and SaO_2) and ventilation (i.e., normal $PaCO_2$)
2. Absence of clinical indications of respiratory distress
3. Absence of clinical indications of hypoperfusion
4. Absence of clinical indications of infection or sepsis
5. Control of pain and discomfort

TABLE 10-2 Management of Laryngeal Trauma

Group	Symptoms	Signs	Management
Group 1	Minor airway symptoms	• Simple hematomas • Small lacerations • No fractures	• Close monitoring of patient • Humidified oxygen • Elevation of head of stretcher
Group 2	Airway compromise	• Swelling or edema • Hematoma • Minor mucosal disruption • No cartilage exposure	• Direct laryngoscopy • Esophagoscopy • Tracheotomy indicated
Group 3	Airway compromise	• Massive swelling or edema • Mucosal tears • Exposed cartilage • Vocal cord immobility	• Tracheotomy immediately • Direct laryngoscopy • Esophagoscopy • Surgical repair
Group 4	Airway compromise	• Massive swelling or edema • Mucosal tears • Exposed cartilage • Vocal cord immobility	• Tracheotomy immediately • Direct laryngoscopy • Esophagoscopy • Surgical repair with stent

Adapted from Pancholi, S. S., Robbins, W. K., & Desai, T. (2009). Laryngeal fractures. Retrieved February 22, 2009, from http://emedicine.medscape.com/article/865277-overview.

Typical disposition: admission for possible surgery

Nasal Fracture

Definition: a fracture of the nasal bones, particularly the nasal pyramid
Predisposing factors
1. Blunt trauma

Pathophysiology: blunt trauma that involves enough force to break bone
1. Most common facial fracture

Clinical presentation
1. Subjective
   a. Pain
   b. Nasal area swollen and tender
2. Objective
   a. Displacement of the nasal bone and asymmetry
   b. Epistaxis
   c. Nasal and periorbital ecchymosis
   d. Subconjunctival hemorrhage
   e. Crepitus with palpation
3. Diagnostic
   a. Nasal speculum examination: to rule out septal hematoma
   b. Nasal radiography: Water's view

Collaborative management
1. Continue assessment
   a. ABCDs
   b. Vital signs: blood pressure, pulse, respiratory rate, and temperature
   c. Oxygen saturation
   d. Respiratory effort and excursion
   e. Pain and discomfort level
   f. Presence of bleeding from nose
   g. Close monitoring for the progression of symptoms
2. Maintain airway, oxygenation, ventilation, and perfusion
   a. Airway with cervical spine immobilization as indicated
   b. Oxygen by nasal cannula at 2 to 6 L/minute or 100% via face mask if indicated to maintain an SpO_2 rate of 95% unless contraindicated; for patients with COPD, use pulse oximetry to guide oxygen administration to an SpO_2 rate of 90%
   c. Rapid-sequence intubation and mechanical ventilation if patient is unable to maintain airway
   d. Replacement of vascular volume
      1) Two large-bore IV catheters
      2) Normal saline for hydration as needed
3. Provide comfort and pain relief
   a. Ice pack to the nose
   b. Nonsteroidal anti-inflammatory drugs
   c. Analgesics
   d. Decongestants
   e. Splint nose as directed

4. Prevent infection
   a. Oral antimicrobials
   b. Tetanus immunization
5. Monitor for complications
   a. Septal hematoma
   b. Bleeding

Evaluation
1. Patent airway, adequate oxygenation (i.e., normal PaO_2, SpO_2, and SaO_2) and ventilation (i.e., normal $PaCO_2$)
2. Absence of clinical indications of respiratory distress
3. Absence of clinical indications of hypoperfusion
4. Absence of clinical indications of bleeding
5. Absence of clinical indications of infection
6. Control of pain and discomfort

Typical disposition: discharge home with instructions
1. Medications as prescribed
2. Use of splint for 1 week
3. Follow up for possible surgical repair 1 to 2 weeks after swelling has resolved

Temporomandibular Joint Dislocation

Definition: the anterior and superior dislocation of the jaw; may be unilateral or bilateral
Predisposing factors
1. Yawning
2. Opening the mouth wide during dental work
3. Mandibular fractures
4. Bruxism (i.e., the grinding of the teeth)
5. Arthritis

Pathophysiology: spasms and muscle contractions prevent the condyles from returning to their normal positions
Clinical presentation
1. Subjective
   a. Pain that worsens with attempts to move the jaw
   b. Spasms and muscle contractions
   c. Inability to close the jaw
   d. Earache
2. Objective
   a. Limited range of motion of mouth
   b. Spasms of the masseter muscle
   c. Inability to close the mouth completely
   d. Drooling
   e. Difficulty speaking
   f. Tenderness of temporomandibular joint with palpation
3. Diagnostic
   a. Panorex oral radiography
   b. Prereduction and postreduction radiography

Collaborative management
1. Continue assessment
   a. ABCDs

b. Vital signs: blood pressure, pulse, respiratory rate, and temperature

c. Oxygen saturation

d. Respiratory effort and excursion

e. Pain and discomfort level

f. Close monitoring for the progression of symptoms

2. Maintain airway, oxygenation, ventilation, and perfusion

a. Airway maintenance with positioning or artificial airway as required

b. Oxygen may be required ; oxygen by nasal cannula at 2 to 6 L/minute or 100% via face mask if indicated to maintain an SpO_2 rate of 95% unless contraindicated; for patients with COPD, use pulse oximetry to guide oxygen administration to an SpO_2 rate of 90%

c. Conscious sedation for the manual reduction of the jaw

3. Control pain and discomfort

a. Nonsteroidal anti-inflammatory drugs

b. Narcotic analgesics

c. Muscle relaxants

d. Anxiolytics

4. Monitor for complications

a. Airway problems

b. Fractured jaw with relocation

Evaluation

1. Patent airway, adequate oxygenation (i.e., normal PaO_2, SpO_2, and SaO_2) and ventilation (i.e., normal $PaCO_2$)

2. Absence of clinical indications of respiratory distress

3. Control of pain and discomfort

4. Successful reduction and mobile jaw

Typical disposition: discharge with instructions

1. Soft diet for 2 to 3 days

2. Avoidance of stress on temporomandibular joint

3. Medications as prescribed

4. Follow up as directed

Facial Emergencies and Facial Nerve Disorders

Definition

1. Bell palsy: a paralysis of the facial muscles on one side of the face

2. Herpes zoster oticus: a viral infection that involves the external, middle, and inner ear

3. Trigeminal neuralgia: brief paroxysms of excruciating facial pain that recur with increasing frequency and severity

4. Temporal arteritis: common systemic vasculitis

Predisposing factors

1. Recent upper respiratory illness: viral or bacterial

2. Trigeminal neuralgia triggered by a cold environment and facial stimulation

a. Seen in women more than men

b. Affects the right side more often than left

Pathophysiology

1. Bell palsy

a. Rapid onset

b. Etiology unknown; possibly a result of polyneuritis

c. Emotional stress and viruses can trigger the condition

2. Herpes zoster oticus

a. Viral infection that involves the external, middle, and inner ear

b. Known as *Ramsay Hunt syndrome* when associated with unilateral facial paralysis

c. Sometimes confused with Bell palsy until vesicles appear

d. Vesicular eruption can occur on the external ear, the tympanic membrane, the soft palate, the oral cavity, the neck, the face, and the shoulders

1) Follows the dermatomes

e. Outcomes worse than Bell palsy

1) Patient may not completely recover from facial paralysis

2) Patient may have permanent hearing loss

3. Trigeminal neuralgia: a disorder of the fifth cranial nerve, which has three divisions: maxillary, mandibular, and ophthalmic

4. Temporal arteritis

a. Unknown etiology

b. Characterized by a granulomatous inflammatory process that is seen primarily along the internal elastic lamina of the arterial walls

c. Can affect any large or medium artery, but symptoms are usually caused by inflammation in the external carotid artery branches

Clinical presentation

1. Subjective

a. Bell palsy: facial discomfort, unilateral facial weakness, drooling, and a loss of taste on one side of the mouth

b. Herpes zoster oticus: presentation that is similar to Bell palsy, but the pain is more severe

c. Trigeminal neuralgia: worsens with cold exposure or the touching of trigger zones

1) Pain-free intervals, but episodes become more frequent and severe with each occurrence

2) Electrical shock feeling in the lower cheek and jaw

d. Temporal arteritis

1) Headache

2) Scalp, jaw, and tongue tenderness

3) Jaw or tongue claudication (i.e., pain while chewing)

4) Hearing loss

5) Vision difficulties: blurred, reduced, or double vision

2. Objective

a. Bell palsy

1) Upward movement of the eyeball on the affected side when closing the eye is known as *Bell phenomenon*

2) Facial drooping and flattening of the nasolabial fold on the affected side
3) Positive corneal sensation on the affected side without blink reflex
4) Eyelid lag on the affected side
5) Inability to wrinkle forehead on the affected side; ask the patient if he or she has had a facial nerve cut or a Botox injection
6) Increased sensitivity to noise

   b. Herpes zoster oticus
   1) Physical examination findings similar to those listed for Bell palsy
   2) Herpetiform vesicles
   c. Trigeminal neuralgia
   1) Facial grimacing during episodes
   2) Minimal to no sensory loss along the trigeminal nerve
   3) Painful paroxysmal tic may be induced with the palpation of the ipsilateral anterior aspect of the face
   d. Temporal arteritis
   1) Scalp tenderness when touching the scalp
   2) Bleeding gums
3. Diagnostic
   a. Bell palsy: diagnosis of exclusion
   1) Schirmer test to evaluate lacrimation
   2) Acoustic reflex testing
   3) Cranial nerve function testing
   4) Audiogram
   b. Lyme titer to rule out Lyme disease
   c. ESR: increased in patients with temporal arteritis
   d. Mastoid radiography to rule out temporal bone fracture
   e. CT with contrast shows a thickening of the arterial walls, stenosis, or occlusion in patients with temporal arteritis

Collaborative management

1. Continue assessment
   a. ABCDs
   b. Vital signs: blood pressure, pulse, respiratory rate, and temperature
   c. Pain and discomfort level
   d. Close monitoring for the progression of symptoms
2. Control pain and discomfort
   a. Nonsteroidal anti-inflammatory drugs
   b. Analgesics
   c. Phenytoin (Dilantin) or carbamazepine (Tegretol) is sometimes beneficial in patients with trigeminal neuralgia to interrupt episodes
   d. Moist heat and passive facial exercises (Bell palsy)
   e. Facial sling (Bell palsy)
   f. Artificial tears to the affected eye
   g. Regional nerve block for trigeminal neuralgia or surgical intervention to relieve pain
3. Medications as prescribed
   a. Antivirals (Ramsay Hunt syndrome)
   b. Corticosteroids (Bell palsy, Ramsay Hunt syndrome)

   c. Antiemetics
   d. Antibiotics for secondary bacterial infections
4. Monitor for complications
   a. Sudden vision loss
   b. Stroke (i.e., temporal arteritis)
   c. Uncontrolled pain

Evaluation

1. Patent airway, adequate oxygenation (i.e., normal PaO_2, SpO_2, and SaO_2) and ventilation (i.e., normal $PaCO_2$)
2. Absence of clinical indications of hypoperfusion
3. Alert and oriented with no neurovascular deficit
4. Control of pain and discomfort

Typical disposition: discharge with instructions

1. Reassurance and support
2. Medications as prescribed
3. Bell palsy and Ramsay Hunt syndrome
   a. Wearing of sunglasses
   b. Avoidance of drafts and keeping the face warm
   c. Moist heat applied to face
   d. Facial exercise and massage
   e. Facial sling as directed
   f. Artificial tears
4. Trigeminal neuralgia: avoidance of cold exposure (e.g., temperatures, fluids with ice)
5. Follow up as directed

Facial Lacerations and Soft-Tissue Injuries

Definitions

1. Laceration: a torn, ragged skin wound
2. Abrasion: a minor injury in which the skin is worn or torn off
3. Puncture wound: a wound that is deeper than it is wide
4. Contusion: an injury that does not break the skin but that causes discoloration (i.e., bruising or ecchymosis)
5. Avulsion: the tearing away of a body part; can be a nerve or a bone

Predisposing factors

1. Trauma

Pathophysiology

1. Injury to the skin, the subcutaneous tissue, or the vascular bed
2. Bleeding
3. Inflammation

Clinical presentation

1. Subjective
   a. Mechanism of injury
   b. Pain
   c. Numbness or loss of sensation
2. Objective
   a. Facial wounds and possible foreign body

b. Bleeding or swelling
c. Facial asymmetry or swelling
d. Motor and sensory deficits
e. Cranial nerve damage
f. Tenderness with palpation
3. Diagnostic
a. Culture open wounds
b. Facial radiography: include the cervical spine if injury is suspected
c. CT

Collaborative management

1. Continue assessment
a. ABCDs
b. Vital signs: blood pressure, pulse, respiratory rate, and temperature
c. Pain and discomfort level
d. Absence of clinical indications of bleeding
e. Close monitoring for the progression of symptoms
2. Maintain airway, oxygenation, ventilation, and perfusion
a. Airway with cervical spine immobilization as indicated
   1) Positioning: high-Fowler position if no indication of spinal injury
b. Oxygen by nasal cannula at 2 to 6 L/minute or 100% via face mask if indicated to maintain an SpO_2 rate of 95% unless contraindicated; for patients with COPD, use pulse oximetry to guide oxygen administration to an SpO_2 rate of 90%
c. Rapid-sequence intubation and mechanical ventilation if patient is unable to maintain airway
d. Replacement of vascular volume
   1) Two large-bore IV catheters
   2) Normal saline for hydration as needed
3. Control pain and discomfort
a. Nonsteroidal anti-inflammatory drugs
b. Narcotic analgesics
c. Ice to the affected area
4. Prevent and treat infection
a. Irrigation and cleansing of wounds with saline
b. Wound closure: sutures, staples, or adhesives
   1) Conscious sedation may be used before the procedure (e.g., Midazolam [Versed], nitrous oxide [Notronox])
   2) Preparation for suturing
      a) Replacement of tissue flaps
      b) Local anesthetics
         i) Lidocaine with epinephrine causes vasoconstriction and helps to decrease bleeding during the procedure
         ii) Lidocaine without epinephrine should be used for the tips of the nose and ears because the epinephrine vasoconstriction could interfere with blood flow in these areas and result in tissue damage
      c) Eyebrows and hairline should not be shaved
      d) Staples should not be used for facial laceration closure

c. Antimicrobials may be ordered, depending on the type and depth of injury
d. Tetanus immunization
5. Monitor for complications
a. Infection
b. Nerve damage
c. Disfigurement

Evaluation

1. Absence of clinical indications of bleeding
2. Control of pain and discomfort
3. Absence of clinical indications of infection

Typical disposition: discharge with instructions

1. Wound care
2. Staple or suture removal as directed
3. Return to the ED if signs of inflammation or infection develop

Mandibular Fracture

Definition: a fracture of the mandible
Predisposing factors: trauma
1. Motor vehicle collisions
2. Altercations
3. Falling forward and landing on the chin

Pathophysiology

1. Common fracture sites include the body of the mandible, the angle adjacent to the wisdom tooth, the subcondylar area, and the condyle
2. Condyle fractures are the most often overlooked
a. Area anterior to the meatus of the ear will be tender to palpation
b. Condyle on the fractured side will not move when the mandible is opened and closed
3. May be life threatening if the tongue is displaced posteriorly, which causes airway obstruction

Clinical presentation

1. Subjective
a. Mechanism of injury
b. Pain with jaw movement
   1) Preauricular pain suggests fracture
c. Bleeding around the mouth
d. Difficulty opening the mouth
e. Numbness of the lower lip or chin
   1) Caused by a disruption of the inferior alveolar nerve and mental branch of that nerve
2. Objective
a. Asymmetry
b. Displacement of two or more lower teeth toward the tongue is indicative of fracture
c. Hematoma
d. Edema
e. Malocclusion
f. Bleeding
g. Trismus
h. Ruptured tympanic membrane or hemotympanum

i. Tenderness with palpation
j. Mobility and crepitus with palpation along the symphysis, angles, or body
k. Intraoral edema and ecchymosis
3. Diagnostic
   a. Face and skull radiography: all views
      1) Water's and Towne views
   b. Panoramic oral radiography (i.e., Panorex)
   c. CT: face and head
   d. Cervical spine films if injury suspected

Collaborative management
1. Continue assessment
   a. ABCDs
   b. Vital signs: blood pressure, pulse, respiratory rate, and temperature
   c. Oxygen saturation
   d. Respiratory effort and excursion
   e. Cardiac rate and rhythm
   f. Bleeding
   g. Pain and discomfort level
   h. Close monitoring for the progression of symptoms
2. Maintain airway, oxygenation, ventilation, and perfusion
   a. Airway with cervical spine immobilization as indicated
   b. Positioning: high-Fowler position unless spinal injury is suspected
   c. Oxygen by nasal cannula at 2 to 6 L/minute or 100% via face mask if indicated to maintain an SpO_2 rate of 95% unless contraindicated; for patients with COPD, use pulse oximetry to guide oxygen administration to an SpO_2 rate of 90%
   d. Rapid-sequence intubation and mechanical ventilation if patient is unable to maintain airway
   e. Suction frequently; give the patient Yankauer suction if he or she is able to use it
   f. Replacement of vascular volume
      1) Two large-bore IV catheters
      2) Normal saline for hydration as needed
      3) Blood and blood products may be needed
   g. Control hemorrhage
      1) Direct pressure as indicated
      2) Ice to mandible to minimize swelling and bleeding
3. Control pain and discomfort: analgesics
4. Stabilize the fracture
   a. Barton bandage: circumferential bandage
   b. Open reduction and internal fixation
5. Treat and prevent infection
   a. Antimicrobials as prescribed
   b. Tetanus immunization
6. Monitor for complications
   a. Airway compromise
   b. Permanent facial deformity
   c. Nerve damage that results in a loss of sensation, facial movement, smell, taste, or vision

d. Infection
e. Hemorrhage

Evaluation
1. Patent airway, adequate oxygenation (i.e., normal PaO_2, SpO_2, and SaO_2) and ventilation (i.e., normal $PaCO_2$)
2. Absence of clinical indications of respiratory distress
3. Absence of clinical indications of hypoperfusion
4. Absence of clinical indications of infection or sepsis
5. Control of pain and discomfort

Typical disposition
1. Most likely: admission for surgery
   a. Nothing to be taken by mouth in preparation for surgery
2. If reduction not required, patient may be discharged home with instructions
   a. Soft diet
   b. Patients with intermaxillary fixation wires or bands in place need to consume high-calorie, high-protein liquids
      1) Carry wire cutters at all times
      2) Avoid overexertion or excessive exercise, because this can increase or facilitate respiratory distress
   c. Instructions to return to the ED immediately if he or she has any difficulty maintaining secretions or airway
   d. Follow up with maxillofacial surgeon as directed

Maxillary Fracture
Definition: a fracture of the maxilla
Predisposing factors
1. High-energy, direct-blow trauma
2. Motor vehicle collisions: rapid deceleration injury

Pathophysiology
1. Frequently massive facial trauma
2. Three types (Figure 10-8)
   a. Le Forte I: transverse fracture above the teeth and across the maxilla
   b. Le Forte II: pyramidal fracture through the nasal bone and down the maxilla
   c. Le Forte III: complete separation from the cranial bones

Clinical presentation
1. Subjective
   a. Mechanism of injury
   b. Pain and swelling
   c. Facial asymmetry
   d. Bruising
   e. Loose teeth
2. Objective
   a. Le Forte I
      1) Crepitus
      2) Bruising
      3) Malocclusion

Lateral view   Frontal view

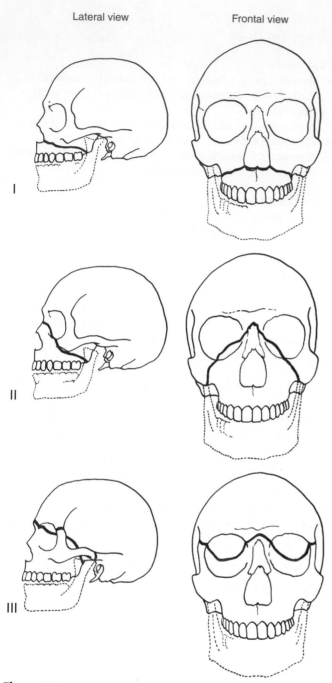

Figure 10-8 Le Fort classification of midface fractures. **I**, Only the lower maxilla. **II**, The infraorbital rim. **III**, Complete detachment of the midface from the skull (i.e., craniofacial dissociation). (From Emergency Nurses Association. [2010]. *Sheehy's emergency nursing: Principles and practice* [6th ed.]. St. Louis: Mosby, p. 360, Figure 27-4.).

4) Epistaxis
5) Numbness of the upper lip
b. Le Forte II
1) Facial elongation (i.e., lengthening)
2) Paresthesia of the anterior cheek
3) Cerebrospinal fluid leakage
4) Decreased extraocular eye movement

c. Le Forte III
1) Massive edema with facial elongation and flattening
2) Anterior open bite may be present as a result of the posterior and inferior displacement of the facial skeleton
3) Movement of all facial bones in relation to the cranial base with manipulation of the teeth and hard palate (i.e., free-floating segment)
4) Epistaxis and rhinorrhea
3. Diagnostic
a. Facial radiography including Waters view
b. CT: head and face
c. Cervical spine radiography: to rule out cervical spine injury

Collaborative management

1. Continue assessment
a. ABCDs
b. Vital signs: blood pressure, pulse, respiratory rate, and temperature
c. Oxygen saturation
d. Respiratory effort and excursion
e. Cardiac rate and rhythm
f. Pain and discomfort level
g. Close monitoring for the progression of symptoms
2. Maintain airway, oxygenation, ventilation, and perfusion
a. Airway with cervical spine immobilization as indicated
b. Positioning: high-Fowler position unless spinal injury is suspected
c. Oxygen by nasal cannula at 2 to 6 L/minute or 100% via face mask if indicated to maintain an Spo_2 rate of 95% unless contraindicated; for patients with COPD, use pulse oximetry to guide oxygen administration to an Spo_2 rate of 90%
d. Rapid-sequence intubation and mechanical ventilation if patient is unable to maintain airway
e. Suctioning frequently; give the patient Yankauer suction if he or she is able to use it
f. Replacement of vascular volume
1) Two large-bore IV catheters
2) Normal saline or lactated Ringer solution by rapid infusion until blood is available; colloids (e.g., albumin, hetastarch, dextran) may also be used
3) Blood and blood products may be needed
g. Control hemorrhage
1) Direct pressure as indicated
2) Ice to the mandible to minimize swelling and bleeding
3. Relieve pain and discomfort
a. Positioning: side lying or in a semi-Fowler position
b. Analgesics
c. Ice to the affected area
4. Stabilize the fracture
a. Traction
b. Surgery

5. Prevent infection
   a. Prophylactic antibiotics intravenously
   b. Tetanus immunization
6. Monitor for complications
   a. Airway compromise
   b. Aspiration
   c. Permanent facial deformity
   d. Nerve damage that results in a loss of sensation, facial movement, smell, taste, or vision
   e. Infection
   f. Hemorrhage

Evaluation

1. Patent airway, adequate oxygenation (i.e., normal PaO_2, SpO_2, and SaO_2) and ventilation (i.e., normal $PaCO_2$)
2. Absence of clinical indications of respiratory distress
3. Absence of clinical indications of hypoperfusion
4. Control of pain and discomfort

Typical disposition: admission for surgery

Zygomatic Fracture

Definition: a fracture of the zygoma, the zygomatic arch, or both; also referred to as a *tripod fracture*
Predisposing factors

1. Trauma: altercations, motor vehicle collisions, direct blows to the zygoma, forward falls in which the patient landed on his or her face
2. Frequently associated with orbital fractures

Pathophysiology

1. Involves all zygomatic suture lines
2. Significant soft-tissue trauma and possible nerve injury

Clinical presentation (Figure 10-9)

1. Subjective
   a. Mechanism of injury
   b. Pain
   c. Swelling, bleeding, and bruising
   d. Limited movement of the lower jaw
   e. Blurred vision, diplopia, and impaired ability to look upward
   f. Paresthesia of the cheek, nose, upper lip, teeth, and gums on the affected side
2. Objective
   a. Obvious deformity
   b. Facial edema and bleeding
   c. Facial and periorbital ecchymosis
   d. Depression of the inferior orbital rim with the downward placement of globe on the affected side
   e. Flattening of the anterior cheek on the affected side
   f. Infraorbital hypesthesia (i.e., a decrease in sensation in response to the stimulation of the sensory nerves)
   g. Tenderness of the arch and the infraorbital rim with palpation
   h. Subcutaneous emphysema: indicates possible sinus injury
3. Diagnostic
   a. Zygomatic radiography: to view the zygoma and the zygomatic arch
      1) Caldwell view provides additional views of the frontal sinus and the superior orbital rim
      2) Submental vertical view: provides six landmarks for the evaluation of facial symmetry
      3) Water's view: best displays the inferior orbital rims, the nasoethmoidal bones, and the maxillary sinuses

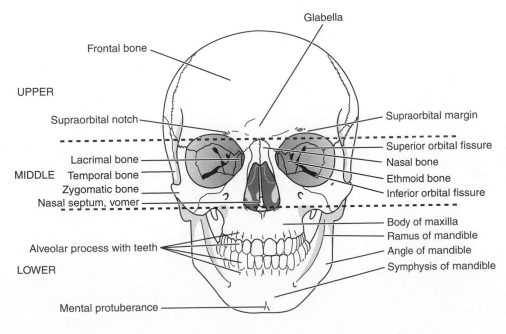

Figure 10-9 Depressed fracture of the zygomatic arch. (From Emergency Nurses Association. [2005]. *Sheehy's manual of emergency care* [6th ed.] St. Louis: Mosby, p. 744, Figure 40-2A.).

b. CT: "gold standard" that will accurately reveal the extent of orbital involvement and the degree of displacement of fractures

Collaborative management

1. Continue assessment
   a. ABCDs
   b. Vital signs: blood pressure, pulse, respiratory rate, and temperature
   c. Oxygen saturation
   d. Respiratory effort and excursion
   e. Cardiac rate and rhythm
   f. Pain and discomfort level
   g. Evidence of bleeding
   h. Close monitoring for the progression of symptoms
2. Maintain airway, oxygenation, ventilation, and perfusion
   a. Airway with cervical spine immobilization as indicated
   b. Positioning: high-Fowler position unless spinal injury is suspected
   c. Oxygen by nasal cannula at 2 to 6 L/minute or 100% via face mask if indicated to maintain an SpO_2 rate of 95% unless contraindicated; for patients with COPD, use pulse oximetry to guide oxygen administration to an SpO_2 rate of 90%
   d. Rapid-sequence intubation and mechanical ventilation if patient is unable to maintain airway
   e. Suctioning frequently; give the patient Yankauer suction if he or she is able to use it
   f. Replacement of vascular volume
      1) Two large-bore IV catheters
      2) Normal saline or lactated Ringer solution by rapid infusion until blood is available; colloids (e.g., albumin, hetastarch, dextran) may also be used
      3) Blood and blood products may be needed
   g. Control hemorrhage
      1) Direct pressure as indicated
      2) Ice to minimize swelling and bleeding
3. Relieve pain and discomfort
   a. Position of comfort
   b. Analgesics
   c. Ice to the affected area
4. Stabilize the fracture: surgery
5. Prevent infection
   a. Prophylactic antibiotics intravenously
   b. Tetanus immunization
6. Monitor for complications
   a. Airway compromise
   b. Permanent facial deformity
   c. Nerve damage that results in a loss of sensation, facial movement, smell, taste, or vision
   d. Infection
   e. Hemorrhage

Evaluation

1. Patent airway, adequate oxygenation (i.e., normal PaO_2, SpO_2, and SaO_2) and ventilation (i.e., normal $PaCO_2$)
2. Absence of clinical indications of respiratory distress
3. Absence of clinical indications of hypoperfusion
4. Absence of clinical indications of infection or sepsis
5. Absence of neurologic injury
6. Control of pain and discomfort

Typical disposition: admission for surgery

1. Ophthalmologic consultation
2. Plastic reconstruction consultation as indicated

LEARNING ACTIVITIES

1. DIRECTIONS: Complete the following crossword puzzle related to maxillofacial and ocular emergencies.

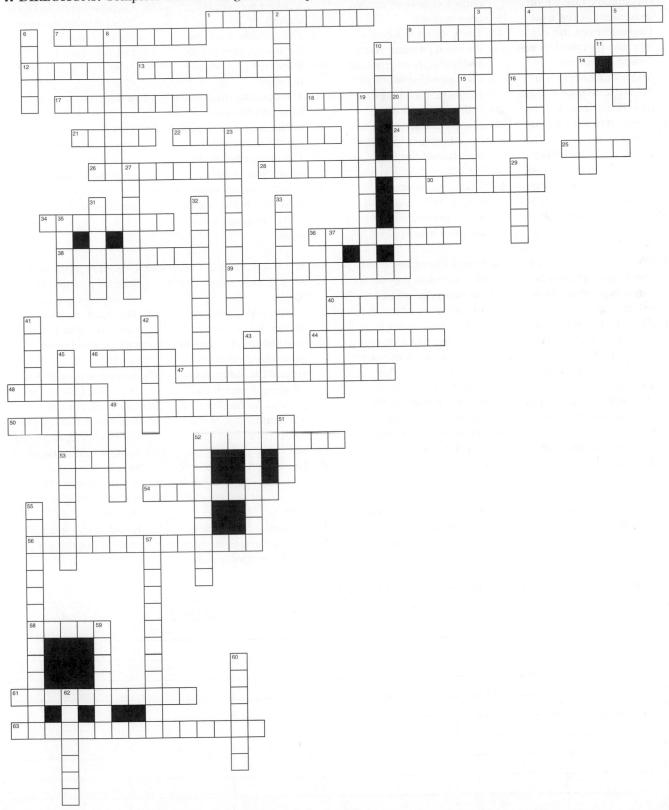

ACROSS

1. Drainage from the nose
4. This muscle closes the mandible for mastication
7. Involuntary, rapid, jerky movement of the eyes
9. Drainage from the ear
11. May also be called *trench mouth* or *Vincent angina* (abbrev)
12. This type of lens is used to irrigate the eye
13. This cerebral lobe controls vision
16. This clear, gelatin-like substance lies between the lens and the retina
17. A type of eyelid retractor
18. May be caused by air travel

21. The cranial nerve that controls visual acuity
22. A sudden unexplained fall without a loss of consciousness or vertigo (two words)
24. These structures inside the nasal passages warm and humidify inspired air
25. The normal color of the tympanic membrane
26. Difficulty swallowing
28. The cranial nerve that has three branches to control sensation of the face
30. Ear pain
34. These are frequently seen in the visual field in the presence of retinal detachment

36. A "sty"
38. A common term for alveolar osteitis (two words)
39. These are also known as *wisdom teeth* (two words)
40. The inability to open the mouth completely
44. Increased intraocular pressure
46. The opening that allows light into the eye
47. Inflammation of the labyrinths of the inner ear
48. The cranial nerve that allows you to smile
49. This type of otoscope is used to test the mobility of the tympanic membrane

50. Tiny hairs in the nasal passages
52. Excessive dilation of the pupil
53. Cranial nerves III, IV, and VI all control the movement of these
54. Double vision
56. "Pink eye" is a form of viral _____
58. A bone of the middle ear
61. This test is used to determine if head movement is the cause of vertigo (two words)
63. The aspiration of middle-ear effusion

DOWN

2. The cranial nerve that controls pupillary constriction
3. This controls pupil size to allow more or less light into the eye
4. This bone houses the lower teeth
5. The most common cause of airway obstruction in infants and children
6. Tonsils are composed of this type of tissue
8. A measurement of intraocular pressure
10. This type of lamp is used to provide a magnified view of the eye

14. Symptoms of this condition are caused by an increase in the volume and pressure of the fluid in the vestibular system
15. The bone that forms the middle third of the face
19. An indication of this condition in an infant is when the infant pulls at the ear (two words)
20. These indicate respiratory distress
23. Strep throat is a form of _____
27. This sinus does not develop until adolescence
29. A tuning fork test for air versus bone conduction of sound

31. The voice box
32. An abnormal sensitivity to light
33. A stain that is used to visualize the cornea
35. This "angina" is a diffuse, generalized cellulitis around the submandibular gland, beneath the jaw, and on the floor of the mouth
37. Tooth pain
41. The external ear
42. To conduct this test, the examiner stands behind the patient and speaks softly
43. Gingival inflammation
45. Also referred to as *swimmer's ear* (two words)

49. Drooping of the eyelid; seen in patients with myasthenia gravis
51. The most common cause of facial injuries in children and older adults
52. A generic drug that is prescribed for vertigo
55. Stiff neck (two words)
57. The use of this drug by the mother during pregnancy could cause pediatric dental abnormalities
59. A visual acuity chart
60. A wick placed into the ear
62. Blood in the anterior chamber of the eye

2. DIRECTIONS: List the cranial nerves, and describe their functions.

Number	Name	Function
I		
II		
III		
IV		
V		
VI		
VII		
VIII		
IX		
X		
XI		
XII		

3. **DIRECTIONS:** Match the assessment finding or treatment with the appropriate dental emergency. Each condition may be used more than once.

____ 1. This is treated by irrigating the socket and applying gauze that is moistened with eugenol (oil of clove)	a. Pericoronitis
____ 2. An inflammation of the gingival tissue that is caused by a tooth eruption or impaction	b. Acute necrotizing ulcerative gingivitis
____ 3. A diffuse generalized cellulitis that can spread from the jaw to the mediastinum	c. Periapical abscess
____ 4. Bleeding and pain after the extraction of a tooth	d. Alveolitis
____ 5. A common dental abscess in children	e. Periostitis
____ 6. A metallic taste in the mouth	f. Periodontal abscess
____ 7. The debridement of the gums	g. Ludwig angina
____ 8. A pus collection in cavity that is formed by the disintegration of tissue	

4. **DIRECTIONS:** Match the clinical presentation with the type of maxillofacial trauma.

____ 1. Pain with jaw movement, malocclusion, edema, ecchymosis, and numbness of the lower lip or chin	a. Le Fort I
____ 2. Malocclusion, ecchymosis, numbness of the upper lip, crepitus, and epistaxis	b. Le Fort II
____ 3. Crepitus, periorbital hematoma, edema, numbness of the cheek, and the inability to look up or down with the affected eye	c. Le Fort III
____ 4. Edema with facial elongation; the movement of all facial bones in relation to the cranial base with the manipulation of the teeth and the hard palate	d. Mandibular
____ 5. Facial elongation, numbness of the anterior cheek, and decreased extraocular eye movement	e. Zygomatic
____ 6. Obvious deformity, bleeding, ecchymosis, and a flattened appearance of the anterior cheek	f. Orbital

5. **DIRECTIONS:** Complete the following chart regarding selected ocular emergencies.

Specific Ocular Emergency	Description	Objective Assessment	Management
Conjunctivitis			
Periorbital cellulitis			
Glaucoma			
Central retinal artery occlusion			
Hordeolum			
Retinal detachment			
Hyphema			

6. DIRECTIONS: Identify the physical findings from the following list that are seen with the listed pathologic conditions. More than one physical finding may be listed for each pathologic condition.

_____ 1. Labyrinthitis	a. Ptosis
_____ 2. Ménière disease	b. Decreased mobility of the temporomandibular joint
_____ 3. Otitis externa	c. Meningeal signs
_____ 4. Otitis media	d. Otalgia
_____ 5. Ruptured tympanic membrane	e. Vertigo
_____ 6. Sinusitis	f. Drop attacks
_____ 7. Cavernous sinus thrombosis	g. Conductive hearing loss
_____ 8. Epistaxis	h. Tenderness of the tragus with palpation
_____ 9. Pharyngitis	i. Ataxias
_____ 10. Peritonsillar abscess	j. Bull-neck appearance
_____ 11. Diphtheria	k. Herpetiform vesicles
_____ 12. Temporal arteritis	l. Bleeding from the nares
_____ 13. Ramsey Hunt syndrome	m. Red, swollen nasal mucosa
	n. "Hot-potato" throat
	o. Tenderness of the scalp with palpation
	p. Cervical lymphadenopathy

7. DIRECTIONS: Match the maxillofacial and ocular emergencies with the appropriate treatments.

_____ 1. Epistaxis	a. Zinc oxide
_____ 2. Mandibular fracture	b. Tracheotomy
_____ 3. Ellis II fracture	c. Pilocarpine (Isopto Carpine) drops
_____ 4. Ramsey Hunt syndrome	d. Continuous pressure applied over the Little area for ≥10 minutes
_____ 5. Larynx fracture	e. Conscious sedation
_____ 6. Central retinal artery occlusion	f. Passive facial exercises
_____ 7. Temporomandibular joint dislocation	g. Systemic acetazolamide
_____ 8. Trigeminal neuralgia	h. Open reduction
_____ 9. Bell palsy	i. Antiviral medication
_____ 10. Glaucoma	j. Carbamazepine (Tegratol)

LEARNING ACTIVITIES ANSWERS

1.

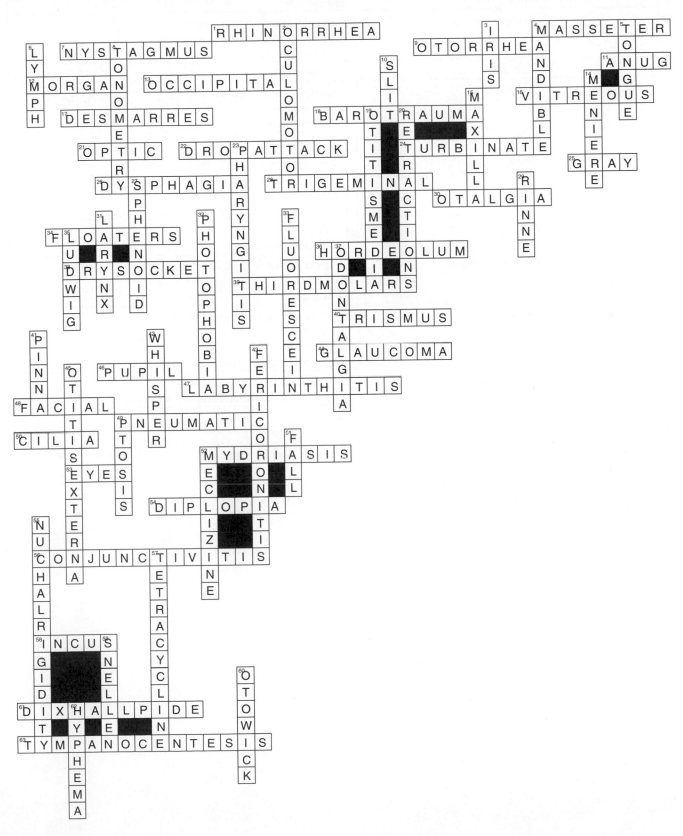

2.

Number	Name	Functions
I	Olfactory	Smell
II	Optic	Vision
III	Oculomotor	Upward lateral eye movement Pupillary constriction Eyelid elevation
IV	Trochlear	Downward medial eye movement
V	Trigeminal	Sensation of scalp and face Sensation of cornea of eye Temporal and masseter muscles
VI	Abducens	Lateral eye movement
VII	Facial	Taste on anterior two thirds of tongue Muscles of facial expression Eyelid closure Lacrimal and salivary glands
VIII	Acoustic	Hearing Equilibrium and balance
IX	Glossopharyngeal	Taste on posterior third of tongue Pharynx Parotid gland
X	Vagus	Pharynx, larynx, neck, and palate Swallowing Cardiac muscle Secretory glands of pancreas and gastrointestinal tract
XI	Spinal accessory	Shoulder and neck movement Sternocleidomastoid and trapezius muscles
XII	Hypoglossal	Tongue

3.

1. d
2. a
3. g
4. e
5. c
6. b
7. a, b
8. c, f

4.

1. d
2. a
3. f
4. c
5. b
6. e

5.

Specific Ocular Emergency	Description	Objective Assessment	Management
Conjunctivitis	Inflammation of the conjunctiva	Burning, itching, watery eyes Hyperemia and mucopurulent drainage	Cool compresses for viral type; nonsteroidal anti-inflammatory drugs Warm compresses for bacterial type; antibiotic drops
Periorbital cellulitis	Infection of the cells around the eyes	Rapid swelling of the eyes Erythema and tenderness of the eyelids without evidence of orbital congestion	Bed rest, warm compresses, antibiotics, antipyretics, and analgesics
Glaucoma	The angle between the iris and the cornea is blocked or insufficient, thereby causing a gradual increase in pressure and the sudden dilation of the eye	Primary open angle glaucoma: usually asymptomatic during the early stages Acute closed angle glaucoma: presents with severe ocular pain Eye redness Headache Decreased vision and halos Nausea and vomiting Excessive tearing Hazy or cloudy cornea	Pilocarpine drops, analgesics, antiemetics, narcotics, and osmotic diuretics
Central retinal artery occlusion	A sudden, painless loss of vision caused by a blocked artery	Sudden unilateral loss of vision Cherry-red spot Afferent pupillary defect, pale and swollen optic nerve with splinter hemorrhages Ground-glass appearance of the retina	β-Blockers, carbogen gas, hyperbaric oxygen chamber, anticoagulants, preparation for possible surgery
Hordeolum	A bacterial infection that develops near the root of an eyelash	Painful swelling of the eye Redness	Warm compresses, analgesics, antibiotic drops or ointment
Retinal detachment	The separation of the two primitive retinal layers	Painless gradual or sudden loss of vision unilaterally Sudden or gradual increase "floaters" in the visual field Light flashes in the eye Appearance of a curtain over the field of vision	Patching of both eyes, bed rest, calm environment
Hyphema	Blood in the anterior chamber of the eye	Blood visualized at the bottom of the iris Pain Afferent pupil defect Decreased extraocular movements	Upright positioning, analgesics, application of a rigid eye shield, cycloplegic drops, bed rest, diuretics; no use of aspirin or nonsteroidal anti-inflammatory drugs

6.

1. d, e
2. e, f
3. d, g, h
4. b, d
5. d, e, i
6. m
7. a, c
8. l, m
9. p
10. d, n, p
11. j, p
12. o
13. k

7.

1. d
2. h
3. a
4. i
5. b
6. g
7. e
8. j
9. f
10. c

References and Suggested Readings

Aung, K., & Ojha, A. (2009). Pharyngitis, viral. Retrieved February 14, 2009, from http://emedicine.medscape.com/article/225362-overview.

Beckstrand, R. L., & Sanders, E. K. (2002). A young girl with missile trauma near the eye. *Journal of Emergency Nursing, 28(3),* 267–269.

Buttaro, T. M., Trybulski, J., Bailey, P. P., & Sandberg-Cook, J. (2003). *Primary care: A collaborative practice.* St. Louis: Mosby.

Calhoun, K., Wax, M., & Eibling, D. E. (2001). Experts guide to otolaryngology. American College of Physicians, American Society of Internal Medicine. Retrieved February 19, 2009, from http://books.google.com/books?id=a4TJ33UHnHMC&printsec=frontcover&dq=sphenopalatine+artery+branches+into+ethmoid#PPA204,M1.

Clark, D. Y., Stocking, J., & Johnson, J. (Eds.). (2006). *Flight and ground transport nursing core curriculum* (2nd ed.). Denver, CO: Air & Surface Transport Nurses Association.

Cleveland Clinic Foundation Website. (1995–2008). Preventing choking in children. Retrieved February 13, 2009, from www.clevelandclinic.org/healthy_living/childrens_health/hic_preventing_choking_in_children.aspx.

Deason, J., & Hope, B. (2005). 23-year-old man with chest pressure, pallor, tachypnea, and tonsillitis. *Journal of Emergency Nursing, 31(2),* 199–202.

Dennison, R. D. (2007). *Pass CCRN!* (3rd ed.). St. Louis: Mosby.

Domino, F. J. (2008). *The 5-minute clinical consultant* (16th ed.). Philadelphia: Lippincott, Williams, & Wilkins.

Echlin, P. & McKeag, D. B. (2004). Maxillofacial injuries in sport. *Current Sports Medicine Reports, 3(1),* 25–32.

Emergency Nurses Association. (2007). *Emergency nursing core curriculum* (6th ed). Philadelphia: Saunders.

Emergency Nurses Association. (2005). *Sheehy's manual of emergency care* (6th ed). St. Louis: Mosby.

Evans, J. A., & Rothenhaus, T. (2007). Epistaxis. Retrieved January 20, 2009, from http://emedicine.medscape.com/article/764719-overview.

Fultz, J. & Sturt, P. A. (2005). *Mosby's emergency nursing reference* (3rd ed.). St. Louis: Mosby.

Graham, R. H., & Ebrahim, S. A. (2009). Central retinal artery occlusion. Retrieved February 13, 2009, from http://emedicine.medscape.com/article/1223625-overview.

Harrahill, M. (2005). Review of a ruptured globe injury: The care for early consult from ophthalmology. *Journal of Emergency Nursing, 31(4),* 408–410.

Haupt, P. S. (2008). Visual acuity testing in the emergency department: Education and competency for emergency nurses. *Journal of Emergency Nursing, 34(3),* 233–235.

Howard, M. L. (2006). Middle ear, tympanic membranes, perforations. Retrieved February 10, 2009, from, http://emedicine.medscape.com/article/858684-overview.

Hoyt, K. S., & Gerhart, A. E. (2008). Mandibular fractures. *Advanced Emergency Nursing Journal, 30(2),* 102–111.

Ing, E. (2007). Lacerations, eyelid. Retrieved February 14, 2009, from http://emedicine.medscape.com/article/1212531-overview.

Jarvis, C. (2008). *Physical examination and health assessment* (5th ed.). St. Louis: Saunders.

Kacker, A. (2001). Foreign body in the nose. *MedlinePlus.* Retrieved February 12, 2009, from http://www.nlm.nih.gov/medlineplus/ency/article/000037.htm.

Mayo Clinic Website (n.d.). Ruptured eardrum. Retrieved February 3, 2009, from http://www.mayoclinic.com/health/ruptured-eardrum/DS00499.

McCleane, G. (2007). Pharmacological pain management in the elderly patient. *Clinical Interventions in Aging, 2(4),* 637–643. Retrieved July 4, 2009, from http://www.pubmedcentral.nih.gov/articlerender.fcgi?artid=2686343.

Mehta, N., & Silverberg, M. A. (2008). Peritonsillar abscess. Retrieved February 20, 2009, from http://emedicine.medscape.com/article/764188-overview.

Merck Manuals Online Medical Library. (n.d.) Mouth and dental emergencies. Retrieved January 25, 2009, from http://www.merck.com/mmhe/sec08.html.

Merriam-Webster Online. (2007–2008). *Merriam Webster's medical dictionary.* Retrieved January 29, 2009, from http://medical.merriam-webster.com.

Pancholi, S. S., Robbins, W. K., & Desai, T. (2009). Laryngeal fractures. Retrieved February 22, 2009, from http://emedicine.medscape.com/article/865277-overview.

Peng, L. F., & Kazzi, A. A. (2007). Dental, fractured tooth. Retrieved January 25, 2009, from http://emedicine.medscape.com/article/763458-overview.

Price, S. A., & Wilson, L. M. (2003). *Pathophysiology: Clinical concepts of disease process* (6th ed.). St. Louis: Mosby.

Proehl, J. A. (2004). *Emergency nursing procedures* (3rd ed.). St. Louis: Saunders.

Roppolo, L. P., Davis, D., Kelly, S. P., & Rosen, P. (2007). *Emergency medicine handbook: Critical concepts for clinical practice.* St. Louis: Mosby.

Sankar, P., Chen, T. C., Grosskreutz, C. L., & Pasquale, L. R. (2002). Traumatic hyphema. International Ophthalmology Clinics. *Ocular Trauma, 42(3),* 57–68.

Schneider, K. (2007). Dental abscess. Retrieved January 25, 2009, from http://emedicine.medscape.com/article/909373-overview.

Scott, I. U., & Luu, K. K. M. (2007). Viral conjunctivitis. Retrieved February 12, 2009, from http://emedicine.medscape.com/article/1191370-overview.

Sharma, R., & Bessman, E. (2008). Cavernous sinus thrombosis. Retrieved January 19, 2009, from http://emedicine.medscape.com/article/791704-overview.

Simon, H. K. (2008). Pediatric, pharyngitis. Retrieved February 14, 2009, from http://medscape.com/article/803258-overview.

Strasnick, B., & Steinberg, A. R. (2008, May). Labyrinthitis. Retrieved January 31, 2009, from http://emedicine.medscape.com/article/792691-overview.

Thomas, J. J., & Edwards, A. R. (2008). Fractured teeth. Retrieved November 8, 2008, from http://www.emedicine.com/proc/topic82755.

Toris, C. B., Yablonski, M. E., Wang, Y. L., & Camras, C. B. (1999). Aqueous humor dynamics in the aging human eye. *American Journal of Ophthalmology, 127*(4), 407–412.

Widell, T. (2008). Fracture, orbital. Retrieved February 14, 2009, from http://emedicine.medscape.com/article/825772-overview.

Wilkerson, R. G., Sinert, R., & Kassutto, Z. (2008). Periorbital infections. Retrieved February 22, 2009, from http://emedicine.medscape.com/article/798397-overview.

Wilkerson, R. G., & Doty, C. I. (2008). Ménière disease. Retrieved February 13, 2009, from http://emedicine.medscape.com/article/792902-overview.

Yamamoto, L. G., Sumida, R. N., Yano, S. S., Derauf, D. C., Martin, P. E., & Eakin, P. J. (2005). Does crying turn tympanic membranes red? *Clinical Pediatrics, 44*(8), 693–697.

Zimmerman, P. G., & Herr, R. (2006). *Triage nursing secrets*. St. Louis: Mosby.

Introduction

Constitutes 15% (10 items) of the CEN examination
The focus is on general medical conditions
commonly encountered in an ED setting
The continuum of age needs to be considered
from infancy to elderly

Age-Related Considerations

Neonates, infants, and children

1. Neonates lose between 5% and 10% of their birth weight
2. Neonates are vulnerable to hypoglycemia because they have decreased glycogen storage
3. Infants are more susceptible to dehydration because their total body weight is approximately 75% water
4. Children have a higher metabolic rate in comparison to adults
5. Infants and children have a compromised immune system since the immune system is not fully developed until around age 8 years
6. Fever is an unreliable indicator of significance of illness in a child

Older adults

1. As the body ages, the body's ability to respond to stressors is decreased
2. With aging, metabolic processes decrease and excretions of fluids, hormones, and medications decrease
3. Total body water composition decreases with age
4. Food and water intake decreases with aging leading to possible malnutrition, dehydration, and electrolyte imbalances
5. Weakness or loss of balance may indicate infection without presence of fever in older adults
6. Changes in mentation, appetite, and activity level may indicate medical problems in older adults

Selected Concepts in Anatomy and Physiology

Endocrine system

1. Function: regulates secretion of hormones that alter metabolic body functions including all of the following:
   a. Chemical reactions and transport of chemicals across cell membranes
   b. Growth and development
   c. Metabolism

d. Fluid and electrolyte balance
e. Acid-base balance
f. Adaptation
g. Reproduction

2. Components of the endocrine system
   a. Glands or glandular tissue that synthesize, store, and secrete hormones
      1) Endocrine glands: ductless but highly vascular
      2) Location of endocrine glands (Figure 11-1)
   b. Hormones
      1) Definition: complex chemical substances produced in one part or organ of the body that initiate or regulate the activity of an organ or a group of cells in another part of the body
         a) Hormones are released by endocrine glands in response to specific signals (e.g., low target gland hormone levels)
         b) Hormones are released directly into the bloodstream to be distributed throughout the body and to the target gland or target organ to initiate a response
      2) Types of hormones include the following
         a) Single amino acids (e.g., epinephrine, dopamine, thyroid hormones)
         b) Proteins (e.g., growth hormone, follicle-stimulating hormone)
         c) Steroids (e.g., androgens, aldosterone, cortisol)
      3) Endocrine glands and hormones are summarized in Table 11-1; hormones are also secreted by the following organs though these organs are not normally considered part of the endocrine system
         a) Gastrointestinal tract (e.g., gastrin, cholecystokinin, somatostatin)
         b) Heart (e.g., atrial natriuretic hormone)
         c) Kidney (e.g., erythropoietin, renin, calcitriol)
   c. Receptor cells: located in an organ or a group of cells in another part of the body
3. Process of hormone synthesis, secretion, effect, suppression (Figure 11-2)
4. Regulation of hormones
   a. The hypothalamus:
      1) The hypothalamus regulates the secretion of hormones through other stimulating hormones called releasing factors
      2) Releasing factors are keyed to cause the release of hormone from the target gland

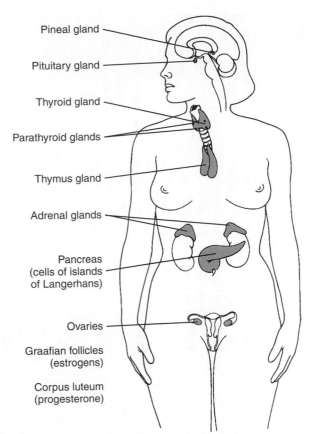

- Pineal gland
- Pituitary gland
- Thyroid gland
- Parathyroid glands
- Thymus gland
- Adrenal glands
- Pancreas (cells of islands of Langerhans)
- Ovaries
- Graafian follicles (estrogens)
- Corpus luteum (progesterone)

Figure 11-1 Location of endocrine glands. (From Dennison, R. D. [2007]. *Pass CCRN!* [3rd ed.]. St. Louis: Mosby.)

b. Neurotransmitters
   1) Sympathetic nervous system: epinephrine, norepinephrine
   2) Parasympathetic nervous system: acetylcholine
c. Feedback regulation
   1) Allows self-regulation
   2) Based on the concentration of the hormone present in the circulation
   3) Also influenced by electrolyte levels, metabolites, osmolality, fluid status, and other hormones
   4) Positive feedback: low hormone levels stimulate release of the releasing factor
   5) Negative feedback: high hormone levels inhibit the release of the releasing factor (Figure 11-3)
5. Endocrine dysfunction
   a. Classification
      1) Based on level of hormone activity
         a) Hyperfunction: increased hormonal activity
         b) Hypofunction: decreased hormonal activity
      2) Based on location of dysfunctional gland or response
         a) Primary disorders: disorder of the target gland (e.g., adrenal or thyroid gland)
         b) Secondary disorder: disorder of the stimulating gland (e.g., hypothalamus or pituitary)
      3) Based on acuity
         a) Acute: beginning abruptly with marked intensity

b) Chronic: developing slowly and persisting for a long period of time, often for the remainder of the lifetime of the individual
   b. Causes of endocrine dysfunction
      1) Dysfunction of a particular gland
      2) Altered secretion of the stimulating hormones for that gland
      3) Altered response to the hormone itself at the target cell

Renal System
1. Functions of the renal system
   a. Regulation of homeostasis and the body's internal environment
      1) Regulation of extracellular fluid volume
      2) Regulation of extracellular fluid osmolality
      3) Regulation of electrolyte balance
      4) Excretion of metabolic wastes
      5) Regulation of acid-base balance (in conjunction with the pulmonary system)
   b. Production and release of hormones
      1) Regulation of blood pressure influenced by aldosterone and antidiuretic hormone (ADH)
      2) Stimulation of red blood cell (RBC) production via erythropoietin
      3) Synthesis and release of prostaglandins
   c. Participation in activation of vitamin D
2. Components of the renal system (Figure 11-4)
   a. Two kidneys
   b. Two ureters
   c. Urinary bladder
   d. Urethra
3. General characteristics of the kidney
   a. Location of kidney
      1) Posterior abdominal wall behind peritoneum
      2) Opposite last thoracic and first three lumbar vertebrae on each side of spine
      3) Right kidney slightly lower than left as a result of liver location
   b. Size, shape, weight of the kidney
      1) Size: approximately 10 × 5 × 2.5 cm or approximately fist-sized
      2) Shape: beanlike with convex lateral border convex and concave medial border; long axis approximately vertical
      3) Weight: 120 to 170 g each kidney
4. Extrarenal structures
   a. Renal capsule
      1) Thin, smooth layer of fibrous membrane that surrounds each kidney
      2) Acts as a protective layer
      3) Prevents kidney swelling
      4) Contains pain receptors
   b. Perirenal fat and renal fascia
      1) Support and protect the kidney
      2) Hold kidney in place
   c. Adrenal gland (also referred to as the suprarenal gland): rests on top of each kidney

TABLE 11-1   Endocrine Glands and Hormones

Hormone	Actions	Releasing Factors	Target	Hypersecretion	Hyposecretion
Pituitary (i.e., Hypophysis)					
Anterior Pituitary (i.e., Adenohypophysis)					
Growth hormone (somatotropin)	Stimulates protein anabolism Mobilizes of fatty acids Conserves carbohydrates Stimulates bone and cartilage growth	Growth hormone releasing hormone (GRH) from hypothalamus in response to exercise, starvation, decreased amino acid levels, stress, hypoglycemia	All body cells capable of growth especially muscle, bone, and cartilage cells	Giantism in children, acromegaly in adults	Dwarfism in children, possible decrease in organ weight in adults
Adrenocorticotropic hormone	Stimulates growth and function of adrenal gland Controls production and release of glucocorticoid hormones Stimulates mineralocorticoid production Stimulates androgen production	Corticotropin releasing hormone (CRH) from hypothalamus in response to hypoglycemia, decrease in cortisol levels, hypoxia, trauma, surgery, physical and/or psychologic stress	Cells of adrenal cortex	Cushing disease	Adrenal insufficiency (chronic) and/or adrenal crisis (acute)
Thyroid-stimulating hormone (thyrotropin)	Increases size and growth of thyroid cells Increases synthesis of thyroid hormones Releases stored thyroid hormones	Thyrotropin-releasing hormone (TRH) from the hypothalamus in response to cold temperature or a decrease in thyroid hormone levels	Cells of the thyroid gland	Hyperthyroidism	Hypothyroidism
Posterior Pituitary (i.e., Neurohypophysis)					
Antidiuretic hormone (vasopressin)	Increases water reabsorption (inhibits diuresis) by kidney tubules and collecting ducts Vasoconstriction of arterioles Abdominal cramping	Increase in serum osmolality, hypernatremia, hypovolemia, hypoxia, hypotension, pain, trauma, stress, nausea, pharmacologic agents	Distal renal tubules and collecting ducts, smooth muscle of arterioles and GI tract	Syndrome of inappropriate anti-diuretic hormone (SIADH)	Diabetes insipidus
Thyroid Gland					
Triiodothyronine (T₃) and thyroxine (T₄) Note: T₃ is more biologically active	Stimulates metabolic rate Increases protein synthesis Increases carbohydrate and fat metabolism Increases bone growth Increases oxygen consumption Increases metabolism and clearance of drugs	Thyroid-stimulating hormone (TSH) from anterior pituitary; TRH from hypothalamus, cold temperature	Most body cells	Hyperthyroidism (chronic), thyroid storm or crisis (acute)	Hypothyroidism (chronic), myxedema coma (acute)
Thyrocalcitonin (calcitonin)	Reduces plasma calcium levels by inhibiting bone lysis and decreasing calcium resorption by the kidney	Increase in serum calcium, magnesium, or glucagon	Bone cells, kidney cells	Not significant	Not significant

	Action	Stimulus	Target	Hypersecretion	Hyposecretion
Parathyroid Gland					
Parathyroid hormone (parathormone)	Increases serum calcium by accelerating bone breakdown with release of calcium into the blood, increasing calcium reabsorption from intestine, and decreasing kidney tubule reabsorption of calcium Decreases blood phosphate levels by increasing phosphate loss in urine Increases reabsorption of magnesium by the renal tubules	Low serum calcium, high serum magnesium or phosphate level, catecholamines, cortisol	Bone cells, cells of GI tract and kidney	Hypercalcemia and hypophosphatemia, possibly renal calculi	Hypocalcemia and bone decalcification, hyperphosphatemia
Adrenal Cortex					
Glucocorticoids, i.e., cortisol	Increases blood glucose by stimulating gluconeogenesis in the liver Inhibits glucose utilization by the cell Inhibits protein anabolism Promotes fatty acid mobilization Inhibits inflammatory response	CRH from hypothalamus, ACTH from anterior pituitary	Most body cells	Cushing syndrome	Addison disease (chronic), adrenal crisis (acute)
Mineralocorticoids, i.e., aldosterone	Increases sodium and water reabsorption and potassium excretion	ACTH from anterior pituitary (minor effect), primary stimulus is renin-angiotensin system, decrease in serum sodium, increase in serum potassium	Distal and collecting tubules of kidney, sweat glands, salivary glands, intestines	Hyperaldosteronism	Addison disease (chronic), adrenal crisis (acute)
Adrenal Medulla					
Catecholamines, i.e., epinephrine, norepinephrine	Dilates pupils Increases heart rate and contractility Dilation of blood vessels to heart, brain and skeletal muscle Constriction of blood vessels to nonessential organs, i.e., skin, kidney, GI tract Bronchodilation Increase in respiratory rate and depth Increase in perspiration, peristalsis and secretion in GI tract Increase in blood sugar	Sympathetic nervous system innervation: insulin, histamine, anxiety, fear, pain, trauma, exercise, temperature extremes, hypoxia, hypotension, hypovolemia, excess thyroid hormone	Most body cells, vascular beds, smooth muscle	Exaggeration or prolongation of normal effects, may be caused by adrenal medulla tumor called pheochromocytoma	May have decrease in stress response or no noticeable effect

Continued

TABLE 11-1	Endocrine Glands and Hormones—cont'd				
Hormone	**Actions**	**Releasing Factors**	**Target**	**Hypersecretion**	**Hyposecretion**
Pancreas					
Glucagon (from α cells)	Stimulates glycogenolysis and gluconeogenesis to increase blood glucose Inhibits glycolysis Increases lipolysis	Decrease in blood glucose, increased blood amino acid, catecholamines, exercise, starvation	Most body cells, especially liver cells	Hyperglycemia	Hypoglycemia
Insulin (from β cells)	Enables glucose to move into the cell Aids in muscle and tissue oxidation of glucose Enhances storage of glycogen Increases protein synthesis Inhibits lipolysis	Increase in blood glucose, gastrin, increase in growth hormone, ACTH, glucagon	Most body cells, especially liver cells	Hypoglycemia	Hyperglycemia (diabetes mellitus)

From Dennison, R. D. (2007). *Pass CCRN!* (3rd ed.). St. Louis: Mosby.

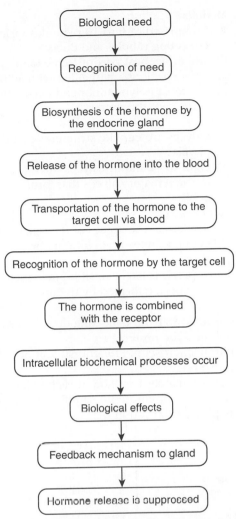

Figure 11-2 Process of hormone systhesis, secretion, effect, and suppression. (From Dennison, R. D. [2007]. *Pass CCRN!* [3rd ed.]. St. Louis: Mosby.)

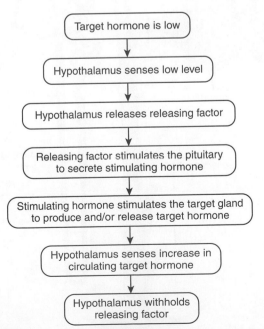

Figure 11-3 Negative feedback mechanism. (From Dennison, R. D. [2007]. *Pass CCRN!* [3rd ed.]. St. Louis: Mosby.)

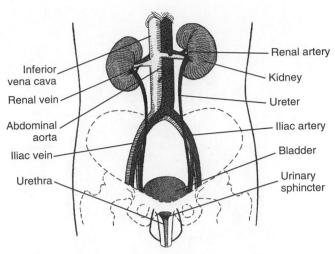

Figure 11-4 The kidneys and other structures. (From Dennison, R. D. [2007]. *Pass CCRN!* [3rd ed.]. St. Louis: Mosby.)

   d. Hilum
     1) Concave notch of medial aspect of kidney
     2) Entry site for renal artery and nerves
     3) Exit site for renal vein and ureter
   e. Ureters
     1) Fibromuscular tubes located behind peritoneum; extend from kidney to posterior part of bladder floor
     2) Ureter walls composed of smooth muscle with mucosal lining and fibrous outer coat
     3) Collect urine from the renal pelvis and propel it to the bladder by peristaltic waves
     4) Ureters enter the superior, posterior bladder at an oblique angle; this angle and the peristaltic action of the ureters prevent reflux of urine
   f. Bladder
     1) Located behind symphysis pubis, below peritoneum
     2) Collapsible bag of smooth muscle
     3) Acts as a reservoir for urine until sufficient amount accumulates for elimination; expels urine from body by way of urethra
   g. Urethra
     1) Located behind symphysis pubis, anterior to the vagina in females; extends through the prostate gland and penis in males
     2) Acts as passageway for expulsion of urine from the urinary bladder to the urinary meatus, where it is expelled from the body
 5. Renal structures (Figure 11-5)
   a. Renal parenchyma
     1) Cortex
       a) Metabolically active portion of kidney where aerobic metabolism occurs and ammonia and glucose are formed
       b) Site of glomerulus, proximal and distal tubules

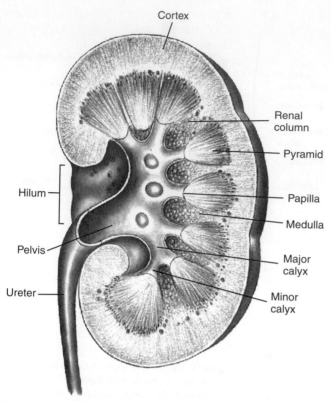

Figure 11-5 Cross section of the kidneys. (From Dennison, R. D. [2007]. *Pass CCRN!* [3rd ed.]. St. Louis: Mosby.)

2) Medulla
   a) Comprised of 6 to 10 pyramids formed by collecting tubules and ducts
   b) Site of deepest part of Henle loop
   b. Renal sinus: spacious cavity filled with adipose tissue, the renal pelvis, minor and major calices, and the origin of the ureter
   1) Calyces
      a) Calyces are cuplike structures that drain the papillae
      b) Eight to 12 minor calyces open into two to three major calyces that form the renal pelvis
   c. Renal pelvis
   1) Papillae are at the apices of the renal pyramids; collecting tubules drain into minor calyces at papillae
   2) Renal pelvis is like a small funnel tapering into the ureter; formed by the union of several calyces
   3) Urine flows from collecting duct to renal pelvis and into the ureter
   d. Nephron: microscopic functional unit of kidney (Figure 11-6)
   1) Approximately 1 million in each kidney
   2) Able to compensate for significant degree of nephron destruction by:

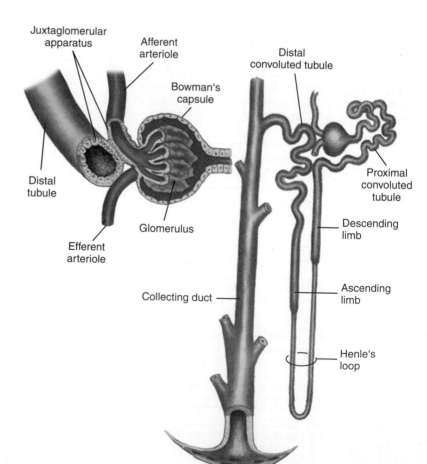

Figure 11-6 Components of the nephron. (From Dennison, R. D. [2007]. *Pass CCRN!* [3rd ed.]. St. Louis: Mosby.)

a) Filtering a greater solute (dissolved substances) load

b) Hypertrophy of remaining functional nephrons

3) Types of nephrons

a) Cortical (85% of nephrons are cortical nephrons)

   i) The glomerulus is located in outer cortex

   ii) Cortical nephrons contain short loops of Henle that dip into the outer edge of the medulla

b) Juxtamedullary (15% of nephrons are juxtamedullary nephrons)

   i) The glomerulus is located in inner cortex

   ii) Juxtamedullary nephrons contain long loops of Henle that penetrate deep into medulla

   iii) These nephrons are important in the kidney's ability to concentrate the urine

4) Functional segments

a) Renal corpuscle: consists of Bowman capsule and glomerulus

   i) The glomerulus is a cluster of tightly coiled capillaries that produces an ultrafiltrate; a portion of this ultrafiltrate eventually becomes urine

   ii) Bowman capsule is the funnel-shaped upper end of the proximal tubule

b) Renal tubules

   i) Segmentally divided into proximal convoluted tubule, loop of Henle, distal convoluted tubule

   ii) Responsible for reabsorption and secretion, which alter the volume and composition of the ultrafiltration to form the final urine volume and composition

c) Collecting duct

   i) Several nephrons converge into a collecting duct

   ii) The collecting duct relays the urine from the tubules to the minor calyx

e. Renal vasculature

1) Pathway of blood supply

a) Renal arteries branch from the aorta

b) The renal arteries branch into interlobar arteries → arcuate arteries → interlobular arteries

c) The interlobular arteries become the afferent arteriole, which forms the glomerulus

d) The efferent arteriole leads out of the glomerulus and forms the peritubular capillary network

e) The efferent arteriole from the juxtamedullary nephron forms a different capillary network called the vasa recta

   i) The vasa recta plays an important role in concentrating interstitial fluid found in the medulla

f) The peritubular capillary network leads to the interlobular vein, which leads to the arcuate vein

g) The arcuate vein leads to the interlobar vein, which leads to the renal vein

h) The renal vein empties into the inferior vena cava

2) Renal blood flow

a) The kidneys receives 20% to 25% of the cardiac output, or approximately 1200 ml/min (600 ml/min for each kidney)

b) Autoregulation maintains constancy in glomerular filtration rate (GFR)

   i) Systemic arterial pressure between 80 and 180 mm Hg prevents large changes in GFR because of the ability of the afferent arteriole to constrict or dilate

   ii) Autoregulation fails at MAP of 60 mm Hg or less

f. Nervous innervation

1) The autonomic nervous system (ANS) supplies the primary innervation of the kidney and the urinary tract

2) Both sympathetic nervous system (SNS) and parasympathetic nervous system (PNS) innervate the kidney but the SNS has the prominent effect on the kidney

6. Formation of urine involves three processes: filtration; reabsorption; and secretion (Figure 11-7)

a. Glomerular filtration: the pressure of the blood within the glomerular capillaries causes blood to be filtered into Bowman capsule, where it begins to pass down to the tubule

1) Filtration is the transfer of water and dissolved substances through a permeable membrane from a region of high pressure to low pressure

2) Filtration depends on hydrostatic pressure, which may be affected by the following:

a) Diminished renal perfusion from hypovolemia

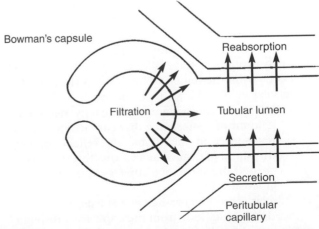

Figure 11-7 Process of filtration. (From Richard, C. J. [1988]. *Comprehensive nephrology nursing*. Copyright © 1986 Little, Brown and Company, Inc. Reproduced with permission of Pearson Education, Inc.)

b) Occlusion of the glomeruli from diabetic neuropathy

c) Alteration in the plasma protein concentration from hypoproteinemia

d) Alterations in the basement membrane from an autoimmune disorder

e) Arteriolar constriction from SNS stimulation or vasopressors

3) GFR

a) Dependent upon the following

i) Permeability of the capillary walls

ii) Vascular pressure

iii) Filtration pressure

b) Clearance: complete removal of a substance from the blood

i) Clearance of a substance equals GFR if the tubules neither reabsorb nor secrete the substance

ii) Clearance of a substance is less than GFR if the tubules secrete the substance

iii) Clearance of a substance is greater than GFR is the tubules secrete the substance

c) Clinically measured by creatinine clearance since creatinine is filtered by the glomeruli and not reabsorbed by the tubules

d) GFR must be maintained at a constant rate and autoregulation ensures this constant rate; systemic mean arterial pressure must be maintained between 80 and 180 mm Hg to maintain regulation

4) The glomerular membrane is a porous but semipermeable membrane

a) Glomerular filtrate (also called ultrafiltrate) is similar in composition to blood except that it lacks blood cells, platelets, and large plasma proteins; water, sodium, glucose, potassium, chloride, phosphate, urea, uric acid, creatinine, ammonia, phenol, calcium, and magnesium pass through the glomerular membrane

b) Glomerular filtrate volume is usually 120 ml/min, but 99% of this will be reabsorbed in the renal tubule

b. Reabsorption: passage of a substance that the body needs from the lumen of the tubules through the tubular cells and into the capillaries

1) Maximal tubular transport capacity: maximum amount of a substance that can be completely reabsorbed in one minute and reflects the renal threshold of a substance; if this threshold is exceeded the substance appears in the urine (e.g., glucosuria)

c. Tubular secretion: passage of a substance not needed by the body from the capillaries through the tubular cells into the lumen of the tubule

d. Countercurrent mechanism uses the juxtamedullary nephrons with their long loops of Henle and occurs within the renal medullary interstitium

1) Countercurrent multiplication is the mechanism that enables the body to excrete urine with an osmolality higher than the osmolality of serum

2) Countercurrent exchange is the maintenance component of the countercurrent mechanism

e. Total of 99% of the glomerular filtrate is reabsorbed from the tubules (especially the proximal limb); the remaining 1% is excreted as urine output

1) Normal urine output is approximately 1500 ml/day

2) Abnormal constituents: glucose, albumin, RBCs, calculi, casts

7. Excretion of metabolic waste products

a. Urea

1) Protein (either ingested or borrowed from protein stores) is broken down into amino acids and nitrogenous wastes

2) Urea nitrogen is the end product of protein metabolism; it circulates in the bloodstream and is excreted in the urine

3) Blood urea nitrogen (BUN) varies with protein intake and hydration status so BUN provides an unreliable evaluation of renal function

b. Creatinine

1) Creatinine is a waste product of muscle metabolism

2) The normal kidney excretes creatinine at a rate equal to the kidney's blood flow or GFR

3) Serum creatinine is a better test for evaluation of renal function than BUN; urine creatinine clearance, which provides a comparison of serum creatinine and 24-hour urine creatinine, is an even better evaluation of renal function

8. Renal regulation of acid-base balance

a. Tubular excretion of H+ ions in exchange for sodium reabsorption

b. Bicarbonate reabsorption into the circulation or excretion into the urine

c. Excretion of H+ ions in the urine as NH_4Cl, H_2PO_4, H_2O

d. Renal response to acidosis

1) Increased hydrogen ion secretion

2) Increased bicarbonate reabsorption

3) Production of ammonia to accommodate hydrogen ion excretion

e. Renal response to alkalosis

1) Decreased hydrogen ion secretion

2) Increased bicarbonate excretion

3) Decreased production of ammonia

9. Fluid balance

a. Body fluids are dilute solutions of water and solutes

b. Measurement methods

1) Milliliter (ml): the unit of measure for fluid volume

2) Milliequivalent (mEq): the unit of measure for chemical combining activity of an electrolyte

3) Milliosmoles (mOsm): the unit of measure for osmotic pressure based on the number of dissolved particles in solution

a) Osmolality and osmolarity: frequently used interchangeably though most calculations of body fluids are based on osmolality
   i) Osmolality: number of osmoles per kilogram of solution; expressed as mOsm/kg
      (a) Normal for blood: 280 to 295 mOsm/kg H_2O
      (b) Normal for urine: 50 to 1200 mOsm/kg H_2O
   ii) Osmolarity: number of osmoles per liter of solution
      (a) Isotonic: the tonicity of body fluids; osmolarity of 280 to 295 mOsm/L
      (b) Hypotonic: lower tonicity than body fluids
      (c) Hypertonic: higher tonicity than body fluids

c. The human body is mostly water
   1) Volume
      a) Adult males: 60% of total body weight in adult males is water
      b) Adult females: slightly less water at 55% of total body weight due to higher percentage of body fat
      c) Older adults: less water at 45% to 55% of total body weight
      d) Obesity: body water decreases with increasing body fat
   2) Distribution (Figure 11-8)
      a) Intracellular
         i) Fluid contained within the cells
         ii) Accounts for 40% of total body weight
      b) Extracellular
         i) Fluid outside the cells
         ii) Accounts for 20% of total body weight

   iii) Distribution
      (a) Interstitial
         i. Fluid surrounding the cells
         ii. Accounts for 15% of total body weight
      (b) Intravascular
         i. Fluid contained within the blood vessels
         ii. Accounts for approximately 4% of total body weight
      (c) Transcellular
         i. Fluid contained within specialized cavities of the body (e.g., cerebrospinal, pericardial, pleural, synovial, intraocular, digestive fluids)
         ii. Accounts for approximately 1% of total body weight
      (d) Homeostasis is the state of internal equilibrium within the body; fluid, electrolyte, and acid-base are in balance

   1) Water and solutes are in constant movement and are exchanged continuously
      a) Most of the membranes of the body are semipermeable, allowing free movement of water and many nonelectrolytes and selective movement of electrolytes according to concentration gradients
      b) Movement of fluids, electrolytes, and other solutes occurs by the following processes
         i) Diffusion: solutes move from an area of higher solute concentration to an area of lower solute concentration
         ii) Osmosis: solutions move from an area of lower solute concentration to an area of higher solute concentration

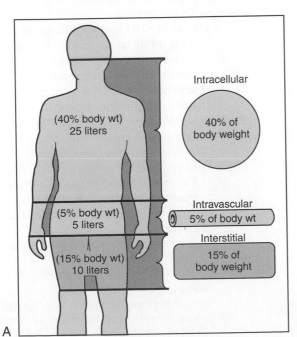
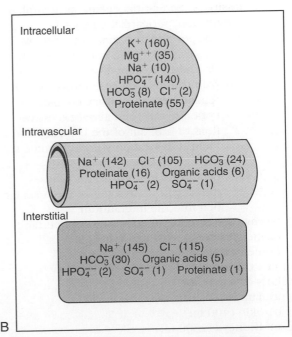

Figure 11-8 Distribution of body fluids. (From Dennison, R. D. [2007]. *Pass CCRN!* [3rd ed.]. St. Louis: Mosby.)

iii) Active transport: use of an energy source to move solutes from an area of lower solute concentration to an area of higher solution concentration

iv) Filtration: use of the pushing pressure of hydrostatic pressure to move water and selected solutes through a semipermeable membrane

c) Movement into and out of the cell occurs by diffusion, osmosis, and active transport

  i) Hydrostatic pressures push

   (a) Capillary hydrostatic pressure pushes fluid out of capillary and into interstitium

   (b) Interstitial hydrostatic pressure pushes fluid out of interstitium and into the capillary

  ii) Colloidal oncotic pressures pull

   (a) Capillary colloidal oncotic pressure pulls and holds fluid in the capillary

   (b) Interstitial colloidal oncotic pressure pulls and hold fluid in the interstitium

  iii) Starling's Law of the Capillaries describes the movement of fluid into and out of the capillaries (for more on capillary dynamics, see Chapter 4)

   (a) Pressure differences at the venous and arterial ends of the capillaries influence the direction and rate of water and solute movement

   (b) Pressures pushing fluid out of the capillary dominate at the arterial end; pressures pushing fluid back into the capillary dominate at the venous end

d) Pathology

  i) Third spacing: fluid accumulation in any space that is not intravascular or intracellular (e.g., interstitial edema, ascites, pleural effusion, pericardial effusion)

   (a) HF: peripheral edema is caused by venous congestion and excessive hydrostatic pressure at the venous end

   (b) Malnutrition: decrease in plasma proteins decrease capillary colloidal oncotic pressure and allow excessive fluid to leak out of the capillary

   (c) Fluid resuscitation with hypotonic solutions (e.g., D_5W): fluids with osmolality less than serum causes movement of fluid out of the vascular bed into the interstitium

2) Normal functioning of cells requires constancy of the body's compartments; imbalances disrupt homeostasis

e. Water exchanges occur continuously

 1) Loss of water: total ~2400 ml/24 hr

  a) Lungs (400 ml)

  b) Skin (400 ml)

  c) Kidneys (1500 ml)

  d) Intestines (100 ml)

e) Losses are increased by any of the following

  i) Increased respiratory rate

  ii) Fever

  iii) Hot, dry environment

  iv) Injury to the skin (e.g., burns)

2) Gains of water: total ~2400 ml/24 hr

  a) Liquids (1500 ml)

  b) Food (500 ml)

  c) Oxidation of food and body tissues (400 ml)

f. Body fluid is regulated by the following mechanisms

 1) Thirst

  a) Thirst mechanism is located in the anterior hypothalamus; osmoreceptor cells sense changes in serum osmolality and initiate impulses to produce the thirst sensation and the release of ADH

  b) The mechanism is stimulated by any of the following

   i) Intracellular dehydration

   ii) Hypertonic body fluids

   iii) Extracellular fluid loss

   iv) Hypotension or decreased cardiac output

   v) Angiotensin

   vi) Dry mouth

  c) The effect of thirst is the conscious desire to drink fluids (NOTE: thirst is unreliable in the elderly or confused patient)

 2) Antidiuretic hormone

  a) ADH is produced by the hypothalamus, stored in and released by the posterior pituitary gland; release may be altered by intracranial processes (e.g., head injury, tumors, craniotomy) and extracranial processes (e.g., mechanical ventilation, tuberculosis)

  b) ADH is stimulated by any of the following

   i) Hyperosmolality of extracellular fluid

   ii) Decrease in extracellular fluid volume

   iii) Hyperthermia

  c) Effects of ADH include the following

   i) Acts on distal and collecting tubules, causing more water to be pulled from the tubule back into the blood

   ii) Increases total volume of body fluid by decreasing urine volume

 3) Renin-angiotensin-aldosterone (RAA) system (see Figure 4-11)

  a) RAA system is stimulated by any of the following

   i) Decreased blood pressure stimulating stretch receptors in juxtaglomerular cells

   ii) Sympathetic nervous system stimulation

   iii) Hyponatremia, hyperkalemia

   iv) Increased adrenocorticotropin hormone (ACTH) levels

  b) Effects of the RAA system include the following

   i) Angiotensin II causes vasoconstriction and secretion of aldosterone, a mineralocorticoid produced by the adrenal cortex

ii) Aldosterone stimulates the renal tubules to reabsorb more sodium and water, which causes sodium retention, water retention, and decreased urine volume

iii) Vasoconstriction and sodium and water retention increases blood pressure, which decreases renin secretion

4) Atrial natriuretic peptide (ANP)

a) ANP is a hormone-like substance that is synthesized and stored by specialized atrial muscle cells

b) ANP secretion is stimulated by the following

i) Volume expansion

ii) Increased cardiac filling pressures

c) Effects of ANP include the following

i) Increased excretion of sodium and water by the kidney

ii) Decreased synthesis of renin and decreased release of aldosterone

5) Countercurrent mechanism of kidney: mechanism for concentration and dilution of urine

10. Electrolyte balance

a. Solutes are substances dissolves in a solution and may be electrolytes or nonelectrolytes

1) Nonelectrolytes (e.g., glucose, proteins, lipids, oxygen, carbon dioxide, urea, creatinine, bilirubin) are solutes without an electrical charge; they stay intact in solution

2) Electrolytes are solutes that dissociate into positive or negative ions when in solution and will generate an electrical charge when in solution

a) Electrical charge

i) Cations are positive charged ions

(a) Major intracellular cation is potassium (K^+)

(b) Major extracellular cation is sodium (Na^+)

(c) Other cations: Ca^{++}; Mg^{++}; H^+

ii) Anions are negative charged electrolytes

(a) Major intracellular anion is chloride (Cl^-)

(b) Major extracellular anion is phosphate (PO_4^{3-})

(c) Other anions: HCO_3^-

b. In each fluid compartment, the various cations and anions balance each other to achieve electrical neutrality; there is no net charge within a fluid compartment (see Figure 11-8)

c. Renal regulation of electrolytes

1) Excretion and/or retention of electrolytes

2) Filter and reabsorb about half of unbound serum calcium and activate vitamin D3, a compound that promotes intestinal calcium absorption

3) Regulates phosphorus excretion

d. Summary of electrolyte normal values, roles, regulation, and food sources (Table 11-2)

11. Renal role in regulation of blood pressure

a. Juxtaglomerular apparatus is a combination of specialized cells located near the glomerulus at the junction of the afferent and efferent arterioles; juxtaglomerular cells contain granules of inactive renin

b. RAA system (see Figure 4-11)

12. RBC synthesis and maturation

a. Erythropoietin secretion

1) Stimulates production of RBCs in bone marrow

2) Prolongs life of RBC

b. Postulated methods of erythropoietin synthesis and stimulus for secretion

1) Normal kidneys either produce erythropoietin or synthesize an enzyme that catalyzes its formation

2) Stimulation for formation is believed to be decreased PO_2 in renal blood

c. Interference in this process causes anemia in patients with chronic renal failure

13. Prostaglandin synthesis

a. Process occurs primarily in the medulla

b. Types of prostaglandins are as follows

1) Vasodilators: PGE_2, PGD_2, PGI_2

2) Vasoconstrictors: PGA_2

c. Release is stimulated by vasoactive substances (e.g., angiotensin, norepinephrine, bradykinins)

d. Effects of prostaglandins include the following

1) Modulate the vasoconstrictive effects of angiotensin and norepinephrine; interference with this process may be one factor contributing to hypertension in patients with renal failure

2) Increase renal blood flow, which results in arterial vasodilation, inhibition of the distal tubule's response to ADH, and promotion of sodium and water excretion

14. Renal role in bone mineralization

a. Vitamin D is metabolized by the kidney from an inactive form to an active metabolite called 1,25-dihydroxycholecalciferol necessary for the absorption of calcium and phosphorus from the intestine

b. Interference in this process causes osteodystrophy in patients with chronic renal failure

Hematology/Immunology

1. Functions of the hematologic and immunologic systems

a. Hematologic

1) Provides the medium for transportation of oxygen, carbon dioxide, and nutrients to the tissues

2) Maintains hemostasis

3) Maintains internal environment, including participation in regulation of temperature and acid-base balance

TABLE 11-2   Electrolyte Functions, Factors Affecting Serum Levels, and Food Sources

Electrolyte	Functions	Regulation and Factors Affecting Serum Level	Food Sources
Sodium: normal 136 to 145 mEq/L	• Maintains extracellular osmolality and volume • Maintains active transport mechanism in conjunction with potassium • Influences the kidney's regulation of the body's water and electrolyte status • Promotes the irritability of nerve tissue and the conduction of nerve impulses • Facilitates muscle contraction • Aids in some enzyme activities • Combines with bicarbonate and chloride to help regulate acid-base balance	• Aldosterone: causes sodium and water retention • Glomerular filtration rate: sodium excretion is increased when GFR is high, decreased when GFR is low • "Third factor": promotes sodium excretion by inhibiting sodium reabsorption; suppression of this factor ensures sodium reabsorption • Increase in sodium concentration stimulates water retention by ADH release diluting sodium back to normal level • Some excretion through skin in perspiration	• Bouillon • Celery • Cheeses • Dried fruits • Frozen, canned, or packaged foods • Monosodium glutamate (MSG) • Mustard • Olives • Pickles • Preserved meat • Salad dressings and prepared sauces • Sauerkraut • Snack foods • Soy sauce
Potassium: normal 3.5 to 5.0 mEq/L	• Promotes transmission of nerve impulses • Maintains intracellular osmolality • Activates several enzymatic reactions • Helps regulate acid-base balance • Influences kidney function and structure • Promotes myocardial, skeletal, and smooth muscle contractility	• Aldosterone: increase in intracellular potassium or decrease in serum sodium causes aldosterone release and potassium excretion • GFR: potassium excretion is directly related to GFR in a normal kidney • Obligatory loss: the kidneys are unable to conserve potassium; it may be flushed out by diuresis even in the presence of a body deficit; 40-50 mEq lost each day • Renal failure: if kidneys fail to excrete potassium normally from the body (e.g., renal failure), toxic levels can occur • pH: potassium shifts into the cell in alkalosis (causing hypokalemia) and out of the cell in acidosis (causing hyperkalemia)	• Apricots • Artichokes • Avocado • Bananas • Cantaloupe • Carrots • Cauliflower • Chocolate • Dried beans, peas • Dried fruit • Mushrooms • Nuts • Oranges, orange juice • Peanuts • Potatoes • Prune juice • Pumpkin • Spinach • Sweet potatoes • Swiss chard • Tomatoes, tomato juice, tomato sauce

Calcium: normal 9.0 to 10.5 mg/dl in adults and 8.8 to 10.8 mg/dl in children (Note: calcium is affected by albumin levels; to correct calcium, add 0.8 mg/dl for each 1 g/dl decrease in albumin)	• Hardens and strengthens bones and teeth • Aids in blood coagulation • Transmits neuromuscular impulses • Maintains cellular permeability • Serves essential role in cardiac contractility	• PTH: stimulated by a decrease in serum calcium; promotes calcium transfer from bone to plasma and aids in renal and intestinal absorption • Phosphorus: inhibits calcium absorption; calcium and phosphorus have an inverse relationship: if calcium goes up, phosphorus goes down and vice versa • Vitamin D: necessary for GI absorption; promotes calcium absorption • Calcitonin: aids transfer of calcium from plasma to bone which directly lowers serum calcium • Albumin: 50% of serum calcium is bound to serum albumin therefore a decrease in serum albumin will lower the total calcium level but not the ionized calcium level and the patient will not have symptoms of hypocalcemia • pH: alkalosis increases binding between albumin and calcium so that the patient will exhibit symptoms of hypocalcemia though total body calcium is normal; acidosis decreases binding between albumin and calcium so that the patient may exhibit symptoms of hypercalcemia • Corticosteroids: contribute to demineralization of the bone and calcium loss, large doses decrease calcium absorption in GI tract • Diuretic effect: calcium is lost along with potassium and magnesium in patient on diuretics	• Brazil nuts • Broccoli • Cheese • Collard, mustard, turnip greens • Cottage cheese • Eggnog • Ice cream • Milk and cream • Milk chocolate • Molasses • Oat flakes • Rhubarb • Seafood especially sardines with bones • Sesame seeds • Soy flour • Spinach • Yogurt
Phosphorus normal 3.0 to 4.5 mg/dl	• Aids in structure of cellular membrane • Essential for glucose metabolism in red cells; produces 2,3-diphosphoglyceric acid (2,3-DPG) as an end product • Regulates the delivery of oxygen to the tissues; 2,3-DPG encourages unloading between hemoglobin and oxygen • Essential for ATP or high energy phosphate formation • May be connected with DNA, RNA, genetic coding • Helps maintain bone hardness • Aids in enzyme regulation (ATPase) • Used by kidney to buffer hydrogen ions (PO_4)	• PTH: inhibits renal reabsorption of phosphates; calcium and phosphorus have an inverse relationship, if calcium goes up, phosphorus goes down and vice versa • Alterations in GFR affect phosphate excretion; increased GFR decreases reabsorption of phosphorus; decreased GFR increases reabsorption of phosphorus	• Dried beans and peas • Eggs and egg products • Fish, poultry • Meats, especially organ meats • Milk and milk products • Nuts • Seeds • Whole grains

Continued

TABLE 11-2   Electrolyte Functions, Factors Affecting Serum Levels, and Food Sources—cont'd

Electrolyte	Functions	Regulation and Factors Affecting Serum Level	Food Sources
Magnesium: normal 1.3 to 2.1 mEq/L in adults, 1.4 to 1.7 mEq/L in children, and 1.4 to 2 mEq/L in infants	• Aids in neuromuscular transmission • Aids in cardiac contractility • Activates enzymes for cellular metabolism of CHO and proteins • Aids in maintaining the active transport mechanism at the cellular level • Aids in the transmission of hereditary information to offspring	• Not completely understood • Factors that influence calcium and potassium balance also affect magnesium • Deficiencies of these electrolytes usually occur together (e.g., diuretics cause the loss of all three) • Availability of sodium: sodium is necessary for the absorption of magnesium • Diuretics: cause the loss of excessive magnesium • PTH: affects magnesium reabsorption as it does calcium	• Bananas • Chocolate • Coconut • Grapefruit • Green, leafy vegetables • Legumes • Milk • Molasses • Nuts and seeds • Oranges • Refined sugar • Seafood • Soy flour • Wheat bran
Chloride: normal 95 to 103 mEq/L	• Maintains serum osmolality (along with sodium) • Combines with major cations to form important compounds (e.g., NaCl, HCl, KCl, CaCl) • Helps maintain acid-base balance through HCl production	• Indirectly affected by aldosterone • Changes almost always linked to sodium • pH: acidosis causes bicarbonate to be reabsorbed while chloride is excreted; alkalosis causes bicarbonate to be excreted while chloride is reabsorbed	• Bananas • Celery • Cheese • Dates • Eggs • Fish • Milk • Spinach • Table salt • Turkey

From: Dennison, R. D. (2007). *Pass CCRN!* (3rd ed.). St. Louis: Mosby.

b. Immunologic
   1) Protects the body's internal milieu against invading organisms and from the development, growth, and dissemination of abnormal cells
   2) Maintains homeostasis by removing damaged cells from the circulation

2. Bone marrow
   a. Most functioning bone marrow in adults is located in flat bones (vertebrae, skull, pelvic and shoulder girdles, clavicle, ribs, sternum) and proximal epiphysis of long bones
   b. The functions of the bone marrow include the following:
      1) Production of the following
         a) Erythrocytes (RBCs)
         b) Leukocytes (white blood cells) including granulocytes, agranulocytes, and lymphocytes
         c) Thrombocytes (platelets)
      2) Recognition and removal of senescent cells
      3) Participation in cellular and humoral immunity

3. Spleen
   a. White pulp: primarily concerned with humoral immunity; performs the following functions
      1) Production of lymphocytes
      2) Stimulation of B cell activity to produce immunoglobulins; therefore, splenectomized patients have a greatly increased risk of sepsis
   b. Red pulp: contains reticuloendothelial tissue; performs the following functions
      1) Storage and release of RBCs into the circulation
         a) Caused by contraction of smooth muscle in the capsule surrounding the spleen and in invaginations of the capsule, called trabeculae
         b) When stimulated by the SNS, as much as 100 ml of concentrated RBCs can be released into the circulation, raising the hematocrit by 1% to 2%
      2) Filtering and destruction (by the process of phagocytosis) of damaged or old erythrocytes (referred to as culling)
         a) Removes particles from intact RBCs without destroying them (referred to as pitting)
         b) Catabolizes hemoglobin released from RBCs that have been destroyed by the spleen; iron returned to the bone marrow for reuse
      3) Filtering and trapping foreign material, including bacteria and viruses
      4) Storage and release of platelets; destruction of damaged or senescent platelets

4. Liver
   a. Filtering of blood as it comes from the gastrointestinal tract
      1) Removal of foreign material including microorganisms, damaged or old RBCs, and other degradation products by the Kupffer cells lining the sinusoidal beds of the liver
      2) Destruction of RBCs produces bilirubin, which the liver converts to bile, necessary for fat digestion
   b. Elimination of immune complexes (e.g., antigen-antibody complexes) from the blood
   c. Detoxification of toxic substances that enter the blood
   d. Manufacture of some clotting factors and anti-thrombin
   e. Storage of blood (e.g., in heart failure, the liver becomes engorged with blood)

5. Lymphatic system
   a. Lymph: pale yellow fluid that transports lymphocytes
      1) Composition: contains lymphocytes, granulocytes, enzymes, and antibodies; deficient in platelets and fibrinogen, so it coagulates very slowly
      2) Function: returns proteins and fat from GI tract, certain hormones, and excess interstitial fluid to the blood
   b. Lymph circulation
      1) Lymphatic capillaries are somewhat larger than blood capillaries and irregular in diameter
      2) Lymphatic vessels are formed by lymphatic capillaries
      3) Lymph ducts drain into subclavian veins
      4) Lymph nodes are small, bean-shaped organs located along lymph vessels
         a) Sites of B- and T-cell lymphocyte production and distribution
         b) Functions
            i) Lymph nodes filter out and allow WBCs to phagocytosize bacteria and foreign material carried by lymph
            ii) Granulocytes, macrophages, and lymphocytes pass through the lymph node to return to the blood
         c) Enlargement of lymph nodes
            i) This occurs with infection or malignancy
            ii) Enlargement of superficial nodes can be palpated; enlarged deep nodes can only be visualized on radiography
   c. Thymus
      1) Location: anterosuperior mediastinum below the thyroid gland; each lobe packed with lymphocytes
      2) Function
         a) Site of maturation and distribution of T lymphocytes
         b) Secretes a hormone, thymosin, which is thought to stimulate immune function

6. Blood
   a. Plasma comprises 55% of total blood volume
      1) Composed of serum and plasma proteins including albumin, serum globulins, fibrinogen, prothrombin, plasminogen
      2) Hematocrit expresses the percentage of RBCs in the total blood volume
   b. All blood cells originate from pluripotential stem cell

1) Erythroid stem cells (pronormoblasts) develop into reticulocytes and finally into erythrocytes
2) Myeloid stem cells (myeloblasts or monoblasts) develop into granulocytes and monocytes
3) Lymphoid stem cells (lymphoblasts) develop into B and T lymphocytes
4) Thrombocytic stem cells (megakaryoblasts) develop into thrombocytes

c. Erythrocytes are also referred to as red blood cells or RBCs
1) Structure
   a) Erythrocytes are nonnucleated round biconcave cell
   b) The inner part of RBC (referred to as stoma) is the location of hemoglobin attachment and contains the antigens that determine ABO and Rh blood type
2) Functions of RBCs
   a) Transport oxygen from lungs to tissues
   b) Participate in maintenance of acid-base balance; highly permeable to hydrogen, chloride, and bicarbonate ions and water
3) Types of RBCs
   a) Reticulocytes: immature RBCs
   b) Erythrocytes: mature RBCs
4) Erythropoiesis
   a) Regulation
      i) Determined by relationship of cellular oxygen requirement and general metabolic activity
      ii) Stimulated by the hormone erythropoietin; erythropoietin is secreted by the kidney in response to hypoxemia
   b) Nutritional requirements for RBC and hemoglobin production: iron, vitamin B_{12}, folic acid
   c) Process
      i) Stem cell
      ii) Erythroblast (has a nucleus)
      iii) Expulsion of nucleus
      iv) Erythrocyte
   d) Hemoglobin synthesis
      i) Synthesis takes place in bone marrow
      ii) Hemoglobin consists of four globin chains and four heme groups per hemoglobin molecule; each hemoglobin molecule has two different types of globin (e.g., normal adult hemoglobin [referred to as HbA]) and has two α chains and two β chains
5) Destruction (hemolysis) of erythrocytes
   a) Destruction of old and immature RBCs occurs in the liver and spleen
   b) Destruction of immature RBCs occurs primarily because they are misshapen or damaged
   c) Presenescent RBCs are removed from the circulation by the spleen, liver, or bone marrow for any of the following reasons
      i) RBC membrane abnormalities
      ii) Hemoglobin abnormalities
      iii) Abnormal metabolic functions
      iv) Physical trauma to the RBC
      v) Antibodies
      vi) Infectious agents and toxins
   d) Hgb and iron are returned to the bone marrow for reuse
   e) Erythrocyte destruction increases bilirubin production; bilirubin is transported to the liver attached to albumin
      i) Indirect bilirubin is unconjugated; this is before the liver has converted it to water-soluble; indirect bilirubin becomes increased in hemolytic states which overwhelm the liver's ability to conjugate or in liver disease where the liver is unable to adequately conjugate
      ii) Direct bilirubin is conjugated; this is after the liver has converted it to a water-soluble substance that will be excreted into the bile; direct bilirubin becomes increased in biliary obstruction

d. Leukocytes: phagocytic and immunologic systems
1) Cytokines: protein hormones synthesized by the various leukocytes
   a) Act as chemical mediators of immunity and inflammation
   b) Important in regulation of normal immune and inflammatory responses
2) Granulocytes: active phagocytes
   a) Neutrophils (also known as polymorphonuclear leukocytes); largest component of circulating WBC mass (40% to 80%)
      i) Neutrophils leave the blood vessel, migrate through the tissues, and search for microorganisms or damaged or old body cells; they then engulf, kill, and digest them through the process of phagocytosis
         (a) After phagocytosis, the neutrophil dies; pus is the end product of neutrophil death
         (b) Neutrophils contain cytoplasmic granules that include lysosomal enzymes, which aid in killing the microorganism
      ii) Maturity
         (a) Bands are immature neutrophils
            i. Phagocytic
            ii. Increase in bands seen in acute infection; frequently referred to as a shift to the left
         (b) Segmented neutrophils (referred to as segs) are mature neutrophils
            i. Phagocytic
            ii. Increase in segs seen in liver disease and pernicious anemia; frequently referred to as a shift to the right
   b) Eosinophils: comprise 0% to 5% of WBC mass

i) Functions
  (a) Ingest immune complexes (antigen-antibody complexes) and inactive mediators of allergic response
  (b) Some phagocytic activity
  (c) Probably most important during parasitic infections and allergic reactions; especially important in helminth infections because these parasitic worms are too large to be phagocytized and eosinophils secrete chemicals that destroy the surface of the helminth
ii) Life span after maturation: half-life in circulation approximately 30 minutes; in tissues, 12 days
iii) Tissue eosinophils are present in large numbers on mucosal surfaces of the respiratory and gastrointestinal systems and the skin because these locations are common entry points for foreign material
c) Basophils: comprise 0% to 2% of WBC mass
  i) Like mast cells, basophils contain heparin and histamine, which are released as the basophils degranulate during acute local or systemic allergic reactions; mast cells stay in the tissue while basophils stay in the circulatory system; if a basophil leaves the circulatory system to stay in the tissue, it becomes a mast cell
3) Agranulocytes
  a) Mononuclear phagocytes
    i) Monocytes: comprise 3% to 8% of WBC mass
      (a) Some phagocytic activity; differentiate into macrophages as they migrate into the tissues
    ii) Macrophages (not measured in WBC count due to their location)
      (a) Greater phagocytic ability than PMNs or monocytes; especially involved in removal or damaged or senescent cells, cellular debris, and mutant or cancer cells
      (b) Fixed (or tissue) macrophages: stay in one organ and phagocytize live and dead debris
        i. Lung: alveolar macrophages
        ii. Brain: microglia
        iii. Liver: Kupffer cells
        iv. Bone: osteoclast
        v. Peritoneum: peritoneal macrophages
        vi. Kidney: mesangial cells
      (a) Mobile macrophages: found primarily at sites of inflammation and in peritoneal, pleural, and synovial spaces; migrate through the circulatory system as monocytes

b) Lymphocytes: comprise 10% to 40% of WBC mass
  i) T cells: comprise approximately 70% to 80% of lymphocytes
    (a) Function: cellular immunity
    (b) Types of T cells
      i. Helper T cells (also referred to as CD4 T lymphocytes, T4 lymphocytes, or TH) detect foreign cells and produce lymphokines to stimulate the production or activation of other cells to fight infection
      ii. Cytotoxic T cells (also referred to as killer cells or Tc) emit chemicals that dissolve the foreign cell's membrane to kill the cell before the invader can use it as a base for multiplication
      iii. Suppressor T cells (also referred to as CD8 T lymphocytes, T8 lymphocytes, or TS) modulate the overall immune system by signaling B cells and T cells to slow down or stop their activity
      iv. Memory T cells circulate in blood and lymph after the initial infection to allow ready response to subsequent invasion by the same organism
      v. Helper T cells typically carry the CD4 surface molecule and suppressor and cytotoxic T cells typically carry the CD8 surface molecule; normally there are twice as many CD4 cells as CD8 cells
  ii) B cells: comprise approximately 10% to 20% of lymphocytes
    (a) Develop and matures in the bone marrow (bursa)
    (b) Function: production of immunoglobulins (humoral immunity)
  iii) Once activated, B cells become plasma cells
  iv) Recognize specific foreign material
  v) Develop specific immunoglobulins to that antigen
  vi) Memory B cells circulate in blood and lymph after the initial infection to allow ready response to subsequent invasion by the same organism
  vii) Natural killer (NK) cells (also referred to as null cells): comprise approximately 10% of lymphocytes
    (a) Large granular cytotoxic lymphocytes that are neither T cells nor B cells (no surface marker exists on these lymphocytes)

(b) Function
  i. Kill nonspecifically and do not need prior exposure for activation
  ii. Involved in surveillance against tumors, some parasites, and viruses

7. Inflammation
  a. Sequential physiologic response the body makes to injuries, immunologic processes, or foreign substances in the body; may be acute or chronic
    1) Occurs at sites of tissue damage irrespective of etiology
    2) May be local only or can become systemic; systemic response is now referred to as systemic inflammatory response syndrome (SIRS) (discussion of SIRS and multiple organ dysfunction syndrome [MODS] is provided in Chapter 13)
  b. Process
    1) Stage I: vascular stage
      a) Phase 1: immediate but temporary vasoconstriction caused by trauma to vascular smooth muscle
      b) Phase 2
        i) Warmth, redness, swelling, pain, and loss of function are the five classic symptoms of the inflammatory response
        ii) Injured tissues and cells secrete chemical mediators; predominant effect is vasodilation and increase in capillary permeability causing warmth, redness, and swelling
          (a) Healing is enhanced by the increase in mobilization of nutrients to the area
          (b) Tissue injury is decreased by diluting toxins or microorganisms that enter the area
          (c) Pain is caused by tissue stretching and histamine and prostaglandin release
          (d) Loss of function is caused by tissue swelling and pain
      c) The major leukocyte in this stage of inflammation is the tissue macrophage
    2) Stage II: cellular stage; major leukocyte in this stage of inflammation is the neutrophil which attacks and destroys foreign material and removes necrotic tissue
    3) Stage III: tissue repair and replacement
      a) Initiated at the time of injury
      b) Regeneration: replacement of lost cells with the same type of cells
      c) Repair: replacement of lost cells with connective tissue cells to form scar tissue; some loss of function occurs with the degree of loss dependent on the percentage of previously functional tissue replaced by scar tissue

8. Immunity
  a. Definition: the protection of the body against pathogenic organisms or other foreign material; dependent on ability to recognize self from nonself

    1) Self is determined genetically; it is anything synthesized by a person's own particular DNA code
    2) Nonself describes anything that is different in its chromosome structure and evokes a response from the immune system; antigens are chemical substances (almost always protein) that are viewed by the body as foreign (nonself)
  b. Lines of defense
    1) First: skin and mucous membranes, acid secretions and enzymes, natural immunoglobulins
    2) Second: macrophages and neutrophils
    3) Third: cellular and humoral immunity
  c. Innate immunity: body's inherent immune mechanisms; present at birth; do not require prior exposure to antigen for activation
    1) Anatomical: skin and mucous membranes
    2) Chemical
      a) Acid secretions in stomach, vagina, mouth
      b) Digestive enzymes in the GI tract
      c) Tears, perspiration
      d) Lysosomes
      e) Natural immunoglobulins
      f) Cytokines
      g) Pyrogen (produced by granulocytes to cause an increase in body temperature)
    3) Cellular
      a) Normal bacterial flora: GI tract, vagina, respiratory tract
      b) Tissue macrophages
      c) Leukocytes and mobile macrophages
      d) Inflammatory process
  d. Acquired immunity: immunity developed by the body through the creation of antibodies and formation of T and B memory cells in response to exposure to foreign material (antigen)
    1) Types
      a) Passive acquired immunity: produced by the injection of antibodies or sensitized lymphocytes
      b) Active acquired immunity: produced by natural exposure to an antigen (e.g., infection)
    2) Cell-mediated immunity
      a) Particularly effective against viruses, parasites, some fungi, and bacteria harbored inside of cells; responsible for delayed hypersensitivity, transplant rejection, and malignancy surveillance and, possibly, destruction
      b) Primarily mediated by T cells
      c) Induced and regulated primarily through the production and activity of cytokines
      d) Process
        i) The macrophage is the first cell to detect most antigens
        ii) The macrophage processes the antigen and "presents" it to both T and B cells
        iii) T cells recognize the antigen when it is on the macrophage cell membrane

iv) The antigen binds with an antigen receptor on the surface of the T cell, sensitizing the T cell

v) Sensitized T cells secrete lymphokines which regulate and coordinate the immune response to combat foreign cells, protect the body against mutant or cancer cells, and destroy foreign tissue; interleukin (IL)-8 is secreted by the macrophage and stimulates T cell division

vi) T cells are programmed to recognize the body's own tissue (self) from nonself (antigenic); autoimmune diseases are caused when the immune system cannot recognize self and the body is damaged by the immune system

vii) Natural killer cells also contribute to cellular immunity especially in relation to cancer cell surveillance

3) Humoral mediated immunity
   a) Primarily effective against bacteria and viruses
   b) Primarily mediated by B cells
   c) Process (Figure 11-9)
      i) Once activated, B cells become plasma cells and recognize specific foreign cells or antigen
      ii) Plasma cells make antibodies (also called immunoglobulins)
         (a) Immunoglobulins (antibodies) are serum proteins that bind to specific antigens; they begin the process that causes lysis or phagocytosis of an offending antigen
      iii) The first exposure to an antigen is followed by a latent phase where no antibody levels are detected
      iv) Primary response follows as serum antibody levels rise rapidly; maximal antibody response takes 3 to 5 days
      v) Levels plateau and finally decline
      vi) Subsequent exposure to the antigen results in more rapid production of antibodies to that antigen and higher concentrations of the antibody; this is the basis for immunizations

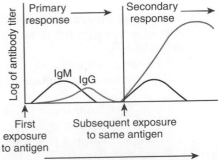

Figure 11-9 Primary and secondary immune response. (From Dennison, R. D. [2007]. *Pass CCRN!* [3rd ed.]. St. Louis: Mosby.)

vii) Inflammation occurs because antigen-antibody complexes (referred to as immune complexes) attract white blood cells

d) Immune complexes activate the complement cascade
   i) Complement is a group of blood proteins: there are more than 20 of these proteins, but 11 are considered the primary complement elements
   ii) When activated, they function as mediators to enhance various aspects of inflammatory response; they also do the following
      (a) Attract and stimulate PMNs
      (b) Kill microorganisms by punching holes in their cell membranes, allowing intracellular fluid to leak out; mononuclear phagocytes and monocytes then clear the debris from the bloodstream
      (c) Agglutinate the bacteria
      (d) Activate basophils and mast cells

4) Hypersensitivity (allergic) reactions
   a) Type I: immediate hypersensitivity reactions ranging from mild reaction with localized response to a severe systemic reaction referred to as anaphylaxis
      i) Reaction occurs within minutes (usually 5 to 20 minutes) of exposure to even a minute amount of the antigen
      ii) Example: anaphylactic reaction to penicillin, insect venom, foods, pollen
   b) Type II: cytotoxic hypersensitivity
      i) Reaction is usually within minutes to days
      ii) Example: mismatched blood transfusion reaction
   c) Type III: immune complex-mediated reaction
      i) Reaction is usually within hours
      ii) Example: environmental antigens (e.g., pollen, some drugs)
   d) Type IV: delayed or cell-mediated hypersensitivity
      i) Reaction is within one or more days
      ii) Example: skin testing for tuberculosis, contact dermatitis

9. Hemostasis
   a. Definition: the termination of bleeding by a complex process that involves integrated interactions among blood vessels, platelets, clotting factors, and the fibrinolytic system
   b. Hemostatic mechanisms
      1) Vascular response
         a) Disruption of vascular integrity causes a sympathetic nervous system response resulting in vasospasm and blood vessel constriction in the injured vessel

b) Thromboxane A2, endothelin, the alpha-adrenergic system, and serotonin are thought to mediate this response

2) Platelet (thrombocytes) aggregation
   a) Process
      i) Endothelial damage exposes the basement membrane of the subendothelial collagen
      ii) Damaged tissues release chemicals (e.g., thromboplastin) to activate platelets
      iii) Activated platelets swell and develop hairlike projections
      iv) Swelling increases the surface area of the platelet for platelet adhesion and makes platelet more likely to aggregate
      v) Granules and components necessary for the clotting process are released from the platelets; adenosine diphosphate (ADP) released by degranulation of the platelet enhances adhesiveness and aggregation
         (a) Adhesiveness: stickiness that aids in ability to stick to vessel walls
         (b) Aggregation: process of platelets adhering or clumping together to form the "platelet plug"
      vi) Activated platelets become adhesive and aggregate
      vii) Platelet aggregation becomes large enough to form a platelet plug (sometimes referred to as a white clot) that seals the damaged blood vessel
      viii) During aggregation of the platelets, platelet factor III (PFIII), an important contributor in the intrinsic pathway, is released
      ix) Platelets contain factor XIII (fibrin stabilizing factor) essential in the formation of a stable fibrin clot
   b) Drugs that decrease the ability of the platelets to aggregate
      i) Alcohol
      ii) Aspirin (ASA)
      iii) Ticlopidine (Ticlid)
      iv) Clopidogrel (Plavix)
      v) GP IIb/IIIa platelet receptor blockers (e.g., abciximab [ReoPro], eptifibatide [Integrilin], tirofiban HCl [Aggrastat])
      vi) Nonsteroidal anti-inflammatory agents (e.g., phenylbutazone [Butazolidin], ibuprofen [Motrin])
      vii) Quinidine (Cardioquin)
      viii) Dextran 40 (low molecular-weight dextran [LMD])
      ix) Heparin
   c) Thrombocytopenia
      i) Significance
         (a) Platelet counts >50,000/mm3: surgery can generally be tolerated

         (b) Platelet counts 20,000 to 30,000/mm3: spontaneous bleeding may occur
         (c) Platelet counts <10,000/mm3: spontaneous intracranial hemorrhages likely
      ii) Causes
         (a) Decreased production (e.g., bone marrow depression, B12 or folic acid deficiency)
         (b) Increased destruction (e.g., idiopathic thrombocytopenia purpura [ITP], disseminated intravascular coagulation [DIC], sepsis)
         (c) Hypersplenism (e.g., portal hypertension)
         (d) Heparin-induced thrombocytopenia and thrombosis (HITT): also called heparin-associated thrombocytopenia and thrombosis (HATT) or white clot syndrome; immune-mediated response caused by heparin
         (e) Dilutional thrombocytopenia: caused by large volumes of fluids that do not contain platelets
   d) Thrombocytosis
      i) Significance: may cause excessive thrombosis or bleeding, depending on the quality of the platelets
      ii) Causes
         (a) Malignancy
         (b) Polycythemia vera
         (c) Leukemia
         (d) Postsplenectomy
         (e) Rheumatoid arthritis
         (f) Trauma

3) Coagulation
   a) Dependent on presence of clotting factors and functioning of the pathways
   b) Blood coagulation factors
      i) Consist of proteins, lipoproteins, and calcium, which is critical in the intrinsic, extrinsic and common pathways
      ii) Circulate as inactive; activated in a cascade fashion
   c) Clotting pathways (Figure 11-10)
      i) Pathways are cascades where one action is dependent on a preceding action or interaction
      ii) A fibrin clot may be produced through activation of either the intrinsic or extrinsic pathway
         (a) Intrinsic pathway
            i. Initiated by damage to RBCs or platelets
            ii. Time from activation through intrinsic pathway and common pathway to a clot: 2 to 6 minutes
            iii. Tested by aPTT
         (b) Extrinsic pathway
            i. Initiated by injured tissue

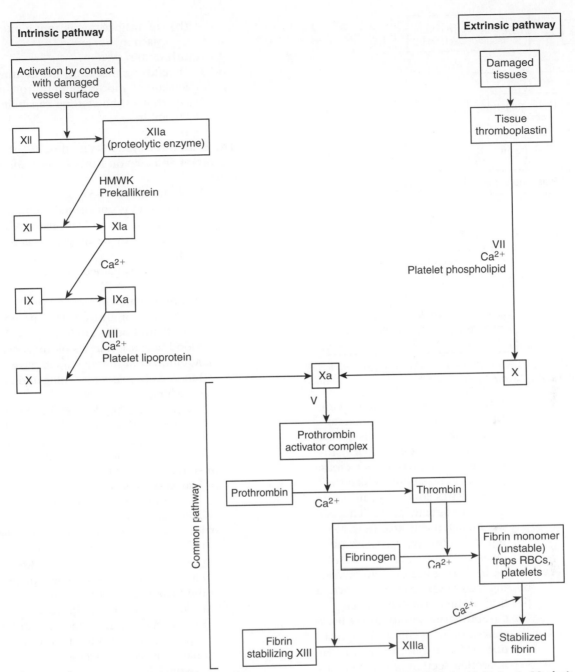

Figure 11-10 The clotting pathways. (From Dennison, R. D. [2007]. *Pass CCRN!* [3rd ed.]. St. Louis: Mosby.)

ii. Time from activation through extrinsic pathway and common pathway to a clot: as short as 15 to 20 seconds
iii. Tested by PT
iii) Common pathway
   (a) Platelet factor III and tissue thromboplastin combine to become a prothrombin activator
   (b) Prothrombin is converted to thrombin
   (c) Fibrinogen is converted to fibrin
   (d) Fibrin clot is formed
   (e) Pathway is tested by aPTT, PT, and thrombin time

4) Anticoagulant mechanisms in normal system
   a) Fibrinolytic system (Figure 11-11)
      i) Activated clotting factors are cleared by the reticuloendothelial system
      ii) Clot-lysing activities maintain blood in fluid state
         (a) Process of clot breakdown takes approximately 7 to 10 days
         (b) Blood (intrinsic pathway) or tissue (extrinsic pathway) plasminogen activators activate plasminogen to plasmin; therefore, once a clot is developed, steps are initiated to eliminate it

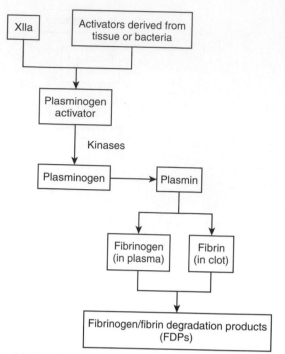

Figure 11-11 The fibrinolytic process. (From Dennison, R. D. [2007]. *Pass CCRN!* [3rd ed.]. St. Louis: Mosby.)

      (c) Plasmin works to lyse fibrin clots producing fibrin split products (FSPs) (also referred to as fibrin degradation products [FDPs]; increased amounts of FSPs increase potential for patient to bleed

      (d) Fibrinolytics speed up this process by either directly providing tissue plasminogen activator (e.g., alteplase [Activase], reteplase [Retavase]), tenecteplase (TNKase) or by triggering the process by adding a complex to cause the activation of the fibrinolytic system (streptokinase [Streptase]) (discussion of these agents and implications is located in the Myocardial Infarction section of Chapter 4)

    iii) Controls of fibrinolysis

      (a) Plasminogen activator inhibitor type 1 inactivates tissue plasminogen activator

      (b) α2-Antiplasmin is an inhibitor of plasmin

    b) Antithrombin system

      i) Defends against excessive clotting

      ii) Release of antithrombin III from mast cells

      iii) Neutralizes the clotting capability of thrombin

10. Blood groups

    a. There are three systems that describe the most important antigens on RBCs, tissues, and other cells

      1) ABO system (Table 11-3)

        a) This system is concerned with antigens on the RBC, which are designated A and B; the presence of these antigens is genetically controlled

        b) Blood type is named for the antigen that is present on the RBC

        c) Antibodies are present in the plasma for the antigen or antigens that are not present (e.g., B antibodies are found in group A blood because B antigens are absent)

        d) Agglutination that occurs in mismatched blood is the basis for typing and cross-matching

          i) Blood typing detects the major antigens: A, B, Rh

          ii) Cross-matching detects the presence of major or minor RBC antigens

      2) Rh system (Table 11-4)

        a) This system is concerned with a series of six common types of Rh antigens, each called an Rh factor

        b) Rh antibodies do not develop spontaneously; they only occur after exposure to Rh antigen (e.g., second exposure to non–Rh-matched blood or Rh-negative mothers pregnant with the second Rh-positive fetus if anti-Rh globin [RhoGAM] was not given); delayed transfusion reactions can occur even after the first exposure to Rh-positive blood and cause a mild transfusion reaction

      3) Uncrossmatched type O negative packed RBCs may be used safely in exsanguinating patient

        a) Whole blood is avoided to decrease the risk of reaction caused by anti-A and anti-B antibodies in type O plasma

TABLE 11-3 ABO Blood Groups

Patient's ABO Group	Percentage of Population	Antigen on RBC	Antibodies in Plasma	Compatible RBCs	Compatible Plasma
O	47%	None	Anti-A; Anti-B	O	O, A, B, AB
A	41%	A	Anti-B	O, A	A, AB
B	9%	B	Anti-A	O, B	B, AB
AB	3%	A and B	None	O, A, B, AB	AB

From: Dennison, R. D. (2007). *Pass CCRN!* (3rd ed.). St. Louis: Mosby.

TABLE 11-4   Rh Compatibility

Patient's Rh Type	RBC Rh Type for Transfusion	Plasma Rh Type for Transfusion
Positive	Positive or negative	Positive or negative
Negative	Negative	Positive or negative

from: Dennison, R. D. (2007). *Pass CCRN!* (3rd ed.). St. Louis: Mosby.

  b) Blood antigen-antibody complexes may complicate later crossmatching and may cause future blood transfusion reaction to own blood type unless it is O negative
  c) Type-specific blood may be preferable, and type matching takes only 5 to 15 minutes

Assessment
Primary and secondary assessment (see Chapter 2)
Focused assessment
1. Chief complaint: why the patient is seeking help and duration of the problem; possible symptoms related to general medical disorders that may be identified as chief complaint may include any of the following:
   a. Changes in mentation
   b. Cough
   c. Dizziness
   d. Dyspnea
   e. Fatigue
   f. Fever
   g. Nausea, vomiting, diarrhea
   h. Pain
   i. Rash
   j. Swelling or edema

History of present illness
1. PQRST
2. Associated symptoms
   a. Specific to endocrine
      1) Fatigue
      2) Weight loss or gain
      3) Dehydration
      4) Polyuria, polydipsia, polyphagia
      5) Palpitations
   b. Specific to renal
      1) Dysuria
      2) Hematuria
      3) Oliguria
      4) Volume overload
   c. Specific to hematology/immunology
      1) Bruising without trauma
      2) Bleeding
      3) Swollen lymph nodes
      4) Fever

Past medical history
1. Current or past illnesses
   a. Recurrent medical infections
   b. Trauma
   c. Bleeding disorders
   d. Cardiovascular disease
   e. Diabetes
   f. Malabsorption syndromes

General survey
1. Airway compromise
2. Apparent health status
3. Level of consciousness
4. Hygiene, odors
5. Discomfort or distress

Inspection
1. Skin: color, lesions, rash
2. Mucous membranes
3. Fontanels
4. Neck veins

Auscultate
1. Lung sounds
2. Heart sounds
3. Bowel sounds

Palpate
1. Abdomen
2. Chest
3. Area that are swollen or appear edematous
4. Areas with erythema or warmth
5. Areas that are tender
6. Pulses
7. Lymph nodes
8. Skin turgor

Vital signs: include orthostatic BP and HR if hemorrhage or dehydration present or suspected
1. Fever
   a. Fever of unknown origin (FUO) (Petersdorf & Beeson as cited in Chan-Tack & Bartlett, 2008)
      1) Temperature greater than 38.3°C (101°F) on several occasions
      2) Illness lasting >3 weeks
      3) After 1 week of inpatient investigation, there is no identification of fever source
   b. History of fever
      1) Onset: sudden or gradual
      2) Recent travel
      3) Immunizations
      4) Exposure to illness, recent surgery or hospitalization
      5) Seizures
   c. Physical examination related to fever
      1) Ability to maintain airway, work of breathing, and clinical signs of oxygenation
      2) Pulses, color of skin, capillary refill

3) Heart sounds
   a) If significantly increased or decreased, place patient on continuous cardiac monitor
4) Hydration status: fontanels, skin turgor, mucous membranes, absence of tears when crying, recent urine output (including reduction in number of wet diapers)
5) Level of consciousness and behavior, meningeal signs
6) Abdominal findings: assess for for distension, bowel sounds, guarding, tenderness (including rebound tenderness if appropriate)
7) Skin assessment; look for bleeding, rashes, bites, bruises, other lesions

d. Diagnostic work up for fever
  1) Lumbar puncture: indications
    a) Adults with nuchal rigidity, severe headache (after CT completed to avoid potential herniation if ICP is increased)
    b) Children with first time febrile seizure before the age of 12 months or children in this age group who have a fever of 41°C (106°F)
    c) Children who are still febrile, irritable, or lethargic after maximal antipyretic therapy (Lazear and Roberts, 2007)
  2) Septic workup: any child under 3 months of age with (FUO) >38°C (100.4°F) requires a septic workup
    a) LP
    b) Blood cultures
    c) Urinalysis with culture
    d) Chest radiography

Diagnostic studies related to endocrine/renal/hematology/immunology systems

1. Serum
  a. Chemistry
   1) Sodium: normal 136 to 145 mEq/L
   2) Potassium: normal 3.5 to 5.0 mEq/L
   3) Chloride: normal 95 to 103 mEq/L
   4) Calcium: normal 9.0 to 10.5 mg/dl in adults and 8.8 to 10.8 mg/dl in children
   5) Phosphorus: normal 3.0 to 4.5 mg/dl
   6) Magnesium: normal 1.3 to 2.1 mEq/L in adults, 1.4 to 1.7 mEq/L in children, and 1.4 to 2 mEq/L in infants
   7) Glucose: normal 65 to 110 mEq/L
   8) Glycosylated hemoglobin: normal 4% to 7%
   9) Bilirubin: normal total bilirubin 0.3 to 1.5 mg/dl
    a) Indirect (before being conjugated by liver): 0.1 to 1.0 mg/dl
    b) Direct (after being conjugated by liver): 0.1 to 0.2 mg/dl
   10) Iron: normal 50 to 150 mcg/dl
   11) Total iron-binding capacity (TIBC): normal 250 to 410 mcg/dl
   12) Total protein: normal 6 to 8 g/dl
   13) Albumin: normal 3.5 to 4.8 g/dl

14) C-reactive protein: normal <1 mg/dl; nonspecific test for evaluating severity and course of inflammatory conditions
15) Serum protein electrophoresis: immunoglobulin analysis
16) Cholesterol: desired 150 to 200 mg/dl
17) Triglycerides: desired 40 to 150 mg/dl
18) Osmolality: normal 280 to 295 mOsm/kg
   a) Measures particles exerting osmotic pull per unit of water
   b) May be calculated: $(Na \times 2) + (BUN/2.6) + (serum\ glucose/18)$
   c) Reflects total body hydration
    i) Increased in dehydration
    ii) Decreased with fluid overload
19) BUN: normal 8 to 23 mg/dl
   a) Reflects difference between rate of urea synthesis and its excretion by the kidneys
    i) Formed in the liver through enzymatic breakdown of protein
    ii) Not as accurate an indicator of renal failure as is creatinine since BUN levels fluctuate greatly with protein intake but creatinine levels are relatively unchanged by protein intake and hydration level
   b) Abnormal values
    i) Increased with decreased renal blood flow or urine production, dehydration, some neoplasms, and certain antibiotics; increased BUN is also referred to as uremia
    ii) Decreased in pregnancy, overhydration, severe liver disease, malnutrition
20) Creatinine: normal 0.6 to 1.1 mg/dl in women and 0.8 to 1.3 mg/dl in men
   a) Nonprotein end-product of muscle metabolism; more accurate than BUN in evaluating renal function since creatinine is normally filtered by the glomerulus and not reabsorbed by the tubule
   b) Unaffected by diet and fluid intake
   c) Abnormal values
    i) Increased
     (a) A twice-normal (~3 mg/dl) creatinine level suggests 50% nephron loss
     (b) If >10 mg/dl indicates end-stage renal disease with less than 10% of nephrons still functioning
    ii) Decreased: muscular dystrophy
21) BUN: creatinine ratio: normal ~10:1
   a) When BUN is increased disproportionately to the creatinine (e.g., BUN: creatinine ratio 20:1), consider an extrarenal cause such as one of the following
    i) Volume depletion (i.e., prerenal)
     (a) Insufficient fluid intake
     (b) Excessive fluid loss

i) Diuresis
ii) Vomiting
iii) Poor renal perfusion
   (a) Shock
   (b) Sepsis
   (c) Decreased cardiac output
   (d) Renovascular disease
iv) Protein catabolism
   (a) Starvation
   (b) Blood in the GI tract
   (c) Corticosteroids
b) When BUN and creatinine are both increased maintaining the normal 10:1 ratio, consider a renal cause such as acute or chronic renal failure
c) When BUN and creatinine is lower than normal
   i) Decreased protein intake
   ii) Liver dysfunction

22) Ketones: negative
23) Anion gap: a calculated parameter (Table 11-5)
   a) Calculated by subtracting the anion from the cation
     i) Anion gap = $Na^+ - (Cl^- + CO_2^-)$
     ii) Normal: 10 to 14 mEq/L
   b) Helpful in determination of cause of metabolic acidosis
     i) A normal anion gap indicates that the reason for the metabolic acidosis is bicarbonate loss
     ii) An increased anion gap indicates that the reason for the metabolic acidosis is an acid gain (e.g., lactic acid, ketoacid, toxins)
b. Hormone levels
   1) Thyroid-stimulating hormone (TSH): normal 2 to 10 mU/ml

TABLE 11-5 Anion Gap

Calculation of Anion Gap	$Na^+ - (Cl^- + CO_2^-)$
Normal value	10 to 14 mEq/L
Causes of metabolic acidosis with normal anion gap: bicarbonate loss	Intestinal loss of bicarbonate • Diarrhea • Pancreatic fistula • Ureterosigmoidostomy Renal loss of bicarbonate • Carbonic anhydrase inhibitors (e.g., acetazolamide [Diamox]) • Aldosterone-antagonists (also referred to as potassium-sparing diuretics) (e.g., triamterene [Dyrenium], spironolactone [Aldactone]) • Renal tubular acidosis • Adrenal insufficiency • Primary hypoaldosteronism Excessive gain of chloride • Large quantities of normal saline • Ammonium chloride • Arginine hydrochloride
Causes of metabolic acidosis with increased anion gap: metabolic acid gain	Renal failure Lactic acidosis • Shock • Hypoxemia/hypoxia • Severe anemia • Status epilepticus • Cyanide poisoning Ketoacidosis • Diabetic ketoacidosis • Starvation • Alcohol Drugs and toxins • Salicylates • Methanol • Ethylene glycol • Paraldehyde • High-dose carbenicillin (Geocillin) Rhabdomyolysis

from: Dennison, R. D. (2007). *Pass CCRN!* (3rd ed.). St. Louis: Mosby.

2) T3: normal 0.2 to 0.3 mcg/dl
3) T4: normal 6 to 12 mcg/dl
4) ACTH: normal 15 to 100 pg/ml in AM, <50 pg/ml in PM
5) Cortisol: normal 6 to 28 mcg/dl at 8 AM, 2 to 12 mcg/dl at 4 PM
6) ADH: normal 1 to 5 pg/ml

c. Arterial blood gases (ABGs)
   1) pH: normal 7.35 to 7.45
   2) $PaCO_2$: normal 35 to 45 mm Hg
   3) HCO_3: normal 22 to 28 mEq/L
   4) PaO_2: normal 80 to 100 mm Hg

d. Hematology
   1) Red blood cells (RBC): normal 4.6 to 6.2×10^6/ml for males; 4.2 to 5.4×10^6/ml for females
      a) Increased in dehydration, chronic hypoxemia, or high altitudes; may temporarily increase after a cold shower or with intense emotions
      b) Decreased in hemorrhage, anemias, leukemias, or hypothyroidism
   2) Reticulocyte count: normal 0.5% to 1.5% of RBCs
      a) Assesses the responsiveness and potential of the bone marrow to respond to bleeding or hemolysis
   3) Erythrocyte sedimentation rate (ESR or sed rate): normal 1 to 9 mm/hr for males, 1 to 20 mm/hr for females
      a) Nonspecific test; measures the amount of RBCs that settle in 1 hour
      b) Increased in inflammatory processes (e.g., rheumatoid arthritis, malignancy, rheumatic fever, hemolytic anemia, thyroid disorders, autoimmune disorders, nephrotic syndrome)
      c) Decreased in polycythemia vera, hypofibrinogenemia, sickle cell anemia, heart failure
   4) Hemoglobin: normal 14 to 18 g/dl for males; 12 to 16 g/dl for females
      a) Increased in polycythemia, which may occur in chronic hypoxia or high altitudes
      b) Decreased in anemia, hemorrhage
   5) Hematocrit: normal 42% to 52% for males; 37% to 47% for females
      a) Measures portion of blood volume occupied by RBCs
      b) Increased in dehydration or polycythemia
      c) Decreased with anemia, leukemia, or with normal hemoglobin and water overload
   6) Red cell indices
      a) Mean corpuscular volume (MCV) (an average of size): normal 80 to 100 fl
      b) Mean corpuscular hemoglobin (MCH) (an average of weight of hemoglobin in an RBC): normal 26.6 to 34 pg
      c) Mean corpuscular hemoglobin concentration (MCHC): normal 31.4 to 36.3 g/dl

7) Peripheral smear: evaluation of blood cell size, shape, and composition
8) White blood cells (WBC): normal 4.8 to 10.8 mm³
   a) Increased in infection, trauma, surgery, acute leukemia, stress, corticosteroid therapy
   b) Decreased in bone marrow depression (e.g., aplastic anemia, agranulocytosis, chronic leukemia, sepsis, autoimmune disorders)
9) Differential
   a) Neutrophils: normal 40% to 80%
      i) Increased in infection, inflammatory processes, malignancy, trauma, hemorrhage, burns, tissue necrosis (e.g., myocardial infarction), ketoacidosis
      ii) Decreased in overwhelming infection, bone marrow depression, vitamin B_{12} or folic acid deficiency, hypersplenism
   b) Eosinophils: normal 0% to 5%
      i) Increased in:
         (a) Allergic conditions
            i. Asthma
            ii. Eczema
         (b) Leukemia
         (c) Autoimmune disorders
         (d) Parasitic infection especially helminthic infections
      ii) Decreased in:
         (a) Adrenocortical stimulation
         (b) Stress
         (c) Cushing syndrome
         (d) Systemic lupus erythematosus
   c) Basophils: 0% to 2%
      i) Increased in allergic conditions, inflammatory processes, graft rejection, acute leukemia, recent splenectomy
      ii) Decreased in hyperthyroidism and long-term corticosteroid therapy
   d) Monocytes: 3% to 8%
      i) Increased in chronic inflammatory conditions, anemia, malignancy, mononucleosis, acute HIV infection
      ii) Decreased in immunodeficiency disorders
   e) Lymphocytes: 10% to 40%
      i) Increased in chronic lymphocytic leukemia, chronic infections: bacterial and viral, multiple myeloma, mononucleosis, Cushing syndrome
      ii) Decreased in immunodeficiency disorders (e.g., AIDS, systemic lupus erythematosus, leukemia, antineoplastic drugs, corticosteroids, sepsis)
      iii) Lymphocyte assays
         (a) T cells
         (b) B cells
         (c) NK cells
   f) Changes in differential
      i) Shift to the left: increased percentage of bands; seen in infection

ii) Shift to the right: increased percentage of segs; seen in pernicious anemia or hepatic disease

iii) Regenerative shift: increased WBC with increased percentage of bands; indicative of stimulation of bone marrow

iv) Degenerative shift: decreased WBC with increased percentage of bands; indicative of bone marrow depression

10) Platelets: normal 150,000 to 400,000/mm^3; decreased in systemic lupus erythematosus, HIV infection, idiopathic thrombocytopenic purpura, DIC

    a) 50,000 to 100,000/mm^3: prolonged bleeding times, increased risk of bleeding after severe trauma or surgery

    b) Below 50,000/mm^3: increased risk of bleeding after minor trauma

    c) Below 20,000/mm^3: risk of spontaneous bleeding, including intracranial bleeding

e. Clotting profile

1) Prothrombin time (PT): normal 11.9 to 18.5. seconds; assesses extrinsic coagulation pathway and the common pathway

2) International normalized ratio (INR): therapeutic INR is usually 2.0 to 3.5 but may be higher depending on indications for anticoagulant therapy

    a) Mathematical calculation that accounts for the differences in sensitivity between reagents; therefore, standardizes PT values

3) Activated partial thromboplastin time (aPTT): normal 24 to 36 seconds; assesses intrinsic coagulation pathway and the common pathway

4) Thrombin time: normal 10 to 15 seconds; assesses time for thrombin to convert fibrinogen to a fibrin clot

5) Bleeding time: normal < 8 minutes; assesses platelet function

6) Fibrinogen: normal 200 to 400 mg/dl

    a) Increased in hypercoagulable states and inflammatory conditions

    b) Decreased in hypocoagulable states with propensity to bleed

7) Fibrin split products (FSPs) (also referred to as fibrin degradation products [FDPs]: normal 0 to 10 mcg/dl; increased in excessive fibrinolysis [e.g., DIC])

8) D-dimer: normal <250 ng/ml; increased in DIC, deep veing thrombosis, pulmonary embolism

9) Specific factor assays: measure amounts of each factor in the blood

f. Type and crossmatch

1) Blood typing: determined by agglutination studies

2) Rh factor determination

3) Coombs' test: detects immune antibodies important in crossmatching

    a) Direct: normal negative; measures antibodies (IgG) attached to RBCs

    b) Indirect: normal negative; measures antibodies (IgG) in the serum

g. HIV antibody screening: normal negative

1) Detects antibodies to HIV; present with exposure to HIV, but absence does not mean that the patient has not been exposed because approximately 6 weeks to 6 months is required for development of antibodies

2) Does not indicate immunity

3) Types of tests

    a) Enzyme-linked immunosorbent assay (ELISA): screening test subject to error; up to 10% false-positive results

    b) Western blot: more specific than ELISA

h. HIV virus screening (e.g., polymerase chain reaction [PCR]: normal negative

2. Urine

a. Visual examination: clear, yellow

b. Glucose: normal negative; glycosuria occurs when renal threshold for glucose is exceeded; renal threshold is variable and patient-specific, so there is no accurate method to predict serum glucose

c. Ketones: normal negative; ketonuria is seen in catabolism (e.g., starvation or diabetic ketoacidosis)

d. Protein: normal 0 to 18 mg/dl

1) Proteinuria may occur after ingestion of a high-protein meal or can accompany renal changes of pregnancy, glomerulonephritis, nephrotic syndrome, and uncontrolled hypertension

e. Myoglobin: normal negative or less than 20 ng/ml; myoglobinuria indicates muscle breakdown

f. Hemoglobin: normal negative; hemoglobinuria indicates free hemoglobin in the urine such as occurs in hemolytic blood transfusion reaction, hemolytic or sickle cell anemia, fresh-water drowning, burns, DIC

g. RBCs: normal 0 to 2/low power field; RBCs in the urine may indicate trauma (e.g., renal calculi), bleeding disorder (e.g., DIC), bladder cancer

h. WBCs: normal 0 to 4/low power field; WBCs in the catheterized urine specimen indicate urinary tract infection

i. Bilirubin: normal negative; urobilinogen indicates biliary obstruction or liver disease

j. Specific gravity: 1.005 to 1.030

1) Increased with any condition causing hypoperfusion of kidneys leading to oliguria (e.g., shock, severe dehydration, proteinuria, glycosuria, contrast media)

2) Decreased in diabetes insipidus, overhydration, and when renal tubules lose their ability to reabsorb water and concentrate urine as in early pyelonephritis

k. Osmolality: normal 50 to 1200 mOsm/L
   1) Measures number of particles per unit of water in urine
   2) Increased in fluid volume deficit due to retention of fluid by the body
   3) Decreased in fluid volume excess due to fluid being excreted by the kidney
l. Culture and sensitivity: normal no bacteria present; if bacteria are present, appropriate antibiotic therapy is identified
m. pH: normal 4.6 to 8
   1) Increased urinary acidity indicates that the body is retaining bicarbonate
   2) Decreased urinary acidity (more alkaline) indicates that the kidney is retaining sodium and acids
      a) Alkaline urine may be associated with urinary tract infection
      b) Alkaline urine and serum acidosis is associated with renal tubular acidosis
n. Spot urine electrolytes
   1) Evaluates the kidney's ability to conserve sodium and concentrate urine
   2) Measures sodium, potassium, and chloride concentrations in the urine
      a) Sodium: normal 40 to 220 mEq/L/day
      b) Potassium: normal 25 to 120 mEq/L/day
      c) Chloride: normal 110 to 250 mEq/day
o. Sediment
   1) Casts: precipitation from the kidney that takes the shape of the tubule where it was formed; normally none or occasional hyaline casts
   2) Bacteria: abnormal in catheterized specimen
   3) Erythrocytes: small numbers normal; large numbers indicative of glomerulonephritis, interstitial nephritis, malignancy, infection, calculi, cystitis, or trauma
   4) Leukocytes: small numbers normal; large numbers indicative of infection, interstitial nephritis
   5) Renal epithelial cells: indicative of acute tubular necrosis, glomerulonephritis, interstitial nephritis
   6) Crystals: indicative of stone formation
   7) Eosinophils: indicative of allergic reaction in kidney
3. Culture and sensitivity: various body secretions (e.g., blood, urine, wound secretions)
   a. Gram stain: identification of gram-positive or gram-negative bacteria
   b. Culture: identification of microorganism
   c. Sensitivity
      1) Minimum inhibitory concentration (MIC): the smallest concentration of antibiotic that effectively inhibits bacterial growth; reported as antibiotic concentration per milliliter of solution necessary for growth inhibition
      2) This is compared with the achievable blood level of the antibiotic
         a) If this level is less than the MIC, the bacterium is considered resistant to that antibiotic
         b) If this level is greater than the MIC, the bacterium is considered sensitive to that antibiotic
         3) Other factors such as known adverse effects of the antibiotic are also considered
4. Stool
   a. Blood: may be grossly bloody or guaiac positive in bleeding disorders
   b. Culture and/or toxins: may show opportunistic infections (e.g., *Clostridium difficile* in immunodeficient patients)
   c. Ova and parasites if parasites are suspected
5. Biopsy
   a. Bone marrow
   b. Lymph node
      1) Open: direct visualization; performed in operating room
      2) Closed or needle: performed at bedside
   c. Synovial
   d. Biopsy of transplanted organs to look for indications of rejection
6. Radiologic studies
   a. Chest radiography
   b. Flat plate of abdomen (KUB)
   c. Computed tomography (CT) of head or abdomen
   d. Magnetic resonance imaging (MRI)
   e. Pancreatic scan
   f. Thyroid scan
   g. Brain scan
   h. Lymphangiography: visualizes the lymph system after injection of a dye; assists in node assessment
   i. Isotopic lymphangiography: uses technetium-99m and is less invasive than radiographic lymphangiography
   j. Scans: liver, spleen, or bone
   k. CT of abdomen for evaluation of liver, spleen, and lymph nodes
7. Other studies
   a. Electrocardiogram
   b. Electroencephalogram
8. Other diagnostic studies (Table 11-6)

Fluid and electrolyte imbalances (Table 11-7)

SPECIFIC ENDOCRINE EMERGENCIES

Hyperglycemic Crises
Definitions
1. Diabetes mellitus: a group of metabolic diseases characterized by hyperglycemia (confirmed fasting serum glucose of greater than or equal to 126 mg/dl) that results from defects in insulin secretion, insulin action, or both
   a. Type 1 diabetes is characterized by β cell destruction, usually leading to absolute insulin deficiency; previously known as juvenile onset, type I, insulin-dependent diabetes mellitus (IDDM)
   b. Type 2 diabetes is a characterized by insulin resistance and a relative (rather than absolute) insulin

Text continues on page 591

TABLE 11-6 Diagnostic Studies

Study	Purposes	Comments
Computed tomography (CT)	• Provides a view of kidneys, retroperitoneal space, bladder, prostate • Evaluates kidney size • Evaluates the kidney for tumors, abscesses, and obstruction	• No special preparation required • Can be safely used in patients with renal failure • Contrast medium may be used

IV pyelogram (IVP)	• Evaluates position, size, shape, and location of kidneys
	• Provides visualization of internal kidney (parenchyma, calyces, pelvis)
	• Evaluates filling of renal pelvis
	• Outlines ureters and bladder
	• Identifies presence of cysts and tumors
	• Identifies obstruction, congenital abnormality
		• Also called excretory urogram
		• Contraindicated in renal insufficiency, multiple myeloma, pregnancy, congestive heart failure, sickle cell disease
		• Bowel preparation (e.g., cathartics) as prescribed
		• NPO prior to the test
		• Contrast media used
		  • Check for allergy to iodine prior to the study
		  • Monitor for allergic reaction postprocedure
		  • Ensure hydration postprocedure

Kidneys, ureters, and bladder (KUB)	• Outlines kidneys, ureters, bladder • Evaluates size, shape, and position of kidneys • Identifies location of calculi	• Also called flat plate of abdomen
Magnetic resonance imaging (MRI)	• Differentiation between cyst and solid mass • Identifies infarction, trauma, obstruction	• More specific than renal ultrasonography or CT as it shows subtle density changes • Cannot be used in patients with any implanted metallic device, including pacemakers • No special preparation required

Renal angiography	• Evaluates renal vasculature
	• Identifies renal artery stenosis
	• Identifies cysts, tumors, infarction, trauma
		• Bowel preparation (e.g., cathartics) as prescribed
		• NPO for 8 hours prior to the test
		• Sedative if usually prescribed prior to the procedure
		• Contrast media used
		  • Check for allergy to iodine prior to the study
		  • Monitor for allergic reaction postprocedure
		  • Ensure hydration postprocedure
		Postprocedure
		• Keep extremity in which catheter was placed immobilized in a straight position for 6-12 hours
		• Monitor arterial puncture point for hemorrhage or hematoma
		• Monitor neurovascular status of affected limb
		• Monitor for indications of systemic emboli

Retrograde pyelogram	• Evaluates position, size, shape, and location of kidneys
	• Outlines ureters and bladder
	• Identifies presence of cysts and tumors
	• Identifies of obstruction
		• Does not require the kidney to excrete the dye so may be used in patients with renal insufficiency
		• Bowel preparation (e.g., cathartics) as prescribed
		• NPO for 8 hours prior to the test
		• Contrast media used
		  • Check for allergy to iodine prior to the study
		  • Monitor for allergic reaction postprocedure
		  • Ensure hydration postprocedure
		• Monitor patient for clinical indications of urinary tract infection or sepsis

Ultrasonography	• Evaluates fluid vs solid mass • Identifies obstructions • Identifies cysts, abscesses, tumors, polycystic kidney disease • Identifies hemorrhage • Identifies urinary tract obstruction and leaks	• No special preparation required • Can be safely used in patients with renal failure • Contrast media may be used

TABLE **11-7** Fluid and Electrolyte Imbalances

Imbalance	Clinical Presentation	Collaborative Management

Hypovolemia due to:
• Insufficient intake
• Inadequate replacement following excess fluid loss
• Excessive fluid losses
  • Hemorrhage
  • GI losses
  • Renal losses
  • Increased insensible losses
  • Draining wounds
• Intravascular to extravascular shift (also called third-spacing)
  • Ascites
  • Intestinal obstruction
  • Peritonitis
  • Burns
	Subjective
	• Weakness
	• Anorexia, nausea, vomiting, constipation
	• Thirst
	• Syncope
	Objective
	• Tachycardia
	• Orthostatic hypotension
	• Low-grade fever
	• Flushed skin (fluid loss) or cool, clammy skin (blood loss)
	• Flat jugular veins
	• Dry, sticky tongue and mucous membranes
	• Poor skin turgor
	• Lethargy, disorientation, coma
	• Oliguria
	• Weight loss >5% of body weight
	• Hemodynamic changes: decreased CVP, PAOP, CO, increased SVR
	Diagnostic
	• Hematocrit and serum osmolality increased if fluid lost; hematocrit decreased if blood lost
	• Urine specific gravity >1.030 if ADH osmoreceptor mechanism is intact
	• BUN increased with normal creatinine (i.e., prerenal)
		• Monitor urine output, input and output, daily weight, laboratory studies
		• Treat the cause
		  • Antiemetics for vomiting
		  • Antidiarrheals for diarrhea
		  • Control of hemorrhage: local pressure, prepare patient for surgery
		  • Antibiotics for infection
		• Replace fluids carefully to prevent hypervolemia
		  • Oral fluids for mild deficits
		  • Parenteral fluids for moderate or severe deficits; replace fluids lost with similar fluids (e.g., blood for hemorrhage, normal saline with electrolytes for excessive diuresis, etc.)
		  • Monitor for clinical indications of fluid overload (e.g., S_3, crackles)
		• Provide frequent oral and skin care

Water loss syndromes: serum osmolality >295 mOsm/L (may be referred to as hyperosmolar hypernatremia) due to water loss without sodium loss due to:
• Inadequate water intake
• Hypertonic fluids or enteral feedings
• Diabetes insipidus
• Diabetes mellitus
• Excess TPN
• Watery diarrhea
	Subjective
	• Weakness
	• Thirst
	• Syncope
	Objective
	• Tachycardia
	• Hypotension
	• Low grade fever
	• Flushed skin
	• Dry, sticky tongue and mucous membranes
	• Poor skin turgor
	• Thirst
	• Mental irritability, confusion
	• Oliguria to anuria (except diabetes insipidus)
	Diagnostic
	• Hematocrit and serum osmolality increased
	• Serum sodium increased (concentration effect)
		• Monitor urine output, I and O, daily weight, laboratory studies
		• Treat the cause
		  • Vasopressin for central diabetes insipidus; chlorpropamide (Diabinese) for nephrogenic diabetes insipidus
		  • Insulin for diabetes mellitus, hyperglycemia
		  • Antidiarrheals for diarrhea
		  • Antiemetics for nausea, vomiting
		  • Appropriate volume replacement and normalize serum osmolality: administer water in excess of sodium (e.g., 1/2NS)
		• Maintain adequate urine output with adequate volume replacement
		• Provide frequent oral and skin care

Medical Emergencies CHAPTER 11   583

TABLE 11-7	Fluid and Electrolyte Imbalances—cont'd	
Imbalance	**Clinical Presentation**	**Collaborative Management**

Imbalance	Clinical Presentation	Collaborative Management

Hypervolemia due to:
• Excessive intake of fluid
• Retention of sodium and water
  • Steroid therapy
  • Heart failure
  • Liver disease e.g., cirrhosis
  • Stress response via ADH secretion, renin-angiotensin-aldosterone system
  • Nephrotic syndrome
  • Acute or chronic renal failure
• Interstitial to intravascular shift
  • Remobilization of fluids after treatment of burns
	Subjective
	• Dyspnea
	• Headache
	Objective
	• Tachycardia
	• Increased blood pressure
	• Jugular venous distention
	• Tachypnea, dyspnea, crackles
	• Peripheral edema
	• Ascites
	• Increased urine output
	• Muscle weakness
	• Confusion, apathy, lethargy, coma
	• Hemodynamic changes: increased CVP, PAOP
	• Weight gain >5% of body weight
	• Clinical indications of pulmonary or cerebral edema
	Diagnostic
	• Hematocrit and serum osmolality decreased
	• BUN decreased
	• Urine specific gravity <1.010 if ADH osmoreceptor mechanism is intact
	• Chest radiography may show pulmonary vascular congestion
		• Monitor urine output, I and O, daily weight, laboratory studies
		• Prevent hypervolemia by closely monitoring IV fluids; volumetric or controller pumps should be used for patients predisposed to hypervolemia
		• Decrease excess volume
		  • Restrict fluids and/or sodium
		  • Administer diuretics as prescribed
		  • Hemodialysis or continuous renal replacement therapy may be utilized especially if renal insufficiency is present
		• Provide frequent oral and skin care

Water excess syndromes: serum osmolality <280 mOsm/L(may be referred to as hypo-osmolar hyponatremia) due to water increased in excess of sodium due to:
• Replacement of isotonic body fluids with hypotonic solution (e.g., D₅W)
• Excess use of tap water enemas
• Psychogenic polydipsia
• GI or GU irrigation with hypotonic fluids (e.g., tap water or distilled water)
• Excessive ice chips
• Syndrome of inappropriate antidiuretic hormone (SIADH)
• Administration of oral hypoglycemic agents, tricyclic antidepressants
	Subjective
	• Anorexia, nausea, vomiting
	• Abdominal and muscle cramps
	• Headache
	• Weakness
	Objective
	• Edema
	• Lethargy
	• Muscle twitching, seizures
	• Confusion
	Diagnostic
	• Serum osmolality <280 mOsm/kg
	• Serum sodium decreased (dilution effect)
	• Hematocrit decreased
		• Monitor urine output, I and O, daily weight, laboratory studies
		• Decrease water and normalize osmolality
		  • Restrict fluids
		  • Administer diuretics as prescribed
		  • Administer hypertonic (3%) saline as prescribed for severe hyponatremia
		    • Usually administered at no more rapidly than 100 ml/hr and no more than 400 ml/24 hr
		    • Monitor closely for clinical indications of fluid overload since it pulls fluid into the vascular space
		  • Initiate CRRT as prescribed
		  • Administer demeclocycline (Declocycline) or lithium (Lithobid) as prescribed for nephrogenic SIADH
		• Provide frequent oral and skin care
		• Monitor for clinical indications of cerebral or pulmonary edema: institute seizure precautions

Continued

Where D_5W appears: serum osmolality <280 mOsm/L

TABLE 11-7 Fluid and Electrolyte Imbalances—cont'd

Imbalance	Clinical Presentation	Collaborative Management

Hyponatremia: sodium <136 mEq/L with normal serum osmolality due to:
• Decreased sodium intake
  • Sodium restricted diet
  • Alcoholism
• Increased sodium excretion
  • Skin losses
  • GI losses
  • Renal losses
  • Adrenal insufficiency
	Subjective
	• Anorexia, nausea, vomiting, abdominal cramps
	• Apprehension
	• Headache
	• Weakness, fatigue
	Objective
	• Tachycardia
	• Postural hypotension
	• Diarrhea
	• Weight loss
	• Decreased skin turgor
	• "Fingerprinting" over sternum
	• Personality changes
	• Mental confusion, disorientation
	• Lethargy progressing to coma
	• Muscle cramps, muscle twitching, increased deep tendon reflexes (DTR)
	• Tremors, seizures
	• Oliguria
	Diagnostic
	• Serum sodium <136 mEq/L with normal serum osmolality
		• Monitor urine output, I and O, daily weight, laboratory studies
		• Restore normal serum electrolyte levels
		  • Encourage sodium in diet in mild deficiency
		  • Administer sodium parenterally for moderate or severe deficiency
		  • Normal saline as prescribed
		  • Hypertonic (3%) saline as prescribed for severe hyponatremia
		    • Usually administered at no more rapidly than 1-2 ml/kg/hr and no more than 400 ml/24 hr
		    • Close monitoring for clinical indications of fluid overload required since it pulls fluid into the vascular space
		  • Potassium replacement may also be needed
		• Monitor for neurologic changes; institute seizure precautions
		• Provide frequent oral and skin care

Hypernatremia: sodium >145 mEq/L with normal serum osmolality due to:
• Excess/rapid administration of normal saline or hypertonic saline solution
• Administration of sodium bicarbonate, sodium polystyrene sulfonate (Kayexalate)
• Heart failure
• Renal failure
• Cirrhosis
• Steroid therapy
• Cushing's syndrome
• Primary hyperaldosteronism
• Salt water near-drowning, ingestion of salt water
	Subjective
	• Thirst
	• Muscle weakness and/or cramps
	Objective
	• Tachycardia
	• Hypertension
	• Low-grade fever
	• Edema
	• Dry, sticky tongue and mucous membranes
	• Flushed, dry skin
	• Muscle rigidity, twitching
	• Increased deep tendon reflexes (DTR)
	• CNS irritability: restlessness, agitation
	• Mental confusion, disorientation
	• Tremors, seizures
	• Oliguria
	• Weight gain
	Diagnostic
	• Serum sodium >145 mEq/L with normal serum osmolality
		• Monitor urine output, I and O, daily weight, laboratory studies
		• Treat the cause
		• Restore normal serum electrolyte levels
		  • Restrict sodium
		    • Mild restriction: 3 to 4 grams/day; commonly referred to as a "no added salt" diet
		    • Moderate restriction: 2 grams/day; consumption of only foods specifically "low sodium"
		    • Severe restriction: 500 mg/day; low sodium foods only with avoidance of shellfish and limitation of dairy and meat
		  • Administer diuretics as prescribed
		• Provide frequent oral and skin care
		• Monitor for change in neurologic status; institute seizure precautions

TABLE 11-7   Fluid and Electrolyte Imbalances—cont'd

Imbalance	Clinical Presentation	Collaborative Management

Hypokalemia: potassium <3.5 mEq/L due to:
• Poor potassium intake (e.g., administration of potassium deficient parenteral fluids or nutrition)
• Increased GI losses
• Increased renal losses
• Skin losses
• Extracellular to intracellular shift
• Alkalosis
• Insulin
• Treatment of diabetic ketoacidosis
	Subjective
	• Anorexia, nausea, vomiting
	• Malaise, fatigue
	• Dizziness
	• Muscle cramps
	Objective
	• Orthostatic hypotension
	• Decreased GI motility and bowel sounds, paralytic ileus, constipation, abdominal distention
	• Muscle weakness, possibly flaccid paralysis
	• Decreased DTR
	• Irritability, mental confusion, drowsiness to coma
	• Respiratory muscle weakness causing shallow ventilation, dyspnea progressing to respiratory paralysis and respiratory arrest
	• Polyuria, polydipsia, inability to concentrate urine
	• Enhanced digitalis effect
	• Decreased cardiac output, dysrhythmias, cardiac arrest may occur
	Diagnostic
	• Serum potassium <3.5 mEq/L
	• ECG changes
	  • Flat T waves and prominent U waves
	  • Depressed ST segment
	  • Prolonged QT and PR intervals
	  • Dysrhythmias (e.g., PVCs, ventricular tachycardia, ventricular fibrillation)
		• Monitor urine output, I and O, daily weight, laboratory studies
		• Treat the cause
		• Correct alkalosis
		  • Correct hypomagnesemia and/or hypocalcemia; hypokalemia that is refractory to treatment is frequently accompanied by hypomagnesemia and/or hypocalcemia
		  • Discontinue causative drug if possible
		• Restore normal serum electrolyte levels
		  • Increase dietary potassium for mild hyperkalemia; encourage use of potassium chloride salt substitute
		  • Administer potassium supplements orally
		    • Decrease gastric irritation by administering with food
		  • Administer potassium parenterally for severe hypokalemia
		    • Never administer potassium IV push
		    • Always use an infusion pump
		  • Do not add to a preexisting infusion; if potassium is to be added to maintenance fluids, a new solution should be mixed to avoid uneven distribution of the potassium
		    • Administer potassium "runs" IV usually via mini-bag (usual safe maximum 10 mEq/100 ml over 1 hour but may be administered at 20 mEq/hr if serum potassium is <2.5 mEq/L)
		    • Administer at no greater concentration than 10 mEq/100 ml if given via peripheral catheter or 20 mEq/100 ml if given via a central venous catheter
		    • Administer in normal saline unless contraindicated; dextrose may stimulate insulin secretion and intracellular shift of potassium
		    • Note: it takes 100-200 mEq of potassium to increase serum potassium by 1 mEq/L
		    • Monitor ECG closely when administering high concentrations of potassium
		• Monitor for clinical indications of digitalis toxicity if patient receiving digitalis preparation
		• Teach patient about adequate potassium replacement if receiving diuretics; potassium-sparing diuretics may be used

Continued

TABLE 11-7   Fluid and Electrolyte Imbalances—cont'd

Imbalance	Clinical Presentation	Collaborative Management

Hyperkalemia: potassium >5.0 mEq/L due to:
 • Increased potassium intake
   • Excessive administration/ingestion of potassium: oral or parenteral
   • Excessive or too rapid potassium replacement
   • Transfusion of banked blood; the longer the blood has been stored, the higher the extracellular potassium content
 • Decreased potassium excretion
   • Acute and chronic renal disease
   • Adrenal insufficiency (Addison disease)
   • Potassium-sparing diuretics
   • ACE inhibitors
 • Cellular disruption with leak of intracellular potassium
   • Hemolysis (e.g., blood transfusion reaction)
   • Trauma or tissue ischemia/necrosis
   • Catabolism
   • Rhabdomyolysis
 • Intracellular to extracellular shift
   • Acidosis
   • Hypertonic glucose with insulin deficiency
   • Muscle paralyzing agents (e.g., succinylcholine)
	Subjective
	 • Nausea, vomiting, abdominal cramping, diarrhea
	 • Numbness, paresthesia of extremities
	 • Weakness, fatigue
	 Objective
	 • Initially tachycardia progressing to bradycardia and cardiac arrest
	 • Decreased contractility, decreased cardiac output, hypotension
	 • Abdominal distention
	 • Hyperactive bowel sounds
	 • Muscle weakness progressing to flaccid paralysis
	 • Increased DTRs initially progressing to decreased to absent DTRs
	 • Respiratory muscle weakness may cause hypopnea, respiratory distress
	 • Lethargy, apathy, mental confusion
	 • Oliguria
	 Diagnostic
	 • Serum potassium >5.5 mEq/L
	   • Mild: 5 to 6 mEq/L
	   • Moderate: 6 to 7 mEq/L
	 • Severe: >7 mEq/L
	 • ECG changes
	   • 5.5 to 6.0 mEq/L: tall, narrow, peaked T waves, shortened QT interval
	   • 6.0 to 7.0 mEq/L: wide QRS complexes, prolonged PR intervals
	   • 7.0 to 7.5: flattened to absent P waves, further widening of QRS complexes
	   • 8.0 or greater: fusion of QRS complexes and T waves, idioventricular rhythm, asystole
		• Monitor urine output, I and O, daily weight, laboratory studies
		   • Check BUN, creatinine levels for data about renal function
		 • Treat the cause
		   • Dialysis for renal failure
		   • Treatment of acidosis
		   • Insulin therapy for hyperglycemia
		   • Discontinuance of any causative drug if possible
		     • Potassium-sparing diuretics
		     • ACE inhibitors or angiotensin receptor blockers (ARB)
		     • Nonsteroidal antiinflammatory drugs
		 • Restore normal serum electrolyte levels
		   • Limit potassium intake
		   • Check medications for potassium content
		 • Administer diuretics as prescribed: usually 40 to 80 mg furosemide (Lasix)
		 • Initiate emergency treatment: potassium is greater than 6.5 mEq/L or dysrhythmias are present, however, patients with chronic renal failure may tolerate high levels of potassium and not be symptomatic until 7.0 mEq/L or greater
		   • Dextrose and insulin as prescribed; this moves potassium back into the cell and the effect lasts about 4-6 hours; sodium polystyrene sulfonate (Kayexalate) should be given during this time
		     • Usual dosage is 50 ml of 50% dextrose and 10 units of insulin
		     • Monitor for increased or decreased serum glucose
		   • Sodium polystyrene sulfonate (Kayexalate), an exchange resin, as prescribed; exchanges sodium for potassium and moves potassium out of the body via the GI tract
		     • Oral or by retention enema
		       • Usual dose is 15 to 50 grams in 50 to 100 ml of 20% sorbitol orally
		       • 50 grams in 200 ml of dextrose as retention enema
		   • Sorbitol (Actidose plus Sorbitol), an osmotic laxative, produces a cathartic effect only when given orally, and may contribute to intestinal necrosis when given by enema
		 • Nebulized albuterol as prescribed
		   • Usual dose is 10 to 20 mg nebulized over 15 minutes
		   • Adverse effect: tachycardia
		 • Bicarbonate as prescribed to correct acidosis
		   • Usual dose 50 mEq IV over 5 minutes
		   • This effect lasts 1-2 hours
		   • Adverse effects: hypernatremia, hyperosmolality
		 • Continuous renal replacement therapy (e.g., continuous venous-venous hemodialysis) if prescribed
		 • Monitor for/prevent cardiac effects of hyperkalemia
		   • IV calcium as prescribed
		     • Usual dose 5 to 10 ml of 10% calcium chloride over 2 to 5 minutes
		     • Blocks the neuromuscular and cardiac effects
		     • Contraindicated if patient is receiving digitalis

TABLE 11-7 Fluid and Electrolyte Imbalances—cont'd

Imbalance	Clinical Presentation	Collaborative Management

Hypocalcemia: calcium <9.0 mg/dl in adults or < 8.8 mg/dl in children due to:
Decreased calcium intake or absorption
• Hypomagnesemia
• Acute and chronic renal failure
• Liver disease
• Post-gastrectomy
• Chronic malabsorption syndrome
• Cushing's syndrome
• Steroid therapy
Increased calcium excretion
• Diuretic therapy
• Chronic diarrhea
• Hyperphosphatemia
Increased calcium binding, decreased ionized calcium
• Citrated blood administration
• Alkalosis
	Subjective
	• Abdominal cramps, biliary colic
	• Muscle cramps
	• Paresthesia of fingertips, circumoral area
	Objective
	• Chvostek sign: facial twitching in response to tapping on the facial nerve
	• Trousseau sign: carpal spasm after 3 minutes of inflation of a blood pressure cuff to a level above systolic pressure
	• Muscle tremors
	• Increased deep tendon reflexes (DTRs), carpopedal spasm
	• Irritability, confusion, psychosis
	• Memory loss
	• Laryngospasm, stridor
	• Tetany (characterized by cramps, twitching of the muscles, sharp flexion of the wrist and ankle joints, seizures)
	• Seizures
	• Decreased contractility, cardiac output
	• Oliguria, anuria if renal calculi obstructive
	• Bruising, bleeding
	Diagnostic
	• Serum calcium less than 8.5 mg/dl (less than 4.5 mEq/L)
	• If albumin is decreased, corrected total calcium can be calculated: measured total calcium + 0.8 × (4.0 − albumin)
	 • Hypocalcemia is present if serum ionized calcium is less than 4.1 mg/dl
	• ECG changes
	 • Prolonged QT interval
	 • Dysrhythmias (e.g., torsades de pointes)
	• Serum phosphate decreased
		• Monitor airway patency and ventilation: cricothyroidotomy may be necessary for severe laryngospasm
		• Monitor urine output, I and O, daily weight, laboratory studies
		• Treat the cause
		 • Phosphate-binding antacids as prescribed for hyperphosphatemia
		 • Calcium administration, phosphate restriction, and phosphate binding agents for renal failure
		• Restore normal serum electrolyte levels
		 • High calcium, low phosphorus diet
		 • Oral calcium with vitamin D supplements as prescribed for mild hypocalcemia
		 • Calcium gluconate or calcium chloride IV as prescribed
		  • Slow administration: dilute in 100 ml of D_5W and administer over 10-30 minutes
		  • Administration through central venous catheter if possible; if administered through a peripheral catheter, prevent extravasation which may cause necrosis and sloughing
		 • Magnesium as prescribed (hypocalcemia unresponsive to treatment may indicate concurrent hypomagnesemia)
		• Monitor for/prevent neurologic complications; institute seizure precautions

Continued

TABLE 11-7 Fluid and Electrolyte Imbalances—cont'd

Imbalance	Clinical Presentation	Collaborative Management

Hypercalcemia: calcium >9.0 mg/dl in adults and > 10.8 mg/dl in children due to:
• Increased calcium intake
• Increased calcium absorption
  • Hypophosphatemia
• Increased mobilization of calcium from bone
  • Hyperparathyroidism
  • Immobility
  • Malignancy especially bone, breast, lung, lymphoma, multiple myeloma
  • Thyrotoxicosis
• Decreased calcium excretion
  • Thiazide diuretics
  • Adrenal insufficiency (Addison disease)
  • Renal tubular acidosis
• Increased ionized calcium (e.g., acidosis)
	Subjective
	• Thirst
	• Anorexia, nausea, vomiting, abdominal pain
	• Malaise, fatigue, weakness
	• Bone and/or flank pain; pathologic fractures may occur
	• Depression
	Objective
	• Decreased bowel sounds, constipation, paralytic ileus
	• Neuromuscular weakness to flaccidity; decreased deep tendon reflexes (DTRs)
	• Agitation, confusion, lethargy, stupor, coma
	• Subtle personality changes progressing to psychosis
	• Renal calculi
	• Polyuria, polydipsia
	• Azotemia
	• Enhanced digitalis effect
	Diagnostic
	• Serum calcium >10.5 mg/dl (>5.8 mEq/L)
	• Serum phosphate decreased
	• ECG changes: shortened QT interval, dysrhythmias and/or blocks
	• Radiography: osteoporosis
		• Monitor urine output, I and O, daily weight, laboratory studies
		• Treat the cause
		  • Discontinuance of causative drugs
		  • Surgery, radiation, antineoplastics for malignancy
		  • Partial parathyroidectomy for hyperparathyroidism)
		• Restore normal serum electrolyte levels
		  • Decrease calcium absorption
		    • Low calcium, high phosphorus diet
		    • Corticosteroids
		  • Increase calcium excretion
		    • Oral or parenteral fluids as prescribed; usually isotonic saline at 100 to 200 ml/hr
		    • Any of the following as prescribed
		      • Loop diuretics (e.g., furosemide [Lasix])
		      • Calcitonin (Miacalcin)
		      • Phosphorus
		      • EDTA (disodium salt)
		    • Dialysis may be utilized
		• Decrease bone resorption of calcium
		  • Weight-bearing activities
		  • Any of the following as prescribed
		    • Etidronate (Didronel)
		    • Pamidronate (Aredia)
		    • Gallium nitrate
		    • Corticosteroids
		    • Plicamycin (formerly known as *mithramycin*) (Mithracin)
		    • Inorganic phosphate
		• Monitor for/prevent cardiac effects of hypercalcemia: calcium channel blockers as prescribed
		• Prevent renal calculi while correcting hypercalcemia: agents to acidification urine may be used because acidification of urine increases solubility of calcium
		• Monitor for clinical indications of digitalis toxicity

TABLE 11-7   Fluid and Electrolyte Imbalances—cont'd

Imbalance	Clinical Presentation	Collaborative Management

Hypophosphatemia: phosphorus <3.0 mg/dl due to:
• Inadequate intake of phosphorus
  • Malnutrition
  • Prolonged low-phosphorus or phosphate-free IV therapy or TPN therapy
• Decreased GI absorption or increased intestinal loss
  • Excessive use of phosphate-binding gels such as aluminum hydroxide (Amphojel)
  • Prolonged vomiting or diarrhea
  • Chronic malabsorption syndrome
• Increased renal excretion of phosphorus
  • Thiazide diuretics
  • Hypomagnesemia
  • Hypokalemia
  • Hyperparathyroidism
• Extracellular to intracellular shifts
  • Parenteral glucose or insulin administration
  • Respiratory alkalosis
  • Large amounts of carbohydrate
  • DKA (before treatment)
	Subjective
	• Anorexia, nausea, vomiting
	• Malaise, fatigue
	• Paresthesia
	• Bone pain
	• Chest pain
	Objective
	• Tachycardia, hypotension
	• Tremors
	• Muscle weakness
	• Nystagmus, anisocoria
	• Incoordination, ataxia
	• Confusion, lethargy, coma
	• Seizures
	• Memory loss
	• Respiratory muscle weakness and decreased respiratory excursion
	• Heart failure: dyspnea, crackles
	• Weight loss
	• Hemolytic anemia
	  • Platelet dysfunction: petechiae, bleeding
	• Immunosuppression
	Diagnostic
	• Serum phosphate <3.0 mg/dl
	• Increased serum and urine calcium
	• ECG: dysrhythmias
	• Radiography: skeletal abnormalities
		• Monitor urine output, I and O, daily weight, laboratory studies
		• Treat the cause
		  • Discontinuance of phosphate binding gels
		  • Correction of hypercalcemia if cause of hypophosphatemia
		• Restore normal serum electrolyte levels
		  • High phosphorus, low calcium diet
		  • Oral phosphate supplements (e.g., Neutra-Phos [sodium and potassium phosphate], Phospho-Soda [sodium phosphate], K-Phos [potassium phosphate]) as ordered and monitor for signs of hypocalcemia when giving supplements
		  • Parenteral sodium phosphate or potassium phosphate IV as ordered and monitor for signs of hypocalcemia
		    • Usual dose
		      • If phosphate <1 mg/dl without adverse effects: usual dose is 0.6 mg/kg/hr
		      • If phosphate <2 mg/dl with adverse effects: usual dose is 0.9 mg/kg/hr
		  • Utilization of central venous catheter if possible
		  • IV phosphate is contraindicated in hypercalcemia
		• Monitor for cardiovascular, pulmonary, neurologic effects of hypophosphatemia

Hyperphosphatemia: phosphate >4.5 mg/dl due to:
• Increased phosphorus intake
• Decreased phosphorus excretion
  • Acute or chronic renal failure
  • Hypoparathyroidism
• Extracellular shifts
  • DKA (before treatment)
  • Respiratory acidosis
• Cellular destruction
  • Neoplastic disease treated with chemotherapy
  • Catabolism
  • Rhabdomyolysis
	Subjective
	• Same as hypocalcemia
	Objective
	• Same as hypocalcemia
	Diagnostic
	• Serum phosphate >4.5 mg/dl
		• Monitor airway patency; cricothyroidotomy may be necessary for severe laryngospasm
		• Monitor urine output, I and O, daily weight, laboratory studies
		• Treat the cause
		  • Correction of hypocalcemia
		  • Dialysis if renal failure is cause
		  • Saline diuresis and urinary alkalization if tumor lysis syndrome or rhabdomyolysis
		• Restore normal serum electrolyte levels
		  • Low phosphorus, high calcium diet
		  • Sucralfate (Carafate) or aluminum antacids to bind with phosphate in the GI tract as prescribed
		  • Glucose and insulin as prescribed to shift phosphate into the cell (transient effect only)
		• Monitor for/prevent neurologic complications; institute seizure precautions

Continued

TABLE 11-7 Fluid and Electrolyte Imbalances—cont'd

Imbalance	Clinical Presentation	Collaborative Management

Hypomagnesemia magnesium <1.5 mEq/L due to:
• Decreased magnesium intake or absorption
  • Protein-calorie malnutrition
  • Starvation
  • Prolonged low-magnesium or magnesium-free IV therapy or TPN therapy
• Impaired absorption
• Increased magnesium loss
  • Diuretics
  • Vomiting, gastric suction, fistula
  • Chronic diarrhea
  • Hyperparathyroidism
  • Hyperaldosteronism
  • Steroids
  • DKA
  • HF
• Increased magnesium binding
  • Citrated blood administration
• Extracellular to intracellular shift
  • Concentrated glucose solutions
  • Amino acid solutions
  • Insulin
	Subjective
	• Anorexia, nausea, vomiting, abdominal distention
	• Paresthesia of fingertips, circumoral area
	• Muscle cramps
	• Syncope
	Objective
	• Tachycardia, hypotension
	• Chvostek and Trousseau signs
	• Tremors, increased DTRs, carpopedal spasm
	• Ataxia, nystagmus
	• Laryngospasm, stridor
	• Tetany
	• Seizures
	• Insomnia
	• Confusion, psychosis
	• Memory loss
	• Decreased contractility, cardiac output
	• Increased digitalis effect
	Diagnostic
	• Serum magnesium <1.5 mEq/L
	• May have concurrent hypocalcemia, hypokalemia, hypophosphatemia
	• ECG changes
	  • Prolonged QT interval
	  • Dysrhythmias especially torsades de pointes
		• Monitor airway patency; cricothyroidotomy may be necessary for severe laryngospasm
		• Monitor urine output, I and O, daily weight, laboratory studies
		• Treat the cause
		  • Nutritional support for malnutrition
		  • Use of potassium-sparing diuretics if diuretics are needed since they spare magnesium
		• Restore normal serum electrolyte levels
		  • High magnesium diet
		  • Oral magnesium supplements in the form of magnesium antacids as prescribed
		  • Magnesium sulfate IV as prescribed
		    • Usually administered in 1-2 grams over 5 to 60 minutes
		      • Usually diluted in 100 ml and administered over 1 hour
		      • May be diluted in 10 ml and administered over 5 to 20 minutes for when life-threatening dysrhythmias (e.g., torsades de pointes) occur
		  • Calcium replacement as prescribed; most patients with hypomagnesemia are also hypocalcemic
		• Monitor for/prevent neurologic complications; institute seizure precautions
		• Monitor for clinical indications of digitalis toxicity for patients on digitalis preparations

TABLE 11-7   Fluid and Electrolyte Imbalances—cont'd

Imbalance	Clinical Presentation	Collaborative Management

Hypermagnesemia: magnesium >2.5 mEq/L due to:
• Increased magnesium intake (e.g., magnesium antacids, magnesium sulfate IV. magnesium-containing laxatives, enemas)
• Decreased magnesium excretion
  • Acute/chronic renal failure
  • Hypoparathyroidism
  • Hypoaldosteronism
• Intracellular to extracellular shift
  • Untreated DKA
  • Rhabdomyolysis
	Subjective
	• Weakness, fatigue
	• Nausea, vomiting
	• Somnolence
	• Diplopia
	Objective
	• Bradycardia, hypotension
	• Facial flushing
	• Muscle weakness progressing to paralysis
	• Decreased DTR: loss of patellar reflex occurs at levels >8 mEq/L
	• Respiratory muscle weakness may cause hypoventilation and dyspnea
	• Respiratory muscle paralysis and apnea may occur with levels >10 mEq/L
	• Confusion, somnolence, lethargy, coma
	• Cardiopulmonary arrest
	Diagnostic
	• Serum magnesium >2.5 mEq/L
	• ECG: prolonged PR, QRS, QT; bradycardias and blocks
		• Monitor and maintain airway and ventilation; intubation and mechanical ventilation may be necessary
		• Monitor urine output, I and O, daily weight, laboratory studies
		• Treat the cause
		  • Discontinuance of magnesium-containing antacids or laxatives, IV magnesium
		• Restore normal serum electrolyte levels
		  • Low magnesium diet
		  • Diuresis
		    • NS or 1/2NS and furosemide (Lasix) (1 mg/kg) as prescribed if normal renal function
		    • Monitor for hypocalcemia, hypokalemia
		  • Dialysis if renal failure is cause of hypermagnesemia
		  • Dextrose and insulin may promote movement of magnesium into the cells (transient effect only)
		• Monitor for/prevent neuromuscular, pulmonary, cardiovascular complications
		• IV calcium as prescribed
		  • Usual dose 5 to 10 ml of 10% calcium chloride over 2 to 5 minutes
		  • Blocks the neuromuscular and cardiac effects
		  • Contraindicated if patient is receiving digitalis

Adapted from: Dennison, R. D. (2007). *Pass CCRN!* (3rd ed.). St. Louis: Mosby.

deficiency; previously known as age-onset, type II, non–insulin-dependent diabetes mellitus (NIDDM)

2. Hyperglycemic crises
   a. Diabetic ketoacidosis (DKA): hyperglycemic crisis associated with metabolic acidosis and increased serum ketones; the most serious metabolic disturbance of type 1 diabetes mellitus
      1) An increase in blood glucose to >250 mg/dl (average ~600 mg/dl) and blood serum ketones >5 mEq/L
   b. Hyperglycemic hyperosmolar nonketotic condition or coma (HHNC): hyperglycemic crisis associated with the absence of ketone formation; most serious metabolic disturbance in type 2 diabetes mellitus
      1) An increase in blood glucose to >600 mg/dl (average ~1100 mg/dl) with normal or only slightly increased serum ketones

Precipitating factors

1. DKA
   a. Undiagnosed type 1 DM
   b. Causes in known type 1 DM
      1) Illness or infection
      2) Omission of exogenous insulin
      3) Trauma
      4) Surgery
   c. Causes in patients with or without diabetes
      1) Cushing syndrome
      2) Hyperthyroidism
      3) Pancreatitis
      4) Pregnancy
      5) Drugs (e.g., glucocorticoids, thiazides diuretics, phenytoin)
2. HHNC: usually seen in patients >50 years with glucose intolerance or type 2 diabetes mellitus; frequently iatrogenic
   a. Pancreatitis
   b. Burns
   c. Infection
   d. Hepatitis
   e. Trauma
   f. Cushing syndrome
   g. Hyperthyroidism
   h. Renal disease
      1) Peritoneal dialysis
      2) Hemodialysis
   i. Hypertonic nutrition: enteral or parenteral
   j. Alcohol
   k. Drugs

1) Glucocorticoids (e.g., prednisone [Delatsone])
2) Thiazide diuretics (e.g., hydrochlorothiazide [Diaxide])
3) Loop diuretics (e.g., furosemide [Lasix])
4) Phenytoin (Dilantin)
5) Diazoxide (Hyperstat)
6) Immunosuppressive drugs
7) β-Blockers (e.g., propranolol [Inderal])
8) Chlorpromazine (Thorazine)
9) Cimetidine (Tagamet)
10) Calcium channel blockers
11) Mannitol
12) Sympathomimetics drugs (e.g., epinephrine)
13) Thyroid preparations

Pathophysiology

1. DKA (Figure 11-12)
   a. Diabetes is the result of an insulin insufficiency or the body's inability to use insulin appropriately to meet the body's needs

1) Type 1 diabetes is characterized by β cell destruction, usually leading to absolute insulin deficiency; previously known as juvenile onset, type I, insulin-dependent diabetes mellitus (IDDM)
2) Type 2 diabetes is a characterized by insulin resistance and a relative (rather than absolute) insulin deficiency; previously known as age-onset, type II, non-insulin-dependent diabetes mellitus (NIDDM)

b. In DKA, insulin production is insufficient or the cells cannot use insulin
c. Without insulin, glucose cannot move into the cell and accumulates in the blood, causing hyperglycemia
d. Insulin deficiency results in the body utilizing triglycerides and muscle
e. Breakdown of glycogen is activated and its synthesis inhibited, gluconeogenesis is stimulated to make new glucose from proteins and fats

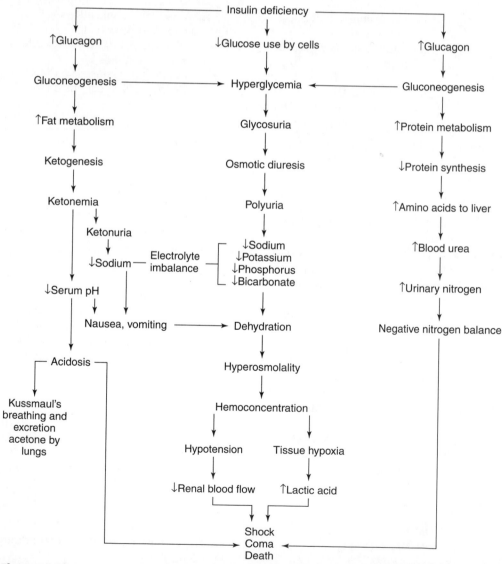

Figure 11-12 Pathophysiology of DKA. (From Dennison, R. D. [2007]. *Pass CCRN!* [3rd ed.]. St. Louis: Mosby.)

f. Hyperglycemia causes an osmotic diuresis as the hypertonic solution goes through the renal tubules and pulls more water into the tubule; this causes glycosuria, dehydration, and electrolyte imbalance
   1) Urinary excretion of ketones causes an additional losses of Na^+ and K^+
2. HHNC (Figure 11-13)
   a. Hyperglycemia and hyperosmolarity lead to osmotic diuresis and an osmotic shift of fluid to the intravascular space, resulting in further intracellular dehydration
   b. Severe dehydration starts a cascade of metabolic derangements resulting in severe dehydration, hyperosmolality, hyperglycemia, and consequent neurologic derangements
   c. Patients make enough insulin to prevent gluconeogenesis, therefore there is no ketoacidosis

Clinical presentation
1. DKA
   a. Subjective
      1) Nausea, vomiting, abdominal pain
      2) Polyphagia initially; may progress to anorexia
      3) Weakness, fatigue
      4) Polydipsia
      5) Polyuria
      6) Headache
      7) Visual disturbances
   b. Objective
      1) Tachycardia, orthostatic hypotension
      2) Slow deep breaths (i.e., Kussmaul respirations)
      3) Flushed, warm, dry skin, poor skin turgor
      4) Sunken eyeballs
      5) Hypothermia or hyperthermia
      6) Acetone (i.e., fruity) odor to breath
      7) Diminished deep tendon reflexes (DTRs)
      8) Lethargy and somnolence indicate severe decompensation
   c. Diagnostic
      1) Glucose: increased >250 mg/dl, but usually < 600 mg/dl
      2) Sodium: normal, increased, or decreased depending on hydration status
      3) Potassium: elevates initially; decreases as pH and dehydration corrected
      4) Anion gap: increased initially and decreases as pH is corrected
      5) Calcium: may be decreased
      6) Phosphorus: decreased
      7) Magnesium: increased initially; then decreases
      8) Ketones: increased
      9) BUN and creatinine: increased (ratio >10:1) due to dehydration
      10) Serum osmolality: increased; usually <350 mOsm/L
      11) CBC
         a) Hematocrit: increased
         b) WBC: may be increased
      12) ABGs: metabolic acidosis frequently with some degree of respiratory compensation

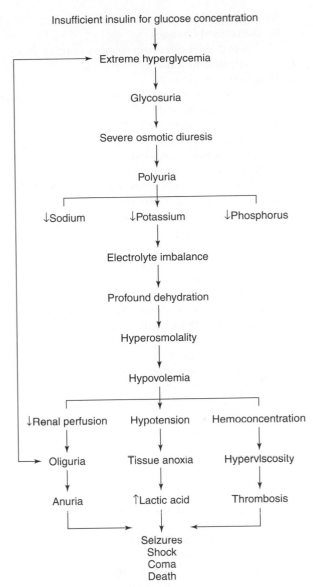

Figure 11-13 Pathophysiology of HHNC syndrome. (From Dennison, R. D. [2007]. *Pass CCRN!* [3rd ed.]. St. Louis: Mosby.)

      13) Urine: positive for glucose and ketones
      14) Electrocardiogram
         a) May show changes associated with potassium levels; high early and then low as pH is corrected and potassium moves from serum back into the cell
         b) Sinus tachycardia is frequently seen
2. HHNC
   a. Subjective
      1) Weakness
      2) Fatigue
      3) Thirst
      4) Polyuria initially; progresses to oliguria
      5) History of taking medications that may inhibit insulin action or cause hyperglycemia
   b. Objective
      1) Tachycardia, orthostatic hypotension
      2) Tachypnea
      3) Flushed, warm, dry skin with poor skin turgor
      4) Dry mucous membranes

5) Decreased deep tendon reflexes
6) Behavioral changes
7) Altered level of consciousness ranging from confusion to lethargy
c. Diagnostic
1) Glucose >600 mg/dl (possible >2000 mg/dl)
2) Sodium: increased
3) Potassium: decreased
4) Calcium: may be decreased
5) Phosphorus: decreased
6) Magnesium: decreased
7) BUN and creatinine: increased with BUN:creatinine ratio >10:1 due to dehydration
8) Serum osmolality increased; usually >350 mOsm/kg
9) CBC
a) Hematocrit: increased
b) WBC: increased
10) ABGs: normal pH or only mildly acidotic (acidosis is lactic acidosis related to hypoperfusion rather than ketoacidosis)
11) Urine
a) Glucose: positive
b) Ketones: negative or slight increase
12) Electrocardiogram
a) May show changes associated with low potassium levels
b) May show sinus tachycardia

Collaborative management

1. Continue assessment
   a. ABCDs
   b. Vital signs: blood pressure, pulse, respiratory rate, and temperature
   c. Oxygen saturations as indicated
   d. Cardiac rate and rhythm
   e. Respiratory effort and excursion
   f. Accurate intake and output
   g. Serum electrolytes and bedside glucose monitoring
      i) Serum glucose and potassium levels are evaluated every 1-2 hours
   h. Level of consciousness
   i. Close monitoring for progression of symptoms
2. Maintain airway, oxygenation, and ventilation
   a. Position of comfort
   b. Oxygen by nasal cannula at 2 to 6 L/min if indicated to maintain SpO$_2$ of 95% unless contraindicated; for patients with COPD, use pulse oximetry to guide oxygen administration to SpO2 of 90%
3. Maintain adequate circulation and perfusion
   a. IV access for fluid and medication administration as indicated
      1) Correction of fluid volume deficit
         a) 0.9% NS IV 1-2 L/hr for 1 to 2 hours then decrease rate to 100 to 500 hr until volume loss corrected; then if hypernatremia still present switch to 0.45% NS
            i) DKA: adult average loss 6 L
            ii) HHNC: adult average loss 8 to 15 L

b) Dextrose 5% to fluids when serum glucose is decreased to 300 mg/dl
2) Monitor for clinical and laboratory indications of dehydration, hypovolemia, and hypoperfusion
b. Regular insulin intravenously as prescribed
1) Adults: 0.1 unit/kg IV injection, then start insulin IV infusion of 0.1 unit/kg/hr
2) In HHNC
a) Smaller amounts of insulin are usually required to normalize serum glucose
b) Usually type 2 DM and sensitive to insulin
3) Check blood glucose every 30 minutes to 1 hour
4. Correct electrolyte imbalance
a. Potassium
1) Replacement required early in HHNC and as pH is normalized in DKA
2) May be administered as KCl or combination of KCl and KPO$_4$
b. Magnesium: may be required
5. Correct acid-base imbalance
a. Correction of cause through hydration and insulin
b. Sodium bicarbonate may be used in severe acidosis (i.e., pH, 7.0)
6. Close monitoring for indications of sepsis (i.e., fever, confusion, widened pulse pressure)
7. Ensure patient safety: seizure precautions especially in HHNC
8. Monitor for complications
a. Hypovolemic shock
b. Dysrhythmias
c. Pulmonary edema
d. Deep vein thrombosis, pulmonary embolism
e. Cerebral edema
f. Seizures
g. Coma
h. Hypoglycemia
i. Electrolyte imbalances: potassium, sodium, phosphorus, magnesium

Evaluation

1. Patent airway, adequate oxygenation (i.e., normal Pao$_2$, Spo$_2$, Sao$_2$) and ventilation (i.e., normal Paco$_2$)
2. Absence of clinical indicators of hypoperfusion
3. Absence of clinical indications of electrolyte imbalances
4. Normal serum glucose
5. Alert and oriented with no neurologic deficit

Typical disposition

1. If evaluation criteria met: discharge with instructions for follow-up
2. If evaluation criteria not met: admission; critical care unit admission may be required

Hypoglycemia

Definition: decrease in the amount of glucose in the blood

1. Serum glucose level <50 mg/dl in males, <45 mg/dl in females, and <40 mg/dl in infants (ENA, 2007)
2. Sudden decrease in serum glucose even though the level is not less than 50 mg/dl

Precipitating Factors

1. Insufficient nutrient intake
   a. Missed or delayed meal
   b. Nausea, vomiting
   c. Interrupted tube feedings or parenteral nutrition
2. Excessive insulin dose
   a. Poor visual acuity causing dose inaccuracy
   b. Injection in area of improved absorption
3. Drugs
   a. Sulfonylurea therapy
      1) Renal insufficiency potentiates effects
      2) Hepatic insufficiency delays metabolism and excretion and impairs gluconeogenesis and glycogenolysis
      3) Potentiated by salicylates, sulfonamides, phenylbutazone, α-glucosidase inhibitors (e.g., acarbose [Precose], miglitol [Glyset])
   b. Ethanol
   c. Quinidine
   d. α-Blockers
   e. Salicylates
   f. Haloperidol
   g. Trimethoprim-sulfamethoxazole (Septra)
4. Inadequate production of glucose
   a. Strenuous physical exercise or stress with inadequate adjustment of food intake and/or insulin dosage
   b. Excessive alcohol intake ingested without adequate food intake
   c. Glucagon deficiency
5. Post-gastrectomy
6. Pancreatic islet cell necrosis: may occur with pentamidine (Pentam) therapy for *Pneumocystis carinii* infection; causes an acute increase in insulin release
7. Adrenal insufficiency
8. Severe liver disease
9. Pregnancy
10. Tumors
    a. Non–β-cell tumors
       1) Malignant: sarcoma, mesothelioma, hepatomas, lymphoma, leukemia, adrenal carcinoma
       2) Benign: carcinoid and carcinoid-like tumors, pheochromocytoma
    b. β-Cell tumors (i.e., insulinomas)

Pathophysiology

1. Too much insulin in relation to amount of glucose
2. Decrease in serum glucose levels to 50 mg/dl or below
3. Release of counterregulatory hormones to insulin
   a. Growth hormone
   b. Cortisol
   c. Glucagon
   d. Epinephrine
      1) SNS stimulation (Note: this stimulation and, therefore, the clinical indications may be blocked by β-blockers)
4. Serum glucose may increase due to glycogenolysis and gluconeogenesis triggered by the counterregulatory hormones and/or food intake
5. Serum glucose may continue to be less than normal causing a decrease in cerebral glucose levels
   a. Neuroglycopenic effects may cause neuronal damage: the brain must have constant supply of glucose (i.e., carbohydrate) and cannot use any other substrates (e.g., protein, fat)
6. Severe neurologic injury, seizures, coma may result with severe and/or prolonged hypoglycemia

Clinical presentation

1. Subjective
   a. Anxiety
   b. Weakness, fatigue
   c. Palpitations
   d. Nausea
   e. Hunger
   f. Paresthesia
   g. Blurred vision, diplopia
   h. Headache
   i. Irritability, difficulty with concentration
2. Objective
   a. Adrenergic (sympathetic) stimulation indicators
      1) Diaphoresis
      2) Pallor, cool skin
      3) Tremors
      4) Piloerection
      5) Tachycardia, tachypnea
   b. Neuroglycopenic indicators
      1) Vasomotor changes: hypotension
      2) Slurred speech
      3) Agitation
      4) Confusion
      5) Staggering gait
      6) Sensory changes: paresthesias
      7) Motor changes: paresis, hemiplegia, paraplegia
      8) Seizures
      9) Coma
   c. Nocturnal hypoglycemia
      1) Restless sleep
      2) Nightmares
      3) Early morning headache
3. Diagnostic
   a. Serum glucose: ≤50 mg/dl
      1) 20 to 40 mg/dl is associated with seizures
      2) <20 mg/dl is associated with coma
   b. Electrocardiogram: sinus tachycardia
   c. Alcohol and serum drug screen as indicated

Collaborative management

1. Continue assessment
   a. ABCDs
   b. Vital signs: blood pressure, pulse, respiratory rate, and temperature
   c. Oxygen saturations as indicated
   d. Cardiac rate and rhythm
   e. Respiratory effort and excursion
   f. Bedside glucose monitoring
   g. Serum electrolytes
   h. Accurate intake and output

i. Level of consciousness

j. Close monitoring for progression of symptoms

2. Maintain airway, oxygenation, and ventilation

a. Position of comfort

b. Oxygen by nasal cannula at 2 to 6 L/min if indicated to maintain SpO_2 of 95% unless contraindicated; for patients with COPD, use pulse oximetry to guide oxygen administration to SpO_2 of 90%

3. Maintain adequate circulation and perfusion

a. Oral fluids and glucose if patient alert and able to swallow

b. IV access for fluid and medication administration as indicated

4. Restore normal serum glucose level

a. Immediate measurement of serum glucose level when clinical indications of hypoglycemia occur

b. 10 to 15 g (40 to 60 calories) of carbohydrates for conscious patients (Box 11-1)

   1) Glucose tablets or gel is required if the patient has been receiving an α-glucosidase inhibitor (e.g., acarbose [Precose], miglitol [Glyset]) since these agents block the conversion of carbohydrates to glucose

c. If unable to administer glucose orally, glucose IV as prescribed

   1) Adults: dextrose 50%

   2) Pediatrics: dextrose 25%

   3) Infants: dextrose 10%

   4) Thiamine 100 mg IV recommended prior to dextrose administration especially in alcoholics to prevent Wernicke encephalopathy

   5) Glucagon IM (0.5 to 2 mg in adults) may be given to unconscious patients if unable to gain IV access

d. Longer acting carbohydrate source (e.g., milk, cheese, crackers) or regularly scheduled meal to avoid recurrence

e. Reassessment of serum glucose 15 minutes after treatment and every 15 minutes until serum glucose is within normal range: an additional 50 ml of $D_{50}W$ may be required for refractory hypoglycemia

f. Anticipation of times when the insulin dependent patient is most likely to exhibit hypoglycemia

   1) Peak times for administered insulin therapy (Table 11-8)

   2) Strenuous exercise

   3) Omission of food

   4) Drugs that the patient is receiving that may potentiate insulin

5. Monitor for complications

a. Myocardial ischemia or infarction

b. Seizures

c. Coma

d. Irreversible neurologic damage

Evaluation

1. Patent airway, adequate oxygenation (i.e., normal PaO_2, SpO_2, SaO_2) and ventilation (i.e., normal $PaCO_2$)

2. Absence of clinical indicators of hypoperfusion

BOX   **11-1   Foods Providing 10 to 15 g of Carbohydrates for Relief of Hypoglycemia**

- 4 ounces of apple or orange juice
- 4 ounces of cola or other carbonated beverage
- 8 ounces of skim or 1% milk
- 4 cubes or 2 packets sugar
- 2 ounces of corn syrup, honey, or grape jelly
- 6 Life Savers or jelly beans
- 10 gumdrops
- 2 tablespoons raisins
- 1/2 cup regular gelatin dessert
- 2-3 squares graham crackers
- 1 small (2 ounces) cake decorating icing
- 3 (5 gram) glucose tablets
- 25 ml of $D_{50}W$ if patient unable to take calories orally

From: Dennison, R. D. (2007). *Pass CCRN!* (3rd ed.). St. Louis: Mosby.

3. Normal serum glucose

4. Alert and oriented with no neurologic deficit

Typical disposition

1. If evaluation criteria met: discharge with instructions

a. Review of medications

b. Glucose monitoring at home

c. Dietary intake

d. Follow-up with primary care provider or endocrinologist

2. If evaluation criteria not met: admission

Hyperthyroidism

Definitions

1. Hyperthyroidism: hyperfunction of the thyroid gland; either increased secretion of thyroid hormones or increased responsiveness to thyroid hormones

---

TABLE   **11-8   Characteristics of Insulin Preparations**

Insulin	Onset (hr)	Peak (hr)	Duration (hr)
Human regular (IV)	Immediate	15 to 30 minutes	1 to 2
Human lispro (SC)	15 minutes	½ to 1½	3 to 5
Human regular (SC)	½ to 1	2 to 3	5 to 7
Human NPH (SC)	2- to 4	4 to 10	14 to 18
Human Lente (SC)	3 to 4	4 to 12	16 to 20
Human Ultralente (SC)	6 to 10	14 to 24	20 to 36

From: Dennison, R. D. (2007). *Pass CCRN!* (3rd ed.). St. Louis: Mosby

2. Thyrotoxic crisis (also referred to as thyroid storm): severe life threatening form of hyperthyroidism

Precipitating factors

1. Graves disease: most common cause
2. Toxic nodular goiter
3. Thyroiditis
4. Iodine excess
5. Pituitary tumors
6. Thyroid cancer
7. Poorly treated hyperthyroidism
8. Patient with hyperthyroidism experiences a physical or emotional stressor that precipitates thyroid storm
   a. Infection
   b. Surgery
   c. Trauma
   d. Radioactive iodine treatment
   e. Pregnancy
   f. Anticholinergic drugs
   g. Adrenergic drugs
   h. DKA

Pathophysiology

1. Graves disease
   a. Autoimmune process leads to thyroid enlargement and over secretion of hormones
   b. Antibodies to TSH receptor stimulate the thyroid to release T3, T4, or both hormones
2. Toxic nodular goiter: nodules secrete thyroid hormones without TSH stimulation; may have one or multiple nodules
3. Thyroiditis
   a. Viral, bacterial, or fungal infections cause inflammation and hypersecretion of thyroid hormones
4. Thyroid storm: extreme hypermetabolic state leading to decompensation resulting in heart failure, central nervous system dysfunction, and GI problems

Clinical presentation: related to the increased metabolism caused by excess circulating thyroid hormones

1. Subjective
   a. Palpitations
   b. Weight loss
   c. Nausea, vomiting, diarrhea
   d. Hair loss
   e. Difficulty focusing eyes
   f. Anxiety, fine tremor of hands
   g. Menstrual irregularities
   h. Heat intolerance
   i. Sleep disturbances, insomnia
2. Objective
   a. Tachycardia; hypertension, bounding pulses
   b. Elevated temperature (>104°F possible in thyroid storm)
   c. Warm, moist velvety skin
   d. Thin nails that are brittle and lifted from nailbed
   e. Visible thyroid goiter with possible thrill or bruits
   f. Exophthalmos (protrusion of the eyeballs) and/or lid lag
   g. Increased bowel sounds
   h. Splenomegaly, hepatomegaly
   i. Dehydration
3. Diagnostic
   a. TSH: decreased
   b. Free thyroxine (free T4): increased
   c. T3: increased
   d. Serum glucose: increased
   e. Liver function studies: increased
   f. ECG: atrial fibrillation/flutter, sinus tachycardia, supraventricular tachycardia

Collaborative management

1. Continue assessment
   a. ABCDs
   b. Vital signs: blood pressure, pulse, respiratory rate, and temperature
   c. Oxygen saturations as indicated
   d. Cardiac rate and rhythm
   e. Respiratory effort and excursion
   f. Pain and discomfort level
   g. Accurate intake and output
   h. Serum electrolytes
   i. Level of consciousness
   j. Close monitoring for progression of symptoms
2. Maintain airway, oxygenation, and ventilation
   a. Position of comfort
   b. Oxygen by nasal cannula at 2 to 6 L/min if indicated to maintain SpO_2 of 95% unless contraindicated; for patients with COPD, use pulse oximetry to guide oxygen administration to SpO_2 of 90%
3. Maintain adequate circulation and perfusion
   a. Increased oral fluids
   b. IV access for fluid and medication administration as indicated: D_5NS preferred
   c. Vasopressors may be required if patient can't tolerate large amounts of fluids, or does not respond to fluid resuscitation
4. Administer drugs and therapies to treat cause and symptoms
   a. Acetaminophen for fever: do not use ASA
   b. β-Blockers to block the effects of sympathetic stimulation
   c. Digoxin (Lanoxin) for HF symptoms
   d. Propylthiouracil (PTU)
   e. Iodine preparations
5. Monitor for complications
   a. Dysthymias
   b. Heart failure

Evaluation

1. Patent airway, adequate oxygenation (i.e., normal PaO_2, SpO_2, SaO_2) and ventilation (i.e., normal $PaCO_2$)
2. Absence of clinical indicators of hypoperfusion
3. Normal body temperature
4. Alert and oriented with no neurologic deficit
5. Control of pain, discomfort

Typical disposition

1. If evaluation criteria met: discharge with instructions
   a. Importance of medications
   b. Followup with primary care provider
2. If evaluation criteria not met: admission; critical care unit admission for thyrotoxic crisis

Myxedema Coma

Definition: severe rare life threatening form of hypothyroidism

Precipitating factors

1. Undiagnosed hypothyroidism
2. Stressors in patients with known hypothyroidism
   a. Infection
   b. Medications (opioids, tranquilizers, barbiturates)
   c. Exposure to cold
   d. Trauma
3. Atrophy due to Hashimoto's thyroiditis or Graves disease

Pathophysiology

1. Occurs in undiagnosed or undertreated patients with hypothyroidism who experience an additional significant stress (e.g., infection, certain medications)
2. A decrease in circulating thyroid hormones leads to slowing down of all body processes
3. Leads to decompensated hypothyroidism in which the body's adaptation attempts are no longer sufficient
4. Alterations in level of consciousness occur due to inadequate circulating thyroid hormone

Clinical presentation

1. Subjective
   a. Fatigue, lethargy
   b. Impaired memory
   c. Decreased activity tolerance
   d. Dyspnea
   e. Cold intolerance
   f. Decreased appetite with nausea, vomiting, constipation, weight gain
   g. Menstrual irregularities
   h. Depression
2. Objective
   a. Bradycardia, hypotension
   b. Bradypnea
   c. Decreased temperature
   d. Coarse sparse hair
   e. Prominent tongue
   f. Periorbital edema, facial swelling
   g. Dry, thick skin
   h. Altered LOC
3. Diagnostic
   a. Sodium: decreased
   b. Chloride: decreased
   c. Glucose: decreased
   d. BUN and creatinine: increased
   e. CBC: anemia, decreased WBC
   f. Thyroid hormones
      1) TSH: increased
      2) Free T4: decreased

Collaborative management

1. Continue assessment
   a. ABCDs
   b. Vital signs: blood pressure, pulse, respiratory rate, and temperature
   c. Oxygen saturations as indicated
   d. Cardiac rate and rhythm
   e. Respiratory effort and excursion
   f. Pain and discomfort level
   g. Accurate intake and output
   h. Serum electrolytes
   i. Level of consciousness
   j. Close monitoring for progression of symptoms
2. Maintain airway, oxygenation, and ventilation
   a. Position of comfort
   b. Oxygen by nasal cannula at 2 to 6 L/min if indicated to maintain SpO_2 of 95% unless contraindicated; for patients with COPD, use pulse oximetry to guide oxygen administration to SpO_2 of 90%
3. Maintain adequate circulation and perfusion
   a. IV access for fluid and medication administration as indicated
   b. Isotonic IV fluids as required for dehydration
4. Control pain and discomfort
   a. Analgesics
   b. Antiemetics; nasogastric tube may be needed for uncontrolled vomiting
   c. Antipyretics and cooling methods to reduce fever
5. Restore normal thyroid hormone levels: thyroid hormone replacement (e.g., levothyroxine [Synthroid])
6. Monitor for complications
   a. Adrenal insufficiency
   b. Hypopituitarism
   c. Hypotension
   d. Shock

Evaluation

1. Patent airway, adequate oxygenation (i.e., normal PaO_2, SpO_2, SaO_2) and ventilation (i.e., normal $PaCO_2$)
2. Absence of clinical indications of hypoperfusion
3. Alert and oriented with no neurologic deficit
4. Control of pain, discomfort

Typical disposition: admission to the critical care unit

Syndrome of Inappropriate ADH (SIADH)

Definition: syndrome causes by either an increase in production and release of ADH despite normal or low plasma osmolarity or an increase in the responsiveness of the renal tubule to ADH

Precipitating factors

1. CNS disorders
   a. Trauma

b. Neoplasms
c. Infection
d. Vascular
2. Pulmonary problems
3. Endocrine disorders
4. Certain medications
5. Malignancies: tumors may release ectopic ADH

Pathophysiology
1. Increase in ADH or responsiveness of the renal tubules to ADH
2. Increase in water reabsorption from renal tubules leading to an increased intravascular volume and preload
3. Dilutional hyponatremia and decreased serum osmolality causing water intoxication
4. ADH regulates water absorption
5. May be self-limiting when caused by an acute process such as head trauma
6. Can be a chronic process when associated with cancer or other metabolic problems

Clinical presentation
1. Subjective
   a. Anorexia
   b. Nausea
   c. Confusion
   d. Irritability
   e. Cold
   f. Weight gain
   g. Recent illness or trauma
2. Objective
   a. Lethargic
   b. Decreased deep tendon reflexes
   c. Oliguria
   d. Edema
   e. Pupils: may be asymmetrical
   f. Cheyne-Stoke respirations
3. Diagnostic
   a. ADH: increased
   b. Sodium: decreased
   c. Serum osmolality: decreased
   d. Specific gravity >1.030

Collaborative management
1. Continue assessments
   a. ABCDs
   b. Vital signs: blood pressure, pulse, respiratory rate, and temperature
   c. Oxygen saturations as indicated
   d. Cardiac rate and rhythm
   e. Respiratory effort and excursion
   f. Pain and discomfort level
   g. Accurate intake and output
   h. Serum electrolytes
   i. Level of consciousness
   j. Close monitoring for progression of symptoms
2. Maintain airway, oxygenation, and ventilation
   a. Position of comfort
   b. Oxygen by nasal cannula at 2 to 6 L/min if indicated to maintain SpO_2 of 95% unless contraindicated; for patients with COPD, use pulse oximetry to guide oxygen administration to SpO_2 of 90%
3. Maintain adequate circulation and perfusion
   a. IV access for fluid and medication administration as indicated
   b. Fluid restrictions
   c. Furosemide (Lasix) to promote water excretion
   d. Hypertonic (3%) saline may be required to prevent seizures; usually prescribed if serum sodium level is <115 mEq/L
4. Monitor for complications
   a. Hypervolemia
   b. Cerebral edema
   c. Seizures

Evaluation
1. Patent airway, adequate oxygenation (i.e., normal PaO_2, SpO_2, SaO_2) and ventilation (i.e., normal $PaCO_2$)
2. Absence of clinical indicators of volume overload
3. Alert and oriented with no neurologic deficit
4. Control of pain, discomfort

Typical disposition: admission to critical care unit

Diabetes Insipidus
Definition: clinical condition characterized by impaired renal conservation of water, resulting in polyuria, low urine specific gravity, dehydration, and hypernatremia; caused either by deficiency of ADH or decreased renal responsiveness to ADH
Precipitating factors
1. Neurogenic (i.e., central) DI: defect in synthesis or release of antidiuretic hormone (ADH) due to defect in hypothalamus, pituitary stalk, or posterior pituitary
   a. Primary: familiar, congenital, idiopathic
   b. Secondary
      1) Intracranial tumors: especially hypothalamic or pituitary; may be primary or metastatic tumor
      2) Extracranial neoplasm: leukemia; breast cancer
      3) CNS trauma: especially basal skull fracture
      4) Intracerebral aneurysm, hemorrhage
      5) CNS infections (e.g., meningitis, encephalitis)
      6) Radiation
      7) Cerebral hypoxia and/or anoxic brain syndrome
      8) Granulomatous diseases (e.g., sarcoidosis, tuberculosis)
      9) Drugs that inhibit the secretion of ADH (e.g., ethanol, phenytoin [Dilantin], chlorpromazine [Thorazine], reserpine [Serpasil])
2. Nephrogenic DI: defect in renal tubular response to ADH; usually less severe than neurogenic DI
   a. Congenital
   b. Renal disease
      1) Renal insufficiency
      2) Pyelonephritis
      3) Renal transplant
      4) Polycystic kidneys

5) Metabolic diseases affecting the kidneys (e.g., amyloidosis, sarcoidosis, multiple myeloma)
   c. Drugs that block the effect of ADH on the renal tubules (e.g., lithium [Lithobid], demeclocycline [Declomycin], α adrenergic agents [e.g., norepinephrine], caffeine, amphotericin B [Amphocin], colchicine [Colcrys], vinblastine [Velban])
   d. Result of electrolyte imbalance (e.g., severe hypokalemia, hypercalcemia)
3. Psychogenic DI
   a. Due to psychiatric disturbances with psychogenic polydipsia
   b. Also referred to as compulsive water drinking

Pathophysiology

1. Deficiency of ADH or inadequate renal tubule response to ADH leading to inadequate antidiuresis
2. Diuresis of large volumes of hypotonic urine
3. Dehydration and hypernatremia
4. Potential shock and/or neurologic effects

Clinical presentation

1. Subjective
   a. Thirst, especially for cold liquids
   b. Fatigue, weakness
2. Objective
   a. Polyuria: 5-15 liters/24 hours; suspect DI if urine output is greater than 200 ml/hour for two consecutive hours
   b. Clinical indications of dehydration and volume depletion
      1) Weight loss
      2) Poor skin turgor
      3) Dry mucous membranes
      4) Sunken eyeballs
      5) Postural hypotension, tachycardia
      6) Decrease in CVP, RAP, and/or PAOP
   c. Neurologic signs resulting from hyperosmolality and hypernatremia
      1) Restlessness, confusion; irritability
      2) Seizures
      3) Lethargy, coma
3. Diagnostic
   a. Serum
      1) Sodium: (elevated >145 mEq/Liter) (hyperosmolar hypernatremia caused by water loss)
      2) BUN: elevated
      3) Increased serum osmolality: elevated, greater than 295 mOsm/kg
      4) Hct: elevated
      5) Serum ADH level: decreased (<1 pg/ml)
   b. Urine
      1) Specific gravity: decreased (<1.005)
      2) Osmolality: less than serum osmolality; less than 200 mOsm/kg

Collaborative management

1. Continue assessments
   a. ABCDs

   b. Vital signs: blood pressure, pulse, respiratory rate, and temperature
   c. Oxygen saturations as indicated
   d. Cardiac rate and rhythm
   e. Respiratory effort and excursion
   f. Pain and discomfort level
   g. Accurate intake and output
   h. Serum electrolytes
   i. Level of consciousness
   j. Close monitoring for progression of symptoms
2. Maintain airway, oxygenation, and ventilation
   a. Position of comfort
   b. Oxygen by nasal cannula at 2 to 6 L/min if indicated to maintain SpO_2 of 95% unless contraindicated; for patients with COPD, use pulse oximetry to guide oxygen administration to SpO_2 of 90%
3. Maintain adequate circulation and perfusion
   a. IV access for fluid and medication administration as indicated
   b. Correct fluid deficit: large volumes of isotonic (0.9% saline) or hypotonic (0.45% saline) solution depending on volume deficit
   c. Close monitoring for electrolyte losses and replace accordingly
4. Treat the cause
   a. Exogenous ADH replacement as prescribed for neurogenic DI
   b. ADH potentiator as prescribed for nephrogenic DI; chlorpropamide (Diabinese) used most often
   c. Pharmacologic agents as prescribed for obsessive compulsive behavior (e.g., serotonin reuptake inhibitors, tricyclic antidepressants, or monoamine oxidase inhibitors) for psychogenic polydipsia
5. Correct electrolyte imbalance: potassium replacement usually required
6. Maintain patient safety
   a. Safe environment: side rails up; call light within reach
   b. Seizure precautions
   c. Frequent reorientation
7. Monitor for complications
   a. Coma
   b. Hypovolemic shock
   c. Thromboembolism

Evaluation

1. Patent airway, adequate oxygenation (i.e., normal PaO_2, SpO_2, SaO_2) and ventilation (i.e., normal $PaCO_2$)
2. Absence of clinical indicators of volume overload
3. Alert and oriented with no neurologic deficit
4. Control of pain, discomfort

Typical disposition: admission to the critical care unit

Acute Adrenocortical Insufficiency (i.e., Adrenal Crisis)

Definition: acute insufficiency of hormones from the adrenal cortex
Precipitating factors
1. Primary (Addison disease)
   a. Autoimmune process (most common cause)

b. Tuberculosis (in developing world)

c. HIV/AIDS

d. Adrenal infarction

e. Fungal infections

f. Metastatic breast and lung cancer

g. Adrenal hemorrhage

2. Secondary:

a. Sarcoidosis

b. Pituitary tumor

c. Chronic steroid use: suppresses adrenal function so crisis precipitated when drug stopped abruptly

d. Postpartum pituitary necrosis (i.e., Sheehan syndrome)

e. Anticoagulants

f. Antineoplastics

g. Bilateral adrenalectomy

h. Head injury with damage to pituitary or hypothalamus

Pathophysiology

1. Deficiency in glucocorticoids, mineralocorticoids, and androgens (Addison disease)

2. Adrenal crisis is a severe acute adrenocortical insufficiency that is usually triggered by an acute illness or stressor

3. Aldosterone deficiency causes excretion of excessive amounts of sodium and water and retention of excessive amounts of potassium; corticosteroid deficiency causes inability to stimulate glycogenosis and glyconeogenesis to mobilize glucose

4. Hypovolemia, hypoglycemia, and dysrhythmias caused by hyperkalemia results

Clinical presentation (usually slow onset)

1. Subjective

a. Pain: abdominal, headache

b. Anorexia, nausea/vomiting/diarrhea/weight loss

c. Salt cravings

d. Amenorrhea in women

e. Weakness and fatigue

f. Recent trauma or stressful event

2. Objective

a. Orthostatic hypotension

b. Tachycardia, dysrhythmias

c. Tachypnea

d. Elevated temperature

e. Hyperpigmentation of the skin in areas exposed to sunlight

3. Diagnostic

a. Sodium: decreased

b. Glucose: decreased

c. Chloride: decreased

d. Potassium: increased

e. Calcium: increased

f. BUN: increased

g. Plasma cortisol: low

h. Adrenocorticotropic hormone (ACTH) stimulation test

1) Primary insufficiency: increased

2) Secondary insufficiency: decreased

i. ECG

1) T waves will appear peaked with hyperkalemia

2) PR and QT intervals may be prolonged

Collaborative management

1. Continue assessment

a. ABCDs

b. Vital signs: blood pressure, pulse, respiratory rate, and temperature

c. Cardiac rate and rhythm

d. Respiratory effort and excursion

e. Oxygen saturations as indicated

f. Pain and discomfort level

g. Accurate intake and output

h. Serum electrolytes

i. Level of consciousness

j. Close monitoring for progression of symptoms

2. Maintain airway, oxygenation, and ventilation

a. Position of comfort

b. Oxygen by nasal cannula at 2 to 6 L/min if indicated to maintain SpO_2 of 95% unless contraindicated; for patients with COPD, use pulse oximetry to guide oxygen administration to SpO_2 of 90%

3. Maintain adequate circulation and perfusion

a. IV access for fluid and medication administration

b. IV fluids: rapid infusion of isotonic fluids, usually 0.9% saline, to correct hypovolemia

c. Dextrose in IV fluids to correct serum glucose as prescribed

d. Vasopressors may be required to maintain blood pressure

4. Control pain and discomfort

a. Analgesics

b. Antiemetics; nasogastric tube may be needed for uncontrolled vomiting

5. Restore normal hormone levels and prevent complications

a. Hormone replacement: usually hydrocortisone (Solu-Cortef) 100 mg IV stat and every 6 hours; has both glucocorticoid and mineralocorticoid properties

b. Dextrose 50% as indicated for hypoglycemia

c. Correction of electrolyte imbalances

6. Monitor for complications

a. Hypovolemia

b. Shock

c. Dysrhythmias

d. Cardiopulmonary arrest

Evaluation

1. Patent airway, adequate oxygenation (i.e., normal PaO_2, SpO_2, SaO_2) and ventilation (i.e., normal $PaCO_2$)

2. Absence of clinical indicators of shock

3. Absence of clinical indicators of hypoperfusion

4. Alert and oriented with no neurologic deficit

5. Control of pain, discomfort

Typical disposition: admission to critical care unit

HEMATOLOGIC EMERGENCIES
Disseminated Intravascular Coagulation
Definition: syndrome characterized by thrombus formation and hemorrhage secondary to overstimulation of the normal coagulation process with resultant decrease in clotting factors and platelets
1. May be acute or chronic
2. DIC is not a primary disease; it is always **secondary**

Precipitating factors: always secondary to another process
1. Vascular disorders (e.g., vasculitis, shock)
2. Infection (e.g., bacterial, viral, protozoal, fungal) and sepsis
3. Hematologic/immunologic (e.g., blood transfusions, sickle cell crisis, lupus)
4. Trauma
5. Burns
6. Heat stroke
7. Surgery
8. Neoplastic disorders
9. Obstetric complications (e.g., abruptio placenta, toxemia, septic abortion)
10. Necrotizing enterocolitis
11. Pancreatitis
12. Hepatic disease (e.g., hepatitis, cirrhosis, hepatic failure)
13. Pulmonary (e.g., ARDS, PE)
14. Toxins

Pathophysiology (Figure 11-14 summarizes pathophysiology and relates therapy to the pathophysiology)
1. The paradox of DIC: bleeding after clotting
2. Triggered by
   a. Intrinsic coagulation system activation: damage to vascular endothelium
   b. Extrinsic coagulation system activation: release of tissue thromboplastin
   c. Red cell or platelet injury
3. Clotting causes ischemia and tissue and organ necrosis; this leads to multiple organ dysfunction syndrome
   a. Tissue damage releases thromboplastin into circulation
   b. Thromboplastin converts prothrombin into thrombin
   c. Abundant intravascular thrombin is produced that both converts fibrinogen to a fibrin clot and enhances platelet aggregation
   d. Excessive blood coagulation creates microvascular thrombi (referred to as microclots) in the microcirculation causing ischemia
4. Bleeding causes loss of hemoglobin and oxygen-carrying capacity; this leads to hypoxia and ischemia
   a. Excessive aggregation of platelets causes a thrombocytopenia and excessive blood coagulation causes depletion of clotting factors (this is why DIC is frequently referred to as a consumptive coagulopathy)

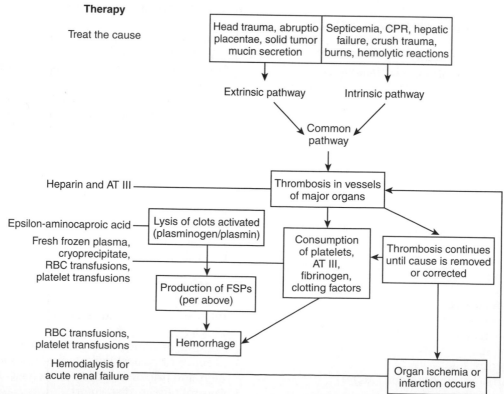

Figure 11-14 Pathophysiology and intended sites of action for therapies in DIC. (From Dennison, R. D. [2007]. *Pass CCRN!* [3rd ed.]. St. Louis: Mosby.)

b. A stable clot, therefore, cannot be formed at injury sites, predisposing patient to hemorrhage

5. Fibrinolysis causes the destruction of once stable clots and more bleeding
   a. Activation of plasminogen to plasmin causes lysis of preexisting clots and surface bleeding
   b. Naturally occurring antithrombins, which inhibit thrombin, are inactivated by plasmin
   c. Fibrinolysis causes production of fibrin split products, also referred to as fibrin degradation products
   d. Fibrin split products are normally cleared by the reticuloendothelial system but overproduction overwhelms the system
   e. Fibrin split products (FSPs) act as an anticoagulant perpetuating bleeding
      1) FSPs coat the platelets and interfere with platelet function
      2) FSPs interfere with thrombin and disrupt coagulation
      3) FSPs attach to fibrinogen which interferes with polymerization process necessary to form a stable clot

Clinical presentation

1. Clinical indications of decreased perfusion
   a. Brain: change in level of consciousness; focal neurologic signs; seizures
   b. Heart: chest pain, ST segment elevation or depression, clinical indications of hypoperfusion
   c. Lung: dyspnea, chest pain, clinical indications of hypoxemia
   d. Kidney: decreased urine output, proteinuria, electrolyte imbalance
   e. GI tract: abdominal pain, diarrhea (may be bloody)
   f. Skin: acral cyanosis of toes, fingers, lips, nose, ears; mottling; coldness; necrosis
2. Clinical indications of platelet dysfunction
   a. Petechiae: frequently the first indication of DIC
   b. Ecchymoses
   c. Purpura
3. Clinical indications of hemorrhage
   a. Tachycardia
      1) Initially postural only then profound tachycardia
   b. Hypotension
      1) Initially narrowed pulse pressure
      2) Then postural hypotension
      3) Then profound hypotension
   c. Tachypnea
   d. Overt bleeding in a patient with no previous bleeding history
      1) Mucosal surfaces: gingival bleeding, epistaxis
      2) GU: Hematuria
      3) GI: Hematemesis, hematochezia, melena, guaiac-positive stool
      4) Pulmonary: hemoptysis
      5) Gynecologic: vaginal bleeding
      6) Skin: prolonged oozing from puncture points, IV sites, and wounds (referred to as surface bleeding), bruising

   e. Occult bleeding
      1) Swollen joints, joint pain may indicate bleeding into the joint
      2) Abdominal distension, rebound tenderness may indicate intraperitoneal bleeding
      3) Back pain, leg numbness, hypotension may indicate retroperitoneal bleeding
      4) Headache, change in level of consciousness, pupillary changes may indicate intracerebral hemorrhage
      5) Visual changes (e.g., blurred vision, loss of visual fields) may indicate retinal hemorrhage
      6) Alterations in hemodynamic parameters: right atrial pressure, pulmonary artery occlusive pressure, cardiac output/cardiac index may be decreased
4. Diagnostic
   a. Platelet count: decreased ($<$150,000/mm^3)
   b. Prothrombin time (PT): prolonged (usually $>$40 seconds)
   c. Activated partial prothrombin time (aPTT): prolonged (usually $>$70 seconds)
   d. Thrombin time: prolonged ($>$15 seconds)
   e. Fibrinogen level: decreased by 50% or more or $<$200 mg/dl
      1) Since fibrinogen is increased in pregnancy, sepsis, and neoplastic conditions, a decrease of 50% is a more accurate indicator of DIC than an absolute value in these patients
   f. Fibrin split products (also referred to as fibrin degradation products: increased (usually $>$40 mcg/ml)
      1) Measures the results of both fibrin and fibrinogen degradation
   g. D-dimer (end-product of fibrin degradation): increased ($>$250 ng/ml)
   h. Hemoglobin and hematocrit: may be decreased if blood loss is significant
   i. ABGs: respiratory alkalosis initially progressing to metabolic acidosis due to lactic acidosis
   j. Urine: may be positive for blood
   k. Stool: may be positive for blood
   l. Sputum: may be positive for blood

Collaborative management

1. Continue assessment
   a. ABCDs
   b. Vital signs: blood pressure, pulse, respiratory rate, and temperature
   c. Cardiac rate and rhythm
   d. Respiratory effort and excursion
   e. Oxygen saturations as indicated
   f. Pain and discomfort level
   g. Accurate intake and output
   h. Serum electrolytes
   i. Level of consciousness
   j. Close monitoring for progression of symptoms
2. Maintain airway, oxygenation, and ventilation
   a. Position of comfort

b. Oxygen by nasal cannula at 2 to 6 L/min if indicated to maintain SpO_2 of 95% unless contraindicated; for patients with COPD, use pulse oximetry to guide oxygen administration to SpO_2 of 90%

3. Maintain adequate circulation and perfusion
   a. IV access for fluid and medication administration as indicated
   b. Normal saline to replace volume until type and crossmatch is completed; blood and blood products as prescribed when available
4. Stop the bleeding by supporting coagulation
   a. Blood products as prescribed to replace clotting factors
      1) Fresh frozen plasma (contains all clotting factors): used for bleeding patients with markedly prolonged PT and aPTT
      2) Cryoprecipitate (contains factors VIII, XIII, and fibrinogen)
      3) Platelets: maintain platelet count above 50,000/mm^3
      4) Packed RBCs: may be needed if blood loss is significant
      5) May potentiate or prolong the clotting, so heparin may be given first
   b. Hemostatic cofactors as prescribed
      1) Vitamin K: needed for liver production of several clotting factors
      2) Folic acid: folic acid deficiency may cause thrombocytopenia
   c. Thrombin-soaked gauze, pressure dressings, and/or ice packs to control bleeding sites
   d. Maintenance of normal body temperature since hypothermia contributes to coagulopathy
5. Stop the microclotting to maintain perfusion and protect vital organ function: IV heparin (usually 5 to 15 units/kg/hr) as prescribed; desirable aPTT is 1.5 to 2 times the control
   a. Controversial as it may potentiate or prolong bleeding but it is thrombosis of small vessels that has the greatest impact on morbidity and mortality in DIC rather than hemorrhage
   b. Contraindicated in CNS or GI hemorrhage, DIC associated with hepatic failure, hemorrhagic obstetric causes (e.g., abruptio placentae), recent surgical procedures
6. Treat ischemic pain
   a. Analgesics as prescribed
   b. Cold compresses for pain caused by bleeding into joints and tissues
7. Provide psychological support and reassurance: reassure patient that treatment is being provided to stop the bleeding (hemorrhage causes extreme anxiety)
8. Monitor for complications
   a. Intracerebral hemorrhage (a major cause of death)
   b. Hemorrhagic shock
   c. ARDS
   d. GI dysfunction
   e. Renal failure
   f. Infection, sepsis

Evaluation

1. Patent airway, adequate oxygenation (i.e., normal PaO_2, SpO_2, SaO_2) and ventilation (i.e., normal $PaCO_2$)
2. Absence of clinical indicators of shock
3. Absence of clinical indications of hemorrhage
4. Alert and oriented with no neurologic deficit
5. Control of pain, discomfort

Typical disposition: admission to critical care unit

Acquired Immunodeficiency Syndrome (AIDS)

Definition: a syndrome of immunodeficiency caused by the human immunodeficiency virus (HIV)

Precipitating factors

1. Exposure to the causative agent: human immunodeficiency virus (HIV), a CD4 cell retrovirus
2. High-risk groups
   a. Participants of high-risk sexual behavior; unprotected sex
   b. Injectable drug users who share needles
   c. Recipients of blood products, especially prior to 1985; hemophiliacs significantly affected
   d. Newborns or breast-fed infants of HIV-infected mothers

Pathophysiology

1. Infection with the human immunodeficiency virus (HIV)
   a. A Lentivirus, a subgroup of retroviruses
      1) Known for the following:
         a) Latency
         b) Persistent viremia
         c) Infection of the nervous system
         d) Weak host immune responses
      2) Two types of HIV that cause AIDS: HIV-1 and HIV-2
         a) There are various subtypes of HIV-1; more than half of all new HIV infections worldwide are caused by subtype C
         b) There are no known subtypes of HIV-2
   b. HIV primarily infects CD4 T lymphocytes and monocytes
      1) CD4 is an antigen on the surface of T helper cells that acts as the primary receptor for HIV
   c. HIV binds to CD4 cells and becomes internalized
   d. HIV replicates itself by generating a DNA copy by reverse transcriptase
   e. Viral DNA becomes incorporated into the host DNA, enabling further replication
   f. Destruction of CD4 cells, CD4 progenitor cells in bone marrow, thymus, and peripheral lymphoid organs, and CD4 cells within the nervous system (e.g., microglia)
   g. Destruction of T4 cells and imbalance between T4 and T8 cells caused by HIV's use of the T4 cells' DNA for reproduction

h. Failure of T-cell production and eventual immune suppression
i. Decrease in cell-mediated immunity T cells' ability to destroy foreign organisms that enter the body
j. General decline in the immune system
k. Presence of opportunistic infections and malignancies

2. Clinical course from exposure to HIV to AIDS
   a. Window period from exposure to seroconversion: approximately 6 weeks to 6 months; may take a year or longer in some persons; therefore repeated testing necessary after suspected exposure
      1) Acute primary infection: lasts 1 to 2 weeks
   b. Asymptomatic phase from seroconversion to symptoms: period is 6 months to 10 years or more; average 2 to 5 years

Clinical presentation

1. Subjective
   a. High-risk group or activity by history
   b. Acute retroviral syndrome: about 70% of patients with primary HIV infection develop a mononucleosis-like syndrome with 2 to 6 weeks after the initial infection
      1) Fever
      2) Fatigue
      3) Headache
      4) Nausea, vomiting, diarrhea
      5) Weight loss
      6) Neurologic symptoms
      7) Sore throat
      8) Muscle and joint discomfort
      9) Night sweats
   c. Fatigue, lethargy, weakness
   d. Anorexia, nausea, vomiting, dysphagia, diarrhea, abdominal pain
   e. Headache, visual changes
   f. Skin dryness, itching
   g. Night sweats, chills
   h. Joint pain
   i. Bruising, bleeding
   j. Dyspnea, cough
   k. Recurrent infections: upper respiratory infection, shingles
   l. Depression, personality change
2. Objective
   a. Acute retroviral syndrome
      1) Lymphadenopathy
      2) Pharyngitis; exudates may be present
      3) Oral ulcers
      4) Maculopapular rash
      5) Oral candidiasis (i.e., thrush)
      6) Hepatomegaly
      7) Genital ulcers
   b. Fever: recurrent
   c. Rash
   d. White spots or sores in mouth
   e. Decrease in visual acuity
   f. Generalized lymphadenopathy

g. Cytomegalovirus (CMV) retinitis, cotton-wool spots noted on funduscopic examination
h. Splenomegaly, hepatomegaly
i. Genital or anal warts

3. AIDS-defining illnesses
   a. Opportunistic infection: infection in the patient with HIV tends to be severe, disseminated, and to recur
      1) Candidiasis: esophagus; trachea; bronchi; lungs
      2) Coccidioidomycosis: disseminated or extrapulmonary
      3) Cryptococcosis: extrapulmonary
      4) *Cryptosporidia* diarrhea for over 1 month
      5) CMV disease or retinitis
      6) Encephalopathy: HIV-related
      7) Herpes simplex: skin ulcers for over 1 month; pneumonia; bronchitis; esophagitis
      8) Histoplasmosis: disseminated or extrapulmonary
      9) Isosporiasis: chronic diarrhea for over 1 month
      10) *Mycobacterium avium-intracellulare* or *M. kansasii*: disseminated or extrapulmonary
      11) *Mycobacterium tuberculosis*: pulmonary or extrapulmonary
      12) *Mycobacterium*: other species disseminated or extrapulmonary
      13) *Pneumocystis juroveci* (formerly known as *Pneumocystis carinii*) pneumonia: most common reason for admission to the critical care unit
      14) Pneumonia: recurrent
      15) Progressive multifocal leukoencephalopathy (PML)
      16) Salmonella septicemia: recurrent
      17) Toxoplasmic encephalitis
   b. Wasting syndrome caused by HIV

4. Diagnostic
   a. Acute retroviral syndrome: leukopenia, elevated liver enzymes
   b. Serum tests for the antibody to HIV
      1) Enzyme-linked immunosorbent assay (ELISA): screening test with high sensitivity so used to rule out HIV
      2) Western blot: high specificity so used to rule in HIV
   c. Hemoglobin and hematocrit: may be decreased
   d. WBC: may be decreased
   e. Platelets: may be decreased
   f. Total protein, albumin, transferrin: decreased in protein malnutrition
   g. Skin tests: may be decreased or absent delayed hypersensitivity reactions to common antigens (e.g., *Candida,* mumps, PPD)
   h. Chest radiography: may reveal pneumonia
   i. Bronchoscopy with lavage and/or biopsy: may be performed for diagnosis of PCP, KS, TB

Collaborative management

1. Continue assessment
   a. ABCDs
   b. Vital signs: blood pressure, pulse, respiratory rate, and temperature
   c. Cardiac rate and rhythm
   d. Respiratory effort and excursion
   e. Oxygen saturation if indicated
   f. Pain and discomfort level
   g. Accurate intake and output
   h. Serum electrolytes
   i. Level of consciousness
   j. Close monitoring for progression of symptoms
2. Maintain airway, oxygenation, and ventilation
   a. Position of comfort
   b. Oxygen by nasal cannula at 2 to 6 L/min if indicated to maintain SpO_2 of 95% unless contraindicated; for patients with COPD, use pulse oximetry to guide oxygen administration to SpO_2 of 90%
3. Maintain adequate circulation and perfusion
   a. Increased oral fluids
   b. IV access for fluid and medication administration as indicated
   c. Treatment of diarrhea if present; may be profuse and lead to dehydration
      1) Fluid and electrolyte replacement
      2) Antidiarrheal medications
4. Prevent infection
   a. Good hand hygiene techniques
   b. All body secretions considered potentially infectious
   c. Clean any contaminated surfaces with 10% bleach solution
5. Monitor for complications
   a. Acute respiratory failure
   b. Septic shock
   c. Coagulopathy
   d. Heart failure
   e. Pulmonary embolism

Evaluation

1. Patent airway, adequate oxygenation (i.e., normal PaO_2, SpO_2, SaO_2) and ventilation (i.e., normal $PaCO_2$)
2. Absence of clinical indicators of respiratory distress
3. Absence of clinical indications of sepsis
4. Alert and oriented with no neurologic deficit
5. Control of pain, discomfort

Typical disposition

1. If evaluation criteria met: discharge with instructions
   a. Importance of followup with primary care provider
   b. Importance of monitoring of immune profile
   c. Prevention of transmission of the virus
2. If evaluation criteria not met: admission, possibly to progressive care unit or critical care unit

Anemia

Definition: decrease in the quantity or quality of circulating RBCs caused by:

1. Decrease in RBC or hemoglobin production
2. Excessive loss of RBCs
3. Excessive lysis of RBCs earlier than the 120-day life expectancy of the RBC

Predisposing factors

1. Iron-deficiency anemia
2. Pernicious anemia: deficiency of intrinsic factor necessary for absorption of vitamin B_{12}
   a. Hereditary affecting primarily people of northern European descent but may also affect people of African and Hispanic descent
   b. Autoimmune disorder
   c. GI disorders (e.g., gastritis, Crohn disease, bowel resection)
   d. Medications such as proton pump inhibitors and antineoplastics
3. Folic acid deficiency anemia
4. Acute blood-loss anemia
   a. GI: esophageal varices, gastric ulcers, lower GI bleed
   b. Genitourinary: renal trauma, menorrhagia
   c. Trauma: bleeding may be overt or occult
   d. Coagulopathies
5. Anemia of chronic illness (e.g., renal failure, cancer)
6. Aplastic anemia: failure of the bone marrow to produce blood cells; some degree of pancytopenia is present
7. Sickle cell anemia: hereditary affecting primarily people of African descent but may also affect people of Hispanic, Mediterranean, or Middle Eastern descent

Pathophysiology

1. General
   a. Reduced oxygen-carrying capacity of the blood
   b. Tissue ischemia
   c. Anaerobic metabolism
   d. Local acidosis
   e. Cellular edema
2. Specific to pernicious anemia
   a. Inherited autoimmune disorder that produces parietal cell antibodies, excessive drinking or smoking, or gastric resection
   b. Defective gastric secretion of the glycoprotein intrinsic factor
   c. Ineffective erythropoiesis
3. Specific to aplastic anemia: stem cell defect or injury or destruction of hematopoietic cells
4. Specific to sickle cell anemia
   a. Hereditary disorder causing presence of hemoglobin S, an abnormal form of hemoglobin A
   b. Crystallization of the abnormal hemoglobin is promoted by deoxygenation, dehydration, acidosis, temperature changes
   c. RBCs become crescent or sickle shaped after they release oxygen

d. These misshapen RBCs get stuck in the blood vessels causing occlusion, tissue injury, and pain

e. Vascular occlusion may cause myocardial infarction, ischemic stroke, splenic or hepatic infarction, blindness, bone necrosis

f. Chronic hemolysis occurs since sickled RBCs are destroyed within 15 days

g. Immunocompromise occurs because spleen function is compromised

Clinical presentation

1. Subjective
   a. Weakness, fatigue
   b. Anorexia, indigestion, epigastric pain, oral pain related to glossitis
   c. Exertional dyspnea
   d. Palpitations
   e. Chest pain
   f. Paresthesia
2. Objective
   a. Pallor
   b. Tachycardia
   c. Tachypnea
   d. Glossitis
   e. Brittle or fine hair
   f. Diarrhea or constipation
   g. Flow murmur (i.e., systolic murmur associated with the turbulence of increased flow of blood through the heart)
   h. Impaired proprioception progressing to ataxia
3. Diagnostic
   a. RBC quantity: less than 4.4 to 5.9 $\times$ 10^6/ml for males or 3.8 to 5.2 $\times$ 10^6/ml for females
   b. RBC quality
      1) Microcytic (i.e., smaller), hypochromic (i.e., RBCs pale in color)
      2) Normocytic, normochromic
      3) Macrocytic (i.e., larger), normochromic
4. Specifics depending on type of anemia
   a. Specifically iron-deficiency anemia: microcytic, hypochromic RBCs
   b. Specific to pernicious anemia
      1) Neurologic changes such as paresthesias and numbness progressing to loss of balance, dementia
      2) Decreased RBC, hemoglobin, and hematocrit
      3) Macrocytic, normocytic RBCs
      4) Increased MCV, normal MCH
      5) Increased serum bilirubin
      6) Decreased fasting serum B_{12}
      7) Normal serum folate (to rule out folate deficiency)
      8) Schilling test: abnormal: indicates impaired B_{12} absorption
   c. Specific to folic acid deficiency anemia: macrocytic, normocytic RBCs
   d. Specific to acute blood-loss anemia: normocytic, normochromic
   e. Specific to anemia of chronic illness: normocytic, normochromic or macrocytic, normocytic

f. Specific to aplastic anemia: normocytic, normochromic

g. Specific to sickle cell crisis
   1) Chest pain
   2) Fever
   3) Jaundice with chronic hemolysis
   4) CBC
      a) Severe reduction in RBC count, hemoglobin, hematocrit
      b) Reticulocyte count: decreased
      c) Presence of nucleated RBCs, sickled RBCs
   5) Chest radiography: pulmonary infiltrates

Collaborative management

1. Continue assessment
   a. ABCDs
   b. Vital signs: blood pressure, pulse, respiratory rate, and temperature
   c. Cardiac rate and rhythm
   d. Respiratory effort and excursion
   e. Oxygen saturations as indicated
   f. Pain and discomfort level
   g. Accurate intake and output
   h. Indications of bleeding
   i. Close monitoring for progression of symptoms
2. Maintain airway, oxygenation, and ventilation
   a. Position of comfort
   b. Oxygen by nasal cannula at 2 to 6 L/min if indicated to maintain SpO_2 of 95% unless contraindicated; for patients with COPD, use pulse oximetry to guide oxygen administration to SpO_2 of 90%
3. Maintain adequate circulation and perfusion
   a. Increased oral fluids
   b. IV access for fluid and medication administration as indicated
   c. Blood and blood products as prescribed (Table 11-9)
      1) Monitor for transfusion reaction (Table 11-10, Box 11-2)
         a) Ask the patient to notify the nurse if he or she develops chills, low back pain, shortness of breath, nausea, sweating, itching, hives, or anxiety
         b) Assess for clinical indications of transfusion reaction (Table 11-10, Box 11-2)
         c) Take appropriate action for transfusion reactions (Table 11-10, Box 11-3) if they occur
         d) Monitor vital signs every 15 minutes for the first hour and then every 30 minutes until transfusion complete or according to hospital policy
      2) Monitor for adverse effects and complications (Table 11-11)
4. Control pain and discomfort
   a. Analgesics
   b. NSAIDs
   c. Antiemetics

TABLE **11-9** Blood and Blood Products

Product	Contents	Compatibility required	Uses	Volume/unit	Comments
Whole blood	RBCs, WBCs, platelets, plasma, and clotting factors	ABO, Rh specific Note: in emergency situations, type-specific blood or O blood may be used	Restores blood volume and oxygen-carrying capacity	Approximately 500 ml	• Must be fresh (<4 hours old) to preserve platelet function • Administer over 2 to 4 hours • Best for hemorrhagic shock
Packed RBCs	RBCs and 20% plasma	ABO, Rh specific preferred; ABO, Rh compatible required	Restores oxygen-carrying capacity	Approximately 250 ml	• Increases hemoglobin by 1 g/dl/unit and hematocrit by 2% to 3%/unit; this change takes at least 6-12 hours • Administer over 2 to 4 hours
Platelets	Platelets, WBCs, plasma	ABO, Rh specific or compatible	Corrects low platelet levels to aid in clotting	Approximately 50 ml	• Administer 1 unit over 10 minutes • Will increase platelet count by 5,000 to 10,000/mm^3 • Agitate often as platelets tend to settle
Fresh frozen plasma	Water, plasma proteins, clotting factors	Rh compatibility required; ABO compatibility preferred	Expands blood volume Restores clotting factor deficiencies Contains no platelets	Approximately 250 ml	• Takes 20 minutes to thaw • Must be given within 6 hours of thawing • Administer 1 unit over 1 to 2 hours or more rapidly if for hemorrhage
Cryoprecipitate	VIII, XIII, fibrinogen, fibronectin	ABO specific or compatible	Replaces clotting factors	Approximately 10 ml; usually 10 bags pooled	• Administer rapidly immediately after thawing • May administer 30 units at one time
Albumin	Albumin from plasma	No compatibility required	Provides volume expansion (no clotting factors)	5%: 200 or 500 ml 25%: 50 ml or 100 ml	• Administer 1 ml/min or more rapidly if patient is in shock • Chemically processed so no risk of hepatitis
Plasma protein fraction	Albumin and globulin in saline solution	No compatibility required	Provides volume expansion (no clotting factors)	5%: 200 to 500 ml	• Administer 10 ml/min • Chemically processed so no risk of hepatitis

From: Dennison, R. D. (2007). *Pass CCRN!* (3rd ed.). St. Louis: Mosby.

5. Administer drugs and therapies to treat cause
  a. Iron supplements (iron-deficiency anemia)
  b. Vitamin B$_{12}$ (pernicious anemia)
  c. Folic acid (folic acid deficiency)
6. Monitor for complications
  a. Shock
  b. Transfusion reactions

Evaluation

1. Patent airway, adequate oxygenation (i.e., normal Pao$_2$, Spo$_2$, Sao$_2$) and ventilation (i.e., normal Paco$_2$)
2. Absence of clinical indicators of hypoperfusion
3. Alert and oriented with no neurologic deficit
4. Control of pain, discomfort

TABLE 11-10   Types of Transfusion Reactions

Type of Reaction	Cause	Clinical Indications	Timing	Treatment
Febrile (nonhemolytic) *Most common type of transfusion reaction	Antigen-antibody reaction to WBCs, platelets, or plasma proteins in the blood product	• Fever (rise in temperature greater than 1°) • Chills • Headache • Nausea, vomiting • Flushing • Anxiety • Muscle pain	Immediately or up to 6 hours after transfusion	Stop transfusion, keep vein open with saline, notify physician and blood bank, send blood specimens to blood bank, antipyretics as indicated, corticosteroids may be prescribed, washed or leukocyte-poor blood should be considered for future transfusions
Mild allergic (Type I hypersensitivity reaction)	Allergic reaction to plasma-soluble antigen in blood product	• Flushing • Itching • Urticaria • Hives	During transfusion or up to 1 hour after transfusion	If febrile, stop transfusion; if afebrile, slow transfusion to keep-vein-open rate until advised by physician, notify physician and blood bank, monitor vital signs, antihistamines as prescribed
Anaphylaxis (Type I hypersensitivity reaction)	Allergic reaction in patients with IgA deficiency sensitized to IgA through previous transfusion or pregnancy	• Anxiety • Urticaria • Facial edema • Dysphagia • Abdominal cramps • Diarrhea • Urinary incontinence • Dyspnea • Stridor • Wheezing • Cyanosis • Chest pain or pulmonary edema may occur • Shock may occur • Cardiopulmonary arrest may occur	Immediately; after transfusion of only a few milliliters of blood	Stop transfusion, keep vein open with saline, notify physician and blood bank; oxygen antihistamines, corticosteroids, and/or aqueous epinephrine as prescribed; emergency airway and/or CPR may be necessary, washed or leukocyte-poor blood or blood from IgA deficient donor should be considered for future transfusions
Acute hemolytic (Type II hypersensitivity reaction)	ABO group incompatibility; antibodies in recipient's plasma attach to antigens in transfused RBCs causing RBC destruction	• Burning sensation along vein • Lumbar pain • Chills, fever, flushing • Nausea, vomiting • Tachycardia, tachypnea • Hypotension (may be only sign in unconscious patient) • May have: dyspnea, chest pain, hemoglobinemia, hemoglobinuria, anuria, disseminated intravascular coagulation • Shock may occur • Cardiopulmonary arrest may occur	Usually within 15 minutes after initiation of transfusion but may occur anytime during transfusion; may be delayed if Rh incompatibility	Stop transfusion, keep vein open with saline, notify physician and blood bank, send blood unit and blood sample from the patient to the blood bank immediately, monitor vital signs and urine output fluids for shock as prescribed, diuretics (usually mannitol) may be prescribed especially if hemoglobinuria occurs, monitor for acute renal failure and shock, request new crossmatch

Continued

TABLE **11-10** Types of Transfusion Reactions—cont'd

Type of Reaction	Cause	Clinical Indications	Timing	Treatment
Delayed hemolytic	Alloimmune response causes slow hemolysis	• Fever • Mild jaundice • Purpura • Anemia	Days to weeks after completion of transfusion	Monitor urine output and hemoglobin and hematocrit levels
Noncardiac pulmonary edema	Donor antibodies react with recipient HLA antigen	• Fever, chills • Dyspnea • Cough • Crackles • Hypoxemia • Shock	During transfusion or shortly after the transfusion	Stop transfusion, administer oxygen, intubation and mechanical ventilation may be necessary, corticosteroids may be prescribed
Circulatory overload	Fluid administered faster that the cardiovascular system can accommodate	• Tachycardia • Hypertension • Headache • Jugular venous distension increased RAP, PA, PAOP • Dyspnea • Cough • Crackles	During transfusion or shortly after the transfusion	Administer RBCs no more rapidly than 4 ml/kg/hr unless severe hemorrhage occurring slow or stop transfusion, continue IV saline slowly if transfusion discontinued, position patient upright with legs over the side of bed, oxygen as indicated, diuretics or venous vasodilators as indicated
Sepsis	Transfusion of contaminated blood components (blood should be infused within 4 hours)	• Chills • Fever • Vomiting • Abdominal pain • Diarrhea (may be bloody) • Hypotension • Shock	During or after transfusion	Stop the transfusion, obtain cultures of patient's blood and send with remaining blood to blood bank, antibiotics as prescribed fluids or corticosteroids as prescribed, vasopressors may be needed

From: Dennison, R. D. (2007). *Pass CCRN!* (3rd ed.). St. Louis: Mosby.

BOX **11-2** Clinical Indications of Blood Transfusion Reaction in an Unconscious or Sedated Patient

• Tachycardia or bradycardia
• Hypotension
• Fever
• Visible signs of hemoglobin in urine
• Oliguria or anuria
• Bleeding

From: Dennison, R. D. (2007). *Pass CCRN!* (3rd ed.). St. Louis: Mosby.

BOX **11-3** Nursing Actions for Suspected Transfusion Reaction

1. Stop transfusion
2. Maintain IV access with normal saline and new administration set
3. Reassure the patient; stay at the bedside
4. Notify physician and blood bank
5. Recheck blood numbers and type
6. Treat symptoms appropriately
7. Return unused portion of blood in blood bag and administration set to the blood bank
8. Collect and send blood and urine samples to the laboratory; send another urine specimen 24 hours after transfusion reaction
9. Document the transfusion reaction and treatment administered

From: Dennison, R. D. (2007). *Pass CCRN!* (3rd ed.). St. Louis: Mosby.

Typical disposition
1. If criteria met, discharge with instructions
   a. Specific to iron-deficiency anemia
      1) Instructions to take oral iron supplements with meals to decrease the GI side effects
   b. Specific to pernicious anemia

TABLE 11-11	Potential Adverse Effects of Blood Transfusion	
Complications	**Clinical Indications**	**Prevention/ Treatment**

Citrate intoxication and hypocalcemia caused by binding of citrate with calcium	• Paresthesia of fingertips, circumoral area
	• Chvostek sign
	• Trousseau sign
	• Muscle cramps, tremors
	• increased deep tendon reflexes (DTRs), carpopedal spasm
	• Abdominal cramps, biliary colic
	• Confusion, psychosis
	• Memory loss
	• Laryngospasm, stridor
	• Tetany (characterized by cramps, twitching of the muscles, sharp flexion of the wrist and ankle joints, seizures)
	• ECG changes
	  • Prolonged QT interval
	  • Dysrhythmias
		• Monitor calcium in patients receiving multiple transfusion and/or patients with hepatic or renal disease
		• Administer 500 mg to 1 g of calcium every 3 to 5 units of blood as prescribed

Hyperkalemia caused by hemolysis of stored blood and liberation of potassium (note: the older the blood, the higher the potassium in the blood)	• Tachycardia progressing to bradycardia and cardiac arrest
	• Nausea, vomiting, intestinal colic, diarrhea
	• Muscle weakness progressing to flaccid paralysis
	• Numbness, tingling of extremities
	• Increased deep tendon reflexes
	• Fatigue
	• Lethargy, apathy, mental confusion
	• Respiratory muscle weakness may cause hypopnea, dyspnea
	• Respiratory distress
	• Oliguria
	• Decreased contractility, cardiac output
	• ECG changes
	  • Tall, peaked T waves
	  • Wide QRS complex
	  • Prolonged PR interval
	  • Flattened to absent P wave
	  • Bradycardia
	  • Dysrhythmia
		• Monitor potassium closely in patients receiving stored blood (especially patients with renal insufficiency)
		• Dextrose and insulin may be prescribed acutely for patients with cardiac effects of hyperkalemia

Loss of 2,3-DPG (2,3-DPG is a byproduct of glucose metabolism on the hemoglobin molecule; banked [refrigerated] blood is low in 2,3-DPG; 2,3-DPG encourages unloading between hemoglobin and oxygen)	• Clinical indications of hypoxia (e.g., tachycardia, dysrhythmias, cyanosis, restlessness, confusion)	• Especially a problem if massive amounts of banked blood are administered • Give fresh whole blood when possible for patients in need of multiple transfusions
Ammonia intoxication Occurs in older blood; especially a problem for patients with hepatic disease	• Decreased cardiac output: hypotension • Confusion • Altered level of consciousness • Increased serum ammonia	• Avoid use of older blood, especially for massive transfusion • Monitor for ammonia intoxication in patients with hepatic disease

Continued

TABLE 11-11   Potential Adverse Effects of Blood Transfusion—cont'd

Complications	Clinical Indications	Prevention/Treatment
Dilutional coagulopathy	• Prolonged PT, aPTT • Bleeding from needle site, wound	• Administer 2 units FFP and/or platelets for every 10 units of packed RBCs as prescribed
Hypothermia	• Decrease in body temperature • Decrease in tissue delivery of oxygen caused by shift of the oxyhemoglobin dissociation curve to the left resulting in increased affinity between hemoglobin and oxygen	• Warm blood to 35-37°C if large quantities of blood are being administered

From: Dennison, R. D. (2007). *Pass CCRN!* (3rd ed.). St. Louis: Mosby.

1) Elimination of cause (e.g., discontinue offending drug)
2) Vitamin B_{12} as prescribed

  c. Specific to folic acid deficiency anemia
    1) Instruction to increase dietary consumption of foods rich in folic acid (e.g., whole grains, legumes, beans, greens)
    2) Folic acid orally as prescribed

  d. Follow up with hematologist or primary care provider as directed

2. If criteria not met: admission

Hemophilia

Definition: rare inherited disease in which blood does not clot normally due to clotting factor deficiency; the four types include the following:
1. Hemophilia A
2. Hemophilia B
3. Hemophilia C
4. von Willebrand disease

Predisposing factors
1. Genetic: X-linked recessive expression (80% to 90%)
  a. Recessive X-linked factor VIII deficiency (classic hemophilia, or hemophilia type A; accounts for about 80% of all cases)
  b. Recessive X-linked factor IX deficiency (hemophilia type B, or Christmas disease; rare; clinically identical to type A, but long-term treatment differs)
2. Autosomal genetic disorder
  a. Lack of functioning factor XI deficiency (hemophilia type C, or Rosenthal syndrome; similar to type A but less severe)
3. Defective platelet adherence and decreased factor VIII (von Willebrand disease, occurs in both males and females) (Hunt, 2007)
4. Genetic mutations
5. Occurs more often in males

Pathophysiology
1. The role of the clotting cascade is to produce a stable fibrin clot at the site of injury
2. There are two pathways in the clotting cascade: intrinsic and extrinsic
3. Lack of factors can significantly alter the clotting cascade pathways and result in bleeding
4. Factor VIII deficiency
  a. Factor VIII is produced in the liver and is needed for the formation of thromboplastin
  b. Decreased thromboplastin leads to decreased blood coagulation
  c. The less factor VIII that is present, the more severe the disease expression
5. Factor IX deficiency
  a. Factor IX is a component of plasma serine proteases required for normal hemostasis

Clinical presentation
1. Subjective
  a. History of bleeding related to a minor trauma or episode of spontaneous bleeding
  b. Pain
  c. Fatigue
  d. Joint stiffness or tingling
  e. Unexplained bruising; large deep bruises
  f. Nose bleeds
2. Objective
  a. Obvious bleeding
  b. Swelling around joints caused by bleeding into joint area
  c. Warmth, redness, swelling, loss of range of motion in joints
  d. Epistaxis
  e. May have signs of obstructed airway if bleeding occurs in the neck, mouth, or thorax
  f. Change in level of consciousness if intracerebral bleeding occurs (Bryant, 2007)
  g. Hematuria
3. Diagnostic
  a. CBC usually normal hematocrit and platelet counts
  b. Coagulation studies:
    1) Factor VIII: decreased in hemophilia A and von Willebrand disease
    2) Factor IX: decreased in hemophilia B
    3) Factor XI: decreased in hemophilia C

c. Radiology
1) May do joint radiography if joint involvement occurs
2) May do head CT if intracranial bleeding suspected or if patient suffered trauma

Collaborative management

1. Continue assessment
   a. ABCDs
   b. Vital signs: blood pressure, pulse, respiratory rate, and temperature
   c. Cardiac rate and rhythm
   d. Respiratory effort and excursion
   e. Oxygen saturations as indicated
   f. Pain and discomfort level
   g. Accurate intake and output
   h. Level of consciousness
   i. Close monitoring for progression of symptoms
2. Maintain airway, oxygenation, and ventilation
   a. Position of comfort
   b. Oxygen by nasal cannula at 2 to 6 L/min if indicated to maintain SpO_2 of 95% unless contraindicated; for patients with COPD, use pulse oximetry to guide oxygen administration to SpO_2 of 90%
3. Maintain adequate circulation and perfusion
   a. Increased oral fluids
   b. IV access for fluid and medication administration as indicated
   c. Warmed cross matched blood if indicated for trauma
   d. Fresh frozen plasma for hemophilia A and von Willebrand disease
   e. Recombinant factor VIII in severe cases
   f. Fresh frozen plasma or factor IX for hemophilia B (Hunt, 2007)
   g. Desmopressin acetate (DDAVP): to increase factor VIIIc
4. Stop active bleeding
   a. Joints
   1) Rest
   2) Ice
   3) Elevation
   4) Splint, elastic wrap, crutches
   b. Soft tissue
   1) Ice
   2) Elevation
   3) Splint or elastic wrap
   c. Muscle
   1) Rest
   2) Ice
   3) Elevation
   4) Splint, elastic wrap, crutches
   5) Complete bed rest for bleeding in ileopsoas muscle
   d. Mucous membranes
   1) Pressure for nose bleed
   2) Topical antifibrinolytic agents
   3) Nasal packing
   e. Laceration
   1) Suture
   2) Monitoring for at least 4 hours after suturing for re-bleed
   3) Anesthetic agent with epinephrine
5. Avoid activities that may lead to bleeding
   a. No intramuscular injections
   b. No aspirin or nonsteroidal anti-inflammatory drugs (NSAIDs)
   c. Avoid injury; safety precautions
6. Monitor for complications
   a. Hematoma
   b. Hemorrhage
   c. Shock
   d. Arthritis (result of bleeding into joints)

Evaluation

1. Patent airway, adequate oxygenation (i.e., normal PaO_2, SpO_2, SaO_2) and ventilation (i.e., normal $PaCO_2$)
2. Absence of clinical indicators of hemorrhage
3. Absence of clinical indicators of hypoperfusion
4. Control of pain/discomfort
5. Alert and oriented with no neurovascular deficit

Typical disposition

1. If evaluation criteria met: discharge with instructions for follow up
2. If evaluation criteria not met (e.g., severe pain, signs of bleeding): admission

GENERAL MEDICAL EMERGENCIES

Acute Renal Failure

Definition: sudden and severe decrease in kidney function that is usually temporary and short term

1. Depending on cause and treatment course, acute renal failure (ARF) may be reversible or cause permanent renal insufficiency and failure
   a. There are three types of renal failure
   1) Prerenal occurs when the kidneys are not properly perfused; may be caused by hypovolemia, shock, or occlusion of the renal artery
   2) Intrarenal failure occurs when there is tissue damage caused by prolonged hypoperfusion, inflammation (e.g., glomerulonephritis), or nephrotoxic agents (e.g., aminoglycosides, NSAIDs)
   3) Postrenal failure occurs when there is obstruction of urinary flow (e.g., stone, tumor, hypertrophied prostate)

Predisposing factors

1. Prerenal
   a. Decreased intravascular volume
   1) Hemorrhage
   2) GI losses: vomiting, diarrhea
   3) Renal losses: osmotic diuresis, diuretics, diabetes insipidus
   4) Skin losses: perspiration, burns, necrotizing fasciitis
   5) Volume shifts: peritonitis, ileus, pancreatitis

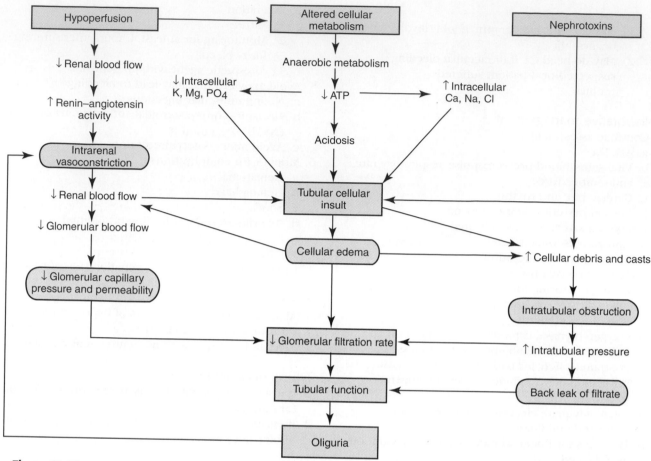

Figure 11-15 Pathophysiology of acute renal failure. (From Dennison, R. D. [2007]. *Pass CCRN!* [3rd ed.]. St. Louis: Mosby.)

b. Decreased cardiac output
   1) Myocardial infarction
   2) Heart failure
   3) Cardiomyopathy
   4) Dysrhythmias
   5) Pulmonary embolism
   6) Vasodilation
   7) Sepsis
   8) Anaphylaxis
   9) Vasodilators
c. Renovascular changes
   1) Renal artery atherosclerosis or thrombosis
   2) Vasopressors
   3) Abdominal aortic aneurysm
2. Intrarenal
   a. Glomerulonephritis
   b. Vasculitis
   c. Interstitial nephritis
      1) Acute pyelonephritis
      2) Allergic nephritis
      3) Severe hypercalcemia
      4) Uric acid nephropathy
      5) Myeloma of the kidney
      6) Malignant hypertension
   d. Acute tubular necrosis

   1) Nephrotoxic agents (e.g., antimicrobials, antineoplastics, NSAIDs, contrast dyes, heavy metals, pesticides, fungicides, heavy pigments [hemoglobin, myoglobin])
   2) Prolonged ischemic injury
      a) MAP <60 mm Hg for 40 minutes or more
      b) Aortic cross-clamping
      c) Bilateral emboli to both kidneys causing renal infarction
      d) Vasopressors (e.g., phenylephrine [Neosynephrine], norepinephrine (Levophed), high dose dopamine [Intropin])
   3) Any of the causes of prerenal failure that is prolonged
3. Post-renal
   a. Mechanical
      1) Ureteral obstruction (e.g., strictures, calculi, neoplasm)
      2) Urethral obstruction (e.g., prostatic hypertrophy)
      3) Bladder outlet obstruction
      4) Edema
   b. Functional
      1) Neurogenic bladder (e.g., diabetic neuropathy, spinal cord injury)
      2) Ganglionic blocking agents

Pathophysiology (see Figure 11-15)
Clinical presentation

1. Subjective
   a. Uremic syndrome: irritability, insomnia, weakness, fatigue, metallic taste
   b. Flank and back pain
   c. Muscle cramps
   d. Dyspnea
   e. Headache
   f. Nausea and vomiting, diarrhea
   g. Weight loss or gain
2. Objective
   a. Decrease in urine volume
   b. Tachycardia
   c. Dysrhythmias occur with electrolyte imbalance
   d. May have pericardial friction rub
   e. Hypertension in volume overloaded states
   f. Kussmaul respirations: deep rapid breathing
   g. Change in behavior (e.g., confusion, altered LOC)
   h. GI symptoms: bleeding gums, constipation, diarrhea
   i. Generalized edema and or ascites
   j. Bruising, petechiae, pruritus, pallor
   k. Halitosis: uremic fetor (i.e., urine like odor to breath)
   l. Jugular vein distention (JVD)
   m. Renal bruits may be audible over left or right midline in periumbilical region in renal vascular disease or renal vascular trauma
   n. Thrill palpated and bruit auscultated over vascular access (e.g., fistula) indicate patency
   o. Asterixis: hand flapping tremors induced by extending the arm and dorsiflexing the wrist (indicates increased ammonia levels in renal and hepatic failure)
3. Diagnostic
   a. Electrolytes: hyperkalemia, hyponatremia, hypocalcemia, hypophosphatemia
   b. BUN increases with decreased renal blood flow and dehydration
   c. Creatinine increases in renal failure (more accurate than BUN in evaluating renal function
   d. Clotting profile: bleeding time may be increased
   e. ABGs: metabolic acidosis with increased anion gap
   f. Urinalysis
      1) Presence of RBCs (casts): if glomerular disease
      2) Uric acid crystals: possible if acute tubular necrosis
      3) Calcium oxalate crystals usually present in acute renal failure
   g. Chest radiography: to evaluate for volume overload, effusions, pulmonary edema, cardiomegaly
   h. Renal ultrasound to identify hemorrhage, obstructions, cysts, abscess, tumors, polycystic kidney disease, urinary tract obstruction
   i. CT: to evaluate kidneys for size, tumors, obstructions, abscesses, calculi
   j. IV pyelogram (IVP) : to identify tumors, cysts, obstructions, and congenital abnormalities

Collaborative management

1. Continue assessment
   a. ABCDs
   b. Vital signs: blood pressure, pulse, respiratory rate, and temperature
   c. Cardiac rate and rhythm
   d. Respiratory effort and excursion
   e. Oxygen saturation if indicated
   f. Pain and discomfort level
   g. Accurate intake and output
   h. Serum electrolytes
   i. Acid-base balance
   j. Level of consciousness and neurologic status
   k. Close monitoring for progression of symptoms
2. Maintain airway, oxygenation, and ventilation
   a. Elevation of head of bed to 30 to 45 degrees; overbed table may be helpful for patient to lean on
   b. Oxygen by nasal cannula at 2 to 6 L/min if indicated to maintain SpO_2 of 95% unless contraindicated; for patients with COPD, use pulse oximetry to guide oxygen administration to SpO_2 of 90%
   c. Artificial airway if ventilation and oxygenation inadequate
   d. Rapid sequence intubation (RSI) and mechanical ventilation if patient unable to maintain airway
3. Maintain adequate circulation and perfusion
   a. IV access with two large-bore catheters for fluid and medication administration
   b. Control of bleeding
4. Prevent and/or treat uremia
   a. Insertion of Foley catheter to allow monitoring of urine output
   b. Treatment of cause
      1) Fluid resuscitation if prerenal failure caused by hypovolemia
      2) Elimination of nephrotoxic agents in intrarenal failure
      3) Removal of obstruction to urine flow in postrenal failure
      4) Pharmacologic agents as prescribed: antihypertensives, inotropic agents, vasopressors, vasodilators, diuretics as prescribed
   c. Preparation for dialysis if indicated
      1) Indications for emergency dialysis: coma, stupor, volume overload, pulmonary edema, hyperkalemia
      2) Insertion of vascular access (e.g., double-lumen central venous catheter) may be done in ED prior to patient receiving dialysis
5. Maintain fluid, electrolyte, and acid-base balance
   a. Fluid resuscitation if hypovolemic cause but otherwise fluid administration should be judicious to prevent fluid overload
   b. Detection and treatment of hyperkalemia
      1) Monitor for large peaked T waves on ECG and/or ventricular dysrhythmias that may indicate hyperkalemia

2) Initiate therapies to decrease serum potassium levels as prescribed
   a) Sodium polystyrene sulfonate (i.e., Kayexalate) by mouth or enema to allow elimination of potassium in the feces
   b) Emergent dialysis
   c) Other treatments allow shifting of potassium from extracellular to intracellular; these treatments are used as a temporizing solution for life-threatening dysrhythmias but the effect on serum potassium only lasts 2 to 4 hours
      i) Dextrose and insulin intravenously
      ii) Sodium bicarbonate intravenously
      iii) Albuterol (Ventolin) by inhalation
3) Administer calcium as prescribed as a cardio-protective agent
6. Monitor for complications
   a. Electrolyte imbalance
   b. Acid-base imbalances
   c. Dysrhythmias
   d. Pericarditis
   e. Cardiac tamponade
   f. Hypertension
   g. Volume overload
   h. Pulmonary edema
   i. Infection
   j. GI hemorrhage
   k. Encephalopathy

Evaluation

1. Patent airway, adequate oxygenation (i.e., normal PaO_2, SpO_2, SaO_2) and ventilation (i.e., normal $PaCO_2$)
2. Absence of clinical indications of respiratory distress
3. Absence of clinical indicators of hypoperfusion
4. Absence of clinical indications of infection/sepsis
5. Alert and oriented with no neurologic deficit
6. Control of pain, discomfort, or dyspnea

Typical disposition

1. If evaluation criteria met: discharge with instructions for follow up with primary care or nephrology
2. If evaluation criteria not met: admission to progressive care unit, critical care unit, or to dialysis

Reye Syndrome

Definition: rare disease that causes swelling in the liver and brain that can result in encephalopathy and acute liver dysfunction
Precipitating factors
1. Viral illness (e.g., influenza, varicella) in children
   a. Though no age group is immune, this disease generally occurs in individuals under 12 years old
2. "Potential association" between aspirin and viral illnesses exists (Bryant & Schultz, 2007, p. 1651)
3. May also be due to drug or toxin exposure or genetic factors
   a. Antiemetics have been implicated in some cases

Pathophysiology

1. Actual pathogenesis is unknown
2. Liver mitochondrial dysfunction leads to an increase in ammonia levels and increased short fatty chains
3. Prolonged vomiting leads to depleted glycogen stores
   a. Glyconeogenesis does not occur because of dysfunction in the process
   b. Fatty acid breakdown does not occur, so the body has no alternative energy source
4. Waste products are not eliminated, so acids continue to accumulate

Clinical presentation: diagnosis is one of exclusion and Reye syndrome should be considered in the differential diagnosis of children who have vomiting and altered mental status
1. Subjective
   a. Recent viral illness followed by abrupt onset of vomiting within 12 hours to 3 weeks (average is 3 days)
   b. Caregiver may relate giving the child aspirin during this illness
   c. Diarrhea is common in children <2 years
   d. Irritability, restlessness
   e. Delirium, seizures
2. Objective
   a. Restlessness, alterations in LOC
   b. Pupils: sluggish or dilated
   c. Vomiting
   d. Dehydration may be present
   e. Hepatomegaly
3. Diagnostic
   a. Serum aminotransferases: increased
   b. Ammonia levels: may increase
   c. Lipase and amylase: increased
   d. Amino and fatty acid levels: increased
   e. Anion gap: increased
   f. Coagulation studies: PT and aPTT increased
   g. BUN may be increased due to dehydration
   h. Glucose may be decreased, especially in children
   i. ABGs: metabolic acidosis initially progressing to respiratory alkalosis
   j. Urine: positive for ketones in most patients
   k. EEG: slowing in early stages and flattened waves as syndrome advances (ENA, 2007)

Collaborative management

1. Continue assessment
   a. ABCDs
   b. Vital signs: blood pressure, pulse, respiratory rate, and temperature
   c. Cardiac rate and rhythm
   d. Respiratory effort and excursion
   e. Oxygen saturation if indicated
   f. Pain and discomfort level
   g. Accurate intake and output
   h. Serum electrolytes
   i. Level of consciousness
   j. Close monitoring for progression of symptoms

2. Maintain airway, oxygenation, and ventilation
   a. Position of comfort
   b. Oxygen by nasal cannula at 2 to 6 L/min if indicated to maintain SpO_2 of 95% unless contraindicated; for patients with COPD, use pulse oximetry to guide oxygen administration to SpO_2 of 90%
3. Maintain adequate circulation and perfusion
   a. Increased oral fluids if tolerated
   b. IV access for fluid and medication administration as indicated
      1) Normal saline bolus as indicated (20 mg/kg for pediatrics)
      2) Albumin as indicated
   c. Close monitoring for prevention/detection of fluid volume overload especially with cerebral edema
4. Protect patient from further injury
   a. Antipyretics, avoiding aspirin, and cooling measures for fever
   b. Seizure precautions
5. Monitor for complications
   a. Seizures
   b. Coma

Evaluation
1. Patent airway, adequate oxygenation (i.e., normal PaO_2, SpO_2, SaO_2) and ventilation (i.e., normal $PaCO_2$)
2. Absence of clinical indicators of hypoperfusion
3. Absence of clinical indications of liver dysfunction
4. Alert and oriented with no neurologic deficit
5. Control of pain, discomfort

Typical disposition: admission, critical care unit admission frequently required to allow intracranial pressure (ICP) monitoring

Hepatic Failure/Encephalopathy
Definitions
1. Hepatic failure: inability of the liver to perform organ functions
2. Hepatic encephalopathy: neurologic impairment as a result of hepatic failure

Etiology
1. Acute liver failure
   a. Viruses
      1) Fulminant viral hepatitis (see Table 11-12)
      2) Herpes simplex
      3) Herpes zoster
      4) Epstein-Barr
      5) Adenovirus
      6) Cytomegalovirus
   b. Hepatotoxic drugs (e.g., acetaminophen [Tylenol], halothane [Fluothane], methyldopa [Aldomet], isoniazid [INH], 3,4-methylenedioxymethamphetamine [Ecstasy]) or toxins (Amanita mushrooms, carbon tetrachloride, sea anemone sting)
   c. Ischemia (e.g., shock and multiple organ dysfunction syndrome [MODS])
   d. Trauma

   e. Reye syndrome
   f. Budd-Chiari syndrome (i.e., hepatic vein obstruction)
   g. Acute fatty liver of pregnancy
   h. Acute hepatic vein occlusion
2. Chronic liver failure with an acute situation (e.g., peritonitis, GI hemorrhage, catabolism)
   a. Cirrhosis
   b. Wilson disease (i.e., genetic disease which causes the accumulation of copper in body tissues which causes damage to the liver and neurologic system)
   c. Primary or metastatic tumors of the liver

Pathophysiology
1. Cirrhosis
   a. Liver parenchymal cells are progressively destroyed and replaced with fibrotic tissue resulting in impaired hepatic function; three-quarters of the liver can be destroyed before symptoms appear
   b. Distortion, twisting, and constriction of central sections cause impedance of portal blood flow and portal hypertension
2. Fulminant hepatitis: liver cells fail to regenerate and necrosis occurs
3. Portal hypertension and impaired hepatic function
   a. Esophageal varices may develop (see GI Hemorrhage section)
   b. Splenomegaly may occur causing thrombocytopenia: thrombocytopenia and vitamin K deficiency cause clotting abnormalities
   c. Inability of the liver to produce adequate amounts of bile and impairment in protein, carbohydrate, and fat metabolism
      1) Serum bilirubin levels become increased since the liver is unable to conjugate the bilirubin and make bile
      2) Deficiency of fat-soluble vitamins may occur since bile salts are required for absorption
      3) Hypoglycemia may occur because the liver cannot perform the functions of glycogenolysis (i.e., breaking down stored carbohydrate to simple sugars) and gluconeogenesis (i.e., converting fat and protein to simple sugars)
   d. Inability of the liver to manufacture plasma proteins and inactivate hormones (e.g., aldosterone, estrogen)
      1) Decreased plasma proteins (albumin being the most important) reduces the capillary oncotic pressure so fluids shift from the vascular space to "third spaces" such as the interstitial space (i.e., peripheral edema), the intraperitoneal space (i.e., ascites), and interpleural space (i.e., pleural effusion)
      2) Increased circulating levels of aldosterone cause continuing retention of sodium and water by the kidney along with increased excretion of potassium; fluid, and electrolyte imbalances occur
         a) Hypokalemia
         b) Hypocalcemia

TABLE **11-12: Types of Viral Hepatitis**

Type	Route	Incubation period	Onset/Chronicity	Comments
A (HAV; infectious hepatitis)	Fecal-oral	2 to 6 weeks	Acute onset Chronicity does not develop	• 99% resolves but 1% becomes fulminant • Treatment is supportive
B (HBV; serum hepatitis)	Parenteral Sexual Perinatal	4 to 24 weeks	Insidious onset Chronicity develops in <5%	• 1% becomes fulminant • 15% to 25% develop liver cancer • Treatment includes interferon alfa-2b (Intron A); antivirals such as lamivudine (Epivir) or famciclovir (Famvir) may also be prescribed
C (HCV; non-A, non-B hepatitis; posttransfusion hepatitis)	Parenteral Sexual Perinatal	2 to 20 weeks	Insidious onset Chronicity develops in 50% to 60%	• 20 to %50% develop cirrhosis • 20% develop liver cancer • 20% develop liver failure • Treatment includes interferon alfa-2b (Intron A) or peginterferon alpha-2b (Peg-Intron) and ribavirin (Virazole); may also include corticosteroids
D (HDV; Delta virus)	Superinfection or coinfection in patient with chronic hepatitis B	4 to 24 weeks	Acute onset Chronicity common with superinfection	• Up to 30% become fulminant • Most have worsening active hepatitis • Treatment is as for hepatitis B
E (HEV; enteric non-A, non-B hepatitis)	Fecal-oral Perinatal	2 to 8 weeks	Acute onset Chronicity does not develop	• Generally benign and self-limiting; however, 10% to 20% mortality when occurs during pregnancy
F (HFV)	Parenteral Sexual Perinatal			• Now considered a variant of hepatitis B
G (HGV)				• Very little known

From: Dennison, R. D. (2007). *Pass CCRN!* (3rd ed.). St. Louis: Mosby.

c) Hypomagnesemia
d) Sodium levels may be increased, normal, or decreased depending on the intravascular volume and serum osmolality
3) Hepatorenal syndrome may develop
  a) Type of renal failure where there is a gradual loss of function but no signs of tissue damage
  b) Associated with cirrhosis of the liver and hepatitis
  c) Cause not completely understood but seems to result from decreased albumin and portal hypertension

e. Inability of the liver to detoxify toxins and drugs and to remove bacteria
  1) Toxins associated with hepatic failure: ammonia, cytokines, endotoxin, tumor necrosis factor-α, bilirubin, and bile acids
  2) Cumulative drug effects frequently occur because the liver is unable to biotransform drugs into inactive and, with some drugs, active metabolites; reduced intravascular volume impairs the ability of the kidney to excrete the active and inactive metabolites
  3) Hepatic encephalopathy may eventually occur

a) Inability to convert ammonia, a byproduct of protein metabolism, to urea causes increased serum ammonia levels

b) Increased cerebral blood flow increases vasoactive peptides which alter the blood-brain barrier allowing neurotoxins (e.g., ammonia) to accumulate in the brain

4) Increased susceptibility to infection and sepsis occurs due to:

   a) Increased amounts of viable bacteria in the circulating blood
   b) Neutrophil malfunction
   c) Complement deficiency
   d) Macrophage deficiency

f. Inability to store vitamins and manufacture clotting factors

   1) Fat-soluble vitamin (A, D, E, K) deficiencies may occur
   2) Clotting abnormalities occur since the liver manufactures all except two of the clotting factors

Clinical presentation

1. Subjective
   a. History of precipitating event
   b. Irritability
   c. Personality change
   d. Confusion, disorientation
   e. Weakness, fatigue
   f. Anorexia, nausea, vomiting
   g. Right upper quadrant dull abdominal pain
   h. Abdominal fullness
   i. Change in bowel habits
   j. Weight loss
2. Objective
   a. General: emaciation, cachectic appearance
   b. Cardiovascular
      1) Tachycardia, dysrhythmias
      2) Bounding pulses
      3) Hypertension or hypotension
      4) Flushed skin
      5) Spider angioma on upper trunk, face, neck, arms
      6) Jugular venous distention
      7) Distended superficial vessels on abdomen (i.e., caput medusae)
   c. Pulmonary
      1) Tachypnea or hyperpnea
      2) Decreased respiratory excursion
   d. Neurologic
      1) Peripheral neuropathy
      2) Slow, slurred speech
      3) Asterixis
      4) Hyperactive reflexes
      5) Seizures
      6) Positive Babinski reflex in encephalopathy
      7) Extreme lethargy or coma in encephalopathy

   e. GI
      1) Fetor hepaticus
      2) Ascites
      3) Hematemesis
      4) Hepatomegaly early; liver atrophy occurs later
      5) Splenomegaly
      6) Ascites
      7) Bowel sounds: diminished
      8) Clay-colored (pale) stools if biliary obstruction
      9) Steatorrhea (i.e., excessive fat in stool, stool floats)
      10) Esophageal varices and/or hemorrhoids
   f. Renal
      1) Oliguria
      2) Dark amber urine
   g. Hematologic/immunologic
      1) Abnormal bruising, bleeding
      2) Susceptibility to infection
      3) Poor wound healing
   h. Integumentary
      1) Jaundice; usually noted in the sclera first
      2) Palmar erythema
      3) Petechiae
      4) Bruises
      5) Edema
      6) Pruritus
      7) Spider angioma
   i. Endocrine changes
      1) Hypogonadism: testicular atrophy and reduced testosterone levels in men
      2) Gynecomastia in men
      3) Altered hair distribution
3. Diagnostic
   a. Sodium: may be decreased or normal
   b. Potassium: may be decreased
   c. Calcium: may be decreased
   d. Magnesium: may be decreased
   e. BUN: may be increased due to dehydration, hepatorenal syndrome, or GI bleeding
   f. Glucose: may be increased or decreased
   g. Creatinine: may be increased due to hepatorenal syndrome
   h. Cholesterol: increased
   i. ALT, AST, LDH: increased
      1) AST/ALT ratio >1 suggests chronic liver failure or tumor
      2) AST/ALT ratio <1 suggests hepatitis
   j. Alkaline phosphatase: increased
   k. Bilirubin: increased
   l. Ammonia: increased in encephalopathy
   m. Total protein, serum albumin, fibrinogen: decreased
   n. Hgb, Hct: may be decreased if hemorrhage or hypersplenism
   o. WBC: decreased; if normal or increased, infection may be present
   p. Platelets: decreased in splenomegaly

q. Clotting studies: PT, aPTT: prolonged
r. ABGs
   1) Respiratory alkalosis
   2) Hypoxemia may be seen
s. Urine
   1) Sodium: decreased
   2) Bilirubin: increased in biliary obstruction
   3) Urobilinogen
      a) Increased in hepatocellular disease
      b) Decreased in complete biliary obstruction
t. Chest radiograph: may show pleural effusion or at-electasis
u. Flat plate of abdomen: may reveal hepatospleno-megaly; abdominal haziness may be seen if ascites is present
v. Abdominal ultrasound: may reveal intra-abdominal fluid if ascites is present
w. Liver scan: may show diffuse changes of cirrhosis
x. Paracentesis: cytologic examination may be done to rule out malignancy; ascites fluid has low specific gravity, low protein concentration, and cell counts
y. EEG: shows abnormal and generalized slowing in patients with encephalopathy
z. Lumbar puncture: may be done to rule out neuro-logic cause of altered consciousness; CSF shows in-crease in glutamine
4. Stages of encephalopathy (Box 11-4)

Collaborative management

1. Continue assessment
   a. ABCDs
   b. Vital signs: blood pressure, pulse, respiratory rate, and temperature
   c. Cardiac rate and rhythm
   d. Respiratory effort and excursion
   e. Oxygen saturation if indicated
   f. Pain and discomfort level
   g. Accurate intake and output
   h. Fluid status and serum electrolytes: serum osmolal-ity, sodium, potassium, calcium, and magnesium
   i. Level of consciousness
   j. Close monitoring for progression of symptoms
2. Maintain airway, oxygenation, and ventilation
   a. Position of comfort
   b. Elevation of head of stretcher 30 to 45 degrees, especially if ascites restricts diaphragmatic excursion
   c. Oxygen by nasal cannula at 2 to 6 L/min if indi-cated to maintain SpO_2 of 95% unless contraindi-cated; for patients with COPD, use pulse oximetry to guide oxygen administration to SpO_2 of 90%
   d. Prevention of aspiration
      1) Artificial airways as necessary in patients with altered consciousness and airway protective mechanisms (e.g., gag reflex)
      2) Intubation usually required at stage III hepatic encephalopathy
3. Maintain adequate circulation and perfusion
   a. IV access for fluid and medication administration as indicated

BOX 11-4	Stages of Encephalopathy
Stage I	• Mild confusion • Decreased attention span • Difficulty performing simple arithmetic computations (e.g., count backward from 100 by 7's) • Decreased response time • Forgetfulness • Mood changes • Slurred speech • Personality changes • Irritability • Disruption in sleep-wake patterns • EEG normal
Stage II	• Lethargy • Confusion • Apathy • Aberrant behavior • Tremor and asterixis (also referred to as *liver flap*) • Inability to reproduce simple designs (constructional apraxia) • Slowing of normal EEG
Stage III	• Somnolent with diminished responsive-ness to verbal stimuli • Severe confusion and incoherence fol-lowing arousal • Speech incomprehensible • Tremor and asterixis • Hyperactive deep tendon reflexes • Hyperventilation • EEG abnormal
Stage IV	• No response to stimuli or abnormal (e.g., decorticate or decerebrate) posturing to stimuli • Areflexia except for pathologic reflexes • Positive Babinski's reflex • Fetor hepaticus • EEG abnormal

From: Dennison, R. D. (2007). *Pass CCRN!* (3rd ed.). St. Louis: Mosby.

b. Colloids as prescribed to improve capillary oncotic pressure and reduce third-spacing; avoid protein-containing colloids (e.g., albumin) in hepatic encephalopathy
c. Crystalloids as prescribed; avoid lactated Ringer so-lution since liver disease impairs the conversion of lactate to bicarbonate
d. Vasopressors may be necessary to maintain vascular tone especially in stage III or IV hepatic encephalopathy
e. Electrolyte replacement as prescribed
f. H_2 receptor antagonists and/or antacids as prescribed to maintain gastric pH 3.5 to 5 to reduce the risk of stress ulcer and GI hemorrhage
4. Prevent and reduce elevated levels of toxins includ-ing ammonia
   a. Lactulose (Cepulac) orally or by nasogastric tube as prescribed

b. Magnesium citrate (Citroma) orally or by enema as prescribed

c. Neomycin by enema as prescribed

5. Prevent/assess for/treat intracranial hypertension and progression of hepatic encephalopathy
   a. Frequent neurologic checks
   b. Avoidance of hepatotoxic agents
   c. Avoidance of sedatives and analgesics and/or reduce dosage if necessary; diphenhydramine (Benadryl) or oxazepam (Serax) may be used for restlessness since they can safely be eliminated
   d. Seizure precautions
   e. Drainage of CSF (if ICP catheter in place) and/or Mannitol (Osmitrol) as prescribed for cerebral edema

6. Decrease portal hypertension: beta-blockers as prescribed

7. Prevent and monitor for bleeding
   a. Avoidance of aspirin and NSAIDs
   b. Avoidance of invasive procedures, including injections, if possible
   c. Vitamin K, fresh frozen plasma, and platelets as prescribed

8. Control pain and discomfort
   a. Analgesics
   b. Antiemetics; nasogastric tube may be needed for uncontrolled vomiting

9. Assess for clinical indications of alcohol withdrawal syndrome (Box 11-5)
   a. Sedatives as prescribed: most of these agents including chlordiazepoxide (Librium) and diazepam (Valium) are hepatotoxic so doses are adjusted and liver enzymes are monitored

10. Monitor for complications
    a. Malnutrition resulting in immunosuppression, poor wound healing, and edema
    b. Coagulopathy
    c. Hemorrhage may be due to:
       1) Esophageal varices
       2) Coagulopathy
       3) DIC
    d. Hypoglycemia
    e. Electrolyte imbalance
    f. Acute respiratory failure related to intrapulmonary shunt or noncardiac pulmonary edema
    g. Pancreatitis
    h. Infection, sepsis
    i. Acute renal failure related to hepatorenal syndrome, acute tubular necrosis, or hypovolemia
    j. Seizures
    k. Cerebral edema

Evaluation

1. Patent airway, adequate oxygenation (i.e., normal Pao_2, Spo_2, Sao_2) and ventilation (i.e., normal $Paco_2$)
2. Absence of clinical indicators of hypoperfusion
3. Absence of clinical indications of sepsis
4. Alert and oriented with no neurologic deficit
5. Control of pain, discomfort

BOX 11-5 Alcohol Withdrawal Syndrome

Early	Late
Mild tachycardia	Marked tachycardia
Mild hypertension	Marked hypertension
Nausea, vomiting	Hyperthermia
Diaphoresis	Dehydration
Pruritus	Delirium
Visual disturbances	Delusions
Time disorientation	Hallucinations
Tremors	Tonic-clonic seizures
Anxiety, agitation	
Sleep disturbances	

Typical disposition: admission, likely to critical care unit

COMMUNICABLE CHILDHOOD DISEASES

Measles

Definition: infection of the respiratory system caused by a virus; two types include:
1. Rubeola
2. Rubella (German measles, 3-day measles)

Precipitating factors
1. Rubeola: exposure to measles virus
2. Rubella: exposure to rubella virus
3. Most often occurs in late winter, early spring

Pathophysiology
1. Rubeola
   a. Highly contagious
   b. A single-stranded RNA virus belonging to the genus Morbillivirus and family Paramyxoviridae
   c. Infects the respiratory epithelium; replicates in regional lymph nodes leading to viremia
   d. Transmitted through respiratory droplets
   e. Incubation: 8 to 12 days
2. Rubella
   a. Not as contagious or severe as rubeola
   b. Transmitted through droplets from the nose and throat
   c. It enters the body by inhalation and infects cells of the respiratory tract
   d. From there it spreads via the lymph nodes to the blood and it induces an immune response, which leads to lasting immunity
   e. Incubation: 14 to 21 days
   f. Fetuses exposed during the first trimester are at risk for specific defects including deafness, blindness, heart defects, or mental retardation

Clinical presentation
1. Rubeola
   a. Subjective
      1) Known exposure
      2) Fever

3) Malaise for approximately 1 day before outbreak of other symptoms
  b. Objective
    1) Classic: the three Cs:
      a) Coryza (i.e., rhinitis)
      b) Cough
      c) Conjunctivitis
    2) Koplik spots (i.e., small gray-blue macules on an erythemic base)
      a) Small irregular bluish spots with red halo may be seen on buccal mucosa opposite premolar teeth starting 2 days before rash appears
    3) Rash
      a) Starts 3 to 4 days after prodrome
      b) Begins on face and behind ears
      c) Later spreads to trunk and extremities in a downward pattern
      d) Erythematous, maculopapular
      e) Palms and soles: maculopapular erythematous rash
      f) Red color fades to purplish, then turns yellow-brown as lesions scale over
      g) Lesion density greater above the shoulders
  c. Diagnostic
    1) CBC may show leukopenia in the latter stages
    2) IgM antibody: positive
    3) IgM enzyme immunoassay if antibody positive
    4) LP for suspected encephalitis
    5) Chest radiograph for suspected pneumonia
2. Rubella
  a. Subjective
    1) Asymptomatic prior to outbreak of rash
    2) History of known exposure
    3) Low-grade fever
    4) Malaise
    5) Headache
    6) Anorexia
    7) Sore throat, coryza, cough, lymphadenopathy that subsides 1 day after the rash appears
  b. Objective
    1) Possible lymphadenopathy
    2) Rash
      a) Begins on face
      b) Rapid downward spread
      c) Discrete, pinkish-red maculopapular lesions
      d) Lesions go away in the same order in which they appeared
      e) Rash usually only lasts 3 days
    3) Mild conjunctivitis
  c. Diagnostic
    1) Serology 4-fold rise in titer of hemagglutination inhibition or complement fixation Ab
    2) Presence of IgM, IgA (indicates infection); IgG (indicates immunity)

Collaborative management
1. Continue assessment
  a. ABCDs

b. Vital signs: blood pressure, pulse, respiratory rate, and temperature
  c. Oxygen saturations as indicated
  d. Pain and discomfort level
2. Maintain airway, oxygenation, and ventilation
  a. Position of comfort
  b. Oxygen by nasal cannula at 2 to 6 L/min if indicated to maintain SpO_2 of 95% unless contraindicated; for patients with COPD, use pulse oximetry to guide oxygen administration to SpO_2 of 90%
3. Prevent transmission: respiratory/droplet isolation; avoidance of pregnant caregivers
4. Control pain and discomfort
  a. Analgesics
  b. Eye care: dim lights for photophobia, wash eyes gently with warm washcloths, monitor for corneal ulceration
  c. Antipyretics if needed
  d. Increased oral fluids
  e. Tepid baths, oatmeal baths, antipruritics for itching
5. Monitor for complications
  a. Rubeola
    1) Otitis media
    2) Pneumonia, bronchiolitis
    3) Obstructive laryngitis and laryngotracheitis
    4) Encephalitis (Hockenberry and Barrera, 2007)
    5) Gangrenous stomatitis (Burnett, 2007)
  b. Rubella
    1) Arthritis
    2) Encephalitis
    3) Purpura (Hockenberry and Barrera, 2007)

Evaluation
1. Patent airway, adequate oxygenation (i.e., normal PaO_2, SpO_2, SaO_2) and ventilation (i.e., normal $PaCO_2$)
2. Absence of clinical indicators of hypoperfusion
3. Absence of clinical indications of sepsis
4. Alert and oriented with no neurologic deficit
5. Control of pain, discomfort

Typical disposition: discharge with instructions
1. Return to the ED for signs of encephalitis
2. High risk contacts should be immunized
  a. Live vaccine within 72 hours of exposure OR
  b. Immune globulin within 6 days of exposure (Peard, 2007)

Mumps
Definition: systemic viral infection involving the salivary and parotid glands; caused by the Paramyxoviridae virus
Predisposing factor: exposure to Paramyxoviridae-family virus
1. Influenza and parainfluenza, types 1 and 3
2. Coxsackieviruses A and B
3. ECHO virus
4. Lymphocytic choriomeningitis virus

Pathophysiology

1. Transmitted by respiratory droplets
2. Incubation: 14 to 25 days
3. Prodromal symptoms start and last between 3 to 5 days
4. Symptoms will depend on the organ affected
   a. Commonly the parotid gland
   b. Can affect testes, pancreas, eyes, ovaries, central nervous system, joints, and kidneys
5. Infectious from 3 days before the onset of symptoms until up to 4 days after the start of active parotitis

Clinical presentation

1. Subjective
   a. Fever
   b. Parotid pain
   c. Earache
   d. Headache
   e. Malaise
   f. Anorexia
2. Objective
   a. Fever 37.8° to 39.4°C (100° to 103°F)
   b. Swollen parotid gland/s; may obscure jawline
   c. Parotid tenderness with palpation
   d. Palpation of Stensen duct may cause pus to emerge from duct opening
   e. Swelling, warmth and tenderness to scrotum or testicles may occur as a complication
3. Diagnostic
   a. CBC with differential: lymphocytosis or leukopenia may be present
   b. Serum amylase: normal or increased
   c. Serum or urine viral isolation for mumps
   d. Polymerase chain reaction (PCR): positive for mumps antigen
   e. Nasopharyngeal or buccal swab: positive 7 days prior to 9 days after parotitis
   f. Testicular ultrasonography if orchitis present to rule out testicular torsion

Collaborative management

1. Continue assessment
   a. ABCDs
   b. Vital signs: blood pressure, pulse, respiratory rate, and temperature
   c. Pain and discomfort level
   d. Accurate intake and output
   e. Close monitoring for progression of symptoms
2. Prevent transmission: airborne precautions
3. Control pain and discomfort
   a. Analgesics
   b. Antipyretics for fever
   c. Increased oral fluids; avoidance of citrus juices as these increase pain
   d. Warm or cold packs to face for comfort
4. Provide treatment for orchitis if present
   a. Bed rest
   b. Scrotal elevation
   c. Ice packs
5. Monitor for complications
   a. Epididymitis
   b. Orchitis
   c. Meningitis
   d. Arthritis
   e. Myocarditis (rare)

Evaluation

1. Patent airway, adequate oxygenation (i.e., normal PaO_2, SpO_2, SaO_2) and ventilation (i.e., normal $PaCO_2$)
2. Absence of clinical indicators of sepsis
3. Control of pain, discomfort

Typical disposition: discharge with instructions

1. Rest
2. Medications as prescribed
3. Follow-up with primary care provider as directed
4. Indications to return to the ED
5. Reassurance to male patients/caregivers that mumps does not cause impotence

Chickenpox

Definition: viral infection; highly contagious

Predisposing factors

1. Exposure to varicella zoster virus
2. More common in children <10 years
   a. Peak incidence in children 2 to 6 years
   b. Affects only about 2% of adults

Pathophysiology

1. Exposure occurs via
   a. Droplets from respiratory tract
   b. Direct contact with fluid from vesicles
2. Incubation period: 10-21 days
3. Patient is contagious until all lesions have crusted over and no new lesions appear

Clinical presentation

1. Subjective
   a. Known exposure
   b. Prodrome of fever, malaise, cough, and anorexia 1 to 3 days prior to lesions
   c. Rash starting on trunk then moving to arms and legs
   d. Anorexia
   e. Headache
2. Objective
   a. Lesions on mucous membranes and skin
      1) Generalized vesicular pruritic rash with 250-500 eruptions
      2) Lesions of many stages in scattered crops: macule, red papule, clear "teardrop" vesicle 1 to 2 mm with pink base, pustule, crust/scab; usually occur around day 6
      3) Necrotic hemorrhagic lesions are more common in elderly
      4) Scarlatiniform rash

b. May show signs of itching; secondary bacterial infections are possible

c. Elevated temperature may be present

d. May show signs of varicella pneumonia/pneumonitis; more common in adults

   1) Cough

   2) Breath sound changes: wheezes, rhonchi

3. Diagnostic

  a. CBC with differential: to rule out other diagnosis

  b. Tzanck smear (scrapings of base of vesicle): if positive will show multinucleated giant cells

  c. Viral culture: positive

  d. Chest radiography: rule out respiratory problems

Collaborative management

1. Continue assessment

  a. ABCDs

  b. Vital signs: blood pressure, pulse, respiratory rate, and temperature

  c. Pain and discomfort level

  d. Close monitoring for progression of symptoms

2. Maintain airway, oxygenation, and ventilation

  a. Position of comfort

3. Prevent spread of infection: contact and respiratory isolation

4. Control pain and discomfort

  a. Analgesics

  b. Antipyretics

  c. Antipruritics

5. Treat infection

  a. Antiviral medications: acyclovir (Zovirax) or famciclovir (Famvir) to lessen disease severity; must be administered within 72 hours of the onset of the rash to have maximal benefits

  b. Increased fluids

  c. Antihistamines for pruritus

  d. Topical anti-itch medications

  e. Skin care: keep skin clean and dry

  f. Referral of high-risk contacts for immunization

6. Monitor for complications

  a. Bacterial infections

  b. Encephalitis

  c. Pneumonia

Evaluation

1. Patent airway, adequate oxygenation (i.e., normal Pao_2, Spo_2, Sao_2) and ventilation (i.e., normal $Paco_2$)

2. Absence of clinical indications of sepsis

3. Control of pain, discomfort

Typical disposition: discharge with instructions

1. Contact precautions

2. Comfort measures: cool compresses, calamine lotion, antihistamines, Aveeno bath

3. Follow-up with primary care provider as directed

4. Indications to return to the ED

Pertussis

Definition: acute tracheobronchitis and paroxysmal cough caused by *Bordetella pertussis;* also known as "whooping cough"

Predisposing factors

1. Exposure to *Bordetella pertussis*

2. Partially immunized children

Pathophysiology

1. Resides in the respiratory tract; affects the ciliated respiratory epithelium of the bronchi

2. Transmission is through contact with airborne droplets from the respiratory tract of an infected person

3. The bacteria attacks the respiratory tract, where they attach to cells and produce toxins that decrease the patient's ability to cough up and clear secretions

4. Highly contagious; contagious from 7 days after exposure up to 3 weeks after onset of symptoms

Clinical presentation

1. Subjective

  a. Known exposure to pertussis

  b. Cough

   1) Hacking cough that ends with a "whooping" sound

   2) May report coughing so hard that they vomit

   3) Worse at night; unable to sleep related to coughing

   4) Productive: copious mucus

  c. Fatigue

2. Objective

  a. Elevated temperature: $>101°F$

  b. Inspiratory "whoop"

  c. May turn blue and take big gulp at the end coughing episode

  d. Petechial rash above the nipple line, conjunctival hemorrhages and facial petechiae caused by forceful coughing

  e. Vomiting

  f. Otitis

  g. Rhinitis (i.e., coryza)

  h. Periorbital edema

3. Diagnostic

  a. CBC with differential: lymphocytosis

  b. Culture and sensitivity: nasal swab from posterior nasopharynx

Collaborative management

1. Continue assessment

  a. ABCDs

  b. Vital signs: blood pressure, pulse, respiratory rate, and temperature

  c. Oxygen saturations as indicated

  d. Pain and discomfort level

  e. Level of consciousness

  f. Close monitoring for progression of symptoms

2. Maintain airway, oxygenation, and ventilation
   a. Position of comfort
   b. Oxygen by nasal cannula at 2 to 6 L/min if indicated to maintain SpO_2 of 95% unless contraindicated; for patients with COPD, use pulse oximetry to guide oxygen administration to SpO_2 of 90%
   c. Suction as needed
3. Maintain adequate circulation and perfusion
   a. Increased oral fluids
   b. IV access for fluid and medication administration as indicated
4. Prevent transmission: respiratory droplet isolation
5. Control pain and discomfort
   a. Analgesics
   b. Antipyretics for fever
6. Prevent/treat infection
   a. Immunization: Tdap (tetanus, diphtheria, pertussis)
      1) Boostrix: 0.5 ml in deltoid IM; ages 11 to 18 years
      2) Adacel: 0.5 ml in deltoid IM; ages 19 to 64 years
   b. Antitussives
   c. Antibiotics (e.g., erythromycin, azithromycin, clarithromycin)
7. Monitor for complications
   a. Pneumonia
   b. Atelectasis
   c. Seizures
   d. Hemorrhage (e.g., subconjunctival, epistaxis)

Evaluation
1. Patent airway, adequate oxygenation (i.e., normal PaO_2, SpO_2, SaO_2) and ventilation (i.e., normal $PaCO_2$)
2. Absence of clinical indicators of respiratory compromise
3. Absence of clinical indications of dehydration
4. Control of pain, discomfort

Typical disposition
1. If criteria met, discharge with instructions
   a. Respiratory isolation until 14 days of antibiotics completed
   b. Close contacts need prophylactic antibiotics
   c. Indications to return to the ED: difficulty breathing, decreased fluid intake, or intolerance of antibiotics
2. If criteria not met (i.e., infants or children who are acutely ill): admission

Diphtheria
Definition: bacterial infection caused by *Corynebacterium diphtheriae* that usually attacks the nose and throat but can affect other organs
Predisposing factors
1. Crowded living conditions
2. Poor sanitation
3. Partially immunized or no immunization

Pathophysiology
1. Highly contagious; spread through respiratory droplets, contaminated food, or surfaces
2. Produces a systemic toxin that affects the respiratory system and can cause widespread organ damage
3. Incubation: 2 to 5 days

Clinical presentation
1. Subjective
   a. History of recent travel out of the country
   b. Fever, chills
   c. Headache
   d. Dyspnea, stridor
   e. Barky cough
   f. Sore throat, difficulty swallowing
2. Objective
   a. Tachycardia, tachypnea
   b. Elevated temperature (>101°F)
   c. Bluish discoloration of skin
   d. Increased work of breathing: nasal flaring, accessory muscle use, stridor
   e. Mucous membranes and pharynx with a dirty, gray-white covering
   f. Swelling of pharynx, tonsils, and surrounding structures
   g. Lymph node enlargement and tenderness
3. Diagnostic
   a. WBC: increased
   b. Thrombocytopenia
   c. Serum antibodies: positive for *C. diphtheriae*
   d. Nasal and/or nasopharyngeal culture: positive for *C. diphtheriae*
   e. Chest radiography: subglottic narrowing
   f. ECG
      1) ST and T wave abnormalities
      2) May have first degree AV block

Collaborative management
1. Continue assessment
   a. ABCDs
   b. Vital signs: blood pressure, pulse, respiratory rate, and temperature
   c. Oxygen saturations as indicated
   d. Cardiac rate and rhythm
   e. Respiratory effort and excursion
   f. Pain and discomfort level
   g. Serum electrolytes
   h. Accurate intake and output
   i. Level of consciousness
   j. Close monitoring for progression of symptoms
2. Maintain airway, oxygenation, and ventilation
   a. Position of comfort
   b. Oxygen by nasal cannula at 2 to 6 L/min if indicated to maintain SpO_2 of 95% unless contraindicated; for patients with COPD, use pulse oximetry to guide oxygen administration to SpO_2 of 90%
   c. Intubation and mechanical ventilation as indicated using RSI

3. Maintain adequate circulation and perfusion
   a. Increased oral fluids
   b. IV access for fluid and medication administration as indicated; IV fluids if dehydrated and/or unable to take oral fluids
4. Prevent transmission: strict respiratory isolation
5. Treat infection and prevent sepsis
   a. Diphtheria antitoxin; sensitivity testing prior to administration
   b. Antibiotics (e.g., penicillin G, erythromycin [E-Mycin])
   c. Close monitoring for indications of sepsis
6. Control pain and discomfort
   a. Analgesics
   b. Antipyretics
   c. Antitussives
   d. Antiemetics as indicated
7. Major complications
   a. Airway obstruction
   b. Myocarditis
   c. Polyneuritis

Evaluation
1. Patent airway, adequate oxygenation (i.e., normal PaO_2, SpO_2, SaO_2) and ventilation (i.e., normal $PaCO_2$)
2. Absence of clinical indications of respiratory distress
3. Absence of clinical indicators of hypoperfusion
4. Absence of clinical indications of infection/sepsis
5. Control of pain/discomfort
6. Alert and oriented with no neurologic deficit

Typical disposition: admission
1. Identify those who have been in close contact with the patient; close contacts need culture and antibiotics prophylactic
2. Education on immunizations
   a. Tetanus, diphtheria booster every 10 years (immunity only lasts 10 years); some sources recommend a booster if it has been over 5 years since the last one (ENA, 2007)
   b. If never immunized, give series of three doses

Encephalitis
Definition: inflammation of the brain
Predisposing factors
1. Older adults and very young are more susceptible
2. Pathogens
   a. Herpes simplex virus (HSV) type 1
   b. Varicella zoster virus (VZV)
   c. Epstein-Barr virus (EBV)
   d. Rabies
3. Transmission can occur from mosquitoes, ticks, animal bites
4. Transmission from human to human occurs through airborne droplets and lesion exudate

Pathophysiology
1. Viruses enter the brain by hematogenous spread or by traveling along the neural and olfactory pathways

2. The virus will cross the blood-brain barrier and enter neural cells, causing a disruption in cell functioning
3. Perivascular congestion and hemorrhage occur
4. The inflammatory response will spread diffusely affecting gray matter disproportionately to white matter

Clinical presentation
1. Subjective
   a. Severe headache
   b. Sudden onset of fever
   c. Drowsiness, confusion
   d. Vomiting
   e. Stiff neck
2. Objective
   a. Elevated temperature
   b. May have rash
   c. Altered LOC
   d. May have abnormal reflexes
3. Diagnostic
   a. Viral serology: to determine causative virus

Collaborative management
1. Continue assessment
   a. ABCDs
   b. Vital signs: blood pressure, pulse, respiratory rate, and temperature
   c. Oxygen saturations as indicated
   d. Cardiac rate and rhythm
   e. Respiratory effort and excursion
   f. Pain and discomfort level
   g. Serum electrolytes
   h. Level of consciousness
   i. Close monitoring for progression of symptoms
2. Maintain airway, oxygenation, and ventilation
   a. Elevation of head of stretcher 30 to 45°C
   b. Oxygen by nasal cannula at 2 to 6 L/min if indicated to maintain SpO_2 of 95% unless contraindicated; for patients with COPD, use pulse oximetry to guide oxygen administration to SpO_2 of 90%
   c. Intubation and mechanical ventilation as indicated utilizing RSI
3. Maintain adequate circulation and perfusion
   a. Increased oral fluids
   b. IV access for fluid and medication administration as indicated; IV fluids if dehydrated and/or unable to take oral fluids
   c. Foley catheter for accurate output measurement
4. Control pain and discomfort
   a. Analgesics
   b. Antipyretics for fever
   c. Antiemetics as indicated
5. Treat infection
   a. Antivirals for viruses
   b. Antibiotics for bacterial causes
   c. Corticosteroids for inflammation and swelling
   d. Osmotic diuretics (e.g., mannitol [Osmitrol]) for increased ICP
6. Maintain safety: seizure precautions

Evaluation

1. Patent airway, adequate oxygenation (i.e., normal PaO_2, SpO_2, SaO_2) and ventilation (i.e., normal $PaCO_2$)
2. Absence of clinical indicators of respiratory compromise
3. Absence of clinical indications of sepsis
4. Alert and oriented with no neurologic deficit
5. Control of pain, discomfort

Typical disposition: admission

Mononucleosis

Definition: viral illness caused by EBV, a member of the Herpes viridae family of viruses
Predisposing factor: exposure to EBV through intimate contact with saliva
Pathophysiology

1. Incubation period is 4 to 6 weeks
2. EB virus is transmitted through contact with infected oropharyngeal secretions, most commonly saliva, which gives rise to the nickname "kissing disease"
3. EB virus infects the epithelial cells of the oropharynx and salivary glands
4. B lymphocytes may get infected, which leads to the virus entering the blood stream and becoming systemic
5. The resulting massive proliferation of T lymphocytes leads to tonsillitis, lymphadenopathy, and hepato-splenomegaly (Omori, 2007)

Clinical presentation

1. Subjective
   a. History of exposure
   b. Chills, fever, malaise, diaphoresis
   c. Fatigue
   d. Nausea/vomiting
   e. Headache
   f. Muscle aching
   g. Sore throat, possible earache
2. Objective
   a. Elevated temperature 38° to 40°C (100° to 104°F)
   b. Pharyngitis: cardinal sign; may be severe and/or exudative
   c. Lymphadenopathy; especially posterior cervical nodes
   d. Splenomegaly may be present
   e. Petechiae of the palate
   f. Rash: if patient treated with amoxicillin [Amocil], will develop a tan or brownish macular rash (Omori, 2007)
   g. Hepatomegaly
3. Diagnostic
   a. Monospot (heterophile antibody titer): positive
   b. Moderate increase in WBCs; may also see thrombocytopenia, lymphocytosis with atypical lymphs
   c. Liver function tests may be increased in hepatomegaly

Collaborative management

1. Continue assessment
   a. ABCDs
   b. Vital signs: blood pressure, pulse, respiratory rate, and temperature
   c. Oxygen saturations as indicated
   d. Cardiac rate and rhythm
   e. Respiratory effort and excursion
   f. Pain and discomfort level
   g. Level of consciousness
   h. Close monitoring for progression of symptoms
2. Maintain airway, oxygenation, and ventilation
   a. Position of comfort
   b. Oxygen by nasal cannula at 2 to 6 L/min if indicated to maintain SpO_2 of 95% unless contraindicated; for patients with COPD, use pulse oximetry to guide oxygen administration to SpO_2 of 90%
   c. Intubation may be required for airway edema
3. Maintain adequate circulation and perfusion
   a. Increased oral fluids
   b. IV access for fluid and medication administration as indicated; IV fluids if dehydrated and/or unable to take oral fluids
4. Control pain and discomfort:
   a. Analgesics
   b. Antipyretics
5. Treat infection and prevent complications
   a. Supportive care: rest, nutrition, stress avoidance
   b. Corticosteroids
   c. Avoidance of vigorous abdominal examination and palpation due to possible splenic rupture
6. Monitor for complications
   a. Airway obstruction
   b. Splenic rupture
   c. Meningitis/encephalitis

Evaluation

1. Patent airway, adequate oxygenation (i.e., normal PaO_2, SpO_2, SaO_2) and ventilation (i.e., normal $PaCO_2$)
2. Absence of clinical indicators of respiratory compromise
3. Alert and oriented with no neurologic deficit
4. Control of pain, discomfort

Typical disposition: discharge with instructions

1. Indications to return to ED for signs of airway obstruction, increased cough or fever, shortness of breath, severe abdominal pain
2. Avoidance of contact sports, heavy lifting, or vigorous activity for 4 weeks if splenomegaly is present
3. Avoidance of sharing of eating utensils, cups, etc and kissing on the mouth
4. Rest
5. Warm salt water gargles for sore throat
6. Follow up with primary care provider as directed

Fibromyalgia Syndrome (FMS)

Definition: "chronic pain illness which is characterized by widespread musculoskeletal aches, pain and stiffness, soft tissue tenderness, general fatigue and sleep disturbances" (National Fibromyalgia Research Foundation, 2009)

1. Can occur in any part of the body; most common areas are neck, back, shoulders, pelvic girdle, and hands

Predisposing factors

1. Unknown
2. May be genetic predisposition
3. May be triggered by a viral illness or Lyme disease
4. Affects females most often

Pathophysiology

1. Pathogenesis not completely understood
2. Generally considered to be a disorder of "central processing with neuroendocrine/neurotransmitter dysregulation" (Roberts, 2007, p. 1727)
3. Pain experienced by the patient is caused by abnormal sensory processing
   a. Abnormalities exist in substance P in the spinal cord, blood flow to the thalamus, the hypothalamic-pituitary-adrenal axis, serotonin and tryptophan levels, and cytokine function
   b. These abnormalities lead to altered pain sensation, sleep abnormalities, and abnormal mood regulation

Clinical presentation

1. Subjective
   a. Pain
      1) Varies in description but burning or aching is common
      2) Widespread deep muscle pain
      3) Varies in intensity
      4) Onset: acute or ongoing >3 months
      5) Duration: constant
   b. Inability to sleep or rest results in tiredness and fatigue
   c. Poor diet and inactivity: can worsen symptoms
   d. Cognitive changes ranging from mild concentration difficulty to severe problems such as memory lapses and difficulty coping
   e. There are many common conditions associated with fibromyalgia (e.g., restless leg syndrome, irritable bowel syndrome, migraines, depression)
2. Objective
   a. Tenderness of more than 11 of 18 tender points
   b. Tender points of fibromyalgia are located at nine bilateral muscle locations: (Figure 11-16)
      1) Low cervical region: anterior aspect of the neck between the transverse processes of C5-C7
      2) Anterior chest: second costochondral junctions
      3) Posterior neck: suboccipital muscle insertions
      4) Trapezius muscle: midpoint upper border
      5) Supraspinatus muscle: above medial border of scapular spine
      6) Lateral epicondyle: 2 cm distal to the lateral epicondyle (just inside elbow area).
      7) Gluteal: upper outer quadrant of the buttocks.
      8) Greater trochanter: posterior to greater trochanteric prominence
      9) Knee: medial fat pad, proximal to joint line
3. Diagnostic
   a. CBC with differential and chemistry to rule out other medical conditions
   b. Rheumatoid arthritis (RA) titer: to rule out RA

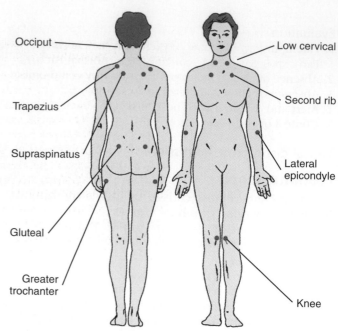

Figure 11-16 Location of specific tender points for diagnostic classification of fibromyalgia.

   c. Dolorimeter: used to test pain tolerance
      1) Fibromyalgia confirmed if test positive in more than 11 or 18 tender points
   d. Antipolymer antibodies: positive in 50%
   e. Serotonin levels: low

Collaborative management

1. Continue assessment
   a. ABCDs
   b. Vital signs: blood pressure, pulse, respiratory rate, and temperature
   c. Pain and discomfort level
   d. Close monitoring for progression of symptoms
2. Maintain airway, oxygenation, and ventilation
   a. Position of comfort
3. Control pain and discomfort
   a. Analgesics
   b. NSAIDs
   c. Antidepressants
   d. Muscle relaxants
4. Medications and therapies to treat or relieve symptoms
   a. Anticonvulsants: gabapentin (Neurontin) for nerve pain
   b. Benzodiazepines in small doses for anxiety
   c. Sedatives (e.g., zolpidem [Ambien] for severe sleep problems
   d. Analgesics (e.g., ibuprofen [Motrin])
5. Monitor for complications
   a. Fatigue
   b. Depression
   c. Substance abuse
   d. Unable to maintain activities of daily living

Evaluation

1. Patent airway, adequate oxygenation (i.e., normal Pao_2, Spo_2, Sao_2) and ventilation (i.e., normal $Paco_2$)

2. Absence of continuing complaints of fatigue
3. Control of pain, discomfort

Typical disposition: discharge home with instructions
1. Medications
2. Well-balanced diet
3. Regular exercise
4. Stress management
5. Sleep hygiene
6. Follow up with primary care provider

Tuberculosis

Definition: bacterial infection caused by *Mycobacterium tuberculosis,* an acid-fast bacillus (AFB)
1. May occur in other parts of the body although the lungs are the most common site
   a. Larynx
   b. Kidneys
   c. Bones
   d. Adrenal gland
   e. Lymph nodes
   f. Meninges
   g. May be widely disseminated (miliary TB)

Predisposing factors
1. Homelessness
2. People who live in inner cities or in crowded conditions
3. Older adults
4. Institutionalized individuals
5. IV drug use
6. Poverty
7. Poor access to health care
8. Immunosuppression, including HIV/AIDS
9. Being of a racial or ethnic minority, or being foreign-born
10. Recent foreign travel

Pathophysiology
1. *M tuberculosis* is spread by droplets
2. Transmission requires repeated episodes of close contact with another infected person to spread
3. The bacteria are inhaled and lodge in small distal airways where they replicate and spread via the lymphatics
4. Cellular immunity is activated and responds by forming granulomas, a cluster of macrophages and bacteria
5. The infection can remain contained in granulomatous tissue and not spread, or it can become a clinically evident disease (Crimlisk, 2007)
   a. Latent TB: patient is noninfectious but has a positive TB skin test
   b. Active TB: patient is infectious

Clinical presentation
1. Subjective
   a. Fatigue and malaise
   b. Unexplained weight loss
   c. Cough for >3 weeks (CDC, 2008)
      1) Productive: mucus may be blood tinged

   d. Chest pain
   e. Fever
   f. Night sweats
   g. Chills
2. Objective
   a. Elevated temperature
   b. Cough
   c. Hemoptysis
   d. Diminished breath sounds
   e. Appears thin or malnourished
3. Diagnostic
   a. AST: obtain prior to initiating isoniazid (INH) in patients older than 35 or in those who have risk of hepatic toxicity
   b. Chest radiography: may show cavitary infiltrates, especially in upper lobes
   c. Skin testing: administer Mantoux tuberculin 0.1 ml superficially in forearm
      1) Must be read in 48 to 72 hours
      2) PPD results >10 mm induration = positive test
      3) In the HIV positive patient, induration >5 mm = positive
   d. Sputum culture: specimen for acid-fast bacilli first thing in the morning three days in a row
   e. Body fluid culture: can obtain fluid for cultures from CSF, gastric washings, effusions, or abscesses

Collaborative management
1. Continue assessment
   a. ABCDs
   b. Vital signs: blood pressure, pulse, respiratory rate, and temperature
   c. Cardiac rate and rhythm
   d. Respiratory effort and excursion
   e. Oxygen saturations as indicated
   f. Pain and discomfort level
   g. Accurate intake and output
   h. Level of consciousness
   i. Close monitoring for progression of symptoms
2. Maintain airway, oxygenation, and ventilation
   a. Position of comfort
   b. Oxygen by nasal cannula at 2 to 6 L/min if indicated to maintain SpO_2 of 95% unless contraindicated; for patients with COPD, use pulse oximetry to guide oxygen administration to SpO_2 of 90%
3. Maintain adequate circulation and perfusion
   a. Increased oral fluids
   b. IV access for fluid and medication administration as indicated; IV fluids if dehydrated and/or unable to take oral fluids
4. Prevent transmission: respiratory isolation
   a. Negative pressure room
   b. Droplet precautions
5. Control pain and discomfort
   a. Position of comfort
   b. Analgesics
6. Treat infection
   a. Antimicrobials
   b. Antipyretics and cooling methods to reduce fever

7. Monitor for complications
    a. Acute respiratory failure
    b. Lung abscess
    c. Bronchiectasis
8. Evaluation
    a. Patent airway, adequate oxygenation (i.e., normal Pao_2, Spo_2, Sao_2) and ventilation (i.e., normal $Paco_2$)
    b. Absence of clinical indications of respiratory distress
    c. Absence of clinical indications of sepsis
    d. Alert and oriented with no neurologic deficit
    e. Control of pain, discomfort

Typical disposition
1. If criteria met: discharge with instructions
    a. Home isolated for the first 14 days of antibiotic therapy
    b. Cough hygiene: cough into a tissue and dispose in a paper bag, burn, or flush down the toilet
    c. Good handwashing for patient and family
    d. Ventilation with fresh air about 20 times per day
    e. No need to boil utensils, dispose of clothes or towels/sheets
    f. Household members and close contacts need to be sent to county health department for prophylactic treatment
    g. Patients can wear surgical masks; family members need special respirators
    h. Good nutrition, rest, hygiene
    i. Follow up with primary care provider as scheduled
2. If criteria not met: admission

Shingles (Herpes Zoster)
Definition: painful or burning rash and/or blisters on the skin caused by varicella-zoster virus
Predisposing factors: expression of the virus, latent in the body, is triggered by immunocompromise, such as the following examples
1. Stress
2. Fatigue
3. Illness or injury
4. Disease that compromises the immune system such as HIV/AIDS, malignancy
5. Medications such as corticosteroids, immunosuppressants

Pathophysiology
1. Highly contagious DNA virus
2. Varicella represents the primary infection and at that time the virus gains entry into the sensory dorsal root ganglia although the exact mechanism is not understood
3. The virus stays latent for years because of varicella-zoster virus-specific cell-mediated immunity acquired during the initial or primary infection
4. Reactivation of the virus occurs following a decrease in virus-specific cell-mediated immunity causing the virus to travel down the sensory nerve
5. This accounts for the dermatomal distribution of pain and blisters

Clinical presentation
1. Subjective
    a. Fever, chills
    b. Numbness or tingling of skin prior to rash breakout
    c. Blisters
    d. Pain
        1) Painful burning
        2) Shooting pain (may be described as a lightning bolt)
    e. Visual changes
2. Objective
    a. Blisters or rash that follows the dermatome but does not cross the midline of the body; blisters may be hemorrhagic
    b. Tenderness along dermatome with palpation
    c. Cranial nerve palsy especially if shingles-type rash involving the nose
        1) Decrease in visual acuity
        2) Hearing loss
3. Diagnostic study: viral culture
    a. Direct fluorescent antibody (DFA): positive for varicella zoster virus
    b. Tzanck smear

Collaborative management
1. Continue assessment
    a. ABCDs
    b. Vital signs: blood pressure, pulse, respiratory rate, and temperature
    c. Oxygen saturations as indicated
    d. Skin integrity
    e. Pain and discomfort level
    f. Close monitoring for progression of symptoms
2. Maintain airway, oxygenation, and ventilation
3. Control pain and discomfort
    a. Position of comfort
    b. Analgesics
    c. Antihistamines
    d. Anesthetics (e.g., lidocaine patch)
    e. Topical anti-itch creams (e.g., hydrocortisone [Westcort], diphenhydramine [Benadryl])
4. Treat infection
    a. Antivirals (e.g., acyclovir [Zovirax], famciclovir [Famvir], valacyclovir hydrochloride [Valtrex])
    b. Corticosteroids
    c. Covering of any oozing lesions
    d. Vaccination for high-risk individuals after symptoms have resolved
5. Major complications
    a. Postherpetic neuralgia
    b. Vision loss
    c. Skin infections
    d. Hearing or balance problems

Evaluation
1. Patent airway, adequate oxygenation (i.e., normal Pao_2, Spo_2, Sao_2) and ventilation (i.e., normal $Paco_2$)
2. Absence of clinical indicators of infection or sepsis

3. Alert and oriented with no neurologic deficit
4. Control of pain, discomfort

Typical disposition

1. If evaluation criteria met: discharge with instructions
   a. Avoidance of public places, school and/or work until lesions crust over to prevent transmission of the virus
   b. Medications
   c. Vaccination for health care workers and high-risk groups (e.g., elderly)
   d. Indications to return to the ED: worsening of symptoms, fever, or signs of infection
   e. Follow up with primary care provider as directed
2. If evaluation criteria not met (e.g., neurologic complications or systemic viremia): admission

Pandemic Illness

Definition: global outbreak of a disease that spreads easily from person to person because there is little or no natural immunity to the causative organism (U.S. Department of Health and Human Service, 2010)

Predisposing factors

1. Disease dependent
2. Exposure to an organism for which the population has little or no immunity

Pathophysiology

1. Disease dependent
2. Organism would need the capacity to replicate and spread quickly and easily through the human population

Clinical presentation

1. Subjective
   a. History of travel to an area of the world where the suspected disease occurs (e.g., Asia: avian flu)
   b. Patient may complain of any of the following
      1) Fever, chills
      2) Nausea/vomiting/diarrhea/anorexia
      3) Fatigue, malaise
      4) Cough, shortness of breath
      5) Pain
         a) Headache
         b) Myalgias, arthralgias
         c) Chest pain
         d) Abdominal pain
         e) Sore throat
      6) Skin eruptions
2. Objective
   a. Elevated temperature
   b. Clinical indications of acute illness
   c. Coughing
   d. Breath sound changes: wheezes, crackles
   e. Lymphadenopathy
   f. Abdominal tenderness with palpation may be present

3. Diagnostic
   a. Disease-dependent
   b. Cultures: blood, urine, sputum, viral isolates
   c. ABGs
   d. Chest radiography: may show pneumonia, infiltrates

Collaborative management

1. Continue assessment
   a. ABCDs
   b. Vital signs: blood pressure, pulse, respiratory rate, and temperature
   c. Cardiac rate and rhythm
   d. Respiratory effort and excursion
   e. Oxygen saturation if indicated
   f. Pain and discomfort level
   g. Accurate intake and output
   h. Serum electrolytes
   i. Level of consciousness
   j. Close monitoring for progression of symptoms
2. Maintain airway, oxygenation, and ventilation
   a. Position of comfort
   b. Oxygen by nasal cannula at 2 to 6 L/min if indicated to maintain SpO_2 of 95% unless contraindicated; for patients with COPD, use pulse oximetry to guide oxygen administration to SpO_2 of 90%
3. Maintain adequate circulation and perfusion
   a. IV access for fluid and medication administration as indicated; IV fluids if dehydrated and/or unable to take oral fluids
   b. Foley catheter may be indicated to monitor closely for impairment in urinary elimination
4. Prevent transmission of infection
   a. Standard precautions
   b. Isolation per CDC guidelines
   c. Vaccination when available
5. Treat infection and prevent sepsis
   a. Antimicrobials (antivirals (e.g., oseltamivir [Tamiflu], antibiotics (i.e., ciprofloxacin [Cipro])
   b. Antipyretics and cooling methods to reduce fever
   c. Corticosteroids may be indicated
   d. Close monitoring for indications or sepsis (i.e., fever, confusion, widened pulse pressure)
6. Control pain and discomfort
   a. Analgesics
   b. Antiemetics; nasogastric tube may be needed for uncontrolled vomiting
7. Monitor for complications
   a. Disease specific, but potentially includes cardiac and respiratory collapse

Evaluation

1. Patent airway, adequate oxygenation (i.e., normal PaO_2, SpO_2, SaO_2) and ventilation (i.e., normal $PaCO_2$)
2. Absence of clinical indicators of cardiopulmonary compromise
3. Absence of clinical indications of sepsis
4. Alert and oriented with no neurologic deficit
5. Control of pain, discomfort

Typical disposition: any patient suspected of having a pandemic illness will be hospitalized unless the community has instituted pandemic plans which call for home isolation

ONCOLOGIC EMERGENCIES

Superior Vena Cava Syndrome

Definition: progressive occlusion of the superior vena cava that leads to venous distention of the head and upper extremities

Predisposing factors: malignancies that commonly cause superior vena cava syndrome include the following:

1. Lung
2. Non-Hodgkin lymphoma
3. Metastatic breast cancer

Pathophysiology

1. Obstruction of the superior vena cava by either a tumor or a thrombosis
2. When the superior vena cava is obstructed, venous return to the heart is decreased
3. This leads to decreased cardiac output and increased venous pressure

Clinical manifestations

1. Subjective
   a. Headache
   b. Dyspnea, worse when lying down
   c. Dizziness
   d. Feeling of fullness or "congestion" in the head, face, and neck
2. Objective
   a. Facial rubor
   b. Conjunctival redness
   c. Swelling of neck and face
   d. Distended veins in the head, neck, and chest
   e. Cyanosis on trunk
   f. Hypotension possible
3. Diagnostic study: usually diagnosed by clinical presentation in a patient with a known thoracic tumor
   a. Chest radiography or CT: mediastinal mass may be evident

Collaborative management

1. Continue assessment
   a. ABCDs
   b. Vital signs: blood pressure, pulse, respiratory rate, and temperature
   c. Cardiac rate and rhythm
   d. Respiratory effort and excursion
   e. Oxygen saturations as indicated
   f. Pain and discomfort level
   g. Accurate intake and output
   h. Serum electrolytes
   i. Level of consciousness
   j. Close monitoring for progression of symptoms

2. Maintain airway, oxygenation, and ventilation
   a. Position of comfort
   b. Oxygen by nasal cannula at 2 to 6 L/min if indicated to maintain SpO_2 of 95% unless contraindicated; for patients with COPD, use pulse oximetry to guide oxygen administration to SpO_2 of 90%
3. Maintain adequate circulation and perfusion
   a. Increased oral fluids
   b. IV access for fluid and medication administration as indicated; IV fluids for dehydration and/or unable to take oral fluids
   c. Close monitoring for indications or sepsis (i.e., fever, confusion, widened pulse pressure)
   d. Anticoagulants
   e. Diuretics and/or glucocorticoids may be prescribed
4. Control pain and discomfort
   a. Analgesics
   b. Antiemetics
5. Monitor for complications
   a. Airway obstruction due to edema
   b. Cardiopulmonary arrest

Evaluation

1. Patent airway, adequate oxygenation (i.e., normal PaO_2, SpO_2, SaO_2) and ventilation (i.e., normal $PaCO_2$)
2. Absence of clinical indications of sepsis
3. Alert and oriented with no neurologic deficit
4. Control of pain, discomfort

Typical disposition: admission

Tumor Lysis Syndrome

Definition: metabolic consequences of rapid tumor destruction by chemotherapy or, less commonly, radiation

Predisposing factors: rapidly growing tumors that are highly sensitive to chemotherapy

Pathophysiology

1. Tumor cells are killed by chemotherapy or radiation therapy
2. Destroyed cells release intracellular components into the circulation
3. Cellular destruction causes
   a. Hyperkalemia
   b. Hyperuricemia
   c. Hyperphosphatemia and hypocalcemia
   d. Acute renal failure can occur

Clinical presentation

1. Subjective
   a. Anorexia, vomiting, abdominal pain
   b. Urinary symptoms: dysuria, oliguria, flank pain, hematuria
   c. Seizures, spasms,
   d. Weakness, paralysis
   e. Dysrhythmias related to hyperkalemia
2. Objective
   a. Abdominal distension
   b. Clinical indications of hypocalcemia: tetany, Chvostek and Trousseau signs

3. Diagnostic
   a. Serum electrolytes: hyperkalemia, hyperuricemia, hyperphosphatemia, and hypocalcemia in patient with recent chemotherapy (especially induction therapy) or, less commonly, radiation therapy
   b. Urinalysis: positive for uric acid crystals
   c. BUN and creatinine: may be elevated

Collaborative management
1. Continue assessment
   a. ABCDs
   b. Vital signs: blood pressure, pulse, respiratory rate, and temperature
   c. Oxygen saturations as indicated
   d. Cardiac rate and rhythm
   e. Respiratory effort and excursion
   f. Pain and discomfort level
   g. Accurate intake and output
   h. Serum electrolytes
   i. Level of consciousness
   j. Close monitoring for progression of symptoms
2. Maintain airway, oxygenation, and ventilation
   a. Position of comfort
   b. Oxygen by nasal cannula at 2 to 6 L/min if indicated to maintain SpO_2 of 95% unless contraindicated; for patients with COPD, use pulse oximetry to guide oxygen administration to SpO_2 of 90%
3. Maintain adequate circulation and perfusion
   a. Increased oral fluids
   b. IV access for fluid and medication administration as indicated: adjust IV rates to maintain urine output of 150 to 200 ml/hr in adults and at least 2 ml/kg/hr in children
   c. Close monitoring for indications or sepsis (i.e., fever, confusion, widened pulse pressure)
4. Control pain and discomfort
   a. Analgesics
   b. Antiemetics
5. Promote excretion of products of cellular destruction
   a. Sodium bicarbonate to maintain urine pH >7.0 and to help decrease uric acid moving into solution
   b. Allopurinol (Zyloprim) to decrease production of uric acid
   c. Treatment of electrolyte imbalances as indicated
6. Monitor for complications
   a. Dysrhythmias
   b. Renal calculi (e.g., uric acid)
   c. Acute renal failure

Evaluation
1. Patent airway, adequate oxygenation (i.e., normal PaO_2, SpO_2, SaO_2) and ventilation (i.e., normal $PaCO_2$)
2. Absence of clinical indicators of hypoperfusion
3. Absence of clinical indications of sepsis
4. Alert and oriented with no neurologic deficit
5. Control of pain, discomfort

Typical disposition: admission

MISCELLANEOUS INFECTIOUS CONDITIONS

Scabies
Definition: contagious skin infection caused by the mite Sarcoptes scabiei
Predisposing factor: direct contact with infected person including even casual contact
Pathophysiology
1. Transmitted through direct contact with infected person, bedding, clothing
2. Eggs are laid in burrows under the skin

Clinical presentation
1. Subjective
   a. Rash
   b. Itching, worse at night
2. Objective
   a. Red rash, visible burrow channel under the skin
      1) Often seen in webs between fingers or toes, or over joints
      2) In smaller children, often seen on soles, palms, face, neck, and scalp
   b. Visible scratch marks
3. Diagnostic study: primarily by clinical presentation
   a. Skin scrapings

Collaborative management
1 Continue assessment
   a. ABCDs
   b. Vital signs: blood pressure, pulse, respiratory rate, and temperature
   c. Pain and discomfort level
   d. Skin integrity
   e. Close monitoring for progression of symptoms
2. Control pain and discomfort
   a. Analgesics
   b. Antihistamines for itching
3. Treat infection
   a. Topical treatments as prescribed;
      1) Lindane 1% (Kwell)
      2) Permethrin 5% cream (Elimite)
4. Prevent disease transmission: contact isolation
5. Monitor for complication: bacterial infection

Evaluation
1. Patent airway, adequate oxygenation (i.e., normal PaO_2, SpO_2, SaO_2) and ventilation (i.e., normal $PaCO_2$)
2. Absence of clinical indicators of infection
3. Control of pain, discomfort

Typical disposition: discharge with instructions
1. Medication administration
2. Instructions related to prevention of recurrence and transmission

a. Washing of all linens and clothing in hot water; not sharing of towels

b. Wiping down surfaces in house

3. Parents of smaller children should be instructed to cover the child's hands at night to prevent damage from scratching

4. Follow up with primary care provider as instructed

Ringworm

Definition: superficial fungal infection of the skin caused by tinea

1. Tinea corporis: fungal infection of the body (limited to arms, legs, trunk)

2. Tinea capitis: fungal infection of the scalp

3. Tinea cruris: fungal infection of the groin (i.e., jock itch)

4. Tinea pedis: fungal infection of the feet (i.e., athlete's foot)

Predisposing factors

1. Contact with infected persons or pets

2. Can be spread by:
   a. Sharing towels, bedding, or clothing with infected person
   b. Public swimming pools, locker rooms
   c. Contact sports

3. Excessive sweating

4. Living in humid moist conditions

5. Wearing tight restrictive clothing

Pathophysiology

1. Superficial dermatophyte infection characterized by either inflammatory or noninflammatory lesions on the glabrous skin

2. Usually inhabits nonliving, cornified layers of the skin, hair, and nail; usually limited to the epidermis

3. Attracted to warm, moist environment, which is conducive to fungal proliferation

Clinical presentation

1. Subjective
   a. Rash
   b. Itching
   c. Known contact with someone who has a fungal infection

2. Objective
   a. Rash
      1) Erythema at edges
      2) Appears scaly or moist and crusted
      3) May have small vesicles or blisters
      4) Center of the rash usually clear with a slightly raised, erythemic, ring-shaped appearance
      5) May be clustering of erythemic raised bumps

3. Diagnostic: primarily by clinical presentation
   a. Skin scrapings: if stained with potassium-hydroxide and examined under a microscope, yeast buds or hyphae can be seen

Collaborative management

1. Continue assessment

a. ABCDs

b. Vital signs: blood pressure, pulse, respiratory rate, and temperature

c. Pain and discomfort level

d. Skin integrity

e. Close monitoring for progression of symptoms

2. Control pain and discomfort
   a. Analgesics
   b. Antihistamines for itching

3. Treat infection
   a. Topical antifungal medications
   b. For severe cases, systemic antifungals
   c. Antibiotics for secondary bacterial infection

4. Monitor for complication: bacterial infection

Evaluation

1. Patent airway, adequate oxygenation (i.e., normal PaO_2, SpO_2, SaO_2) and ventilation (i.e., normal $PaCO_2$)

2. Absence of clinical indicators of infection

3. Control of pain, discomfort

Typical disposition: discharge with instructions

1. Medications as prescribed

2. Examination and treatment of pets

3. Good hand washing

4. Follow up as instructed

Lice

Definitions

1. Body lice: infection with *Pediculus humanus var corporis*

2. Head lice: infection with *Pediculus humanus*

3. Pubic lice: infection with *Pthirus pubis*

Predisposing factors

1. Body lice
   a. Overcrowded living conditions
   b. Unsanitary conditions

2. Head lice
   a. Close personal contact
   b. Sharing hats, combs, brushes

3. Pubic lice
   a. Primarily a sexually transmitted infestation
   b. May be transferred with close, but not sexual, contact
   c. Often seen in conjunction with other STIs

Pathophysiology

1. Ectoparasites that live off of human hosts

2. Once they pierce the skin and inject saliva, they feed off human blood

3. The lice saliva can cause pruritus

4. Lice die of starvation within 10 days without a human host

5. Mature female lice will lay 3 to 6 eggs (nits) each day

6. Nits appear white, <1 mm long; hatch in 8 to 10 days

Clinical presentation

1. Subjective

a. Reported exposure to lice
b. Itching
  1) Itching from head lice can be particularly severe
2. Objective
  a. Scratch marks on arm
  b. Small red macules and/or small gray-blue macules on patient's trunk
  c. Nits or mature lice in hair
  d. Swelling and redness: possible cellulitis
3. Diagnostic
  a. Use of magnifying glass will aid in identify and diagnosing lice
  b. Woods lamp: nits appear fluorescent
  c. For pubic lice, consider testing for other STIs

Collaborative management
1. Continue assessment
  a. ABCDs
  b. Vital signs: blood pressure, pulse, respiratory rate, and temperature
  c. Pain and discomfort level
  d. Skin integrity
  e. Close monitoring for progression of symptoms
2. Control pain and discomfort
  a. Analgesics
  b. Antihistamines for itching
  c. Corticosteroids (e.g., hydrocortisone [Westcort]) may be used for severe cases
3. Treat infection and prevent spread of infestation
  a. Contact isolation
  b. Topical treatments
    1) Lindane 1% (Kwell)
    2) Permethrin 5% cream (Elimite)
  c. Antibiotics as indicated for secondary skin infection
4. Monitor for complication: bacterial infection

Evaluation
1. Patent airway, adequate oxygenation (i.e., normal PaO_2, SpO_2, SaO_2) and ventilation (i.e., normal $PaCO_2$)
2. Absence of clinical indicators of infection
3. Control of pain, discomfort

Typical disposition: discharge with instructions
1. Medication administration
2. Instructions related to prevention of recurrence and transmission
  a. Nit removal; incomplete nit removal is the most common cause of "resistant" or "recurrent" lice
  b. Washing of all clothes, bedding in hot water and dry in hot dryer; clothing and bedding that cannot be washed should be sealed in plastic for at least 2 weeks
  c. Small children should wear socks or mittens at night to reduce tissue trauma from scratching
  d. For pubic lice, patient needs education on STIs and partner needs treatment (Peard, 2007)
3. Follow-up with primary care provider as instructed

Myiasis
Definition: skin infestation caused by larvae (maggots)
Predisposing factors
1. Ulcerated or nonintact skin
2. Crowded, unsanitary living conditions
3. Self-care deficit
4. Substance abuse
5. Homelessness

Pathophysiology
1. Pathophysiology depends on the type of fly
2. Adult flies are not parasitic, but female flies can deposit their eggs near or in open wounds or breaks in the skin
  a. The eggs hatch into their larval stage (i.e., maggots)
  b. Larvae can feed on live or necrotic tissue
3. Maggots can enter through the mouth, nose, ear, or open skin
4. Larvae may be ingested by eating contaminated meat or food causing stomach or gastrointestinal myiasis

Clinical presentation
1. Subjective
  a. Lesions or boils
  b. Painful swelling
  c. Discharge from open wound
  d. Facial swelling or nose blocked or stopped up
  e. Crawling sensation or buzzing in ears
2. Objective
  a. Unkempt appearance
  b. Skin lesions
  c. Visible maggots in the skin or appearance or a "creeping eruptions" from lesion
  d. Obstruction of nasal passage and facial edema with nasal myiasis
3. Diagnostic study: microscopic identification

Collaborative management
1. Continue assessment
  a. ABCDs
  b. Vital signs: blood pressure, pulse, respiratory rate, and temperature
  c. Pain and discomfort level
  d. Skin integrity
  e. Close monitoring for progression of symptoms
2. Control pain and discomfort
  a. Analgesics
  b. Antihistamines for itching
3. Control infestation and eliminate myiasis
  a. Contact isolation
  b. Covering of wounds with petroleum jelly to reduce oxygen supply and force maggots to the skin's surface, where they are easily removed (Peard, 2007)
  c. Dressing of any open wounds
  d. Antibiotics for bacterial superinfection
4. Monitor for complication: bacterial infection

Evaluation

1. Patent airway, adequate oxygenation (i.e., normal PaO_2, SpO_2, SaO_2) and ventilation (i.e., normal $PaCO_2$)
2. Absence of clinical indicators of infection
3. Control of pain, discomfort

Typical disposition

1. If evaluation criteria met: discharge with instructions
   a. Medications as prescribed
   b. Instructions related to prevention of recurrence and transmission
      1) Apply petroleum jelly and dressing as directed
      2) Improve sanitation in living situation
      3) Stay indoors
   c. Follow up with primary care provider or wound management as instructed
2. If evaluation criteria not met (e.g., sepsis or other complications): admission

Intestinal Parasites

Giardiasis
Definition: infection by the protozoan *Giardia lamblia*

Predisposing factors

1. Attending daycare centers for lengthy periods of time
2. Low family income
3. Foreign travel to areas where the infection is endemic

Pathophysiology

1. Patient ingests cysts, which are the parasites in non-motile stage
2. Stomach acid activates the cysts, which then travel on to the duodenum
3. The parasites then enter their feeding stage in the distal duodenum and proximal jejunum
4. Cysts are passed via the feces into the environment where they can live for months
5. Transmission is via the fecal-oral route, drinking contaminated water, eating contaminated food, and from pets (Hockenberry and Barrera, 2007)

Clinical presentation

1. Subjective
   a. Diarrhea
   b. Anorexia, vomiting
   c. Failure to thrive in infants
   d. Older children (>5 years) often complain of abdominal pain and diarrhea alternating with constipation
2. Objective
   a. Stools
      1) Malodorous, watery, pale, and greasy
      2) Stools may float
   b. Ill appearance to child
3. Diagnostic: stool culture
   a. Difficult to isolate, may need several specimens over a period of weeks

Collaborative management

1. Continue assessment
   a. ABCDs
   b. Vital signs: blood pressure, pulse, respiratory rate, and temperature
   c. Pain and discomfort level
   d. Skin integrity
   e. Close monitoring for progression of symptoms
2. Maintain airway, oxygenation, and ventilation
   a. Position of comfort
   b. Oxygen by nasal cannula at 2 to 6 L/min if indicated to maintain SpO_2 of 95% unless contraindicated; for patients with COPD, use pulse oximetry to guide oxygen administration to SpO_2 of 90%
3. Maintain adequate circulation and perfusion
   a. Increased oral fluids
   b. IV access for fluid and medication administration as indicated
4. Control pain and discomfort
   a. Analgesics
   b. Antihistamines for itching
5. Treat infection
   a. Metronidazole (Flagyl) is the treatment of choice
   b. Other drug options include furazolidone (Furoxone), albendazole (Albenza) tinidazole (Tindamax) nitazoxanide (Alinia)
6. Monitor for complications: hypovolemia

Evaluation

1. Patent airway, adequate oxygenation (i.e., normal PaO_2, SpO_2, SaO_2) and ventilation (i.e., normal $PaCO_2$)
2. Absence of clinical indicators of infection
3. Control of pain, discomfort

Typical disposition

1. If criteria met, discharge with instructions
   a. Medications as prescribed
   b. Instructions related to prevention of recurrence and transmission: sanitary measures
   c. Indications to return to the ED for worsening condition or signs of dehydration
2. If criteria not met (e.g., dehydration or other other complications): admission

Enterobiasis (Pinworm)
Definition: intestinal infection with the nematode *Enterobius vermicularis;* most common helminthic infection in the United States
Predisposing factor: crowded conditions such as classrooms, daycare, pets

Pathophysiology

1. Nematode eggs are ingested or inhaled (they float in the air)
2. After hatching in the upper intestine, the eggs mature after 2 to 8 weeks and migrate to the cecum
3. Mating occurs and the female migrates out the anus and lays eggs, as many as 17,000

4. This process causes intense anal itching, and the eggs stick to the child's hands and under the fingernails
5. When the child puts his/her fingers in his/her mouth, the cycle begins again (Hockenberry & Barrera, 2007)
6. Otherwise transmission occurs with direct contact with common household surfaces, such as doorknobs, furniture, and from contaminated clothing

Clinical presentation
1. Subjective
   a. Perianal itching
   b. Irritability, restlessness
   c. Sleep disturbances, short attention span, and bed-wetting (in children)
   d. Diarrhea (uncommon but due to inflammation of bowel wall [Huh, 2006])
2. Objective
   a. Perianal scratch marks
   b. Female patients can have vaginal and urethral involvement
   c. Worm may be visible on anal area
3. Diagnostic: "tape test"
   a. A piece of transparent tape is wrapped, sticky side outward, around a tongue depressor and pressed firmly against the patient's anus
   b. This should be done in the morning when the child wakes up, prior to bathing or having a bowel movement
   c. Tongue depressors should be collected and placed in a plastic bag or glass jar and brought to the care provider for examination
   d. It may take more than one attempt to capture eggs or worms

Collaborative management
1. Continue assessment
   a. ABCDs
   b. Vital signs: blood pressure, pulse, respiratory rate, and temperature
   c. Pain and discomfort level
   d. Skin integrity
   e. Close monitoring for progression of symptoms
2. Maintain airway, oxygenation, and ventilation
   a. Position of comfort
3. Maintain adequate circulation and perfusion
   a. Increased oral fluids
   b. IV access for fluid and medication administration as indicated
4. Control pain and discomfort
   a. Analgesics
   b. Antihistamines for itching
5. Treat infection and prevent spread of infestation
   a. Drug therapy: single dose, repeated at 3-week intervals
      1) Mebendazole (Vermox)
      2) Piperazine citrate (Antepar)
      3) Pyrantel pamoate (Antiminth)
      4) Pyrvinium pamoate (Vanquin)
   b. Reinfection is highly likely because the worm can live on environmental surfaces for 2 weeks

6. Monitor for complications
   a. Bacterial superinfection
   b. Ectopic infection (rare)

Evaluation
1. Patent airway, adequate oxygenation (i.e., normal PaO_2, SpO_2, SaO_2) and ventilation (i.e., normal $PaCO_2$)
2. Absence of clinical indications of infection or sepsis
3. Control of pain, discomfort

Typical disposition: discharge with instructions
1. Medications asa prescribed
2. Instructions related to prevention of recurrence and transmission
   a. Good handwashing (especially before meals)
   b. Short fingernails to help with scratching and to decrease egg adherence under the nails (Hockenberry & Barrera, 2007)
   c. Good sanitary habits at home
3. Follow-up with primary care provider as instructed

Tapeworm Infestation
Definition: intestinal infestation by a worm of the Cestoda class
Predisposing factors
1. Poor cooking/storage of meat
2. Poor handwashing

Pathophysiology
1. Tapeworms are long, segmented, parasitic worms that absorb nutrients through their integumentary system
2. Eggs enter the soil from their primary host
3. An intermediate host ingests the eggs and they hatch, after which they migrate to gastrointestinal tissues and encyst
4. The primary host then ingests the intermediate host as a food source
5. Humans can be either the primary or the intermediate host
6. In most infestations, humans are the primary host and fecal contamination passes the eggs into the soil

Clinical presentation
1. Subjective
   a. Usually asymptomatic
   b. When symptoms do occur, they are often vague
      1) Abdominal pain
      2) Anorexia
      3) Weight loss
      4) Malaise
2. Objective
   a. Tapeworms on feces, toilet paper, or anus
   b. In severe cases, effects on vital organs, malnutrition, anaphylaxis, or severe inflammatory response can be seen
3. Diagnostic
   a. Direct visualization
   b. Stool sample for ova and parasites: need two or three samples

Collaborative management

1. Continue assessment
   a. ABCDs
   b. Vital signs: blood pressure, pulse, respiratory rate, and temperature
   c. Pain and discomfort level
   d. Skin integrity
   e. Close monitoring for progression of symptoms
2. Maintain airway, oxygenation, and ventilation
   a. Position of comfort
3. Maintain adequate circulation and perfusion
   a. Increased oral fluids
   b. IV access for fluid and medication administration as indicated
4. Control pain and discomfort
   a. Analgesics
   b. Antihistamines for itching
5. Treat infection and prevent spread of infestation
   a. Definitive treatment in the ED is not likely unless the worm is detected in the ED
   b. Generally patients will be referred for further diagnostic studies
   c. Anti-helminthic drug determined by worm type
      1) Albendazole (Albenza, Zentel)
      2) Paromomycin (Humatin)
      3) Praziquantel (Biltricide, Droncit)
      4) Mebendazole (Vermox)
   d. Corticosteroids may be prescribed
6. Monitor for complications
   a. Systemic infection
   b. B_{12} deficiency (can be mistaken for pernicious anemia)
   c. Iron deficiency anemia

Evaluation

1. Patent airway, adequate oxygenation (i.e., normal PaO_2, SpO_2, SaO_2) and ventilation (i.e., normal $PaCO_2$)
2. Absence of clinical indications of infection or sepsis
3. Control of pain, discomfort

Typical disposition: discharge with instructions

1. Medications as prescribed
2. Instructions related to prevention of recurrence and transmission
   a. Good handwashing (especially before meals)
   b. Proper meat cooking and storage
   c. Sanitary practices
   d. Assessment of dogs for the infestation (Irizarry and Phan, 2007)
   e. Follow up with primary care provider as directed

LEARNING ACTIVITIES

1. DIRECTIONS: Complete the following crossword puzzle related to medical emergencies.

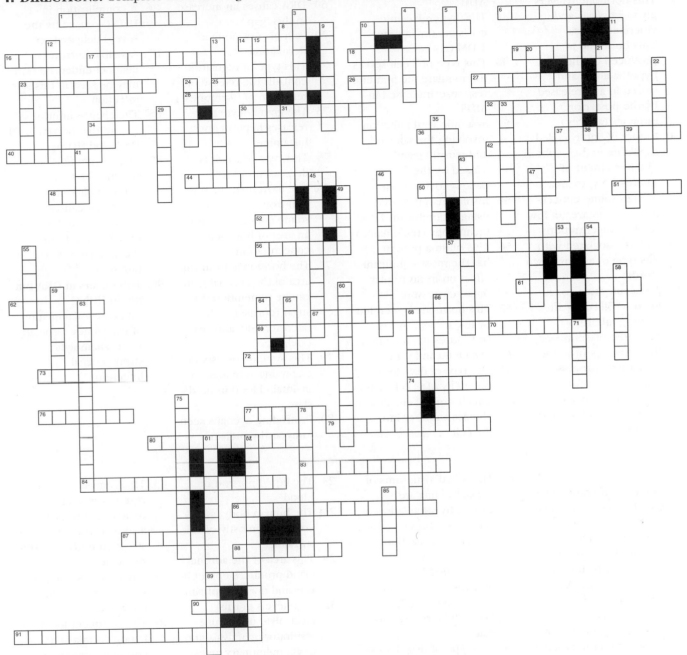

ACROSS

1. An ion exchange agent used to decrease serum potassium (brand)
6. Severe hypothyroidism may cause _____ coma, which results in hypothermia, hypotension, bradycardia, and coma
8. This hyperglycemic crisis occurs in type 2 diabetes mellitus or in patients with glucose intolerance (abbrev)
10. Global outbreak of a disease that spreads easily from person to person because there is little or no natural immunity to the causative organism
14. This system is concerned with antigens on the RBC
16. This syndrome is associated with a viral illness and aspirin
17. The movement of solutes and solutions from an area of high pressure to an area of low pressure
18. Increased levels of urea in the blood
19. This organ produces glucagon and insulin
23. High levels of this electrolyte occur in renal failure; low levels occur in malnutrition
25. Significant changes in serum levels of this electrolyte causes T-wave changes and dysrhythmias

26. This lab value is normally 10 times the creatinine value (abbrev)
27. This hormone triggers glycogenolysis and gluconeogenesis
28. This hormone is produced by the hypothalamus and stored in and released by the posterior pituitary (abbrev)
30. Cluster of tightly coiled capillaries in the nephron
32. The movement of solutes from an area of high solute concentration to an area of low solute concentration
34. HBS is associated with this type of anemia (two words)
36. A consumptive coagulopathy; bleeding after clotting (abbrev)
38. Activated plasminogen; the active agent in the fibrinolytic process
40. A deficiency of this electrolyte may cause paresthesia, tetany, and seizures

42. The color of the skin in a patient with Addison disease
44. This is another name for ADH
48. This hyperglycemic crisis occurs in type 1 DM (abbrev)
50. This type of T cell serves to modulate the immune response; increased in AIDS
51. Systemic viral infection involving the salivary and parotid gland; caused by the paramyxoviridae virus
52. Insulin manufactured using recombinant DNA technology (trade name)
56. This plasma protein has the most significant effect on intravascular oncotic pressure
57. This hormone is secreted by the adrenal cortex and causes the retention of sodium and water
61. This type of diabetes is caused by ADH deficiency
62. This hormone enables glucose to move into the cell

67. A term for infections that are more likely when the immune system is compromised
69. DKA causes an increase in this "gap"
70. Pain occurs along a dermatome
72. This type of regulation controls the release or retention of hormones
73. The granulocyte that releases heparin and histamine
74. This type of T cell is decreased in AIDS
76. The movement of solution from an area of low solute concentration to an area of high solute concentration
77. The hormones from this area of the adrenal gland can be remembered as sugar (cortisol), salt (aldosterone), and sex (androgen)
79. This system consists of clot-lysing activities to maintain blood in fluid state
80. Protruding eyeballs seen in hyperthyroidism

83. A mature RBC
84. These hypoglycemic effects are caused by low brain glucose
86. A complication in HHNC caused by the severe dehydration
87. A visible burrow channel under the skin may be seen in this skin infection
88. The change in urine output that occurs in DI, DKA, and HHNC
89. This hormone is produced by the anterior pituitary gland that causes the production and release of hormones from the adrenal cortex (abbrev)
90. This occurs in DKA but not in HHNC
91. An acute inflammation of the kidney associated with β-hemolytic streptococcal infection

DOWN

2. The type of granulocyte, which is significant in allergic reactions
3. This is given with glucose for hypoglycemia in patients with substance abuse to prevent Wernicke encephalopathy
4. _____ disease is caused by a deficiency of hormones from the adrenal gland
5. This is an immune-mediated response caused by heparin (abbrev)
7. The clotting pathway that is initiated by tissue injury
9. _____ respirations are seen in DKA due to the metabolic acidosis
10. Acute tracheobronchitis and paroxysmal cough caused by *Bordetella pertussis*

11. The initial symptoms of hypoglycemia are caused by stimulation of the _____ (abbrev)
12. The type of reaction that occurs with mismatched blood transfusion
13. This is an example of Type I hypersensitivity reaction
15. This type of drug blocks the early symptoms of hypoglycemia
20. A drug frequently administered to decrease platelet aggregation (abbrev)
21. This endocrine gland is located on top of the kidney
22. This endocrine glad is located in the neck and produces hormones that control metabolic rate

23. The liquid portion of blood
24. The human body is composed mostly of this substance
29. This area of the adrenal gland produces epinephrine and norepinephrine
31. High levels of this electrolyte may cause respiratory paralysis and cardiopulmonary arrest
33. The clotting pathway that is initiated by endothelial injury
35. The product of erythrocyte destruction
37. Increase in the number of bands causes a shift to the _____
39. Levels of this electrolyte are greatly affected by water balance
41. The end product of protein metabolism

43. This is most likely the result of insulin deficiency but may also be caused by stress, steroids, or insulin resistance
45. The body's sequential physiologic response to injury or invasion
46. The treatment for hypoglycemia in a conscious patient is 10 to 15 g of _____
47. A cascading system that can result in direct killing of invading organism
49. The substance is secreted by the juxtaglomerular apparatus in response to low perfusion
53. This hormone is considered a stress hormone and is produced by the adrenal cortex

54. This type of diabetes is caused by insulin deficiency
55. A condition characterized by cramps, convulsions, twitching of the muscles, and sharp flexion of the wrist and ankle joints
58. The filtering and destruction of damaged or old erythrocytes
59. German (3-day) measles is caused by this virus

60. The electrolyte imbalance that occurs with crush injury, renal failure, and hemolysis
63. A synonym for antibody; made by B cells
64. _____ disease is the most common cause of thyrotoxicosis
65. This space includes interstitial, intraperitoneal, intrapericardial, interpleural

66. This serum value goes down in overhydration and up in dehydration
68. Another term for the posterior pituitary
71. A screening test for HIV
75. A serum glucose less than 50 mg/dl
78. Mononucleosis is caused by this virus

81. This electrolyte imbalance occurs with insulin therapy in DKA since glucose moves into the cell and increased amounts of ATP are produced
82. Another term for the anterior pituitary
85. Pain in this area is frequently associated with renal conditions

2. **DIRECTIONS:** Complete the following statements related to the movement of solutes and solutions.

Water moves by the process of _____.

Electrolytes move by the process of _____.

The sodium-potassium pump is an example of _____.

The use of a pushing pressure, such as hydrostatic pressure, is called _____.

3. **DIRECTIONS:** A 72-year-old woman is brought to the ED from a long-term care facility. She had recently been started on enteral feedings. She has had a change in level of consciousness. Her sodium level is 150 mEq/L, her BUN is 80 mg/dl, and her serum glucose is 1000 mg/dl. Calculate her serum osmolality and identify what this serum osmolality indicates. What is the most likely cause of this abnormal serum osmolality?

4. **DIRECTIONS:** Identify whether these signs and symptoms are indicative of electrolyte deficit or excess.

Sign/Symptom	Excess (hyper)	Deficit (hypo)
Sodium		
Weight gain		
Abdominal cramps		
Flushed, dry skin		
Postural hypotension		
Headache		
Hypertension		
Potassium		
Flat T waves, prominent U waves		
Decreased GI motility, paralytic ileus		
Intestinal colic, diarrhea		
Muscle cramps → flaccid paralysis		
Decreased cardiac contractility		
Tall, peaked T waves, widened QRS complex		
Calcium		
Tetany		
Decreased deep tendon reflexes		
Neuromuscular weakness, flaccidity		
Seizures		
Bone or flank pain		
Laryngospasm		

Continued

Sign/Symptom	Excess (hyper)	Deficit (hypo)
Phosphorus		
Tetany		
Fatigue		
Chest pain		
Dyspnea		
Increased deep tendon reflexes		
Abdominal cramps		
Magnesium		
Decreased deep tendon reflexes		
Anorexia, nausea, vomiting		
Cardiopulmonary arrest		
Lethargy		
Dysrhythmias, especially torsades de pointes		
Facial flushing		

5. DIRECTIONS: Complete this table.

	DKA	HHNC
Age		
Type of diabetes mellitus		
Serum glucose range		
Presence of ketosis		
pH		
Anion gap		
Respiratory pattern		
Breath odor		
Serum osmolality		
Serum sodium		
Serum potassium		
BUN		
Average fluid deficit		

6. DIRECTIONS: Identify the following clinical indications as DKA, HHNC, or both.

Serum glucose >300 mg/dl	
Kussmaul respirations	
pH <7.30	
Positive serum and urine ketones	
Abdominal pain	
Dehydration	
Lethargy → coma	
Serum glucose >600 mg/dl	

7. DIRECTIONS: Identify the following clinical indications as DKA, hypoglycemia, or both.

Headache	
Serum glucose >300 mg/dl	
Abdominal pain	
Cold, clammy skin	
Nervousness, tremors	
Polyuria	
Lethargy → coma	
Seizures	
Glycosuria	
Tachycardia	
Agitation, inability to concentrate	
Weakness, fatigue	
Fruity breath	
Serum glucose <50 mg/dl	

8. DIRECTIONS: Match the type of anemia to the possible cause.

___ 1. Iron-deficiency anemia	a. Esophageal varices
___ 2. Pernicious anemia	b. Radiation or drugs
___ 3. Folic acid deficiency anemia	c. Hereditary
___ 4. Sickle cell anemia	d. Malignancy
___ 5. Aplastic anemia	e. Lead-poisoning
___ 6. Acute blood-loss anemia	f. Crohn disease
___ 7. Anemia of chronic illness	g. Anorexia nervosa

9. DIRECTIONS: Identify the appropriate actions to take for suspected transfusion reaction.

a.
b.
c.
d.
e.
f.
g.
h.
i.

10. DIRECTIONS: Identify the direction of change of the following laboratory values in DIC.

Platelets	
PT	
aPTT	
Fibrin split products	
Factors V, VIII	
Fibrinogen	

11. DIRECTIONS: Match the following clinical manifestations of hepatic failure with the pathophysiologic change (answers may be used more than once).

___ 1. Splenic engorgement	a. Petechiae, purpura, bleeding
___ 2. Stretching of the liver capsule	b. Jaundice

Continued

____ 3. Decrease in the metabolism of testosterone	c. Third-spacing
____ 4. Decrease in metabolism of aldosterone	d. Testicular atrophy
____ 5. Decrease in production of plasma proteins	e. Gynecomastia
____ 6. Decrease in metabolism of estrogen	f. Anemia. leukopenia, thrombocytopenia
____ 7. Decrease in production of clotting factors	g. Dull RUQ pain
____ 8. Decrease in conjugation and excretion of bilirubin	

12. DIRECTIONS: Fill in the blanks related to Reye syndrome.

a. _____ are injured, by a virus, toxin, or drug

b. Prolonged vomiting leads to decreased _____.

c. Waste products are not eliminated so _____ build up.

d. Liver damage leads to accumulated _____.

e. Fatty infiltrates are found in the _____, _____, and _____.

13. DIRECTIONS: Match the infections with the appropriate statements. Infections may be used once, more than once, or not at all.

____ 1. This infection causes prolonged immunosuppression	a. Pertussis
____ 2. This infection poses a special danger to a fetus	b. Mononucleosis
____ 3. Patients with this infection have a decreased ability to clear secretions	c. Rubella
____ 4. There may be as many as 500 lesions in this infection	d. Rubeola
____ 5. There is often no prodrome in children who have this infection	e. Mumps
____ 6. This infection is usually treated with clarithromycin [Biaxin] or erythromycin [Ery-Tab]	f. Chickenpox
____ 7. This infection is a historic killer of children	
____ 8. Symptoms of this infection include earache and pain in parotid gland	
____ 9. This infection has three stages: catarrhal, paroxysmal, convalescent	
____ 10. The "3 Cs" are cardinal signs in this infection	
____ 11. Antiviral medications are often prescribed to treat this infection	
____ 12. This infection may involve the testes	
____ 13. The fluid in the characteristic vesicles spreads this infection	
____ 14. Koplik spots are diagnostic for this infection	
____ 15. Patients often report overwhelming fatigue when ill with this infection	
____ 16. Splenic rupture is a rare but possible complication with this infection	
____ 17. Instruct patients with this infection to avoid drinking citrus juices	
____ 18. Complications of any type are rare in this childhood infection	
____ 19. Exudative pharyngitis may be noted in patients with this infection	

14. DIRECTIONS: Fill in the blanks.
A child undergoing septic workup for a fever of unknown origin will have diagnostic testing consisting of _____, _____
_____, _____, and _____.

15. DIRECTIONS: List the medications that can be used for adrenocortical insufficiency.
a.
b.
c.

16. DIRECTIONS: List infection control measures a patient convalescing at home with TB should be taught.
a.
b.
c.
d.
e.
f.
g.

17. DIRECTIONS: Match the miscellaneous infectious skin conditions with the appropriate treatment or assessment finding. Some may have more than one answer.

_____ 1. An intestinal parasite	a. Scabies
_____ 2. Lindane 1% (Kwell) is used for treatment	b. Ringworm
_____ 3. Instructions to the patient should include the proper storage and cooking of meat	c. Lice
_____ 4. Metronidazole (Flagyl) is the treatment of choice	d. Myiasis
_____ 5. Skin infestation caused by larvae	e. Giardiasis
_____ 6. Small red macules and/or small gray-blue macules on patient's trunk	f. Enterobiasis
_____ 7. In small children, often seen on soles, palms, face, neck, and scalp	g. Tapeworm
_____ 8. Also known as pinworms	
_____ 9. Presents with rash that usually has a clear center with slightly raised erythremic ring-shaped appearance	
_____10. Treatment includes covering skin wounds with petroleum jelly	
_____11. Burrow channel is visible under the skin	
_____12. "Tape test" is used for diagnosis	
_____13. A complication is development of B_{12} deficiency (can be mistaken for pernicious anemia)	
_____14. This skin infection usually inhabits nonliving, cornified layers of the skin, hair, and nail	
_____15. In this condition, eggs stick to the child's hands and under the fingernails which lead to re-infestation	
_____16. This appears fluorescent when examined using a Woods light	
_____17. Definitive treatment in the ED is not likely unless confirmation made in the ED	
_____18. Caused by itch mites	
_____19. Also known as jock itch	
_____20. Lesions in this condition have a "creeping eruption" appearance	

LEARNING ACTIVITIES ANSWERS

1.

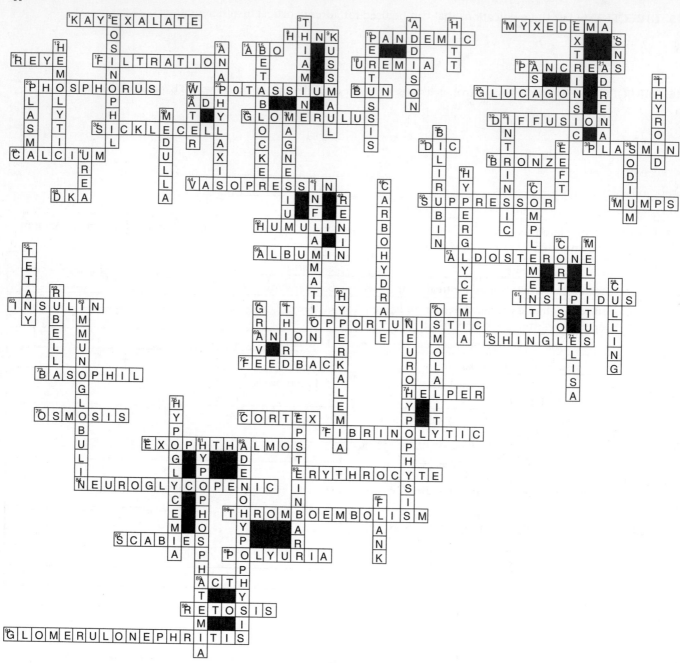

2.

Water moves by the process of <u>osmosis</u>.

Electrolytes move by the process of <u>diffusion</u>.

The sodium-potassium pump is an example of <u>active</u> <u>transport</u>.

The use of a pushing pressure, such as hydrostatic pressure, is called <u>filtration</u>.

3. Serum osmolality is 433 mOsm/kg, which indicates severe dehydration. This is an example of hyperglycemic hyperosmolar nonketotic condition caused by glucose intolerance associated with recent initiation of high glucose enteral feedings.

4.

Sign/Symptom	Excess (hyper)	Deficit (hypo)
Sodium		
Weight gain	✖	
Abdominal cramps		✖
Flushed, dry skin	✖	
Postural hypotension		✖
Headache		✖
Hypertension	✖	
Potassium		
Flat T waves, prominent U waves		✖
Decreased GI motility, paralytic ileus		✖
Intestinal colic, diarrhea	✖	
Muscle cramps → flaccid paralysis		✖
Decreased cardiac contractility	✖	
Tall, peaked T waves, widened QRS complex	✖	
Calcium		
Tetany		✖
Decreased deep tendon reflexes	✖	
Neuromuscular weakness, flaccidity	✖	
Seizures		✖
Bone or flank pain	✖	
Laryngospasm		✖
Phosphorus		
Tetany	✖	
Fatigue		✖
Chest pain		✖
Dyspnea		✖
Increased deep tendon reflexes	✖	
Abdominal cramps	✖	
Magnesium		
Decreased deep tendon reflexes	✖	
Anorexia, nausea, vomiting		✖
Cardiopulmonary arrest	✖	
Lethargy	✖	
Dysrhythmias, especially torsades de pointes		✖
Facial flushing	✖	

5.

	DKA	HHNC
Age	Young	Old
Type of diabetes mellitus	1 (IDDM)	2 (NIDDM) or none
Average serum glucose	600 mg/dl	1100 mg/dl
Presence of ketosis	Positive	Negative
pH	May be very acidotic	Normal or minimally acidotic
Anion gap	Increased	Normal
Respiratory pattern	Kussmaul (rapid and deep)	Normal or tachypneic (rapid and shallow)
Breath odor	Acetone (fruity)	Normal
Serum osmolality	295 to 330 mOsm/kg	330 to 450 mOsm/kg
Serum sodium	Decreased, normal, or increased	Normal or increased
Serum potassium	Increased initially; drops with rehydration and correction of acidosis	Decreased
BUN	Mildly increased	Severely increased
Average fluid deficit	4 to 8 L	8 to 15 L

6.

Serum glucose >300 mg/dl	Both
Kussmaul respirations	DKA
pH <7.30	DKA
Positive serum and urine ketones	DKA
Abdominal pain	DKA
Dehydration	Both
Lethargy → coma	Both
Serum glucose >600 mg/dl	HHNC

7.

Headache	Hypoglycemia
Serum glucose >300 mg/dl	DKA
Abdominal pain	DKA
Cold, clammy skin	Hypoglycemia
Nervousness, tremors	Hypoglycemia
Polyuria	DKA
Lethargy → coma	DKA
Seizures → coma	Hypoglycemia
Glycosuria	DKA
Tachycardia	Both
Agitation, difficulty with concentration	Hypoglycemia
Weakness, fatigue	DKA
Fruity breath	DKA
Serum glucose <50 mg/dl	Hypoglycemia

8.

__e__ 1. Iron-deficiency anemia	a. Esophageal varices
__f__ 2. Pernicious anemia	b. Radiation or drugs
__g__ 3. Folic acid deficiency anemia	c. Hereditary
__c__ 4. Sickle cell anemia	d. Malignancy
__b__ 5. Aplastic anemia	e. Lead poisoning
__a__ 6. Acute blood-loss anemia	f. Crohn disease
__d__ 7. Anemia of chronic illness	g. Anorexia nervosa

9.

a. Stop transfusion

b. Maintain IV access with normal saline and new administration set

c. Reassure the patient; stay at the bedside

d. Notify physician and blood bank

e. Recheck blood numbers and type

f. Treat symptoms appropriately

g. Return unused portion of blood in blood bag and administration set to the blood bank

h. Collect and send blood and urine samples to the laboratory; send another urine specimen 24 hours after transfusion reaction

i. Document the transfusion reaction and treatment administered

10.

Platelets	↓
PT	↑
aPTT	↑
Fibrin split products	↑
Factors V, VIII	↓
Fibrinogen	↓

11.

__f, a__ 1. Splenic engorgement Remember that splenic engorgement causes thrombocytopenia and, therefore, clotting abnormalities	a. Petechiae, purpura, bleeding
__g__ 2. Stretching of the liver capsule	b. Jaundice
__d__ 3. Decrease in the metabolism of testosterone	c. Third-spacing
__c__ 4. Decrease in metabolism of aldosterone	d. Testicular atrophy
__c, a__ 5. Decrease in production of plasma proteins Remember that many plasma proteins are actually clotting factors	e. Gynecomastia
__e__ 6. Decrease in metabolism of estrogen	f. Anemia. leukopenia, thrombocytopenia
__a__ 7. Decrease in production of clotting factors	g. Dull RUQ pain
__b__ 8. Decrease in conjugation and excretion of bilirubin	

12.

a. Mitochondria	
b. Glycogen	
c. Acids	
d. Ammonia	
e. Liver, renal tubules, heart	

13.

b	1. Exudative pharyngitis may be noted in patients with this infection	a. Pertussis
c	2. This infection poses a special danger to a fetus	b. Mononucleosis
a	3. Patients with this infection have a decreased ability to clear secretions	c. Rubella
f	4. There may be as many as 500 lesions in this infection	d. Rubeola
c	5. There is often no prodrome in children who have this infection	e. Mumps
a	6. This infection is usually treated with clarithromycin or erythromycin	f. Chickenpox
e	7. Instruct patients with this infection to avoid drinking citrus juices	
e	8. Symptoms of this infection include earache, pain in parotid gland	
b	9. Splenic rupture is a rare but possible complication with this infection	
d	10. The "3 Cs" are cardinal signs in this infection	
f	11. Antiviral medications are often prescribed to treat this infection	
e	12. This infection may involve the testes	
f	13. The fluid in the characteristic vesicles spreads this infection	
d	14. Koplik spots are diagnostic for this infection	
b	15. Patients often report overwhelming fatigue when ill with this infection	

14. LP, blood cultures, urinalysis with culture, chest radiography

15.

a. Hydrocortisone (Westcort)

b. Dexamethasone (Decadron)

c. Fludrocortisone (Florinef)

16.

a. Patient to remain at home isolated for the first 14 days of antibiotic therapy

b. Cough hygiene: cough into a tissue and dispose in a paper bag, burn, or flush down the toilet

c. Good handwashing for patient and family

d. Provide ventilation with fresh air about 20 times per day

e. No need to boil utensils, dispose of clothes or towels/sheets

f. Household members and close contacts need prophylactic treatment as well

g. Patients can wear surgical masks; family members need special respirators

17.

e, f	1. An intestinal parasite	a. Scabies
a, c	2. Lindane 1% (Kwell) is used for treatment	b. Ringworm
g	3. Instructions to the patient should include the proper storage and cooking of meat	c. Lice
e	4. Metronidazole (Flagyl) is the treatment of choice	d. Myiasis

__d__ 5. Skin infestation caused by larvae	e. Giardiasis
__c__ 6. Small red macules and/or small gray-blue macules on patient's trunk	f. Enterobiasis
__a__ 7. In small children, often seen on soles, palms, face, neck, and scalp	g. Tapeworm
__f__ 8. Also known as pinworms	
__b__ 9. Presents with rash that usually has a clear center with slightly raised erythremic ring-shaped appearance	
__d__ 10. Treatment includes covering skin wounds with petroleum jelly	
__a__ 11. Burrow channel is visible under the skin	
__f__ 12. "Tape test" is used for diagnosis	
__g__ 13. A complication is development of B_{12} deficiency (can be mistaken for pernicious anemia)	
__b__ 14. This skin infection usually inhabits nonliving, cornified layers of the skin, hair, and nail	
__f__ 15. In this condition, eggs stick to the child's hands and under the fingernails which lead to re-infestation	
__c__ 16. This appears fluorescent when examined using a Woods light	
__g__ 17. Definitive treatment in the ED is not likely unless confirmation made in the ED	
__a__ 18. Caused by itch mites	
__b__ 19. Also known as jock itch	
__d__ 20. Lesions in this condition have a "creeping eruption" appearance	

References and Suggested Readings

Burton, M., & Krusinski, P. (2007). Measles, rubeola. Retrieved November 29, 2009, from http://emedicine.medscape.com/article/1132710-overview.

Buttaro, T. M., Trybulski, J., Bailey, P. P., & Sandberg-Cook, J. (2003). *Primary care: A collaborative practice*. St. Louis: Mosby.

Carmody, K. A., & Sinert, R. H. (2009). Mumps. Retreived November 29, 2009, from http://emedicine.medscape.com/article/784603-overview.

Centers for Disease Control and Prevention. (2008). Tuberculosis. Retrieved Novemebr 23, 2009, from http://www.cdc.gov/Features/TBsymptoms/.

Chan-Tack, K. M., & Bartlett, J. (2008). Fever of unknown origin. *eMedicine*. Retrieved November 22, 2009, from http://emedicine.medscape.com/article/217675-overview.

Citkowitz, E. (2008). Myxedema coma or crisis. Retrieved November 21, 2009, from http://emedicine.medscape.com/article/123577-overview.

Dennison, R. D. (2007). *Pass CCRN!* (3rd ed.). St. Louis: Mosby.

Domino, F. J. (2008). *The 5-minute clinical consultant* (16th ed.). Philadelphia: Lippincott, Williams, and Wilkins.

Dyne, P. L., Sawtelle, S., & DeVore, H. K. (2009). Pediatrics, measles. Retrieved November 29, 2009, from http://emedicine.medscape.com/article/802691-overview.

Emergency Nurses Association. (2007). *Emergency nursing core curriculum* (6th ed.). Philadelphia: Saunders.

Emergency Nurses Association. (2005). *Sheehy's manual of emergency care* (6th ed.). St Louis: Mosby.

Ferry, R. J., & Pascual-y-Baralt, J. F. (2009). Syndrom of inappropriate anti-diuretic hormone secretion. Retrieved November 29, 2009, from http://emedicine.medscape.com/article/924829-overview.

Gilliland, R. P. (2009). Fibromyalgia. Retrieved November 22, 2009, from http://emedicine.medscape.com/article/312778-overview.

Hamdy, O. (2009). Diabetic ketoacidosis. Retrieved November 21, 2009, from http://emedicine.medscape.com/article/118361-overview.

Jarvis, C. (2008). *Physical examination and health assessment* (5th ed.). St. Louis: Saunders.

Klauer, K. M. (2008). Adrenal insufficiency and adrenal crisis. Retrieved November 21, 2009, from http://emedicine.medscape.com/article/765753-overview.

Krause, R. S. (2009). Herpes zoster. Retrieved November 29, 2009, from http://emedicine.medscape.com/article/788310-overview.

National Fibromyalgia Research Foundation. (2009). Retrieved November 23, 2009, from http://www.nfra.net/fibromyalgia_definition.php.

Price, S. A., & Wilson, L. M. (2003). *Pathophysiology: Clinical concepts of disease process* (6th ed.). St. Louis: Mosby.

Rushing Lott, M. E., Zember, G., & Lesher, J. L. (2008). Tinea corporis. Retreived Novemebr 29, 2009, from http://emedicine.medscape.com/article/1091473-overview.

U.S. Department of Health and Human Service. (2010). About the flu. Retrieved July 2, 2010, from http://www.pandemicflu.gov/individualfamily/about/index.html.

Weiner, D. L. (2009). Pediatrics, Reyes syndrome. Retrieved November 29, 2009, from http://emedicine.medscape.com/article/803683-treatment.

Wolfram, W. (2009). Pediculosis (lice). Retreived November 29, 2009, from http://emedicine.medscape.com/article/910321-overview.

CHAPTER 12

Substance Abuse, Toxicologic, and Environmental Emergencies

Introduction

This content constitutes 6.5% (10 items) of the CEN examination

The focus is on substance abuse, toxicologic, and environmental emergencies that are commonly encountered in an ED setting

The continuum of age needs to be considered from infancy through older adulthood

Age-Related Considerations

Neonates, infants, and children

1. Substances can be secreted by lactating mothers and passed to infants
2. Infants and toddlers have small airways that occlude faster with edema if the inhalation of chemicals or hot air occurs
3. Multiple factors increase the risk for toxicities
   a. Infants and toddlers are curious by nature and explore the environment with the use of the visual, touch, and oral senses; they are attracted to brightly colored pills and substances, and they frequently pick up items and put them in their mouths
   b. Infants and children have a larger surface-area-to-volume ratio, so they will absorb more topical solutions and medications, thus increasing their risk for toxicity
      1) Caution must be exercised when using iodine and other solutions with neonates
      2) This also makes them more susceptible to thermal changes
   c. Neonates have immature renal function, which means that toxicity can occur easily with drugs that are eliminated by the kidneys
   d. Infants have fewer binding sites for medications, so more drug is free in the blood and active, thus increasing the risk for toxicity (Emergency Nurses Association [ENA], 2004)
4. Multiple factors increase the risk for environmental emergencies
   a. Children are less likely to attempt to avoid obstacles in the environment
   b. The autonomic nervous system in children is immature, thus making children at risk in the presence of temperature extremes
   c. Neonates and infants <3 months old are unable to dissipate heat through shivering, which makes them more susceptible to cold stress

Older adults

1. Degenerative changes that occur with aging may mask neurologic symptoms or cause them to be missed during an assessment for a toxicologic or environmental emergency
2. Decreased metabolic rate
   a. Delays the onset of symptoms of toxicity
   b. Diminishes the metabolism of drugs and toxins
3. Impaired renal function diminishes the elimination of drugs and toxins
4. Loss of subcutaneous tissue with aging may cause thermal and chemical injuries to be more severe
5. Decreased reflexes make the older adult more susceptible to environmental injuries
6. Older adults are more likely to have chronic medical problems that can complicate environmental and toxicologic emergencies

Toxicologic Emergencies

Definitions

1. Drug toxicity: the ingestion of a drug in an amount that is more than the recommended amount; the ingestion or absorption of a substance that is toxic to the human body
2. Poisoning: accidental exposure to a toxic substance
   a. Pharmaceutical exposures tend to be more toxic than plant and chemical exposures
3. Overdose: the consumption of a substance that results in toxic blood levels of that substance; an overdoes is usually intentional, but it may be inadvertent

Predisposing factors

1. The accidental or intentional overdosage of prescribed medication
   a. Intentional overdosage often involves more than one agent; it frequently includes alcohol, illegal drugs, or both
   b. Intentional overdosage may be a suicide attempt or an attention-seeking behavior (i.e., suicide gesture)
   c. Accidental overdosage may be caused by any of the following:
      1) Deficient knowledge or confusion regarding drug dosing
      2) Impaired metabolism or excretion caused by hepatic or renal insufficiency
      3) Food or drug (including herbal supplements) interactions

4) Electrolyte imbalances, especially involving cardiac drugs
2. Accidental overdosage of illegal drugs
   a. Overdosage is frequently caused by changes in drug purity
   b. Patients may have a psychiatric illness and have the tendency to be violent
3. Ingestion or absorption of poisons or toxins
4. Use of drugs (especially sedating drugs) with alcohol

Pathophysiology: depends on the following:

1. Drug-ingested
   a. Fatal drug intoxications are most likely to be caused by analgesics, antidepressants, carbon monoxide, and cardiovascular drugs
2. Amount of drugs or toxins ingested or absorbed
3. Time from ingestion to treatment
4. Preexisting condition of patient: cardiovascular, hepatic, or renal disease may increase drug effect by impairing biotransformation and excretion

Clinical presentation

1. Primary assessment
   a. ABCDs (see Chapter 2)
   b. Baseline assessment allows for the determination of changes that have occurred during care
2. Subjective
   a. Suspect poisoning or overdose if any of the following are present:
      1) History of psychiatric illness
      2) Trauma
      3) Patient rescued from a fire, especially if he or she was in an enclosed space
      4) Unexplained symptoms, such as the following:
         a) Coma of unknown cause
         b) Life-threatening dysrhythmias, especially in a young person
         c) Metabolic acidosis
         d) Seizures
         e) Gastrointestinal disturbances
         f) Suspicious or unusual behavior
   b. History of drug ingestion or exposure to toxins
      1) The history provides an important way to identify the toxic substance and to determine the likelihood of significant toxicity
      2) Patients are frequently inaccurate with regard to the amount of drug that they have ingested; they may minimize or exaggerate the amount of the drug taken; verify information provided by patients with family, friends, police officers, and paramedics
      3) Identify the following:
         a) The five Ws (ENA, 2004)
            i) Who? (i.e., were other family members, adults, or children exposed?)
            ii) What and how much?
               (a) Evidence of exposure

(b) Route and amount of exposure; if no history is available, look for clues such as bottles or containers
               (c) Treatment before arrival at the ED
            iii) When? (i.e., time and duration of exposure)
            iv) Where? (i.e., location of patient and how he or she was found)
            v) Why? (i.e., dose confusion, suicide attempt, or inadvertent exposure to toxin)
         b) Previous exposure to drug or toxin
            i) Drugs regularly taken
            ii) Alcohol regularly consumed
         c) Source
            i) Prescription
            ii) Over the counter
            iii) Street
      4) Weight and age of a pediatric patient
   c. May have a history of depression or psychiatric illness
   d. May have a history of previous drug overdosage or toxin ingestion
   e. May have a history of chemical dependency
   f. May have a history of a complicated drug regimen with or without confusion
   g. Note any history of cardiovascular, renal, or hepatic disease
3. Objective
   a. Vital signs
   b. Mental status
   c. Seizures
   d. Pupils
   e. Ventilation
   f. Skin and mucous membranes
   g. Peristalsis
   h. Odors
   i. Urine color
   j. Also note the presence of the following:
      1) Needle marks
      2) Evidence of self-injury (e.g., cutting on the forearms)
   k. Physiologic grading of the severity of the poisoning (Table 12-1)
   l. Appearance can provide clues regarding the type of poison; initial clues that can help to identify the type of poisoning if it is unknown before the secondary assessment are listed in Table 12-2
   m. Breath odors
      1) Sweet (acetone): diabetic ketoacidosis, ethanol, camphor, glue, chloroform, or lacquer
      2) Bitter almond: cyanide, apricot pits, or laetrile
      3) Coal gas: carbon monoxide
      4) Garlic: arsenic, phosphorus, organophosphates, or thallium
      5) Rotten eggs: hydrogen sulfide or a sulfur-containing substance
      6) Pears: chloral hydrate or paraldehyde
      7) Wintergreen: methyl salicylate
4. Mental status: hyperactive to obtunded, depending on drug or toxin ingested

TABLE 12-1 Physiologic Grading of the Severity of Poisoning

	Signs and Symptoms	
Severity	Stimulant Poisoning	Depressant Poisoning
Grade 1	Agitation, anxiety, diaphoresis, hyperreflexia, mydriasis, tremors	Ataxia, confusion, lethargy, weakness, verbal, able to follow commands
Grade 2	Confusion, fever, hyperactivity, hypertension, tachycardia, tachypnea	Mild coma (nonverbal but responsive to pain), brainstem and deep tendon reflexes intact
Grade 3	Delirium, hallucinations, hyperpyrexia, tachydysrhythmias	Moderate coma (respiratory depression, unresponsive to pain), some but not all reflexes absent
Grade 4	Coma, cardiovascular collapse, seizures	Deep coma (apnea, cardiovascular depression), all reflexes absent

From Irwin, R. S., & Rippe, J. M. (2003). *Irwin and Rippe's intensive care medicine* (vol. 5). Philadelphia: Lippincott Williams & Wilkins.

TABLE 12-2 Initial Clues to the Type of Poisoning

Substance	Pupils	Blood Pressure	Heart Rate	Respiratory Rate	Temperature	Dysrhythmias
Alcohol	Mydriasis		↑	↓	↓	
Amphetamines	Mydriasis	↑	↑	↑	↑	
Anticholinergics	Mydriasis	↑	↑	↑	↑	+
Atropine	Mydriasis	+	+			+
Barbiturates	Mydriasis (early); miosis (late)		↓	↓	↓	+ / −
β-Blockers		↓ or normal	↓			+
Calcium-channel blockers		↓ or normal	↓			+ / −
Cholinergics	Miosis	↓	↓			+ / −
Cocaine	Mydriasis	↑	↑			+
Cyanide		↓				
Digitalis		↓	↓			+ / −
Ecstasy		↑	↑			
γ-Hydroxybutyric acid		↓	↓	↓		
Hallucinogenics	Mydriasis	↑	↑	↑	↑	+ / −
Hydrocarbons		↓	↑	↑		
Narcotics	Miosis (except with meperidine)	↓ or normal	↓	↓	↓	+ / −
Organophosphates	Miosis		↓	↑		+
Salicylates						
Early			↑	↑		+ / −
Late			↓	↓		+ / −
Sedatives/hypnotics		↓	↓	↓	↓	
Tricyclic antidepressants			↓		↓	+

Key: + = Present; − = absent; ↓ = decreased; ↑ = increased.

5. Urine color (Terris, n.d.)
   a. Blue or blue green
      1) Methylene blue (also can turn stool bluish)
      2) Medications: amitriptyline (Elavil), indometha-cin (Indocin), cimetidine (Tagamet), prometha-zine (Phenergan), rifampin (Rifadin), or sildena-fil (Viagra)
      3) Blue dyes or food dyes
   b. Brown, brown black, or red brown
      1) Excessive levodopa or melanin excretion
      2) Copper or phenol poisoning
      3) Large amount of rhubarb, fava beans, or aloe ingested
      4) Medications: furazolidone (Furadantin), metroni-dazole (Flagyl), nitrofurantoin (Macrodantin), senna laxatives, methocarbamol (Robaxin), or sorbitol
   c. Orange
      1) Medications: phenazopyridine (Pyridium), ethoxazene (Serenium), rifampin (Rifadin), or sulfasalazine (Azulfidine)
      2) Vitamin C or riboflavin
      3) Carrots
   d. Red or pink
      1) Hematuria or hemoglobinuria
      2) Free hemoglobin can cause urine to turn pinkish
      3) Mercury or lead
      4) Red dye: food coloring or diagnostic contrast dye
      5) Acid urine will turn red from the ingestion of blackberries or beets, which contains a dye called anthocyanin
      6) Alkali urine can turn red with the ingestion of rhubarb or anthraquinone laxatives
      7) Medications: phenothiazines, phenytoin (Dilantin), or pyrvinium (Vanquin)
6. Diagnostic
   a. Toxicology
      1) Rapid drug screens (qualitative)
         a) Serum
            i) Acetaminophen
            ii) Ethanol
            iii) Salicylates
            iv) Tricyclic antidepressants
         b) Urine
            i) Amphetamines
            ii) Barbiturates
            iii) Benzodiazepines
            iv) Cannabinoids
            v) Cocaine
            vi) Methadol (ORLAAM)
            vii) Opiates
            viii) Phencyclidine (Sernyl)
            ix) Propoxyphene (Darvon)
      2) Quantitative drug levels may be required to determine appropriate treatment
         a) Carbamazepine (Tegratol)
         b) Carbon monoxide

   c) Digoxin (Lanoxin)
   d) Ethylene glycol
   e) Lithium (Lithobid)
   f) Methanol
   g) Methemoglobin
   h) Phenytoin (Dilantin)
   i) Theophylline (Theodur)
   b. ABGs
      1) Respiratory acidosis caused by hypoventilation when drugs or toxins depress ventilation
      2) Metabolic acidosis
         a) With increased anion gap
            i) Paraldehyde, ethylene glycol, methanol, toluene, or salicylates
            ii) Agents that cause hypoxia (e.g., cyanide, carbon monoxide) result in an increase in the serum lactate level
         b) With decreased anion gap: lithium, bromide, or iodide
   c. Electrocardiography (ECG): dysrhythmias are fre-quently seen, depending on the drug or toxin
   d. Flat plate of abdomen: to assess for the presence of radiopaque agents
   e. CT may be done to rule out pathology
   f. LP: may be done to rule out pathology
7. Clinical presentation specific to drug or toxin (Tables 12-3 and 12-4)

Collaborative management: General
1. Continue assessment
   a. ABCDs
   b. Vital signs: blood pressure, pulse, respiratory rate, and temperature
   c. Oxygen saturation if indicated
   d. Psychiatric status, especially suicidal ideation
   e. Respiratory effort and excursion
   f. Breath sounds
   g. Cardiac rate and rhythm
   h. Level of consciousness
   i. Serum electrolyte levels
   j. Accurate intake and output
   k. Safety
   l. Pain and discomfort levels
   m. Close monitoring for the progression of symptoms
2. Maintain airway, oxygenation, and ventilation
   a. Oxygen, dextrose, thiamine, and naloxone (Narcan)—sometimes referred to as a *coma cocktail*—as prescribed for altered mental status with no known cause
      1) Oxygen to reverse hypoxemia as a cause of loss of consciousness
         a) Oxygen to maintain SpO$_2$ of 95% unless contraindicated; for patients with COPD, use pulse oximetry to guide oxygen administra-tion to SpO$_2$ of 90%
            i) Contraindicated if the herbicide paraquat is ingested, because it would likely in-crease the alveolar injury caused by oxy-gen free radicals

TABLE 12-3   Clinical Presentation and Collaborative Management of Selected Drugs and Toxins

Drug or Toxin	Clinical Presentation of Intoxication	Specific Collaborative Management

Acetaminophen (Tylenol)
• Also found in many over-the-counter medications, including Comtrex, Contac, Coricidin D, Dristan Cold, Robitussin Cold and Flu, Sinutab Sinus, Theraflu, Nyquil, Alka-Seltzer Plus, and multisymptom liquid gels
• Also found in many prescription analgesics, including acetaminophen/butalbital/caffeine (Fioricet), hydrocodone/acetaminophen (Lortab), and acetaminophen/dichloralphenazone/isometheptene (Midrin)
• The ingestion of >7.5 g or 150 mg/kg has the potential to cause toxicity
	Stage 1: 30 min–24 hr
	• May be asymptomatic
	• Anorexia, nausea, and vomiting
	• Diaphoresis
	• Malaise
	• Pallor
	Stage 2: 24–48 hr
	• Nausea, fatigue, and malaise
	• Signs of hepatotoxicity may occur: liver enzymes and bilirubin may be elevated, prothrombin time may be prolonged, and there may be right upper quadrant pain
	• A gradual return to normal may occur
	Stage 3: 72–96 hr
	• Anorexia, nausea, and vomiting
	• Hepatic failure
	  • More likely if there has been ethanol consumption, malnutrition, or short-term fasting
	  • Jaundice and elevated bilirubin level
	  • Hepatosplenomegaly
	  • Prolonged prothrombin time
	  • Gastrointestinal bleeding
	  • Hypoglycemia
	  • Metabolic acidosis
	  • Hepatic encephalopathy: confusion that leads to coma
	• Acute tubular necrosis and renal failure may develop
	• Dysrhythmias and shock may occur
	• Death may result from severe metabolic disturbances, cerebral edema, or coagulopathy
	Stage 4: 4 days–2 weeks
	• Gradual return of liver function in patients who recover
		• Gastric lavage only if ≤1 hr since ingestion
		• Activated charcoal (single dose) if the patient arrives within 4–6 hr after ingestion; although activated charcoal does adsorb N-acetylcysteine and reduces its peak serum levels, the loading dose of N-acetylcysteine does not need to be increased
		• N-acetylcysteine (Mucomyst) 140 mg/kg initially and then 70 mg/kg every 4 hr for 17 doses for a total of 1330 mg/kg
		  • If given PO, dilute in juice or a carbonated beverage; if given via NG or duodenal tube, dilute 3-to-1 with juice or a carbonated beverage
		  • May cause anorexia, nausea, vomiting, diarrhea; repeat the dose if vomiting occurs in ≤1 hr
		  • If given IV (Acetadote): 140 mg/kg initially and then 70 mg/kg every 4 hr for a total of 12 doses over 48 hr
		• Treatment of vomiting with metoclopramide (Reglan); use ondansetron (Zofran) or droperidol (Inapsine) for refractory vomiting
		• Monitoring for bleeding; vitamin K may be prescribed, especially if hepatic failure occurs
		• $D_{50}W$ may be needed for hypoglycemia
		• Antidysrhythmics may be needed
		• Registration for hepatic transplantation if indicated

Continued

TABLE 12-3   Clinical Presentation and Collaborative Management of Selected Drugs and Toxins—cont'd

Drug or Toxin	Clinical Presentation of Intoxication	Specific Collaborative Management

Amphetamines
• Prescription examples include dextroamphetamine (Dexedrine), methamphetamine (Desoxyn), methylphenidate (Ritalin), phentermine (Adipex-P), and amphetamine mixture (Adderall)
  • May be prescribed for weight control, narcolepsy, or attention-deficit/hyperactivity disorder
  • Usually oral but may be crushed and snorted or injected
• Illegal examples
  • Methamphetamine (crank), methamphetamine crystals (crystal meth, ice): may be snorted, injected, smoked, or instilled rectally (i.e., "booty bumping" or "butt whacking")
  • Ecstasy (3-4 methylenedioxy-methamphetamine): may be in tablet, capsule, powder, or liquid form; usually ingested via mixing with caffeine beverages but may be snorted or injected intravenously
	• Tachycardia
	• Hypertension or hypotension
	• Tachypnea
	• Dysrhythmias
	• Chest pain or palpitations
	• Dyspnea or respiratory distress
	• Hyperthermia, diaphoresis, and flushing
	• Dilated but reactive pupils, decreased visual acuity, and nystagmus
	• Dry mouth
	• Abdominal pain or cramps
	• Urinary retention
	• Nausea, vomiting, and diarrhea
	• Headache
	• Muscle spasms or pain
	• Weight loss
	• Formication: the sensation of insects crawling on the skin
	• Painful rash, needle marks, or abscesses
	• Trismus, grinding of teeth, and enamel erosion
	• "Meth mouth" and bad breath caused by decaying teeth with methamphetamine (Handly, 2007)
	• Paranoid-type psychotic behavior
	• Hallucinations
	• Hyperactivity, anxiety, and panic attacks
	• Hyperactive deep tendon reflexes, tremor, and seizures
	• Confusion, stupor, and coma
	• May have hypoglycemia, hyponatremia, or hypokalemia
		• Calm, quiet environment
		  • Avoid overstimulation of the patient
		  • Do not speak loudly or move quickly
		  • Do not approach the patient from behind
		  • Avoid touching the patient unless you are sure that it is safe
		  • Do not leave the patient alone
		• Gastric lavage only if ≤1 hr of ingestion
		• Activated charcoal (single dose); best if given ≤30 min of ingestion and of little use if >4 hr since ingestion
		• Diazepam (Valium) or lorazepam (Ativan) for agitation
		• Sedatives, nitroglycerin (Tridil), or nitroprusside (Nipride) as prescribed for hypertension
		• Anticonvulsants (e.g., diazepam [Valium], phenytoin [Dilantin], phenobarbital [Luminol]) for seizures
		• Antidysrhythmics (e.g., lidocaine, amiodarone [Cordarone]), cardioversion, or defibrillation for ventricular dysrhythmias
		• Haloperidol (Haldol) may be prescribed for acute psychotic reactions, but this is controversial because the drug lowers the seizure threshold and interferes with thermoregulation (Handly, 2007)
		• Hypothermia blanket, ice packs, ice-water sponge baths, ice-bath immersion, or sedatives for hyperthermia
		  • Dantrolene (Dantrium) may be prescribed for malignant hyperthermia

TABLE **12-3**   Clinical Presentation and Collaborative Management of Selected Drugs and Toxins—cont'd

Drug or Toxin	Clinical Presentation of Intoxication	Specific Collaborative Management
Barbiturates • Examples include pentobarbital (Nembutal), phenobarbital (Luminal), and secobarbital (Seconal)	• Bradycardia and cardiac dysrhythmias • Hypotension • Hypothermia • Respiratory depression that leads to respiratory arrest • Headache • Nystagmus, dysconjugate eye movements, and sluggish pupil reaction to light • Dysarthria • Ataxia • depressed deep tendon reflexes • Confusion, stupor, and coma • Vesicles or bullae at pressure points (i.e., barb burns) • Serum glucose level may be decreased if combined with alcohol • Gastric irritation (chloral hydrate [Somnote]) • Pulmonary edema (meprobamate [Miltown]) • Hypertonicity, hyperreflexia, myoclonus, and seizures (methaqualone [Quaalude])	• Gastric lavage only if ≤1 hr since ingestion • Multiple doses of activated charcoal with cathartic added to first dose • Phenobarbital (Luminal): sodium bicarbonate to alkalinize the urine and to increase the rate of barbiturate excretion; maintain a urine of pH >7.50 • Monitor potassium, calcium, and magnesium levels • Anticonvulsants (e.g., diazepam [Valium], phenytoin [Dilantin], phenobarbital [Luminal]) for seizures • Hemodialysis or hemoperfusion may be required

Benzodiazepines
• Examples include diazepam (Valium), lorazepam (Ativan), clonazepam (Klonopin), and midazolam (Versed)
• Frequently used in combination with alcohol or other central nervous system depressants
	• Hypotension
	• Respiratory depression
	• Diminished or absent bowel sounds
	• Decreased deep tendon reflexes
	• Confusion, drowsiness, stupor, or coma
		• Gastric lavage only if ≤1 hr since ingestion
		• Activated charcoal (single dose)
		• Flumazenil (Romazicon), a benzodiazepine receptor antagonist, may be prescribed
		  • Contraindicated if the patient has also ingested tricyclic antidepressants; use cautiously if the patient has history of the long-term use of benzodiazepines, because seizures may occur with acute withdrawal
		  • Dose is typically 0.2 mg by IV injection; may be repeated every 1 min to a maximum dose of 2 mg
		  • Monitor for seizures, agitation, flushing, nausea, and vomiting as side effects of flumazenil
		• Intubation and mechanical ventilation may be necessary

Continued

TABLE **12-3** Clinical Presentation and Collaborative Management of Selected Drugs and Toxins—cont'd

Drug or Toxin	Clinical Presentation of Intoxication	Specific Collaborative Management
β-Blockers • Examples include propranolol (Inderal), nadolol (Corgard), and metoprolol (Lopressor)	• Sinus bradycardia, arrest, or block • Junctional escape rhythm • Atrioventricular nodal block • Bundle branch block (usually right) • Hypotension • Heart failure • Cardiogenic shock • Cardiac arrest • Decreased level of consciousness • Seizures • Respiratory depression or apnea • Bronchospasm • Hyperglycemia or hypoglycemia	• Gastric lavage only if ≤1 hr since ingestion • Multiple doses of activated charcoal with cathartic added to first dose • Bowel irrigation if sustained-release preparations are ingested • Atropine, epinephrine (Adrenalin), dopamine (Intropin), or isoproterenol (Isuprel) for bradycardia and hypotension; temporary pacing may be required • Glucagon 3-5 mg IV, IM, or subcutaneously; may repeat in 5 min if necessary or initiate an infusion of 1-5 mg/hr as prescribed • Monitor for hypoglycemia, hyperglycemia, and hypokalemia • Anticonvulsants (e.g., diazepam [Valium], phenobarbital [Luminal]) for seizures; phenytoin is contraindicated
Calcium-channel blockers • Examples include nifedipine (Procardia), diltiazem (Cardizem), and verapamil (Calan)	• Sinus bradycardia, arrest, or block • Sinoatrial blocks (diltiazem) • Atrioventricular blocks (verapamil) • Hypotension • Heart failure • Confusion, agitation, dizziness, lethargy, and slurred speech • Seizures • Nausea and vomiting • Paralytic ileus • Hyperglycemia	• Gastric lavage only if ≤1 hr since ingestion • Activated charcoal; multiple doses with cathartic added to the first dose if massive ingestion or ingestion of sustained-release preparations • Bowel irrigation if sustained-release preparations ingested • Calcium chloride 5-10 ml (500 mg-1 g) of 10% solution; may repeat every 5-10 min up to four doses • Atropine, epinephrine, dopamine (Intropin), or isoproterenol (Isuprel) for bradycardia and hypotension; temporary pacing may be required • Glucagon 3-5 mg IV, IM, or SQ, followed by an infusion of 1-5 mg/hr • Anticonvulsants (e.g., diazepam [Valium], phenytoin [Dilantin], phenobarbital [Luminal]) for seizures

12-3 Clinical Presentation and Collaborative Management of Selected Drugs and Toxins—cont'd

Drug or Toxin	Clinical Presentation of Intoxication	Specific Collaborative Management
Cannabinoids • Examples include hashish and marijuana	• Euphoria • Slowed thinking and reaction time • Confusion • Impaired balance and coordination	• Supportive care

Carbon monoxide
• Note: The affinity between carbon monoxide and hemoglobin is approximately 200× the affinity between oxygen and hemoglobin
	• Dysrhythmias
	• Impaired hearing or vision
	• Pallor; cherry-red skin coloring may also be seen
	• Elevated carbon monoxide levels; normal is 0%–3% for nonsmokers and 3%–8% for smokers
	  • 10%–20%: mild headache, flushing, dyspnea or angina on vigorous exertion, nausea, and dizziness
	  • 20%–30%: throbbing headache, nausea, vomiting, weakness, dyspnea on moderate exertion, and ST segment depression
	  • 30%–40%: severe headache, visual disturbances, syncope, and vomiting
	  • 40%–50%: tachypnea, tachycardia, chest pain, and worsening syncope
	  • 50%–60%: chest pain, respiratory failure, shock, seizures, and coma
	  • 60%–70%: respiratory failure, shock, coma, and death
		• Removal from the contaminated area
		• Oxygenation
		  • 100% oxygen via mask initially; continuous positive airway pressure by mask may be used
		  • Intubation and mechanical ventilation until carbon monoxide level is <5%; positive end-expiratory pressure may be used
		  • Hyperbaric oxygen (at 3 atmospheres) as soon as available if the following conditions are present:
		    • Carboxyhemoglobin level of >25%
		    • Carboxyhemoglobin level of >15% if history of cardiovascular disease, acute electrocardiogram changes, or central nervous system symptoms
		• Fluids, diuretics, and urine alkalinization to treat myoglobinuria if present
		• Anticonvulsants (e.g., diazepam [Valium], phenytoin [Dilantin], phenobarbital [Luminal]) for seizures

Caustic poisoning • Acids (e.g., battery acid, drain cleaners, hydrochloric acid) • Alkalis (e.g., drain cleaners, refrigerants, fertilizers, photographic developers)	• Burning sensation in the oral cavity, the pharynx, and the esophageal area • Dysphagia • Respiratory distress: dyspnea, stridor, tachypnea, and hoarseness • Soapy-white mucous membranes **Acid** • Oral ulcerations or blisters • May have signs of gastric perforation (e.g., abdominal pain, distention, absent bowel sounds, rebound tenderness) • May have signs of shock **Alkali** • May have signs of esophageal perforation (e.g., chest pain, subcutaneous emphysema)	• Diluent: flush the mouth with copious volumes of water; have the patient drink water or milk (≈250 ml) • Do not induce vomiting or perform gastric lavage • Esophagogastroscopy to assess damage • Corticosteroids may be prescribed for alkali poisoning

Continued

TABLE 12-3   Clinical Presentation and Collaborative Management of Selected Drugs and Toxins—cont'd

Drug or Toxin	Clinical Presentation of Intoxication	Specific Collaborative Management

Cholinergic agents
• May be prescribed for myasthenia gravis; too much pyridostigmine (Mestinon) causes cholinergic crisis
• Most likely toxic exposure is organophosphate poisoning (e.g., agricultural workers, anyone working with pesticides); may also result from exposure to nerve agents
	• Vital sign changes depend on whether muscarinic or nicotinic signs predominate
	  • Muscarinic: bradycardia, hypotension, or respiratory depression
	  • Nicotinic: tachycardia, hypertension, or tachypnea
	• Anxiety, agitation, and restlessness
	• Rhinorrhea, cough, dyspnea, crackles, and respiratory distress
	• Blurred vision, miosis, and watering eyes
	• Ototoxicity: inner ear damage caused by toxicity
	• Increased oral secretions
	• Nausea, vomiting, diarrhea, and abdominal pain and cramping
	• Impaired memory and confusion
	• Slurred speech
	• Headache
	• Poor motor control, muscle cramps, muscle pain, and twitching
	• Dizziness and unsteady gait
	• Cogwheel rigidity: tension in a muscle that gives way in little jerks when the muscle is passively stretched (often seen with Parkinson disease)
	• Urinary incontinence
	• Seizures may occur
	• Decreased level of consciousness
	• Possible flaccid paralysis
	  • Type I
	    • Acute paralysis as a result of ongoing depolarization at the neuromuscular junctions
	  • Type II
	    • Occurs 24-48 hr after exposure
	    • Often results in respiratory distress and mechanical ventilation
	    • Central muscles involvement, with relative sparing of the distal muscle groups
	    • May be the result of inadequate treatment
	    • Lasts for 4-18 days
	  • Type III
	    • Organophosphate-induced polyneuropathy begins 2-3 weeks after exposure to some organophosphates
	    • Distal muscle involvement, with sparing of the central muscles
	    • May take 12 months for complete recovery (Katz et al., 2008)
	• Guillain-Barré–like syndrome may be present
	• Serum cholinesterase level increased
	• Leukocytosis
	• Metabolic acidosis
	• Hyperglycemia, hypokalemia, or hypomagnesaemia
	• Amylase level and liver function studies elevated
	• Electrocardiogram: prolonged QT wave, ST elevation, and inverted T waves
	• SLUDGE: salivation, lacrimation, urination, diarrhea, gastrointestinal upset, and emesis (i.e., cholinergic crisis)
	• DUMBELS: diaphoresis/diarrhea, urination, miosis, bradycardia/bronchospasm/bronchorrhea, emesis/excess lacrimation, and salivation
		• Prevention of exposure to health-care providers
		  • Protective gear: health-care workers should wear neoprene gloves and gowns because hydrocarbons can penetrate nonpolar substances such as latex and vinyl (Katz, Brooks, Furtado, & Chan, 2008)
		• Removal and disposal of all clothing and leather products; these are considered hazardous waste
		• If on skin: cleansing with soap and water because organophosphates are readily hydrolyzed in aqueous solutions with high pH levels (Katz et al., 2008)
		• If ocular exposure: irrigation of the eye with saline or lactated Ringer solution; may use a Morgan lens
		• Gastric lavage for ingestion only if ≤1 hr since ingestion
		• Activated charcoal if ingested
		• Atropine 1-4 mg IV initially in adults and 0.01-0.04 mg/kg initially in children; repeat as required
		• Pralidoxime chloride (Protopam) 1-2 g IV over 15-30 min followed by an infusion of 10-20 mg/kg in adults and 20-40 mg/kg in children over 15-30 min may be used for organophosphates; may be repeated if required in 2-4 hr
		• Anticonvulsants (e.g., diazepam [Valium], phenytoin [Dilantin], phenobarbital [Luminal]) for seizures
		• Antidysrhythmics (e.g., lidocaine, amiodarone, magnesium), cardioversion, or defibrillation for ventricular dysrhythmias

TABLE 12-3 Clinical Presentation and Collaborative Management of Selected Drugs and Toxins—cont'd

Drug or Toxin	Clinical Presentation of Intoxication	Specific Collaborative Management
Cocaine (benzoylmethylecgonine), including "crack" cocaine • Cocaine hydrochloride salt is a water-soluble substance that can be swallowed, snorted, smoked, or injected intravenously • Chemically altered alkaloid "free-base" cocaine is soluble in acetone and alcohol and is smoked • Crack: a solid, preprocessed, free-base cocaine that is a purer form and that is smoked • Causes arterial spasms, which may cause ischemia	• Tachycardia, dysrhythmias, and conduction defects • Hypertension or hypotension • Palpitations • Tachypnea or hyperpnea • Fever, cough, difficulty breathing, and severe chest pain; known as "crack lung" • Cocaine-induced myocardial infarction • Pallor or cyanosis • Euphoria, hyperexcitability, and anxiety • Headache • Hyperthermia and diaphoresis • Nausea, vomiting, and abdominal pain • Dilated but reactive pupils and photophobia • Feeling of impending doom and flight of ideas • Confusion, delirium, tactile or visual hallucinations, and paranoia • Track marks or skin abscesses if injecting • Perforated nasal septum if snorting • Seizures • Coma • Respiratory arrest • Insomnia, chronic fatigue, epistaxis, anxiety, depression, and paranoia with long-term use • Withdrawal symptoms may include lethargy, depression, and suicide attempts	• Swabbing of inside of nose to remove any residual drug if cocaine was snorted • Activated charcoal (single dose); best if given ≤30 min since ingestion and of little use if >4 hr since ingestion • Bowel irrigation for "body packers" • Anxiolytics (e.g., lorazepam [Ativan], diazepam [Valium]) • Anticonvulsants (e.g., benzodiazepines, phenytoin [Dilantin], phenobarbital [Luminal]) for seizures • Antidysrhythmics; usually calcium-channel blockers are used (they may also help with coronary artery spasm) • Antihypertensives: vasodilators (e.g., nitroprusside [Nipride]) • Vasopressors (e.g., norepinephrine [Levophen]) for hypotension • Hypothermia blanket, ice packs, ice-water sponge baths, and benzodiazepines for hyperthermia • Dantrolene (Dantrium) may be prescribed for malignant hyperthermia • Fluids, diuretics for urine alkalinization to treat myoglobinuria if present

Continued

TABLE 12-3   Clinical Presentation and Collaborative Management of Selected Drugs and Toxins—cont'd

Drug or Toxin	Clinical Presentation of Intoxication	Specific Collaborative Management

Cyanide
• Although it is present in many plant species, the concentration is not high enough to be toxic
• Possible causes of toxic exposure include smoke inhalation, laetrile treatments, intentional poisoning, sodium nitroprusside, and bioterrorism
• Effects include hypoxia, lactic acidosis, and rapid deterioration
	• Anxiety, restlessness, weakness, and dizziness
	• Hyperventilation initially with bradypnea and apnea later
	• Tachycardia followed by bradycardia
	• Hypertension followed by hypotension
	• Dysrhythmias
	• Bitter-almond odor to breath
	• Cherry-red mucous membranes
	• Nausea and vomiting
	• Dyspnea
	• Headache
	• Dizziness
	• Pupil dilation
	• Confusion
	• Stupor, seizures, coma, and death
	• Metabolic (i.e., lactic) acidosis
	• Elevated serum lactate level
	• Elevated cyanide level
	  • $\leq$0.5 mcg/ml: asymptomatic
	  • 0.5–1.0 mcg/ml: tachycardia and flushing
	  • 1.0–2.5 mcg/ml: agitation or decreased level of consciousness
	  • 2.5–3.0 mcg/ml: coma
	  • >3.0 mcg/ml: potentially fatal
		• 100% oxygen initially by facemask
		  • Avoidance of mouth-to-mouth ventilation to avoid the exposure of providers; barriers should be used during cardiopulmonary resuscitation to avoid provider exposure
		  • Hyperbaric oxygen may be needed
		  • Rapid-sequence intubation and mechanical ventilation are frequently necessary
		• Supportive care if only anxiety, restlessness, or hyperventilation present
		• Elimination of source
		  • Removal of any liquids on the skin or clothing
		  • Activated charcoal for ingestion
		  • Flushing the skin with water if dermal contamination; removal and isolation of clothing
		  • Irrigation of eyes for at least 15 min in a case of eye exposure
		  • Discontinuance of causative agent (e.g., nitroprusside [Nipride])
		• Antidotes for more serious symptoms; monitor closely for hypotension with these drugs
		  • Amyl nitrite (Aspiral) by inhalation
		  • Sodium nitrite (PARAS) IV (contraindicated if fire victim with carbon monoxide exposure)
		  • Sodium thiosulfate IV
		• Fluids and vasopressors for blood pressure support
		• Anticonvulsants (e.g., diazepam [Valium], phenytoin [Dilantin], phenobarbital [Luminal]) for seizures
		• Antidysrhythmics (e.g., lidocaine) for ventricular dysrhythmia and atropine for bradydysrhythmias
		• Sodium bicarbonate for severe metabolic acidosis
		• Vitamin B_{12} may be prescribed

TABLE 12-3   Clinical Presentation and Collaborative Management of Selected Drugs and Toxins—cont'd

Drug or Toxin	Clinical Presentation of Intoxication	Specific Collaborative Management

Digitalis preparations
• Examples include digoxin (Lanoxin) and digitoxin (Crystodigin)
• Electrolyte imbalances, herbal preparations (i.e., kyushin, licorice, plantain, uzara root, hawthorn and ginseng), and other cardiac drugs (i.e., quinidine [Cardioquin], verapamil [Calan]) increase the risk of toxicity
	• Anorexia
	• Nausea
	• Vomiting
	• Headache
	• Restlessness
	• Visual changes
	  • Disturbed color perception (i.e., yellow vision)
	  • Scotomata (i.e., the loss of a portion of the visual field surrounded by normal vision)
	• Sinus bradycardia, block, or arrest
	• Paroxysmal atrial tachycardia with atrioventricular block
	• Junctional tachycardia
	• Atrioventricular blocks: first, second (Type 1), or third
	• Premature ventricular contractions: bigeminy, trigeminy, or quadrigeminy
	• Ventricular tachycardia (especially bidirectional)
	• Ventricular fibrillation
		• Treatment of cause (e.g., replacement of electrolytes, evaluation of drug interactions
		• Gastric lavage only if ≤1 hr since ingestion
		• Multiple doses of activated charcoal with cathartic added to first dose
		• Cholestyramine (Questran)
		• Bowel irrigation for large ingestions
		• Correction of hypoxia and electrolyte imbalance (especially potassium)
		• Treatment of dysrhythmias
		  • Do not attempt cardioversion
		  • For symptomatic bradydysrhythmias and blocks
		    • Atropine
		    • External pacemaker
		  • For symptomatic tachydysrhythmias
		    • Lidocaine
		    • Phenytoin (Dilantin)
		    • Magnesium if hypomagnesemia or hyperkalemia present
		    • Cardioversion at lowest effective voltage and only if life-threatening dysrhythmias exist
		    • Defibrillation for ventricular fibrillation
		    • Verapamil if supraventricular tachycardia
		• Digoxin immune FAB (Digibind, DigiFab) if >10 mg was ingested by an adult, if the serum digoxin level is >10 ng/ml, or if they serum potassium level is >5.0 mEq/L
		• Monitor closely for the exacerbation of the condition for which the digitalis was being used (i.e., increase in heart rate, heart failure)

Continued

TABLE 12-3 Clinical Presentation and Collaborative Management of Selected Drugs and Toxins—cont'd

Drug or Toxin	Clinical Presentation of Intoxication	Specific Collaborative Management
Ethanol (i.e., alcohol) • One of the most commonly abused substance • Found in many forms (e.g., beverages, cold preparations, mouthwashes, antiseptics) • Abuse occurs 5× more frequently among men than women • Predisposing factors include a family history of alcoholism, peer pressure, stress, low self-esteem, and a history of psychiatric illness	• Increased serum ethanol concentration (i.e., blood alcohol concentration) affected by amount of alcohol ingested, body size and composition, drinking rate, hormonal levels, and alcohol concentration in the drinks consumed (O'Brien, 2007); Table 12-4 describes the typical clinical presentation at various blood levels; however, note that there is wide variability among these signs and symptoms and serum ethanol levels; the signs and symptoms described are for a person who is not alcohol dependent) **Also:** • Alcohol odor to breath (Note: The individual may also have a breath odor of breath mints being used to cover the odor of alcohol) • Hypoglycemia • Seizures • Metabolic acidosis **Also may be present if the individual is a chronic user of ethanol:** • Elevated liver enzyme studies • Abnormal clotting profile • Clinical indications of liver cirrhosis	• Gastric lavage if ≤1 hr since ingestion • Fluid and electrolyte replacement (i.e., potassium, magnesium, calcium) may be needed • Anticonvulsants (e.g., diazepam [Valium], phenytoin [Dilantin], phenobarbital [Luminal]) for seizures • Monitor blood glucose; administer $D_{50}W$ for hypoglycemia as well as multivitamins that include thiamine and folic acid (Note: Thiamine is necessary for the brain to make use of glucose; thiamine deficiency in alcoholic patients may cause Wernicke encephalopathy) • Hemodialysis may be necessary
Ethylene glycol • Possible sources include antifreeze, detergents, paints, polishes, and coolants • Ingestion may be accidental, recreational, suicidal, or for the provision of ethanol-like effect in alcoholic individuals • Metabolism by alcohol dehydrogenase forms glycoaldehyde, which is then metabolized to glycolic, glyoxylic, and oxalic acids; these cause severe metabolic acidosis, renal damage, and hypocalcemia	**First 12 hr after ingestion** • Appears "drunk" without the odor of ethanol on the breath • Nausea, vomiting, and hematemesis • Focal seizures or coma • Nystagmus, depressed reflexes, and tetany • Metabolic acidosis with increased anion gap **12–24 hr after ingestion** • Tachycardia • Mild hypertension • Pulmonary edema • Heart failure **24-72 hr after ingestion** • Flank pain or costovertebral tenderness • Acute renal failure • Hypocalcemia with tetany, dysrhythmias, and seizures	• Gastric lavage only if ≤1 hr since ingestion • 10% ethanol in D_5W IV to maintain a serum ethanol level of 100–200 mg/dl • Fomepizole (Antizol) IV may be used instead of ethanol for ethylene glycol • Fluid and electrolyte replacement (particularly calcium but also potassium and magnesium) may also be needed • Sodium bicarbonate for severe metabolic acidosis • Glucose for hypoglycemia as well as multivitamins that include thiamine, folic acid, and pyroxidine (Note: thiamine is necessary for the brain to make use of glucose; thiamine deficiency in alcoholic patients may cause Wernicke encephalopathy) • Anticonvulsants (e.g., diazepam [Valium], phenytoin [Dilantin], phenobarbital [Luminal]) for seizures • Hemodialysis may be needed

TABLE 12-3   Clinical Presentation and Collaborative Management of Selected Drugs and Toxins—cont'd

Drug or Toxin	Clinical Presentation of Intoxication	Specific Collaborative Management
Flunitrazepam (Rohypnol) • Also referred to as the *date-rape drug* or *roofies* • Oral; individuals may not be aware that this drug has been added to their drinks	• Similar to other benzodiazepines • Amnesia; may awaken but not know where they are or how they got there • Feel "hungover" when awakening • Does not show on routine benzodiazepine screen; must screen urine specifically for flunitrazepam • Sexually transmitted infection testing for date-rape cases	• Treatment as for other benzodiazepines • Assist with sexual assault examination and evidence collection as indicated
γ-Hydroxybutyric acid (i.e., liquid ecstasy, liquid X) • Oral; usually mixed with a sweet liquid; has a salty or soapy flavor • Popular in clubs, at "raves," and as a date-rape drug • May be used for weight loss • Increased toxicity when taken with alcohol	• Similar to flunitrazepam (Rohypnol) • Bradycardia or hypotension • Respiratory distress and possibly arrest • Euphoria that progresses with higher doses to dizziness • Hypersalivation, nausea, and vomiting • Hypotonia • Amnesia • Agitation • Flailing activity (i.e., like trying to swim or get air) • Seizures • Withdrawal syndrome: anxiety, insomnia, tremors, and possibly treatment-resistant psychoses • Positive urine screen	• Calm, quiet environment • Activated charcoal (single dose); best if given ≤30 min since ingestion and of little use if >4 hr since ingestion • Diazepam (Valium) or lorazepam (Ativan) for agitation • IV fluids as prescribed • Atropine for bradycardia as prescribed • Anticonvulsants (e.g., diazepam [Valium], phenytoin [Dilantin], phenobarbital [Luminal]) for seizures • Assist with sexual assault examination and evidence collection as indicated
Hallucinogens (e.g., D-lyscrgic acid diethylamide) • Available as liquid (most common form), tablets (called *microdots*), or applied to blotting paper, sugar cubes, or gelatin squares (called *window panels*); can also be absorbed through the skin • After the drug is taken, the experience or "trip" lasts ≈12 hr • Individuals can experience flashbacks or recurrences of certain aspects of the drug experience; flashbacks occur suddenly without warning and have been reported to occur a few days to more than a year after use • Often taken in conjunction with other drugs and substances; ingestion may be unknown if the drug is added to drinks or food at parties, clubs, or raves	• Tachycardia and hypertension • Hyperthermia • Diaphoresis • Dry mouth • Anorexia or nausea • Headaches • Dizziness • Agitation and anxiety • Impaired judgment • Dreaming without a loss of consciousness • Distortion and intensification of sensory perception • Hallucinations, vivid colors, distorted perceptions, and crossing senses (e.g., tasting colors) • Changes in behavior that run from paranoia, psychosis, and panic to euphoria • Toxic psychosis and paranoia • Dilated pupils • Rambling speech • Polyuria	• Reassurance • Quiet environment with soft lighting • If ingested orally: activated charcoal may be used • Benzodiazepines (e.g., diazepam [Valium], lorazepam [Avitan]) for anxiety and agitation • Anticonvulsants (e.g., phenytoin [Dilantin], phenobarbital [Luminal]) for seizures • Antipsychotics (e.g., haloperidol [Haldol] may be prescribed • Restraints only if necessary to protect the patient

Continued

TABLE 12-3   Clinical Presentation and Collaborative Management of Selected Drugs and Toxins—cont'd

Drug or Toxin	Clinical Presentation of Intoxication	Specific Collaborative Management

Heavy metals
• Include iron, zinc, mercury, arsenic, and lead (most common)
• Possible causes
  • Iron: overdosage of iron-containing vitamins or iron preparations
  • Lead: lead paint or occupational exposure for plumbers or steel workers
  • Zinc: occupational exposure for metal workers
  • Mercury: broken mercury thermometers, fluorescent lights, or mercury-contaminated seafood
  • Arsenic: poisons (e.g., rat poison); occupational exposure for exterminators, copper workers, or lead smelters; or suicide or homicide
• Effects include alterations in enzymatic activity, mitochondrial dysfunction, and cellular death
	Iron
	• Tachycardia and hypotension possible
	• Nausea, vomiting, abdominal pain, and abdominal tenderness with palpation
	• Hematochezia
	• Dry mucous membranes and poor skin turgor
	• Hypoglycemia that eventually progresses to hyperglycemia
	• Three stages of symptoms
	  • Stage 1: Nausea and vomiting, abdominal pain, bloody stools, and hyperglycemia
	  • Stage 2: Gastrointestinal symptoms continue, and dehydration symptoms develop
	  • Stage 3: acidosis, hypoglycemia, and coagulopathies
	• Serum iron levels: >350 mcg/100 ml
	Lead
	• Any combination of neurologic dysfunction, gastrointestinal complaints, and anemia in a child should raise the suspicion of lead poisoning
	• Gastrointestinal complaints (more common among adults)
	• Neurocognitive effects: developmental delays, lower intelligence quotient, speech and language problems, reading deficits, visual–spatial problems, visual–motor problems, and learning disabilities
	• Behavioral effects: aggression, hyperactivity, impulsiveness, delinquency, disinterest, and withdrawal
	• Central nervous system dysfunction, including encephalopathy (more common among children)
	• "Lead lines": purple–black discoloration seen at the gingival border
	• Serum lead level: >10 mcg/dl is toxic
	• Anemia
	• Dense metaphyseal bands in children that indicate radiopaque bone at the metaphysic of growing bone (these bands are more prominent at the wrist and knees); also known as *dense metaphyseal lines, transverse bands,* or *lead lines*
	  • Lead lines in general indicate past lead toxicity; they can take ≤4 years to disappear (Raber, 1999)
	• Retained foreign bodies found in abdominal films (e.g., lead bullets from previous gunshot wounds) can cause lead toxicity and should be removed
	Zinc
	• Fever
	• Headache
	• Shortness of breath or coughing
	• Metallic taste in mouth
	• Nausea, vomiting, diarrhea, abdominal pain, and abdominal tenderness with palpation
	• Hypoxemia (decreased SpO_2)
	• Elevated serum zinc levels: normal range is 0.6–1.1 mg/L (plasma) and 10–14 mg/L (red cells)
	• Anemia can occur as the patient develops a copper deficiency
		• IV access and fluid
		• May require large volumes of crystalloids if there have been significant gastrointestinal losses (i.e., vomiting, diarrhea)
		• Adequate hydration required before chelation therapy
		• Antidysrhythmics (e.g., lidocaine, amiodarone [Cordarone]), cardioversion, or defibrillation for ventricular dysrhythmias
		• Decrease absorption and promote excretion
		  • Gastric lavage only if immediately after ingestion
		  • Bowel irrigation may be helpful
		  • Chelation therapy
		    • Iron: deferoxamine (Desferal); note that this medication will turn the urine pink
		    • Lead
		      • Dimercaprol (British anti-Lewisite; BAL); monitor for hypertension and nephrotoxicity
		      • Calcium chelate of disodium ethylenediaminetetraacetate (EDTA): administered IV after BAL has been initiated; may worsen neurologic status if given before BAL; monitor for hypoglycemia in patients with diabetes mellitus
		      • Succimer (Chemet) : should not be given with EDTA or penicillamine
		    • Zinc: EDTA and dimercaprol
		    • Mercury
		      • Dimercaprol
		      • Penicillamine: monitor for thrombocytopenia, agranulocytosis, and aplastic anemia
		    • Arsenic: dimercaprol and penicillamine
		  • Hemodialysis for acute renal failure
		• Anticonvulsants (e.g., benzodiazepine) for seizures
		• Analgesics as required for headache
		• Antipyretics as required for fever (especially with zinc poisoning)

TABLE 12-3	Clinical Presentation and Collaborative Management of Selected Drugs and Toxins—cont'd	
Drug or Toxin	**Clinical Presentation of Intoxication**	**Specific Collaborative Management**
	Mercury • Nausea, vomiting, and watery diarrhea • Chronic exposure causes stomatitis, tremors, and hypersensitivity (i.e., Pink disease) • Clinical signs of dehydration: tachycardia, hypotension, and dry mucous membranes • Altered neurologic status, from lethargy to extreme excitability • Hematochezia • Rash with desquamation (i.e. shedding of skin) on the face, palms, and soles • Increased serum mercury levels (normal limits: 10 μg/L in whole blood) • 24-hr urine for heavy metals (may be started in the ED); normal limit for mercury is 20 μg/L • Chest radiography: may show pneumomediastinum Arsenic • Anorexia, nausea, vomiting, and abdominal pain • Diarrhea that looks like "rice water" • Painful neuropathy • Edema of the eyelids • May see ascending paralysis (often mistaken for Guillain-Barré syndrome) • Central and peripheral neuropathies • Microcytic hypochromic anemia is common • Urine spot test may detect arsenic • 24-hr urine clearance: >50 mcg is unusual • Hair and fingernail clippings may be sent for arsenic levels • Abdominal radiographs may show the presence of radiopaque densities caused by heavy-metal deposits • Nerve conduction studies may show peripheral neuropathy as a result of arsenic	• Monitor for complications • Lead: encephalopathy (poor prognosis) and seizures • Zinc: hypoxia • Mercury: renal or hepatic failure; bone or teeth deterioration • Arsenic: renal failure and ascending flaccid paralysis

Continued

TABLE 12-3   Clinical Presentation and Collaborative Management of Selected Drugs and Toxins—cont'd

Drug or Toxin	Clinical Presentation of Intoxication	Specific Collaborative Management

Inhalants
• Types
  • Volatile solvents: liquids that vaporize at room temperature; examples include paint thinner, gasoline, and glue
  • Aerosols: sprays that contain propellants and solvents; examples include paint, spot remover, and spray adhesive
  • Gases: include medical anesthetic agents and substances found in household products; examples include butane, propane, aerosol propellants, and nitrous oxide
  • Nitrites: a special class of inhalants that are used mainly for sexual enhancement; examples include amyl nitrate, butyl nitrate, and cyclohexyl nitrate
• The inhaling of vapors is also known as *huffing, bagging,* or *snorting*
• Popular with school-aged children (especially those in middle school)
• Rapid absorption and short duration
	• Mood swings
	• Red, watery, itchy eyes and itchy nose
	• Nausea and vomiting
	• Headache
	• Dizziness and syncope
	• Behavior changes: irritable, anxious, and belligerent
	• Unsteady gait, staggering, or stuporous
	• Muscle weakness and lack of coordination
	• Slurred speech
	• Rash around the nose and mouth
	• Inflamed nostrils and nosebleeds
	• Mydriasis
	• Memory impairment
	• Central nervous system damage
	• Chemical pneumonitis may occur
	• Cardiopulmonary arrest
	  • Asphyxiation can occur from repeated inhalations, which lead to high concentrations of inhaled fumes displacing the available oxygen in the lungs
	  • Suffocation can occur when air is blocked from entering the lungs while inhaling fumes from a plastic bag placed over the head
		• Oxygen
		• Supportive care

TABLE 12-3   Clinical Presentation and Collaborative Management of Selected Drugs and Toxins—cont'd

Drug or Toxin	Clinical Presentation of Intoxication	Specific Collaborative Management
Isopropanol (i.e., isopropyl alcohol, rubbing alcohol) • Sources include rubbing alcohol, disinfectants, cleansers, and nail polish removers • Ingestion may be accidental, recreational, suicidal, or for the provision of ethanol-like effects in alcoholic individuals • Metabolism by alcohol dehydrogenase forms acetone	• Similar to ethanol • Gastrointestinal distress (e.g., nausea, vomiting, abdominal pain) • Acetone odor to breath • Headache • Central nervous system depression, areflexia, and ataxia • Respiratory depression • Hypothermia • Hypotension • Hypoglycemia may occur	• Gastric lavage only if ≤1 hr since ingestion • Gastric suction • Hemodialysis may be needed • Fluids and vasopressors for hypoperfusion • $D_{50}W$ for hypoglycemia
Lithium • Prescribed for bipolar disorder	**Mild** • Vomiting and diarrhea • Lethargy and weakness • Polyuria and polydipsia • Nystagmus • Fine tremors **Severe** • Hypotension • Severe thirst • Tinnitus • Hyperreflexia • Coarse tremors • Ataxia • Seizures • Confusion • Coma • Dilute urine or renal failure • Heart failure	• Gastric lavage only if ≤1 hr since ingestion • Hydration with normal saline • Anticonvulsants (e.g., phenytoin [Dilantin], phenobarbital [Luminal]) for seizures • Bowel irrigation • Hemodialysis may be necessary • Treatment of nephrogenic diabetes insipidus with amiloride (Midamor)
Methanol (i.e., wood alcohol) • Possible sources include windshield wiper fluid, canned fuel (Sterno), copy fluids, brake fluids, and paint removers • Ingestion may be accidental, recreational, suicidal, or for the provision of ethanol-like effects in alcoholic individuals • Metabolism by alcohol dehydrogenase forms formaldehyde, which is then metabolized to formate, which causes severe metabolic acidosis and ocular toxicity	• Similar to ethanol • Nausea and vomiting • Hyperpnea and dyspnea • Visual disturbances that range from blurring to blindness • Speech difficulty • Headache • Central nervous system depression • Motor dysfunction with rigidity, spasticity, and hypokinesis • Metabolic acidosis with anion gap	• Gastric lavage only if ≤1 hr since ingestion • 10% ethanol in D_5W IV to maintain a serum ethanol level of 100–200 mg/dl • Sodium bicarbonate for severe metabolic acidosis • Hemodialysis if visual impairment, a base deficit of >15, renal insufficiency, or a blood methanol concentration of > 30 mmol/L

Continued

TABLE 12-3　Clinical Presentation and Collaborative Management of Selected Drugs and Toxins—cont'd

Drug or Toxin	Clinical Presentation of Intoxication	Specific Collaborative Management
Methemoglobinemia • Caused by nitrites, nitrate, sulfa drugs, local anesthetics such as benzocaine, and others	• Tachycardia • Fatigue • Nausea • Dizziness • Cyanosis in the presence of a normal PaO_2 level; failure of cyanosis to resolve with oxygen therapy • Dark red or brown blood • Elevated methemoglobin levels 　• 15%-30%: nausea, headache, dizziness, fatigue, headache, and cyanosis 　• 30%-50%: tachycardia, tachypnea, dyspnea, weakness, and marked cyanosis 　• 50%-70%: dysrhythmias, respiratory depression, seizures, and coma 　• >70%: potentially fatal	• Oxygen • Removal of cause 　• Stop nitroglycerin, nitroprusside, sulfa drugs, anesthetic agents, or other causative agents 　• Gastric lavage only if ≤1 hr since ingestion if ingested 　• Multiple doses of activated charcoal with cathartic added to the first dose if agent was ingested • Methylene blue 　• If stupor, coma, angina, or respiratory depression or if the serum level is >30% 　• Administered at 1-2 mg/kg over 5 min; repeated at 1 mg/kg if the patient is still symptomatic after 30-60 min; total dose should not exceed 7 mg/kg • Ascorbic acid may be administered in large doses
Opioids • Prescription drug examples include fentanyl (Sublimaze), morphine, hydromor-phone (Dilaudid), methadone, oxycodone (Percocet, Oxycodone), and hydrocodone/acetaminophen (Lortab); administered orally or by injection • Illegal drug example is heroin; adminis-tered by sniffing, snorting, smoking, or injection • Many prescription opiates are misused or abused • Prescription opiates or heroin may be used in combination with alcohol or other drugs	• Bradycardia • Hypotension • Nausea and vomiting • Respiratory depression that leads to respiratory arrest • Decreased level of consciousness • Hypothermia • Miosis • Diminished bowel sounds • Needle tracks and abscesses • Seizures • Pulmonary edema (especially with heroin)	• Gastric lavage only if ≤1 hr since ingestion • Activated charcoal • Bowel irrigation for "body packers" • Naloxone (Narcan) 0.4-2 mg IV, IM, or transtracheally or nalmefene (Revex) 0.5 mg IV; use caution because these drugs cause acute withdrawal 　• Duration of action of naloxone is 1-2 hr, whereas nalmefene has a duration of action of 4-8 hr (heroin and morphine have durations of 4-6 hr, and meperi-dine's duration is 2-4 hr) • Anticonvulsants (e.g., diazepam [Valium], phenytoin [Dilantin], phenobarbital [Luminal]) for seizures • Rapid-sequence intubation and mechanical ventilation may be required; positive end-expiratory pressure may be required for pulmonary edema

TABLE 12-3   Clinical Presentation and Collaborative Management of Selected Drugs and Toxins—cont'd

Drug or Toxin	Clinical Presentation of Intoxication	Specific Collaborative Management

Hydrocarbons
• Examples include gasoline, kerosene, paint thinner, dry cleaning solvents, spot removers, motor oil, and furniture polish
• Causes include accidental exposure (i.e., occupational exposure, ingestion by young children) or intentional exposure (i.e., suicide or homicide)
• Toxicity is affected by the properties of the product, including viscosity, volatility, surface tension, and chemical activity
  • High-viscosity substances are thicker and not readily absorbed in the gastrointestinal tract, so they have a lower toxicity (e.g., motor oil)
  • Low-viscosity substances are thin and easily absorbed by the gastrointestinal tract, so they have a higher toxicity (e.g., gasoline, kerosene)
  • Substances with a low viscosity and that are highly volatile are more likely to be inhaled or aspirated
  • Substances with a high volatility quickly change into a gaseous form and displace oxygen, which leads to hypoxia
• High risk of aspiration pneumonitis
• Some of these substances cross the blood–brain barrier, which causes direct chemical brain injury
	• Tachypnea
	• Flushed skin
	• Hyperthermia
	• Vomiting, diarrhea, and abdominal pain
	• Dyspnea
	• Cyanosis
	• Coughing
	• Breath-sound changes: crackles, rhonchi, wheezes, and diminished breath sounds
	• Staggering gait
	• Confusion
	• Central nervous system depression or excitation
	• Gagging or choking sensation
	• Syncopal episodes
	• Nausea, vomiting, sore throat, and throat or mouth burning
	• Headache and complaints of weakness
	• Tachypnea and cyanosis
	• Tachycardia, dysrhythmias, or hypotension
	• Altered level of consciousness, from lethargy to seizures and coma
	• May appear euphoric or experience hallucinations
	• Leukocytosis or anemia
	• Anion gap: most often normal but can be elevated with toluene exposure
	• Creatine kinase level: elevated if rhabdomyolysis
	• Liver function studies: may be elevated
	• Chest radiography: abnormal if aspiration; may show changes typical of acute respiratory distress syndrome
		• Washing of skin with soap and water if dermal contamination; removal and isolation of clothing
		• Oxygen
		• Positioning the patient on his or her left side
		• Bronchodilators may be required
		• Antiemetics

Continued

TABLE 12-3 Clinical Presentation and Collaborative Management of Selected Drugs and Toxins—cont'd

Drug or Toxin	Clinical Presentation of Intoxication	Specific Collaborative Management

Phencyclidine (PCP)
• Also referred to as *angel dust, ozone, wack,* and *rocket fuel;* administered orally, snorted, or smoked
• Considered a dissociative anesthetic, like ketamine
	• Vital sign changes
	  • Mild ingestion: increased temperature, blood pressure, heart rate, and respiratory rate
	  • High-dose ingestion: decreased blood pressure, heart rate, and respiratory rate
	• Flushed skin and diaphoresis
	• May be amnesic to recent events
	• Agitation and hyperactivity
	• Violent, psychotic behavior
	  • Symptoms that mimic schizophrenia: delusions, hallucinations, paranoia, and disordered thinking
	• Blank stare
	• Nystagmus or flicking up and down of the eyes
	• Blurred vision
	• Tremors, muscle rigidity, and ataxia
	• Loss of coordination and numbness in the extremities
	• Nausea and vomiting
	• Drooling
	• Seizures
	• Lethargy or coma
	• Cardiac arrest
	• May have signs of traumatic injury but the patient may not be aware of them as a result of anesthesia for pain
	• Hypoglycemia
	• Myoglobinuria or renal failure
		• Quiet environment
		• Activated charcoal if ingested
		• Gastric suction
		• Benzodiazepines (e.g., diazepam [Valium]) for anxiety and agitation
		• Antidysrhythmics if required
		• Antihypertensives: vasodilators (e.g., nitroprusside [Nipride]) as prescribed
		• Hypothermia blanket, ice packs, and ice-water sponge baths for hyperthermia
		  • Dantrolene (Dantrium) may be prescribed for malignant hyperthermia
		• Anticonvulsants (e.g., diazepam [Valium], phenytoin [Dilantin], phenobarbital [Luminal]) for seizures
		• Haloperidol (Haldol) for acute psychotic reactions
		• Fluids and diuretics for myoglobinuria; sodium bicarbonate is contraindicated because urinary alkalinization interferes with the urinary elimination of PCP
		• Caregiver should wear gloves to avoid having PCP absorbed through his or her own skin

TABLE 12-3	Clinical Presentation and Collaborative Management of Selected Drugs and Toxins—cont'd	
Drug or Toxin	**Clinical Presentation of Intoxication**	**Specific Collaborative Management**
Salicylates • Types • Acetylated (e.g., aspirin): inhibit platelet aggregation and increase bleeding time • Nonacetylated (e.g., choline magnesium trisalicylate [Trilisate]): less effect on platelets and thus on bleeding • Common in many over-the-counter preparations, including topical creams and oil of wintergreen (98% methyl salicylate)	**Severity depends on the serum salicylate level 6 hr after ingestion** • <35 mg/dl: asymptomatic (therapeutic levels are 15-30 mg/dl) • 35-70 mg/dl: mild to moderate symptoms • 70-100 mg/dl: severe symptoms • >120 mg/dl: potentially fatal **Initially** • Hyperthermia • Burning sensation in the mouth or throat • Change in the level of consciousness • Petechiae **Progressive** • Hyperventilation (respiratory alkalosis) • Nausea, vomiting, epigastric pain, and gastrointestinal bleeding • Thirst • Tinnitus • Diaphoresis **Late** • Hearing loss • Motor weakness • Vasodilation and hypotension • Oliguria and renal failure • Pulmonary edema • Respiratory depression that leads to respiratory arrest • Dysrhythmias may occur **Diagnostic** • Metabolic acidosis with an increased anion gap • Prolonged prothrombin time and bleeding time • Hypokalemia or hypocalcemia	• Gastric lavage only if ≤1 hr since ingestion • Multiple doses of activated charcoal with cathartic added to first dose • Bowel irrigation if enteric-coated salicylates ingested • Fluids with dextrose (e.g., $D_5\frac{1}{2}$ NS) to maintain urine output at 2 ml/kg/hr • Hypothermia blanket, ice packs, and ice-water sponge baths for hyperthermia • Dantrolene (Dantrium) may be prescribed for malignant hyperthermia • Sodium bicarbonate to alkalinize the urine and to increase the rate of salicylate excretion; maintain a urine pH of >7.5 • Usually 44 mEq/L of bicarbonate in $D_5\frac{1}{2}$ NS at 300 ml/hr • Monitor potassium, calcium, and magnesium levels • Hemodialysis may be necessary • Monitoring for bleeding; vitamin K may be needed • Monitoring and correction of potassium and calcium levels • Anticonvulsants (e.g., diazepam [Valium], phenytoin [Dilantin], phenobarbital [Luminal]) for seizures • Antidysrhythmics as indicated • H_2-receptor blocker or proton-pump inhibitor for gastric ulcer prophylaxis

Continued

TABLE 12-3 Clinical Presentation and Collaborative Management of Selected Drugs and Toxins—cont'd

Drug or Toxin	Clinical Presentation of Intoxication	Specific Collaborative Management

Tricyclic antidepressants
• Examples include amitriptyline (Elavil), desipramine (Norpramin), doxepin (Sinequan), imipramine (Tofranil), nortriptyline (Aventyl), and trimipramine (Surmontil)
	Anticholinergics
	• Tachycardia and palpitations
	• Dysrhythmias
	• Hyperthermia
	• Headache
	• Restlessness
	• Mydriasis
	• Dry mouth
	• Nausea and vomiting
	• Dysphagia
	• Decreased bowel sounds
	• Urinary retention
	• Decreased deep tendon reflexes
	• Restlessness or euphoria
	• Hallucinations
	• Seizures
	• Coma
	Anti-α-adrenergics
	• Hypotension
	• QT prolongation and quinidine-like dysrhythmias, including torsades de pointes
	• Atrioventricular and bundle-branch blocks
	• Clinical indications of heart failure
	• Respiratory or metabolic acidosis
		• Syrup of ipecac contraindicated
		• Gastric lavage only if ≤1 hr since ingestion
		• Activated charcoal if agent ingested
		• Sodium bicarbonate to alkalinize the urine and to increase the rate of tricyclic antidepressant excretion; maintain a urine pH of >7.5
		  • Usually 44 mEq/L of bicarbonate in $D_5\frac{1}{2}$ normal saline at 300 ml/hr
		  • Monitor potassium, calcium, and magnesium levels
		• Hyperventilation may be used to produce alkalosis
		• Physostigmine (Antilirium) may be prescribed
		• Cardioversion, defibrillation, and pacemaker as needed for dysrhythmias; avoid quinidine (Cardioquin), lidocaine, and digitalis; phenytoin (Dilantin) or β-blockers may be used to shorten QRS duration; overdrive pacing for torsades de pointes
		• Anticonvulsants (e.g., diazepam [Valium], phenytoin, phenobarbital [Luminal]) for seizures
		• Fluids and vasopressors for hypotension
		• Bethanechol (Urecholine) for urinary retention

Adapted from: Dennison, R. D. (2007). *Pass CCRN!* (3rd ed.). St. Louis: Mosby.

D_5W, $D_{50}W$, Dextrose; IM, intramuscularly; IV, intravenously; NG, nasogastric; PO, by mouth; SQ, subcutaneously.

2) Dextrose to reverse possible hypoglycemia as the cause of a loss of consciousness
  a) Usual dose is 50 to 100 ml of 50% dextrose intravenously
3) Thiamine to prevent Wernicke encephalopathy, especially if there is a history of alcoholism or chronic drug abuse
  a) Usual dose is 50 to 100 mg IV or IM
  b) Also helpful for patients with ethylene glycol intoxication because thiamine may aid in prevention of the formation of toxic metabolites
4) Naloxone (Narcan) to reverse possible opiate intoxication as the cause of a loss of consciousness
  a) Usual dose is 1 to 2 mg IV, IM, or transtracheally; a dose of ≤10 mg may be required
  b) The goal is to reverse the central nervous system and respiratory depression, not to restore full consciousness

c) Sudden narcotic withdrawal occurs in patients with opiate intoxication, so caution must be exercised to prevent patients from injuring themselves or health-care providers
b. Positioning: maintain head-tilt–chin-lift position to maintain an open airway; use a jaw-thrust technique if cervical spine injury may exist
c. Artificial airway
  1) Use an oropharyngeal or nasopharyngeal airway to keep the tongue away from the hypopharynx
    a) Choose an appropriate airway: oropharyngeal airways should not be used in conscious patients because of their propensity to cause vomiting by stimulating the gag reflex in these patients
    b) Place the patient in a left side-lying position
    c) Have suction equipment available

TABLE 12-4 Serum Ethanol Levels and Typical Signs and Symptoms

Serum Level (mg/dl)	Percentage	Typical Signs and Symptoms
20	0–0.02	• Light to moderate drinkers begin to feel effects
40	0.04	• Relaxed, having fun
60	0.06	• Judgment is mildly impaired
80	0.08	• Impairment of muscle coordination • Driving skills affected
100	0.1	• Deterioration of reaction time and control • Giddy, decreased inhibitions • Legally intoxicated in most states
120	0.12	• May start vomiting unless this level is reached slowly
150	0.15	• Balance and movement impaired • Decreased sensory awareness • Slurred speech, vertigo, ataxia, and tachycardia
200	0.2	• Sensory awareness significantly decreased • Reaction times are greatly reduced • Trouble ambulating • Nausea and vomiting
300	0.3	• May lose consciousness
400	0.4	• Decreased deep tendon reflexes • Hypotension, tachycardia, and cool, clammy skin • Seizures • May be fatal
400–500	0.45–0.5	• Respiratory arrest • Death

From: Dennison, R. D. (2007). *Pass CCRN!* (3rd ed.). St. Louis: Mosby.

2) Assist with endotracheal intubation if the patient's gag and cough reflexes are depressed or if gastric lavage is initiated in a lethargic patient

   d. Mechanical ventilation may be required for situations that involve respiratory failure and respiratory acidosis or respiratory arrest

3. Maintain cardiovascular function
   a. Monitor the ECG rhythm for conduction changes or dysrhythmias, especially in the presence of tricyclic antidepressant overdosage
   b. Antidysrhythmic agents as prescribed
   c. Treatment of hypotension if required
      1) Insertion of intravenous catheter
      2) Treatment of hypovolemia with the infusion of isotonic crystalloids
      3) Administration of vasopressors for vasodilation
         a) α-Stimulants for tricyclic antidepressants
         b) α- and β-stimulants for β-blocker or calcium-channel blocker intoxication
         c) Calcium may be administered for calcium-channel blocker intoxication
   d. Treatment of hypertension if required
      1) Sedation with benzodiazepine as prescribed
      2) α-/β-Blocker (e.g., labetalol [Normodyne]) as prescribed for hypertension with tachycardia
      3) Peripheral vasodilator (e.g., nitroprusside [Nipride], nitroglycerin [Tridil]) if patient is hypertensive with a normal heart rate or bradycardia
   e. Blankets and radiant heat lamps if needed for hypothermia
4. Prevent further absorption of the drug or toxin depending on the route of absorption
   a. Eye: immediate irrigation of the eyes with large quantities of isotonic saline
      1) At least 15 to 20 minutes
      2) At least 1 hour or until pH is normal (i.e., 6.5–7.5) if alkaline substance
   b. Skin
      1) Protection of yourself with gloves, gown, and goggles
      2) Brushing or blowing of substance from skin
      3) Removal and disposal of clothing
      4) Water rinse until skin pH is normal if toxin is a strong acid or alkaline
      5) Washing of body with soap and water
   c. Ingestion
      1) Phoenix position: placing patient in the left lateral decubitus position can help to prevent absorption
      2) Induced emesis with the use of ipecacuanha (i.e., ipecac); may be used if it has been <1 hour since ingestion; contraindicated in the presence of any of the following:
         a) Ingestion of acid, alkali, or hydrocarbons
         b) Airway compromise or absence of gag reflex
         c) Decreased level of consciousness or comatose
         d) Infants <6 months old
         e) Seizures or ingestion of a substance that may cause seizures
      3) Gastric lavage: especially helpful if the patient arrives within 60 minutes of ingestion of the drug or toxin
         a) Endotracheal intubation before gastric lavage in patients who have a decreased level of consciousness and a diminished gag reflex

b) Contraindications
  i) Ingestion of hydrocarbons or caustic or corrosive substances: in this situation, use dilution, and give the patient water or milk (usually ≈250 ml)
  ii) Airway cannot be protected
  iii) Seizures
c) Insertion of a large-bore orogastric tube (e.g., Ewald tube)
  i) Size
    (a) Adults: 36 Fr to 40 Fr Ewald oral tube
    (b) Pediatric patients: 28 Fr to 32 Fr Ewald oral tube
  ii) Viscous lidocaine on the tube may decrease the gag reflex
  iii) Placement confirmed by aspirating gastric contents
d) Placement of the patient in a left side-lying, head-down position; have suction equipment available
e) Approximately 5 to 10 L of warm tap water injected 150 to 200 ml at a time and then aspirated completely before injecting any more lavage fluid
f) Potential complications: esophageal or gastric perforation, aspiration pneumonitis, laryngospasm, epistaxis, hypothermia, hyponatremia
g) Tube is not removed until after activated charcoal has been given
4) Adsorbent therapy: activated charcoal as prescribed
  a) Especially helpful if the patient arrives within 60 minutes of ingestion of the drug or toxin, but may be used if it has been >1 hour since ingestion if a significant overdosage of a drug that slows gastric emptying
  b) Contraindications
    i) Substances that do not bind to charcoal including the following:
      (a) Metal salts: iron, lithium, and potassium
      (b) Alcohols: ethanol, ethylene glycol, glycol, and methanol
      (c) Hydrocarbons, solvents, corrosives, acids, and alkalis
      (d) Pesticides
      (e) Cyanide
    ii) Airway cannot be protected
    iii) Oral antidote is given
  c) Caution: may induce vomiting, so ensure that the patient has an adequate airway and that a suction setup is ready
    i) Delay giving if ipecac has been given: wait 60 to 90 minutes after vomiting has subsided
  d) Administration

  i) Initial dose
    (a) Adults: 1 to 2 gm/kg (Dart, 2004)
    (b) Pediatric patients: 0.5 gm/kg; not recommended for children <2 years old
  ii) Multiple doses: may repeat every 2 to 6 hours (ENA, 2005)
    (a) Adults: 20 to 50 g
    (b) Pediatric patients: half of the initial dose
  iii) Route: orally or by nasogastric tube
  e) Cathartics: sorbitol with the first dose of activated charcoal as prescribed
    i) Not included in subsequent doses if giving multiple doses because this may cause intractable diarrhea
5) Bowel irrigation: nonabsorbable, osmotically active solution (e.g., polyethylene glycol lavage electrolyte solution [GoLYTELY, Colyte]) as prescribed
  a) Indications
    i) Large ingestions of drugs or toxins not adsorbed with the use of activated charcoal
    ii) Large ingestions of sustained-release or enteric-coated drugs
    iii) Formed concretions of drugs in the gastrointestinal tract
    iv) "Body packers" and "body stuffers"; surgical intervention may also be required in these situations
      (a) "Body packers" swallow condoms or balloons filled with a drug to smuggle it
      (b) "Body stuffers" swallow drugs to prevent detection by police; these drugs are not specially prepared to prevent absorption in the gastrointestinal tract, so they present a great risk of overdosage
  b) Contraindicated if the patient has significant gastrointestinal pathology or dysfunction
  c) Cautions: monitor for vomiting
  d) Administration
    i) Route: orally or by nasogastric tube
    ii) Rate: usually 1 to 2 L/hour for 4 to 6 hours or until the patient is having clear stools
6) Gastroscopy if indicated: may be necessary to remove a coalesced mass of pills
5. Facilitate the removal of the drug
  a. Chelation: used for heavy-metal poisonings
    1) A chelating agent is an organic compound that forms bonds with metals
  b. Forced diuresis: IV fluids and osmotic or loop diuretics used to cause a forced diuresis in a patient with ethanol, methanol, or ethylene glycol intoxication in the past; rarely used today
    1) Urine alkalization
      a) Intravenous sodium bicarbonate used

b) Indicated for overdosage of salicylates, tricyclic antidepressants, phenobarbital (Luminol), or chlorpropamide (Diabinese)

c) Goal is a urine pH of 7.5 to 8.5

d) Monitoring of potassium required

2) Urine acidification was previously used for phencyclidine and amphetamine overdosage, but it is currently avoided because of the associated incidence of rhabdomyolysis and resultant myoglobinuria, which may cause acute renal failure

c. Hemoperfusion or hemodialysis as prescribed

1) Both require a double-lumen central venous catheter

2) Both use either a hemodialysis machine or a machine designed specifically for continuous venous–venous hemodialysis (e.g., Prisma)

3) Hemoperfusion involves the use of a charcoal filter and is more effective for drugs that are bound to plasma proteins, but it is not effective for correcting acid–base imbalances

4) Hemodialysis is indicated for the following:

a) Heavy-metal intoxication

b) Salicylate intoxication with a severe acid–base imbalance or seizures that are unresponsive to treatment

c) Severe poisoning of a dialyzable drug, such as acetaminophen (Tylenol), amphetamines, most antibiotics, barbiturates, lithium (Eskalith), phenobarbital (Luminal), salicylates, Amanita (mushrooms), carbamazepine (Tegretol), colchicine (Colcrys), or theophylline (Theo-dur)

d) Ingestion of an agent that is known to produce delayed toxicity

e) May also be indicated for the following:

i) Drug-induced renal or hepatic toxicity

ii) Severe electrolyte imbalance

iii) Metabolic acidosis

d. Appropriate antidote if available and prescribed (see Table 12-3)

6. Maintain renal function

a. IV fluids to maintain urine output at 0.5 to 1 ml/kg/hour

b. Close monitoring for myoglobinuria; administer fluids and diuretics as prescribed

7. Monitor hepatic function: liver function studies and coagulation studies

8. Provide comfort and decrease anxiety

a. Cool, quiet room to reduce sensory stimulation and to help prevent hallucinations

b. Avoidance of stress and limited activity

c. If possible, a responsible friend or family member should stay with the patient (as long as he or she does not agitate the patient)

d. Protection of patient and others from injury; use chemical, soft, or leather restraints as required and prescribed

9. Protect the patient from injury and complications during seizure

a. Patient should not be left alone

b. Patient's clothing should be loosened to avoid constriction

c. Pillow under the patient's head should be removed

d. Patient should be turned to the side and the airway maintained; an artificial airway may be required

e. Gentle guiding of the extremities is acceptable, but the limbs should not be restrained

f. Side rails should be padded with blankets or pillows

g. Careful assessment for injury after seizure

10. Ensure appropriate psychologic counseling

a. Encouragement of expression of feelings with a noncondemning approach

b. Environment that is free of safety hazards and that includes suicide precautions if indicated

c. Referral of the patient to a substance abuse program if appropriate

d. Psychiatric consultation for destructive behaviors if appropriate

11. Monitor for complications (depending on the drug or toxin)

a. Acute respiratory failure or respiratory arrest

b. Aspiration pneumonitis

c. Dysrhythmias

d. Hypotension or hypertension

e. Heart failure or pulmonary edema

f. Nephrotoxicity or acute renal failure

g. Hepatotoxicity or acute hepatic failure

h. Gastrointestinal ileus, bleeding, or perforation

i. Seizures

j. Cerebral edema, coma, or neurologic injury

k. Hyperthermia or hypothermia

l. Fluid and electrolyte imbalance

m. Acid–base imbalance

n. Repeat overdosage

Collaborative management: Specific to the drug or toxin (see Table 12-3)
Evaluation

1. Patent airway, adequate oxygenation (i.e., normal PaO_2, SpO_2, SaO_2) and ventilation (i.e., normal $PaCO_2$)

2. Absence of clinical indications of respiratory distress

3. Absence of clinical indications of hypoperfusion

4. Absence of clinical indications of renal failure

5. Absence of clinical indications of hepatic failure or bleeding

6. Control of pain and discomfort

7. Alert and oriented with no neurovascular deficit

Typical disposition

1. If evaluation criteria met: discharge with instructions for follow up, which should include psychiatric consultation if the overdosage was intentional

2. If evaluation criteria met but overdosage was intentional: a psychiatric consultation is required and the patient may be placed on a 72-hour hold

3. If evaluation criteria not met: admission to progressive care unit or critical care unit

ENVIRONMENTAL EMERGENCIES

Frostbite and Frostnip

Definitions
1. Frostbite: the freezing of tissues
   a. Predominantly affects the hands and feet, but the shins, cheeks, nose, ears, and corneas may also be involved
   b. Divided into four classifications
      1) First degree involves only the epidermis
      2) Second degree involves the epidermis and the dermis
      3) Third degree is a partial-thickness burn that involves the epidermis, the dermis, and the subcutaneous tissue
      4) Fourth degree is a full-thickness burn that involves the epidermis, the dermis, the subcutaneous tissue, the muscle, the tendons, and possibly the bone
2. Frostnip: superficial frostbite

Predisposing factors
1. Debilitation
2. Not being acclimatized to high altitudes
3. Racial predisposition (e.g., African-Americans)
4. Constrictive clothing or other interference with blood supply to an extremity
5. Previous cold injury to the exposed body part
6. Unconsciousness
7. Insufficient clothing
8. Other risk factors
   a. Malnourishment
   b. Peripheral vascular disease
   c. Raynaud disease
   d. Cryoglobulinemia or cold agglutinin disease
   e. Heavy tobacco use
   f. Peripheral neuropathy, especially with diabetes
   g. Alcoholism or drug use

Pathophysiology
1. Degree of injury is affected by the following:
   a. Temperature and length of exposure
   b. Wetness or dryness of clothing
   c. Contact with metal
   d. Wind chill factor (Figure 12-1)
2. Exposure to cold leads to peripheral vasoconstriction and decreased blood flow
3. Vascular stasis occurs
4. Ice crystals begin to form in the intracellular space
5. Sodium and chloride increase in the intracellular space
6. Cells are destroyed as crystals enlarge and as metabolic processes are interrupted
7. The release of histamine causes increased capillary permeability, which leads to red blood cell aggregation and occlusions in the microvasculature and the formation of edema
8. Systemic hypothermia is possible
9. Rewarming will cause cells to swell
   a. Erythrocyte and platelet aggregation occur and lead to cell damage, thrombosis, and tissue edema
   b. The pressure within the compartment space then increases, which causes the formation of blebs and localized ischemia that can result in tissue death

Clinical presentation
1. Subjective
   a. History of exposure to cold as well as other contributing factors
   b. Tingling, numbness, or burning of the affected area
   c. May experience warm stinging or an electrical current-like feeling as the tissue thaws or is rewarmed

Estimated wind speed (in mph)	Actual Thermometer Reading (F)											
	50	40	30	20	10	0	−10	−20	−30	−40	−50	−60
	EQUIVALENT CHILL TEMPERATURE (F)											
CALM	50	40	30	20	10	0	−10	−20	−30	−40	−50	−60
5	48	37	27	16	6	−5	−15	−26	−36	−47	−57	−68
10	40	28	16	4	−9	−24	−33	−46	−58	−70	−83	−95
15	36	22	9	−5	−18	−32	−45	−58	−72	−85	−99	−112
20	32	18	4	−10	−25	−39	−53	−67	−82	−96	−110	−124
25	30	16	0	−15	−29	−44	−59	−74	−88	−104	−118	−133
30	28	13	−2	−18	−33	−48	−63	−79	−94	−109	−125	−140
35	27	11	−4	−21	−35	−51	−67	−82	−98	−113	−129	−145
40	26	10	−6	−21	−37	−53	−69	−85	−100	−116	−132	−148
(Wind speeds greater than 40 mph have little additional effect)	LITTLE DANGER in <5 hr with dry skin Maximum danger of false sense of security				INCREASING DANGER Danger from freezing of exposed flesh within one minute				GREAT DANGER Flesh may freeze within 30 seconds			
	Trenchfoot and immersion foot may occur at any point on this chart.											

Figure 12-1 The cooling power of wind on exposed flesh expressed as equivalent temperature. (From the Emergency Nurses Association [2005]. *Sheehy's manual of emergency care* [6th ed.] St. Louis: Mosby, p. 500.)

d. Joint pain
e. Cold or shivering
2. Objective
   a. First degree: paleness or redness, possible waxy appearance, and decreased sensation
   b. Second degree: erythema, edema, blisters (may take ≤24 hours to form), and decreased sensation
   c. Third degree: pale with significant blue coloring, edema, numbness at the site, nonpliable skin, and blood-filled blisters that progress to eschar over the course of a few weeks
   d. Fourth degree: pale, blue, necrotic, or gangrenous skin; edema; and numbness
   e. Hyperemia possible
3. Diagnostic
   a. CBC with differential
   b. Clotting studies: may be abnormal since hypothermia can cause coagulopathy
   c. Serum chemistries, including BUN, creatinine, and glucose
   d. Radiography: to rule out injury of the affected area

Collaborative management

1. Continue assessment
   a. ABCDs
   b. Oxygen
   c. Vital signs: blood pressure, pulse, respiratory rate, and temperature
   d. Oxygen saturations as indicated
   e. Cardiac rate and rhythm
   f. Pain and discomfort levels
   g. Level of consciousness
   h. Neurovascular checks
   i. Motor function and sensation of the affected area or part
2. Maintain airway, oxygenation, and ventilation
   a. Oxygen by nasal cannula at 2 to 6 L/minute as indicated to maintain an SpO_2 level of 95% unless contraindicated; for patients with COPD, use pulse oximetry to guide oxygen administration to an SpO_2 level of 90%
   b. Positioning or artificial airway to ensure a patent airway
   c. Rapid-sequence intubation and mechanical ventilation if required
3. Maintain adequate circulation and perfusion: IV access and fluids as prescribed
4. Initiate warming measures
   a. Removal of jewelry and wet clothing
   b. Rewarming of any area that could be re-exposed to cold should not be started because this could cause further tissue damage
      1) Most damage to tissue occurs during the rewarming, freezing, and rewarming again of tissue (ENA, 2007)
   c. Submersion of the affected area into a whirlpool or agitated bath with a temperature of between 100.8°F and 106°F; when flushing of the skin appears, rewarming is adequate

5. Prevent further injury to the tissue
   a. Gentle handling of the tissue; avoidance of rubbing or massage of the affected area
   b. Application of bulky sterile dressings and splints to reduce movement of thawed part
   c. Elevation of extremity to decrease swelling
   d. Application of splint to affected extremity
6. Prepare patients and assist with procedures as indicated
   a. Assistance with the debridement of nonhemorrhagic blisters
   b. Assistance with emergent escharotomy as indicated
7. Treat infection and prevent sepsis
   a. Tetanus immunization as indicated
   b. Antipyretics
   c. Antibiotics
8. Control pain and discomfort: analgesics
9. Monitor for complications
   a. Hypothermia
   b. Compartment syndrome

Evaluation

1. Patent airway, adequate oxygenation (i.e., normal PaO_2, SpO_2, SaO_2) and ventilation (i.e., normal $PaCO_2$)
2. Absence of clinical indications of neurovascular compromise
3. Absence of clinical indications of infection or sepsis
4. Control of pain and discomfort

Typical disposition

1. If evaluation criteria met (i.e., frostbite is superficial or first or second degree without serious complications): discharge with instructions
   a. Proper layering of clothes for cooler temperatures
   b. Cold exposure risks and symptoms
   c. Frostbite and hypothermia prevention
   d. Follow up with primary care provider as directed
2. If evaluation criteria not met: admission

Hypothermia

Definition: a state in which body temperature regulation is overwhelmed by cold factors, thereby causing a drop in the core body temperature to <95°F (35°C)
1. Occurs when heat loss exceeds the body's heat production
2. Classified into three categories
   a. Mild hypothermia: 93.2°F to 96.8°F (34–36°C)
   b. Moderate hypothermia: 86°F to 93.2°F (30–34°C)
   c. Severe hypothermia: <86°F (<30°C)

Predisposing factors

1. Environmental temperatures: this condition is usually seen during cold periods, but it can also be seen in warm environments (e.g., as a result of submersion or contact with cold surfaces for extended periods)
2. Age: older adults and children have higher risk
3. Medications and drugs that inhibit shivering

4. Trauma
5. Shock states
6. Chronic systemic diseases, particularly diabetes

Pathophysiology

1. Thermoregulation is controlled by the hypothalamus
   a. Heat is conserved by peripheral vasoconstriction
      1) Heat preservation may be overwhelmed in the face of cold stress, and the core temperature can drop as a result of fatigue or glycogen depletion
   b. Heat production in the body is accomplished through metabolism in the cells, shivering, muscle activity, and increasing levels of thyroxine and epinephrine
   c. Any injury to the central nervous system can alter thermoregulation
   d. The body loses more heat to the environment than it can compensate for, which results in the body not being able to maintain an adequate temperature
2. Heat loss can occur by four mechanisms
   a. Conduction: heat conducted through another object (e.g., patient lying on cold stretcher)
   b. Convection: transfer of heat by automatic circulation (e.g., cold intravenous fluids)
   c. Radiation: seen mainly in dry conditions
   d. Evaporation: the evaporation of sweat is the primary way that the body cools down and maintains body temperature; this process requires heat (e.g., breathing)
3. When the body responds to a dropping core temperature by shivering and peripheral vasoconstriction, it causes a decrease in tissue perfusion, which can affect all systems
   a. Basal metabolic rate drops, and the myocardium becomes irritable
   b. Kidneys lose blood flow and the glomerular filtration rate drops, which leads to decreased water reabsorption and dehydration, thereby causing hemoconcentration
   c. Lactic acid builds up as oxygenation decreases; the body then uses anaerobic metabolism, which causes acidosis
   d. Hypoglycemia occurs as all metabolic processes slow down and glucose is no longer being converted
4. Hypothermia shifts the oxyhemoglobin dissociation curve to the left at 34°C, thus impairing oxygen delivery to the tissues
5. Apnea and arrest can occur at temperatures of 21°C to 24°C

Clinical presentation

1. Subjective
   a. History of exposure
      1) Ambient temperature
      2) Amount of time exposed
      3) Injuries or events surrounding exposure
      4) Treatment before arrival
      5) Complaints of pain and decreased sensation
   b. Paradoxic undressing: bizarre behavior in which a decrease in body temperature causes an alteration in consciousness and judgment that results in the patient starting to remove clothing; this is a classic sign
2. Objective
   a. Body temperature of <95°F (35°C)
   b. Hypotension, bradycardia, and decreased respiratory rate; vital signs may be hard to detect in severe cases
   c. Shivering
      1) Initial response to heat loss
      2) Stops when body temperature is <31°C
   d. Skin can appear pale, mottled, or cyanotic
   e. Reflexes are diminished
   f. Patient appears clumsy
   g. Altered level of consciousness: lethargy, irritability, confusion, or coma
   h. Pupils: may be nonreactive
   i. Dysrhythmias: atrial fibrillation, premature ventricular contractions, ventricular tachycardia or fibrillation
3. Diagnostic
   a. Diagnosis by core temperature (i.e., not oral or axillary)
   b. Serum analysis is not accurate, because metabolism slows with hypothermia
      1) CBC with differential
      2) Coagulation panel
      3) BUN, creatinine, and glucose levels
      4) Liver panel
      5) Alcohol and drug screening
   c. ABGs: blood analysis machines warm blood to 37°C, which may cause higher Pao_2 and CO_2 levels and a lower pH than patient's actual values (Edelstein, 2007)
   d. ECG: J wave (i.e., Osborne wave) may occur
      1) Also referred to as *camel hump* (Figure 12-2)
      2) Appears as a positive reflection between the QRS complex and the ST segment that looks like a hump on the back side of the QRS complex
      3) More prominent with temperatures of <26°C
   e. Radiology
      1) As indicated by clinical condition
      2) CT of head may be requested

Collaborative management

1. Continue assessment
   a. ABCDs
   b. Vital signs: blood pressure, pulse, respiratory rate, and temperature
   c. Respiratory effort and excursion
   d. Oxygen saturations as indicated
   e. Cardiac rate and rhythm
   f. Pain and discomfort levels
   g. Serum electrolytes
   h. Sensation and movement of affected extremities
   i. Level of consciousness
   j. Close monitoring for the progression of symptoms

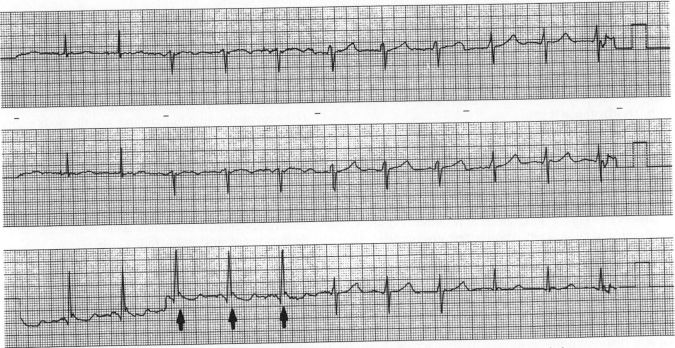

Figure 12-2 Hypothermic J waves with QT prolongation. (From the Emergency Nurses Association [2009]. *Sheehy's emergency nursing: Principles & practice* [6th ed.] St. Louis: Mosby, p. 540.)

2. Manage cardiopulmonary arrest if required with the use of basic or advanced cardiac life support
   a. Defibrillation is limited to one attempt until rewarming has been achieved
   b. Advanced cardiac life support measures may not be effective until the patient's temperature reaches ≥86°F (28°C)
   c. No medications are given during advanced cardiac life support if the patient's temperature is <30°C, because the medications will not be metabolized; when the patient's temperature is >30°C, medications are given at lower doses and over longer intervals until the temperature normalizes
3. Maintain airway, oxygenation, and ventilation
   a. Oxygen by nasal cannula at 2 to 6 L/minute as indicated to maintain an Spo₂ level of 95% unless contraindicated; for patients with COPD, use pulse oximetry to guide oxygen administration to an Spo₂ level of 90%
   b. Positioning or artificial airway to ensure a patent airway
   c. Rapid-sequence intubation and mechanical ventilation if required
4. Maintain circulation and perfusion
   a. IV access and warmed normal saline
      1) Adults: 1 to 2 L as indicated
      2) Pediatric patients: 20 ml/kg as indicated
5. Prepare patient and begin rewarming
   a. Removal of wet clothing and drying of patient occur first
   b. Rewarming until the patient's temperature reaches 96.8°F (36°C)

1) Three types of rewarming: one, two, or all three are used according to degree of hypothermia
   a) Passive external rewarming if patient's temperature is less than 96.8°F (36°C)
      i) Warm environment
      ii) Warm blankets
   b) Active external rewarming delivers heat on the external body surfaces
      i) Heat packs to body (e.g., axilla, groin, neck)
      ii) Forced warm-air blankets
      iii) Radiant-heat lamps
   c) Active internal rewarming if patient's temperature is less than 86°F (30°C): delivers heat to the body core
      i) Warmed intravenous solutions
      ii) Warmed humidified oxygen
      iii) Warmed peritoneal lavage
      iv) Warmed gastric lavage via nasogastric tube
      v) Warmed pleural lavage via chest-tube insertion
      vi) Cardiopulmonary bypass for patients with extreme hypothermia
      vii) Continuous hemodialysis
2) Cautions with rewarming
   a) Vasodilation which may lead to a relative hypovolemia and hypotension
   b) Afterdrop
      i) Occurs when acidotic cold blood is shunted to the body's core during rewarming
      ii) Caused by warming too quickly; blood moves from the central circulation to the

extremities, which causes a drop in blood pressure and possible dysrhythmias

  iii) Prevented by warming of >2°C per hour

6. Assist with other procedures as needed (e.g., Foley catheter)
7. Monitor for complications
   a. Afterdrop
   b. Dysrhythmias
   c. Cardiopulmonary arrest

Evaluation

1. Patent airway, adequate oxygenation (i.e., normal PaO_2, SpO_2, SaO_2) and ventilation (i.e., normal $PaCO_2$)
2. Absence of clinical indications of hypoperfusion
3. Absence of clinical indications of respiratory distress
4. Absence of clinical indications of neurovascular compromise
5. Alert and oriented with no neurologic deficit
6. Absence of clinical indications of infection or sepsis
7. Alert and oriented with no neurologic deficit
8. Control of pain and discomfort

Typical disposition

1. Patient with mild hypothermia exposure without complications: discharge with follow-up instructions
2. Patient with moderate to severe hypothermia: admission to the hospital

Heat-Related Emergencies

Definition: injuries that are caused when compensatory mechanisms (e.g., sweating, tachypnea, vasodilation) do not fully compensate for exposure to heat and humidity; the four types of heat-related emergencies include the following:

1. Heat cramps
2. Heat exhaustion
3. Heat stroke
4. Malignant hyperthermia: chemical-induced hyperthermia; this is rarely seen in the ED

Predisposing factors

1. Failure to replace fluids during warm weather (heat cramps)
2. Strenuous activity in a warm environment (heat exhaustion)
3. Not being acclimated to hot weather

Pathophysiology

1. Heat cramps result form a loss of fluids and electrolytes from sweating and inadequate replacement during activity
   a. Often seen in athletes or people who are in good physical condition
2. Heat exhaustion is more severe than heat cramps and results from a loss of water and salt in the body
   a. Heavy exertion in hot weather leads to peripheral vasodilation to enhance cooling but leads to a relative hypovolemia
   b. More fluid and electrolytes are lost via profuse sweating

   c. Core body temperature begins to rise because cooling is ineffective
3. Heat stroke is a medical emergency in which the body's thermoregulatory mechanisms in the hypothalamus fail
   a. Dehydration and hypernatremia occur as a result of sweating, hyperventilating, and vasodilation
   b. Sweat glands stop functioning, and the body's core temperature rises rapidly
   c. As the temperature increases, cerebral alterations occur, and cardiovascular collapse eventually follows
4. Malignant hyperthermia: a biochemical chain reaction response that is triggered by commonly used general anesthetics and the paralyzing agent within the skeletal muscles of susceptible individuals
   a. A hypermetabolic state occurs that involves increased oxygen consumption, hyperventilation, and respiratory acidosis
   b. An intracellular calcium accumulation results in sustained muscle contractions
   c. Temperature elevates (>105°F)

Clinical presentation

1. Subjective
   a. History of exposure to warm environment, strenuous activity, or both
   b. Nausea and vomiting
   c. Frontal headache
   d. Dizziness
   e. Diaphoresis with heat exhaustion
   f. Complaints of severe thirst with heat exhaustion
   g. Heat cramps: mild symptoms
2. Objective
   a. Tachycardia, hypotension, and tachypnea with heat exhaustion and heat stroke.
   b. Temperature elevation
      1) Heat exhaustion (99.6–102.2°F [37.5–39°C])
      2) Heat stroke (<102.5–106°F [<39.2–41°C])
   c. Skin changes
      1) Pale, cool, wet skin from heavy perspiration
      2) Pale, ashen, dry skin with heat stroke
   d. Muscle cramps may be intermittent with heat cramps
   e. Pupil changes
      1) Dilated pupils with heat exhaustion
      2) Pupils may be fixed and dilated with heat stroke.
   f. Altered mental status and level of consciousness, from confusion to coma; patient may hallucinate or be combative with heat stroke
   g. May see posturing with heat stroke
3. Diagnostic
   a. WBC: increased
   b. Clotting panel: prolonged clotting times
   c. Serum chemistries
      1) Sodium level: decreased
      2) Glucose level: decreased
      3) Potassium level: increased or decreased
      4) BUN: increased

d. Liver function studies: may see elevations in aspartate transaminase (AST) and alanine transaminase (ALT) levels
e. ABGs: metabolic acidosis and respiratory alkalosis
f. Blood and urine drug screening as indicated
g. Urinalysis: to check for myoglobinuria
h. Radiology: chest radiography and head CT
i. ECG: ST elevation, T-wave abnormalities, and widening of the QRS

Collaborative management

1. Continue assessment
   a. ABCDs
   b. Vital signs: blood pressure, pulse, respiratory rate, and temperature
   c. Oxygen saturation
   d. Respiratory effort and excursion
   e. Cardiac rate and rhythm
   f. Pain and discomfort levels
   g. Accurate intake and output
   h. Serum electrolytes
   i. Level of consciousness
   j. Close monitoring for the progression of symptoms
2. Maintain airway, oxygenation, and ventilation
   a. Oxygen by nasal cannula at 2 to 6 L/minute as indicated to maintain an SpO_2 level of 95% unless contraindicated; for patients with COPD, use pulse oximetry to guide oxygen administration to an SpO_2 level of 90%
   b. Positioning or artificial airway to ensure a patent airway
   c. Rapid-sequence intubation and mechanical ventilation if required
3. Maintain adequate circulation and perfusion
   a. Oral fluids if patient is able to drink: 0.1% saline
   b. IV access as indicated
   c. Intravenous fluids: 0.9% saline as prescribed
   d. Electrolyte replacement as indicated
4. Prepare patient for rapid cooling: the goal for heat stroke is to cool the patient to 102°F (39°C) during the first hour (the patient should not be cooled to <102°F to prevent complications)
   a. Cool environment
   b. Removal of restrictive clothing
   c. Fluid replacement as indicated previously
   d. Cooling methods:
      1) Damp sheet placed on the patient to allow for evaporative cooling
      2) Luke warm baths with a fan blowing over the patient
      3) Ice packs along the patient's trunk, axilla, and groin; monitor for the following:
         a) Avoid allowing the patient to shiver, which increases the metabolic rate and leads to an increase in temperature; low intravenous doses of chlorpromazine (Thorazine) or meperidine (Demerol) may be used to reduce shivering
         b) Frostbite and tissue injury

   e. Aggressive methods of cooling as prescribed for extreme situations
      1) Cool peritoneal dialysis
      2) Gastric lavage with cool water
   f. Antipyretics are not effective, because the temperature is not related to an inflammatory process
5. Reduce cerebral edema: intravenous mannitol (Osmitrol) as prescribed
6. Manage pain and discomfort
   a. Elevation and gentle massage of painful areas
   b. Mild analgesics
7. Monitor for complications
   a. Dehydration
   b. Electrolyte imbalances
   c. Dysrhythmias
   d. Rhabdomyolysis

Evaluation

1. Patent airway, adequate oxygenation (i.e., normal PaO_2, SpO_2, SaO_2) and ventilation (i.e., normal $PaCO_2$)
2. Absence of clinical indications of hypoperfusion
3. Absence of clinical indications of respiratory distress
4. Normal core body temperature
5. Alert and oriented with no neurologic deficit
6. Control of pain and discomfort

Typical disposition

1. If evaluation criteria met: discharge with instructions
   a. Patients with heat cramps: discharge after hydration with instructions for prevention after hydrated
      1) Do not overexert in hot weather
      2) Stay hydrated and drink plenty of fluids (e.g., Gatorade) when exercising or working outdoors
      3) Rest in a cool place if you feel like you are getting hot
      4) Massage painful areas
      5) If symptoms return or worsen, return to the ED
   b. Patients with heat exhaustion without complications: discharge with instructions as previously listed
2. If evaluation criteria not met: admission
   a. Patients with complications or who do not stabilize are admitted to the hospital; older adults, infants, and patients with other chronic illnesses are often admitted for observation
   b. Patients with heat stroke: admission to the critical care unit

Radiation Exposure and Acute Radiation Syndrome

Definitions

1. Radiation: energy that travels in waves or high-speed particles
   a. Examples from nature: sunlight and sound waves
   b. Manmade examples: radiography, nuclear weapons, and cancer radiation treatments

2. Acute radiation syndrome (also known as *acute radiation sickness*): a condition that occurs when a person is exposed to a high dose of radiation that penetrates the body, usually over a short time; radiation from radiographic films is too low to cause this syndrome, but radiation from cancer treatment can cause it

Predisposing factors

1. Cancer treatments
2. Exposure as a result of working with nuclear weapons or nuclear reactors
3. Exposure to a radiologic dispersal device (i.e., a dirty bomb)

Pathophysiology

1. Energy is transferred through space in the form of waves or particles
2. The higher the frequency, the higher the energy and the more destruction that can occur
3. Exposure leads to the depletion of immature parenchymal stem cells in target tissues (Centers for Disease Control and Prevention [CDC], 2005)
4. Most common types of radiation particles are alpha, beta, and gamma
   a. Alpha particles: have a positive charge, lose their energy quickly
      1) Do not penetrate skin so therefore not as hazardous; hazardous when ingested or inhaled or when they enter through breaks in the skin
      2) Can be stopped by skin or clothing
   b. Beta particles: have a negative charge and are fast moving
      1) Can penetrate tissue a few millimeters before losing energy
      2) Can be stopped by wood
   c. Gamma rays: have no charge
      1) Can pass through body tissue at the speed of light
      2) Can be stopped with lead or concrete
5. Three types of classic acute radiation syndromes
   a. Bone-marrow syndrome (CDC, 2005)
      1) Causes destruction of the bone marrow, which leads to hemorrhage, infection, and death
      2) Survival depends on the dose of radiation received: the higher the dose, the less likely the patient is to survive
   b. Gastrointestinal syndrome
      1) Causes destruction of the bone marrow and the gastrointestinal tract, which leads to infection, dehydration, and electrolyte imbalances
      2) Survival is not likely; death usually occurs within 2 weeks
   c. Cardiovascular and central nervous system syndromes
      1) Causes circulatory collapse and increased intracranial pressure as a result of cerebral edema, vasculitis, and meningitis
      2) Death usually occurs within 3 days

Clinical presentation

1. Subjective
   a. History of exposure
      1) Severity depends on the amount of time that the patient was exposed, how far away from the source the patient was, and whether there was any shielding
   b. Anorexia, nausea, vomiting, and diarrhea occur after exposure but then resolve and the patient feels better; nausea, vomiting, and diarrhea reoccur
   c. Fatigue
   d. Bruising or bleeding
   e. Fever
2. Objective
   a. Elevated temperature
   b. Change in level of consciousness
   c. Vomiting (possible hematemesis)
   d. Ataxia
   e. May have clinical indications of overt or covert bleeding
   f. May have signs of shock: tachycardia, hypotension, or hypoperfusion
   g. May have an overt radiation burn
   h. Seizures may occur
3. Diagnostic
   a. CBC with differential: decreased absolute neutrophil count
   b. Serum chemistries: may be abnormal
   c. Amylase: may be increased
   d. Radiation contamination monitor: shows exposure

Collaborative management

1. Continue assessment
   a. ABCDs
   b. Vital signs: blood pressure, pulse, respiratory rate, and temperature
   c. Respiratory effort and excursion
   d. Oxygen saturations as indicated
   e. Cardiac rate and rhythm
   f. Pain and discomfort levels
   g. Accurate intake and output
   h. Serum electrolytes
   i. Level of consciousness
   j. Close monitoring for the progression of symptoms
2. Maintain airway, oxygenation, and ventilation
   a. Oxygen by nasal cannula at 2 to 6 L/minute as indicated to maintain an SpO_2 level of 95% unless contraindicated; for patients with COPD, use pulse oximetry to guide oxygen administration to an SpO_2 level of 90%
   b. Positioning or artificial airway to ensure a patent airway
   c. Rapid-sequence intubation and mechanical ventilation if required
3. Maintain adequate circulation and perfusion
   a. IV access with one or two large-bore intravenous catheters
   b. Vasopressors as required to maintain perfusion

4. Prepare the patient for decontamination
   a. Use of institutional protocols for decontamination (see Chapter 2)
      1) Staff safety is a priority
      2) Decontamination should be performed outside if possible
5. Treat any concurrent injuries (e.g., blast injuries from the detonation of a weapon)
6. Monitor for complications
   a. Hemorrhage
   b. Aplastic anemia
   c. Hypovolemic or septic shock
   d. Intracranial hypertension or herniation

Evaluation

1. Patent airway, adequate oxygenation (i.e., normal PaO_2, SpO_2, SaO_2) and ventilation (i.e., normal $PaCO_2$)
2. Absence of clinical indications of respiratory distress
3. Absence of clinical indications of bleeding
4. Absence of clinical indications of hypoperfusion
5. Absence of clinical indications of infection or sepsis
6. Alert and oriented with no neurologic deficit
7. Control of pain and discomfort

Typical disposition: admission

Food Poisoning

Definition: the ingestion of infectious organisms or noninfectious substances; infection can occur from a variety of sources, including *Staphylococcus aureus, Clostridium perfringens,* and *Salmonella typhimurium*

Predisposing factors

1. Improper food handling, cooking, storing, and hand hygiene
2. Recent travel
3. Farming
4. Pet contact
5. Recent camping
6. Group picnic or family reunion

Pathophysiology

1. Ingestion of pathogens
2. Production of toxins by the pathogens and the invasion and inflammation of the gastrointestinal mucosa lining
3. Villus atrophy and malabsorption
4. Gastroenteritis (see Chapter 7)

Clinical Presentation (Table 12-5)

1. Subjective
   a. Nausea, vomiting, and crampy abdominal pain
   b. Watery or bloody diarrhea
   c. Numbness
   d. Muscle weakness and soreness
   e. Blurred vision
   f. Headache and dizziness
   g. Neck stiffness and meningeal signs

2. Objective
   a. Orthostatic tachycardia and hypotension
   b. Elevated temperature
   c. Vomiting and diarrhea
   d. Abdominal tenderness with palpation
   e. Hyperactive bowel sounds
   f. Flushing
   g. Lymphadenopathy
   h. Anaphylactic response may occur: angioedema, urticaria, stridor or wheezing, tachycardia, and hypotension
3. Diagnostic
   a. WBC: increased
   b. Serum chemistry: may show increased BUN level as a result of dehydration or electrolyte imbalance
   c. Stool: white blood cells, ova, parasites, occult blood, frank blood, or mucus may be present

Collaborative management

1. Continue assessments
   a. ABCDs
   b. Vital signs: blood pressure, pulse, respiratory rate, and temperature
   c. Respiratory effort and excursion
   d. Oxygen saturations as indicated
   e. Cardiac rate and rhythm
   f. Pain and discomfort levels
   g. Fluids and electrolytes
   h. Accurate intake and output
   i. Vomiting, stools, or both: color, consistency, and frequency
   j. Close monitoring for the progression of symptoms
2. Maintain airway, oxygenation, and ventilation
   a. Oxygen by nasal cannula at 2 to 6 L/minute as indicated to maintain an SpO_2 level of 95% unless contraindicated; for patients with COPD, use pulse oximetry to guide oxygen administration to an SpO_2 level of 90%
   b. Positioning or artificial airway to ensure a patent airway
      1) If the patient is vomiting, place on his or her side
      2) Have suction equipment available
   c. Rapid-sequence intubation and mechanical ventilation if required
3. Maintain adequate circulation and perfusion
   a. IV access with one or two large-bore intravenous catheters; administer crystalloid fluids as ordered
   b. Nothing-by-mouth status; may attempt oral rehydration when vomiting stops
4. Control pain and discomfort
   a. Antiemetics
   b. Non-narcotic analgesics as prescribed
   c. Anticholinergics
5. Treat inflammation and infection and prevent sepsis
   a. Antimicrobials as prescribed
   b. Corticosteroids to reduce inflammation and for parasitic infection
   c. Antipyretics and cooling methods to reduce fever if required

TABLE 12-5 Bacterial Food Poisoning

Type of Illness	Staphylococcal	Clostridial	Salmonella	Shigella
Causative agent	*Staphylococcus aureus*	*Clostridium perfringens*	*Salmonella typhimurium*	Four subspecies of the genus *Enterobacteriaceae*
Sources	Meat, seafood, bakery products, cream fillings, salad dressings, milk, and the skin and respiratory tracts of food handlers	Meat, seafood, or poultry dishes that are cooked at lower temperatures, reheated leftover meat and poultry dishes, gravies, and improperly canned vegetables	Improperly cooked meat of all types, seafood, and eggs	Food contaminated by improperly washed hands; flies can contaminate food if they have landed on infected feces; this type may also be acquired from swimming in or drinking contaminated water
Onset of symptoms	30 min–7 hr after ingestion	8–24 hr after ingestion	8 hr–several days after ingestion	24 hr after ingestion
Manifestations	Nausea, vomiting, diarrhea, and abdominal cramping	Diarrhea, nausea, vomiting (rare), abdominal cramps, and midepigastric pain	Nausea, vomiting, diarrhea, abdominal cramps, fever, and chills	Watery stools that contain blood and mucus, tenesmus, urgency, severe abdominal cramping, and fever
Treatment	Symptomatic; fluid and electrolyte replacement as well as antiemetics	Symptomatic; fluid and electrolyte replacement	Symptomatic; fluid and electrolyte replacement	Symptomatic; fluid and electrolyte replacement
Prevention	Proper refrigeration of food and proper hand hygiene	Correct preparation of meat and poultry dishes; serve food immediately after cooking or cool rapidly	Correct preparation of meat and egg dishes; serve food immediately after cooking or cool rapidly	Proper hand hygiene; keep flies away from food; do not drink or swallow water from swimming pools

Adapted from Lewis, S. M., Heitkemper, M., Dirksen, S., O'Brien, P., & Butcher, L. (2007). *Medical-surgical nursing* (7th ed.) St. Louis: Mosby.

6. Monitor for complications
   a. Dehydration
   b. Electrolyte imbalance
   c. Sepsis or multiorgan failure
   d. Hypovolemic shock

Evaluation

1. Patent airway, adequate oxygenation (i.e., normal PaO_2, SpO_2, SaO_2) and ventilation (i.e., normal $PaCO_2$)
2. Absence of clinical indications of hypoperfusion
3. Absence of clinical indications of infection or sepsis
4. Control of pain and discomfort
5. Decrease in nausea and number of stools

Typical disposition

1. If evaluation criteria met: discharge with instructions
   a. Clear liquids for 24 hours, then BRAT diet: bananas, rice, applesauce, and toast and tea
   b. Small feedings that are gradually increased; continue to increase fluid intake
   c. Indications to return to the ED: bloody vomitus or diarrhea, weakness or fainting, intractable vomiting or diarrhea, or severe abdominal pain
2. If evaluation criteria not met: admission

Rabies

Definition: a viral illness of the central nervous system that produces encephalitis and possibly death in humans after they become symptomatic

Predisposing factors

1. Contact with an infected animal or human
   a. Bites are most common, but rabies can be spread through scratches, mucus membrane contact, and inhalation
   b. Mammals such as bats, raccoons, foxes, and wild dogs are frequent carriers
2. Rare cases of rabies being spread via organ transplantation (Merlin et al., 2009)

Pathophysiology

1. After inoculation, the virus attaches to the acetylcholine receptors of the skeletal muscle
2. Deposition on mucous membranes, primary replication in muscles or connective tissues at site of bite, neurogenic (intraneural) spread, and secondary replication in the dorsal horn nerve cell body
3. Viral replication occurs by budding and destroys nerve cells; virus uses the acetylcholine receptors
4. The virus replicates and then enters the nervous system through sensory and motor terminals
5. After the virus has entered the nervous system, vaccination will not be effective
6. After rabies reaches the spinal cord, it will continue to spread throughout the central nervous system
7. Virus is shed in saliva when it has spread through the central nervous system
8. Incubation period is 5 days to several years after the initial exposure, depending on the length of the nerve (i.e., the distance from the bite to the central nervous system); the usual progression occurs over 7 to 14 days, with death occurring in an average of 16.2 days (Merlin et al., 2009)
9. Almost always fatal without prophylactic management before or after exposure
10. Three phases
    a. Prodrome: occurs 2 to 10 days after exposure and lasts ≤2 weeks; flu-like symptoms or sore throat
    b. Neurologic: begins about 7 days after the prodrome phase; involves neurologic changes such as numbness, aphasia, diplopia, and vertigo
    c. Late: usually occurs about 7 days after neurologic changes occur; changes in level of consciousness, seizures, coagulopathy, and cardiopulmonary arrest

Clinical presentation

1. Subjective
   a. History of contact with a rabid or unknown animal that involved either a bite or a scratch
   b. Odynophagia: painful spasms with swallowing
   c. May also have tingling and numbness at the bite site
      1) Dysarthria
   d. Diplopia
   e. Coordination and balance problems
   f. Vertigo
2. Objective
   a. Elevated temperature
   b. Hypersalivation and spasming of the pharyngeal muscles at the taste, sound, or sight of water (hydrophobia; i.e., frothing at the mouth)
   c. Increased lacrimation
   d. Agitation
   e. Aphasia
   f. Hyperactive reflexes
   g. Nuchal rigidity
   h. Positive Babinski sign

   i. Late stage
      1) Changes in level of consciousness
      2) Flaccidity
      3) Seizures
      4) Apnea
      5) Shock
      6) Disseminated intravascular coagulation
      7) Cardiopulmonary arrest
3. Diagnostic
   a. Culture for the isolation of the rabies virus
      1) Saliva culture
      2) Cerebrospinal fluid culture
      3) Central nervous system tissue culture
   b. Skin biopsy: used to detect rabies in the hair follicles
   c. CT of the head to rule out other causes

Collaborative management

1. Continued assessment
   a. ABCDs
   b. Vital signs: blood pressure, pulse, respiratory rate, and temperature
   c. Respiratory effort and excursion
   d. Oxygen saturations as indicated
   e. Cardiac rate and rhythm
   f. Pain and discomfort levels
   g. Accurate intake and output
   h. Serum electrolytes
   i. Level of consciousness
   j. Close monitoring for the progression of symptoms
2. Maintain airway, oxygenation, and ventilation
   a. Oxygen by nasal cannula at 2 to 6 L/minute as indicated to maintain an SpO_2 level of 95% unless contraindicated; for patients with COPD, use pulse oximetry to guide oxygen administration to an SpO_2 level of 90%
   b. Positioning or artificial airway to ensure a patent airway; suctioning as required
   c. Rapid-sequence intubation and mechanical ventilation if required
3. Maintain adequate circulation and perfusion
   a. IV access; administer fluids as prescribed
   b. Vasopressors as required to maintain perfusion
4. Prevent infection and sepsis
   a. Wound care: clean area with thoroughly with soap and water
   b. Tetanus immunization as indicated
   c. Rabies vaccination per protocol
      1) If the patient was bitten by an animal with a known vaccination status, the animal is quarantined and observed for 2 weeks, and prophylactic vaccination is withheld
      2) If the vaccination status is unknown or the animal has signs of rabies, the head of the animal will be sent for testing if the animal is captured, and prophylactic vaccination will be started until the results are known or the vaccination series is completed
      3) Rabies immune globulin will provide immediate passive immunity that lasts for 21 days and is

given only if patient has not been previously immunized with rabies vaccine

    4) Rabies vaccine provides active immunity

       a) Human diploid cell vaccine (Imovax) and RabAvert

       b) Active immune response occurs 7 to 10 days after vaccine administration and will last for about 2 years

       c) Vaccine is given in the deltoid muscle

       d) Dosage: 1 ml given on days 0, 3, 7, 14, and 28 after initial exposure (ENA, 2007)

  d. Bites must be reported to the local health department

5. Monitor for complications

  a. Paralysis

  b. Seizures

  c. Encephalitis

  d. Flaccid paralysis with respiratory arrest

  e. Coma

Evaluation

1. Patent airway, adequate oxygenation (i.e., normal Pao_2, Spo_2, Sao_2) and ventilation (i.e., normal $Paco_2$)
2. Absence of clinical indications of respiratory distress
3. Absence of clinical indications of hypoperfusion
4. Absence of clinical indications of infection or sepsis
5. Alert and oriented with no neurologic deficit
6. Control of pain and discomfort

Typical disposition

1. If evaluation criteria met: discharge with instructions
  a. Wound care as directed
  b. Follow up with primary care provider as directed
  c. If the patient is receiving the rabies vaccination, he or she will be given a schedule of dates to return for injections
    1) May experience erythema at the site of injection
    2) If other symptoms or concerns occur, return to the ED
2. If evaluation criteria not met: admission to the critical care unit

Tick-Borne Illnesses

Definitions

1. Tick-borne illnesses: spirochetal infections caused by tick bites
2. Lyme disease: an infection caused by a bite from a deer tick infected with *Borrelia burgdorferi*
3. Rocky Mountain spotted fever: vasculitis caused by *Rickettsia rickettsii*

Predisposing factors

1. Being outdoors during the warmer months (i.e., April–September) in tick-infested areas
2. Children, outdoor workers, hikers, and campers
3. Exposure to pets that wander outdoors in infested areas

4. Lyme disease: exposure to white-tailed deer, small mammals (e.g., white-footed mouse), and lizards on the U.S. West Coast
5. Rocky Mountain spotted fever: exposure to dog ticks

Pathophysiology

1. Ticks are vectors of disease; illnesses are spread through their saliva while they are attached to humans and animals
2. Lyme disease
  a. *B. burgdorferi*: a spirochete that was identified in 1982; it has two major outer surface proteins, a flagellar antigen, and an endotoxin lipopolysaccharide (Wormser et al., 2005)
  b. The spirochete enters its victim along with the saliva of the tick; the tick usually has to feed for 72 hours to transmit the disease (Wormser et al., 2005)
  c. Factors in the saliva prevent a normal immune response to the invasion and create a protective environment in which the spirochete can replicate
  d. As the spirochetes replicate, they migrate into the victim's dermis, and the characteristic lesion is seen
  e. An immune response starts, but neutrophils do not appear at the site, which allows the spirochete to continue to multiply and spread through the bloodstream to other organs, including the joints, the heart, the central and peripheral nervous systems, and distant skin sites (Pachner & Steiner, 2007)
  f. Three stages
    1) Stage 1: manifested by an expanding annular skin lesion (erythema migrans) with or without minor symptoms (e.g., mild fever, aches, fatigue, malaise, headache, regional adenopathy)
    2) Stage 2: musculoskeletal manifestations (e.g., oligoarthritis of large joints [usually the knee]); may have months of remission then recurrence; limp may occur; severe fatigue and sore throat may be present
    3) Stage 3: chronic arthritis, chronic cutaneous and neurologic sequelae, subacute encephalopathy, cognitive deficits, disturbed mood, disturbed sleep, and fatigue
3. Rocky Mountain spotted fever
  a. *R. rickettsii* lives in dogs and rodents and can be spread by bird migration
  b. Transmission occurs by tick bite and usually requires 6 to 10 hours of attachment
  c. The spirochete enters its victim along with the saliva of the tick
  d. The spirochetes live and multiply inside the cells that line the small and medium-sized blood vessels; they can be found mostly in the cytoplasm or nuclei of these cells
  e. As the spirochetes multiply, they damage and eventually kill their host cells, which leads to blood seeping out of the cell and into adjacent tissues, which serves to spread the infection (CDC, 2005)
  f. Incubation period is 2 to 14 days, with an average of 5 to 7 days

Clinical presentation

1. Subjective
   a. Exposure to tick or tick bite
   b. Lyme disease
      1) Usually presents with headache and stiff neck
      2) Viral illness symptoms: fever, chills, fatigue, swollen and tender lymph nodes, and joint and muscle pain
   c. Rocky Mountain spotted fever
      1) Early:
         a) Sudden onset of fever and chills
         b) Pain: headache and muscle aches
         c) Anorexia, nausea, and vomiting
      2) Late:
         a) Abdominal pain, abdominal distention, and diarrhea
         b) Joint pain
2. Objective
   a. A tick may be present on the patient
   b. Lyme disease
      1) Erythema migrans is the hallmark; this is an annular enlarging red rash with a clear central area (i.e., bull's-eye rash)
      2) Lymphadenopathy or lymphocytoma
      3) Diffuse erythema and urticaria
      4) Splenomegaly
      5) Conjunctivitis
      6) Keratitis
      7) Nerve palsies, cranial neuritis, or Bell palsy
      8) Motor or sensory radiculoneuritis
      9) Generalized scleroderma-like lesions
   c. Rocky Mountain spotted fever
      1) Rash that appears 2 to 5 days after fever
         a) Early: small, rose-colored, blanching maculae that become papules
         b) Seen on the arms, wrists, palms, ankles, and soles of the feet
         c) Later: a red, maculopapular rash that looks like petechiae that spreads to cover the entire body, including the palms and soles
      2) Hepatosplenomegaly with palpation
      3) Lymphadenopathy
      4) Meningismus: a state of meningeal irritation
      5) Myocarditis
      6) Altered level of consciousness (late sign)
3. Diagnostic
   a. Lyme disease: equivocal enzyme-linked immunoassay or immunofluorescent assay; if positive, follow up with a confirmatory Western blot
   b. Rocky Mountain spotted fever
      1) Rule out measles
      2) Weil-Felix test: a type of agglutination test in which a patient's serum is tested for agglutinins to the O antigens of certain rickettsial strains
      3) CBC count
         i) WBC: normal or decreased
         ii) Platelets: decreased
      4) Serum sodium: decreased

5) Liver function studies: elevated
6) Serology: indirect immunofluorescent assay looks for immunoglobulin G or M; however, this test is not usually used because it takes 7 to 10 days to obtain results

Collaborative management

1. Continue assessment
   a. ABCDs
   b. Vital signs: blood pressure, pulse, respiratory rate, and temperature
   c. Respiratory effort and excursion
   d. Oxygen saturations as indicated
   e. Cardiac rate and rhythm
   f. Pain and discomfort levels
   g. Accurate intake and output
   h. Serum electrolytes
   i. Level of consciousness
   j. Close monitoring for the progression of symptoms
2. Maintain airway, oxygenation, and ventilation
   a. Oxygen by nasal cannula at 2 to 6 L/minute as indicated to maintain an SpO_2 level of 95% unless contraindicated; for patients with COPD, use pulse oximetry to guide oxygen administration to an SpO_2 level of 90%
   b. Positioning or artificial airway to ensure a patent airway; suctioning as required
   c. Rapid-sequence intubation and mechanical ventilation if required
3. Maintain adequate circulation and perfusion
   a. IV access and fluids as prescribed
   b. Vasopressors as required to maintain perfusion
4. Prevent infection and sepsis
   a. Removal of the tick if present
      1) Grasp the tick firmly as close to the skin surface as possible with tweezers
      2) Pull upward with steady, even pressure, and ensure that you have removed the entire tick
      3) Do not damage the body of the tick as you are removing it
      4) Do not heat the tick with a match or other heat source because burns can occur
      5) Wash the bite site with soap and water
   b. Antimicrobials as indicated
      1) Lyme disease: doxycycline (Vibramycin), cefuroxime (Ceftin), or amoxicillin (Amoxil)
      2) Rocky Mountain spotted fever: doxycycline (Vibramycin)
5. Monitor for complications
   a. Lyme disease
      1) Neurologic problems (i.e., Bell palsy, headaches, poor coordination)
      2) Arthritis
   b. Rocky Mountain spotted fever
      1) Focal neurologic deficits
      2) Coma
      3) Gangrene of distal extremities and scrotum
      4) Renal failure
      5) Disseminated intravascular coagulation
      6) Shock

Evaluation

1. Patent airway, adequate oxygenation (i.e., normal Pao_2, Spo_2, Sao_2) and ventilation (i.e., normal $Paco_2$)
2. Absence of clinical indications of hypoperfusion
3. Absence of clinical indications of infection or sepsis
4. Alert and oriented with no neurologic deficit
5. Control of pain and discomfort

Typical disposition

1. If evaluation criteria met: discharge with instructions
   a. Importance of completing medication prescriptions
   b. General wound care instructions
   c. General precautions to avoid ticks
      1) Wear long pants and long-sleeved shirts when outside in tall grass or wooded areas
      2) Tuck pants into socks
      3) Use tick repellents
      4) Check regularly and thoroughly for ticks and promptly remove any attached ticks
      5) Wear closed-toe shoes
      6) Avoid areas in which ticks maybe found
   d. Follow up with primary care provider as directed
2. If evaluation criteria not met: admission

Hantavirus Infection

Definition: a viral infection that is spread by rodents

1. Two causative types of hantavirus
   a. Hantavirus causes hemorrhagic fever with renal syndrome, which is also known as *hantavirus disease*
   b. Sin Nombre virus (literally "unnamed virus" in Spanish) causes hantavirus pulmonary syndrome

Predisposing factors

1. Rodent bite
2. Food or water contaminated with rodent droppings or urine
3. Contact with dried rodent (e.g., deer mouse) droppings, which become aerosolized

Pathophysiology

1. Rodents shed the virus in their urine, droppings, and saliva
2. Virus is transmitted to people usually by air when they breathe
3. Hantavirus disease
   a. Multisystem damage occurs to capillaries and small-vessel walls, which results in vasodilation and congestion with hemorrhage
   b. Results in severe hypotension and oliguria, which may result in nephritis
4. Hantavirus pulmonary syndrome
   a. Basically a capillary leak syndrome in which there is widespread edema in the retroperitoneum, the pleura, and the lungs
   b. Endothelial cells in the lungs swell, which leads to interstitial pneumonitis
   c. Alveolae become fibrotic
   d. The spleen becomes engorged and infiltrated with blood cells
   e. In severe cases, the patient develops noncardiac pulmonary edema

Clinical presentation

1. Subjective
   a. Three phases (Table 12-6)
   b. Difficult to distinguish from upper respiratory infections
   c. Typical viral complaints
      1) Fatigue
      2) Fever and chills
      3) Muscle aches, usually in the back and legs
      4) Headaches
   d. Dizziness
   e. Nausea, vomiting, and diarrhea
   f. Dyspnea
2. Objective
   a. Tachycardia and tachypnea
   b. Elevated temperature

TABLE 12-6   Signs and Symptoms of Hantavirus Infection

Prodromal Phase	Cardiopulmonary Phase	Convalescent Phase
• Occurs within 1–4 weeks of exposure • Lasts 3–5 days • Symptoms are primarily gastrointestinal in nature: nausea, vomiting, and diarrhea • Other symptoms include headache, fever, and myalgia • Often misdiagnosed at this stage as a viral gastroenteritis	• Occurs after the prodromal phase • Lasts only 24–48 hr • Dyspnea • Nonproductive cough that becomes productive when pulmonary edema forms • Shock • Death may occur	• Occurs after the cardiopulmonary phase • Significant diuresis • Usually no sequelae if the patient survives the cardiopulmonary phase

From Cunha, B. A. (2009). Hantavirus pulmonary syndrome. Retrieved August 4, 2009, from http://emedicine.medscape.com/article/236425-overview

c. Breath sound changes: crackles or diminished breath sounds
d. Abdominal tenderness with palpitation
3. Diagnostic
   a. Serum blood for virus detection
      1) Immunoglobulins M and G: present
      2) Rapid immunoblot strip assay: positive
   b. CBC count with differential
      1) WBC count: increased with a left shift
      2) Atypical lymphocytes
      3) Hematocrit : increased
   c. aPTT increased with a normal fibrinogen level maybe seen
   d. Liver function studies: elevated
   e. Albumin: decreased in patients with pulmonary edema because the fluid leaking from the capillaries is rich in protein
   f. Lactic acid level: increased
   g. ABGs: hypoxemia and hypercapnia
   h. Chest radiography: pulmonary edema
   i. ECG: dysrhythmias may be present

Collaborative management
1. Continue assessment
   a. ABCDs
   b. Vital signs: blood pressure, pulse, respiratory rate, and temperature
   c. Respiratory effort and excursion
   d. Oxygen saturations as indicated
   e. Cardiac rate and rhythm
   f. Pain and discomfort levels
   g. Accurate intake and output
   h. Serum electrolytes
   i. Level of consciousness
   j. Close monitoring for the progression of symptoms
2. Maintain airway, oxygenation, and ventilation
   a. Oxygen by nasal cannula at 2 to 6 L/minute as indicated to maintain an SpO_2 level of 95% unless contraindicated; for patients with COPD, use pulse oximetry to guide oxygen administration to an SpO_2 level of 90%
   b. Positioning or artificial airway to ensure a patent airway; suctioning as required
   c. Rapid-sequence intubation and mechanical ventilation if required
3. Maintain adequate circulation and perfusion
   a. IV access and fluids as prescribed
   b. Vasopressors as required to maintain perfusion
   c. Antidysrhythmics as needed
   d. Foley catheter to monitor intake and output
4. Prevent the transmission of the virus: strict universal precautions
5. Treat infection and prevent sepsis
   a. Antimicrobials as prescribed
   b. Antipyretics and cooling methods to reduce fever
6. Monitor for complications
   a. Dysrhythmias
   b. Respiratory failure

c. Acute tubular necrosis and acute renal failure
d. Cardiopulmonary arrest

Evaluation
1. Patent airway, adequate oxygenation (i.e., normal PaO_2, SpO_2, SaO_2) and ventilation (i.e., normal $PaCO_2$)
2. Absence of clinical indications of hypoperfusion
3. Absence of clinical indications of respiratory distress
4. Absence of clinical indications of infection or sepsis
5. Alert and oriented with no neurologic deficit
6. Control of pain and discomfort

Typical disposition: admission

Plague
Definition: an infectious disease caused by the bacterium *Yersinia pestis* that can affect animals and humans; there are three types:
1. Bubonic: the most common of the three types
2. Pneumonic: a more virulent type that is less common than the bubonic type
3. Septicemic: this type usually occurs as a complication of the other two types when the plague multiplies within the blood stream; it is rarely seen otherwise, but it may result from a direct bite

Predisposing factors
1. Contact with vector, which is usually a rat flea (e.g., veterinarians)
2. Breathing air droplets from an infected person (i.e., pneumonic type)
3. Handling or eating plague-contaminated animals (i.e., septicemic type)

Pathophysiology
1. Transmitted through the bite of a vector (usually the rat flea), which was infected by its host; hosts are usually rats but can include other mammals, such as dogs, cats, camels, raccoons, squirrels, and chipmunks
2. Bubonic plague
   a. Infection enters the skin through a cutaneous lesion or a flea bite and travels through the lymphatic system
   b. The bacillus actually blocks the flea's esophagus, which leads to starvation
   c. The flea goes from host to host trying to find food; the flea deposits the bacillus in the skin of the host when the flea's esophagus distends and recoils
   d. The bacillus enters the host's lymphatic system, where it produces the bubo (i.e., an inflamed, necrotic, hemorrhagic lymph node)
   e. Eventually the bacteria enter the bloodstream, which leads to multiorgan involvement and sepsis
   f. Plague kills about half of infected patients within 3 to 7 days without treatment; the mortality rate is 1% to 15% for treated cases but 40% to 60% for untreated cases

3. Pneumonic plague
   a. Occurs via direct inhalation of the bacillus either through close contact with an infected person or through weaponization; the incubation period is 1 to 3 days
   b. When the bacteria enter the lungs, they rapidly spread to the bloodstream and are highly contagious
   c. Rapidly progressive, multilobar bronchopneumonia develops and leads to sepsis
   d. Mortality rate is 40% if treated, 100% if not treated
4. Septicemic plague
   a. Usually secondary to bubonic or pneumonic plague but may be caused by bacillus invading the bloodstream directly without entering the lymphatic system
   b. It is thought that these cases result from bites to the oral and pharyngeal cavities because of their vascularity; the incubation period is 1 to 4 days
   c. Mortality rate is 100% if not treated within 24 hours of infection

Clinical presentation
1. Subjective
   a. History of exposure to someone with plague or exposure to a possible host (e.g., prairie dogs in the western and midwestern United States)
   b. Fever and chills
   c. Malaise and weakness
   d. Sore throat
   e. Headache
   f. Gastrointestinal complaints: nausea, vomiting, diarrhea or constipation, and abdominal pain; may have black or tarry stools
2. Objective
   a. Bubos (i.e., the inflamed lymph nodes caused by *Y. pestis*): inguinal nodes are most commonly affected
   b. Cough: may have hemoptysis
   c. Breath sound changes: diffuse crackles with pneumonic plague
   d. Abdominal tenderness to palpation
   e. Nuchal rigidity
   f. Ecchymosis, petechiae, and gangrene with septicemic plague
   g. Change in level of consciousness or seizures
   h. Clinical indications of shock
3. Diagnostic
   a. WBC: increased with a left shift
   b. Urine dip: positive for *Y. pestis*
   c. Urinalysis: hematuria, red blood cell casts, and proteinuria
   d. Cultures and gram staining: positive for *Y. pestis;* cultures can be taken of blood, bubo aspirate, and sputum
   e. Florescent antibody stains and antibody titers are available at some labs and at the CDC

Collaborative management
1. Continue assessment
   a. ABCDs
   b. Vital signs: blood pressure, pulse, respiratory rate, and temperature
   c. Respiratory effort and excursion
   d. Oxygen saturations as indicated
   e. Cardiac rate and rhythm
   f. Pain and discomfort levels
   g. Accurate intake and output
   h. Serum electrolytes
   i. Level of consciousness
   j. Close monitoring for the progression of symptoms
2. Maintain airway, oxygenation, and ventilation
   a. Oxygen by nasal cannula at 2 to 6 L/minute as indicated to maintain an SpO_2 level of 95% unless contraindicated; for patients with COPD, use pulse oximetry to guide oxygen administration to an SpO_2 level of 90%
   b. Positioning or artificial airway to ensure a patent airway; suctioning as required
   c. Rapid-sequence intubation and mechanical ventilation if required
3. Maintain adequate circulation and perfusion
   a. IV access and fluids as prescribed
   b. Antidysrhythmic medications as prescribed
   c. Vasopressors if needed to maintain blood pressure
4. Treat infection and prevent sepsis
   a. Prevention of the spread of infection
      1) Strict respiratory and contact isolation are required
      2) Prompt reporting to the CDC
   b. Antibiotics (e.g., gentamicin [Garamycin], streptomycin [Kantrex], doxycycline [Vibramycin], ciprofloxacin [Cipro], co-trimoxazole [Bactrim]) as prescribed; close contacts of infected person should be treated prophylactically
5. Monitor for complications
   a. Meningitis
   b. Sepsis or septic shock
   c. Disseminated intravascular coagulation
   d. Necrosis of the skin
   e. Pericarditis
   f. Death

Evaluation
1. Patent airway, adequate oxygenation (i.e., normal Pao_2, Spo_2, Sao_2) and ventilation (i.e., normal $Paco_2$)
2. Absence of clinical indications of hypoperfusion
3. Absence of clinical indications of respiratory distress
4. Absence of clinical indications of infection or sepsis
5. Alert and oriented with no neurologic deficit
6. Control of pain and discomfort

Typical disposition: admission to the critical care unit; strict isolation must be maintained in the ED and during transport for admission

Cat-Scratch Fever
Definition: an infection caused by the bacterium *Bartonella henselae*
Predisposing factors
1. Exposure to an infected cat via scratches, bites, or saliva
2. Contact with another animal that has been infected

Pathophysiology

1. Cats are a primary host
2. Typically the inoculation of pathogen occurs through the skin at site of a cat scratch; other animals (e.g., monkeys) can also be vectors
3. After inoculation via the scratch occurs, an acute inflammatory reaction occurs the site of the bite or scratch, and the bacteria spreads to the regional lymph nodes
4. Splenomegaly occurs
5. The infection is benign and self-limiting unless the person is immunosuppressed

Clinical presentation

1. Subjective
   a. History of a bite or scratch from a cat about 2 to 3 weeks before the onset of the lymphadenopathy
   b. Fever and sore throat
   c. Anorexia and weight loss
   d. Abdominal pain
   e. Fatigue and weakness
   f. Headache
   g. Arthralgia
2. Objective
   a. Elevated temperature
   b. Papule or pustule at the site of injury; maculopapular rash
   c. Unilateral tender regional lymphadenopathy
   d. Spleen may be palpable
   e. Abdominal tenderness with palpation
   f. Atypical presentation can include altered mental status, prolonged fever, vision loss, seizures, transverse myelitis, encephalitis, and joint pain
3. Diagnostic
   a. Usually based on history and presentation
   b. Polymerase chain reaction assay
   c. Aspiration of infected joint fluid for microscopy

Collaborative management

1. Continue assessment
   a. ABCDs
   b. Vital signs: blood pressure, pulse, respiratory rate, and temperature
   c. Oxygen saturation levels as indicated
   d. Pain and discomfort levels
   e. Accurate intake and output
   f. Serum electrolytes
   g. Level of consciousness
   h. Close monitoring for the progression of symptoms
2. Maintain airway, oxygenation, and ventilation
   a. Oxygen by nasal cannula at 2 to 6 L/minute as indicated to maintain an SpO_2 level of 95% unless contraindicated; for patients with COPD, use pulse oximetry to guide oxygen administration to an SpO_2 level of 90%
   b. Positioning or artificial airway to ensure a patent airway; suctioning as required
3. Maintain adequate circulation and perfusion; IV access and fluids as prescribed

4. Treat infection and prevent sepsis
   a. Antibiotics as prescribed
      1) Painful lymph nodes in a healthy person: azithromycin (Zithromax)
      2) Immunocompromised individuals: trimethoprim-sulfamethoxazole (Bactrim DS), gentamicin (Garamycin), ciprofloxacin (Cipro), and rifampin (Rifadin)
   b. Wound cleansing
   c. Antipyretics and cooling methods to reduce fever if indicated
5. Control pain and discomfort: analgesics as prescribed
6. Monitor for complications
   a. Sepsis
   b. In immunocompromised patients, serious sequelae are possible
      1) Seizures
      2) Encephalitis
      3) Severe systemic illness

Evaluation

1. Patent airway, adequate oxygenation (i.e., normal PaO_2, SpO_2, SaO_2) and ventilation (i.e., normal $PaCO_2$)
2. Absence of clinical indications of hypoperfusion
3. Absence of clinical indications of infection or sepsis
4. Alert and oriented with no neurologic deficit
5. Control of pain and discomfort

Typical disposition

1. If evaluation criteria met: discharge with instructions
   a. General wound care
   b. Importance of completing medication prescriptions
   c. Follow up with primary care provider as instructed
2. If evaluation criteria not met (most likely in patients with compromised immune systems): admission

Snake Bites

Definition: bites from snakes and particularly bites from venomous snakes

1. Types of venomous snakes found in the United States
   a. Crotalidae (also called pit vipers): copperheads, cottonmouths, rattlesnakes, and water moccasins
      1) Pit vipers have a triangular head with a pit between their eyes and nostrils
      2) Pupils are like those of a cat's eye
      3) Two fangs leave characteristic fang marks with or without accessory teeth marks when they bite
   b. Elapidae: coral snakes
      1) Coral snakes have a black head and a slender body with characteristic black, red, and yellow bands
      2) Eyes are black and round
      3) Fangs are fixed and leave scratch marks or tiny puncture marks when they bite

Predisposing factors

1. Handling, teasing, or playing with snakes
2. Hiking

3. Camping
4. Outdoor activities

Pathophysiology

1. Snake venom contains proteins that are cardiotoxic, neurotoxic, and hemolytic
2. Reactions vary from mild local irritation to severe, overwhelming, and life-threatening systemic reactions

Clinical presentation

1. Subjective
   a. History of snake bite
   b. Pain at the site of the bite
   c. Metallic taste in the mouth
   d. Dyspnea
   e. Nausea and vomiting
   f. Paresthesias and loss of limb function
   g. Syncope
2. Objective
   a. Local edema and redness at the site of the bite; tissue necrosis may occur later
   b. Petechiae or bruising at the site
   c. Vital sign changes: tachycardia and tachypnea; hypertension initially with hypotension later
   d. Diaphoresis
   e. Pupil and eye changes: constriction, ptosis, and diplopia
   f. Muscle twitching
   g. Excess salivation
   h. Difficulty speaking
   i. Confusion
   j. Hematochezia and other signs of bleeding
   k. Paralysis
3. Diagnostic
   a. Serum chemistries: BUN, creatinine, glucose, and electrolytes may be abnormal
   b. WBC: may be increased
   c. Clotting panel: may show coagulopathy
   d. Typing and cross-matching
   e. D-dimer
   f. Other diagnostics on the basis of presentation

Collaborative management

1. Continue assessment
   a. ABCDs
   b. Vital signs: blood pressure, pulse, respiratory rate, and temperature
   c. Respiratory effort and excursion
   d. Oxygen saturations as indicated
   e. Cardiac rate and rhythm
   f. Pain and discomfort levels
   g. Accurate intake and output
   h. Serum electrolytes
   i. Level of consciousness
   j. Close monitoring for the progression of symptoms
2. Maintain airway, oxygenation, and ventilation
   a. Oxygen by nasal cannula at 2 to 6 L/minute as indicated to maintain an SpO_2 level of 95% unless contraindicated; for patients with COPD, use pulse oximetry to guide oxygen administration to an SpO_2 level of 90%
   b. Positioning or artificial airway to ensure a patent airway; suctioning as required
   c. Rapid-sequence intubation and mechanical ventilation if required
3. Maintain adequate circulation and perfusion
   a. IV access and fluids as prescribed
   b. Antidysrhythmics as prescribed
   c. Vasopressors if required to maintain blood pressure
4. Prevent or slow the spread of venom
   a. Removal of constrictive clothing and jewelry
   b. Immobilization of the extremity no higher than the level of the heart to slow envenomation
   c. Avoidance of factors (e.g., caffeine, nicotine) that cause an increase in the heart or metabolic rate)
   d. Ice or tourniquets should not be used
5. Provide wound care and prevent infection or sepsis
   a. Antibiotics as indicated
   b. Wound care: wash with soap and water; a dressing is not usually required
   c. Tetanus prophylaxis as needed
6. Prepare and administer antivenin for patients with severe or progressive symptoms as prescribed
   a. Antivenin type is specific, depending on the type of snake
      1) CroFab (Crotalidae antivenom): antivenin for pit vipers; most commonly available in ED
         a) Administered in large doses (i.e., 5–20 vials)
         b) May repeat dose at 6, 12, and 18 hours after bite occurs
         c) Requires close monitoring for anaphylaxis; there is a potential for life-threatening reactions
7. Relieve pain and discomfort
   a. Non-narcotic analgesics
      1) Acetaminophen (Tylenol) for pain
      2) Avoidance of aspirin and nonsteroidal anti-inflammatory drugs because of the increased risk for bleeding
   b. Narcotics (e.g., acetaminophen with codeine [Tylenol #3 or #4], morphine) as prescribed
8. Monitor for complications
   a. Pulmonary edema
   b. Coagulopathies, hemorrhage, and shock
   c. Renal failure
   d. Seizures
   e. Paralysis

Evaluation

1. Patent airway, adequate oxygenation (i.e., normal PaO_2, SpO_2, SaO_2) and ventilation (i.e., normal $PaCO_2$)
2. Absence of clinical indications of respiratory compromise
3. Absence of clinical indications of hypoperfusion
4. Absence of clinical indications of infection/sepsis
5. Alert and oriented with no neurologic deficit
6. Control of pain and discomfort

Typical disposition

1. If evaluation criteria met: discharge with instructions for follow up after observation in the ED
   a. Indications to return for evaluation: increased redness or swelling
   b. Preventive measures
      1) Wear boots or high-top shoes when hiking or in areas of tall grass
      2) Know the types of snakes that are likely to be encountered in the camping area
2. If evaluation criteria not met or if treated with antivenin: admission

Diving Emergencies

Definitions

1. Arterial gas embolism: a complication that occurs during diving in which gas bubbles form in the arterial circulation and obstruct blood flow; it has a sudden onset and usually occurs as soon as the diver resurfaces
2. Decompression sickness: a complication that occurs during diving in which nitrogen is not able to be reabsorbed during a rapid ascent; this causes bubbles to form, and these enter the joints, the pulmonary system, the central nervous system, and possibly the skin

Predisposing factors

1. Smoking
2. Obesity
3. Flying soon after diving
4. Environmental factors
   a. Cold water can cause vasoconstriction, which prevents nitrogen offloading
   b. Excessive exercise or work can have a vacuum effect on the tendons and cause actual gas pockets
   c. Diving in turbulent waters
   d. Heated diving suits can increase the chance of dehydration, which will lead to decompression symptoms and problems
5. Rapid ascent while holding the breath, which causes barotrauma
6. Diving without stopping to rest and let the body adjust to pressure changes

Pathophysiology

1. Arterial gas embolism
   a. Overinflation of the lungs occurs, which causes free gas to enter into the pulmonary vessels; this is followed by the embolization of the cerebral vessels
   b. Air enters either the pulmonary arterial circulation by way of an alveoli rupture or the arterial circulation itself in severe decompression sickness
2. Decompression sickness as a result of diving
   a. Gases in the hollow spaces and the viscous organs and those dissolved in the blood are subject to pressure changes
   b. Mechanisms by which barometric pressure affects the body during diving follow Henry's gas law
      1) Gas dissolved in the blood is released, which results in abnormal tissue concentrations of various gases (see Chapter 15 for more information about gas laws)
   c. Nitrogen dissolved in the blood and tissues by high pressure comes out of solution and forms bubbles as pressure decreases
   d. These bubbles can form in the joints, the lungs, the central nervous system, and under the skin
   e. Gas bubbles accumulate in joint spaces as a result of local negative pressure created by movement and peripheral circulation
   f. When bubbles form in the blood, they may activate early phase reactants that are vasoactive and that promote blood coagulation
3. Decompression sickness
   a. The "creeps": mottled to diffuse rash and sensation as though tiny insects are moving underneath the skin; thought to be caused by tiny bubbles of gas evolving under the skin
   b. The "bends": pain located around or near the articulating joints; this pain immobilizes the affected joint and descends
   c. The "chokes": nitrogen gas bubbles in the blood vessels of the lungs cause deep, sharp pain and a burning sensation under the sternum
   d. The "staggers": central nervous system symptoms occur, including headache, numbness, vertigo, and staggering about

Clinical presentation

1. Arterial gas embolism
   a. Subjective
      1) History of diving or another precipitating factor
      2) Chest pain or tightness
      3) Vertigo
      4) Paresthesias
   b. Objective
      1) Cyanosis
      2) Focal pallor of the tongue
      3) Sensory or motor deficits
      4) Altered level of consciousness
      5) Hematuria
      6) Seizures
      7) Apnea
   c. Diagnostic
      1) Urine dip: positive for blood and protein
      2) Echocardiography: air in the cardiac chambers
      3) Ventilation–perfusion scan: probable pulmonary emboli
      4) CT
         a) Chest: local lung injury or hemorrhage
         b) Head: intravascular gas and diffuse edema
2. Decompression sickness
   a. Subjective
      1) Tingling under skin (creeps)
      2) Pain in the joints (bends)
         a) Deep massaging of muscles toward the affected joint increases pain because it

moves nitrogen bubbles toward the joint (ENA, 2007)

    b) Inflating a blood-pressure cuff over the painful area to ≥150 mm Hg will decrease pain because it pushes the nitrogen bubbles away from the area (ENA, 2007)

   3) Chest pain or tightness, dyspnea, or burning in the chest (chokes)

   4) Vertigo, paresthesias, and headache (staggers)

  b. Objective

   1) Mottled to diffuse rash (creeps)

   2) Tenderness in affected joint (bends)

   3) May be able to palpate subcutaneous emphysema in the sternal area

   4) Altered level of consciousness

  c. Diagnostic

   1) No specific test for decompression sickness

   2) Chest radiography: to evaluate for pressure-related injuries (e.g., pneumothorax)

   3) CT to rule out causes of neurologic symptoms

Collaborative management

1. Continue assessment
   a. ABCDs
   b. Vital signs: blood pressure, pulse, respiratory rate, and temperature
   c. Respiratory effort and excursion
   d. Oxygen saturations as indicated
   e. Cardiac rate and rhythm
   f. Pain and discomfort levels
   g. Accurate intake and output
   h. Level of consciousness
   i. Close monitoring for the progression of symptoms
2. Maintain airway, oxygenation, and ventilation
   a. Oxygen by nasal cannula at 2 to 6 L/minute as indicated to maintain an SpO_2 level of 95% unless contraindicated; for patients with COPD, use pulse oximetry to guide oxygen administration to an SpO_2 level of 90%
   b. Positioning or artificial airway to ensure a patent airway; suctioning as required
   c. Rapid-sequence intubation and mechanical ventilation if required
   d. Needle decompression if pneumothorax is present or suspected
3. Maintain adequate circulation and perfusion
   a. IV access and fluids; crystalloids to maintain a moderate urine output that will help to flush out nitrogen
   b. Aspirin for platelet aggregation inhibition; rule out possibility of active bleeding before the initiation of aspirin
4. Control pain and discomfort
   a. Antiemetics as indicated
   b. Non-narcotic analgesics are used to avoid further central nervous system depression
5. Prepare the patient and assist with procedures as indicated

  a. Positioning: supine on left side
  b. Foley catheter and nasogastric tube as prescribed
  c. Hyperbaric oxygen chamber as indicated; recompression rapidly alleviates symptoms
  d. Heliox (i.e., a helium and oxygen mixture with helium replacing nitrogen) as prescribed for decompression sickness

6. Monitor for complications
   a. Respiratory depression
   b. Barotraumas
   c. Myocardial necrosis or other ischemic injuries
   d. Residual paralysis
   e. Dysbaric osteonecrosis: a form of avascular necrosis
   f. Seizures

Evaluation

1. Patent airway, adequate oxygenation (i.e., normal PaO_2, SpO_2, SaO_2) and ventilation (i.e., normal $PaCO_2$)
2. Absence of clinical indications of respiratory distress
3. Absence of clinical indications of hypoperfusion
4. Alert and oriented with no neurologic deficit
5. Control of pain and discomfort

Typical disposition: admission

1. If hyperbaric oxygen is not available, prepare the patient for transfer to a facility with hyperbaric oxygen as indicated

Burns

Definition: tissue injury that occurs as a result of exposure to a burning process

1. Types of burns include thermal, chemical, electrical, and radiation
2. Smoke and inhalation injuries are discussed in the pulmonary chapter (see Chapter 5)
3. The severity of a burn is determined by the type of burn, the extent of tissue involvement, the depth and location of the burn, and the patient's health status

Predisposing factors

1. Occupational: working with tar, chemicals, heated metal, steam, fuels, fertilizers, or electricity
2. Developmental: poor supervision of children who can play with matches, pull pots off of the stove, and so on
3. Exposure to household hazards (e.g., hot water, grills, space heaters, frayed electrical cords)
4. Intentional: suicide or homicide
5. Firefighters and rescue workers

Pathophysiology

1. Thermal
   a. The burning process occurs in three distinct zones
      1) Zone of coagulation: tissue has become necrotic and has died or will die
      2) Zone of stasis: surrounds the zone of coagulation and consists of tissue with capillary occlusion, decreased perfusion, and edema; regeneration is possible if treated early

3) Zone of hyperemia: surrounds the zone of stasis; has signs of the inflammatory response, such as increased blood flow and redness
b. The inflammatory process is initiated and biochemical mediators are released, including vasoactive substances
c. Vasoactive substances lead to changes in the permeability of the capillary; the capillaries become "leaky"
d. Hyperemia increases pressure within the capillaries, thus further forcing proteins and fluids out; the patient becomes severely fluid depleted despite the appearance of edema
e. Other inflammatory mediators include the following:
   1) Histamine: causes vasodilation and increased capillary permeability
   2) Prostaglandins: causes vasodilation and increased permeability; thromboxane A2 causes platelet aggregation
   3) Leukotrienes and cytokines: propagate the inflammatory process
   4) Bradykinin: leads to vasodilation
   5) Oxygen free radicals: damage the endothelial cells of the smaller vessels
f. The result is hemoconcentration, increased blood viscosity, increased peripheral vascular resistance, and a higher percentage of red blood cells in the serum (despite their absolute numbers being decreased)
g. The patient also becomes hypermetabolic as a result of the effects of catecholamines and neurohormones
h. Hypoxemia and asphyxiation occur when victims are in an enclosed space as the fire uses up all the oxygen
i. Carbon monoxide poisoning can also occur
j. Pulmonary injury can occur as a result of the inhalation of toxic fumes created from the byproducts of incomplete combustion

2. Specific to electrical burns
a. Damage depends on the voltage, the type of current, the source, and the duration of contact
   1) Voltage: low-voltage (<1000 watts) and high-voltage (>1000 watts) burns occur
   2) Type of current
      a) Alternating current changes direction and produces more explosive wounds
      b) Direct current moves in one direction and produces a more discrete exit wound
b. Electricity enters the body and travels along the path of least resistance, damaging organs and tissues in its path and making it difficult to determine the true extent of the injury
   1) Injury becomes more significant as the voltage increases
   2) Current follows the path of least resistance and collects at a grounding site
      a) Passing through the head and thorax will affect the heart and the respiratory center

c. Direct contact burns occur when the person becomes part of the circuit
   1) Appears to be a crush-like injury
   2) The sizes of the entrance and exit wounds are not good indicators of the amount of internal damage
d. Arc burns occur when current leaves body; temperatures may reach 3000 to 20,000°F
e. Lightning strike: a type of direct current electrical injury
   1) The intensity is greater than that of electrical exposure, but the duration is much shorter; the burns are less severe than those that occur with electrical injuries
   2) Serious injury is a result of the paralysis of the respiratory center causing temporary respiratory arrest
   3) Only reverse triage situation: treat those who appear dead first because they are usually in respiratory arrest; if cardiac arrest occurs, it is ventricular fibrillation, and defibrillation usually restores the normal rhythm
f. Consequences
   1) Rhabdomyolysis can occur as a result of damaged muscles and may result in myoglobinuria and acute renal failure (ENA, 2007)
   2) Damage to blood vessels can include vascular disruption, thrombi, or hemorrhage
   3) May also cause long-bone fractures, dysrhythmias, metabolic acidosis, and cardiac arrest

3. Specific to chemical burns
a. Severity is related to several factors: the pH of the agent, the concentration of the agent, the length of contact time, the volume of the offending agent, and the physical form of the agent (Cox, 2008)
b. Acids produce a coagulation necrosis; this occurs by protein denaturing, which causes eschar to form and which limits the penetration of the acid
c. Alkalis cause liquefaction necrosis, which causes a burn that is deeper and more severe
   1) Proteins are denatured and the saponification of fats occurs, which is how the burn can penetrate deep into tissue
   2) Hydrofluoric acid produces a liquefaction necrosis (Cox, 2008)
d. In concentrated forms, acids and bases can generate significant heat when diluted, thereby causing significant thermal and caustic injury
e. Ocular chemical burns can result in the opacification of the cornea and a complete loss of vision
f. Esophageal and gastric chemical burns can result in stricture formation
g. Dermal chemical burns can result in significant scarring

Clinical presentation
1. Subjective
   a. History of exposure: mechanism, time of burn, and treatment before arrival

b. Pain; with severe burns, there may be no pain, because the nerve endings have been damaged

c. Dyspnea, especially if smoke inhalation has occurred

d. Complaints of other injuries

2. Objective

a. Tachycardia and hypotension

b. Airway changes

   1) Carbonaceous sputum

   2) Singed facial hair

   3) Face, neck, or oropharynx burns

   4) Blisters in the oral cavity or the nares

c. Respiratory distress

   1) Stridor

   2) Breath sound changes: crackles

d. Change in level of consciousness

e. Burn surface area: use the rule of nines or the rule of palms for estimating the total body surface area (TBSA) that was burned

   1) Rule of nines: 9% head, 18% anterior trunk, 18% posterior trunk, 9% each upper extremity, 18% each lower extremity, and 1% genitalia (Figure 12-3)

   2) Rule of palms: the palm of the patient's hand equals 1% TBSA for every time you can put the palm over the burned area; this is used mostly with pediatric patients or for irregular burns

   3) Other charts (e.g., Lund and Browder) are available for calculating TBSA and fluid requirements, but they are not used routinely in the ED, because you need the actual chart in front of you to do the calculations

f. Depth of burn (Table 12-7 and Figure 12-4)

g. Location of burn

   1) Special problems are related to burns in these areas

      a) Face, including the eyes and ears

      b) Neck

      c) Circumferential around the extremities or the trunk

      d) Hands and feet

      e) Over the joints

      f) Perineum

3. Diagnostic

a. ABGs: respiratory acidosis and metabolic acidosis

b. Carboxyhemoglobin level: >10% significant

c. Typing and cross-matching: to prepare for potential blood transfusion requirement

d. Coagulation panel: to assess for any coagulopathy

e. Urine

   1) Screen for drugs

   2) Assess for myoglobinuria or hematuria

f. Radiology

   1) Chest radiography: to assess for changes related to smoke inhalation or acute respiratory distress syndrome

   2) Cervical spine and other radiographs related to history and clinical presentation

g. ECG: may have dysrhythmias

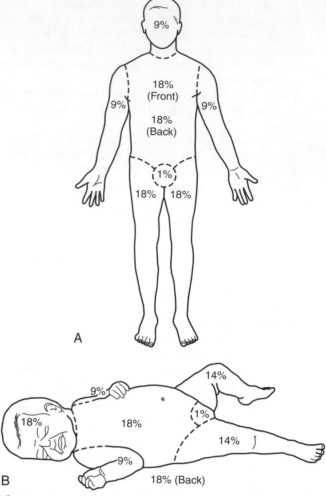

Figure 12-3 Rule of nines: percentages of total body surface area. A, Adult. B, Infant. (From the Emergency Nurses Association [2005]. *Sheehy's manual of emergency care* [6th ed.] St. Louis: Mosby, p. 765.)

Collaborative management

1. Continue assessment

a. ABCDs

b. Vital signs: blood pressure, pulse, respiratory rate, and temperature

c. Respiratory effort and excursion

d. Oxygen saturations as indicated

e. Cardiac rate and rhythm

f. Pain and discomfort levels

g. Accurate intake and output

h. Neurovascular status distal to burn area

i. Level of consciousness

j. Close monitoring for the progression of symptoms

2. Stop the burning process (this is the first priority if active burning is occurring)

a. Removal of clothing and jewelry

b. Logrolling of patient to check for smoldering clothing under the patient

c. Cool areas immediately

TABLE 12-7   Depth of Burn

	Superficial Partial Thickness	Deeper Partial Thickness	Full Thickness
Previously called	First degree	Second degree	Third and fourth degree
Depth	• Epidermis	• Epidermis and the upper layers of the dermis	• All of the layers of the skin and into the subcutaneous tissue (third degree); may even be into the muscle or bone (fourth degree) • All skin appendages (e.g., hair follicles, sweat glands, sebaceous glands) are destroyed
Skin appearance	• Pink or red • Blanches with pressure • Little or no edema • Dry and intact • May be small blisters	• Red • Blanches with pressure • Edematous • Wet, weeping, and shiny surface • Fluid-filled blisters	• Deep red, brown, black, or white leathery appearance • Edematous • Exposed subcutaneous layer may be visible • Does not blanch to pressure • Thrombosed blood vessels appear as brownish streaks • Sunken as a result of the loss of underlying fat or muscle
Pain	• Painful at first but decreases with cooling; itches later	• Very painful • Extremely sensitive to touch, temperature, and air currents	• Complete superficial anesthesia; deep pain (e.g. ischemia, inflammation) is intact
Healing time	• <1 week	• 1 week–1 month	• > 1 month
Healing process	• Heals spontaneously without scarring	• May heal spontaneously • If it converts to a full-thickness burn, may require skin grafting	• If < 4 cm in diameter granulation and migration of healthy epithelium from wound edges occur; grafting is required for wounds ≥ 4 cm

From: Dennison, R. D. (2007). *Pass CCRN!* (2nd ed.). St. Louis: Mosby.

    d. If a tar burn:
      1) Cool the tar with cool water and then cover with a tar solvent, mineral oil, or Vaseline
      2) Gently loosen the tar off of the skin
      3) Treat the underlying burns as thermal burns
    e. If a chemical burn:
      1) Remove contaminated clothing
      2) Neutralize or dilute chemicals
        a) Dry chemicals: brush affected area off and then flush with large amounts of saline
        b) Wet chemicals: flush with copious amounts of saline
      3) Flush the eyes for ≥15 minutes for acids and for ≥1 hour for alkalis (see Chapter 10)
3. Maintain airway, oxygenation, and ventilation
    a. Oxygen by nasal cannula at 2 to 6 L/minute as indicated to maintain an SpO_2 level of 95% unless contraindicated; for patients with COPD, use pulse oximetry to guide oxygen administration to an SpO_2 level of 90%
      1) Humidification required
      2) If elevated carbon monoxide: 100% oxygen by nonrebreather mask; hyperbaric oxygenation may be required, depending on carbon monoxide levels
    b. Coughing should be encouraged to expel mucus and soot if the patient is capable of effective coughing
    c. Positioning or artificial airway to ensure a patent airway; suctioning as required
      1) Close monitoring for delayed airway obstruction for 24 to 48 hours as a result of progressive swelling; suspect this condition if the patient was burned in a confined space, sustained a facial burn or singed facial hair, has charring or carbon particles in the oropharynx, expels carbonaceous sputum, or has circumferential burns of trunk (especially with thick eschar)
      2) Elective intubation with the use of rapid-sequence intubation may be performed if the patient has airway edema before the airway becomes obstructed; cricothyrotomy may be necessary
    d. Mechanical ventilation with positive end-expiratory pressure may be required to maintain alveolar ventilation
    e. Pharmacologic agents

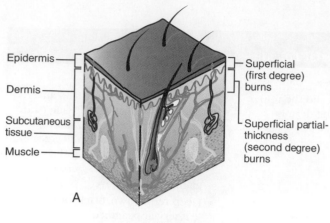

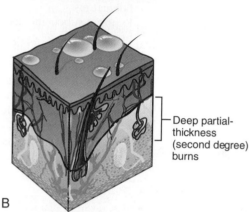

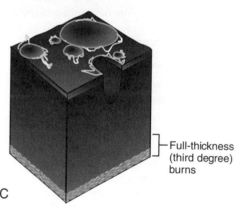

Figure 12-4 Burn depth. (From Carlson, K. K. [Ed.]. [2009]. *AACN Advanced Critical Care Nursing.* St. Louis: Saunders.)

1) Racemic epinephrine for upper airway obstruction
2) Bronchodilators for lower airway obstruction
4. Maintain adequate circulation and perfusion
   a. IV access with two large-bore (14- or 16-gauge) catheters
     1) May be inserted through burn tissue if necessary
     2) Insertion in lower extremities should be avoided
   b. Warmed lactated Ringer solution or normal saline 0.9%

1) Determine the volume with the use of the Parkland formula for burn resuscitation (Box 12-1):
   a) Adult formula: 2–4 ml × kg × % TBSA = Total fluid needed for 24 hours
   b) Pediatric formula: 3–4 ml × kg × % TBSA = Total fluid needed for 24 hours
2) Give half of the fluid volume during the first 8 hours after the burn; note that the first 8 hours starts from the time of the initial burn rather than from the time that the patient arrived in the ED
3) Give the other half over the remaining 16 hours
  c. Foley catheter to monitor output and assess the color of urine
   1) Use of urine output to gauge the adequacy of fluid resuscitation
     a) Goal urine output
       i) 1 ml/kg/hour for adults and for children who weigh >30 kg
       ii) 1 to 2 ml/kg/hour for children who weigh <30 kg
   2) Monitor urine output for myoglobinuria
     a) Urine will appear dark red or brown
     b) Intravenous fluids at a rate to maintain a urine output of ≥100 ml/hour if indications of myoglobinuria present
     c) Sodium bicarbonate as prescribed to facilitate the excretion of myoglobin

---

BOX 12-1 Fluid Resuscitation Calculation Example

- An adult patient was burned at noon and arrives to the ED at 3 pm. The first half of the fluid requirement will need to be completed by 8 pm.
- Do not forget to subtract any fluid given by prehospital personnel before the patient arrived at the ED.
- The patient weighs 76 kg and has a burn that covers 35% of the total body surface area (TBSA).
- To calculate the fluid requirement for the first 24 hours: 4 (from the Parkland formula) × 76 kg × 35 TBSA = 10,640 ml. Do not convert the TBSA percentage (i.e., 35%) to a decimal number.
- To calculate the fluid requirement for the first, second, and third 8-hour periods, do the following: If the patient need is 10,640 ml in 24 hours and half of that is to be given within the first 8 hours, give the patient 5320 ml. A quarter of the total amount (2660 ml) will then be given during each of the two following 8-hour periods of the first 24 hours for a total of 10,640 ml.
- If emergency medical personnel gave the patient 1000 ml of fluid, the remainder of the 5320 ml (i.e., 5320 − 1000 = 4320 ml) must be given before the end of the first 8 hours after the time of injury.
- Because the burn occurred at noon and it is now 3 p.m., that 4320 ml must be given within the next 5 hours, so the infusion should set at 864 ml/hour.

d. Antidysrhythmics as prescribed; dysrhythmias are more likely with electrical burns

e. Assistance with escharotomy as required for compartment syndrome related to swelling and compression

5. Relieve pain and discomfort
   a. Narcotics given intravenously for comfort and before painful procedures and treatments
   b. Temperature regulation with the use of blankets, a Bair Hugger, or radiant heat lamps as indicated
6. Prepare the patient and assist with procedures
7. Prevent infection and sepsis
   a. Wound care as directed
      1) Avoidance of ice directly on skin because this may cause further tissue damage and increase the risk of hypothermia
      2) Gentle cleansing of the wound with saline or a mild antiseptic solution
      3) Assistance with debridement as requested (this is not usually done in the ED)
      4) Topical medications as prescribed
         a) Water-based ointments to the head, face, neck, and perineum as prescribed (e.g., bacitracin-polymixin B [Polysporin])
         b) Silver sulfadiazine (Silvadene)
      5) Dressing
         a) Small burns (<10% TBSA): cool dampened saline dressing
         b) Large burns (>10% TBSA): dry dressing to decrease the risk of hypothermia or a sterile sheet applied over burned areas

b. Tetanus prophylaxis as indicated
8. Monitor for complications
   a. Airway compromise
   b. Respiratory distress
   c. Hypovolemic shock
   d. Infection or sepsis
   e. Compartment syndrome
   f. Rhabdomyolysis
   g. Cardiopulmonary arrest

Evaluation
1. Patent airway, adequate oxygenation (i.e., normal PaO_2, SpO_2, SaO_2) and ventilation (i.e., normal $PaCO_2$)
2. Absence of clinical indications of respiratory distress
3. Absence of clinical indicators of hypoperfusion
4. Absence of clinical indications of infection or sepsis
5. Alert and oriented with no neurologic deficit
6. Control of pain and discomfort

Typical disposition
1. If small burn (<10% TBSA) and evaluation criteria met: discharge with instructions
   a. Wound care
   b. Follow-up with primary care provider or plastic surgery as directed
2. If larger burn (>10% TBSA), electrical or chemical burn, or evaluation criteria not met: admission; may require admission to the critical care unit

LEARNING ACTIVITIES

1. DIRECTIONS: Complete the following crossword puzzle related to substance abuse, toxicologic, and environmental emergencies.

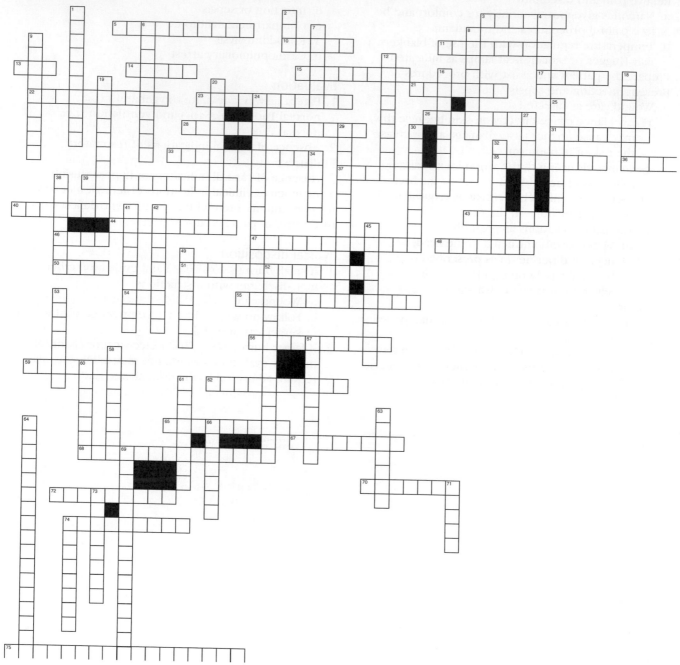

ACROSS

3. Pinpoint pupils
5. This type of syndrome may cause generalized seizures
10. The breath odor of an individual with choral hydrate intoxication smells like this
11. Drug used to treat the bradycardias (generic)
13. Carbon monoxide poisoning causes the skin to be very _____
14. This organ is most likely to be injured by acetaminophen overdose
15. Antidotes for opiates (generic)
17. This "gap" is increased with alcohol intoxication
21. Dilution is used rather than gastric lavage if this type of chemical is ingested
22. This is the greatest risk with the ingestion of petroleum distillates
23. This syndrome is a complication of frostbite, burns, and fractures
26. This antidote is given if the digoxin level is >10 ng/ml (trademarked name)
28. This blood-cleansing procedure is more effective than hemodialysis for plasma-protein–bound drugs

31. This drug may cause necrosis and perforation of the nasal septum (generic)
33. This type of consult should always be requested for patients with drug overdosage
35. This drug is given for elevated prothrombin time
36. This disease is associated with a bite from a deer tick infected with *Borrelia burgdorferi*
37. This type of fever is caused by the bacterium *Bartonella henselae* (two words)
39. Sedative–hypnotic toxidromes are usually caused by this type of drug
40. Drug intoxication in an effort to get attention is referred to as a suicide _____
43. This condition occurs when nitrogen gas bubbles are in the pulmonary blood vessels; associated with decompression
44. This type of hyperthermia is chemically induced
46. This heavy-metal poisoning may be found in metal workers

47. A blood-cleansing procedure that may be used to remove some drugs or toxins from the blood
48. This type of behavior is a danger to health-care staff; it may occur with the rapid reversal of sedating drugs
50. Hypothermia shifts the oxyhemoglobin dissociation curve to the _____, thus impairing oxygen delivery to the tissues
51. The affinity between hemoglobin and this substance is much greater than the affinity between hemoglobin and oxygen (two words)
54. This radiologic procedure may be used to identify the presence of radiopaque agents (abbrev)
55. The antidote for methemoglobinemia (generic; two words)
56. This antidote for benzodiazepines should not be given if the patient has also ingested tricyclic antidepressants
59. This drug can stimulate β-receptors even in the presence of β-blockade; used to treat β-blocker overdosage

62. This drug is used for malignant hyperthermia that occurs with some drug overdosages (generic)
65. A type of antidepressant that may cause torsades de pointes, especially at toxic levels
67. Bowel irrigation with this solution is used to treat overdosage with sustained-release drugs (trademarked name)
68. Medication that is given for shivering in a patient with hypothermia (generic)
70. This is the most common of the three types of plague
72. This calcium-channel blocker is most frequently used for cocaine-induced coronary artery spasms (generic)
74. Accidental exposure to a toxic substance
75. Hemoglobin that is saturated with carbon monoxide rather than oxygen

DOWN

1. This virus is spread by rodents
2. This dissociative agent is associated with violent behavior (abbrev)
4. Induced vomiting, which was previously stimulated by this drug, is no longer recommended, especially in the hospital setting (trademarked name)
6. This type of blood screening is done to determine which drugs have been ingested

7. A procedure that is used to flush a drug or toxin from the stomach; this is indicated if the patient arrives within 1 hour of the ingestion of most substances
8. Superficial frostbite (two words)
9. This therapy may be used to detoxify heavy-metal poisoning
12. A category of toxins that includes aerosol propellants, paint thinner, and glue
16. A reason that children are often exposed to toxic substances

18. This drug may be used intravenously to treat methanol or ethylene glycol intoxication
19. This type of overdose causes metabolic acidosis and respiratory alkalosis
20. An abnormal sensation that feels like insects running over or into the skin; it is associated with cocaine intoxication
24. The drug that is most often involved with intentional and unintentional drug overdose in the United States

25. The antidote for acetaminophen (Tylenol) (trademarked name)
27. A coma cocktail consists of oxygen, _____, thiamine, and naloxone (Narcan)
29. Ocular burns can result in this injury to the cornea
30. Dilated pupils
32. The usually intentional but possibly inadvertent exposure to toxic levels of a substance
34. This quality of the urine may be helpful to identify the drug consumed

38. A new antidote used for ethylene glycol intoxication (trademarked name)

41. This device may be required for the bradycardia seen with the overdosage of β-blockers or calcium-channel blockers

42. This is increased during stage 2 or 3 of acetaminophen overdose

45. This type of high-pressure oxygen therapy is used for the treatment of carbon monoxide poisoning

49. This is known as the "hug drug"

52. An antiemetic that is frequently used to treat acetaminophen overdose (generic)

53. Toxicity caused by this drug causes nystagmus, tremors, ataxia, seizures, and nephrogenic diabetes insipidus (generic)

57. This may occur when patients are warmed too rapidly

58. This osmotic laxative is added to the first dose of activated charcoal if multiple doses are going to be given

60. This heavy-metal poisoning may be seen in exterminators

61. This adsorbent agent is used to treat drug overdose

63. This electrolyte is given for calcium-channel blocker overdosage

64. A condition that may be caused by nitrates, nitrates, sulfa drugs, and local anesthetics

66. A toxin that may cause a bitter almond odor of the breath

69. Insecticides are frequently of this type, which causes a cholinergic effect

71. This mnemonic identifies decontamination products to consider when treating a patient with hydrocarbon poisoning

73. This B vitamin must be given with dextrose to malnourished patients to prevent Wernicke encephalopathy

74. This type of snake has cat-like pupils (two words)

2. DIRECTIONS: Match the toxicity with the specific antidote.

____ 1. Methemoglobinemia	a. Glucagon
____ 2. Cyanide	b. 100% oxygen or hyperbaric oxygen if possible
____ 3. Methanol	c. Digoxin Immune Fab (Digibind)
____ 4. Organophosphates	d. Fomepizole (Antizol)
____ 5. Carbon monoxide	e. Ethanol
____ 6. Acetaminophen	f. Methylene blue
____ 7. Benzodiazepines (e.g., diazepam [Valium])	g. Calcium
____ 8. Opiates (e.g., morphine sulfate)	h. Amyl nitrate
____ 9. Ethylene glycol	i. Atropine
____ 10. β-Blockers	j. Acetylcysteine (Mucomyst)
____ 11. Digoxin	k. Flumazenil (Romazicon)
____ 12. Calcium-channel blockers	l. Naloxone (Narcan)

3. DIRECTIONS: List the main effects of hydrocarbon toxicity on each body system.

Pulmonary	
Heart	
Brain	
Gastrointestinal tract	
Liver	

4. DIRECTIONS: Explain the acronym *SLUDGE* that is used to assess patients with organophosphate poisoning.

S	
L	
U	
D	
G	
E	

5. DIRECTIONS: Name and describe the main effects of the antidotes for organophosphate poisoning.

6. DIRECTIONS: Match the statement with the disease. Answers may be used once, more than once, or not at all.

___	1. The disruption of acetylcholine produces paralytic effects in this disease	a. Botulism
___	2. Poor food handling and personal hygiene help spread this	b. Hemolytic–uremic syndrome
___	3. This disease is spread by fleas	c. Salmonella
___	4. The biggest clue to this disease is a rapid serious illness in a healthy person	d. Rabies
___	5. The major risk factor for this is eating improperly home-canned food	e. Lyme disease
___	6. CroFab is the medication of choice to treat this problem	f. Hantavirus infection
___	7. Exposure to bats, foxes, and raccoons can lead to this	g. Plague
___	8. The eating of undercooked meat seems to precipitate this disease	h. Snake bites
___	9. Infected deer ticks spread this disease	i. Rocky Mountain spotted fever
___	10. Common problems associated with this condition are related to neurotoxicity, cardiotoxicity, and hemolytic effects	j. Cat-scratch disease
___	11. Two less-well-known types of this disease are pneumonic and septicemic	
___	12. This condition is best diagnosed with the mouse bio-assay test	
___	13. The only really effective treatment for this condition is early hemodialysis	
___	14. This disease is severe, so a two-drug regime is recommended	
___	15. Encephalitis is the final outcome of this problem	
___	16. The cardinal sign of this condition the bull's-eye rash	
___	17. Suspect this disease for any child who has acute renal failure, hemolytic anemia, and thrombocytopenia	
___	18. This is the most common spirochetal infection in the United States	
___	19. After the patient becomes symptomatic, this disease is always fatal	
___	20. This disease is not usually diagnosed in the laboratory because of concerns with biosafety	
___	21. Pulmonary edema is possible with this disease	

7. DIRECTIONS: What is the preferred treatment for diving emergencies?

8. DIRECTIONS: Calculate the fluid resuscitation needed for a 125-kg man who sustained a full thickness burn of 65% of the total body surface area, and describe how it would be given.

Total volume to be given during the first 24 hours	
Volume to be given during the first 8 hours after the burn	
Volume to be given during the second 8 hours after the burn	
Volume to be given during the third 8 hours after the burn	

9. DIRECTIONS: Complete the following table about burns.

Classification	Clinical Appearance	Cause	Structures Involved
Partial-thickness burn Superficial (first degree)			
Deep (second degree)			
Full-thickness burn (third and fourth degree)			

LEARNING ACTIVITIES ANSWERS

1.

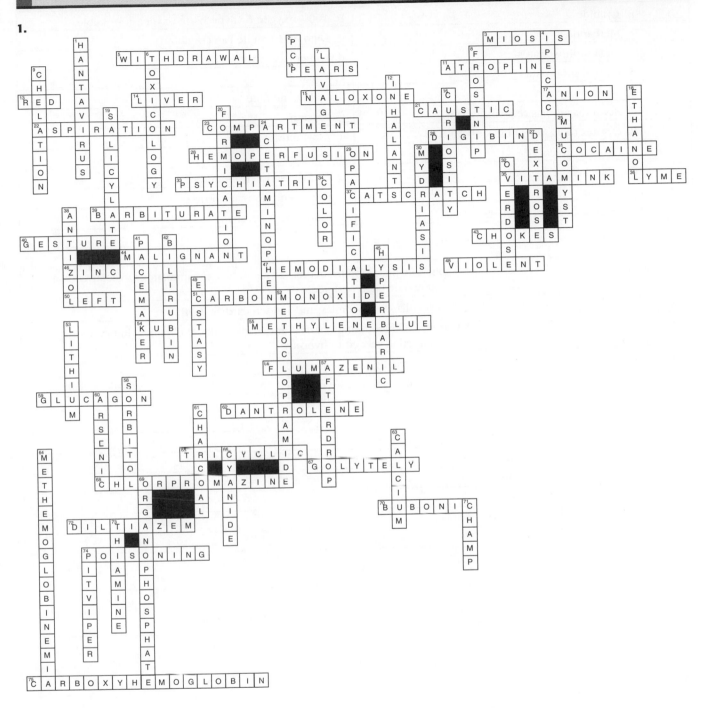

2.

_f_ 1. Methemoglobinemia	a. Glucagon
_h_ 2. Cyanide	b. 100% oxygen or hyperbaric oxygen if possible
_e_ 3. Methanol	c. Digoxin Immune Fab (Digibind)
_i_ 4. Organophosphates	d. Fomepizole (Antizol)
_b_ 5. Carbon monoxide	e. Ethanol
_j_ 6. Acetaminophen	f. Methylene blue
_k_ 7. Benzodiazepines (e.g., diazepam)	g. Calcium
_l_ 8. Opiates (e.g., morphine sulfate)	h. Amyl nitrate
_d or e_ 9. Ethylene glycol	i. Atropine
_a_ 10. β-Blockers	j. Acetylcysteine (Mucomyst)
_c_ 11. Digoxin	k. Flumazenil (Romazicon)
_g_ 12. Calcium-channel blockers	l. Naloxone (Narcan)

3.

Pulmonary	Aspiration, pneumonitis, decreased surfactant, inflammation, alveolar edema and hemorrhage, and necrosis
Heart	Tachycardia, dysrhythmias, and sudden cardiac death
Brain	Crosses the blood–brain barrier and leads to direct chemical injury and dysfunction related to hypoxia
Gastrointestinal tract	Mucosal irritation
Liver	Lipid peroxidation of hepatocytes

4.

S	Salivation
L	Lacrimation
U	Urination
D	Diarrhea
G	Gastrointestinal upset
E	Emesis

5.

Atropine: decreases cholinergic effect Pralidoxime: reverses the muscle paralysis that occurs with organophosphate poisoning

6.

_a_	1. The disruption of acetylcholine produces paralytic effects in this disease	a. Botulism
_c_	2. Poor food handling and personal hygiene help spread this	b. Hemolytic–uremic syndrome
_g_	3. This disease is spread by fleas	c. Salmonella
_f_	4. The biggest clue to this disease is a rapid serious illness in a healthy person	d. Rabies
_a_	5. The major risk factor for this is eating improperly home-canned food	e. Lyme disease
_h_	6. CroFab is the medication of choice to treat this problem	f. Hantavirus infection
_d_	7. Exposure to bats, foxes, and raccoons can lead to this	g. Plague
_b_	8. The eating of undercooked meat seems to precipitate this disease	h. Snake bites
_e_	9. Infected deer ticks spread this disease	i. Rocky Mountain spotted fever
_h_	10. Common problems associated with this condition are related to neurotoxicity, cardiotoxicity, and hemolytic effects	j. Cat-scratch disease
_g_	11. Two less-well-known types of this disease are pneumonic and septicemic	
_a_	12. This condition is best diagnosed with the mouse bioassay test	
_b_	13. The only really effective treatment for this condition is early hemodialysis	
_g_	14. This disease is severe, so a two-drug regime is recommended	
_d_	15. Encephalitis is the final outcome of this problem	
_e_	16. The cardinal sign of this condition the bull's-eye rash	
_b_	17. Suspect this disease for any child who has acute renal failure, hemolytic anemia, and thrombocytopenia	
_e_	18. This is the most common spirochetal infection in the United States	
_d_	19. After the patient becomes symptomatic, this disease is always fatal	
_f_	20. This disease is not usually diagnosed in the laboratory because of concerns with biosafety	
_f_	21. Pulmonary edema is possible with this disease	

7.

Recompression in a hyperbaric oxygen chamber

8.

The formula is 2–4ml/kg/%TBSA burned. Since the burns are full thickness, initial resuscitation attempts should be at 4 ml/kg/%TBSA and then adjusted according to urine output and hemodynamic status.

	2 ml/kg	4 ml/kg
Total volume to be given during the first 24 hours	16,250 ml	32,500 ml
Volume to be given during the first 8 hours after the burn	8125 ml	16,250 ml
Volume to be given during the second 8 hours after the burn	4625 ml	8125 ml
Volume to be given during the third 8 hours after the burn	4625 ml	8125 ml

9.

Classification	Clinical Appearance	Cause	Structures Involved
Partial-thickness burn Superficial (first degree)	Erythema; blanches with pressure; pain and mild swelling; no vesicles or blistering, although, after 24 hours, blisters may occur and skin may peel	Superficial sunburn, quick heat flash	Superficial epidermal damage with hyperemia; tactile and pain sensation are intact
Deep (second degree)	Fluid-filled vesicles that are red, shiny, and wet (if they have ruptured); severe pain caused by nerve injury; mild to moderate edema	Flame, flash, scald, contact burns, chemicals, tar	Epidermis and dermis are involved to varying depths; skin elements from which epithelial regeneration occurs remain viable
Full-thickness burn (third and fourth degree)	Dry, waxy white, leathery, or hard skin; visibly thrombosed vessels; no pain because of nerve destruction (although the surrounding area may have a second-degree burn and thus involve severe pain); possible involvement of muscles, tendons, and bones	Flame, scald, chemicals, tar, electric current	All skin elements and local nerve endings are destroyed; coagulation necrosis is present; surgical intervention required for healing

References and Suggested Readings

Aehlert, B. (2007). *ACLS study guide* (3rd ed.). St. Louis: Mosby JEMS.

American Psychiatric Association. (2000). *Diagnostic and statistical manual of mental disorders.* Washington, D.C.: Author.

Antosia, R. E., & Cahill, J. D. (2006). *Handbook of bioterrorism and disaster medicine.* New York: Springer.

Armed Forces Radiobiology Research Institute. (2007) AFRRI pocket guide: Emergency radiation medicine response. Retrieved July 2, 2008, from http://www.afrri.usuhs.mil/www/outreach/pdf/pcktcard.pdf.

Barnett, G. (2005). Alcohol emergencies. In L. Newberry & L. M. Criddle (Eds.). *Sheehy's manual of emergency care* (6th ed.). St. Louis: Mosby.

Bishop, C. R., Dargan, P. I., Greene, S. L., Garnham, F., & Wood, D. M. (2009). Emergency department presentations with suspected acute coronary syndrome—frequency of self-reported cocaine use [short report]. *European Journal of Emergency Medicine, 17,* 164–166.

Blume, W. T. (2006). Drug effects on EEG. *Journal of Clinical Neurophysiology, 23(4),* 306–311.

Brashear, A. (2007). Botulinum toxin poisoning. Retrieved July 14, 2008, from http://pier.acponline.org/physicians/public/d995/diagnosis/d995-g3.3-rec.html.

Brenner, S. & Dribben, B (2009). Toxicity, hallucinogenic—LSD. Retrieved August 1, 2009, from http://emedicine.medscape.com/article/1011615-overview

Bruns, J. J. (2008). Toxicity, anticholinergics. Retrieved May 27, 2009, from http://emedicine.medscape.com/article/812644-overview.

Buajordet, I., Naess, A., Jacobsen, D., & Brors, O. (2004). Adverse events after naloxone treatment of episodes of suspected acute opioid overdose. *European Journal of Emergency Medicine, 11(1),* 19–23.

Bucher, L. (2007). Emergency and disaster nursing. In S. L. Lewis, M. M. Heitkemper, S. R. Dirksen, P. G. O'Brien, & L. Bucher (Eds.). *Medical-surgical nursing: Assessment and management of clinical problems* (7th ed.). St. Louis: Mosby.

Burnett, L. B., & Adler, J. (2008). Toxicity, cocaine. Retrieved June 21, 2009, from http://emedicine.medscape.com/article/813959-overview

Buttaro, T. M., Trybulski, J., Bailey, P. P., & Sandberg-Cook, J. (2003). *Primary care: A collaborative practice.* St. Louis: Mosby.

Caldwell, J. D. (2009). Hantavirus cardiopulmonary syndrome Retrieved August 4, 2009, from http://emedicine.medscape.com/article/788980-overview.

Capape, S., Mora, E., Mintegui, S., Garcia, S., Santiago, M., & Benito, J. (2008). Prolonged sedation and airway complications after administration of an inadvertent ketamine overdose in emergency department. *European Journal of Emergency Medicine, 15(2),* 92–94.

Carlson, K. K. (Ed.). (2009). *AACN Critical Care Nursing.* St. Louis: Saunders.

Centers for Disease Control and Prevention. (2006). *Acute radiation sickness.* Retrieved August 2, 2009, from http://www.bt.cdc.gov/radiation/ars.asp

Centers for Disease Control and Prevention. (2006). Acute radiation syndrome: A fact sheet for physicians. Retrieved Jul 2, 2008, from http://www.bt.cdc.gov/radiation/arsphysicianfactsheet.asp.

Centers for Disease Control and Prevention. (2005). Rocky mountain spotted fever. Retrieved July 15, 2008, from http://www.cdc.gov/ncidod/dvrd/rmsf/index.htm.

Clark, D. Y., Stocking, J., & Johnson, J. (Eds.). (2006). *Flight and ground transport nursing core curriculum* (2nd ed.). Denver, CO: Air & Surface Transport Nurses Association.

Cox, R. D. (2008). Burns, chemical. Retrieved August 9, 2009, from http://emedicine.medscape.com/article/769336-overview.

Cunha, B. A. (2008). Hantavirus pulmonary syndrome Retrieved August 4, 2009, from http://emedicine.medscape.com/article/236425-overview

Daram, S. R. & Hayashi, P. H. (2005). Acute liver failure due to iron overdose in an adult. *Southern Medical Journal, 98(2),* 241-244.

Denke, N. J. (2005). Environmental emergencies. In L. Newberry & L. M. Criddle (Eds.). *Sheehy's manual of emergency care* (6th ed.). St. Louis: Mosby.

Dennison, R. D. (2000). *Pass CCRN!* (2nd ed.). St. Louis: Mosby.

Dennison, R. D. (2007). *Pass CCRN!* (3rd ed.). St. Louis: Mosby.

Digibind Prescribing Information. Retrieved July 3, 2008 from http://us.gsk.com/products/assets/us_digibind.pdf.

Diver's Alert Network. Retrieved July 21, 2008, from http://www.diversalertnetwork.org.

Domino, F. J. (2008). *The 5-minute clinical consultant* (16th ed.). Philadelphia: Lippincott Williams & Wilkins.

Drugs.com. Rohypnol information. Retrieved July 3, 2008, from http://www.drugs.com/rohypnol.html.

Duncan, R. A., Armstrong, P. A. R., & Paterson, B. (2008). Severe hypoglycaemia in citalopram overdose. *European Journal of Emergency Medicine, 15(4),* 234-235.

Edelstein, J. A., Li J., Silverberg, M. A., & Decker, W. (2007). Hypothermia. *Emedicine.* Retrieved July 27, 2009, from http://emedicine.medscape.com/article/770542-overview

Emergency Nurses Association. (2007). *Emergency nursing core curriculum* (6th ed). Philadelphia: Saunders.

Emergency Nurses Association. (2004). *Emergency nursing pediatric course provider manual* (3rd ed.). Des Plaines, IL: Author.

Emergency Nurses Association. (2005). *Sheehy's manual of emergency care* (6th ed.). St. Louis: Mosby.

Emergency Nurses Association (2007). *TNCC trauma nursing core course provider manual.* Des Plaines, IL: Author.

Farrell, S. E. (2007). Toxicity, acetaminophen. Retrieved August 1, 2009, from http://emedicine.medscape.com/article/820200-overview

Fasano, C. J., O'Malley, G. F., Lares, C., & Rowden, A. K. (2009). Pediatric ziprasidone overdose. *Pediatric Emergency Care, 25(4),* 258-259.

Flarity, K. (2007). Environmental emergencies. In K. S. Hoyt & J. Selfridge-Thomas (Eds.). *Emergency nursing core curriculum* (6th ed.). St. Louis: W.B. Saunders.

Freudenthal, W., & Ralston, M. (2008). Toxicity-organophosphates. Retrieved July 19, 2008, from http://www.emedicine.com/ped/topic1660.htm.

Furlanut, M., Franceschi, L., Poz, D., Silvestri, L., & Pecorari, M. (2006). Acute oxcarbazepine, benazepril, and hydrochlorothiazide overdose with alcohol. *Therapeutic Drug Monitoring, 28(2),* 267-268.

Gahlinger, P. M. (2004). Club drugs: MDMA, gamma-hydroxybutyrate (GHB), Rohypnol, and ketamine. *American Family Physician.* Retrieved June 22, 2009, from http://www.aafp.org/afp/20040601/2619.html.

Gentry, T. (2005). Toxicologic emergencies. In L. Newberry & L. M. Criddle (Eds.). *Sheehy's manual of emergency care* 96th ed.). St. Louis: Mosby.

Graziano, C. (2008). Toxicity, arsenic. Retrieved July 17, 2008, from http://www.emedicine.com/med/topic168.htm.

Hahn, I. & Yew, D. (2009). Toxicity, MDMA. Retrieved June 24, 2009, from http://emedicine.medscape.com/article/821572-overview.

Hall, A., Logan, J. E., Toblin, R. L., Kaplan, J. A., Kraner, J. C., Bixler, D., et al. (2008). Patterns of abuse among unintentional pharmaceutical overdose fatalities *Journal of the American Medical Association, 300(22),* 2613-2620.

Handly, N. (2007, July). Toxicity, amphetamines Retrieved June 21, 2009, from http://emedicine.medscape.com/article/812518-overview.

Heitkemper, M. M. (2007). Upper gastrointestinal problems. In S. L. Lewis, M. M. Heitkemper, S. R. Dirksen, P. G. O'Brien, & L. Bucher (Eds.). *Medical-surgical nursing: Assessment and management of clinical problems* (7th ed.). St. Louis: Mosby.

Hockenberry, M. J., & Berrera, P. (2007). Health problems of early childhood. In M. J. Hockenberry & D. Wilson (Eds.). *Wong's nursing care of infants and children* (8th ed.). St. Louis: Elsevier.

Irwin, R. S., & Rippe, J. M. (2003). *Irwin and Rippe's intensive care medicine* (vol. 5). Philadelphia: Lippincott Williams & Wilkins.

Jones, K. R. (2008). Hydroxocobalamin (Cyanokit): A new antidote for cyanide toxicity. *Advanced Emergency Nursing Journal, 30(2),* 112-121.

Kapitanyan, R., Su, M., & Landry, D. R. (2006). Plant poisoning, glycosides-cardiac. Retrieved July 21, 2008, from http://www.emedicine.com/emerg/topic439.htm.

Katz, K. D. & Brooks, D. E., Furtado, M. C., & Chan, L. (2009). Toxicity, organophosphate Retrieved June 30, 2009, from http://emedicine.medscape.com/article/167726-overview

Kaufman, T. & Jauch, E. C. (2007). Inhalants. Retrieved June 30, 2009, from http://emedicine.medscape.com/article/1174630-overview

Kearney, J., & Chiang, W. K. (2007). Plant poisoning-oxalates. Retrieved July 21, 2008, from http://www.emedicine.com/emerg/topic444.htm.

Keyes, D. C. (2007). Toxicity-ethylene glycol. Retrieved July 20, 2008, from http://www.emedicine.com/emerg/topic177.htm.

Korabathina, K., Benbadis, S. R., & Likosky, D. (2007). Methanol. Retrieved July 20, 2008, from http://www.emedicine.com/neuro/topic217.htm.

Lairez, O., Cournot, M., Minville, V., Roncalli, J., Austruy, J., Elbaz, M., et al. (2009). Risk of neurological decompression sickness in the diver with a right-to-left shunt: Literature review and meta-analysis. *Clinical Journal of Sport Medicine, 19(3),* 231-235.

Laskowski-Jones, L. (2007). Peripheral nerve and spinal cord problems. In S. L. Lewis, M. M. Heitkemper, S. R. Dirksen, P. G. O'Brien, & L. Bucher (Eds.). *Medical-surgical nursing: Assessment and management of clinical problems* (7th ed.). St. Louis: Mosby.

Levine, M. D., Johnson, J. J., & Barron, T. P. (2006). Toxicity-hydrocarbons. Retrieved July 19, 2008, from http://www.emedicine.com/emerg/topic873.htm.

Lewis, S. M., Heitkemper, M. M., Dirksen, S. R., O'Brien, P. G., & Bucher, L. (2007). *Medical-surgical nursing: Assessment and management of clinical problems* (7th ed.). St. Louis: Mosby.

Mason, D. (2005). Substance abuse. In L. Newberry & L. M. Criddle (Eds.). *Sheehy's manual of emergency care* (6th ed.). St. Louis: Mosby.

Mechem, C. C. (2009). Frostbite. Retrieved July 25, 2009, from http://emedicine.medscape.com/article/770296-overview.

Medline Plus. Cat scratch disease. Retrieved July 21, 2008, from http://www.nlm.nih.gov/medlineplus/ency/article/001614.htm.

Merlin, M. A., Pryor, P. W., & Bertolini, J. (2009). Rabies. Retrieved August 3, 2009, from http://emedicine.medscape.com/article/785543-overview.

Mirghani, R. A. (2008). Current status of point-of-care testing in clinical toxicology: Focus on drugs of abuse. *Point of Care: The Journal of Near-Patient Testing & Technology, 7(4)*, 266-270.

Morgan, D. L., Borys, D. J., Stanford, R., Kjar, D., & Tobleman, W. (2007). Texas coral snake (micrurus tener) bites. *Southern Medical Journal, 100(2)*, 152-156.

National Institute on Drug Abuse. (2009). *NIDA InfoFacts: Hallucinogens—LSD, peyote, psilocybin, and PCP*. Retrieved June 25, 2009, from http://www.drugabuse.gov/Infofacts/hallucinogens.html

National Institute on Drug Abuse. (2005). *Inhalant abuse*. Retrieved June 25, 2009, from http://www.nida.nih.gov/researchreports/inhalants/Inhalants.html

National Institutes of Health. (2006). NIDA Infofacts: LSD. Retrieved July 3, 2008, from http://www.nida.nih.gov/infofacts/LSD.html.

National Institutes of Health. (2006). NIDA Infofacts: Rohypnol and GHB. Retrieved July 4, 2008, from http://www.nida.nih.gov/infofacts/RohypnolGHB.html.

O'Brien, B., Quigg, C., & Leong, T. (2005). Severe cyanide toxicity from vitamin supplements. *European Journal of Emergency Medicine, 12(5)*, 257-258.

O'Brien, P. G. (2007). Addictive behaviors. In S. L. Lewis, M. M. Heitkemper, S. R. Dirksen, P. G. O'Brien, & L. Bucher (Eds.). *Medical-surgical nursing: Assessment and management of clinical problems* (7th ed.). St. Louis: Mosby.

Pachner A. R., & Steiner, I. (2007). Lyme neuroborreliosis: Infection, immunity, and inflammation. *Lancet Neurology. 6(8)*, 544-552.

Peddy, S. B., Rigby, M. R. & Shaffner, D. H. (2006). Acute cyanide poisoning. *Pediatric Critical Care Medicine, 7(1)*, 79-82.

Phillips, M. (2007). Toxicologic emergencies. In K. S. Hoyt & J. Selfridge-Thomas (Eds.). *Emergency nursing core curriculum* (6th ed.). St. Louis: W.B. Saunders.

Pulley, S. A. (2007). Decompression sickness. Retrieved August 7, 2009, from http://emedicine.medscape.com/article/769717-overview.

Raber, S. A. (1999). The dense metaphyseal band sign. *Radiology, 211(3)*, 773-774. Retrieved June 30, 2009, from http://radiology.rsnajnls.org/cgi/content/full/211/3/773.

Roberts, D. (2007). Arthritis and connective tissue disease. In S. L. Lewis, M. M. Heitkemper, S. R. Dirksen, P. G. O'Brien, & L. Bucher (Eds.). *Medical-surgical nursing: Assessment and management of clinical problems* (7th ed.). St. Louis: Mosby.

Sahjian, M., and Frakes, M. A. (2008). Where there is smoke … Inhalation injuries, carbon monoxide, and cyanide poisoning. *Advanced Emergency Nursing Journal, 30(2)*, 180-187.

Salyer, S. W. & Battista, R. (2001). Managing the acutely poisoned patient. *Physicians Assistant, 256*, 41-42, 45-49.

Schrage, E. D. (2008). Cat scratch disease. Retrieved July 21, 2008, from http://www.emedicine.com/emerg/topic84.htm.

Smith, D. H. (2006). About brown recluse spider bites. *Nursing 2006. 36(4)*, 71.

Spiller, H. A. & Schaeffer, S. E. (2008). Multiple seizures after bupropion overdose in a small child. *Pediatric Emergency Care, 24(7)*, 474-475.

Soghoian, S. & Seinert, R. (2008). Toxicity, heavy metals. Retrieved June 30, 2009, from http://emedicine.medscape.com/article/814960-overview

Sood, S. K. (2009). Food poisoning. Retrieved August 2, 2009, from http://emedicine.medscape.com/article/964048-overview

Stopford, B. M., & Colon, W. L. (2007). Weapons of mass destruction. In K. S. Hoyt & J. Selfridge-Thomas (Eds.). *Emergency nursing core curriculum* (6th ed.). St. Louis: W.B. Saunders.

Tenenbein, M. S., & Tenenbein, M. (2005). Acute pancreatitis due to erythromycin overdose. *Pediatric Emergency Care, 21(10)*, 675-676.

Terris, M. K. (n.d.). *The significance of urine color*. Retrieved June 30, 2009 from http://urology.stanford.edu/about/articles/abnormal_urine.html.

Theodorou, S., & Haber, P. S. (2005). The medical complications of heroin use. *Current Opinion in Internal Medicine, 4(4)*, 346-352.

Todar, K. (2008). Shigella and shigellosis. Retrieved July 14, 2008, from http://www.textbookofbacteriology.net/Shigella.html.

Turk, D. C., Swanson, K. S., & Gatchel, R. J. (2008). Predicting opioid misuse by chronic pain patients: A systematic review and literature synthesis. *Clinical Journal of Pain, 24(6)*, 497-508.

University of California Davis (2006). SafetyNet#71: Radiation and human health. Retrieved July 3, 2008, from http://www.safetynets/master-list-1/safetynet-71-radiation-and-human-health.

Velendzas, D. G., & Dufel, S. (2007). CBRNE-Plague. Retrieved July 16, 2008, from http://www.emedicine.com/emerg/topic428.htm.

Washington State Department of Health. The basics of radiation and radiation health effects. Retrieved July 3, 2008, from http://www.doh.wa.gov/handford/publications/health/mon2.htm.

Wilkes, J. M., Clark, L. E., & Herrera, J. L. (2005). Acetaminophen overdose in pregnancy. *Southern Medical Journal, 98(11)*, 1118-1122.

Wormser, G. P., McKenna, D., Carlin, J., Nadelman, R. B., Cavaliere, L. F., Holmgren, D., et al. (2005). Brief communication: Hematogenous dissemination in early Lyme disease. *Annals of Internal Medicine, 142(9)*, 751-755.

Introduction

This content constitutes 7% (11 items) of the CEN examination
The focus is on shock and multiple system trauma with an emphasis on management within the ED setting
The continuum of age needs to be considered from infancy to elderly
Represents a very diverse group of patients, all ages from infancy to elderly and of all socioeconomic levels and preexisting health status

Age-Related Considerations

Neonates, infants, children

1. Trauma is the leading cause of death, especially motor vehicle collisions, bicycle collisions, and when struck by vehicle
2. Since the skeletal system of a child is flexible, it provides less protection to underlying structures and serious injury may occur in the absence of fracture (Fultz & Sturt, 2005)
3. Thermoregulation is inadequate and accidental hypothermia may occur during treatment of trauma and/or shock; prevention of heat loss is a priority (Fultz & Sturt, 2005; Holleran, 2007)
4. Allowing the parent to remain present is helpful to aid in emotional coping with the trauma (Fultz & Sturt, 2005)
5. Since a greater percentage of a child's weight is water, a relatively small blood loss can cause significant hemodynamic compromise
6. Hypovolemia may be masked for a prolonged period of time (Fultz & Sturt, 2005; Holleran, 2007)
7. Because a child's myocardial fibers are shorter and less compliant, they cannot significantly increase stroke volume; cardiac output is increased by an increase in heart rate (Holleran, 2007)
8. Unlike adults, infants and young children may become hypovolemic as a result of intracranial hemorrhage or hematoma due to presence of fontanels (Holleran, 2007)
9. The size and weight of the head in relation to the body weight increases the risk of drowning and falls
10. Physical (child) abuse must be considered as a cause of trauma

Older adults

1. Trauma is a growing problem in older adults since the 65 years and older age group is the fastest growing segment of the U.S. population (CDC, 2007); these older adults are particularly at risk of motor vehicle collisions and falls
2. Falling is the leading cause of trauma and more than one third of adults aged 65 years or older fall every year (CDC, 2007); factors include the following
   a. Posture changes such as kyphosis
   b. Rugs
   c. Pets
   d. Clutter
   e. Medications
      1) Antihypertensives may cause postural blood pressure (BP) changes
      2) Sedating drugs such as anxiolytics, sedatives, and narcotics may affect balance or cause dizziness
3. Motor vehicle collision: physiologic factors such as limited vision, hearing, cervical spine mobility contribute to motor vehicle collisions in older adults
4. Mortality is higher than in younger patients
   a. Limited resilience due to the effects of aging and the presence of comorbidities
   b. Sepsis is the most serious complication; contributing factor is the effect of aging on the immune system causing immunocompromise (i.e., immunosenescence)
5. Fractures are more likely, especially in women, due to osteoporosis
6. Brain injury is associated with high mortality
   a. Clinical indications of intracranial hemorrhage/hematoma may be late since cerebral atrophy of aging allows for larger space for formation
   b. Neurologic signs such as alertness, motor activity, and pupillary changes may be unreliable in older adults
7. Cardiovascular reserve and ability to compensate for blood loss is limited in older adults, especially if the patient is on β-blockers
8. Pulmonary reserve and ability to increase tidal volume are limited in older adults, especially when kyphosis or kyphoscoliosis is present
9. The fragility of the older adult's skin necessitates extra care such as padding bony prominences and removal of spine board as soon as possible

10. Physical (elder) abuse must be considered as a cause of trauma
11. Older adults may have advance directives or power of attorney; end-of-life issues need to be considered

Trauma

Definitions

1. Trauma: injury to the body caused by acute exposure to mechanical, thermal, electrical, or chemical energy
   a. Unintentional causes include vehicular collision; falls; burns; or firearm, recreational, or occupational mishaps
   b. Intentional: deliberate acts of violence such as shootings, stabbings, assaults, and child or elder abuse
2. Mechanism of injury: circumstances and energy forces that produced the trauma
   a. Blunt trauma
      1) Caused by the following forces
         a) Acceleration or deceleration: occurs with increased velocity or speed of a moving object followed by a sudden decrease
         b) Shearing: occurs when two oppositely directed parallel forces are applied to tissue
         c) Compression: occurs when a squeezing inward pressure is applied to tissues
      2) Results in more injuries and more types of injury such as contusions, lacerations, fractures, or ruptures of solid tissue masses
      3) Tend to be more difficult to manage because more structures are injured, frequently occult presentation so diagnosis may be delayed, and results in more significant complications
   b. Penetrating trauma
      1) Caused by direct contact with an instrument that cuts the skin, such as stabbing with a sharp object, bullet wound, high-pressure injections, or foreign object impalement
      2) Results in injury to fewer body structures
3. Kinematics: the physics of trauma; the relationship between energy and trauma
   a. Newton's first law of motion: a body at rest will remain at rest unless acted upon by an outside force (i.e., principle of inertia) and a body in motion will remain in motion traveling in a straight line unless acted upon by an outside force (i.e., principle of momentum)
   b. Energy can be changed from one form to another but it can neither be created nor destroyed
      1) Consider that the transformation of the kinetic energy of a moving object (e.g., motor vehicle) that suddenly stops causes damage to the motor vehicle and occupants
         a) Four collisions occur in vehicle collisions
            i) A: auto collision
            ii) B: body collision
            iii) C: cavity contents collision
            iv) D: debris collision

c. Kinetic energy: the energy of motion
   1) Formula: $(mass \times velocity^2)/2$
   2) Consider that doubling the size of an object results in doubling the kinetic energy while doubling the velocity quadruples the kinetic energy; this explains why a bullet (small mass with significant velocity) can cause such tissue damage
   3) Force applies slowly over a large surface area results in less tissue destruction than that same force applied to a small surface area

Predisposing factors

1. Blunt trauma
   a. Vehicular collision: motor vehicle, motorcycle, bicycle, watercraft, pedestrian struck by motor vehicle
   b. Falls
   c. Assault
   d. Industrial mishaps
   e. Blast force
   f. Sports-related injuries
2. Penetrating trauma
   a. Gunshot wounds
   b. Stab wounds
   c. Impalement
   d. Projectiles
3. Alcohol is a major factor in both intentional and nonintentional trauma; in 40% of all traffic-related fatalities, the driver has an elevated blood alcohol concentration (Schulman, 2007)
4. Another risk to vehicular safety is talking on cellular phones or texting while driving

Mechanism of injury

1. Motor vehicle collision
   a. Useful information
      1) Speed of vehicle(s)
      2) Size of vehicle(s)
      3) Location of impact
         a) Head on
         b) Rear impact
         c) Lateral
         d) Ejection
         e) Rollover
      4) Position of patient in vehicle before and after the impact
         a) If thrown from the vehicle, distance from the vehicle
      5) Use of safety devices
         a) Lap belt
         b) Shoulder belt
         c) Child car seat
         d) Airbags
            i) Whether or not the airbag(s) deployed
            ii) Location: front or side
      6) Damage to vehicle
         a) Indications of impact
            i) Bent steering wheel
            ii) Broken windshield

iii) Broken rearview mirror
iv) Broken gearshift
7) Smoke or fumes on scene
8) Condition of other occupants
b. Anticipated injury
1) By type of collision (Table 13-1)
2) By position in vehicle
a) Driver may strike steering column, instrument panel, gearshift, rearview mirror, windshield, pillar between windshield and door, and door

TABLE 13-1	Anticipated Injuries in Motor Vehicle Collisions	
Type of Collision	**Anticipated Injuries**	
Head-on: up-and-over pathway	• Cervical spine compression injury • Skull fractures, traumatic brain injury • Rib, sternal fractures, flail chest • Pulmonary contusion, pneumothorax, hemothorax • Myocardial contusion • Liver, spleen, duodenum, diaphragmatic lacerations • Great vessel tear	
Head-on: down-and-under pathway	• Cervical spine flexion injury • Laryngeal trauma • Carotid shearing • Rib, sternal fractures, flail chest • Pulmonary contusion, pneumothorax, hemothorax • Myocardial contusion • Aortic tears • Pelvic or acetabular fractures • Femur, tibia, fibula fractures	
Read-end	• Whiplash • Rib, sternal fractures, flail chest • Pulmonary contusion, pneumothorax, hemothorax	
Lateral	• Cervical ligamentous injuries • Lateral rib fractures, flail chest • Pulmonary contusion, pneumothorax, hemothorax • Spleen or liver lacerations • Pelvic, hip, acetabular fractures • Humerus and clavicle fractures	
Ejections	• Skull fractures, traumatic brain injury • Cervical and thoracic spine compression fractures • Rib fracture, pneumothorax, hemothorax • Liver, spleen, pancreas lacerations • Aortic tears • Pelvic fractures, straddle fractures	

Adapted from: Schulman, C. S. (2009). Trauma. In K. K. Carlson (Ed.), *Advanced Critical Care Nursing* (pp. 1134-1188). St. Louis: Saunders Elsevier.

i) Facial laceration, facial bone fractures
ii) Scalp lacerations, skull fracture, traumatic brain injury
iii) Spinal injuries
iv) Chest wall lacerations, pulmonary contusion, rib, clavicle or sternal fractures, pneumohemothorax
v) Thoracic aorta tear
vi) Abdominal wall lacerations, rupture or avulsion of liver, spleen, kidney, pancreas, bowel, and bladder
vii) Fractured humerus, radius, ulna, wrist, hand
viii) Fractures pelvis, hip dislocation, fractured femur, tibia, fibula, ankle, foot, ligamentous injury to knee
b) Front seat passenger: higher incidence of head, abdominal injuries and upper torso fractures but fewer thoracic injuries and lower torso fractures
c) Rear seat passenger: similar to front seat passenger if not restrained
c. Injury caused by protective devices (Shulman, 2009)
1) Lap belt only worn
a) Fractured ribs, sternum, clavicle
b) Myocardial contusion
c) Aortic tear
d) Mesenteric tear, bowel perforation
e) Bladder rupture
f) Lower thoracic or lumbar vertebral fracture
2) Shoulder harness only
a) Cervical spine injuries
b) Abrasions to neck, chest, abdomen
c) Carotid artery injuries
d) Laryngeal injuries
3) Air bag deployment
a) Cervical spine injuries
b) Bag slap injuries to face and neck
c) Temporary hearing deficit
d) Corneal abrasion, corneal burns, retinal detachment
e) Respiratory distress or anaphylaxis from inhaled particles from within the bag and propellant
f) Upper extremity contusion
g) Fracture or dislocation of thumb or wrist
2. Motorcycle collision
a. Useful information
1) Deformity of the motorcycle
2) Stationary objects impacted
3) Helmet: cracks in helmet are likely to be associated with significant brain injury
b. Anticipated injury
1) Traumatic brain injury is the leading cause of death, especially if rider is not wearing a helmet
2) Tibial and radial injuries are the most common injury
3) Facial fractures

4) Spinal injuries, especially thoracic
5) Pulmonary injuries (i.e., pulmonary contusion, pneumothorax, hemothorax)
6) Pelvic fractures result from straddling position; may have coexisting bladder or urethral injury
7) Traumatic amputation
8) Specific to type of impact
   a) Head on: bike flips forward so rider strikes or travels over the handlebars
      i) Injury to abdomen, chest as rider strikes handlebars
      ii) Bilateral femur fractures
      iii) Head and neck injuries
   b) Angular: cycle hit at an angle and collapses on the rider
      i) Tibia, fibula fractures, may be open
      ii) Crushed legs
      iii) Ankle dislocation
   c) Ejection: rider is thrown off motorcycle
      i) Serious injury likely, especially head injury
   d) Laying the bike down
      i) Fractures, abrasions, crush injuries, road burns to lower leg
3. Bicycle collision
   a. Useful information: forward, sideward, or backward unseating
   b. Anticipated injury
      1) If over the handlebars, facial injuries and/or fractures, head injury
      2) Blunt trauma caused by handlebars
         a) Serious abdominal injury may not be apparent until later in children
      3) Fractures of the feet from spokes of wheel
      4) Straddle injuries such as vaginal tears, scrotal injuries, perineal contusions, anal or rectal injuries
      5) Injury to rider from rearview mirror extending from truck or van can cause serious, even fatal, injury to the head, neck, face
4. Watercraft collision
   a. Useful information
      1) Description of event: collision with another boat or obstruction with an object in the water or on shore
   b. Anticipated injury
      1) Drowning
      2) Hypothermia
      3) Other injuries as for ejection from a vehicle
5. Pedestrian struck by motor vehicle
   a. Useful information: type of vehicle
   b. Anticipated injury: three points of impact
      1) Bumper
         a) Adult: impact to lower leg
            i) Tibia, fibula fractures
         b) Child: leg
            i) Femur, tibia, fibula fractures
      2) Hood

   a) Adult: as the person bends, impact to lower abdomen, pelvis, or upper femur
      i) Thoracic injuries
      ii) Abdominal injuries
      iii) Spinal fractures
      iv) Hip, pelvis, or femur fractures
   b) Child: head, chest, or abdominal injury; very small children are knocked down and under the vehicle and then run over
      3) Ground: head, cervical spine, chest, or abdominal injuries
   c. Waddell triad: the combination of injuries that often occurs when a child is struck by a car
      1) Chest
      2) Head
      3) Femurs
6. Falls
   a. Useful information
      1) Distance of fall: a fall from more than 3 times the person's height results in significant injury (McSwain et al., 2000)
      2) Surface of impact
      3) Area of body that made initial impact
      4) If objects were struck during the fall
      5) Patient's activity before and after fall
   b. Anticipated injury
      1) Compression fractures: os calcis (i.e., heel), femur, tibia, fibula, pelvis, lumbar spine; may be referred to as Don Juan syndrome
      2) Bilateral wrist (Colles) fractures if arms are put forward for protection in forward propulsion
      3) Vascular injuries: pelvis and thorax
      4) Renal injury
7. Sports-related injuries
   a. Useful information
      1) Impact to patient
      2) Damaged equipment
      3) Previous training (or lack of training) of patient
      4) Use of protective equipment
   b. Anticipated injury: dependent upon sport (Table 13-2)
8. Penetrating injury
   a. Useful information
      1) Wounding agent (e.g., knife, bullet, arrow, ice pick)
      2) Number and location of wounds
      3) Size and length of the agent
      4) If gunshot, caliber and distance of the weapon form the patient
         a) Low velocity bullets travel at <1000 feet per second (fps)
         b) Medium velocity bullets travel at 1000 to 2000 fps
         c) High-velocity bullets travel at >2000 fps
      5) Trajectory
      6) Contaminants
   b. Anticipated injury: dependent upon above indicated factors

TABLE 13-2   Anticipated Injuries in Sports

Sport	Anticipated Injuries
Baseball	• Skull fracture, traumatic brain injury • Ocular injuries • Extremity fractures • Lacerations • Sprains • Strains
Basketball	• Lower extremity sprains, strains, fractures • Lacerations • Contusions
Boxing	• Skull fracture, traumatic brain injury (cumulative) • Ocular injuries • Nasal fractures • Hand fractures • Lacerations
Bungee jumping	• Impact-related injuries (may be major) • Intraocular hemorrhages • Spinal fractures, spinal cord injury • Peroneal nerve injury • Soft tissue injury
Football	• Spinal fractures, spinal cord injuries • Skull fracture, traumatic brain injury • Knee strains, ligament tears • Fractures • Lacerations
Gymnastics	• Spinal fractures, spinal cord injuries • Extremity fractures • Sprains • Strains
Horseback riding	• Skull fracture, traumatic brain injury • Crush wounds
Ice hockey	• Facial fractures • Soft tissue injuries • Lacerations
Inline skating	• Skull fracture, traumatic brain injury • Wrist fractures • Lower extremity fractures
Running	• Lower extremity injuries • Sprains • Strains
Skiing	• Skull fracture, traumatic brain injury • Lower extremity fractures • Hypothermia, frostbite

Adapted from Revere, C. (2002). Mechanisms of injury. In L. Newberry (Ed.), *Sheehy's emergency nursing. Principles and practice* (5th ed.). St. Louis: Mosby.

9. Injury related to machinery
   a. Useful information
      1) Location of injury
      2) Length of time since injury/extrication
      3) Function of the machine
      4) Potential contaminants
   b. Anticipated injury: depends on above information

Pathophysiology

1. Hemorrhage: may be overt or occult
   a. Caused initially by injury and potentially secondarily by coagulopathy
   b. Results in decrease in decreased oxygen delivery to tissues (DO_2)
      1) Decrease in cardiac output due to loss of circulating blood volume
      2) Loss of hemoglobin to carry oxygen
2. Hypoperfusion
   a. Caused by decrease in hemoglobin and cardiac output which results in a decrease in DO_2
   b. Results in the following
      1) Organ ischemia and, possibly, organ failure
      2) Rhabdomyolysis with muscle ischemia, necrosis, or crush injury potentially causing acute renal failure
      3) Bowel ischemia with resultant translocation of intestinal bacteria into lymphatics or vascular bed potentially causing sepsis
      4) Acidosis
3. Hypothermia: most trauma patients arrive in the ED with hypothermia, but treatments may also contribute to hypothermia
   a. Caused by the following
      1) Exposure: lack of clothing
      2) Open body cavities especially if lengthy surgery required
      3) Administration of refrigerated blood
      4) Administration of room temperature intravenous fluids
      5) Possible alcohol intoxification
   b. Results in the following
      1) Shift in oxyhemoglobin dissociation curve, which impairs tissue oxygen delivery
      2) Shivering, which increases oxygen consumption
      3) Impaired platelet function causes coagulopathy, which perpetuates hemorrhage
      4) Increased blood viscosity
      5) Myocardial depression
      6) Acidosis
4. Hypertension (compartment)
   a. Potential intracranial hypertension and brain herniation
   b. Abdominal hypertension and abdominal compartment syndrome
   c. Compartment syndrome related to fracture, tissue injury
5. Specific pathophysiology is included with each emergency in appropriate chapter (e.g., closed head injury in Chapter 6)

Clinical presentation: see specific emergencies in appropriate chapter
Collaborative management

1. Initiate primary survey to identify and treat life-threatening conditions (see Chapter 2 for detailed description of primary survey)
   a. **A:** airway

b. **B**: breathing
c. **C**: circulation
d. **D**: disability
e. **E**: exposure

2. Provide resuscitation measures (Talbert, 2005)
  a. **A**: airway and **B**: breathing
    1) Maintain airway, oxygenation, and ventilation
      a) Jaw-thrust until cervical spine has been cleared either clinically or radiologically; then may use head-tilt, chin lift
        i) Note that any patient with blunt or penetrating trauma above the nipple line must have the cervical spine immobilized with assessment of the airway (Fultz and Sturt, 2005)
      b) Oropharyngeal (if no gag reflex) or nasopharyngeal (if basal skull fracture is not suspected) airway adjunct to hold the tongue away from the hypopharynx in patients with altered LOC
      c) Intubation may be required; RSI methods should be used and performed by most experienced provider
      d) Oxygen by whatever delivery method necessary to maintain SpO_2 of 95%: may be nasal cannula, 100% nonrebreathing mask, or intubation with mechanical ventilation with PEEP
  b. **C**: circulation
    1) Control of bleeding
      a) Pressure on site or artery above site
      b) Reinforcement and stabilization of impaled object before surgical procedure for removal
      c) Emergent surgery may be required
    2) Maintain adequate circulation and perfusion
      a) IV access with two large-bore catheters for fluid and medication administration
    3) Fluid replacement
      a) Crystalloids: usually 0.9% saline or lactated Ringer solution
      b) Red packed cells or other blood products as prescribed
      c) Should be given early if significant blood loss is suspected to prevent tissue hypoxia; replacement of platelets, clotting factors, and calcium should be considered especially if multiple transfusions are given
      d) Colloids are not generally recommended in trauma
  c. **D**: disability
    1) Neurologic assessment, including Glasgow Coma Scale score, and protection of the cervical spine
  d. **E**: environment
    1) Expose: remove all clothing but do not leave patient uncovered; care must be taken to prevent or treat hypothermia
    2) Evacuate if necessary: prompt transfer should be achieved if the patient's needs are beyond the resources available at the facility

3. Conduct secondary survey to identify serious threats that may require emergency surgery or emergency procedures (see Chapter 2 for detailed description of secondary survey)
  a. **F**
    1) Full set of vital signs
    2) Focused adjuncts
      a) Cardiac monitoring
      b) Pulse oximetry to measure SpO_2
      c) Calculate trauma score (Table 13-3)
      d) Nasogastric or orogastric tube to low suction if indicated and not contraindicated
      e) Foley catheter if indicated and not contraindicated
      f) Diagnostic
        i) Serum
          (a) CBC with differential, hemoglobin, hematocrit
          (b) Chemistry profile including glucose, BUN, creatinine
          (c) Coagulation profile
          (d) Serum lactate
          (e) Toxicology including alcohol
          (f) Type and cross-match
        ii) Urine
          (a) Pregnancy test if female of childbearing age
          (b) Toxicology
        iii) Diagnostic imaging
          (a) Spine
          (b) Chest
          (c) Pelvis
          (d) Focused assessment sonography for trauma (FAST)
        iv) CT
          (a) Head
          (b) Chest
          (c) Abdomen
        v) Diagnostic peritoneal lavage (DPL) or diagnostic peritoneal aspiration (DPA)
    3) Family presence
      a) Facilitate and support family's involvement
      b) Provide explanations about procedures
      c) Support family's emotional and spiritual needs
  b. **G**: give comfort measures
    1) Positioning for comfort
    2) Anxiolytics
    3) Analgesics: nonsteroidal anti-inflammatory drugs (NSAIDs), narcotics, anesthetics
    4) Ice if appropriate
    5) Splinting and stabilization of fractures
    6) Cutaneous stimulation (e.g., massage)
    7) Distraction (e.g., music)
  c. **H**
    1) History
      a) Prehospital: MIVT
        i) Mechanism of injury
        ii) Injuries sustained

TABLE **13-3** Revised Trauma Score

Measurement	Numeric Score	Probability of Survival	
		Total Score	Percent Survivors
Systolic blood pressure (mm Hg)			
>89	4	12	99.5%
76-89	3	11	96.9%
50-75	2	10	87.9%
1-49	1	9	76.6%
0	0		
Respiratory rate (spontaneous inspirations per minute)*			
10-29	4	8	66.6%
>29	3	7	63.6%
6-9	2	6	63%
1-5	1	5	45.5%
0	0		
Glasgow Coma Scale score			
13-15	4	3 or 4	33.3%
9-12	3	2	28.6%
6-8	2	1	25%
4-5	1	0	3.7%
3	0		

Data from Emergency Nurses Association (2000). *Trauma nursing core course* (5th ed.). Des Plaines, IL: The Association.
*Patient initiated breaths, not mechanically ventilated

iii) Vital signs
iv) Treatment initiated and response
  b) Past medical history
 2) Head-to-toe assessment
  d. **I**: inspect posterior surfaces while maintaining cervical spine protection; assist with rectal exam as indicated
  e. Focused assessment related to mechanism of injury
4. Continue assessment throughout ED stay
  a. ABCDs
  b. Vital signs: blood pressure, pulse, respiratory rate, and temperature
  c. Oxygen saturation
  d. Respiratory effort and excursion
  e. Cardiac rate and rhythm
  f. Pain and discomfort level
  g. Accurate intake and output
  h. Serum electrolytes
  i. Level of consciousness
  j. Close monitoring for progression of symptoms
5. Reverse or prevent hypothermia
  a. Passive warming
   1) Removal of wet linens, clothing
   2) Application of warm blankets including convection blankets
  b. Active external warming: convection blankets
  c. Active internal warming as indicated
   1) Warm IV fluid

  2) Warm humidified oxygen
  3) Lavage of stomach, chest, colon, and/or bladder with warm isotonic fluids
  4) Peritoneal lavage with warm isotonic fluids
  5) Extracorporeal systems such as hemodialysis, cardiopulmonary bypass, or continuous arteriovenous or venovenous warming
  d. Monitoring for afterdrop (i.e., decrease in core body temperature that occurs with redistribution of cold blood returning from peripheral tissues)
  e. Monitoring for hypotension caused by vasodilation with rewarming
6. Reverse acidosis
  a. Measures to treat underlying cause of decrease in tissue delivery (DO_2)
   1) Hemoglobin
    a) Stop the bleeding: apply pressure, prepare patient for surgery, etc.
    b) Administer blood and blood products as prescribed
   2) Cardiac output
    a) Administer isotonic fluids and blood and blood products
    b) Administer vasopressors (e.g., phenylephrine [Neo-Synephrine], norepinephrine [Levophed], dopamine [Intropin]) as prescribed

i) Vasopressors should be used only when hypotension persists despite adequate fluid resuscitation

ii) Phenylephrine (Neo-Synephrine) causes the least tachycardia of these vasopressors; norepinephrine (Levophed) causes less tachycardia than does dopamine (Intropin)

c) Administer inotropic agents (e.g., dobutamine [Dobutrex]) to improve contractility as prescribed

3) SaO$_2$

a) Ensure airway, oxygenation, and ventilation to maintain SaO$_2$ at least 95%

b. Treatment of hypothermia which can impair oxygen delivery to the tissues

c. Avoidance of the use of sodium bicarbonate unless the pH is less than 7.0; adverse effects of sodium bicarbonate include the following

1) Shifts the oxyhemoglobin dissociation curve to the left impairing the dissociation of oxygen from the hemoglobin at the tissue level, which may worsen metabolic acidosis

2) Increased CO_2 production, which may cause or worsen respiratory acidosis

3) Hypokalemia by shifting potassium from serum to intracellular space

4) Hypocalcemia by increasing the amount of calcium bound to albumin thereby reducing ionized calcium

7. Correct coagulopathy

a. Treatment of hypothermia, which can adversely affect platelet function

b. Replacement of clotting factors as prescribed

8. Assist with measurement and treatment of compartment hypertension (e.g., intracranial hypertension, abdominal hypertension, compartment syndrome)

9. Treat infection (if present) and prevent sepsis

a. Antimicrobials as prescribed

b. Tetanus prophylaxis if indicated

c. Dressing of wounds

d. Stabilization of fractures

10. Identify, prevent, and treat rhabdomyolysis

a. Identification of high-risk patient (e.g., crush injuries, muscle ischemia/necrosis, electrical burns, sustained generalized seizures)

b. Detection of change in color of urine (e.g., brownish, tea-colored); laboratory confirmation of myoglobinuria

c. Isotonic fluids, diuretics (e.g., mannitol [Osmitrol]), and alkalinization of the urine using intravenous sodium bicarbonate as prescribed

d. Hemodialysis or continuous renal replacement therapy (e.g., continuous venovenous hemodialysis) may be required

11. Monitor for complications

a. Shock

b. Multiple organ dysfunction syndrome (MODS)

1) Acute respiratory distress syndrome (ARDS)

2) Disseminated intravascular coagulation (DIC)

3) Renal failure

4) Hepatic failure

5) Myocardial failure

6) Cerebral failure

c. Infection/sepsis/septic shock

d. Deep vein thrombosis (DVT) and pulmonary embolism (PE)

e. Other complications specific to organ injury (see specific emergency in appropriate chapter)

Evaluation

1. Patent airway, adequate oxygenation (i.e., normal PaO$_2$, SpO$_2$, SaO$_2$) and ventilation (i.e., normal PaCO$_2$)

2. Absence of clinical indications of respiratory distress

3. Absence of clinical indicators of hypoperfusion

4. Absence of clinical indications of bleeding

5. Absence of clinical indications of infection/sepsis

6. Control of pain, discomfort, or dyspnea

7. Alert and oriented with no neurovascular deficit

Typical disposition

1. If evaluation criteria met (i.e., minor trauma): discharge with instructions

2. If evaluation criteria not met: admission to the progressive care unit or the critical care unit; may require emergent surgery and go directly to operating room

Shock

Definitions

1. Shock: the condition of insufficient perfusion of cells and vital organs, causing tissue hypoxia; perfusion is inadequate to sustain life; results in cellular, metabolic, and hemodynamic derangements

2. Systemic inflammatory response syndrome (SIRS): the systemic response to a variety of insults that begin as local inflammation; consider the vasodilation and increased capillary permeability of local inflammation as a normal healing process while the more global vasodilation and increased capillary permeability of SIRS as being life-threatening

3. MODS: failure of more than one organ in an acutely ill patient with SIRS to such an extent that homeostasis cannot be maintained without intervention

Predisposing factors

1. Hypovolemic: caused by inadequate intravascular volume

2. Cardiogenic: caused by impaired ability of the heart to pump blood effectively

3. Distributive: caused by massive vasodilation and a resultant relative hypovolemia

a. Septic: resulting from massive vasodilation caused by release of mediators of the inflammatory process in response to overwhelming infection

b. Anaphylactic: resulting from massive vasodilation caused by release of histamine in response to a severe allergic reaction

c. Neurogenic: resulting from massive vasodilation caused by suppression of the sympathetic nervous system

Pathophysiology

1. Stages of shock
   a. Initial stage: subclinical hypoperfusion caused by inadequate delivery and/or inadequate extraction of oxygen
      1) Shock is initiated by decreased tissue oxygenation caused by any of the following
         a) Decrease in circulating blood volume (hypovolemic)
         b) Decrease in ability of the heart to pump blood (cardiogenic)
         c) Decrease in vascular tone (distributive, may also be referred to as vasogenic)
      2) Cardiac output and index are decreased but there are no clinical indications of hypoperfusion; this decrease in cardiac output and index would be detected by invasive hemodynamic monitoring
   b. Compensatory stage: attempts of the neuroendocrine systems to compensate and restore tissue perfusion to vital organs
      1) Sympathetic nervous system (SNS) stimulation
         a) Baroreceptor reflex: decrease in blood pressure stimulates the baroreceptors, which then stimulate the vasomotor center in the medulla to activate the SNS
         b) SNS: epinephrine and norepinephrine released from adrenal medulla cause the following physiologic responses
            i) Cardiac effects
               (a) Positive chronotropic (i.e., increase in heart rate)
               (b) Positive inotropic (i.e., increase in contractility)
               (c) Positive dromotropic (i.e., increase in conductivity)
            ii) Vascular effects
               (a) Arterial vasoconstriction
            i) Systemic response increases SVR and blood pressure
            ii) Constriction of afferent and efferent arterioles of kidneys decreases glomerular filtration rate (GFR) and urine output
               (b) Venous vasoconstriction
            i) Widespread reflex venoconstriction increases venous return to the heart, which increases preload
            ii) Increased venous return and preload increases myocardial contractility by increasing myofibril stretch (Starling's Law of the Heart)

iii) Redistribution of blood flow from nonessential (e.g., skin, bowel, kidney) to essential (e.g., heart and brain) organs

c) CNS ischemic response
   i) Low oxygen levels stimulate chemoreceptors to increase rate and depth of ventilation
   ii) Hyperventilation causes respiratory alkalosis and cerebral vasoconstriction and, potentially, cerebral ischemia
   iii) Also, a CNS ischemic response occurs when MAP falls to less than 50 mm Hg
   iv) CNS ischemia causes powerful stimulation of the SNS

2) Hormonal compensation
   a) Hypoperfusion of the kidney causes the activation of renin-angiotensin-aldosterone system (see Figure 4-11, Chapter 4)
      i) Vasoconstriction of arteries and arterioles caused by angiotensin II
      ii) Increase in reabsorption of sodium and water by the renal tubule caused by aldosterone
   b) Hypothalamic stimulation causes release of antidiuretic hormone (ADH) from posterior pituitary gland and adrenocorticosteroid hormone (ACTH) from anterior pituitary gland
      i) ADH causes vasoconstriction and retention of water at renal tubules
      ii) ACTH stimulates the adrenal cortex to release the following
         (a) Glucocorticoids: stimulate glycogenolysis and gluconeogenesis to mobilize glucose for cellular energy
         (b) Aldosterone: stimulates the reabsorption of sodium and water at the renal tubules

c. Progressive stage: the inability of the compensatory mechanisms to maintain tissue perfusion
   1) Myocardial depression
      a) Coronary artery perfusion pressure is dramatically reduced by decrease in MAP to less than 60 mm Hg, which causes myocardial ischemia
      b) Myocardial depressant factor (MDF) is released by the ischemic pancreas
   2) Vasomotor center depression caused by severe cerebral ischemia
      a) Increases capillary permeability
      b) Decreases circulating volume
      c) Results in decreased flow to vital organs
   3) Deterioration of microcirculation
      a) Spasm of the precapillary sphincter and venules
      b) Continuing ischemia and local acidosis causes dilation of the precapillary sphincters, whereas the venules are more resistant to the effects of acidosis and remain constricted

c) Blood enters capillaries and pools

d) Stagnant blood increases capillary hydrostatic pressure and increases tissue edema

4) Thrombosis of small vessels

a) Microcirculation is sluggish

b) Microclots develop, which lead to organ ischemia, anoxia, and consumption of clotting factors, potentially leading to DIC

5) Cellular deterioration

a) Reduced delivery of oxygen to tissues

b) Change from aerobic to anaerobic metabolism

   i) Metabolic acidosis occurs since lactic acid is produced as a byproduct of anaerobic metabolism and accumulates in the blood

   ii) Depletion of cellular adenosine triphosphate (ATP) reserves occurs since anaerobic metabolism results in significantly less ATP than does aerobic metabolism

c) Failure of sodium-potassium pump, an active transport system that requires ATP causes excessive sodium and water to enter cell

d) Organelle edema

   i) Lysosomes may rupture releasing active enzymes into the cell

   ii) Mitochondria can no longer use glucose and oxygen to make ATP, worsening the ATP deficiency

e) Cellular destruction

   i) Cellular edema caused by failure of sodium-potassium pump

   ii) Apoptosis (i.e., preprogrammed cellular suicide) activated by injury

f) Organ failure

6) Massive ischemia of tissues leading to the release of mediators of the inflammatory process and SIRS (see next section on SIRS)

7) Effects of shock on specific organs and organ systems

a) Heart

   i) Dysrhythmias occur because of the failure of the sodium-potassium pump resulting from decreased ATP, hypoxemia, ischemia, and acidosis

   ii) Cardiac failure may occur because of ischemia, acidosis, and MDF

b) Lung

   i) Endothelial damage in the capillary bed and precapillary arterioles along with damage to the type II pneumocytes may cause acute lung injury or acute respiratory distress syndrome (ARDS)

   ii) Hypoxemia causes hypoxemic vasoconstriction of pulmonary circulation and pulmonary hypertension

   iii) Ventilation-perfusion mismatch occurs because of disturbances in both ventilation and perfusion

   iv) Pulmonary edema may result from disruption of the alveolar-capillary

membrane, ARDS, heart failure, or from overaggressive fluid resuscitation

c) Brain

   i) Loss of autoregulation and brain ischemia occur when cerebral perfusion pressure is <50 mm Hg

   ii) SNS dysfunction, depression of cardiac and respiratory centers, and impaired thermoregulation occur

   iii) Cerebral infarction may occur

d) Kidney

   i) Renal vasoconstriction and hypoperfusion of the kidney decrease glomerular filtration rate

   ii) Prolonged ischemia causes acute tubular necrosis (ATN) and renal failure

   iii) Metabolic acids accumulate in the blood, worsening the metabolic acidosis caused by lactic acid production during anaerobic metabolism

e) Liver

   i) Hypoperfusion damages the reticuloendothelial cells, which causes recirculation of bacteria and cellular debris and predisposes to bacteremia and sepsis

   ii) Damage to the hepatocytes causes the liver to be unable to detoxify drugs, toxins, or hormones or conjugate bilirubin

   iii) Hepatic dysfunction causes a decreased ability to mobilize carbohydrate, protein, and fat stores, which results in hypoglycemia

f) Pancreas

   i) Pancreatic enzymes are released by the ischemic and damaged pancreas

   ii) Pancreatic ischemia causes the release of MDF, which results in depression of cardiac contractility

   iii) Hyperglycemia occurs as the result of endogenous and/or exogenous corticosteroids and insulin resistance; hyperglycemia results in the following

      (a) Dehydration and electrolyte imbalances related to osmotic diuresis

      (b) Impairment of leukocyte function causing decreased phagocytosis and increased risk of infection

      (c) Depression of the immune response

      (d) Impairment in gastric motility

      (e) Shifts in the substrate availability from glucose to free fatty acids or lactate

      (f) Negative nitrogen balance and decreased wound healing

g) Gastrointestinal

   i) Ischemia and increased gastric acid production caused by glucocorticoids increase risk of stress ulcer

ii) Prolonged vasoconstriction and ischemia lead to the inability of the intestinal walls to act as intact barriers to prevent the migration of bacteria out of the gastrointestinal tract; this may allow translocation of bacteria from the GI tract into the lymphatic and vascular beds increasing the risk for sepsis

h) Hematologic/immunologic

   i) Hypoxia and release of inflammatory cytokines impair blood flow and result in microvascular thrombosis

   ii) Sluggish blood flow, massive tissue trauma, and consumption of clotting factors may cause DIC

   iii) The bone marrow mobilizes the release of white blood cells (WBCs)

     (a) Causes leukocytosis early in shock

     (b) Causes leukopenia as depletion of WBCs in blood and in bone marrow occurs

   iv) Massive tissue injury caused by widespread ischemia stimulates a systemic inflammatory response syndrome with massive release of mediators of the inflammatory process

2. Refractory stage is irreversible and refractory to conventional therapy

  a. Clinical indications of profound hypoperfusion and profound hypotension unresponsive to potent vasopressors

  b. Clinical indications of MODS (i.e., failure of two or more body systems)

   1) ARDS

   2) DIC

   3) Hepatic dysfunction/failure

   4) ATN/renal failure

   5) Myocardial ischemia/infarction (MI)/failure

   6) Cerebral ischemia/infarction

  c. Death from ineffective tissue perfusion due to failure of the circulation to meet the oxygen needs of the cell

Clinical presentation (Table 13-4)

1. Initial stage: no clinical indications; expert nurse may detect that "something is different"

2. Compensatory stage: SNS stimulation

  a. Subjective

   1) Anxiety, fear, feeling of impending doom

   2) Thirst

  b. Objective

   1) Tachycardia

   2) Blood pressure (BP) changes

    a) Systolic BP increases or stays the same while diastolic BP increases resulting in a decrease in pulse pressure

     i) Since diastolic BP is a reflection of arterial elasticity, the vasoconstriction caused by the SNS causes an elevation in diastolic BP and a narrowing of the pulse pressure earlier than a decrease in systolic BP or MAP

    b) Orthostatic effects with the BP decreasing when the patient is repositioned from lying to sitting

   3) Tachypnea

   4) Skin: cool, pale, clammy

   5) GI: decreased bowel sounds

   6) Renal: oliguria (i.e., <0.5 ml/kg/hr)

   7) CNS: irritability, restlessness, confusion

    a) Since the CNS is very sensitive to changes in oxygen and glucose, neurologic signs and symptoms occur early

3. Progressive stage: hypoperfusion

  a. Subjective

   1) Anorexia, nausea

   2) Chest pain, palpitations may occur

   3) Dyspnea may occur

  b. Objective

   1) Tachycardia, dysrhythmias

   2) Hypotension

   3) Hypothermia (except early septic)

   4) Tachypnea

   5) Skin

    a) Bluish, mottled appearance

    b) Peripheral cyanosis

   6) GI: vomiting, absent bowel sounds

   7) Renal: anuria (i.e., negligible or <100 ml/24 hr)

   8) CNS: lethargy, coma

4. Refractory stage: profound hypoperfusion and evidence of MODS

  a. ARDS: clinical indications of respiratory distress; crackles; decreased Pao_2, Sao_2; decreased pulmonary compliance; diffuse pulmonary infiltrates on chest radiograph

  b. DIC: bleeding in a patient without a prior history of bleeding; petechiae; blood in sputum, vomitus, nasogastric aspirate, urine, stool; elevated PT, aPTT, decreased platelets, elevated FSP, positive D-dimer

  c. Hepatic dysfunction/failure: jaundice; elevated bilirubin; elevated AST, ALT, LDH; hypoglycemia

  d. Gastrointestinal: paralytic ileus; gastrointestinal bleeding

  e. ATN/renal failure: oliguria or anuria; elevated BUN, creatinine; decreased urine creatinine clearance

  f. Myocardial ischemia/infarction/failure: chest pain; ECG indicators of myocardial infarction; positive CK-MB and troponin; clinical indicator of left ventricular and/or right ventricular failure

  g. Cerebral ischemia/infarction: change in level of consciousness, change in Glasgow Coma Scale score of ≥1, focal signs (e.g., hemiparesis or hemiplegia, aphasia)

5. Hemodynamic parameters (Table 13-5)

  a. Decreased oxygen delivery to the tissues (DO_2): common to all forms of shock except early septic shock, in which DO_2 is increased but extraction and utilization are impaired

TABLE 13-4 Clinical Presentation of the Stages of Shock

Initial: Subclinical Hypoperfusion	Compensatory: SNS	Progressive: Hypoperfusion	Refractory: Profound Hypoperfusion
CI 2.2 to 2.5 L/min/m²	CI 2.0 to 2.2 L/min/m²	CI <2.0 L/min/m²	CI <1.8 L/min/m²
• No clinical indications of hypoperfusion but "something is different" • Detected by invasive hemodynamic monitoring	• Tachycardia • Narrowed pulse pressure • Tachypnea • Cool skin • Oliguria • Diminished bowel sounds • Restlessness → confusion	• Dysrhythmias • Hypotension • Tachypnea • Cold, clammy skin • Anuria • Absent bowel sounds • Lethargy → coma	• Life-threatening dysrhythmias • Hypotension despite potent vasopressors • ARDS • DIC • Hepatic dysfunction/ failure • ATN • Mesenteric ischemia/ infarction • Myocardial ischemia/ infarction/failure • Cerebral ischemia/ infarction

From: Dennison, R. D. (2007). *Pass CCRN!* (3rd ed.). St. Louis: Mosby.

1) Oxygen delivery $(DO_2) = CO \times (Hgb \times 1.34 \times Sao_2) \times 10$
2) Normal: approximately 1000 ml/min

6. Diagnostic
   a. Serum
      1) Sodium: increased early, increased or decreased late
      2) Potassium: decreased early, increased late
      3) Chloride: decreased early, increased late
      4) Bicarbonate: normal early, decreased late
      5) CO_2: normal early, decreased late
      6) Glucose: increased early, decreased late
      7) BUN: increased
      8) Creatinine: increased
      9) Total protein, albumin: decreased
      10) Bilirubin: increased late
      11) Amylase, lipase: increased late
      12) Ammonia: increased late
      13) CK: increased
      14) Liver enzymes (AST, ALT, LDH): increased
      15) Lactate: increased (should be done on arterial blood)
         a) Correlates with the degree of hypoperfusion
         b) Above 2 mmol/L is associated with increased mortality
      16) Hemoglobin, hematocrit: decreased if due to hemorrhage
      17) Hematocrit: increased is due to cause other than hemorrhage
      18) WBC: increased early, decreased late
      19) PT, aPTT: may be prolonged
      20) Platelets: may be decreased
      21) ABGs: respiratory alkalosis progressing to metabolic acidosis; Pao_2 and Sao_2 may be decreased
      22) Blood cultures: may identify organism if septic shock
   b. Urine
      1) Urine creatinine clearance: decreased
      2) Urine specific gravity: increased early, decreased late

TABLE 13-5 Hemodynamic Alterations in Shock

	Hypovolemic	Cardiogenic	Early Septic	Late Septic	Anaphylactic	Neurogenic
HR	High	High	High	High	High	Normal or low
BP	Normal → low	Normal → low	Normal → low	Low	Normal → low	Normal → low
CO	Low	Low	High	Low	Normal → Low	Normal → low
CVP or PAOP	Low	High	Low	High	Low	Low
SVR	High	High	Low	High	Low	Low
Svo_2 or $Scvo_2$	Low	Low	High	Low	Low	Low

3) Urine osmolality: increased early, decreased late
4) Urine sodium: decreased
5) Presence of heavy pigments
   a) Myoglobinuria occurs with muscle tissue destruction (e.g., crush injuries, muscle ischemia/necrosis, electrical burns, prolonged seizures [i.e., status epilepticus])
   b) Hemoglobinuria occurs with mismatched blood transfusion reaction and fresh water drowning
c. Other diagnostic studies may be done to evaluate the reason for shock

Collaborative management

1. Continue assessment
   a. ABCDs
   b. Vital signs: blood pressure, pulse, respiratory rate, and temperature
   c. Oxygen saturation
   d. Respiratory effort and excursion
   e. Cardiac rate and rhythm
   f. Hemodynamic parameters as available
   g. Pain and discomfort level
   h. Accurate intake and output
   i. Serum electrolytes
   j. Level of consciousness
   k. Close monitoring for progression of symptoms
2. Maximize oxygen delivery to the tissues (Hgb, Sao$_2$, CO/CI)
   a. Maintain optimal hemoglobin and vascular volume: monitor and use central venous pressure (CVP) or pulmonary artery occlusive pressure (PAOP) when available
      1) Two IV catheters should be inserted immediately, especially in cases of hemorrhage; these catheters should be short and large-gauge
      2) Volume replacement for hypovolemic and vasogenic; may be necessary even in cardiogenic shock to achieve optimal CVP and MAP
         a) Types of fluids used for fluid resuscitation (Table 13-6)
            i) Crystalloids: solutions with dextrose or electrolytes; safe, effective, inexpensive and usually the initial fluid type (Table 13-7)
            ii) Colloids: large molecule (protein or starch) solutions; considered when the patient's response to initial efforts are insufficient
               (a) Stay in the vascular space better than crystalloids and contribute to intravascular colloidal oncotic pressure to pull more fluid into the vascular space
               (b) May be used in hypovolemic shock (except early burns) or neurogenic shock; since septic and anaphylactic shock are both associated with increased capillary permeability, colloids should be avoided at least initially

TABLE 13-6   Types of Fluids Used for Fluid Resuscitation

Crystalloids	Colloids	Blood and Blood Products
Isotonic: NS; LR (D$_5$NS, D$_5$LR) Hypotonic: ½NS (D$_5$½NS, D$_5$W) Hypertonic: 3% saline; D$_{10}$W; TPN	Albumin Dextran 70/75 Hetastarch (Hespan)	Whole blood Packed RBCs Fresh frozen plasma

NS, normal (0.9%) saline; LR, lactated Ringer; D$_5$NS, 5% dextrose in normal saline; D$_5$LR, 5% dextrose in lactated Ringer; ½NS, 0.45% saline; D$_5$½NS, 5% dextrose in 0.45% saline; D$_5$W, 5% dextrose in water; D$_{10}$W, 10% dextrose in water; TPN, total parenteral nutrition (usually 25% dextrose)

*Dextrose solutions are in parentheses because even though 5% dextrose adds to osmolality in the bottle or bag, this small amount of dextrose is metabolized so quickly when in the body that it should not be considered in the osmolality of the solution. So consider D$_5$NS as NS, D5½NS as ½NS, and D$_5$W as water. This last example is why D$_5$W is avoided except in extreme hyperosmolar conditions. In significant volumes, D$_5$W will dilute electrolytes, particularly sodium, and potentially cause neurologic changes including seizures.

            (c) Examples
               (1) Albumin: plasma protein component; costly
               (2) Dextran: contains polymers of high-molecular-weight polysaccharides; may cause coagulopathy or ATN
               (3) Hetastarch: contains polymers of hydroxyethyl starch; may cause coagulopathy
               (4) Blood and blood products: used only to achieve a specific physiologic goal, such as to increase oxygen delivery or clotting capability
                  (a) Contains plasma proteins present to add to intravascular colloidal oncotic pressure; only solution that increases the Cao$_2$ (content of oxygen in arterial blood) since 97% of all oxygen is carried on the hemoglobin molecule
                  (b) Indicated when the patient has lost blood and there are clinical indications of hypoperfusion
                  (c) Hematocrit of 30% to 32% is probably a reasonable goal since no significant increase in oxygen delivery is achieved and blood flow may become sluggish with a greater hematocrit
                  (d) Major disadvantages of blood and blood products: cost and risk of blood transfusion reaction or blood transmitted disease

TABLE **13-7** Crystalloids

	Isotonic	Hypotonic	Hypertonic
Osmolality	• 250 to 350 mOsm/L (which is similar to blood osmolality of 280 to 295 mOsm/L)	• <250 mOsm/L	• >350 mOsm/L
Uses	• Tend to stay in the vascular space better than other crystalloids • Require replacement with 3 ml for every 1 ml lost since they do equilibrate across fluid compartments	• Tend to leave the vascular space and replace the interstitial space better than the vascular space	• Pull fluid from the interstitial space into the intravascular space • Expands intravascular volume over isotonic crystalloid without the adverse effects of colloids • Monitor closely for clinical indications of fluid overload when these solutions are administered

Examples	0.9% saline
	• Composition
	  • 154 mEq of sodium
	  • 154 mEq of chloride
	  • Water
	• Osmolality is 289 mOsm/L
	• pH is 5.7
	• Large volumes may cause metabolic (hyperchloremic) acidosis
	Lactated Ringer
	• Composition
	  • 130 mEq/L
	  • 109 mEq/L chloride
	  • 4 mEq/L potassium
	  • 3 mEq/L of calcium
	  • 28 mEq/L of lactate
	  • Water
	• Osmolality is 273 mOsm/L
	• pH 6.7
	• Lactate is added as a buffer to make the solution less acidic (than without the lactate)
	• Lactate is converted to bicarbonate by the liver so large volumes may cause metabolic alkalosis and this solution should be avoided in patients who have liver disease
		Half-normal (0.45%) saline
		• Composition
		  • 77 mEq of sodium
		  • 77 mEq of chloride
		  • Water
		D_5W
		• Composition
		  • 50 grams of dextrose
		  • Water
		• Note that though D_5W is isotonic in the bottle, the body quickly metabolizes the dextrose and free water is left; avoid this solution except in extremely hyperosmolar patients (e.g., HHNC, DI)
			Hypertonic (3% saline)
			• Composition
			  • 513 mEq of sodium
			  • 513 mEq of chloride
			$D_{10}W$ (10% dextrose in water)
			• Composition
			  • 100 grams of dextrose/L
			  • Water
			$D_{50}W$ (50% dextrose in water)
			• Composition
			  • 25 grams of dextrose/ 50 ml ampule
			  • Water
			Total parenteral nutrition solution
			• Central
			  • 250 grams of dextrose/L
			  • Protein, electrolytes, vitamins vary
			  • Water
			• Peripheral
			  • 100 grams of dextrose/L
			  • Protein, electrolytes, vitamins vary
			  • Water

(e) For more information on blood and blood products and administration of blood, see Chapter 11

b) Selection of solution for replacement
   i) Colloids should not be used in situations with increased capillary permeability (e.g., burns during first 24 to 48 hours, sepsis, anaphylaxis)
   ii) In other situations, there is no difference in effectiveness (Anderson et al., 2004) and colloids are considerably more costly
   iii) Blood should be used when the patient has lost blood and shows clinical indications of hypoperfusion

c) Volume
   i) Typical fluid challenge is 250 to 500 ml of normal saline over 5 minutes (Figure 13-1)
   ii) BP and hemodynamic monitoring (e.g., CVP, PAOP) as available
   iii) Monitoring for clinical indicators of fluid overload (e.g., dyspnea, jugular venous distention, S_3, systolic flow murmur, crackles)

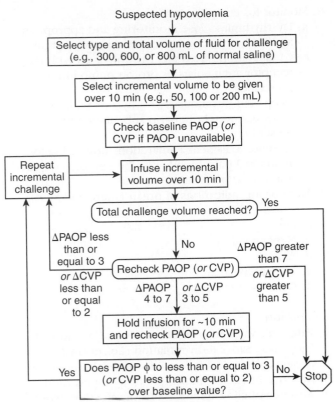

Figure 13-1 Fluid challenge algorithm. (From Kruse, J.A., Fink, M.P., & Carlson, R.W. [2003]. *Saunders manual of critical care*. Philadelphia: Saunders.)

3) Intraosseous infusions if IV access is unobtainable
   a) Sites
      i) Adult: sternum
      ii) Children: proximal tibia
         (a) Palpate the tibial tuberosity just below the knee
      iii) Consistent flat area of bone ~2 cm distal and slightly medial to the tibial tuberosity
      iv) Identification of landmarks to decrease the chance of insertion into the growth plate
         (a) Distal tibia or femur are alternative sites to be used if tibia is fractured
      v) Application of dressing with antibiotic ointment and 4×4 pads
   b) All medications and blood products can be given via an intraosseous line
      i) Onset and peak drug levels are comparable to doses given IV
   c) Complications (ACS, 2004)
      i) Infection
         (a) Intraosseous needles left in the marrow for >72 hours increase the risk of infection
      ii) Through-and-through penetration of bone
      iii) Subcutaneous or subperiosteal infiltration
      iv) Pressure necrosis of the skin

v) Physeal plate injury
vi) Hematoma
4) Type and cross-match immediately if patient is hemorrhaging; type specific blood or O negative may be given in severe hemorrhage but may make future crossmatching more difficult
5) Prevention of hypothermia during fluid resuscitation; fluids may need to be warmed if the patient's body temperature is low (≤35°C) at the initiation of fluid resuscitation or if multiple units of blood or multiple L of IV fluids are needed
6) Venous vasodilators and/or diuretics as prescribed to decrease the preload (CVP/PAOP) in cardiogenic shock
   b. Maintain optimal cardiac contractility and cardiac output
      1) Inotropes (e.g., dobutamine [Dobutrex]) as prescribed
      2) Diuretics (e.g., furosemide [Lasix]) as prescribed
      3) Vasoactive agents
         a) Arterial vasodilators (e.g., nitroprusside [NTP]), to decrease afterload (SVR) and/or venous vasodilators (e.g., nitroglycerin [NTG]) to decrease preload (PAOP) as prescribed; these agents are typically needed in cardiogenic shock
         b) Vasopressors (e.g., norepinephrine [Levophed], dopamine [Intropin]) as prescribed and in the lowest doses necessary to achieve desired effects
            i) Vasopressors are generally contraindicated in patients with cardiogenic shock as they increase afterload (SVR) and myocardial oxygen consumption
            ii) Vasopressors may be used in an effort to maintain MAP >60 mm Hg to maintain perfusion pressure but by constricting the vessels they may actually decrease blood flow to organs, even through the MAP is higher
      4) Correction of metabolic acidosis because it affects cardiac contractility
         a) Improvement of oxygenation and perfusion by improving Hgb, SaO_2, Hgb to decrease lactic acid production
         b) Sodium bicarbonate as prescribed; indicated only if pH 7.0 or less
      5) Avoidance of overheating, which may cause vasodilation and decrease in preload
   c. Maintain optimal oxygen saturation
      1) Monitoring of SpO_2, SvO_2, ABGs
      2) Artificial airway as indicated; endotracheal intubation frequently necessary
      3) Oxygen at 5 to 6 L/min initially
         a) Higher concentrations may be necessary depending on SpO_2 and ABG values
         b) CPAP or PEEP may be required for refractory hypoxemia

4) Mechanical ventilation as prescribed for respiratory muscle fatigue, respiratory acidosis, and/or refractory hypoxemia

5) Monitoring for changes in SpO_2, ABGs, pulmonary vascular resistance, chest radiograph, and lung compliance indicative of ARDS

3. Minimize oxygen consumption of the tissues
   a. Patient comfort
      1) Bedrest and provide adequate rest periods
      2) Analgesics and anxiolytics as required but be cautious to avoid cumulative effect
   b. Control of body temperature
      1) Treatment of hyperthermia with cooling blankets as necessary: set at 1°C below patient's temperature to avoid drift and resultant shivering
      2) Avoidance of overheating, which may increase myocardial oxygen consumption
   c. Monitoring of work of breathing; initiate mechanical ventilation as prescribed for respiratory fatigue
   d. Control of pain and anxiety
      1) Analgesics and/or anxiolytics as prescribed and indicated
      2) Patient and family support
         a) Effective communication to keep patient and family informed
         b) Encouragement of the patient and family to discuss fear, concerns
4. Prevent injury caused by decreased perfusion
   a. Sedatives and other central nervous system (CNS) depressants are limited
   b. Drugs are administered only IV because peripheral perfusion and drug absorption is impaired; central venous catheter with multiple-lumen catheter is preferred
5. Maintain renal perfusion and glomerular filtration rate (GFR)
   a. Foley catheter to monitor hourly urine output
   b. Monitoring of BUN, creatinine, urine creatinine clearance, urine sodium
   c. Adequate volume replacement as indicated by CVP or PAOP
   d. Monitoring for change in color of urine which may indicate myoglobinuria, hemoglobinuria
6. Maintain glycemic control
   a. Recognition that hyperglycemia is related to stress and insulin resistance and occurs in patients without diagnosis of diabetes mellitus
   b. Goal is a serum glucose <150 mg/dl
      1) IV insulin adjusted according to serum glucose level
      2) $D_{10}W$ for hypoglycemia
7. Provide emotional support to the patient and family
   a. Effective communication to inform the patient or family regarding what is going to occur and why
      1) Provide with accurate information
      2) Maintain hope but do not give false reassurance

8. Monitor for complications
   a. Dysrhythmias: close monitoring and appropriate antidysrhythmic agents depending on rhythm
   b. GI ulceration: stress ulcer prophylaxis with H_2 receptor antagonists or proton pump inhibitors as prescribed
   c. Deep vein thrombosis: prophylaxis with low-molecular-weight heparin subcutaneously as prescribed
   d. Mesenteric ischemia, infarction: monitoring for abdominal pain, bloody diarrhea; surgery required if intestinal perforation occurs
9. Monitor for indications of organ failure and MODS
   a. ARDS
   b. DIC
   c. Hepatic failure
   d. ATN
   e. Myocardial infarction
   f. Cerebral infarction

Evaluation

1. Patent airway, adequate oxygenation (i.e., normal PaO_2, SpO_2, SaO_2) and ventilation (i.e., normal $PaCO_2$)
2. Absence of clinical indications of respiratory distress
3. Absence of clinical indicators of hypoperfusion
4. Absence of clinical indications of infection/sepsis
5. Control of pain/discomfort/dyspnea
6. Alert and oriented with no neurovascular deficit

Typical disposition: admission to critical care unit

Hypovolemic Shock

Definition: shock caused by inadequate intravascular volume

Predisposing factors

1. External losses
   a. Blood
      1) Gastrointestinal (e.g., esophageal varices, peptic ulcer, hemorrhoids)
      2) Genitourinary (e.g., antepartal or postpartum bleeding, hematuria)
      3) Amputations
      4) Major blood vessel disruption (may also be occult)
      5) Coagulopathy
         a) Congenital coagulopathy (e.g., hemophilia)
         b) Acquired coagulopathy (e.g., DIC, excessive anticoagulation)
   b. Fluid
      1) Gastrointestinal losses (e.g., vomiting, diarrhea, nasogastric suction)
      2) Renal losses
         a) DKA
         b) HHNC
         c) Diabetes insipidus
         d) Hypoaldosteronism (Addison disease)
         e) Diuretics
         f) Osmotic dyes
      3) Cutaneous losses
         a) Burns

b) Exudative wounds

c) Excessive perspiration (e.g., heat exhaustion)

2. Internal sequestration

  a. Blood

    1) Hemoperitoneum or retroperitoneal (e.g., hemorrhagic pancreatitis, ruptured spleen, lacerated liver)

    2) Thoracic trauma with hemothorax, hemomediastinum

    3) Dissecting aortic aneurysm

    4) Pelvic or long bone fractures

  b. Fluid

    1) Ascites: peritonitis, pancreatitis, cirrhosis, intra-abdominal malignancies (e.g., liver, ovarian)

    2) Pleural effusion

    3) Intestinal obstruction

Pathophysiology (Figure 13-2)
Clinical presentation (as for shock as well as the following)

1. Subjective: history of precipitating factor

2. Objective

  a. Flat neck veins

  b. Intake and output: 1 L is equal to 1 kg

    1) Consider insensible losses

    2) Weigh dressings and convert to volume using 1 kg equal to 1000 ml

    3) Include drainage from all tubes

  c. Parameters used for evaluation of severity of hemorrhagic shock (Table 13-8)

3. Hemodynamics (see Table 13-5)

4. Diagnostic

  a. Hct

    1) Elevated if due to dehydration

    2) Decreased if due to blood loss

  b. Diagnostic peritoneal lavage to detect intra-abdominal bleeding

  c. CT of chest or abdomen to detect source of bleeding

Collaborative management: as for shock as well as the following

1. Identify high-risk patient and monitor for clinical indications of hypoperfusion

2. Continue assessment

  a. ABCDs

  b. Vital signs: blood pressure, pulse, respiratory rate, and temperature

  c. Oxygen saturation

  d. Respiratory effort and excursion

  e. Cardiac rate and rhythm

  f. Hemodynamic parameters as available

  g. Pain and discomfort level

  h. Accurate intake and output

  i. Serum electrolytes

  j. Level of consciousness

  k. Close monitoring for progression of symptoms

3. Treat the cause

  a. Compression of any compressible vessels

  b. Surgery may be necessary to control bleeding

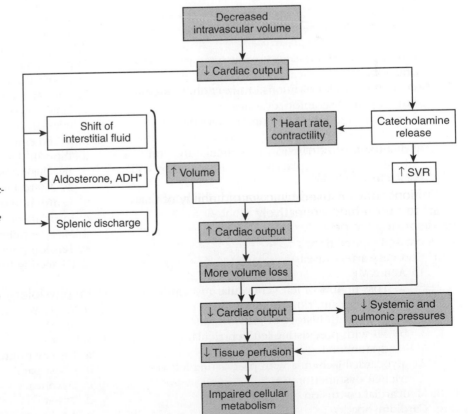

Figure 13-2 Pathophysiology of hypovolemic shock. (From McCance, K. L., & Huether, S. E. [2006]. *Pathophysiology: The basis of disease in adults and children* (5th ed.). St Louis: Mosby.)

TABLE 13-8   Severity of Hemorrhagic Shock

Class	I	II	III	IV
Blood loss (% of blood volume)	<15%	15% to 30%	30% to 40%	>40%
Blood loss (ml)	<750 ml	750 to 1500 ml	1500 to 2000 ml	>2000 ml
Heart rate, beats/min	<100	>100	>120	≤140
Blood pressure	Normal	Normal	Decreased	Decreased
Pulse pressure	Widened or normal	Narrowed	Narrowed	Narrowed
Capillary refill	Normal	Delayed	Delayed	Delayed or absent
Ventilatory rate, /min	14 to 20	20 to 30	30 to 40	>35
Urine output (ml/hr)	≤30	20 to 30	<20	Negligible
Skin appearance	Cool, pink	Cool, pale	Cold, moist, pale	Cold, clammy, cyanotic
Neurologic status	Slightly anxious	Mildly anxious	Anxious, confused	Confused, lethargy

Adapted from American College of Surgeons' Committee on Trauma. (2004). *Advanced Trauma Life Support for Doctors (ATLS) student manual* (7th ed.). Chicago: American College of Surgeons.

   c. Antidiarrheal agents for diarrhea, insulin for hyperglycemia, etc.
4. Administer appropriate volume replacement
   a. Two large-gauge IV catheters
   b. Normal saline at rapid rate initially
   c. Monitoring for fluid overload (e.g., heart sounds for S_3, breath sounds for crackles)
5. Use autotransfusion if appropriate; used primarily in chest trauma or chest surgery to decrease the risk of transfusion transmitted disease

Evaluation
1. Patent airway, adequate oxygenation (i.e., normal Pao_2, Spo_2, Sao_2) and ventilation (i.e., normal $Paco_2$)
2. Absence of clinical indications of respiratory distress
3. Absence of clinical indicators of hypoperfusion
4. Absence of clinical indications of infection/sepsis
5. Control of pain/discomfort/dyspnea
6. Alert and oriented with no neurovascular deficit

Typical disposition: admission to critical care unit

Cardiogenic Shock
Definition: shock caused by impaired ability of the heart to pump blood effectively
Predisposing factors
1. Decreased contractility
   a. Coronary artery disease
      1) Acute MI
         a) Loss of 40% of left ventricular myocardium
            i) Large anterior MI
            ii) MI with history of previous MI
         b) MI with preexisting left ventricular dysfunction
      2) Myocardial ischemia with preexisting left ventricular dysfunction
   b. Myocardial contusion
   c. Cardiomyopathy

   d. Myocarditis
   e. Severe heart failure
   f. Ventricular aneurysm
   g. Overdosage of myocardial depressant drugs (e.g., β-blockers, calcium channel blockers, barbiturates)
   h. Stunned myocardium: transient cardiogenic shock
      1) Cardiac surgery: related to hypothermia, cardioplegic arrest, surgical incisions
      2) Reperfusion injury
      3) Post CPR
      4) Hypoxemia
      5) Acidosis
      6) Hypoglycemia
      7) Electrolyte imbalance
   i. Acute rejection of cardiac transplant
2. Impaired filling
   a. Dysrhythmias
   b. Cardiac tamponade
   c. Noncompliant ventricle (e.g., left ventricular hypertrophy, right ventricular hypertrophy)
3. Impaired emptying (may be referred to as obstructive)
   a. Valvular dysfunction
      1) Chronic: stenosis or regurgitation
      2) Acute: papillary muscle rupture
   b. Ventricular septal rupture
   c. Intracardiac tumor
   d. Massive pulmonary embolism
   e. Tension pneumothorax
   f. Dissecting thoracic aortic aneurysm

Pathophysiology (Figure 13-3)
Clinical presentation (as for shock as well as the following)
1. Subjective
   a. History of precipitating factor
   b. Chest pain
   c. Dyspnea
   d. Thirst
   e. Anxiety, fear, feeling of impending doom

2. Objective
   a. Clinical indicators of LVF
      1) Tachycardia
      2) Dysrhythmias
      3) Pulsus alternans
      4) Tachypnea
      5) Heart sound changes: S_3
      6) Breath sound changes: crackles
   b. Clinical indicators of RVF
      1) Jugular venous distention
      2) Peripheral edema
      3) Hepatosplenomegaly
3. Hemodynamics (see Table 13-5)
4. Diagnostic
   a. Serum
      1) Enzymes and troponin: elevated if acute MI
      2) Electrolytes: note any abnormality
      3) ABGs: may reveal significant hypoxemia in pulmonary edema, respiratory acidosis as patient fatigues and acute respiratory failure occurs, and eventually metabolic acidosis as tissue hypoxia causes lactic acidosis
   b. ECG
      1) May reveal acute (i.e., ST-segment elevation, pathologic Q waves) or old MI (pathologic Q waves without ST segment elevation)
      2) May reveal ventricular aneurysm (i.e., persistent ST-segment elevation in anterior leads)
      3) May reveal dysrhythmias
   c. Chest radiography: may show pulmonary vascular congestion
   d. Cardiac catheterization
      1) May reveal cause of cardiogenic shock
      2) May reveal abnormal intracardiac pressures
   e. Echocardiography: may reveal cause of cardiogenic shock
      1) Ventricular wall motion abnormality
         a) Regional myocardial wall motional abnormality in myocardial ischemia or infarction
         b) Global wall motion abnormality in cardiomyopathy or myocarditis
      2) Valvular abnormality (e.g., ruptured ventricular septum, ruptured papillary muscle with acute mitral regurgitation)
      3) Cardiac tamponade

Collaborative management: as for shock as well as the following

1. Identify high-risk patients and monitor for clinical indications of hypoperfusion; invasive hemodynamic monitoring if appropriate for early detection of changes in cardiac index
2. Continue assessment
   a. ABCDs
   b. Vital signs: blood pressure, pulse, respiratory rate, and temperature
   c. Oxygen saturation
   d. Respiratory effort and excursion
   e. Cardiac rate and rhythm
   f. Hemodynamic parameters as available
   g. Pain and discomfort level
   h. Accurate intake and output
   i. Serum electrolytes

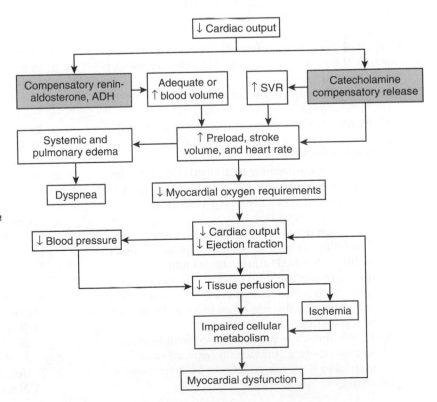

Figure 13-3 Pathophysiology of cardiogenic shock. (From McCance, K. L., & Huether, S. E. [2006]. *Pathophysiology: The basis of disease in adults and children* (5th ed.). St Louis: Mosby.)

j. Level of consciousness

k. Close monitoring for progression of symptoms

3. Prevent/treat the cause

a. Early reperfusion for acute MI

b. Pericardiocentesis for cardiac tamponade

c. Fibrinolytics, anticoagulants for pulmonary embolus

d. Surgery for removal of intracardiac tumors, valve replacement, septal repair, etc.

e. Emergency decompression followed by chest tube for tension pneumothorax

4. Improve oxygenation

a. Oxygen by nasal cannula to achieve SaO_2 of at least 95%; nonrebreathing face mask may be required to achieve this SaO_2 but is likely to increase dyspnea

b. Mask CPAP may be helpful to improve oxygenation, especially for patients with significant pulmonary edema, but is likely to increase dyspnea

c. Intubation and mechanical ventilation may be required to decrease the work of breathing as well and improve ventilation and oxygenation

5. Improve myocardial perfusion

a. Nitrates for ischemia while being careful not to decrease blood pressure or coronary artery perfusion pressure; since one nitroglycerin sublingually is 400 mcg, titratable intravenous nitroglycerin is preferred

b. Prompt evaluation for emergency reperfusion options if acute MI

1) Primary Percutaneous coronary intervention PCI: preferred if facilities available

2) Fibrinolytics may be used

3) Coronary artery bypass graft (CABG)

6. Optimize cardiac output and improve tissue perfusion

a. Inotropes (e.g., dobutamine [Dobutrex]) to increase contractility

b. Diuretics (e.g., furosemide [Lasix]) or venous vasodilators (e.g., nitroglycerin [NTG]) to decrease preload (PAOP)

c. Arterial vasodilators (e.g., nitroprusside [NTP]) to decrease afterload if no contraindications

1) Nitroprusside is contraindicated in acute myocardial ischemia due to the risk of coronary artery steal with shunting of blood from ischemic areas to nonischemic areas

2) Caution must be exercised with all arterial vasodilators in acute myocardial ischemia since they are likely to decrease aortic root pressure and coronary artery perfusion pressure

3) Careful titration of all vasodilators is required to maintain the MAP above the 60 mm Hg required to perfuse vital organs; afterload reduction may need to be achieved nonpharmacologically through the use of an intra-aortic balloon pump (IABP)

d. Antidysrhythmics as required to control heart rate

1) Anxiolytics (e.g., lorazepam [Ativan]) may be helpful to decrease heart rate by decreasing anxiety

2) β-Blockers are contraindicated during cardiogenic shock states since they do decrease contractility

e. Mechanical supports (e.g., IABP)

1) IABP is especially helpful in patients who have very high afterload but are too hypotensive to use arterial vasodilators to reduce afterload

2) IABP or ventricular assist devices may also serve as a bridge to transplant if the patient is a candidate for cardiac transplantation

7. Registration of the patient for cardiac transplantation if appropriate

Evaluation

1. Patent airway, adequate oxygenation (i.e., normal PaO_2, SpO_2, SaO_2) and ventilation (i.e., normal $PaCO_2$)

2. Absence of clinical indications of respiratory distress

3. Absence of clinical indicators of hypoperfusion

4. Absence of clinical indications of infection/sepsis

5. Control of pain/discomfort/dyspnea

6. Alert and oriented with no neurovascular deficit

Typical disposition: admission to critical care unit

Anaphylactic Shock

Definition: shock resulting from massive vasodilation caused by release of histamine in response to a severe allergic reaction

Predisposing factors

1. Foods, especially the following

a. Fish

b. Shellfish

c. Eggs

d. Milk and milk products

e. Wheat

f. Strawberries

g. Legumes (e.g., peanuts, soybeans)

h. Nuts (e.g., walnuts, pecans)

i. Chocolate

j. Food additives

1) Artificial coloring

2) Preservatives: sulfites, MSG

2. Drugs

a. ACE inhibitors (e.g., captopril [Capoten], enalapril [Vasotec])

b. Acetylcysteine (Mucomyst)

c. Allergic extracts in hyposensitization therapy

d. Anesthetics

1) Local anesthetics: lidocaine, cocaine

2) General anesthetics: thiopental (Pentothal), etomidate (Amidate), ketamine (Ketalar)

e. Animal serums: antitoxins, antivenins

f. Antibiotics

1) β-Lactam antibiotics

a) Penicillin

b) Cephalosporins

2) Tetracycline (Sumycin, Achromycin)

3) Macrolides

g. Barbiturates

h. Blood and blood products: blood transfusion incompatibilities, γ-globulin, albumin

i. Dextran

j. Enzymes
1) Pancreatic
2) Papaya enzyme
a) Chymopapain (Chimodiactin) (used in chemical discectomy)
b) Meat tenderizer

k. Insulin: pork or beef

l. Iodine-containing contrast media (e.g., Renografin)

m. Narcotics: morphine, meperidine (Demerol), codeine

n. Neuromuscular blocker

o. NSAIDs: acetylsalicylic acid (aspirin), ibuprofen (Motrin), indomethacin (Indocin)

p. Protamine sulfate

q. Thiazide diuretics (e.g., hydrochlorothiazide [Diazide])

3. Venoms
a. Snakes
b. Hymenoptera: wasps, hornets, bees, yellow jackets, fire ants
c. Spiders
d. Jellyfish
e. Stingrays
f. Deer flies
g. Scorpions

4. Other chemicals or biologicals
a. Materials (e.g., latex)
b. Hand lotions
c. Soap
d. Perfume
e. Iodine-containing solutions (e.g., Betadine)
f. Animal dander

Pathophysiology (Figure 13-4)

1. Anaphylactic reaction requires previous exposure to the antigen
a. With first exposure to the antigen, specific IgE antibody is formed
b. The antibody binds to the mass cells and basophils
c. Repeat exposure triggers a response by the IgE antibodies
d. Mast cells are triggered to degranulate
e. Bioactive mediators are released

Clinical presentation (for shock as well as the following)

1. Subjective
a. History of precipitating factor
b. Anxiety, vague uneasiness
c. Warmth
d. Nausea, abdominal cramping, abdominal pain
e. Chest tightness, palpitations
f. Dyspnea

g. Dizziness, vertigo

h. Pruritus

i. Feeling of a lump in throat

2. Objective
a. Cutaneous
1) An identifiable site of allergen exposure, bite, sting, or envenomation may be evident as localized redness, swelling, and pruritus
2) May be generalized
a) Angioedema (edema of membranous tissues): swelling of eyes, lips, tongue, hands, feet, and genitalia
b) Flushing
c) Warm to hot skin
d) Urticaria
e) Conjunctival injection, tearing
f) Watery rhinorrhea, sneezing
g) Erythema more in upper extremities

b. Cardiovascular
1) Tachycardia
2) Hypotension
3) Dysrhythmias
4) ST,T wave changes consistent with ischemia
5) Shock
6) Cardiac arrest may occur

c. Pulmonary
1) Hoarseness
2) Cough
3) Prolonged expiration
4) Breath sound changes: stridor, wheezing, crackles, rhonchi
5) Respiratory arrest may occur

d. Neurologic
1) Restlessness
2) Headache
3) Paresthesia
4) Change in level of consciousness
5) Seizures

e. Genitourinary
1) Urinary incontinence
2) Urine output: may be decreased
3) Vaginal bleeding

f. Gastrointestinal
1) Dysphagia
2) Vomiting
3) Hyperactive bowel sounds
4) Diarrhea

3. Hemodynamics: (see Table 13-5)

4. Diagnostic
a. Serum
1) IgE levels may be used to confirm allergic origin
2) Eosinophils elevated
3) ABGs: initially respiratory alkalosis with hypoxemia, eventually respiratory and metabolic acidosis as hypoventilation and tissue hypoxia occur

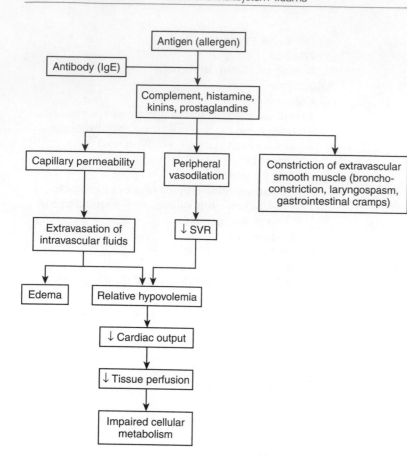

Figure 13-4 Pathophysiology of anaphylactic shock. (From McCance, K. L., & Huether, S. E. [2006]. *Pathophysiology: The basis of disease in adults and children* [5th ed.]. St Louis: Mosby.)

Collaborative management: as for shock as well as the following

1. Identify high-risk patients and monitor for clinical indications of allergic reaction and hypoperfusion
2. Continue assessment
   a. ABCDs
   b. Vital signs: blood pressure, pulse, respiratory rate, and temperature
   c. Oxygen saturation
   d. Respiratory effort and excursion
   e. Cardiac rate and rhythm
   f. Hemodynamic parameters as available
   g. Pain and discomfort level
   h. Accurate intake and output
   i. Serum electrolytes
   j. Level of consciousness
   k. Close monitoring for progression of symptoms
3. Maintain airway, oxygenation, and ventilation
   a. Airway
      1) Assess airway for clinical indications of angioedema (i.e., edema of uvula, respiratory distress, stridor, hypoxemia)
      2) If angioedema is present, assist with endotracheal tube insertion early to prevent complete airway obstruction; cricothyrotomy may be necessary because of laryngeal edema
   b. Oxygen at 5 to 6 L initially; adjust to maintain SpO_2 at 95% unless contraindicated; 100% nonrebreathing mask may be required but the mask may increase the sensation of dyspnea
   c. Mechanical ventilation as prescribed
4. Remove the offending agent or slow absorption of antigen
   a. Removal of stinger if anaphylaxis is due to a sting and the stinger can be removed easily without squeezing
   b. Ice if due to sting or bite
   c. Discontinuance of infusion of dye, drug, or blood
   d. Dermal decontamination with soap and water if skin exposure to allergen
   e. Gastric lavage not recommended to remove an ingested antigen
5. Modify or block the effects of biochemical mediators
   a. Sympathomimetic agents
      1) Epinephrine
         a) IV
            i) IV injection: 0.1 mg (100 mcg) IV over 5 to 10 minutes initially if clinical indications of cardiovascular compromise are present: stop injection if dysrhythmias or chest pain occur
            ii) IV infusion: 1 to 4 mcg/min if inadequate response to IV injection
         b) Intramuscular: 0.3 to 0.5 mg every 5 to 10 minutes for patients with less severe symptoms; thigh injection preferred over upper arm

2) Glucagon 1 mg IV every 5 minutes for patients taking β-blockers with hypotension refractory to epinephrine and fluids
   a) Glucagon can stimulate an increase in heart rate and contractility even with beta-blockade
   b) Care should include monitoring for nausea, vomiting, hypokalemia, hyperglycemia
b. Crystalloids: 1 to 2 L of normal saline
c. Antihistamines as prescribed to block histamine receptors
   1) H_1: Diphenhydramine (Benadryl) 25 to 50 mg IV, IM, or PO
   2) H_2: Ranitidine (Zantac) 50 mg IV or cimetidine (Tagamet) 150 mg IV
d. Steroids as prescribed to stabilize mast cells, decrease capillary permeability, prevent delayed reaction
   1) Methyl prednisolone sodium succinate (Solu-Medrol): 125 mg IV or hydrocortisone sodium succinate (Solu-Cortef) 100 to 200 to 500 mg IV
   2) Prednisone 40 to 60 mg PO daily
e. Bronchodilators as prescribed to reverse the bronchoconstriction caused by histamine, SRS-A, and bradykinin
   1) Albuterol (Ventolin), intermittent or continuous nebulizer for wheezing refractory to epinephrine
   2) Ipratropium bromide (Atrovent) or magnesium may also be used
6. Maintain MAP and tissue perfusion: fluids, inotropes, and/or vasopressors may be necessary

Evaluation
1. Patent airway, adequate oxygenation (i.e., normal Pao_2, Spo_2, Sao_2) and ventilation (i.e., normal $Paco_2$)
2. Absence of clinical indications of respiratory distress
3. Absence of clinical indicators of hypoperfusion
4. Absence of clinical indications of infection/sepsis
5. Control of pain/discomfort/dyspnea
6. Alert and oriented with no neurovascular deficit

Typical disposition: admission to critical care unit

Neurogenic Shock
Definition: shock resulting from massive vasodilation caused by suppression of the sympathetic nervous system
Predisposing factors
1. Spinal cord injury
2. Head injury
3. Insulin shock
4. General anesthesia
5. Spinal anesthesia
6. Epidural block
7. Drugs
   a. Barbiturates
   b. Phenothiazines
   c. Sympathetic blocking agents (e.g., antihypertensives)

8. Exposure to unpleasant circumstances (e.g., fright, pain)

Pathophysiology (Figure 13-5)
Clinical presentation
1. Subjective: history of precipitating factor
2. Objective
   a. Bradycardia
   b. Hypotension
   c. Hypothermia
   d. Skin warm, dry, flushed
   e. Definite neurologic deficit
3. Hemodynamics: (see Table 13-5)

Collaborative management: as for shock as well as the following
1. Identify high-risk patients and monitor for clinical indications of hypoperfusion
2. Continue assessment
   a. ABCDs
   b. Vital signs: blood pressure, pulse, respiratory rate, and temperature
   c. Oxygen saturation
   d. Respiratory effort and excursion
   e. Cardiac rate and rhythm
   f. Hemodynamic parameters as available
   g. Pain and discomfort level
   h. Accurate intake and output
   i. Serum electrolytes
   j. Level of consciousness
   k. Close monitoring for progression of symptoms
3. Prevent/treat the cause
   a. Suspected spinal cord injury

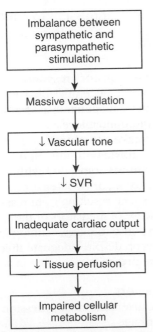

Figure 13-5 Pathophysiology of neurogenic shock. (From McCance, K. L., & Huether, S. E. [2006]. *Pathophysiology: The basis of disease in adults and children* [5th ed.]. St Louis: Mosby.)

1) Early immobilization of the spine with suspected spinal injury
   2) Elevation of the head of the bed to 30 degrees
   b. Anesthesia: reverse anesthesia, gradually rewarm
   c. Insulin shock
   1) Monitoring for clinical indications of hypoglycemia, measure serum glucose as required
   2) Administration of 10 to 15 g of carbohydrate if the patient is conscious or 50 ml of $D_{50}W$ if unconscious
4. Maintain MAP and tissue perfusion
   a. Interventions to maintain MAP >70 mm Hg
   1) Fluids
      a) Crystalloids: hypertonic saline may be used
      b) Colloids: albumin has been traditionally advocated but recent studies and a meta-analysis show no benefit to the use of colloids including in patients with neurologic problems
      c) Monitoring closely for pulmonary or cerebral edema
   2) Inotropes and/or vasopressors may be necessary
   b. Interventions to maintain heart rate 60-100/min: atropine and/or pacemaker may be necessary
5. Prevent venous stasis and deep vein thrombosis: anticoagulants (e.g., mini-heparin) as prescribed

Evaluation

1. Patent airway, adequate oxygenation (i.e., normal Pao_2, Spo_2, Sao_2) and ventilation (i.e., normal $Paco_2$)
2. Absence of clinical indications of respiratory distress
3. Absence of clinical indicators of hypoperfusion
4. Control of pain/discomfort/dyspnea
5. Alert and oriented with no neurovascular deficit

Typical disposition: admission to critical care unit

Septic Shock

Definitions
1. Infection: an inflammatory response to microorganisms
2. Bacteremia: the presence of viable bacteria in the blood
3. Sepsis: systemic state generalized by the presence of invading microorganisms and their toxins in blood and tissues; systemic inflammatory response syndrome associated with infection
4. Severe sepsis: sepsis associated with organ dysfunction, hypoperfusion, or hypotension
5. Septic shock: shock resulting from massive vasodilation caused by release of mediators of the inflammatory process in response to overwhelming infection; sepsis with hypotension despite adequate fluid resuscitation along with the presence of perfusion abnormalities

Predisposing factors
1. Factors that cause immunosuppression
   a. Extremes of age
   b. Malnutrition
   c. Alcoholism or drug abuse
   d. Debilitation
   e. Malignancy
   f. AIDS
   g. History of splenectomy
   h. Chronic health problems (i.e., diabetes mellitus, liver disease, heart disease [e.g., coronary artery disease or heart failure], renal failure)
   i. Bone marrow suppression
   j. Immunosuppressive therapies (e.g., immunosuppressive drugs, antineoplastic drugs, antibiotic therapy, corticosteroids)
2. Factors that cause bacteremia, septicemia
   a. Invasive procedures and devices
   b. Pulmonary procedures
   c. Diagnostic procedures
   d. Surgical procedures or wounds
   e. Traumatic wounds or burns
   f. Genitourinary infection
   g. Untreated GI disease (cholelithiasis, intestinal obstruction, appendicitis, diverticulitis)
   h. Peritonitis
   i. Food poisoning
   j. Prolonged hospitalization
   k. Translocation of GI bacteria: NPO status, decreased peristalsis, and GI ischemia contribute to proliferation of gastrointestinal bacterial and translocation of these bacterial into blood or lymph
3. Microorganisms
   a. Gram-negative bacteria (*most likely)
   1) *Escherichia coli**
   2) *Klebsiella enterobacter**
   3) *Pseudomonas aeruginosa**
   4) *Proteus mirabilis*
   5) *Enterococcus*
   6) *Serratia marcescens*
   7) *Bacteroides* organisms
   8) *Haemophilus influenzae*
   b. Gram-positive organisms
   1) *Staphylococcus aureus*
   2) *Staphylococcus epidermidis*
   3) *Streptococcus pneumoniae*
   4) *Clostridium* organisms
   5) *Pneumococcus*
   c. Less likely
   1) Viruses
   2) Fungi
   3) Rickettsiae
   4) Spirochaeta
   5) Protozoa
   6) Parasites

Pathophysiology (Figure 13-6)
1. Triad of inflammation, hypercoagulability, and impaired fibrinolysis (Figure 13-7)

Clinical presentation
1. Severe sepsis
   a. Known or suspected infection
   b. Two or more clinical indications of SIRS
   1) Heart rate >90 beats/min (sinus rhythm)

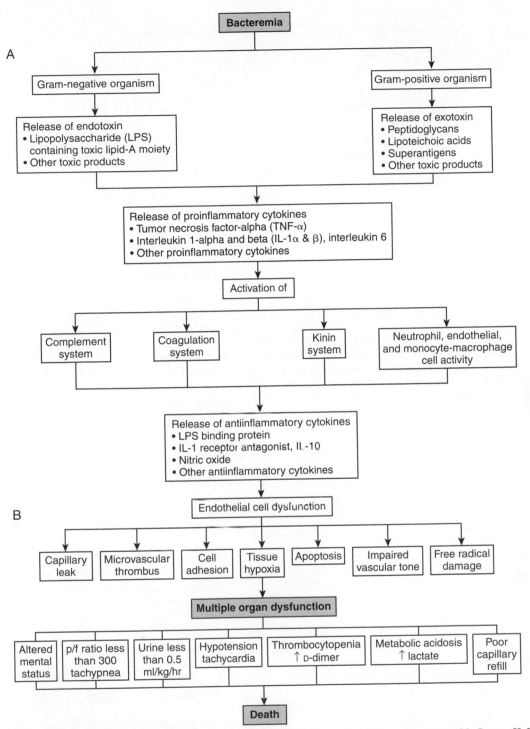

Figure 13-6 Pathophysiology of septic shock. p/f (Pao₂/FiO₂) = oxygenation ratio. (From McCance, K. L., & Huether, S. E. [2006]. *Pathophysiology: The basis of disease in adults and children* [5th ed.]. St Louis: Mosby; **A** from Larson, V., and Barke, R. A. [1999]. *Urol Clin North Am, 26[4],* 687; **B**, ©2003, Eli Lilly and Company. Reprinted with permission from Eli Lilly and Company.)

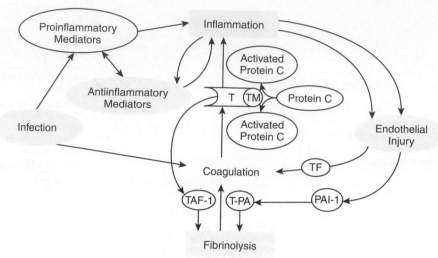

Figure 13-7 Severe sepsis is associated with three integrated components: (**1**) Infection with the systemic activation of inflammation. During progression of sepsis, a wide variety of proinflammatory cytokines is released. Endotoxin induces rapid increases in the levels of tumor necrosis factor (TNF), interleukin-1 (IL-1), and interleukin-6 (IL-6) in experimental models of sepsis. These proinflammatory cytokines are linked to the development of the clinical signs of sepsis. Release of proinflammatory cyto- kines is associated with endothelial injury and vascular bed–specific changes in the thrombogenicity of the endothelium. These can include increased tissue factor (TF) expression in a subset of endothelial cells and release of plasminogen activator inhibitor-1 (PAI-1). (**2**) Activation of coagulation. Inflammatory changes trigger the extrinsic pathway of coagulation. Activation of coagulation in patients with sepsis is not always disseminated intravascular coagulation. Instead, in most patients, activation of coagulation is a subclinical activation of the hemostatic system as indicated by changes in commonly measured hemo- static parameters. Experimentally, there are increases in thrombin-antithrombin (TAT) complexes. Clini- cal laboratory findings include significant increases in D-dimer, a marker of coagulation and associated fibrinolysis. (**3**) Impairment of fibrinolysis. In patients with sepsis, plasminogen levels fall rapidly while antiplasmin levels remain normal. This decreases the normal fibrinolytic response. Fibrinolysis is im- paired further by release of PAI-1 and the generation of increased amounts of thrombin-activatable fibri- nolysis inhibitor (TAFI). Although the plasminogen/antiplasmin ratio and PAI-1 levels remain abnormal in nonsurviving patients, they tend to normalize in survivors. (Courtesy Eli Lilly.)

2) Hyperthermia (temperature >38°C or 100.4°F) or hypothermia (temperature <36°C or 96.8°F) (note that hypothermia is more common in elderly patients)
3) Respiratory rate >20/min or $Paco_2$ <32 mm Hg
4) WBCs >12,000 cells/mm³, <4000 cells/mm³, or >10% bands

c. Evidence of at least one organ dysfunction (Figure 13-8)
2. Septic shock (Table 13-9)
3. Hemodynamics (see Table 13-5)

Collaborative management: as for shock as well as the following

1. Identify high-risk patients and monitor for clinical indi- cations of infection and sepsis; note any of the following:
   a. Hyperthermia
   b. Increase in respiratory rate
   c. Elevated glucose caused by insulin resistance
   d. Poor gastric motility and retention of enteral feedings
   e. Elevated serum lactate despite clinical picture of increased cardiac output

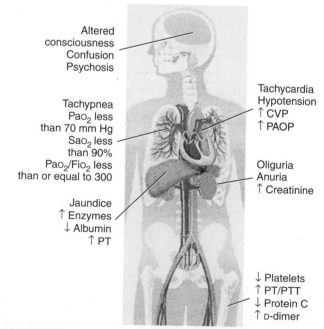

Figure 13-8 Acute organ dysfunction as a marker of severe sepsis.

Labels in figure:
Altered consciousness Confusion Psychosis
Tachypnea Pao_2 less than 70 mm Hg Sao_2 less than 90% Pao_2/Fio_2 less than or equal to 300
Jaundice ↑ Enzymes ↓ Albumin ↑ PT
Tachycardia Hypotension ↑ CVP ↑ PAOP
Oliguria Anuria ↑ Creatinine
↓ Platelets ↑ PT/PTT ↓ Protein C ↑ D-dimer

TABLE 13-9   Stages of Septic Shock

Early (Hyperdynamic)	Late (Hypodynamic)
LOOKS LIKE INFECTION	**LOOKS LIKE SHOCK**
Objective	
• Tachycardia	• Tachycardia
• Pulses bounding	• Pulses weak and thready
• Blood pressure: normal or low	• Hypotension
• Wide pulse pressure	• Narrow pulse pressure
• Skin warm, flushed	• Skin cool, pale
• Hyperpnea	• Bradypnea or tachypnea
• Change in mental status (e.g., irritability, confusion)	• Decreased level of consciousness (e.g., lethargy, coma)
• Oliguria	• Anuria
• Hyperthermia	• Hypothermia
Hemodynamic	
• CO/CI increased	• CO/CI decreased
• CVP/RAP/PAP/PAOP decreased	• CVP/RAP/PAP/PAOP variable
• SVR decreased	• SVR increased
• Svo$_2$ increased	• Svo$_2$ decreased
Diagnostic	
• ABGs: respiratory alkalosis with hypoxemia	• ABGs: metabolic acidosis with hypoxemia
• PT, aPTT increased	• PT, aPTT increased
• Platelets decreased	• Platelets decreased
• WBCs increased	• WBCs decreased
• Glucose increased	• Glucose decreased
	• BUN, creatinine increased
	• Serum arterial lactate increased
	• Amylase, lipase increased
	• AST, ALT, LDH increased

CO, Cardiac output; *CI*, cardiac index; *RAP*, right atrial pressure; *PAP*, pulmonary artery pressure; *PAOP*, pulmonary artery occlusive pressure; *SVR*, systemic vascular resistance; *Svo₂*, oxygen saturation of venous blood; *PT*, prothrombin time; aPTT, activated partial thromboplastin time; *WBC*, white blood cell; *BUN*, blood urea nitrogen; *AST*, aspartate aminotransferase (formerly called SGOT), *ALT*, alanine aminotransferase (formerly called SGPT); *LDH*, lactic dehydrogenase

2. Continue assessment
   a. ABCDs
   b. Vital signs: blood pressure, pulse, respiratory rate, and temperature
   c. Oxygen saturation
   d. Respiratory effort and excursion
   e. Cardiac rate and rhythm
   f. Hemodynamic parameters as available
   g. Pain and discomfort level
   h. Accurate intake and output
   i. Serum electrolytes
   j. Level of consciousness
   k. Close monitoring for progression of symptoms
3. Prevent infection and sepsis
   a. Good hand-washing techniques and prevent cross-contamination
   b. Avoidance of invasive procedures if possible
   c. Early identification of focus of infection
      1) Monitor color, characteristics of sputum, urine, stools, wounds, etc.
      2) Culture secretions and wounds as indicated
   d. Preparation of patient for surgery as indicated for any of the following
      1) Removal of all necrotic tissue
      2) Drainage of abscess
      3) Early débridement of burn eschar
      4) Prompt stabilization of fractures to minimize soft tissue damage, inflammation, infection
   e. Meticulous oral and airway care; silent aspiration of oral, nasopharyngeal, sinus secretions around the endotracheal tube cuff occurs and is a cause of nosocomial pneumonia
   f. Meticulous intravenous, intraarterial, pulmonary arterial, and urinary catheter care according to CDC guidelines or hospital policy

g. Meticulous wound care as indicated by type and appearance of wound

h. Prophylactic antibiotic therapy as prescribed

  1) Controversial today as an increasing number of microorganisms become resistant to available antibiotic therapy

4. Restore tissue perfusion and normalize cellular metabolism

a. Early goal-directed therapy during first 6 hours after severe sepsis or septic shock are recognized (STOP Sepsis Bundle Toolkit, 2006) (Figure 13-9)

  1) Indications

    a) Two or more indications of SIRS

    b) Suspected or confirmed infection

    c) MAP <65 mm Hg after 20 ml/kg fluid bolus OR serum lactate of $\geq$4 mmol/L

  2) Goals include the following

    a) CVP of 8 to 12 mm Hg

    b) MAP of $\geq$65 mm Hg

    c) $ScvO_2$ or SvO_2 of $\geq$70%

    d) Urine output >0.5 ml/kg/hr

  3) Initial treatment includes the following

    a) Intubation and mechanical ventilation when require for respiratory distress; use the following setting to avoid ventilator-induced lung injury (VILI)

      i) Tidal volume at 6 ml/kg

      ii) Peak inspiratory plateau pressure of no $\leq$30 cm H_2O

    b) Antimicrobial agents following blood cultures

      i) Cultures

        (a) One blood draw should be percutaneous

        (b) One blood draw should be through each vascular access device that has been in place more than 48 hours

        (c) Other cultures from other sites (e.g., CSF, pulmonary secretions, urine, wound) may be indicated

      ii) Antimicrobials

        (a) Initiated within 1 hour of recognition of severe sepsis

        (b) One or more antimicrobials active against the likely pathogens

        (c) Reassess after 48 to 72 hours

    c) Preload correction

      i) If CVP less than 8 mm Hg: crystalloid fluid boluses until CVP 8 to 12 mm Hg

        (a) Colloids are not indicated and may be harmful

        (b) Hypertonic crystalloid are also not recommended at this time

      ii) If CVP more than 15 mm Hg and MAP greater than 110 mm Hg: NTG until CVP less than 12 or MAP less than 90 mm Hg

    d) Afterload correction

      i) If MAP is less than 65 mm Hg after 20 ml/kg of crystalloids, vasopressors as necessary to maintain a MAP of at least 65 mm Hg

        (a) The preferred agent is still debatable; norepinephrine (Levophed) (2 to 20 mcg/min) is frequently advocated as the initial agent; dopamine (Intropen) (5 to 20 mcg/kg/min) may also be used

          i. Low-dose dopamine (Intropin) (previously thought to provide renal protection) is not advocated

        (b) Phenylephrine (Neo-Synephrine) is preferred if heart rate is greater than 120 beats/min

        (c) Vasopressin (Pitressin)

          i. Very low doses (0.01 to 0.04 unit/min) of vasopressin have been shown to improve MAP in septic shock

        (d) Arterial catheter for continuous monitoring of blood pressure is indicated

      ii) Corticosteroids should be considered if patient is vasopressor dependent

    e) Optimize oxygen delivery

      i) If $ScvO_2$ is <70% after above listed therapies and hemoglobin is <10 g/dl, red blood cells (RBCs) are indicated

        (a) Platelets are indicated if platelet counts are less than $5000/mm^3$ or when $<30,000 mm^3$ if there is significant risk for bleeding

      ii) If $ScvO_2$ is <70% after above listed therapies and hemoglobin is >10 g/dl, dobutamine (Dobutrex) or dopamine (Intropin) is indicated

      iii) If heart rate is >120 beats/min, digoxin (Lanoxin) may be considered

b. Interventions to decrease inflammation and antithrombotic aspects of sepsis

  1) Activated protein C (drotrecogin alfa [Xigris] for patients with severe sepsis who have a high risk of death (i.e., severe sepsis with evidence of organ dysfunction)

    a) Actions

      i) Antiinflammatory

      ii) Anticoagulant

      iii) Profibrinolytic

    b) Dose: 24 mcg/kg/hr for a total infusion duration of 96 hours

    c) Contraindications: the primary contraindication is bleeding or increased risk of bleeding, especially intracranial or intraspinal bleeding

    d) Adverse effect: bleeding

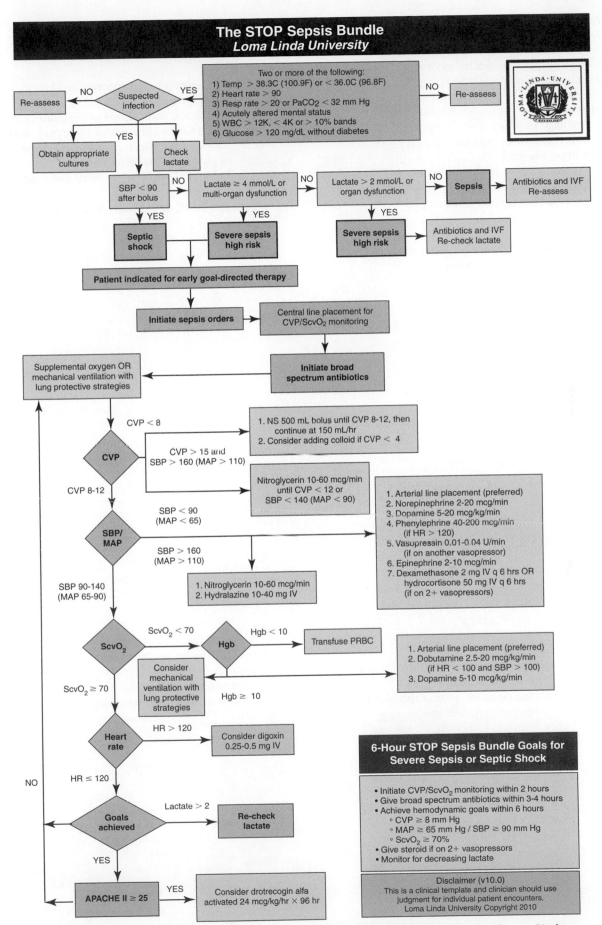

Figure 13-9 Early goal-directed therapy for sepsis. (From STOP Sepsis Working Group of Loma Linda University Medical Center, Loma Linda, California.)

2) Corticosteroids as prescribed

3) Control of serum glucose as described in the general discussion of shock

5. Treat infection and neutralize toxins
   a. Antimicrobials as prescribed
   b. Preparation of the patient for surgery as requested
      1) Drainage of abscess
      2) Debridement of wound

6. Control hyperthermia
   a. Monitoring of core body temperature
   b. Antipyretics as indicated
   c. Cooling blankets, tepid soaks

7. Monitor for complications of shock and clinical indications of organ failure

Evaluation

1. Patent airway, adequate oxygenation (i.e., normal Pao_2, Spo_2, Sao_2) and ventilation (i.e., normal $Paco_2$)
2. Absence of clinical indications of respiratory distress
3. Absence of clinical indicators of hypoperfusion
4. Absence of clinical indications of infection/sepsis
5. Control of pain/discomfort/dyspnea
6. Alert and oriented with no neurovascular deficit

Typical disposition: admission to critical care unit

LEARNING ACTIVITIES

1. DIRECTIONS: Complete the following crossword puzzle related to trauma.

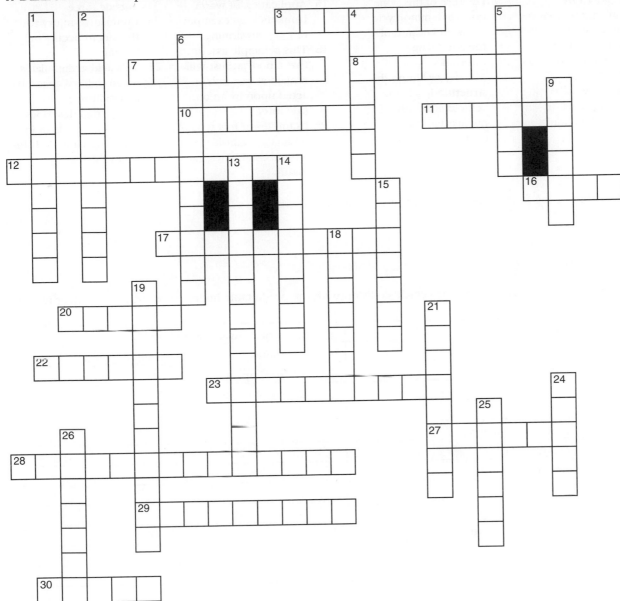

ACROSS

3. Air bag deployment may temporarily cause this sensory loss
7. Since the bones of a child are _____, they provide less protection to underlying structures
8. Drug frequently involved in intentional and nonintentional trauma
10. The E of the primary survey that requires unclothing the patient
11. Warming of IV fluids and peritoneal lavage with warm isotonic fluid is an example of _____ rewarming
12. A contributing factor to fractures in older adults, especially females
16. Acronym for documentation of prehospital care
17. The physics of trauma
20. This type of trauma results in more injuries and more types of injury
22. This type of fracture occurs when a person holds arms out in front to break a fall
23. A cause of intentional trauma in children (2 words)
27. Injury to the body caused by acute exposure to mechanical, thermal, electrical, or chemical energy
28. This potential cause of acute renal failure occurs in severe crush injury
29. Recurrent hypothermia after rewarming caused by perfusing cold areas
30. Patients with significant hemorrhage require the intravenous administration of _____

DOWN

1. Occurs when a squeezing inward pressure is applied to tissues
2. This is caused by exposure and may cause coagulopathy
4. This type of motor vehicle collision is most likely to cause whiplash (2 words)
5. The leading cause of trauma in older adults adult

6. This type of trauma is caused by direct contact with an instrument that cuts the skin
9. Fracture of this bone occurs in motorcycle collision because of the straddling position
13. The driver hitting this structure inside the vehicle is a cause of myocardial contusion (2 words)

14. Occurs when two oppositely directed parallel forces are applied to tissue
15. Application of warm blankets is an example of _____ rewarming
18. This principle asserts that a body at rest will remain at rest unless acted upon by an outside force
19. Examples of this type of trauma are gunshot wounds, stabbings, and assault

21. This principle asserts that a body in motion will remain in motion unless acted upon by an outside force
24. Cumulative injury to this organ occurs in boxing
25. This acid accumulates when there is anaerobic metabolism
26. _____ triad describes the three points of impact when a child is hit by a vehicle

2. DIRECTIONS: List the four collisions that occur in a vehicular collision.

A:

B:

C:

D:

3. DIRECTIONS: Match the type of motor vehicle collision with the predictable injury. More than one answer may be correct.

_____ 1. Traumatic brain injury		___ a. Frontal impact: up-and-over pathway	
_____ 2. Aortic or pulmonary artery tear		___ b. Frontal impact: down-and-under pathway	
_____ 3. Liver lacerations		___ c. Rear impact	
_____ 4. Whiplash		___ d. Lateral impact	
_____ 5. Hip fracture		___ e. Ejection	
_____ 6. Cervical spine flexion injury			
_____ 7. Myocardial contusion			
_____ 8. Rib fractures, pneumothorax			
_____ 9. Pelvic fracture			
_____ 10. Cervical spine compression			
_____ 11. Splenic laceration or rupture			
_____ 12. Lower extremity fractures			
_____ 13. Upper extremity fractures			

4. DIRECTIONS: List the three points of impact when a pedestrian is hit by a motor vehicle.

a.

b.

c.

5. DIRECTIONS: Complete the following crossword puzzle related to shock.

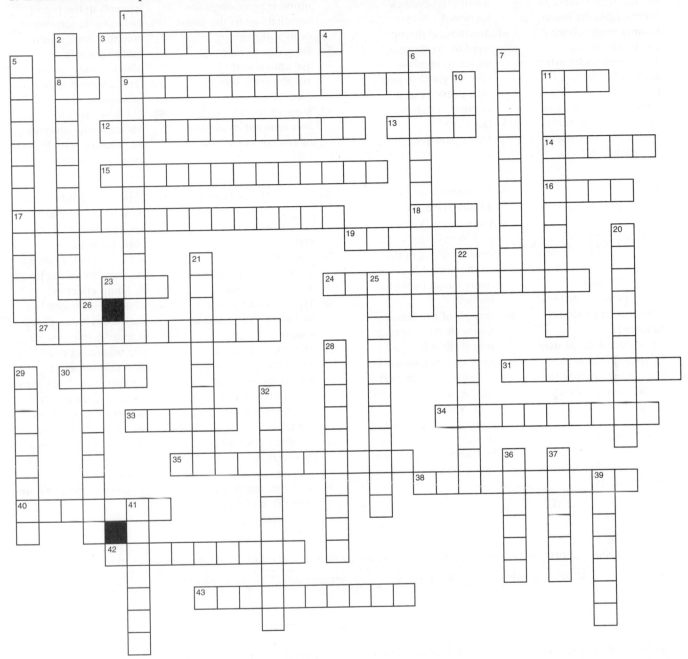

ACROSS

3. Mediator seen in ana- phylactic shock which causes vasodilation and increased capillary permeability

8. Most common cause of cardiogenic shock (abbrev)

9. Consequence of hemo- lytic blood transfusion reaction; may cause renal failure

11. This hemodynamic pa- rameter differentiates between hypovolemic from cardiogenic shock

12. This type of shock is caused by antigen- antibody response, IgE and the release of histamine and other mediators

13. Frequently fatal result of SIRS; previously referred to as multisystem organ failure (abbrev)

14. Condition of insufficient perfusion of cells and vital organs

15. Consequence of muscle destruction; may cause renal failure

16. Type of acute respiratory failure seen in MODS (abbrev)

17. Method of returning the patient's hemor- rhaged blood to his or her intravascular volume; greatest risks are infection and coagulopathy

18. Hemodynamic parame- ter that is increased in hypovolemic and cardiogenic shock (abbrev)

19. Systemic response of the immune system to microorganism, tissue trauma, toxins, burns, etc. (abbrev)
23. Type of coagulopathy seen in MODS (abbrev)
24. This stage of shock is associated with fever, increased CO/CI, and decreased SVR

DOWN

1. H_1 receptor antagonist (generic)
2. The stage of shock dominated by neuroendocrine responses to hypoperfusion
4. The type of acute renal failure seen in MODS (abbrev)
5. This type of drugs may be used to decrease preload or afterload in cardiogenic shock (plural)
6. This type of drugs may be used in vasogenic shock to restore normal vascular tone (plural)

27. First-line drug for anaphylactic shock (generic)
30. Mechanical therapy used in cardiogenic shock to increase coronary artery perfusion pressure and decrease afterload (abbrev)
31. DO_2 is oxygen _____

7. A complication of administering large volumes of IV fluid and blood which may cause shifting of the oxyhemoglobin dissociation curve to the left
10. Branch of the autonomic nervous system responsible for the early compensatory response to hypoperfusion in shock (abbrev)
11. This type of IV fluid contains solutes and may be categorized as hypotonic, isotonic, or hypertonic

33. This type of intravenous infusion is required for hemorrhage to the point of hypoperfusion
34. Drug most common associated with anaphylactic shock (generic)
35. Stage of septic shock is also referred to as late or cold septic shock

20. Type of shock caused by suppression of the sympathetic nervous system
21. Stage of shock associated with irreversible organ damage
22. Type of shock caused by loss of intravascular volume
25. The stage of shock when compensatory mechanisms are no longer effective in maintaining tissue perfusion
26. Alkaline buffer used for severe metabolic acidosis
28. Inotropic agent used most often in cardiogenic shock (generic)

38. Presence of viable bacteria in the blood
40. Colloid solution that contains large starch molecules; affects platelet aggregation
42. Oral antiprostaglandin (generic)
43. The term for the edema of the mucous membranes seen in anaphylactic shock

29. Type of IV fluids that are used to increase intravascular colloidal oncotic pressure
32. Type of shock caused by the inability of the heart to pump effectively
36. This type of shock is associated with mediator release in response to overwhelming infection
37. Infection with SIRS
39. This stage of shock is associated with a decrease in tissue oxygenation but no clinical indications of hypoperfusion
41. Plasma protein with the greatest effect on plasma oncotic pressure

6. DIRECTIONS: Identify which type of shock the following pathologic conditions or procedures may cause.

Condition	Hypovolemic	Cardiogenic	Septic	Anaphylactic	Neurogenic
Myocardial infarction					
Bee sting					
Head injury					
Diarrhea					
Pulmonary embolus					
Ruptured gallbladder					
Esophageal varices					
Insulin shock					
Ascites					
IVP dye					
Spinal cord injury					

Condition	Hypovolemic	Cardiogenic	Septic	Anaphylactic	Neurogenic
Invasive procedures					
Burns					
Blood transfusion reaction					
Spinal anesthesia					
Trauma					
Malnutrition					
Chemotherapy					

7. DIRECTIONS: Match the pathophysiology with the type of shock.

_____ 1. Cardiogenic	a. Vasodilation resulting from stimulation of the inflammatory and immune systems by endotoxins
_____ 2. Septic	b. Inability of the heart to effectively pump
_____ 3. Anaphylactic	c. Inadequate amount of circulating volume
_____ 4. Neurogenic	d. Vasodilation resulting from the release of histamine from mast cells caused by major allergic reaction
_____ 5. Hypovolemic	e. Vasodilation resulting from suppression or loss of the sympathetic nervous system

8. DIRECTIONS: Identify the following signs/symptoms of shock as occurring during the compensatory, progressive, and/or refractory stages of shock.

Sign/Symptom	Compensatory	Progressive	Refractory
Tachycardia			
Dysrhythmias			
Cool, pale skin			
Uncontrollable bleeding (DIC)			
Mottling of extremities			
Neurologic changes: lethargy, coma			
Oliguria			
Anuria			
Profound hypoxemia, increased PVR, decreased lung compliance (ARDS)			
Narrow pulse pressure			
Profound hypotension despite vasopressors			
Dysrhythmias			
Hypotension			
Decreased bowel sounds			
Thirst			
Neurologic changes: irritability confusion			
Nausea			
Neurologic changes: coma; focal signs			

9. DIRECTIONS: List two fluids in each category.

Crystalloids		
Isotonic		
Hypotonic		
Hypertonic		
Colloids		
Blood or blood products		

10. DIRECTIONS: Identify the three factors that affect oxygen delivery.

LEARNING ACTIVITIES ANSWERS

1.

The completed crossword puzzle:

Across:
3. HEARING
7. FLEXIBLE
8. ALCOHOL
10. EXPOSURE
11. ACTIVE
12. OSTEOPOROSIS
16. MIVT
17. KINEMATICS
20. BLUNT
22. COLLES
23. CHILDABUSE
27. TRAUMA
28. RHABDOMYOLYSIS
29. AFTERDROP
30. BLOOD

Down:
1. COMPRESSION
2. HYPOTHERMIA
4. REAREND
5. FALLING
6. PENETRATING
9. PELVIS
13. STEERINGWHEEL
14. SHEARING
15. PASSIVERTI
18. INERTI
19. INTENTI
21. MOMENTUM
24. BRAIN
25. LACTIC
26. WADDELL

2.

A: Auto collision

B: Body collision

C: Cavity contents collision

D: Debris collision

3.

a, e 1. Traumatic brain injury	a. Frontal impact: up-and-over pathway
a, b, c, e 2. Aortic or pulmonary artery tear	b. Frontal impact: down-and-under pathway
a, d, e 3. Liver lacerations	c. Rear impact
c 4. Whiplash	d. Lateral impact
d 5. Hip fracture	e. Ejection
b 6. Cervical spine flexion injury	
a, b 7. Myocardial contusion	
a, b, d, e 8. Rib fractures, pneumothorax	
b, d, e 9. Pelvic fracture	
a, e 10. Cervical spine compression	
a, d, e 11. Splenic laceration or rupture	
b 12. Lower extremity fractures	
d 13. Upper extremity fractures	

4.

a. Bumper
b. Hood
c. Ground

5.

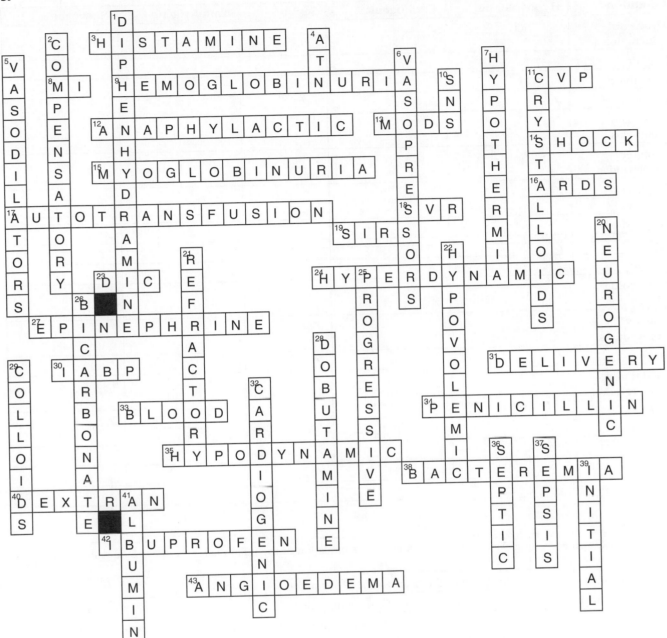

6.

Condition	Hypovolemic	Cardiogenic	Septic	Anaphylactic	Neurogenic
Myocardial infarction		✓			
Bee sting				✓	
Head injury					✓
Diarrhea	✓				
Pulmonary embolus		✓			
Ruptured gallbladder			✓		
Esophageal varices	✓				
Insulin shock					
Ascites	✓				✓
IVP dye	✓			✓	
Spinal cord injury					✓
Invasive procedures			✓		
Burns	✓		✓		
Blood transfusion reaction				✓	
Spinal anesthesia					✓
Trauma	✓		✓		
Malnutrition			✓		
Chemotherapy			✓		

7.

_b_	1. Cardiogenic	a. Vasodilation resulting from stimulation of the inflammatory and immune systems by endotoxins.
_a_	2. Septic	b. Inability of the heart to effectively pump.
_d_	3. Anaphylactic	c. Inadequate amount of circulating volume.
_e_	4. Neurogenic	d. Vasodilation resulting from the release of histamine from mast cells caused by major allergic reaction.
_c_	5. Hypovolemic	e. Vasodilation resulting from suppression or loss of the sympathetic nervous system.

8.

Sign/Symptom	Compensatory	Progressive	Refractory
Tachycardia	✓	✓	
Dysrhythmias		✓	✓
Cool, pale skin	✓		
Uncontrollable bleeding (DIC)			✓
Mottling of extremities		✓	✓
Neurologic changes: lethargy, coma		✓	✓
Oliguria	✓		
Anuria		✓	✓
Profound hypoxemia, increased PVR, decreased lung compliance (ARDS)			✓
Narrow pulse pressure	✓		
Profound hypotension despite vasopressors			✓
Dysrhythmias		✓	✓
Hypotension		✓	✓
Decreased bowel sounds	✓	✓	
Thirst			
Neurologic changes: irritability confusion	✓		
Nausea		✓	
Neurologic changes: coma; focal signs			✓

9.

Crystalloids		
Isotonic	Normal (0.9%) saline	Lactated Ringer's
Hypotonic	Half-normal (0.45%) saline	5% Dextrose in water
Hypertonic	3% Saline	10 % Dextrose in water
Colloids	Albumin	Dextran 70
Blood or blood products	Whole blood	Red blood cells

10.

Sao$_2$	Hgb	Cardiac output

References and Suggested Readings

Ahrens, T. (2006). Hemodynamics in sepsis. *AACN Advanced Critical Care, 17(4)*, 435–445.

Ahrens, T. (2007). Sepsis: Stopping the insidious killer. *American Nurse Today, 2(1)*, 36–39.

American College of Surgeons' Committee on Trauma. (2004). *Advanced Trauma Life Support for Doctors (ATLS) student manual* (7th ed.). Chicago: American College of Surgeons.

Atkinson, M., & Ryzner, D. (2007). Sepsis signposts: Can you spot them? *American Nurse Today, 2(10)*, 20–22.

Cain, J. E., Daly, M. L., & Powers, J. (2007). Act fast against anaphylaxis. *American Nurse Today, 2(2)*, 30.

Carlson, K. K. (Ed.). (2009). *AACN Advanced critical care nursing.* St. Louis: Saunders Elsevier.

Center for Disease Control and Prevention. (2007). Preventing injuries in America: Public health in action. Retrieved October 24, 2009, from www.cdc.gov/.../Preventing%20Injuries%20in%20America%20Public%20Health%20in%20Action-2006.pdf

Cottingham, C. (2006). Resuscitation of traumatic shock. A hemodynamic review. *AACN Advanced Critical Care, 17(3)*, 317–326.

Crum, E., & Valenti, J. (2007). Can a bloodless surgery program work in the trauma setting? *Nursing2007, 37(3)*, 54–56.

Cunha, B. A. (2008). Sepsis and septic shock: Selection of empiric antimicrobial therapy. *Critical Care Clinics, 24*, 313–334.

Cunneen, J., & Cartwright, M. (2004). The puzzle of sepsis. Fitting the pieces of the inflammatory response with treatment. *AACN Clinical Issues, 15(1)*, 18–44.

Danis, D., Blansfield, J., & Gervasini, A. (2007). *Manual of clinical trauma care* (4th ed.). St. Louis: Elsevier Mosby.

Dennison, R. D. (2007). *Pass CCRN!* (3rd ed.). St. Louis: Mosby.

Ecklund, M. M., & Ecklund, C. R. (2007). How to recognize and respond to hypovolemic shock. *American Nurse Today, 2(2)*, 28–31.

Frakes, M. A. (2007). Emergency department management of severe sepsis. *Advanced Emergency Nursing Journal, 29(3)*, 228–238.

Fultz, J., & Sturt, P. A. (2005). *Mosby's emergency nursing reference* (3rd ed.). St. Louis: Elsevier Mosby.

Gessner, P. (2006). The effect of vasopressin on the renal system in vasodilatory shock. *Dimensions of Critical Care Nursing, 25(1)*, 1–8.

Giuliano, K. K. (2006). Continuous physiologic monitoring and the identification of sepsis: What is the evidence supporting current clinical practice? *AACN Advanced Critical Care, 17(2)*, 215–223.

Holleran, R. S. (2007). Shock emergencies. In K. S. Hoyt & J. Selfridge-Thomas (Eds.). *Emergency nursing core curriculum* (6th ed., pp. 721–737). St. Louis: Saunders Elsevier.

Hoyt, K. S., & Selfridge-Thomas, J. (Eds.). (2007). *Emergency nursing core curriculum* (6th ed.). St. Louis: Saunders Elsevier.

King, K. J., & Olson, D. M. (2007). What you should know about neurogenic shock. *American Nurse Today, 2(2)*, 36–37.

Kleinpell, R. M., Graves, B. T., & Ackerman, M. H. (2006). Incidence, pathogenesis, and management of sepsis. *AACN Advanced Critical Care, 17(4)*, 385–393.

Kortgen, A., Niederprum, P., & Bauer, M. (2006). Implementation of an evidence-based "standard operating procedure" and outcome in septic shock. *Critical Care Medicine, 34(3)*, 943–949.

Lauzier, F., Levy, B., Lamarre, P., & Lesur, O. (2006). Vasopressin or norepinephrine in early hyperdynamic septic shock: A randomized clinical trial. *Intensive Care Medicine, 32(11)*, 1782–1789.

McSwain, N. E. (2000). Kinematics of trauma. In K. L. Mattox, D. V. Feliciano & E. E. Moore (Eds.). *Trauma* (pp. 127–152). New York: McGraw-Hill.

Newberry, L., & Criddle, L. M. (Eds.). (2005). *Sheehy's manual of emergency care* (6th ed.). St. Louis: Elsevier Mosby.

Nguyen, H. B., Corbett, S. W., Steele, R., Banta, J., Clark, R. T., Hayes, S. R., et al. (2007). Implementation of a bundle of quality indicators for the early management of severe sepsis and septic shock is associated with decreased mortality. *Critical Care Medicine, 35(4)*, 1105–1112.

O'Brien, J. M., Ali, N. A., Aberegg, S. K., & Abraham, E. (2007). Sepsis. *The American Journal of Medicine, 120*, 1012–1022.

Picard, K. M., O'Donoghue, S. C., Young-Kershaw, D. A., & Russell, K. J. (2006). Development and implementation of a multidisciplinary sepsis protocol. *Critical Care Nurse, 26(3)*, 43–54.

Pirrung, J. M. (2009). An upward trend in motorcycle crashes. *Nursing 2009, 39(2)*, 28–34.

Powers, J., & Jacobi, J. (2006). Pharmacologic treatment related to severe sepsis. *AACN Advanced Critical Care, 17(4)*, 423–432.

Rizoli, S. B., Rhind, S. G., Shek, P. N., Inaba, K., Filips, D., Tien, H., et al. (2006). The immunomodulatory effects of hypertonic saline resuscitation in patients sustaining traumatic hemorrhagic shock: A randomized, controlled, double-blinded trial. *Annals of Surgery, 243(1)*, 47–57.

Talbert, S. (2005). Trauma. In J. Fultz & P. A. Sturt (Eds.). *Mosby's emergency nursing reference* (3rd ed., pp. 682–723). St. Louis: Elsevier Mosby.

Sakr, Y., Reinhart, K., Vincent, J. L., Sprung, C. L., Moreno, R., Ranieri, V. M., et al. (2006). Does dopamine administration in shock influence outcome? Results of the Sepsis Occurrence in Acutely Ill Patients (SOAP) Study. *Critical Care Medicine, 34(3)*, 589–597.

Schulman, C. S. (2009). Trauma. In K. K. Carlson (Ed.), *Advanced critical care nursing* (pp. 1134–1188). St. Louis: Saunders Elsevier.

Shapiro, N. I., Howell, M. D., Talmor, D., Lahey, D., Ngo, L., Buras, J., et al. (2006). Implementation and outcomes of the Multiple Urgent Sepsis Therapies (MUST) protocol. *Critical Care Medicine, 34(4)*, 1025–1032.

Singh, A., Carlin, B. W., Shade, D., & Kaplan, P. D. (2009). The use of hypertonic saline for fluid resuscitation in sepsis. A review. *Critical Care Nursing Quarterly, 32(1)*, 10–3.

Spaniol, J. R., Knight, A. R., Zebley, J. L., Anderson, D., & Pierce, J. D. (2007). Fluid resuscitation therapy for hemorrhagic shock. *Journal of Trauma Nursing, 14(3)*, 152–162.

STOP Sepsis Working Group (2006). The STOP Sepsis Bundle Toolkit. Retrieved April 24, 2006, from http://www.llu.edu/llumc/emergency/patientcare/documents/patientcare-sepsis.pdf?PHPSESSID= 0ec53300a00d8305710882972d9e9706

Volles, D. F., & Strickland, B. C. (2007). Role of recombinant human activated protein C (drotrecogin alfa, activated, Xigris) for severe sepsis. *Advanced Emergency Nursing Journal, 29(3)*, 198–208.

Zeitzer, M. B., & Ulrich, C. M. (2008). Using physiologic criteria to determine emergency trauma care: Necessary, but sufficient? *Journal of Emergency Nursing, 34(3)*, 270–271.

CHAPTER 14

Psychosocial Emergencies

Introduction

The content constitutes 4% (6 items) of the CEN examination

The focus is on psychosocial emergencies that are commonly encountered in an emergency department setting

The continuum of age needs to be considered from infancy through older adulthood

Age-Related Considerations

Neonates, infants, and children

1. Developmental and age appropriateness
   a. The pediatric patient can regress to the previous developmental stage when he or she is frightened or ill
   b. The pediatric patient may act out or throw a tantrum when he or she is stressed and confronted with an unknown situation and environment
   c. Appropriateness of interaction between parent and child should be noted
2. Stress and anxiety
   a. In infants and small children, anxiety occurs with separation from the caregiver
   b. During adolescence, peer pressure can cause stress and influence substance abuse
      1) Adolescents should be assessed for signs of substance abuse and suicidal tendencies or ideas
      2) Adolescents should be assessed for isolation and changes in behavioral patterns

Older adults

1. Depression is common with personal loss, the inability to maintain activities of daily living, and loss of independence
2. Abuse and neglect should be considered
3. Health problems may be the result of medications
   a. Polypharmacy is common; when many drugs are prescribed—frequently by different providers—interactions are likely, and these may include psychosocial effects
   b. Intentional overdose or substance abuse may occur as a result of loneliness
   c. Accidental overdose may occur as a result of declining cognitive function or poor eyesight
   d. Medications take longer to be eliminated as a result of aging's effects on renal function and may cause the patient to appear depressed or exhibit flat affect

Physical Assessment

Chief complaint

1. History of present illness: current symptoms
2. Medical history
3. Previous illnesses or injuries
4. Previous hospitalizations
5. Allergies
6. Review of body systems
7. Current medications

Social history

1. Family structure
2. Substance abuse history

Mental status examination that includes the following:

1. Presentation
   a. Dress (e.g., is the patient's clothing appropriate for the season?)
   b. Eye contact
   c. General appearance (e.g., hygiene)
   d. Motor activity
2. Social history
   a. Family
   b. Significant others
   c. Education level
   d. Job history
   e. Major family traumas
3. Affect
   a. Anxious
   b. Flat
   c. Inappropriate
   d. Labile
   e. Guarded
   f. Normal
4. Mood
   a. Hostile
   b. Depressed
   c. Elated
   d. Anxious
   e. Agitated
5. Speech
   a. Pressured
   b. Slurred
   c. Loud
   d. Soft
   e. Patterns
   f. Idiosyncrasies

757

6. Thought processes
   a. Blocking: a cessation of the flow of thought or speech
   b. Flight of ideas: a leap from one idea to another unconnected idea as a result of being distracted by thoughts and things in the environment
   c. Looseness of association: a loss of normal thought patterns
   d. Circumstantial: thoughts connect to each other and come back to the original topic, but in a roundabout way (e.g., lots of details that circle the point and an extensive explanation to answer a question)
   e. Tangential: there is some connection between the preceding thought and the following thought but there is very little association between them as a whole
7. Thought content
   a. Suspicious
   b. Hopeless
   c. Guilty
   d. Delusion: a persistent belief or perception held by a person despite evidence to the contrary; examples include the following:
      1) Being controlled
      2) Grandeur
      3) Persecution
      4) Nihilistic
      5) Somatic
   e. Ideation: persistent thoughts regarding either of the following:
      1) Suicide
      2) Homicide
8. Perceptual disturbances
   a. Hallucinations: sensory perceptions that do not result from an external stimulus and that occur when the patient is in an awake state (Table 14-1)
      1) Normal hallucinations
         a) Hypnagogic: associated with the semiconsciousness that immediately precedes sleep
         b) Hypnopompic: associated with the semiconsciousness that precedes waking
      2) Abnormal hallucinations (see Table 14-1)
   b. Illusion: false interpretations of an external sensory stimulus

9. Cognition
   a. Orientation: to person, place, and time
   b. Memory: recent and past
   c. Intelligence
   d. Concentration
10. Judgment and insight

Diagnostic studies to rule out medical conditions and substance abuse

1. CBC
2. Hemoglobin level
3. Hematocrit level
4. Thyroid panel
5. Liver and renal function tests
6. Drug toxicology
7. Pregnancy tests for women between the ages of 10 and 60 years
8. Urinalysis

General Principles of Care

Focus on the initial signs and symptoms, the methods of assessment for specific disorders, principles of safe care, and the use of pharmacologic agents appropriate to the presentation

1. Emergency personnel are frequently confronted by individuals or families who appear to be out of control, in a state of extreme distress, confused, or numb
2. It is the job of the clinician to assess the reason behind the distress; to diagnose any accompanying disorders and treat them effectively; and to release, refer, or hospitalize the involved individuals for additional care

Therapeutic milieu

1. An environment in which the focus is designed to heal
   a. Healthy social interactions
   b. Respect for all persons
   c. Recognition of client's rights
   d. Freedom of speech
   e. Sense of support
   f. Honesty in interactions
2. Staff responsibilities
   a. Adherence to schedules
   b. Maintenance of safety at all times
   c. Activities that focus on growth and understanding
   d. Responsibility is encouraged
   e. Clients are informed about all changes
   f. Clients are incorporated into the government of the environment

Ethical care

1. Fundamental concept used when making decisions regarding patient care
   a. Each patient must be treated equally, fairly, and with dignity
   b. Do no harm (i.e., nonmaleficence) and do what is in the patient's best interest (i.e., beneficence)

TABLE **14-1** Types of Abnormal Hallucinations	
Type	**Perceptions Involved**
Auditory	Voices or other sounds
Visual	Images
Gustatory	Tastes
Tactile	Touches
Olfactory	Odors
Kinesthetic	Bodily movements
Somatic	Things occurring within one's own body

c. Be honest with the patient and build a trusting relationship

d. Provide impartial treatment of all patients (i.e., justice)

e. Patients have the independence and freedom to select their treatment (i.e., autonomy)

2. Patients with psychiatric emergencies have the same rights as other patients to make decisions; it is the health care provider's responsibility to intervene in the freedom of decision making if the patient's safety is at risk (Hamilton, 2007)

3. Care should be provided in accord with the provider's standards of care as defined on a state-by-state basis

Confidentiality

1. Health care agencies and providers must provide confidentiality and privacy for an individual's health care information that is collected and maintained; only those who require the information to provide further care are permitted to have access to it

2. Health Insurance Portability and Accountability Act (HIPAA) of 1996

   a. Protects the privacy of an individual's identifiable health information and identifiable personal information

   b. Requirements must be followed by each institution

Civil rights

1. Civil rights protect an individual from unfair treatment or discrimination on the basis of race, color, national origin, disability, age, gender, or religion

2. Civil rights laws ensure that everyone has equal access to and opportunities to participate in certain health care and human services programs without facing unlawful discrimination

3. Patients with mental illness have the same patient rights as any other patient

4. Hospitalization of the Mentally Ill Act of 1964: all patients in public or private hospitals have a right to treatment (Hamilton, 2007)

Crisis

Definition: a state that occurs when one's usual ways of coping are inadequate to deal with the current level of stress (Caplan, 1970)

Types of crises

1. Situational crisis

   a. Occurs suddenly

   b. Can be devastating

   c. Is not part of normal development

      1) Motor vehicle collision

      2) Acts of nature (e.g., tornado, flood)

      3) Sexual assault

      4) Robbery

      5) Legal difficulties

      6) Separation or divorce

      7) Unemployment

      8) Diagnosis of a terminal illness

2. Maturational crisis

   a. Occurs over time

   b. Is recognized as common and occurs as part of normal development

   c. Includes the following:

      1) Pregnancy

      2) Childbirth

      3) Adolescence

      4) Leaving home

      5) Marriage

      6) Midlife events

      7) Aging

      8) Death

Clinical indications

1. Crying or screaming

2. Anger, pacing, or striking out at others

3. Silence, being unresponsive to questions, appearing to be in shock

Crisis intervention

1. Alleviate the crisis state

   a. Many will abate over time without interventions

   b. Problem-solving techniques can be implemented for others

   c. The goal is to return the person to his or her precrisis level of functioning

2. Use interventions that have been shown to be helpful

   a. Listen to the patient's story

   b. Offer empathy

   c. Ask about attempts to cope

      1) Coping behaviors that have been used successfully in the past

      2) Current attempts at coping, such as turning to friends and family, prayer, crying, and substance abuse

      3) Suicidal thoughts or plans

   d. Help the patient with the organization of the next few hours or days

   e. Connect the patient to support services or family members

Family Support and End-of-Life Issues

Family presence should be encouraged throughout the resuscitation process in the emergency department

Bereavement: a state of sorrow regarding the loss of a loved one

1. Attempts should be made to keep the family informed; family members should be allowed to visit with patient

2. After the patient has died, the family should be given time to sit with the body and mourn

3. Cultural behaviors that have been shown to be supportive should be acknowledged; personnel (e.g., social worker, counselor, chaplain) should be provided as the family requires

4. Do not rush the family through the process

Sudden infant death syndrome: provide privacy for parents and family members to hold the baby, and place the family in contact with relevant support groups

Do-not-resuscitate order: a medical order to provide no resuscitation to an individual who has an advanced directive requesting this or for whom resuscitation is not warranted

Withdrawal of staff support only when the family has another person available to continue as a supportive presence

SPECIFIC PSYCHIATRIC DISORDERS

Anxiety Disorders

Definition

1. Anxiety: a state of uneasiness and apprehension
   a. A subjective experience that differs from one individual to another
   b. Both physiologic and psychologic components
   c. Person often does not know cause
   d. Unpleasant emotional state with increased feelings of tension and helplessness
2. Types of anxiety disorders include the following:
   a. Panic disorder: sudden-onset anxiety in the form of fear and panic (e.g., panic attack)
   b. Phobia: an irrational or illogical fear of an object, situation, or event
   c. Obsessive–compulsive disorder: recurrent, persistent thoughts and feelings coupled with behaviors that are ritualistic and repetitive
   d. Posttraumatic stress disorder: persistent or repetitive thoughts and memories that occur as a result of exposure to a traumatic event or experience and that induce an anxiety disorder response
   e. Substance-induced anxiety disorder: anxiety symptoms that develop with substance withdrawal or within a month of substance abuse cessation

Predisposing factors

1. Genetic predisposition
2. Preexisting diseases
3. Developmental causes
   a. Children: separation from parents, perceived loss of love
   b. Adolescents: peer pressure related to appearance, substance abuse, pressure to achieve, puberty
   c. Adults: life changes, such as marriage, divorce, childbirth, menopause, career pressures, or loss of parents
   d. Older adults: loss of spouse/significant others/friends, diminished independence and health
4. Exposure to high levels of stress over time
5. Sleep deprivation
6. Acute changes in health status
7. Often coexists with depression
8. Related to a decrease in substance abuse

Pathophysiology (Yates, 2009)

1. Not well understood
2. Thought to be caused by a disruption of modulators within the central nervous system
3. Several neurotransmitter systems are thought to be involved
   a. Serotonin
   b. Norepinephrine
   c. γ-Aminobutyric acid
   d. Peptides
   e. Corticotropin
4. The autonomic and sympathetic nervous systems mediate the majority of the symptoms

Clinical presentation

1. Subjective
   a. May have history of the following:
      1) Excessive anxiety or worry for >6 months
      2) Inability to control feelings
      3) Fatigue
      4) Difficulty concentrating
      5) Irritability
      6) Muscle tension
      7) Sleep disturbances
      8) Sexual problems
   b. Apprehensiveness, fearfulness, or helplessness
   c. Tightness in chest or shortness of breath
   d. Dizziness
   e. Choking feeling
2. Objective
   a. Tachycardia or tachypnea; may have elevated blood pressure
   b. Pallor
   c. Tremors
   d. Dilated pupils or nystagmus
3. Diagnostic
   a. Serum blood and urine drug screening as indicated
   b. ECG: may show dysrhythmias, particularly sinus tachycardias, premature atrial contractions (PACs), or premature ventricular contractions (PVCs)
   c. Other diagnostic studies to rule out medical conditions

Collaborative management

1. Continue assessment
   a. ABCDs
   b. Vital signs: blood pressure, pulse, respiratory rate, and temperature
   c. Oxygen saturation if indicated
   d. Psychiatric status, especially in the presence of suicidal ideation or a significant agitation level
   e. Environmental safety
   f. Close monitoring for the progression of symptoms
2. Maintain airway, oxygenation, and ventilation
   a. Oxygen by nasal cannula at 2 to 6 L/minute if to maintain an SpO_2 level of 95% unless contraindicated; for patients with chronic obstructive

pulmonary disease (COPD), use pulse oximetry to guide oxygen administration to an SpO$_2$ level of 90%

   b. IV access for fluid and medication administration if indicated

3. Establish a trusting relationship
   a. Quiet room that allows for continuous observation
   b. Calm manner when approaching the patient; calm tone and eye contact when speaking with the patient
   c. Acknowledgement of the patient's feelings and fears
   d. Honesty when communicating with patient
   f. Assistance with problem solving
4. Reduce anxiety
   a. Anxiolytics as directed (e.g., diazepam [Valium], lorazepam [Ativan], alprazolam [Xanax])
     1) Because benzodiazepines are synergistic with alcohol, assess for recent use
   b. β-Blockers may also be prescribed
   c. Antidepressants as prescribed
5. Monitor for complications
   a. Dysrhythmias
   b. Suicide

Evaluation
1. Patent airway, adequate oxygenation (i.e., normal SaO$_2$) and ventilation (i.e., normal PaCO$_2$)
2. Absence of patient injury
3. Patient report of lessened anxiety

Typical disposition
1. If evaluation criteria met and no indications of suicidal ideation: discharge with instructions
   a. Medications to reduce anxiety
   b. Outpatient psychiatric consultation
2. If patient at risk for injury to self or others: admission or transfer to another facility

Depression
Definition: a disturbance of mood that is associated with an increase in sadness, negative thinking, and a loss of interest in usual activities; it is not associated with medication withdrawal or bereavement

Predisposing factors
1. Genetic predisposition
2. Severe psychosocial stressors
3. Hormonal imbalance
4. Sudden decrease in substance use
5. Coexistence with medical conditions
6. Medication side effects

Pathophysiology (Bhalla, Moraille-Bhalla, & Aronson, 2009)
1. Not well defined but thought to be a disturbance in central nervous system serotonin activity
2. Dysregulation of neurotransmitter system
3. Serotonin deficiency
4. Norepinephrine and dopamine are also thought to be involved

Clinical presentation
1. Subjective
   a. Expressions of the following:
     1) Guilt, worthlessness, or hopelessness
     2) Feelings of suicide
     3) Recurrent thoughts of death
   b. History of attempted suicide
   c. Insomnia or hypersomnia
   d. Low energy or fatigue
   e. Inability to concentrate
   f. Changes in appetite
   g. Weight loss
   h. Decreased libido
   i. Amenorrhea
   j. Constipation
   k. Psychomotor symptoms
   l. Depressed mood daily
   m. Psychomotor agitation or retardation
   n. Symptoms that last >2 months
2. Objective
   a. Appearance that is indicative of poor hygiene or of a lack of concern regarding the appearance
   b. Flat affect
   c. Tearful
   d. Quiet speech
   e. Little eye contact
   f. Psychomotor retardation (i.e., a visible generalized slowing down of movements, physical reactions, and speech)
   g. Evidence of psychotic symptoms (e.g., hallucinations, delusions)
3. Diagnostic studies
   a. Serum blood and urine drug screenings
   b. Serum alcohol screening
   c. Thyroid function test: to rule out hypothyroidism
   d. CBC with differential: to rule out anemia
   e. CT and possible MRI of the head to rule out a medical cause

Collaborative management
1. Continue assessment
   a. ABCDs
   b. Vital signs: blood pressure, pulse, respiratory rate, and temperature
   c. Oxygen saturation if indicated
   d. Psychiatric status, especially in the presence of suicidal ideation
   e. Environmental safety
   f. Close monitoring for the progression of symptoms
2. Maintain airway, oxygenation, and ventilation
   a. Oxygen by nasal cannula at 2 to 6 L/minute if to maintain an SpO$_2$ level of 95% unless contraindicated; for patients with COPD, use pulse oximetry to guide oxygen administration to an SpO$_2$ level of 90%
   b. IV access for fluid and medication administration if indicated

3. Provide safe environment
    a. Quiet room with minimal stimulation to allow for continuous observation
    b. Nonjudgmental approach
    c. Frequent contacts to reassure the patient regarding the staff's concern
    d. If suicide is a concern, someone must stay with the patient at all times
4. Assist with the treatment of depression
    a. Antidepressant therapy
    b. Counseling
    c. Electroconvulsant therapy
5. Monitor for complications
    a. Violent behavior
    b. Suicide

Evaluation

1. Patent airway, adequate oxygenation (i.e., normal SaO_2) and ventilation (i.e., normal $PaCO_2$)
2. Absence of patient injury
3. Absence of suicidal thoughts

Typical disposition

1. If evaluation criteria met and no indications of suicidal ideation: discharge with instructions
    a. Antidepressants
    b. Outpatient psychiatric consultation
2. If patient at risk for injury to self or others: admission or transfer to another facility

Mania
Definitions

1. Mania: elevated, irritable, or expansive mood
    a. Episode of irritable or elevated mood of ≥ 1 week
    b. Marked impairment of functioning
    c. Symptoms are not the result of substance abuse or a general medical condition
2. Bipolar: a combination of mood swings from mania to depression

Predisposing factors

1. Genetic predisposition
2. Severe psychosocial stressors
3. Hormonal imbalance
4. Sudden decrease in substance use
Pathophysiology: thought to involve the dysregulation of neurotransmitters

Clinical presentation

1. Subjective
    a. History of manic or hypomanic episodes
    b. Racing thoughts
    c. Little need for sleep
    d. Increased use of prescribed or illegal drugs to calm down
    e. Risky behaviors
        1) Abuse of credit cards and reckless spending
        2) Multiple sex partners
        3) Arrests

f. Interference with job performance
    g. Unrealistic future plans
    h. Previous suicide attempts: past and current plans
2. Objective
    a. Fidgeting or pacing
    b. Difficulty staying on topic, flight of ideas
    c. Elation or euphoria, laughing
    d. Grandiosity
    e. May have injuries
3. Diagnostic
    a. Serum blood and urine drug screenings
    b. Serum alcohol screening
    c. ECG: tachycardias, PACs, or PVCs
    d. Other diagnostic studies to rule out other causes

Collaborative management

1. Continue assessment
    a. ABCDs
    b. Vital signs: blood pressure, pulse, respiratory rate, and temperature
    c. Oxygen saturation if indicated
    d. Psychiatric status, especially in the presence of suicidal or homicidal ideation
    e. Environmental safety
    f. Close monitoring for the progression of symptoms
2. Maintain airway, oxygenation, and ventilation
    a. Oxygen by nasal cannula at 2 to 6 L/minute if to maintain an SpO_2 level of 95% unless contraindicated; for patients with COPD, use pulse oximetry to guide oxygen administration to an SpO_2 level of 90%
    b. IV access for fluid and medication administration if indicated
3. Provide safe environment
    a. Quiet room with minimal stimulation to allow for continuous observation
    b. Nonjudgmental approach
    c. Restraints should be avoided if possible but may be required to ensure patient safety
4. Control mania
    a. Antipsychotics for psychosis (if present) until mood stabilizers take effect
    b. Anticonvulsants for the regulation of mood; these drugs help stabilize mania and depression in patients who are bipolar
    c. Antidepressants for depression
    d. β-Blockers to block the effects of catecholamines
    e. Counseling to deal with the cycling of moods, behaviors, and interpersonal relationships
5. Monitor for complications: self-injury or suicide

Evaluation

1. Patent airway, adequate oxygenation (i.e., normal SaO_2) and ventilation (i.e., normal $PaCO_2$)
2. Absence of patient injury
3. Absence of suicidal thoughts
4. Reduction in indications of mania

Typical disposition

1. If evaluation criteria met and no indications of suicidal ideation: discharge with instructions
   a. Medications to control mania, depression, or both
   b. Outpatient psychiatric consultation
2. If patient at risk for injury to self or others: admission or transfer to another facility

Psychosis

Definition: a severe psychiatric disorder that is characterized by personality derangement, a loss of contact with reality, and a deterioration of normal social functioning

1. Acute or chronic: lasting from a few days to several months
2. May be functional or organic

Predisposing factors

1. Functional type: severe depression, mania, schizophrenic disorder, or a brief psychotic episode
2. Organic type
   a. Ingestion of a toxic substance
   b. Shock or trauma
   c. Dementia: slow onset
   d. Delirium: rapid onset

Pathophysiology: poorly understood
Clinical presentation

1. Subjective: may report any of the following:
   a. History of psychotic episodes
   b. Confusion or amnesia
   c. Paranoid ideation
   d. Fears about safety
   e. Loss of energy
   f. Self-medication
2. Objective
   a. Positive symptoms
      1) Delusions
      2) Hallucinations: usually auditory
   b. Negative symptoms
      1) Avolition: inability to initiate activities, including self-care
      2) Alogia: absence of speech
      3) Anhedonia: lack of pleasure
      4) Flat affect: absence of emotional responses
   c. Disorganized speech or incoherence
   d. Conversation shows confusion, loss of touch with reality, and loss of orientation to time, place, and person
   e. Increased agitation or bizarre behavior
   f. Grossly exaggerated behaviors
   g. Psychomotor retardation (i.e., the visible generalized slowing down of movements, physical reactions, and speech)
3. Diagnostic
   a. Urinalysis, especially if the patient is an older woman
   b. Urine and serum drug screenings
   c. CT if changes have been rapid
   d. Other diagnostic studies to rule out other causes

Collaborative management

1. Continue assessment
   a. ABCDs
   b. Vital signs: blood pressure, pulse, respiratory rate, and temperature
   c. Oxygen saturation if indicated
   d. Psychiatric status, especially in the presence of suicidal or homicidal ideation, lack of orientation to present circumstances, or significant agitation level
   e. Environmental safety
   f. Close monitoring for the progression of symptoms
2. Maintain airway, oxygenation, and ventilation
   a. Oxygen by nasal cannula at 2 to 6 L/minute if to maintain an SpO_2 level of 95% unless contraindicated; for patients with COPD, use pulse oximetry to guide oxygen administration to an SpO_2 level of 90%
   b. IV access for fluid and medication administration if indicated
3. Provide safe environment
   a. Quiet room with minimal stimulation to allow for continuous observation
   b. Nonjudgmental approach
   c. Conversations should be kept simple and short; delusions or hallucinations should not be supported, but avoid agitating the patient
   d. Frequent reorientation to person and place
   e. Restraints should be avoided if possible but may be required to ensure patient safety
4. Assist with the management of psychosis
   a. Antipsychotic medications to reduce psychosis
   b. Anxiolytic medications to reduce anxiety or induce sleep
   c. Consultation with the patient's current psychiatrist or referral to a psychiatrist if the patient has not been previously treated for psychosis
5. Monitor for complications
   a. Neuromuscular malignant syndrome
   b. Incontinence
   c. Coma

Evaluation

1. Patent airway, adequate oxygenation (i.e., normal SaO_2) and ventilation (i.e., normal $PaCO_2$)
2. Absence of patient injury
3. Reduction in agitation
4. Alert and oriented with no neurologic deficit

Typical disposition

1. If evaluation criteria met and no indications that the patient is at risk for injury to self or others: discharge with instructions
   a. Medications
   b. Outpatient psychiatric consultation
2. If patient is at risk for injury to self or others: admission or transfer to another facility

Dementia

Definition: a deterioration of intellectual functioning (e.g., memory, concentration, judgment)
1. Results from a disorder of the brain or an organic disease
2. May be accompanied by personality changes and emotional disturbances
3. Chronic or progressive in nature

Predisposing factors
1. Aging
2. Cerebrovascular disease
3. Brain tumors
4. Alzheimer disease
5. Hypothyroidism
6. Hypercalcemia
7. Neurosyphilis
8. Human immunodeficiency virus infection
9. Substance abuse
10. Normal pressure hydrocephalus
11. Subdural hematoma
12. Deficiency of any of the following:
    a. Folic acid
    b. Vitamin B_{12}
    c. Niacin

Pathophysiology: dependent on cause
1. A chronic global deterioration of cognition
2. Cognitive malfunctioning preceded by deterioration of the following:
    a. Emotional control
    b. Social behavior
    c. Motivation
3. Cognitive malfunctioning of the following:
    a. Memory
    b. Intellect
    c. Learning
    d. Orientation
    e. Comprehension
    f. Calculation
    g. Language
    h. Judgment

Clinical presentation
1. Subjective
    a. Memory loss
    b. Confusion
    c. Decline in cognitive functioning or judgment
2. Objective
    a. Lack of orientation to time, place, and person
    b. Aphasia
    c. Apraxia
    d. Agnosia
    e. Behavioral disturbances
    f. Shallow to flat affect
    g. Focal neurologic signs
        1) Exaggeration of deep tendon reflexes
        2) Extensor plantar response
        3) Pseudobulbar palsy
        4) Gait abnormalities
        5) Weakness of an extremity
3. Diagnostic
    a. Mini-Mental State Examination (Folstein, Folstein, & McHugh, 1975)
    b. Other diagnostic studies to rule out other causes

Collaborative management
1. Continue assessment
    a. ABCDs
    b. Vital signs: blood pressure, pulse, respiratory rate, and temperature
    c. Oxygen saturation if indicated
    d. Level of consciousness and orientation
    e. Sensory deficits (e.g., hearing, vision)
    f. Psychiatric status, especially in the presence of suicidal ideation
    g. Environmental safety
    h. Close monitoring for the progression of symptoms
2. Maintain airway, oxygenation, and ventilation
    a. Oxygen by nasal cannula at 2 to 6 L/minute if to maintain an SpO_2 level of 95% unless contraindicated; for patients with COPD, use pulse oximetry to guide oxygen administration to an SpO_2 level of 90%
    b. IV access for fluid and medication administration if indicated
3. Provide a safe environment
    a. Quiet room with minimal stimulation to allow for continuous observation
    b. Use of the patient's name during conversation
    c. Conversations should be kept simple and short
    d. Frequent reorientation to person and place
    e. Determination of additional information to ensure safety
        1) Interview the family for additional information
        2) Evaluate the risk of the patient making unsafe decisions
        3) Evaluate the potential for the patient to wander and fall
    f. Restraints should be avoided if possible but may be required to ensure patient safety
4. Monitor for complications
    a. Violence
    b. Falls

Evaluation
1. Patent airway, adequate oxygenation (i.e., normal SaO_2) and ventilation (i.e., normal $PaCO_2$)
2. Absence of patient and staff injury
3. Reduction in agitation
4. Alert and oriented with no neurologic deficit

Typical disposition
1. If evaluation criteria met and no indications that the patient is at risk for injury to self or others: discharge with instructions
    a. Further diagnostic testing
    b. Medications as prescribed
    c. Outpatient psychiatric consultation

2. If patient is at risk for injury to self or others: admission or transfer to another facility

Eating Disorders

Definitions

1. Eating disorder: a life-threatening disturbance in the patterns of eating that can occur across the life span
2. Anorexia nervosa
   a. Deliberate weight loss
   b. Induced or sustained by the person
   c. Most commonly seen among young people of both sexes
3. Bulimia nervosa
   a. Repeated bouts of overeating
   b. Excessive preoccupation with controlling body weight that causes the person to adopt extreme measures to mitigate the fattening effects of ingested food (e.g., inducing vomiting, consuming laxatives)
   c. Usually seen at a later age than anorexia nervosa
   d. Behaviors have to have occurred ≥2 times a week for ≥3 months
4. Pica
   a. The persistent eating of nonnutritive substances for ≥1 month
   b. Inappropriate to developmental level
   c. Not part of a culturally sanctioned practice
5. Rumination disorder of infancy
   a. Repeated regurgitation or rechewing food for ≥1 month
   b. Not caused by esophageal reflux
   c. Not occurring with anorexia or bulimia

Predisposing factors

1. Sociocultural and biologic factors are more prevalent than psychological ones
2. Attempts to counteract the fattening effects of food by vomiting, laxatives, appetite suppressants, diuretics, and other drugs
3. Intense fear of becoming fat

Pathophysiology

1. Anorexia nervosa
   a. Fear of eating and gaining weight that can cause potentially life-threatening physiologic effects and long-lasting psychological disturbances
   b. Exhibited either by restrictions or binging and purging behaviors
   c. Malnutrition occurs and affects all organ systems, although the cardiovascular and endocrine systems are primarily affected
2. Bulimia nervosa (Kalapatapu, Walsh, Uwaifo, & Daly, 2008)
   a. Frequent episodes of binge eating that are associated with emotional distress
   b. Sense of loss of control and compensatory behavioral patterns to prevent weight gain
   c. Repeated vomiting that causes electrolyte imbalances, seizures, cardiac arrhythmias, tetany, and discoloration of the teeth

d. Metabolic derangements that include low plasma insulin, C peptide, triiodothyronine, and glucose values
   e. May have increased β-hydroxybutyrate and free fatty acid levels
3. Pica (Ellis & Schnoes, 2009)
   a. The nature and amount of the ingested substance determine the medical sequelae
   b. Can lead to toxicity
4. Rumination disorder of infancy: specific origin is unclear

Clinical presentation (DSM-IV TR, 2000)

1. Subjective
   a. History of fasting, frequent vomiting, or excessive exercise after eating
   b. History of weight loss
   c. Palpitations
   d. Amenorrhea
   e. Irritability
   f. Signs of depression
   g. Suicidal ideation
2. Objective
   a. Weight changes
      1) Anorexia nervosa: <85% of normal weight for height
      2) Bulimia: usually overweight but may be in poor nutritional state
   b. Dysrhythmias
   c. Lanugo hair on body
   d. Discoloration or erosion of teeth and bleeding gums
   e. Signs of dehydration
      1) Tachycardia and possible hypotension
      2) Dry skin
      3) Poor skin turgor
      4) Dry and brittle hair
      5) Weak pulses
3. Diagnostic
   a. Electrolytes: may have hypokalemia
   b. CBC: may have anemia
   c. Serum and urine drug screenings
   d. Other diagnostic studies to rule out other causes

Collaborative management

1. Continue assessment
   a. ABCDs
   b. Vital signs: blood pressure, pulse, respiratory rate, and temperature
   c. Oxygen saturation if indicated
   d. Presence of vomiting or diarrhea
   e. Accurate intake and output
   f. Serum electrolyte levels
   g. Level of consciousness
   h. Psychiatric status, especially in the presence of suicidal ideation
   i. Environmental safety
   j. Close monitoring for the progression of symptoms

2. Maintain airway, oxygenation, and ventilation
   a. Oxygen by nasal cannula at 2 to 6 L/minute if to maintain an SpO_2 level of 95% unless contraindicated; for patients with COPD, use pulse oximetry to guide oxygen administration to an SpO_2 level of 90%
   b. IV access for fluid and medication administration if indicated
   c. Crystalloids as prescribed
3. Provide adequate fluid and nutritional intake
   a. Electrolytes as prescribed
   b. Enteral or parenteral nutrition as prescribed
4. Monitor for complications
   a. Cardiac dysrhythmias
   b. Malnutrition
   c. Electrolyte imbalance
   d. Dehydration or shock

Evaluation
1. Patent airway, adequate oxygenation (i.e., normal SaO_2) and ventilation (i.e., normal $PaCO_2$)
2. Absence of clinical indications of malnutrition
3. Absence of cardiac dysrhythmias
4. Absence of electrolyte imbalances
5. Alert and oriented with no neurologic deficit

Typical disposition
1. If evaluation criteria met and no indications that the patient is at risk for injury to self or others: discharge with instructions
   a. Nutritionist referral
   b. Psychiatric referral
2. If evaluation criteria not met or patient is at risk for injury to self or others: admission or transfer to another facility

Substance Use Disorders
Definitions
1. Substance dependence: a maladaptive pattern of substance use that leads to clinically significant impairment or distress as manifested by three or more of the following occurring at any time during the same 12-month period (DSM IVTR Diagnostic Criteria):
   a. Tolerance
   b. The substance being taken in larger amounts or over a longer period than intended
   c. Persistent desire or unsuccessful efforts to cut down or control the use of the substance
   d. Much time spent participating in the activities necessary to obtain the substance
   e. Important social, occupational, or recreational activities given up or reduced as a result of the use of the substance
   f. Use is continued despite knowledge of physical or psychologic problems caused by such use
2. Substance abuse: a maladaptive pattern of substance use that leads to clinically significant impairment or distress as manifested by one or more of the following occurring within a 12-month period (DSM-TR Diagnostic Criteria):

   a. Recurrent substance use that results in a failure to fulfill major role obligations at work, home, or school
   b. Recurrent substance use in situations in which it is physically hazardous
   c. Recurrent substance-related legal problems
   d. Continued substance use despite having persistent or recurrent social or interpersonal problems caused or exacerbated by the effects of the substance

Predisposing factors
1. Family history of substance abuse or dependence
2. Inability to cope effectively
3. Group modeling, especially during adolescence

Clinical presentation
1. Subjective
   a. Related history of use
   b. Request for help with addiction
   c. Emotionally distressed or weeping
2. Objective
   a. Person exhibits intoxication or erratic behavior, including impaired judgment, aggression, and mood lability
   b. Speech can be slurred or rambling
   c. Unsteady gait
   d. Nystagmus
   e. Impaired memory or attention
   f. Stupor or coma
3. Diagnostic studies: serum and urine drug screenings

Collaborative management
1. Continue assessment
   a. ABCDs
   b. Vital signs: blood pressure, pulse, respiratory rate, and temperature
   c. Oxygen saturation if indicated
   d. Level of consciousness
   e. Psychiatric status, especially in the presence of suicidal ideation
   f. Environmental safety
   g. Close monitoring for the progression of symptoms
2. Maintain airway, oxygenation, and ventilation
   a. Oxygen by nasal cannula at 2 to 6 L/minute if to maintain an SpO_2 level of 95% unless contraindicated; for patients with COPD, use pulse oximetry to guide oxygen administration to an SpO_2 level of 90%
   b. IV access for fluid and medication administration if indicated
3. Provide a safe environment
   a. Quiet room with minimal stimulation to allow for continuous observation
   b. Determination of suicidal ideation or plan for suicide
   c. Restraints should be avoided if possible but may be required to ensure patient safety
4. Prevent seizures: benzodiazepines as prescribed

5. Monitoring for complications
   a. Cardiac dysrhythmias
   b. Hypertension or hypotension
   c. Respiratory depression
   d. Seizures
   e. Coma

Evaluation

1. Patent airway, adequate oxygenation (i.e., normal SaO_2) and ventilation (i.e., normal $PaCO_2$)
2. Absence of clinical indications of respiratory distress
3. Absence of clinical indications of hypoperfusion
4. Absence of clinical indications of seizures
5. Alert and oriented with no neurologic deficit

Typical disposition

1. If evaluation criteria met and no indications that the patient is at risk for injury to self or others: discharge with instructions
   a. Support groups
   b. Psychiatric consultation
2. If evaluation criteria not met or patient is at risk for injury to self or others: admission or transfer to another facility

Substance Abuse/Withdrawal

Definition: the development of a substance-specific syndrome as a result of the cessation of (or a reduction in) substance use that has been heavy and prolonged (DSM-TR Diagnostic Criteria)
1. Causes clinically significant distress or impairment
2. Unrelated to a general medical condition or another mental disorder

Predisposing factors: the cessation of the use of a substance that has been heavy and prolonged
Clinical presentation: two or more of the following develop within hours to a few days after cessation:
1. Autonomic hyperactivity
2. Hand tremors
3. Insomnia
4. Nausea or vomiting
5. Visual, tactile, or auditory hallucinations
6. Psychomotor agitation
7. Anxiety
8. Seizures

Collaborative management

1. Continue assessment
   a. ABCDs
   b. Vital signs: blood pressure, pulse, respiratory rate, and temperature
      1) Monitor the vital signs every 15 to 30 minutes until the patient is stable
   c. Oxygen saturation if indicated
   d. Respiratory effort and excursion
   e. Cardiac rate and rhythm
   f. Level of consciousness and neurologic status
   g. Psychiatric status, especially in the presence of suicidal ideation

   h. Environmental safety
   i. Close monitoring for the progression of symptoms
2. Maintain airway, oxygenation, and ventilation
   a. Oxygen by nasal cannula at 2 to 6 L/minute if to maintain an SpO_2 level of 95% unless contraindicated; for patients with COPD, use pulse oximetry to guide oxygen administration to an SpO_2 level of 90%
   b. IV access for fluid and medication administration if indicated
3. Provide a safe environment
   a. Quiet room with minimal stimulation to allow for continuous observation
   b. Nonjudgmental attitude
   c. Conversations should be kept simple and short
   d. Frequent reorientation to person and place
   e. Restraints should be avoided if possible but may be required to ensure patient safety
4. Prevent seizures: benzodiazepines as prescribed
5. Monitoring for complications
   a. Delirium tremens
   b. Death

Evaluation

1. Patent airway, adequate oxygenation (i.e., normal SaO_2) and ventilation (i.e., normal $PaCO_2$)
2. Absence of clinical indications of respiratory distress
3. Absence of clinical indications of hypoperfusion
4. Absence of clinical indications of seizures
5. Alert and oriented with no neurologic deficit
6. Absence of patient injury

Typical disposition

1. If evaluation criteria met and no indications that the patient is at risk for injury to self or others: discharge with instructions
   a. Support groups
   b. Psychiatric consultation
2. If evaluation criteria not met or patient is at risk for injury to self or others: admission or transfer to a residential treatment center

Trauma, Violence, and Abuse

Definition: injury caused by violence, accidental injuries, or criminal activity
1. Abuse: the mistreatment of another; this can be physical, mental, or emotional
2. Neglect: an individual's physical, mental, or emotional well-being has not been cared for
3. Sexual assault (see Chapter 9)

Predisposing factors

1. Substance abuse
2. Stress reactions
3. Inability to cope
4. Direct intent to injure (e.g., assault)

Clinical presentation

1. Subjective
   a. Pain related to injury

b. Extreme emotional distress
   1) May be unable to report symptoms
   2) Injury and history of incident may not seem to match
   3) Inconsistency with the report of what happened before coming in to the emergency department or changes in the story
c. Collaborative information provided by family, friends, or significant others

2. Objective
   a. Sudden unexpected physical or emotional injury
      1) Injury can be obvious or not obvious
   b. Clinical presentation related to the location and severity of the injury
   c. Bruises in various stages of healing may indicate physical abuse
   d. Injury with an identifiable pattern (e.g., scald by immersion)

3. Diagnostic
   a. Serum laboratory work to rule out medical concerns
   b. Forensic testing as indicated (e.g., DNA)
   c. Evidence collection if associated with a crime (see Chapter 9); photos as indicated
   d. Radiographic films of injured areas; radiographic films that show old fractures may indicate abuse
   e. CT as indicated; noncontrast head scanning if internal bleeding is suspected
   f. Other diagnostic studies to rule out other causes

Age-related considerations

1. Adults: gunshot wounds, lacerations, fractures, rape, penetrating injuries, and domestic violence
2. Children: blunt traumas, shaken baby syndrome, burns, fractures, sexual and physical abuse, accidental injuries, failure to thrive, and neglect
3. Older adults: fractures, nutritional deficits, domestic violence, self-injury, and neglect and physical abuse

Collaborative management

1. Continue assessment
   a. ABCDs
   b. Vital signs: blood pressure, pulse, respiratory rate, and temperature
   c. Oxygen saturation if indicated
   d. Psychiatric status, especially in the presence of suicidal ideation
   e. Environmental safety
   f. Close monitoring for the progression of symptoms
2. Maintain airway, oxygenation, and ventilation
   a. Oxygen by nasal cannula at 2 to 6 L/minute if to maintain an SpO_2 level of 95% unless contraindicated; for patients with COPD, use pulse oximetry to guide oxygen administration to an SpO_2 level of 90%
   b. Artificial airway and mechanical ventilation may be necessary depending on the severity of the injury
   c. IV access for fluid and medication administration if indicated

3. Ensure patient safety
   a. Clothing and other personal articles must be secured as a protection of the chain of evidence if there are potential legal ramifications
   b. Notification of authorities if abuse or neglect is suspected
   c. Maintenance of safe environment for patient
   d. Protection against unwanted visitors or potential abusers who may attempt to control care
   e. Documentation of what patient reports with the use of exact quotations
   f. Awareness of Duty to Protect regulations for health care providers

4. Control pain and discomfort
   a. Position of comfort
   b. Analgesics
   c. Complementary therapies (e.g., heat, cold)

5. Prepare the patient and assist with procedures as indicated by the type, location, and severity of the injury
   a. Determination of what the patient wishes if able to comprehend situation
   b. Determination of parent or guardian wishes if the patient is a child

6. Monitor for complications: dependent on the type, location, and severity of injury
   a. Homicide
   b. Suicide

Evaluation

1. Patent airway, adequate oxygenation (i.e., normal SaO_2) and ventilation (i.e., normal $PaCO_2$)
2. Absence of clinical indications of respiratory distress
3. Absence of clinical indications of hypoperfusion
4. Alert and oriented with no neurologic deficit

Typical disposition

1. If evaluation criteria are met, the patient is medically stable, and the environment is safe: depending on the type of injury and the vulnerability of patient, discharged to home or a protective environment
   a. Support groups
   b. Protective authorities if the need is apparent
2. If evaluation criteria are not met or the patient is at risk for suicide or homicide: admission or transfer to another facility

Suicide and Homicide

Definitions

1. Suicide: the willful taking of one's own life
2. Homicide: the taking of another's life
3. Either may be premeditated or impulsive

Predisposing factors

1. Family history
2. Prior attempts at suicide
3. Substance abuse
4. Depression
5. Physical illnesses
6. Violent environmental factors

Clinical presentation

1. Subjective
   a. Suicidal or homicidal thoughts (note that these may be unconscious)
2. Objective: dependent on the mechanism of injury, if method is substance overdose need to elicit both time and type of substance if possible
3. Diagnostic study: serum toxicology to determine serum levels if overdose

Collaborative management

1. Continue assessment
   a. ABCDs
   b. Vital signs: blood pressure, pulse, respiratory rate, and temperature
   c. Oxygen saturation
   d. Respiratory effort and excursion
   e. Cardiac rate and rhythm
   f. Psychiatric status
      1) Suicidal ideation
      2) Agitation
   g. Environmental safety
   h. Level of consciousness
   i. Close monitoring for the progression of symptoms
2. Maintain airway, oxygenation, and ventilation
   a. Oxygen by nasal cannula at 2 to 6 L/minute if to maintain an SpO_2 level of 95% unless contraindicated; for patients with COPD, use pulse oximetry to guide oxygen administration to an SpO_2 level of 90%
   b. Artificial airway and mechanical ventilation may be necessary depending on the severity of the injury
   c. IV access for fluid and medication administration if indicated
3. Provide a safe environment
   a. Quiet room with minimal stimulation to allow for continuous observation; however, if space allowing continuous observation is not available, ensure the following:
      1) Patient should not be left in closed area
      2) Provide suicide/homicide checks every 15 minutes and document
   b. Nonjudgmental approach
   c. Restraints should be avoided if possible but may be required to ensure patient safety
   d. Immediate medical crisis needs to be resolved before dealing with mental health issues
   e. Support to family members
4. Prepare for surgery or other treatment if indicated
5. Monitor for complications
   a. Injury
   b. Death

Evaluation

1. Patent airway, adequate oxygenation (i.e., normal SaO_2) and ventilation (i.e., normal $PaCO_2$)
2. Absence of suicidal or homicidal intent
3. Absence of patient injury

Typical disposition

1. If evaluation criteria are met, the patient is medically stable, and the environment is safe: depending on the type of injury and the vulnerability of patient, discharge home or to a protective environment is the focus
   a. If charges have been filed, notification of police before discharge
   b. Notification of protective authorities if need is apparent
   c. Referral to primary care provider if known
   d. Notification of family as permitted by patient if over age of 18 years
   e. Referral to community resources for follow-up services
   f. Medications
2. If evaluation are criteria not met or the patient is at risk for suicide, homicide, or serious injury: admission or transfer to another facility

LEARNING ACTIVITIES

1. DIRECTIONS: Complete the following crossword puzzle related to psychosocial emergencies.

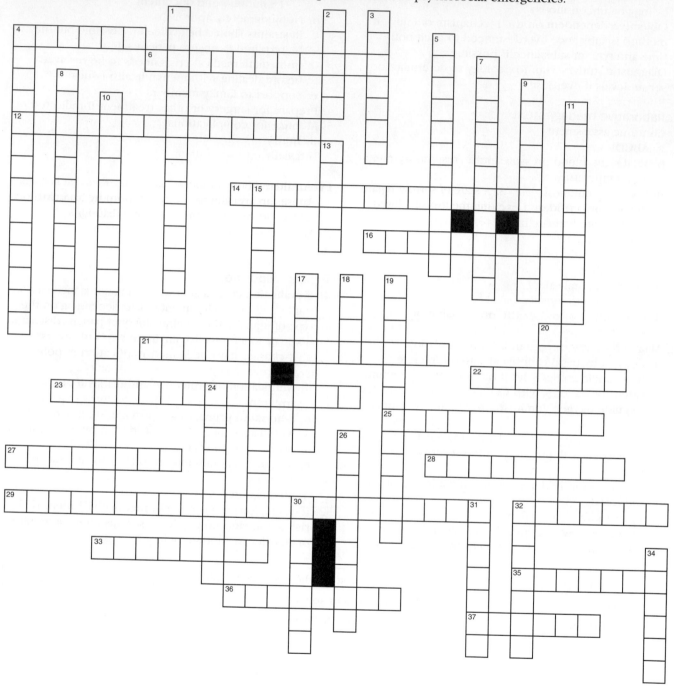

ACROSS

4. Absence of speech
6. This type of crisis occurs suddenly
12. Thoughts that connect to each other and come back to the original topic but in a round-about way
14. These are a distortion of the perception of reality; however, they are usually accompanied by a powerful sense of being real

DOWN

1. Leaping from one idea to another and being easily distracted by environment (three words)
2. Elevated or irritable mood that has lasted for ≥1 week
3. Frequent binge eating is associated with this condition
4. Drugs that are used to treat mania may also be used as an _____
5. Medications that decrease anxiety
7. A vivid, dream-like hallucination

16. Hallucinations are this type of disturbance
21. Recurrent substance use that results in the failure to fulfill major role obligations at work, home, or school (two words)
22. The inability to recognize or identify objects despite intact sensory function
23. This type of drug is administered to decrease the risk of seizures during substance withdrawal

8. A state of sorrow regarding the loss of a loved one
9. An alteration in mood that is characterized by sadness and a negative self-concept
10. Tolerance to a substance or the use of a substance for longer than it was intended to be used (two words)
11. This examination is performed in patients with dementia to determine their mental state
13. The physical, mental, or emotional mistreatment of another

25. A thought that has some connection between the preceding and following thoughts but with little association among these ideas as a whole
27. A chronic global deterioration of cognition
28. Fixed false beliefs
29. The loss of normal thought patterns (three words)
32. This disorder is characterized by feelings of helplessness and tension

15. An altered body image causes an aversion to eating in patients with this condition (two words)
17. A cessation in the flow of thought or speech
18. This disorder is characterized by the eating of chalk, paper, or other nonfood objects
19. This type of crisis occurs over time
20. The inability to initiate activities that is seen in patients with psychosis
24. A lack of pleasure

33. There is an increase in this type of thinking with depression
35. The inability to perform motor activities despite intact motor function
36. The willful taking of another person's life
37. The state that occurs when one's usual ways of coping are inadequate to deal with the current level of stress

26. A disorder that is characterized by hallucinations and delusions
30. The willful taking of one's own life
31. Not attending to the emotional, physical, or mental care needs of another who cannot care for himself or herself
32. A language disturbance that is seen in patients with dementia
34. Patients with mania have these type of thoughts

2. DIRECTIONS: Match the following hallucinations with the correct definition.

_____ 1. Auditory	a. Feeling sensations when not being touched
_____ 2. Visual	b. Seeing images that are not present
_____ 3. Gustatory	c. Smelling odors that are not present
_____ 4. Hypnopompic	d. Perceiving a taste without an identifiable cause
_____ 5. Tactile	e. Hearing voices or sounds that are not there
_____ 6. Olfactory	f. Vivid, dream-like hallucinations that occur upon awakening
_____ 7. Kinesthetic	g. Perceiving movement of the body without cause
_____ 8. Somatic	h. Feeling that something is occurring within one's own body

3. DIRECTIONS: List at least five significant age-related differences to consider when caring for patients with psychosocial emergencies.

Pediatric Patients	Older Adult Patients
1.	1.
2.	2.
3.	3.
4.	4.
5.	5.

4. DIRECTIONS: Identify the assessment findings for each of the following conditions that would help you to distinguish it from the others.

Condition	Subjective Assessment	Objective Assessment
Anxiety disorder		
Depression		
Mania		
Hallucinations		
Psychosis		
Dementia		
Anorexia nervosa		
Bulimia		

LEARNING ACTIVITIES ANSWERS

1.

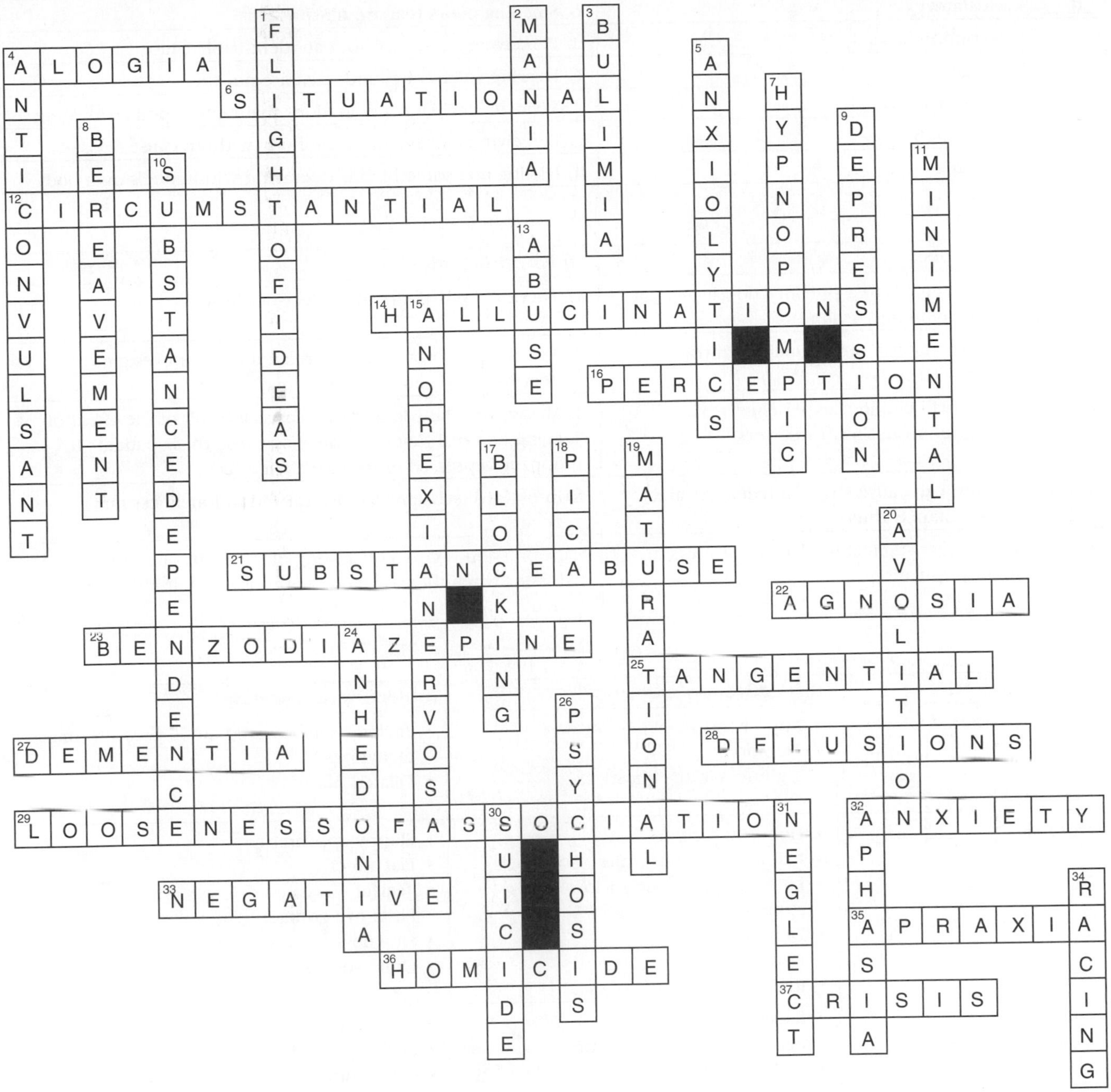

1 FLIGHTOFIDEAS
2 MANIA
3 BULIMIA
4 ALOGIA
4 ANTICONVULSANT
5 ANXIOLYTICS
6 SITUATIONAL
7 HYPNOPOMPIC
8 BEREAVEMENT
9 DEPRESSION
10 SUBSTANCEDEPENDENCE
11 MINIMENTAL
12 CIRCUMSTANTIAL
13 ABUSE
14 HALLUCINATIONS
15 ANOREXIANERVOSA
16 PERCEPTION
17 BLOCKING
18 PICA
19 MATURATIONAL
20 AVOLITION
21 SUBSTANCEABUSE
22 AGNOSIA
23 BENZODIAZEPINE
24 ANHEDONIA
25 TANGENTIAL
26 PSYCHOSIS
27 DEMENTIA
28 DELUSIONS
29 LOOSENESSOFASSOCIATION
30 SUICIDE
31 NEGLECT
32 ANXIETY
32 APHASIA
33 NEGATIVE
34 RACING
35 APRAXIA
36 HOMICIDE
37 CRISIS

2.

_e_	1. Auditory	a. Feeling sensations when not being touched
_b_	2. Visual	b. Seeing images that are not present
_d_	3. Gustatory	c. Smelling odors that are not present
_f_	4. Hypnopompic	d. Perceiving a taste without an identifiable cause
_a_	5. Tactile	e. Hearing voices or sounds that are not there
_c_	6. Olfactory	f. Vivid, dream-like hallucinations that occur upon awakening
_g_	7. Kinesthetic	g. Perceiving movement of the body without cause
_h_	8. Somatic	h. Feeling that something is occurring within one's own body

3.

Pediatric Patients	Older Adult Patients
1. Children can regress to a previous developmental stage when frightened or ill.	1. There is a possibility of neglect or abuse.
2. Pediatric patients may throw temper tantrums when faced with stress.	2. Accidental substance abuse related to poor eyesight or decreasing cognitive function may occur.
3. Infants and small children experience anxiety when separated from their caregivers.	3. Medications take longer to clear as a result of the effect of aging on renal function; this may cause these patients to appear depressed or to have a flat affect.
4. Peer pressure can cause stress in teenagers and influence substance abuse.	4. Intentional substance abuse related to loneliness may occur.
5. Stress can trigger suicidal tendencies or ideas in this patient population.	5. Depression is common among older adults after a personal loss or when they are faced with losing their independence.

4.

Condition	Subjective Assessment	Objective Assessment
Anxiety disorder	• Apprehension or nervousness • Tremors • Tightness in the chest • Dizziness	• Tachycardia, elevated blood pressure, or tachypnea • Dilated pupils
Depression	• Hopeless feeling • Inability to concentrate • Low energy, fatigue, or loss of appetite • Depressed mood • Decreased libido • Recurrent thoughts of death	• Sloppy appearance • Flat affect • Tearful • Little eye contact • Slowness of movement • Quiet speech
Mania	• Racing thoughts • Risky or reckless behaviors • Little need for sleep	• Increased activity • Flight of ideas • Distractibility • Elation • Grandiosity
Hallucinations	• Patient reports having visions or hearing voices	• Patient is talking or responding to voices or other perceptual disturbances
Psychosis	• Paranoid ideas • Confusion or amnesia • Fears about safety	• Delusions or hallucinations • Agitation or bizarre behavior • Appears to be out of touch with reality • Lack of pleasure • Disorganized speech

Dementia	• Memory loss • Speech impairment • Decline in cognitive function	• Decrease in orientation and judgment • Aphasia • Apraxia • Agnosia • Shallow affect
Anorexia nervosa	• Perception of being overweight • Constantly trying to lose weight	• Weighs <85% of normal body weight for height • Malnourished • Dehydrated
Bulimia	• Sense of loss of control to prevent weight gain • Frequent binge eating	• Binge eating and purging

References and Selected Readings

Bernstein, B. E. (2008). Eating disorders: Anorexia. Retrieved on November 14, 2009, from http://emedicine.medscape.com/article/912187-overview.

Bhalla, R. N., Moraille-Bhalla, P., & Aronson, S. C. (2009). Depression. Retrieved on November 14, 2009, from http://emedicine.medscape.com/article/286759-overview.

Caplan, A. I. (1970). Effects of the nicotinamide-sensitive teratogen3-acetylpyridine on chick limb cells in culture. *Experimental Cell Research, 62(2),* 341-355.

Ellis, C. R., & Schnoes, C. J. (2009) Eating disorder: Pica. Retrieved on November 15, 2009, from http://emedicine.medscape.com/article/914765-overview.

Emergency Nurses Association. (2007). *Emergency nursing core curriculum* (6th ed). Philadelphia: Saunders.

Emergency Nurses Association. (2005). *Sheehy's manual of emergency care* (6th ed.). St. Louis: Mosby.

Fawcett, J. (2008). Bipolar disorder: Manic-depressive illness. Merck Manuals Online. Retrieved on November 15, 2009, from http://www.merck.com/mmhe/sec07/ch101/ch101c.html.

Folstein, M. F., Folstein, F. E., & McHugh, P. R. (1975). "Mini-mental state." A practical method for grading the cognitive state of patients for the clinician. *Journal of Psychiatric Research,* 12(3), 189-198.

Hamilton, P. M. (2007). Psychiatric emergencies: Caring for people in crisis. Retrieved on November 15, 2000, from http://www.nursingceu.com/courses/198/index_nceu.html.

Kalapatapu, R. K., Walsh, K. H., Uwaifo, G. I., & Daly, R. C. (2008, August). Bulimia. Retrieved on November 14, 2009, from http://emedicine.medscape.com/article/286485-overview.

Merriam Webster Online. (2007-2008). Merriam Webster's medical dictionary. http://medical.merriam-webster.com.

U.S. Department of Health and Human Services Website. (nd). Civil rights. Retrieved on November 15, 2009, from http://www.hhs.gov/ocr/civilrights/index.html.

Yates, W. R. (2009, October). Anxiety disorders . Retrieved on November 14, 2009, from http://emedicine.medscape.com/article/286227-overview.

Common Abbreviations and Acronyms

2,3-DPG	2,3-diphosphoglyceric acid
A	Alveolar
a	Arterial
AAA	Abdominal aortic aneurysm
AACN	American Association of Critical-Care Nurses
AAL	Anterior axillary line
ABCD	Airway, breathing, circulation, disability
ABD	Abdomen
ABG	Arterial blood gas
ABI	Ankle-brachial index
AC	Assist-control
AC	Alternating current
ACC	American College of Cardiology
ACE	Angiotensin converting enzyme
ACLS	Advanced cardiac life support
ACS	Acute coronary syndrome
ACS	Anticholinergic syndrome
ACT	Activated clotting time
ACTH	Adrenocorticotropic hormone
ADD	Attention deficit disorder
ADH	Antidiuretic hormone
ADHD	Attention deficit/hyperactivity disorder
ADL	Activities of daily living
ADP	Adenosine diphosphate
AED	Automated external defibrillator
AF	Atrial fibrillation
AFB	Acid-fast bacillus
AGREE	Appraisal of Guidelines for Research and Evaluation
AHA	American Heart Association
AHA	American Hospital Association
AHRQ	Agency for Healthcare Research and Quality
AICD	Automatic implantable cardiac defibrillator
AIDS	Acquired immune deficiency syndrome
AIVR	Accelerated idioventricular rhythm
ALI	Acute lung injury
ALP	Alkaline phosphatase
ALS	Amyotrophic lateralizing sclerosis
ALT	Alanine aminotransferase
AMA	Against medical advice
AMP	Applied Measurement Professionals

Continued

ANA	Antinuclear antibody
ANA	American Nurses Association
ANS	Autonomic nervous system
ANUG	Acute necrotizing ulcerative gingivitis
AP	Anteroposterior
APA	American Psychiatric Association
APAP	Paracetamol and N-acetyl-p-aminophenol (i.e., Tylenol)
APR	Air purifying respirator
aPTT	Activated partial thromboplastin time
AR	Aortic regurgitation
ARB	Angiotensin receptor blocker
ARDS	Acute respiratory distress syndrome
ARF	Acute respiratory failure
AS	Aortic stenosis
ASA	Acetylsalicylic acid (aspirin)
AST	Aspartate aminotransferase
ATM	Atmospheric pressure
ATN	Acute tubular necrosis
ATP	Adenosine triphosphate
ATPase	Adenosine triphosphatase
ATSDR	Agency for Toxic Substances and Disease Registry
AV	Atrioventricular
AVM	Arteriovenous malformation
BAC	Blood alcohol concentration
BAL	British anti-lewisite
BBB	Bundle branch block
BCCTPC	Board of Critical Care Transport Paramedic Certification
BCEN	Board of Certification for Emergency Nursing
BCLS	Basic cardiac life support
Bi-PAP	Positive airway pressure on both inspiration and expiration
Bi-PAP	Combination of pressure support ventilation and continuous positive airway pressure
Bi-VAD	Biventricular assist device
BLS	Basic life support
BNP	Brain-type natriuretic peptide
BP	Blood pressure
BPH	Benign prostatic hypertrophy
BSA	Body surface area
BTLS	Basic trauma life support
BUN	Blood urea nitrogen
BVM	Bag valve mask
C	Celsius (also referred to as centigrade)
Ca++	Calcium
CABG	Coronary artery bypass graft
CAD	Coronary artery disease
CaO_2	Oxygen content in arterial blood
CAP	Community-acquired pneumonia
CAPP	Coronary artery perfusion pressure
CAVH	Continuous arteriovenous hemofiltration
CBC	Complete blood count
CBF	Cerebral blood flow
CC	Chief complaint

CCB	Calcium channel blocker
CCO	Continuous cardiac output
CCU	Critical care unit
CDC	Centers for Disease Control and Prevention
CEN	Certified Emergency Nurse
CFRN	Certified Flight Registered Nurse
CHB	Complete heart block
CHO	Carbohydrate
CHP	Capillary hydrostatic pressure
CI	Cardiac index
CK	Creatinine kinase
CK-MB	Creatinine kinase-myocardial band
Cl^-	Chloride
cm	Centimeter
cm H_2O	Centimeters of water
CMP	Complete metabolic panel
CMV	Cytomegalovirus
CN	Cranial nerve
CNS	Central nervous system
CO	Cardiac output
CO	Carbon monoxide
CO_2	Carbon dioxide
COBRA	Consolidated Omnibus Budget Reconciliation Act
COP	Colloidal oncotic pressure
COPD	Chronic obstructive pulmonary disease
CPAP	Continuous positive airway pressure
CPD	Citrate phosphate dextrose
CPG	Clinical practice guidelines
CPP	Cerebral perfusion pressure
CPP	Calcium pyrophosphate
CPR	Cardiopulmonary resuscitation
CRAO	Central retinal artery occlusion
CRH	Corticotropin-releasing hormone
CRM	Crew resource management
CRP	C-reactive protein
CRRT	Continuous renal replacement therapy
CSF	Cerebrospinal fluid
CST	Cavernous sinus thrombosis
CT	Computerized tomography
cTnI	Cardiac troponin I
cTnT	Cardiac troponin T
CTRN	Critical Care Transport Registered Nurse
CVA	Costovertebral angle
CVA	Cerebrovascular accident
CvO_2	Oxygen content in venous blood
CVP	Central venous pressure
D_5LR	5% dextrose in lactated Ringer
D_5NS	5% dextrose in normal saline
D_5W	5% dextrose in water
DAI	Diffuse axonal injury
db	Decibels

Continued

DBP	Diastolic blood pressure
DC	Direct current
DCA	Directional coronary atherectomy
DCS	Decompression sickness
DDAVP	Desmopressin acetate
DFA	Direct fluorescent antibody
DHS	Department of Homeland Security
DI	Diabetes Insipidus
DIC	Disseminated intravascular coagulation
DKA	Diabetes ketoacidosis
Dl	Deciliter
DM	Diabetes mellitus
DNA	Deoxyribonucleic acid
DNR	Do not resuscitate
DO_2	Oxygen delivery to the tissues
DO_2I	Delivery of oxygen to the tissue index
DPA	Diagnostic peritoneal aspiration
DPD	Deoxypyridinoline
DPL	Diagnostic peritoneal lavage
DSM	Diagnostic and Statistical Manual of Mental Disorders
DTR	Deep tendon reflexes
DUB	Dysfunctional uterine bleeding
DVT	Deep vein thrombosis
e.g.	For example
EBP	Evidence-based practice
EBV	Epstein Barr virus
$ECCO_2OR$	Extracorporeal carbon dioxide removal
ECF	Extracellular fluid
ECG	Electrocardiogram (may also be abbreviated EKG)
ECMO	Extracorporal membrane oxygenator
ED	Emergency department
EDC	Expected date of confinement
EDH	Epidural hematoma
EDTA	Edetate calcium sodium
EEG	Electroencephalogram
EF	Ejection fraction
ELCA	Excimer laser coronary arthrectomy
ELISA	Enzyme linked immuno sorbent assay
ELT	Emergency locator transmitter
EMG	Electromyogram
EMI	Electromagnetic interference
EMS	Emergency Medical Services
EMTLA	Emergency Medical Treatment and Active Labor Act
EMV	Eye response, motor response, verbal response
ENA	Emergency Nurses Association
ENT	Ear, nose, throat
EOM	Extra ocular movement
EPA	Environmental Protection Agency
E-PAP	Expiratory positive airway pressure
EPS	Electrophysiology studies
ERCP	Endoscopic retrograde cholangiopancreatography

ERV	Expiratory reserve volume
ESR	Eosinophil sedimentation rate
ET	Endotracheal
ETC	Esophageal tracheal Combitube
ETCO$_2$	End tidal carbon dioxide
ETOH	Alcohol
F	Fahrenheit
f	Frequency of ventilation
FAA	Federal Aviation Administration
FAR	Federal Aviation Regulations
FAST	Focused abdominal sonography for trauma
FB	Foreign body
FBO	Foreign body object
FCC	Federal Communications Commission
FEV	Forced expiratory capacity
FFP	Fresh frozen plasma
FHT	Fetal heart tones
Fio$_2$	Fraction of inspired oxygen
FMS	Fibromyalgia syndrome
FP-C	Flight Paramedic Certified
FPS	Feet per second
FRC	Functional residual capacity
FSH	Follicle stimulating hormone
FSP	Fibrin split products (also referred to as *fibrin degradation products*)
FUO	Fever of unknown origin
FVC	Forced vital capacity
G	Gram
GABH	Group A beta-hemolytic streptococci
GAS	Group A streptococcus
GCS	Glasgow Coma Scale
GERD	Gastroesophageal reflux disease
GFR	Glomerular filtration rate
GHB	Gamma-hydroxybutyric acid
GI	Gastrointestinal
GP	Glycoprotein
GRH	Growth releasing hormone
GU	Genitourinary
GYN	Gynecology
H$^+$	Hydrogen ion
H$_2$O	Water
HAP	Hospital-acquired pneumonia
HAPE	High altitude pulmonary edema
HBO	Hyperbaric oxygen chamber
HBV	Hepatitis B virus
HCO$_3$	Bicarbonate
Hct	Hematocrit
HDL	High-density lipoprotein
HDVC	Human diploid cell vaccine
HF	Heart failure
Hg	Mercury
Hgb	Hemoglobin

Continued

HHNC	Hyperglycemic hyperosmolar nonketotic (condition or coma)
HIPAA	Health Insurance Portability and Accountability Act (of 1996)
HITT	Heparin-induced thrombosis and thrombocytopenia; also referred to as heparin-associated thrombosis and thrombocytopenia or white clot syndrome
HIV	Human immunodeficiency virus
HLA	Human leukocyte antigen
HOB	Head of bed
HPS	Hantavirus pulmonary syndrome
HPV	Human papillomavirus
HR	Heart rate
HRFS	Hemorrhagic fever with renal syndrome
HSV	Herpes simplex virus
HVD	Hantavirus disease
HVS	Hyperventilation syndrome
Hz	Hertz
I&O	Intake and output
i.e.	That is
I:E	Inspiration: expiration
IABP	Intra-aortic balloon pump
IC	Inspiratory capacity
ICH	Intracranial hematoma
ICOP	Interstitial colloidal oncotic pressure
ICP	Intracranial pressure
ICS	Intercostal space
ICU	Intensive care unit
IDDM	Insulin-dependent diabetes mellitus
IFA	Immunofluorescent assay serology
IFR	Instrument flight rules
Ig	Immunoglobulin
IHP	Interstitial hydrostatic pressure
IHSS	Idiopathic hypertrophic subaortic stenosis
IL	Interleukin
IM	Intramuscular
IMC	Instrument meteorological conditions
IMV	Intermittent mandatory ventilation
INH	Isonicotinic acid hydrazide (isoniazid)
INR	International normalized ratio
IPPB	Intermittent positive pressure breathing
IQ	Intelligence quotient
IRA	Infarct-related artery
IRV	Inspiratory reserve volume
ITP	Idiopathic thrombocytopenia Purpura
IU	International units
IUD	Intrauterine device
IV	Intravenous
IVP	Intravenous pyelogram
JCAHO	Joint Commission on Accreditation of Healthcare Organizations
JVD	Jugular venous distention
K+	Potassium
KCL	Potassium chloride
Kg	Kilogram

KS	Kaposi sarcoma
KUB	Kidneys, ureters, bladder (same as flat plate of abdomen)
L	Liter
LA	Left atria
LAAL	Left anterior axillary line
LAD	Left anterior descending (artery)
LAP	Left atrial pressure
LBB	Left bundle branch
LBBB	Left bundle branch block
LCA	Left circumflex artery
LDH	Lactic dehydrogenase
LDL	Low density lipoproteins
LES	Lower esophageal sphincter
LFT	Liver function test
LGL	Long-Ganong-Levine
LH	Luteinizing hormone
LICS	Left intercostal space
LLQ	Left lower quadrant
LMA	Laryngeal mask airway
LMAL	Left midaxillary line
LMCL	Left midclavicular line
LMN	Lower motor neuron
LMP	Last menstrual period
LMWD	Low molecular weight dextran
LMWH	Low molecular weight heparin
LOC	Level of consciousness
LP	Lumbar puncture
LPAL	Left posterior axillary line
LPM	Liters per minute
LR	Lactated Ringer's (solution)
LSB	Left sternal border
LSD	Lysergic acid diethylamide
LUQ	Left upper quadrant
LV	Left ventricle
LVEDP	Left ventricular end-diastolic pressure
LVEDV	Left ventricular end-diastolic volume
LVF	Left ventricular failure
LVH	Left ventricular hypertrophy
LVMI	Left ventricular myocardial infarction
LZ	Landing zone
M_1	Mitral (first) component of S_1
mA	Milliampere (unit of measurement for electrical current)
MAL	Midaxillary line
MALT	Mucosal associated lymphoid tissues
MAO	Monoamide oxidase (as in MAO inhibitors)
MAP	Mean arterial pressure
MAST	Military antishock trousers
Max	Maximum
Mcg	Microgram (unit of measurement for weight)
MCH	Mean corpuscular hemoglobin
MCHC	Mean corpuscular hemoglobin concentration

Continued

MCI	Mass causality incident
MCL	Midclavicular line
MCV	Mean corpuscular volume
MDF	Myocardial depressant factor
MDMA	Methylenedioxymethamphetamine (i.e., Ecstasy)
mEq	Milliequivalent (unit of measurement for solutes in solution)
METTAG	Medical Emergency Triage Tag
Mg	Milligram (unit of measurement for weight)
Mg++	Magnesium
MI	Myocardial infarction
MIC	Minimum inhibitory concentration
Min	Minimum
Min	Minute
ml	Milliliter (unit of measurement for volume)
mm	Millimeter (unit of measurement for length)
mm Hg	Millimeters of mercury
MODS	Multiple organ dysfunction syndrome
MOI	Mechanism of injury
mOsm/kg	Milliosmols per kilogram (unit of measure for osmolality)
MR	Mitral regurgitation
MRA	Magnetic resonance angiography
MRI	Magnetic resonance imaging
MS	Mitral stenosis
MSC	Monosodium urate crystals
MSG	Monosodium gluconate
MSL	Midsternal line
MUGA	Multiple-gated acquisition scan
MV	Mechanical ventilation
MVC	Motor vehicle collision
N/V	Nausea and vomiting
N/V/D	Nausea, vomiting, and diahrrea
Na+	Sodium
NAC	N-acetylcysteine (i.e., mucomyst)
NALS	Neonatal Advanced Life Support
NASPE	North American Society of Pacing and Electrophysiology
NCLEX	National Council Licensure Examination (for Registered Nurses)
NDNQI	National Database of Nursing Quality Indicators
NFRA	National Fibromyalgia Research Association
NG	Nasogastric
NHAP	Nursing home acquired pneumonia
NHTSA	National Highway Traffic Safety Administration
NIBP	Noninvasive blood pressure
NIDA	National Institute on Drug Abuse
NIF	Negative inspiratory force
NIHSS	National Institutes of Health Stroke Scale
NIMS	National Incident Management System
NK	Natural killer
NPO	Nothing by mouth
NPPV	Noninvasive positive pressure ventilation
NRB	Non-rebreather
NRF	National Response Framework

NRP	National Response Plan
NRP	Neonatal resuscitation provider
NS	Normal saline
NSAID	Nonsteroidal anti-inflammatory drugs
NSR	Normal sinus rhythm
NTG	Nitroglycerin
NTP	Nitroprusside
O_2	Oxygen
OCD	Obsessive-compulsive disorder
OD	Overdose
OSHA	Occupational Safety and Health Administration
OTC	Over the counter
P_2	Pulmonic (second) component of S_2
PA	Pulmonary artery
PA	Posteroanterior
PAC	Premature atrial contraction
$PaCO_2$	Partial pressure of carbon dioxide in arterial blood
PAd	Pulmonary artery diastolic pressure
PAL	Posterior axillary line
PALS	Pediatric Advanced Life Support
PAm	Pulmonary artery pressure mean
Pao_2	Pressure of oxygen in arterial blood
PAO_2	Pressure of oxygen in alveolar blood
PAOP	Pulmonary artery occlusive pressure (previously referred to as pulmonary capillary wedge pressure or pulmonary artery wedge pressure)
PAP	Pulmonary artery pressure
Pap	Papanicolaou test
PAs	Pulmonary artery systolic pressure
PAT	Paroxysmal atrial tachycardia
P_B	Barometric pressure
PC/IRV	Pressure controlled/inverse ratio ventilation
PCA	Patient controlled analgesia
PCI	Percutaneous coronary intervention
PCP	*Pneumocystis carinii* pneumonia (now referred to as *Pneumocystis jiroveci*)
PCP	Phencyclidine
PCR	Polymerase chain reaction
PCV	Pressure-controlled ventilation
PCWP	Pulmonary capillary wedge pressure
PD	Postural drainage
PE	Pulmonary embolism
PEA	Pulseless electrical activity
PEARL	Pupils equal and reactive to light
PEEP	Positive end-expiratory pressure
PEFR	Peak expiratory flow rate
PET	Positron emission tomography
$PETCO_2$	Partial pressure of carbon dioxide in end-tidal air
pH	Hydrogen ion concentration
PHTLS	Prehospital trauma life support
PID	Pelvic inflammatory disease
PIH	Pregnancy induced hypertension
PIP	Peak inspiratory pressure

Continued

PJC	Premature junctional contraction
PMI	Point of maximal impulse
PMS	Palpable pulses, movement, and sensation
PND	Paroxysmal nocturnal dyspnea
PNS	Parasympathetic nervous system
PO	Oral
PO_4^{3-}	Phosphate
PPD	Purified protein derivative
PPE	Personal protective equipment
PPF	Plasma protein fraction
PPI	Proton pump inhibitor
PPN	Peripheral parenteral nutrition
PROM	Premature rupture of membranes
PSA	Procedural sedation and analgesia
PSV	Pressure support ventilation
PSVT	Paroxysmal supraventricular tachycardia
PT	Prothrombin time
PT	Physical therapy
PTCA	Percutaneous transluminal coronary angioplasty
PTH	Parathyroid hormone
PTL	Preterm labor
PTSD	Post-trauma stress disorder
PTSMA	Percutaneous transluminal septal myocardial ablation
PTT	Partial prothrombin time
PTU	Propylthiouracil
PV	Peak velocity
PVC	Premature ventricular contraction
PVR	Pulmonary vascular resistance
Q	Perfusion
QI	Quality improvement
QM	Quality management
QT_c	QT interval corrected for rate
R/T	Related to
RA	Right atrium
RA	Rheumatoid arthritis
RAA	Renin-angiotensin-aldosterone
RAAL	Right anterior axillary line
RAD	Right axis deviation
RAM	Radiometer for atmospheric measurements
RAP	Right atrial pressure
RAS	Reticular activating system
RBB	Right bundle branch
RBBB	Right bundle branch block
RBC	Red blood cell
RCA	Right coronary artery
RDD	Radiologic dispersal device
REF	Right (ventricular) ejection fraction
REM	Rapid eye movement
Rh	Rhesus
RHD	Rheumatic heart disease
RIBA	Rapid immunoblot strip assay

RICS	Right intercostal space
RIG	Rabies immune globulin
RLQ	Right lower quadrant
RMAL	Right midaxillary line
RMCL	Right midclavicular line
RN	Registered nurse
RNA	Ribonucleic acid
ROM	Range of motion
r-PA	Recombinant plasminogen activator
RPAL	Right posterior axillary line
RQ	Respiratory quotient
RR	Respiratory rate
RSB	Right sternal border
RSI	Rapid sequence intubation
RSV	Respiratory syncytium virus
rt-PA	Recombinant tissue plasminogen activator
RUQ	Right upper quadrant
RV	Right ventricle
RV	Residual volume
RVF	Right ventricular failure
RVH	Right ventricular hypertrophy
RVMI	Right ventricular myocardial infarction
SA	Sinoatrial
SAED	Semiautomatic external defibrillator
SAH	Subarachnoid hemorrhage
SaO_2	Oxygen saturation of arterial blood
SC	Subcutaneous
SCI	Spinal cord injury
SCIWORA	Spinal cord injury without radiographic abnormality
$ScvO_2$	Oxygen saturation of central venous blood
SDH	Subdural hematoma
SI	Stroke index
SIADH	Syndrome of inappropriate antidiuretic hormone
SIDS	Sudden infant death syndrome
SIMV	Synchronized intermittent mandatory ventilation
SIRS	Systemic inflammatory response syndrome
SK	Streptokinase
SLE	Systemic lupus erythematosus
SNS	Sympathetic nervous system
SpO_2	Oxygen saturation in plasma (e.g., pulse oximetry)
SRS-A	Slow reacting substance of anaphylaxis
START	Simple triage and rapid transport
STEMI	ST-segment elevation MI
STI	Sexually transmitted infection
SV	Stroke volume
SvO_2	Oxygen saturation of mixed venous blood
SVR	Systemic vascular resistance
SVT	Supraventricular tachycardia
T	Temperature
TAA	Thoracic aortic aneurysm
TB	Tuberculosis

Continued

TBSA	Total body surface area
TCA	Tricyclic antidepressants
Td	Tetanus immunization
Tdap	Tetanus, diphtheria, pertussis immunization
TEC	Transluminal extraction catheter
TECP	Totally encapsulating chemical-protective
TENS	Transcutaneous electrical nerve stimulation
TIA	Transient ischemic attack
TIBC	Total iron-binding capacity
TLC	Total lung capacity
TLC	Total lymphocyte count
TM	Tympanic membrane
TMJ	Temporomandibular joint
TMP-SMX	trimethoprim-sulfamethoxazole
TN	Trigeminal neuralgia
TNCC	Trauma nursing core course
TNF	Tumor necrosis factor
TPN	Total parenteral nutrition
TR	Tricuspid regurgitation
TRH	Thyrotropin releasing hormone
TSH	Thyroid stimulating hormone
TTP	Thrombotic thrombocytopenia purpura
TUMT	Transurethral microwave therapy
TURP	Transurethral resection of prostate
U	Units
UES	Upper esophageal sphincter
UMN	Upper motor neuron
UOP	Urine output
UTI	Urinary tract infection
UVB	Ultraviolet B
V	Ventilation
V/Q	Ventilation/perfusion ratio
V_A	Alveolar minute ventilation
VC	Vital capacity
V_D	Anatomical deadspace
VDRL	Venereal Disease Research Laboratory
V_E	Minute ventilation
VF	Ventricular fibrillation
VFR	Visual flight rules
VMC	Visual meteorological conditions
VO_2	Oxygen consumption by the tissues
VO_2I	Consumption of oxygen by the tissue index
VPR	Volume pressure response
VSD	Ventricular septal defect
VT	Ventricular tachycardia
V_T	Tidal volume
VZV	Varicella zoster virus
WBC	White blood cell
WPW	Wolff-Parkinson-White syndrome

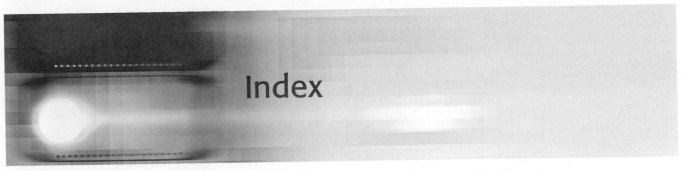

Index

Page number followed by b indicates box; f, figure; t, table.